AJN / MOSBY

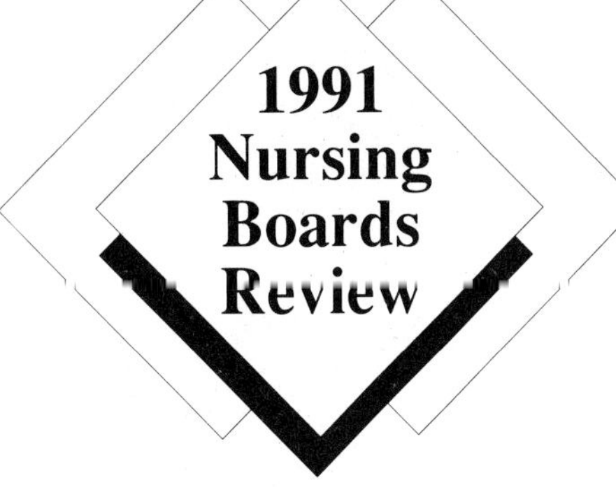

For the NCLEX-RN Examination

Coordinators for this Edition

Patricia E. Downing, MN, RN. *Formerly with School of Nursing, University of California, San Francisco, CA*

Susan Droske, MN, RN. *Independent Nurse Consultant, Texarkana, TX*

Alene Harrison, EdD, RN. *Assistant Professor, Idaho State University, Pocatello, ID*

Paulette D. Rollant, MSN, RN, CCRN. *President, Education Consultant, Multi-Resources, Inc., Grantville, GA*

Marybeth Young, MSN, RNC. *Assistant Professor, Maternal-Child Nursing, Niehoff School of Nursing, Loyola University, Chicago, IL*

Contributing Authors

Quilla D. Bell-Turner, PhD, RN. *Assistant Professor, University of Colorado School of Nursing, Denver, CO*

Karen S. Bernardy, MSN, RN. *Atlanta, GA*

Carolyn V. Billings, MSN, RN, CS. *Nurse Therapist in Independent Practice, Raleigh, NC*

Suzette Cardin, MS, RN, CCRN. *Nurse Manager, Coronary Care Unit/ Coronary Observation Unit, UCLA Medical Center, Los Angeles, CA*

Virginia L. Cassmeyer, PhD, MSN, RN. *Associate Professor, Medical-Surgical Nursing, University of Kansas School of Nursing, Kansas City, KS*

Robin Donohoe Dennison, MSN, RN, CS. *Cardiopulmonary Nursing Consultant, Continuing Education for Health Professionals, Inc., Huntington, WV*

Gita L. Dhillon, MEd, RNC. *Associate Professor, The American University, Washington, DC*

Deborah Ennis, MSN, RN, CCRN. *Assistant Professor of Nursing, Harrisburg Area Community College, Harrisburg, PA*

Sharon Golub, MN, RN. *Instructor of Nursing, Mount St. Mary's College, Los Angeles, CA*

Ann Jessop, MSN, RN. *Waco, TX*

Stephen Jones, MSN, RNC. *Pediatric Clinical Nurse Specialist, The Children's Hospital at Albany Medical Center, Albany, NY*

Roberta Kordish, MSN, RN. *Owner, Director, and Corporate Treasurer, Professional Nurse Associates, Inc., Cleveland, OH*

Janet Elizabeth Bloomer Kristic, MSN, RN. *Assistant Professor of Nursing, University of Oklahoma, Oklahoma City, OK*

Alma J. Labunski, PhD, MSN, RN. *Associate Professor of Nursing, St. Xavier College, Chicago, IL*

Judith K. Leavitt, MEd, RN. *Professor of Nursing, Tompkins Cortland Community College, Dryden, NY*

Mariann C. Lovell, MS, RN. *Assistant Professor of Nursing, Wright State University, Dayton, OH*

Susan McCabe, MS, RN. *Instructor Psychiatric Mental Health Nursing, Crouse Irving Memorial Hospital School of Nursing, Syracuse, NY*

Michele A. Michael, PhD, RN. *Assistant Professor, University of Maryland, School of Nursing, Baltimore, MD*

B. Patricia Nix, MSN, RN. *Instructor of Nursing, Henry Ford Community College, Dearborn, MI*

Kathleen Deska Pagana, PhD, RN. *Assistant Professor of Nursing, Lycoming College, Williamsport, PA*

Tamra Parsons, MSN, RN. *Associate Professor, Dekalb College, Clarkston, GA*

Judith K. Sands, EdD, RN. *Assistant Professor, University of Virginia School of Nursing, Charlottesville, VA*

Karen Stefaniak, MSN, RN. *Divisional Director Obstetrical Nursing, University of Kentucky Adjunct Faculty, Lexington, KY*

Deborah L. Ulrich, PhD, RN. *Associate Professor, Miami University, Oxford, OH*

Bernadette Mazurek Vulcan, MSN, RN, C, PNP. *Doctoral Student, University of Rochester, Rochester, NY; Pediatric Nurse Practitioner Consultant, Children's Unit, Elmira Psychiatric Center, Elmira, NY*

Gail D. Wegner, MSN, RN. *Associate Professor, Purdue University, Calumet, Hammond, IN*

Janet Sullivan Wilson, MEd, RN. *Assistant Professor and Consultant, University of Oklahoma College of Nursing, Oklahoma City, OK*

Contributors Previous Editions

Ida M. Androwich, MS, RN
Janis P. Bellack, PhD, MN, RN
Kay Bensing, MA, RN
Cecily Lynn Betz, PhD, RN
Phyllis Gorney Cooper, MN, RN
Olivian De Souza, MSN, RN
Cynthia Dunsmore, MSN, RN
Jackie Flaskerud, PhD, RN
Carolyn Vas Fore, MSN, RN
Elizabeth Anne Gomez, MSN, RN
E. Ingvarda Hanson, MSN, RN
Anne C. Holland, MSN, RN
Esther Matassarin-Jacobs, PhD, RN
Michele M. Kamradt, EdD, RN
Carol W. Kennedy, PhD, RN
Deborah Koniak, EdD, RN
Beverly Kopala, MS, RN
Karen Krejci, MSN, RN
Edwina A. McConnell, PhD, MS, RN
Jerry R. Myhan, MSN, RN
Joan Reighley, MN, RN
Constance M. Ritzman, MSN, RN
Mary Charles Santopietro, EdD, MS, EdM, RN, CS
Ann M. Schofield, MS, RN
Victoria Schoolcraft, MSN, RN
Diane S. Smith, MSN, RN, CS
Diane M. Taylor Snow, MSN, RN
Deborah L. Ulrich, MA, RN
Francene Weatherby, MSN, RNC

AJN / MOSBY

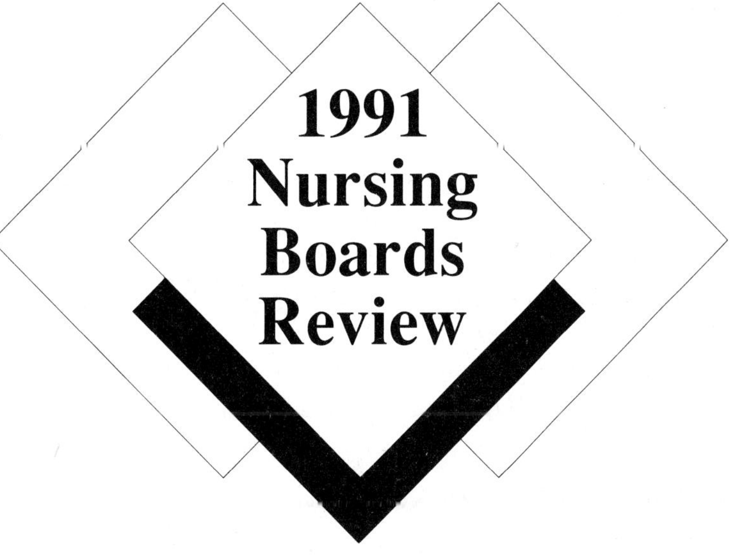

For the NCLEX-RN Examination

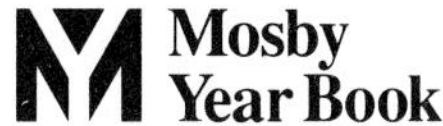

St. Louis Baltimore Boston Chicago London Philadelphia Sydney Toronto

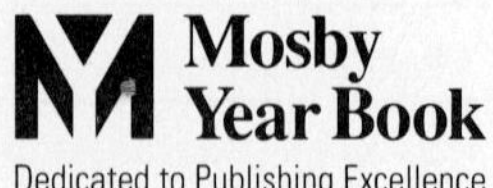

Accurate indications, adverse reactions, and dosage schedules for drugs are provided in this book, but it is possible that they may change. The reader is urged to review the package information data of the manufacturers of the medications mentioned.

Printed in the United States of America

Mosby-Year Book, Inc.
11830 Westline Industrial Drive
St. Louis, MO 63146

ISBN: 0-8016-0018-9

HG / MV / MV 9 8 7 6 5 4 3 2

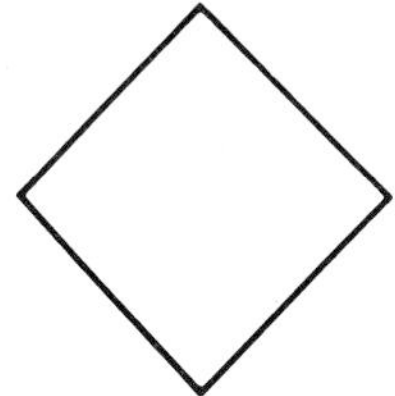

Contents

Section 1: Preparing for the NCLEX-RN 1

Section 2: Nursing Care of the Client with Psychosocial, Mental Health/ Psychiatric Problems 13

INTRODUCTION 15

Overview 15
Scope of the Profession 15
Interpersonal Relationships 15
Roles Assumed by the Nurse 16
Locations of Practice 16
Psychosocial Characteristics of the Healthy Client 16

THERAPEUTIC USE OF SELF 21

Theoretical Knowledge Base 21
Nurse-Client Relationship 22
Nursing Process 24
Interpersonal Treatment Modalities 25

LEGAL ASPECTS OF PSYCHIATRIC NURSING 28

Civil Procedures 28
Criminal Procedures 28
Recent Judicial Precedents 29
Role of the Nurse 29

LOSS, DEATH AND DYING 30

General Concepts 30
Overview 30
Application of the Nursing Process to the Client Experiencing a Loss 31
Selected Health Problems 31
Loss (other than death and dying) 31
Death and Dying 32

ANXIOUS BEHAVIOR 36

General Concepts 36
Overview 36
Application of the Nursing Process to the Client Experiencing Anxious Behavior 37
Selected Health Problems 40
Phobias 40
Dissociative Reactions 41
Obsessive-Compulsive Disorders 42
Anorexia Nervosa 43
Bulemia 43
Psychosomatic Disorders 44
Conversion Disorders 45
Post-Traumatic Stress Disorder 46

CONFUSED BEHAVIOR 48

General Concepts 48
Overview 48
Application of the Nursing Process to the Client Exhibiting Confused Behavior 48
Selected Health Problem 48
Chronic Confusion 48

ELATED-DEPRESSIVE BEHAVIOR 50

General Concepts 50
Overview 50
Application of the Nursing Process to the Client with an Affective Disorder 52
Selected Health Problems 53
Depression 53
Elation and Hyperactive Behavior 58

SOCIALLY MALADAPTIVE BEHAVIOR 62

General Concepts 62
Overview 62
Application of the Nursing Process to the Client Exhibiting Socially Maladaptive Behavior 62
Selected Health Problems 63
Violence in the Family 63
Hostile and Agressive Behavior 66
Sexual Acting Out 67
Antisocial Behavior 68

SUSPICIOUS BEHAVIOR 70

General Concepts 70
Overview 70
Application of the Nursing Process to the Client Exhibiting Suspicious Behavior 70
Selected Health Problem 70
Paranoia 70

WITHDRAWN BEHAVIOR 72

General Concepts 72
Overview 72
Application of the Nursing process to the Client Exhibiting Withdrawn Behavior 76
Selected Health Problem 80
Schizophrenic Disorders 80

SUBSTANCE USE DISORDERS 81

General Concepts 81
Overview 81
Application of the Nursing Process to the Client with a Substance Use Disorder 82
Selected Health Problems 83
Alcohol 83
Drugs other than Alcohol 87

GLOSSARY 91

REPRINTS 95

Horsely, G. "Baggage from the Past" 97
Harris, E. "Lithium" 101
DiMotto, J. "Relaxation" 106
Harris, E. "Extrapyramidal Side Effects of Antipsychotic Medications" 111
Harris, E. "Antipsychotic Medications" 116
Harris, E. "Drugs and Depression" 124
Campbell, E., Williams, M., & Mlynarczyk, S. "After the Fall—Confusion" 126
Harris, E. "Sedative-Hypnotic Drugs" 130
Hoff, L. & Resing, M. "Was This Suicide Preventable" 136
Acee, A. & Smith, P. "Crack" 142

Section 3: Nursing Care of the Adult 147

THE HEALTHY ADULT 151

Characteristics of the Healthy Young and Middle-Aged Adult 151
Characteristics of the Elderly Healthy Adult 153

SURGERY 157

Overview 157
Perioperative Period 157
Discharge 160

OXYGENATION 162

General Concepts 162
Overview/Physiology 162
Application of the Nursing Process to the Client Experiencing Oxygenation Problems 164
Selected Health Problems Resulting in Interference with Cardiac Functioning 169
Cardiopulmonary Arrest 169
Shock 170
Angina Pectoris 171
Myocardial Infarction 173
Pacemaker 177
Congestive Heart Failure 178
Hypertension 182
Circulatory Problems 183
Selected Health Problems Resulting in Interference with Respiration 185
Chronic Obstructive Pulmonary Disease 185
Pneumonia 188
Tuberculosis 190
Pulmonary Embolus 192
Chest Tubes and Chest Surgery 193
Cancer of the Lung 195
Cancer of the Larynx 196

NUTRITION AND METABOLISM 199

The Digestive Tract 199
General Concepts 199
Overview/Physiology 199
Application of the Nursing Process to the Client with Digestive Tract Problems 201
Selected Health Problems Resulting in Problems with Digestion 205
Hiatal Hernia 205
Gastritis 205
Peptic Ulcer Disease 206
Diverticulosis/Diverticulitis 210
Cholecystitis with Cholelithiasis 210
Pancreatitis 211
Hepatitis 212
Cirrhosis 213
Complications of Liver Disease: Esophageal Varices, Ascites, Hepatic Encephalopathy 214
The Endocrine System 216
General Concepts 216
Overview/Physiology 216
Application of the Nursing Process to the Client with Endocrine System Problems 218
Selected Health Problems 219
Hyperpituitarism 219
Hypopituitarism 220
Hyperthyroidism 220
Hypothyroidism 222
Hyperparathyroidism 222
Hypoparathyroidism 223
Hyperfunction of the Adrenal Glands 223
Hyposecretion of the Adrenal Glands 225
Hypofunction of the Pancreas: Diabetes Mellitus 225

ELIMINATION 232

The Kidneys 232
General Concepts 232
Overview/Physiology 232
Application of the Nursing Process to the Client with Kidney Problems 236
Selected Health Problems Resulting in Alteration in Urinary Elimination 242
Cystitis/Pyelonephritis 242
Urinary Calculi 243
Cancer of the Bladder 244
Acute Renal Failure 245
Chronic Renal Failure 247
Dialysis 249
Kidney Transplantation 252
Benign Prostatic Hypertrophy 254
Cancer of the Prostate 256
The Large Bowel 257
General Concepts 257
Overview/Physiology 257
Application of the Nursing Process to the Client with Large Bowel Problems 258
Selected Health Problems Resulting in Alteration in Large Bowel Elimination 259
Alteration in Normal Bowel Evacuation 259
Inflammatory Bowel Disease (Regional Enteritis, Ulcerative Colitis) 261
Total Colectomy with Ileostomy 263
Mechanical Obstruction of the Colon 264
Cancer of the Colon 265
Hemorrhoids or Anal Fissure 266

SAFETY AND SECURITY 269

General Concepts 269
Overview/Physiology 269
Application of the Nursing Process to the Client with Problems of Safety and Security 270
Selected Health Problems Resulting in an Interference with Senation and Perception 275
Acute Head Injury 275
Intracranial Surgery 276
Cerebrovascular Accident 277
Spinal Cord Injuries 279
Parkinson's Syndrome 281
Multiple Sclerosis 283
Amyotrophic Lateral Sclerosis 284
Myasthenia Gravis 285
Cataracts 286
Retinal Detachment 289
Glaucoma 290
Nasal Problems Requiring Surgery 291
Epistaxis 291

ACTIVITY AND REST 293

General Concepts 293
Overview/Physiology 293
Application of the Nursing Process to the Client with Activity and Rest Problems 293
Selected Health Problems Resulting in an Interference with Activity and Rest 295
Fractures 295
Fractured Hip 297
Amputation 299
Arthritis 300
Collagen Disease 302
Herniated Nucleus Pulposus 302

CELLULAR ABERRATION 306

General Concepts 306
Overview/Physiology 306
Application of the Nursing Process to the Client with Cancer 307

Selected Health Problems 311
Hodgkin's Disease 311
Cancer of the Cervix 312
Cancer of the Endometrium of the Uterus 313
Cancer of the Breast 313
Acquired Immune Deficiency Syndrome 315

REPRINTS 317

''CE Pain'' 319
Cohen, S. ''How to Work with Chest Tubes'' 331
Caine, R. & Bufalino, P. ''The Patient Receiving Total Parenteral Nutrition'' 351
Gavin, J. ''Diabetes and Exercise'' 352
Chambers, J. ''Bowel Management in Dialysis Patients'' 359
Larrabee, J. & Pepper, G. ''The Person with a Spinal Cord Injury'' 361

Section 4: Nursing Care of the Childbearing Family 379

FEMALE REPRODUCTIVE ANATOMY AND PHYSIOLOGY 383
General Concepts 383
Overview/Physiology 383
Application of the Nursing Process to Reproductive Health Maintenance and Health Promotion of Adult Women 385

ANTEPARTAL CARE 390
General Concepts 390
Normal Childbearing 390
Overview of Management 395
Application of the Nursing Process to Normal Childbearing, Antepartal Care 395
High-Risk Childbearing 399
Application of the Nursing Process to the High-Risk Pregnant Client 403
Selected Health Problems in the Antepartal Period 404
Abortion 404
Incompetent Cervical Os 404
Ectopic Pregnancy 405
Hydatidiform Mole 405
Placenta Previa 406
Abruptio Placentae 407
Pregnancy-Induced Hypertension (Hypertensive Disorders) 408
Diabetes 410
Cardiac Disorders 412
Anemia 413
Hyperemesis Gravidarum (Pernicious Vomiting of Pregnancy) 414
Infections 414
Multiple Gestation 416
Adolescent Pregnancy 416

INTRAPARTAL CARE 419
General Concepts 419
Normal Childbearing 419
Ongoing Management and Nursing Care 422
Application of the Nursing Process to Normal Childbearing, Intrapartal Care 426
Application of the Nursing Process to the High-Risk Intrapartal Client 431
Selected Health Problems in the Intrapartal Period 432
Dystocia 432
Premature Labor 434
Emergency Birth 435
Episiotomy 436
Forceps 436
Vacuum Extraction 437
Cesarean Birth 438
Vaginal Birth After Cesarean Delivery (VBAC) 439
Rupture of the Uterus 439
Amniotic Fluid Embolism 440

POSTPARTAL CARE 441
General Concepts 441
Normal Childbearing 441
Application of the Nursing Process to Normal Childbearing, Postpartal Care 443
Application of the Nursing Process to the High-risk Postpartal Client 446
Selected Health Problems in the Postpartal Period 447
Postpartum Hemorrhage 447
Hematoma 448
Pulmonary Embolus 448
Puerperal Infection 448
Mastitis 449
Postpartum Cystitis 450
Psychological Maladaptations 450
Selected Long-term Problems Associated with Childbearing 451
Uterine Prolapse with or without Cystocele or Rectocele 451
Uterine Fibroids 452

NEWBORN CARE 454
The Normal Newborn 454
General Characteristics 454
Specific Body Parts: usual findings and common variations 455
Systems Adaptations 458
Gestational Age Variations Based on Neuromuscular Responses and External Physical Characteristics 460
Application of the Nursing Process to the Normal Newborn 463
Application of the Nursing Process to the Newborn at Risk 466
Selected Health Problems in the Newborn 466
Hypothermia 466
Neonatal Jaundice 467
Respiratory Distress 469
Neonatal Necrotizing Enterocolitis (NEC) 470
Hypoglycemia 471
Newborn Infection 472
Neonatal Drug and Alcohol Addiction 472
Acquired Immune Deficiency Syndrome (AIDS) 473
Birth Injuries/Congenital Anomalies 474
Parental Reaction to a Sick, Disabled, or Malformed Newborn 475

REPRINTS 477

Devore, N. & Baldwin, K. ''Ectopic Pregnancy on the Rise'' 479
Smith, J. ''The Danger of Prenatal Cocaine Use'' 484
Hoffmaster, J. ''Detecting and Treating Pregnancy-Induced Hypertension'' 490
Whitaker, C. ''Death Before Birth'' 498
Fullar, S. ''Care of Postpartum Adolescents'' 500
Wilkerson, N. ''A Comprehensive Look at Bilirubinemia'' 506

Section 5: Nursing Care of the Child 513

THE HEALTHY CHILD 517
General Concepts 517
Infant 517
Toddler 520
Preschooler 522
School Age 523
Adolescent 524
Application of the Nursing Process to the Healthy Child 525

THE ILL AND HOSPITALIZED CHILD 529
Overview 529
Application of the Nursing Process to the Ill and Hospitalized Child 530

SENSATION, PERCEPTION, AND PROTECTION 535
General Concepts 535
Overview/Physiology 535
Application of the Nursing Process to the Child with a Sensory Problem 535
Selected Health Problems: Interference with Sensation 535
Otitis Media 535
Tonsillectomy and Adenoidectomy 537
Strabismus 537
Application of the Nursing Process to the Child with an Interference with Protection: Communicable Disease 538
Selected Health Problems: Communicable Diseases, Skin Problems, Infestations 538
Communicable Diseases 538
Sexually Transmitted Diseases 541
Common Skin Problems and Infestations 543
Pinworms 543
Application of the Nursing Process to the Child with an Interference with Protection: Safety 545
Selected Health Problems Resulting in an Interference with Protection: Safety 545
Poisonous Ingestions 545
Burns 548
Application of the Nursing Process to the Child with Developmental or Neurologic Disabilities 553
Selected Health Problems: Developmental or Neurologic Disabilities 555
Mental Retardation 555
Attention Deficit Disorder 556
Down Syndrome 556
Cerebral Palsy 557
Hydrocephalus 558
Spina Bifida 559
Seizure Disorders 560
Meningitis 563

OXYGENATION 565
General Concepts 565
Overview/Physiology 565
Application of the Nursing Process to the Child with Respiratory Problems 565
Selected Health Problems Resulting in an Interference with Respiration 567
Sudden Infant Death Syndrome 567
Acute Spasmodic Laryngitis (Spasmodic Croup) 568
Acute Epiglottis 568
Laryngotracheobronchitis 568
Bronchiolitis 568
Bronchopulmonary Dysplasia 568
Bronchial Asthma 569
Application of the Nursing Process to the Child with Cardiovascular Dysfunction 571
Selected Health Problems Resulting in an Interference with Cardiac Functioning 572
Congenital Heart Disease 572
Rheumatic Fever and Rheumatic Heart Disease 578
Application of the Nursing Process to the Child with Hematologic Problems 579
Selected Health Problems Resulting in an Interference with Formed Elements of the Blood 579
Iron-Deficiency Anemia 579
Sickle Cell Anemia 580
Hemophilia 582

NUTRITION AND METABOLISM 584
General Concepts 584
Overview/Physiology 584
Application of the Nursing Process to the Child with Problems of Nutrition and Metabolism 584
Selected Health Problems Resulting in an Interference with Nutrition and Metabolism 585
Vomiting and Diarrhea 585
Nonorganic Failure to Thrive 587
Pyloric Stenosis 588
Celiac Disease 589
Cleft Lip and Palate 590
Congenital Hypothyroidism 592
Insulin-Dependent Diabetes Mellitus 593
Cystic Fibrosis 595

ELIMINATION 598
General Concepts 598
Overview/Physiology 598
Application of the Nursing Process to the Child with Elimination Problems 598
Selected Health Problems Resulting in an Interference with Urinary or Bowel Elimination 598
Hypospadias 598
Urinary Tract Infection 599
Vesicourethral Reflux 600
Nephritis 601
Nephrosis 602
Lower GI Tract Obstruction 603

MOBILITY 605
General Concepts 605
Overview/Physiology 605
Application of the Nursing Process to the Child with an Interference with Mobility 605
Selected Health Problems Resulting in an Interference with Mobility 609
Congenital Clubfoot 609
Congenital Hip Dysplasia 609
Legg-Calvé-Perthes Disease 610
Scoliosis 610
Osteomyelitis 611

CELLULAR ABERRATION 613
General Concepts 613
Overview/Physiology 613
Application of the Nursing Process to the Child with Cancer 613
Selected Health Problems Resulting from Cellular Aberration 613
Leukemia 618
Solid Tumors 619

REPRINTS 621
Reynolds, E. & Ramenofsky, M. "The Emotional Impact of Trauma on Toddlers" 623
Rimar, J. "Shock in Infants and Children: Assessment and Treatment" 627
Meier, E. "Evaluating Head Trauma in Infants and Children" 635
Sheredy, C. "Factors to Consider When Assessing Responses to Pain" 639

Section 6: Questions and Answers (Sample NCLEX-RN Test) 643

Part One 645
Questions 645
Answers and Rationales 655
Part Two 663
Questions 663
Answers and Rationales 673
Part Three 681
Questions 681
Answers and Rationales 692
Part Four 700
Questions 700
Answers and Rationales 712
Nursing Process/Client Needs Categories 720

Appendix A 725
Approved Nursing Diagnoses from the North American Nursing Diagnosis Association, June 1988 725
Appendix B 727
Common Laboratory Values—Adult 727
Appendix C 729
Information for Foreign Nurse Graduates Who Wish to Practice in the United States 729
Index 733

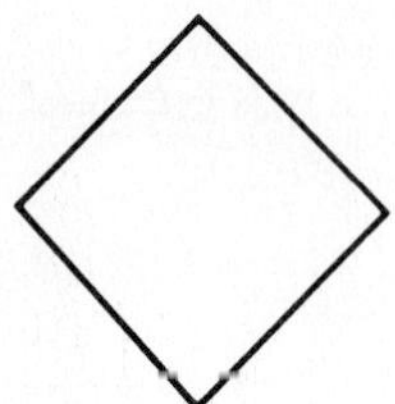

Tables and Figures

SECTION 1

Tables

1.1 Test Item Focus Suggested by the Nursing Process 4
1.2 Categories of Human Needs 5
1.3 Test Item Focus Suggested by Categories of Human Needs 5
1.4 Cognitive Strategies for Success 6
1.5 Focus of Communication Test Items 8
1.6 Keys to Success on the NCLEX-RN 10

SECTION 2

Tables

2.1 Life Cycle Stages 17
2.2 Theoretical Models 22
2.3 Social Determinants of Mental Health and Illness 23
2.4 Communication Skills in the Nurse-Client Relationship 24
2.5 Manifestations of Anxiety 37
2.6 Stress Management 39
2.7 Antianxiety Agents (Minor Tranquilizers) 41
2.8 Medications Used to Treat Affective Disorders 51
2.9 Suicide Methods 56
2.10 Major Tranquilizers (Neuroleptics) 75
2.11 Side Effects of Major Tranquilizers 76
2.12 Selected Problem Behaviors and Interventions 77
2.13 Types of Withdrawn Behavior (Schizophrenia) 80
2.14 Signs and Symptoms of Withdrawal and Overdose of Common Drugs of Abuse 89

SECTION 3

Tables

3.1 Basic Four Food Groups 152
3.2 US Recommended Daily Nutrition for An Average Health Adult 153
3.3 Stages of General Anesthesia 159
3.4 General Points Regarding Anesthetic Agents 160
3.5 Calculating IV Rates 160
3.6 Postoperative Diet Modifications 160
3.7 Classes of Analgesics 161
3.8 Emergency Drugs 170
3.9 Angina Pectoris Drugs 173
3.10 Blood Tests for Myocardial Infarction 175
3.11 Anticoagulant and Thrombolytic Drugs 176
3.12 Approximate Sodium Content in Selected Food Items 177
3.13 Cholesterol and Saturated Fat Content in Selected Items 177
3.14 Congestive Heart Failure 179
3.15 Cardiac Glycosides 179
3.16 Antihypertensive Drugs 180
3.17 Foods High in Potassium 182
3.18 Bronchodilators 187
3.19 Expectorants 187
3.20 Antibiotics 189
3.21 Antituberculosis Drugs 191
3.22 Gastrointestinal Hormones 200
3.23 Digestive Enzymes 200
3.24 Drug Therapy for Peptic Ulcer Disease 207
3.25 High Fiber/Roughage Diet 210
3.26 Principles of a Low Fat Diet 210
3.27 Hormones 217
3.28 Steroids 226
3.29 Hypoglycemic Drugs 227
3.30 Diabetic Meal Planning with Exchange Lists 229
3.31 Differentiating Hypoglycemia from Ketoacidosis (Hyperglycemia) 230
3.32 Fluid Imbalance 234
3.33 Electrolyte Imbalances 234
3.34 Acid-Base Imbalance 237
3.35 Laboratory Tests Used to Evaluate Renal Function 237
3.36 Drug Therapy for Kidney Problems 241
3.37 Diuretics 246

3.38 Low Protein Diet Sample Menu 247
3.39 Immunosuppressive Drugs 253
3.40 Prostatectomies 255
3.41 Drug Therapy for Bowel Management 260
3.42 Comparison of Crohn's Disease and Ulcerative Colitis 262
3.43 Foods to be Avoided on a Low Residue Diet 263
3.44 Cranial Nerves 269
3.45 Parasympathetic and Sympathetic Effects 269
3.46 Spinal Cord 280
3.47 Drugs Used to Treat Parkinsonism .. 282
3.48 Drugs Used to Treat Myasthenia Gravis 286
3.49 Eye Medications 287
3.50 Anti-inflammatory Drugs 301
3.51 Antigout Medications 303
3.52 Antiemetics 310
3.53 Staging of Hodgkin's Disease 312

Figures

3.1 The Normal Heart 163
3.2 Pressures in the Vascular System 164
3.3 Areas of Auscultation of Heart Valves 165
3.4 Pulmonary Volumes and Capacities of an Adult 166
3.5 Components of a Normal Electrocardiogram 167
3.6 Distribution of Typical Angina Pain 172
3.7 Coronary Blood Supply 174
3.8 Myocardial Infarction 174
3.9 Typical Enzyme Patterns 175
3.10 Pattern for Rotating Tourniquets 181
3.11 Common Manifestations of Chronic Arterial and Venous Peripheral Vascular Disease 184
3.12 Water-Seal Chest Drainage 194
3.13 Pleur-evac System 195
3.14 Components of the Kidney 233
3.15 Components and Functions of the Nephron 233
3.16 Schematic Representation of Dialysis 249
3.17 Normal Male Anatomy 254
3.18 Types of Prostatectomies 256
3.19 The Eye 270
3.20 Decorticate Posturing 272
3.21 Decerebrate Posturing 273
3.22 Areas of the Brain that Control Certain Motor and Sensory Functions 278

SECTION 4

Tables

4.1 Assessment of Fertility/Infertility 386
4.2 Family Planning 387
4.3 Interpretation of Pap Test Results ... 389
4.4 Health Teaching to Reduce Risk of Osteoporosis 389
4.5 Signs and Symptoms of Pregnancy .. 393
4.6 Naegele's Rule 395
4.7 McDonald's Rule 396
4.8 Recommended Dietary Allowances for Females aged 11–50 398
4.9 Selected Nutrients Essential for Health in Pregnancy and Lacatation 399
4.10 Pregnant Woman's Daily Food Intake 399
4.11 Childbirth Preparation 400
4.12 Laboratory Studies of Fetal Well-Being 403
4.13 Classification of Pregnancy-Induced Hypertension 409
4.14 Anticonvulsive Agent 410
4.15 Baseline Fetal Heart Rate 422
4.16 Decelerations in Fetal Heart Rate 424
4.17 Stages and Phases of Labor 425
4.18 Uterine Smooth Muscle Stimulants .. 431
4.19 Uterine Dysfunction in Labor 432
4.20 Oxytocin 433
4.21 Tocolytic Agent 436
4.22 Lochia Changes 442
4.23 Maternal Psychological Adaptation .. 443
4.24 Rh O (D) Human Immune Globulin 444
4.25 Lactation Suppressant Drugs 445
4.26 Postpartum Depression 451
4.27 Nutritional Comparison of Human and Cow's Milk 460
4.28 High Risk Conditions for Newborns by Gestational Age and Growth Classifications 462
4.29 Apgar Scoring Chart 464

Figures

4.1 Female Pelvis 384
4.2 Female Internal Reproductive Organs 384
4.3 Basal Body Temperature 386
4.4 Common Site of Ectopic Pregnancy 405
4.5 Hydatidiform 405
4.6 Placenta Previa 406
4.7 Abruptio Placentae 407
4.8 Selected Categories of Presentation .. 420

4.9 Tracing of Normal Fetal Heart Rate 421
4.10 Acceleration of Fetal Heart Rate in Response to Uterine Activity 422
4.11 Types of Deceleration in Fetal Heart Rate 423
4.12 Assessment of Uterine Contraction .. 426
4.13 Leopold's Maneuvers 427
4.14 Site of Auscultation of FHR with Fetus in ROA Position 429
4.15 Friedman Curve 434
4.16 Types of Episiotomies 437
4.17 Types of Cesarian Incisions 438
4.18 Bones, Fontanels, and Sutures of Newborn's Skull 456
4.19 Fetal Circulation 459
4.20 Newborn Maturity Rating and Classification 461
4.21 Rh Sensitization 467
4.22 Silverman-Anderson Scale 470

SECTION 5

Tables

5.1 Vital Sign Ranges in Children 518
5.2 Average Daily Caloric Needs of Infants and Children 519
5.3 American Academy of Pediatrics Recommended Immunization Schedule 520
5.4 Commonly Used Pediatric Restraints 532
5.5 Medication and Temperature Guide . 532
5.6 Medication Administration for Young Children 533
5.7 Estimating Pediatric Drug Doses 534
5.8 Types of Isolation 540
5.9 Sexually Transmitted Diseases 542
5.10 Common Skin Problems and Infestations 544
5.11 Commonly Ingested Poisonous Substances 546
5.12 Systemic Responses to Burn Injury .. 549
5.13 Levels of Retardation 555
5.14 Signs and Symptoms of Increased Intracranial Pressure in Infants and Children 557
5.15 Medications Used to Treat Seizure Disorders 562
5.16 Hematology Values in Children 566
5.17 Comparison of Croup and Bronchiolitis 568
5.18 Medications Used to Treat Asthma .. 569
5.19 Cardiac Catherization in Children: Nursing Considerations 571
5.20 Comparison of Type 1 (Insulin Dependent) and Type 2 (Non-insulin Dependent) Diabetes Mellitus 593
5.21 Types of Traction 606
5.22 Commonly Used Chemotherapeutic Agents 614
5.23 Child's Conception of Death 617
5.24 Common Solid Tumors in Children 628

Figures

5.1 Estimation of Burn Surface Area 550
5.2 Normal and Abnormal Hearts 573
5.3 Common Modes of Genetic Transmission 581
5.4 Types of Traction 607
5.5 Petaled Cast Edges 609

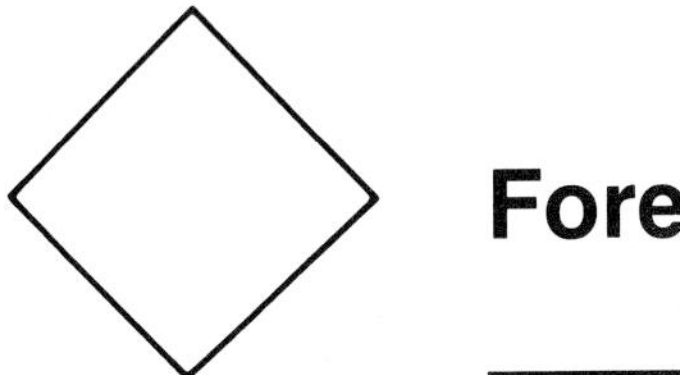

Foreword

One day when I was in the clinical setting talking with staff nurses about the changes in nursing practice, the conversation turned to the state board examinations we took to become licensed registered nurses. Although most of us recalled the long hours of sitting at a desk in a heavily monitored room, one of the nurses close to retirement described her very different experience. Her exam was a test of her ability to assemble the right equipment on the right tray for procedures such as an enema or catheterization. One of the more difficult "test items" was to assemble a Bunsen burner and then to use it to bend a glass tube to the angle correct for use by a bedridden patient. I think back to that conversation periodically as something of a benchmark that describes how far both our society and the profession of nursing have progressed.

Today's nurses are knowledge workers in that their primary service generates from the ability to use their unique body of knowledge to the benefit of the clients they serve. The fact that nurses are knowledge workers does not minimize the requirement that they must also be able to implement procedures safely; it simply means that their knowledge is the primary ingredient in their performance. I like to think of today's nurse as a **THOUGHT-FULL DOER**; that is, everything a nurse does reflects a fullness of knowledge regarding that individual client and potential nursing actions.

The *AJN 1990 Nursing Boards Review* is an excellent compilation of the knowledge base required by today's nurse. It is organized to highlight the facts, concepts, and guiding principles required to implement the nursing process with a broad range of clients and settings. It provides readings to supplement critical points. It allows you to test yourself and compare the rationale for your response with the rationale for the correct and the incorrect answers for over 350 test questions. And it gives you as a test taker, guidance on how to be effective. Before writing this foreword, I read the content and took the test, and the design of this review worked for me. It is an excellent review.

To those of you about to embark on a career in nursing, my wish is that you will find nursing the stimulating and fulfilling career it can and should be. Each day you will find yourself confronted with the familiar and the unfamiliar but never anything that is "just routine." You have the privilege to be part of a profession that offers essential, irreplaceable services to human beings. Today, review and refresh your knowledge base to ensure attainment of the license required for you to offer nursing services to the public. Tomorrow and tomorrow and forever, review and refresh your knowledge base to ensure those services are the best they can be.

Carol Lindeman, PhD, RN, FAAN
Dean, School of Nursing
Oregon Health Sciences University
Portland, Oregon

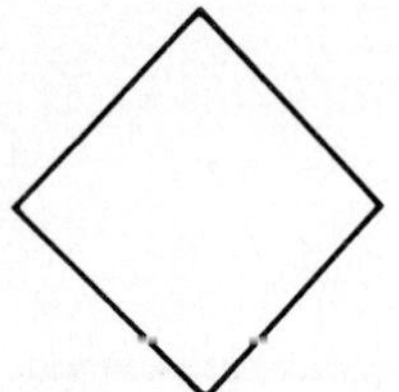

Introduction

Congratulations! You have achieved a goal you set for yourself by completing your nursing program. Now you are about to embark on a new and exciting career but you have one more challenge to meet to become a registered nurse: to pass the NCLEX-RN examination. Here, in one single volume, the *AJN/Mosby 1991 Nursing Boards Review* book provides you with a comprehensive review of the essential content needed to pass your state board examination. Your courses have given you the information you need, however a vital component in helping to ensure your success on the boards is the process of review and study.

The examination has two foci: the nursing process and client needs. Emphasis is also placed on the care of the healthy as well as the ill client. Content areas covered by the examination include the care of the adult, child, childbearing family, and the client with an emotional disturbance.

This book is divided into three parts. Part one introduces you to the format of the NCLEX-RN including the scoring methods. The specific framework of the test, including information on the nursing process, client needs, and areas of human functioning, is presented with explanations and examples of how these might be tested. To help with your test-taking skills, strategies to increase your competence and confidence are reviewed. Techniques for stress reduction on the day of the examination are also presented. As you study, refer to this section frequently to reinforce principles you will need to remember during the examination.

Part two covers the content areas. Review one clinical area at a time. You may choose to start with the one in which you feel least comfortable. A highlighter pen is helpful to underline areas you may want to return to for more study, or you may choose to make notes in the margins. Use your nursing texts to look up unfamiliar material or to broaden your knowledge base. At the end of each content area in this review book, timely articles from the *American Journal of Nursing* and *MCN*: the American Journal of Maternal/Child Nursing are included to further enhance your knowledge.

Part three consists of one sample NCLEX-type examination. The items in each of the four test booklets are deliberately mixed because the NCLEX exam is integrated. Set aside time each day to answer the questions in one test booklet. Time yourself so that you can complete the questions in 90 minutes. The goal is to be able to answer one question per minute.

In the appendixes of the book, the test questions have been coded according to the nursing process and type of client need. If you wish to strengthen your skill in answering questions on a particular step of the nursing process or a particular category of client need, you will be able to locate specific questions to help you become more familiar and comfortable with that subject area.

These tests can also be used as pretests before you begin your study to identify areas on which you need to spend more time. After you have reviewed the material in the book, retake the tests to see how much you improved your score. Answers and rationales are given for all test items. The rationales can be used to clarify information. To determine the percentage of items you answered correctly in each test, divide the number of your correct answers by the total number of questions on the test. If your score is less than 75%, you need to spend more time reviewing.

You may also want to take an intensive review course such as the AJN/Mosby Nursing Boards Review. The opportunity to listen to an instructor who is not only a specialist in a content area but also experienced in the review process can be very helpful to you in structuring your own review.

Whether you decide to study on your own or to use this book in conjunction with a review course, the instructors who contributed to this edition as well as the staff of the AJN and Mosby–Year Book, Inc. wish you success on the NCLEX-RN and a stimulating and rewarding nursing career.

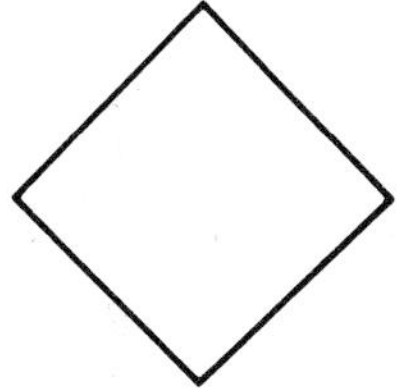

Preface

We know that you will be as pleased as we are that you have selected the *AJN/Mosby 1991 Nursing Boards Review*. With this excellent review book, you can prepare to successfully take the NCLEX-RN exam.

You will note the long and impressive list of faculty contributors and contributing authors who have developed this book. These top national nursing specialists are experienced educators and clinicians who have personally taught and continue to teach the AJN/Mosby Nursing Boards Review course. Their knowledge and experience, and their skill at helping students trigger memory of knowledge gained in nursing education, make them eminently qualified to help you through this book and through the AJN/Mosby Nursing Boards Review course.

We at the AJN Company and Mosby–Year Book, Inc., thank the talented and conscientious faculty contributors who have honed the focus of this book on the NCLEX format. We know their efforts will help you approach the NCLEX-RN exam with confidence.

To achieve a greater sense of security about your exam, consider taking the AJN/Mosby Nursing Boards Review course. For more information on this course, please call Resource Applications, Inc., toll-free 800-826-1877; in Maryland, call 301-796-9010.

Our sincere best wishes to you for success in the exam and throughout your nursing career.

Maryanne Shanahan, RN
Chief Operating Officer
The AJN Company

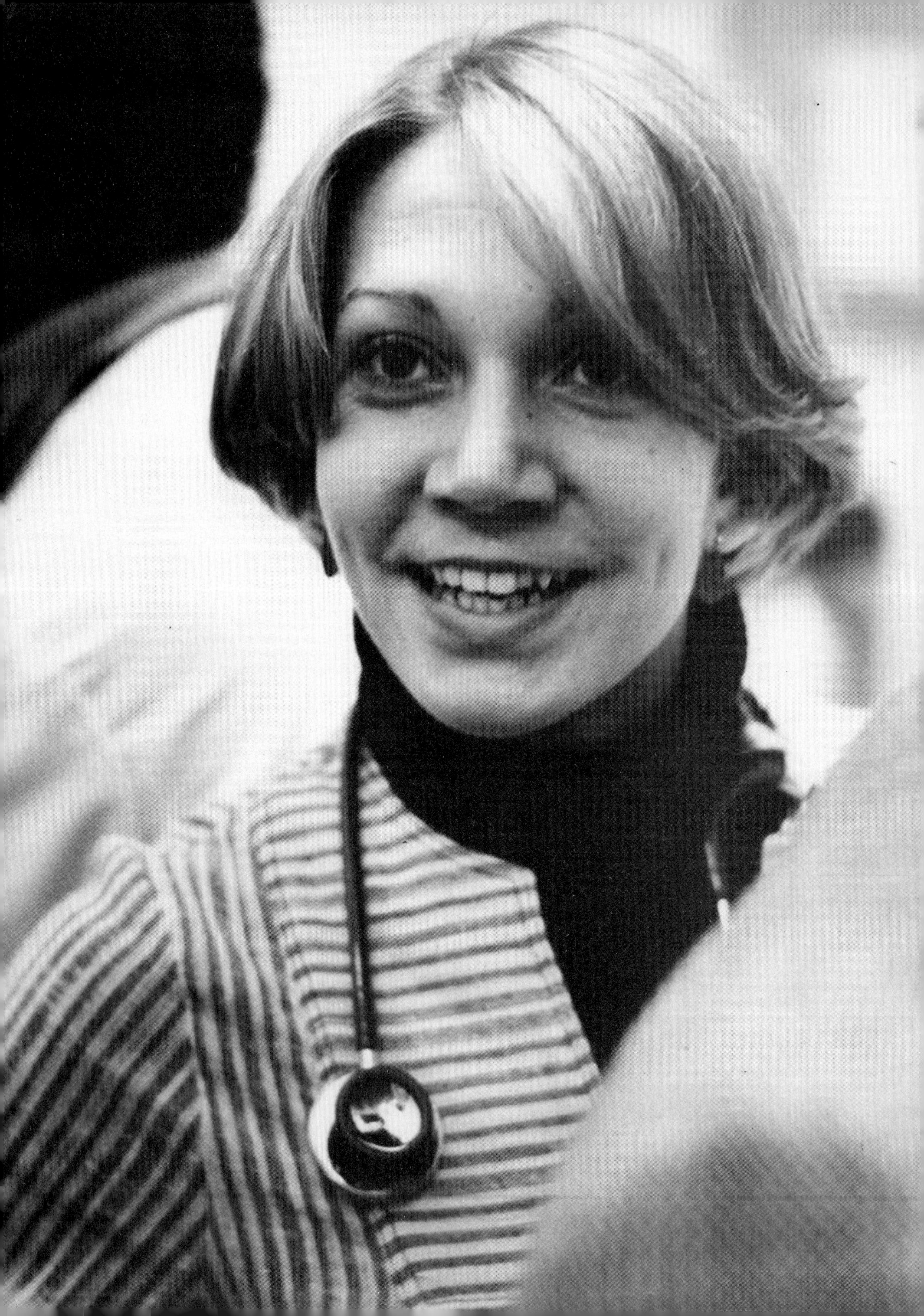

Preparing for the NCLEX-RN

Marybeth Young, MSN, RNC

Section 1: Preparing for the NCLEX-RN

TABLES

1.1 Test Item Focus Suggested by the Nursing Process 4
1.2 Categories of Human Needs 5
1.3 Test Item Focus Suggested by Categories of Human Needs 5
1.4 Cognitive Strategies for Success 6
1.5 Focus of Communication Test Items 8
1.6 Keys to Success on the NCLEX-RN 10

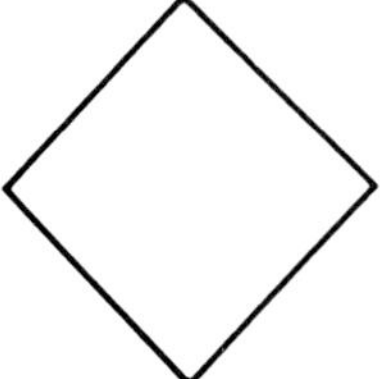

Pretest

1. Test items on the NCLEX-RN are based on case studies
   a. describing actual or potential health problems.
   b. integrating knowledge of physiologic and psychosocial needs.
   c. focusing on situations encountered by entry level nurses.
   d. All of the above choices are correct.
2. The examination requires that the graduate nurse select
   a. one single correct response.
   b. answers from "multiple-multiple" options.
3. Time allotted for each of the approximately 92 items in each section is
   a. 20 seconds.
   b. 30 seconds.
   c. 45 seconds.
   d. 60 seconds.
4. The integrated nursing exam contains about the same number of questions measuring knowledge and application of
   a. pediatric, maternity, and medical–surgical nursing.
   b. assessment, analysis, planning, implementation, and evaluation.
   c. acute illnesses and chronic health problems.
   d. identification of risk factors and health promotion needs.
5. Which of the following test taking hints is *not* useful in taking the licensure examination?
   a. "Try to narrow the possible answers to two choices."
   b. "Focus on key words such as *initially* or *never*."
   c. "If you do not know an answer, avoid guessing."
   d. "Be careful when erasing responses and changing them."

After completing the above pretest, you may find that you want more accurate information about the licensure examination ahead. Reading the following information may contribute to your success.

Preparing for the Licensure Exam

Planning for Review: Unique Features of This Text

You made a career choice that has required long-range planning and an investment of time, energy, and money. Now, your preparation for the NCLEX-RN examination (state boards) requires the same thoughtful preparation. *Passing* will be confirmation of your nursing competence, allowing entry into a profession eagerly awaiting new graduates. This section of the book is designed to help you achieve the goal of success.

A summary of the exam format, suggested cognitive testing strategies, and approaches to reduce tension should help you to develop an individualized plan for preparation and review. You will then be able to use the material in this text to better organize your nursing knowledge and understand the many aspects of safe practice.

While the content in the review book is basic, there are many unique features; take a few moments to familiarize yourself with the layout. Notice that the *nursing process* is the basis for organizing client health needs. Each assessment and implementation is in *priority sequence*. Goals are patient centered. Evaluation statements reflect the goals. In several chapters of each section, possible nursing diagnoses are suggested using the latest approved list of the North American Nursing Diagnosis Association (NANDA). You will need to individualize a nursing diagnosis based on analysis of assessed data for each patient suggested in a case study, as you do in actual clinical practice.

The content in each section is supplemented by tables, summaries, and illustrations to clarify information and reinforce your knowledge of specific health problems, pharmacology, growth and development, and nutrition. Examine these carefully; they may help you to recall content, promote understanding, and lead to synthesis of knowledge as you begin to see connections.

The page format includes margin space so you can mark any topic area that needs further study or clarification. Use a systematic coding system throughout the book, to guide you in later study. For example, you may wish to ** an area to refer back to notes or school texts.

Reprints of articles are collected at the end of each section. These provide a convenient reference source to supplement some content and may be especially useful if many months have separated one clinical rotation from your exam preparation.

Section 6 contains a practice test, simulating the actual NCLEX-RN exam. You may use this test separately or complete one section of it at a time. Further suggestions for using exam questions are included later in this section.

Know the Test Format

Just as the novice driver needs to know what to expect on the state driving test, each graduate nurse needs a clear idea of the professional licensure exam format. Knowing that you have some questions about the test itself, or are unsure of your responses on the pretest, the following brief summary will provide answers.

Success on the national examination is required for entry into professional practice. The same multiple-choice test is currently administered simultaneously throughout the United States twice each year. Future plans include individualized computer testing at selected sites in each state. This proposed change will eliminate the stress often experienced in a massive testing environment, allowing graduates to demonstrate nursing knowledge in a quiet setting. If your state is involved in pilot testing this new approach, information will be shared with you in advance.

There are approximately 93 test items in each of four separate, integrated sections. (Some questions are ''pilot items'' and are not counted towards the pass/fail score. However, since these are not identified as such, respond to each item with equal attention.) Situations and questions represent a variety of patient health needs and problems. One case study describing a plan for health promotion of a young family may be followed by another case study focusing on the safe care environment of an adolescent in an acute-care setting. Test items focus on critical requirements for competent practice rather than on separate specialty content, such as pediatric nursing or care of the adult.

The National Council of State Boards of Nursing organizes the licensure examination around a broad framework comprised of the *Nursing Process* and *Categories of Human Needs*. Each part of this plan is summarized briefly; implications for review are suggested.

Nursing Process

The nursing process provides organization for the test as it does for care planning in every clinical setting. Each nursing process phase is equally important in resolving health problems. This consistency is immediately evident to test takers who perceive this equal emphasis. These same graduates are quick to point out that the numbers of items testing maternity or psychiatric nursing are not equal. Table 1.1 suggests a possible test item focus for each phase of the nursing process.

Table 1.1 Test Item Focus Suggested by the Nursing Process

Phase	Possible Item Focus
Assessment	• Identifying data base • Selecting appropriate means to gather data • Gathering information from patient/family • Noting significant observations/data • Considering environmental factors • Recognizing patient/family strengths, limitations
Analysis	• Prioritizing potential/actual problems • Selecting an appropriate nursing diagnosis • Interpreting meaning of test results
Planning	• Setting measurable long/short term goals • Prioritizing goals • Involving patient/family in goal setting • Examining/modifying existing plan • Sharing plan with patient/family/staff
Implementation	• Carrying out nursing actions safely • Understanding rationale for care • Prioritizing care • Assisting with self-care • Calculating/administering medications safely • Suggesting diet modifications • Ensuring safety/comfort • Preventing infection/injury • Promoting mobility/independence • Responding to emergencies • Recording/sharing information • Teaching to intellectual level • Communicating appropriately to patient/family/staff • Teaching/supervising staff
Evaluation	• Comparing outcomes to goals • Examining response to therapy • Asking for/interpreting feedback • Identifying learning outcomes • Recognizing risks/problems of therapy • Communicating outcomes to staff/family • Reassessing/revising plan

Categories of Human Needs

Concepts basic to understanding human needs are another exam focus. Among these are Maslow's hierarchy of needs, the teaching-learning process, therapeutic communication, crisis intervention, and developmental theory. Knowledge of anatomy-physiology and pathophysiology, asepsis, nutrition, accountability, the group process, and mental health concepts are basic to the practice of nursing and are also incorporated into many test items. The organization of patient needs based on these concepts is identified by the National Council of State Boards of Nursing as Categories of Human Needs and is part of the test format. These four categories are based on the ANA Nursing Social Policy Statement and current research on job analysis for beginning practitioners. The greatest NCLEX-RN exam emphasis is on the categories of physiologic integrity (42%–48%) and a safe care environment (25%–31%). Health promotion and maintenance (12%–18%) and psychosocial integrity (9%–15%) are also incorporated (see Tables 1.2 and 1.3).

Some overlap is evident as you look at the nursing process framework and the categories of client needs. For example, the nursing process phase of planning addresses both physiologic and psychosocial needs of any patient based on priority setting. If an individual has a severe deficit in fluid volume related to dehydration, emotional needs are attended to *after* setting a goal to resolve life-threatening physiologic problems.

Use your knowledge of the test format to help you identify and review concepts learned throughout your nursing education, and to prepare thoughtfully for the examination. However, as you take the NCLEX-RN exam, do not attempt to identify what is being tested in a particular item.

Applied knowledge, rather that mere recall of facts, is measured in most test questions. Case studies present a description of a patient or family with emphasis on health needs, followed by six or more questions. In order to answer these, you will need to transfer knowledge from clinical experience and classroom learning to identify and resolve patient problems. Expect to find test questions challenging, and of varied difficulty levels. Application of knowledge may be subtle, such as selecting a toy appropriate for a hospitalized toddler in a body cast, or handling an emergency birth at a roadside. Remember that standards for care are based on general principles. While problems implied in the

Table 1.2 Categories of Human Needs

Categories	Nursing Focus
Safe, effective care environment	Coordinating care Ensuring quality Setting goals Promoting safety Preparing client for treatments/procedures Implementing care
Physiologic integrity	Promoting adaptation Identifying/reducing risks Fostering mobility Ensuring comfort Providing care
Psychosocial integrity	Promoting adaptation Facilitating coping
Health promotion/maintenance	Promoting growth and development Directing self-care Fostering support systems Preventing/early treatment of disease

Table 1.3 Test Item Focus Suggested by Categories of Human Needs

Human Needs Category	Possible Test Item Focus
Safe, effective care environment	• Understanding basic principles • Using management skills • Implementing protective measures • Promoting safety • Ensuring client/family rights • Preventing spread of infection
Physiological integrity	• Recognizing altered body function • Using body mechanics • Providing comfort measures • Using equipment safely • Understanding effects of immobility • Recognizing untoward responses to therapy/medication/procedures • Documentation of emergency actions
Psychosocial integrity	• Identifying mental health concepts • Recognizing behavior changes • Referring to resources • Communicating appropriately
Health promotion maintenance	• Understanding family systems • Teaching nutrition • Promoting wellness • Fostering immune responses • Recognizing adaptive changes to health alterations • Considering cultural/religious impact on childbearing • Supporting the dying/family

environment may affect client needs, priorities for safe care are based on those general principles.

How the Test Is Scored

The exam grading method differs significantly from standardized achievement or aptitude tests. For example, instructions given prior to college placement exams urge students to avoid guessing. Directions given to you before the nursing licensure exam stress that guessing is not penalized. An educated guess may thus contribute to success! If you can narrow the four options to two possibilities, the probability is 50% for making a correct choice. Completing all questions becomes a critical goal because the grading process results in a pass/fail score (without a numerical grade) based on the number of correct responses.

There is no separate answer sheet, and responses are marked by filling in circles at the left of each option. All stray pencil marks and underlining must be erased before turning in the test booklet, so that the scanner does not pick them up during the grading process. A blank page is provided for mathematical calculations of medication doses and IV flow rates. This is also an ideal "scratch sheet" on which to note items you skip initially and then plan to re-examine after completing the rest of the exam. (Such noting of specific questions saves time and eliminates the need to scan the entire booklet to locate omitted responses.)

Remember, the NCLEX-RN test plan has been developed to measure critical thinking and nursing competence. Knowing the framework of the exam should dispel some of your fears and help you to anticipate and prepare for the testing reality. When the actual date arrives, do not think about the "test plan" but concentrate on the challenge of each case study and its questions. Just as the driver attends to the road test without wondering, "What is being tested now?" you need only address the problem-solving task.

Where Should You Begin?

When you are familiar with this text and the test format, map out a personal plan for preparation and review. If independent study is planned, set realistic goals within the time available. Ideally, review of content over several months is preferable to "cramming" in a few weeks. Studying regularly, over time, helps to reinforce knowledge and improves your ability to apply that knowledge.

Begin your review plan by focusing on content that is less familiar to you, or about which you feel insecure. Your results on standardized national tests could serve as a guide, or you may select several case studies from Section 6 and answer the questions that follow after reviewing that content. After completing the test items, refer to the correct responses, rationale, and test format classification, then compare your problem-solving abilities to those of content experts. You may find it helpful to return to the review book outline, to a nursing specialty or fundamentals text, or to your class notes to resolve doubts or increase understanding. Look for patterns of test-taking difficulties as you review responses. Awareness of your strengths and weaknesses in test taking is an important phase of review and gives more meaningful feedback than counting correct and incorrect responses. By beginning with the greatest challenge and reinforcing understanding, your confidence is renewed as the date for the exam approaches.

Cognitive and Affective Keys to Success

There are three factors that are important in your achievement of success: *reading*, which affects both reviewing and test taking; *test wiseness*, which has been defined as the ability to use a test and situation to demonstrate learning, and the ability to *control tension* in a major examination, freeing the mind to concentrate on the written questions. While each of these factors is interrelated, they are discussed separately. Suggestions and strategies are offered for use during your licensure exam experience (Table 1.4).

Cognitive Strategies to Promote Success

Reading with concentration is a learned skill that is critical for study, review, and successful examination performance. When preparing for the NCLEX-RN, select an environment that is well lighted and suits your learning style. Avoid reading on a bed—its comfort may induce sleep rather than reinforce knowledge. Gather all materials in advance for the planned study session, including this review book,

Table 1.4 Cognitive Strategies for Success

• Prepare	for safe practice
• Plan a review	to broaden knowledge
• Read carefully	for understanding
• Identify key words	to focus attention
• Narrow options	by critical thinking
• Use an educated guess	not random choice
• Set priorities	based on health risk
• Trust decisions	avoid many erasures

other appropriate texts, notes, and marker pens to highlight content needing subsequent review.

Skim the review text material, then read for understanding. Look up any unfamiliar terms. Make a note for further questions that come to mind as you review information. Use your knowledge of anatomy/physiology, and pathophysiology to visualize the impact of a specific health alteration. Review the disease process, preventive measures, restoration, and rehabilitation. Refresh your memory on procedures specifically used in treatment. Think about ways in which health might be improved.

While reading test items as practice or in a real situation, be especially observant for *key words*. Notice cues such as *age*, *risk factors*, and *coping mechanisms* used. Clearly identify the question focus (e.g., the concerned parent, the ill child, or the care giver). Use your knowledge of nursing to think through the question and consider possible responses even before reading all possible options.

As you consider each situation and question, be sure to control the time spent. During each 90-minute test section you will not have the luxury of time to thoughtfully reread and reflect. For this reason, it is wise to omit the very complex problems that may take several minutes to resolve. Return to those challenges after completing the less difficult items.

While you must read carefully to understand the questions, avoid reading into the words more than is actually stated. Assume that the health care agency described is ideal and well-staffed. If you feel that the patient's needs would be met by a midnight snack of milk and crackers, do not qualify this with, ". . . but it may be impossible to provide this at night."

During the exam, you have no resource for defining vocabulary. Use the sentence context to deduce the meaning of unfamiliar words. Refer back to the case study for insight and clarification. And remember to apply your understanding of pathophysiology throughout the exam.

One word of caution about rereading prior questions as you complete a test section. Occasionally, a series of items describes a patient's progress over several days of treatment. Do not alter care priorities for the day of admission based on results of later diagnostic tests.

One approach to the complexity of priority setting is to treat a test item and options as a set of true/false statements. This is particularly helpful if all nursing implementations suggested are appropriate but you are asked to select a BEST or FIRST action. When reading, ask yourself, "Is the life or well-being of the patient at risk if this action is *not* performed *initially*?" If gas exchange is altered, physiologic integrity clearly dictates priority assessments, an emergency plan, and immediate interventions. Consider the following test item example:

1. Mrs. Lee is injured in a bicycle accident and appears to have injured her neck and left leg. A nurse driving past the scene stops to offer assistance and asks another driver to phone for an ambulance. Which of the following emergency interventions is an appropriate first action?

- ○ **1.** Ask Mrs. Lee if she can bear weight on the leg.
- ○ **2.** Carry Mrs. Lee away from the traffic on a board.
- ○ **3.** Set flares so that passing cars avoid the area.
- ○ **4.** Use rolled newspapers for splinting the leg.

Using the "true/false" approach, ask yourself, is option #1, 2, 3, or 4 an appropriate *first* action? Asking the victim to bear weight shows poor judgment, and thus can be "eliminated." Splinting the leg is not an essential first action. The priority for this woman is to provide a safe environment so that further injuries are not inflicted. Responses 2 and 3 are possible correct emergency actions. However, because she has a neck injury, any movement could be dangerous and increase the risk of spinal cord injury. Until the ambulance arrives, directing traffic away from the scene is the critical action.

Communication test items present a special challenge. As in actual practice, nonverbal cues and the environment affect the communication process. When reading case studies and questions focusing on nurse/patient/family interactions, consider all information presented in the case study very carefully. A reference to an interaction or the presence of quotation marks does not automatically signal therapeutic use of self. Table 1.5 lists suggested ways in which communication test items might vary with interaction types. Apply basic principles and be aware of possible communication blocks. Base choices on sound rationale rather than selecting a response that "sounds like" what you might actually say.

Consider the following communication test items:

2. The nurse employed in an outpatient clinic has a varied practice that includes health maintenance. While completing a precollege health assessment, a student asks the nurse why males must be immunized against rubella. Select an appropriate response to the question.

- ○ **1.** "Each school sets its own rules."
- ○ **2.** "The policy follows national guidelines."
- ○ **3.** "Elimination of rubella depends on 'herd' immunity."

Table 1.5 Focus of Communications Test Items

Type of Interaction	Approach
Interview	• Asking purposeful questions • Identifying risk factors • Using appropriate vocabulary • Listening to responses • Maintaining confidentiality
Information-giving	• Describing tests/procedures • Clarifying data • Explaining treatment to patient/family
Teaching/learning	• Assessing health/learning needs • Using developmentally appropriate terms • Giving instructions to promote safety • Demonstrating self care • Reinforcing group learning • Observing a return demonstration • Involving family in basic care • Evaluating learning outcome
Therapeutic use of self	• Establishing trust • Identifying own communication skills • Developing goal direction • Listening actively • Clarifying, reflecting • Sharing observations • Anticipating needs • Reinforcing positive coping styles • Supporting in loss • Referring for help

○ **4.** "There have been outbreaks of rubella each year."

3. A young woman asks the nurse about the tuberculin test administered during a routine physical exam. In addition to explaining the purpose of the test, which statement indicates teaching based on sound rationale?

○ **1.** "Keep your arm dry today and check back in 48 hours if redness develops."

○ **2.** "Do not scratch the area; stop in to have the test read in 48–72 hours."

○ **3.** "Place an adhesive bandage on the site; call if there is itching or swelling."

○ **4.** "Avoid direct sun today; let me know if there is bruising or inflammation."

4. After a community seminar on AIDS awareness, a young man approaches the nurse-speaker and asks to discuss a personal matter. "I know my 22-year-old brother is using IV drugs; I'm very worried about him, and the possibility that he or my family members could get hepatitis or AIDS." Which of the following statements is an appropriate first response to the questioner?

○ **1.** "Your brother needs to see a drug rehabilitation counselor."

○ **2.** "Casual contact is not a factor in AIDS transmission."

○ **3.** "Here are several pamphlets on protective measures."

○ **4.** "Let's find a quiet place to talk about your concerns."

5. Therese White paces the halls outside the emergency room. As a staff nurse stops to ask what the problem is, she responds with tears, "My 2-year-old daughter swallowed half a bottle of antihistamines, but I was on the phone and didn't realize it until she became very sleepy. I feel so guilty! They tell me she will be alright, but I could have killed her! How can I forgive myself?" Which comment made by the nurse is appropriate?

○ **1.** "You surely have learned a difficult lesson about safe storage of medication."

○ **2.** "All children get into things that are left within reach."

○ **3.** "You must be feeling very upset. Let's see if you can be with her."

○ **4.** "Yes, she could have died; be relieved that all is well."

Each of these questions explores nurse-patient interactions. Question 2 focuses on *information giving*, based on knowledge of health promotion through community-wide immunizations. While each option is partially correct, only option #3 responds to the specific question asked by the young man and is based on physiologic principles of active immunity.

Teaching as communicating is illustrated in question 3. Three responses offer inaccurate information and advice. The tuberculin skin test site should not be covered, and must be interpreted in 48–72 hours (option #2). In teaching the patient who participates in routine health screening, potential risks of the spread of tuberculosis are reduced.

Question 4 identifies a need for therapeutic communication by the nurse-speaker. While identification of risk factors associated with contact is important, only option #4 meets the man's psychosocial needs to express feelings and concerns. The nurse must go beyond information giving in this situation.

Therapeutic use of self in a crisis situation (question 5) is reflected in option #3. Although health promotion and teaching for maintaining a safe home environment are critical, the young mother's feelings must be acknowledged. In addition, inquiring about reuniting the family shows that the nurse is sensitive to the toddler's and parent's needs.

Affective Strategies for Success

It is difficult to separate cognitive from emotional factors in test performance. There are, however, distinctly separate ways to prepare for the mental and emotional challenges of the examination.

Long-range goal setting must include realistic life plans. Anticipate the time that study and review demand; avoid a major life change that increases tension. While a wedding date may be difficult to reschedule, consider delaying other emotionally charged events, such as a three-week hiking trip through Europe just before the exam.

Realistically evaluate your personal responses to test challenges. Look at past successes and ways you maintain energy and confidence under stress. How have you reacted to past major examinations? What physiologic or psychological responses to stress are common for you? Many graduates report that tension headaches or gastrointestinal distress occur during the two days of testing. Some suggest that lapses of concentration are frequent during a tiring day of problem-solving. Expect that your thoughts may "drift" or that you may experience a "failure fantasy," as many other nurses have described. Expect some anger about a specific test item. You may feel that you could have written "better answers than those!"

In order to use your mind to its fullest and to demonstrate your competence as a nurse, you need to control the effects of anxiety. Several effective ways exist to reduce tension, including

- progressive muscle relaxation and contraction from head to toe
- slow deep breathing and deliberate calming
- guided imagery with focus on a peaceful scene
- meditation, prayer, positive thoughts
- focus on a confident self.

Select the method of stress reduction that has worked for you in the past, learn new approaches and practice them during times of tension while studying. For example, to use imagery, see yourself in the setting that is most peaceful for you. Close your eyes and visualize the quiet, the scents, the scenery around you. Feel the warmth and energy. Enjoy the calm. Revisit the imaged scene many times before the examination. Change the setting as you need to, until it is the perfect relaxing pause. Recall these images during difficult moments in the exam when you need a brief recharge. You will feel your spirits lift and experience clearer thinking.

Close to the test date, plan your travel to the exam site. If distance allows, visit the area in advance so that you know the best route and alternatives. Consider seasonal problems that may affect travel time. It is critical to arrive at the testing site ahead of time, or entry to the building may be refused.

Anticipate that the massive test setting may be overwhelming. Plan ways that you can block out environmental distractions such as a noisy lobby, classmates who desire a last minute review of content, or friends who wish to hold a lunch hour test item postmortem. Replace those stimuli with a walk during the noon break, a brief nap on the steps, or reminiscence about school experiences. This is one time in your professional life that *your* needs are a priority. Do what you must to remain calm and confident.

On the exam days, consider your own comfort and nutritional needs. Dress in nonconstricting and attractive clothing that helps you to feel good about yourself. It is wise to carry a jacket in anticipation of temperature changes within the testing room. Eat a high protein breakfast, but avoid excessive caffeine and fluids so that repeated trips to the restroom can be avoided during the examination period. Carry fruit, a can of juice, and other quick energy sources for breaks.

If you know that you often have a tension headache during a long day of concentration, carry a remedy with you. Prepare for other problems by bringing cough drops or antacids. However, do not take medications that might cause drowsiness, since you need to remain attentive during the 90-minute test periods.

Expect to encounter at least one unfamiliar health problem in the NCLEX-RN exam. Remain confident that you can use your knowledge of anatomy/physiology, pathophysiology, and nursing to transfer knowledge and related concepts. Do not allow anger to destroy your concentration with thoughts such as, "Why didn't we learn about that condition in school?" Rather, think to yourself, "I can try to solve this problem," or, "Maybe this set of questions doesn't count!", or just omit the entire set of items and return to it later.

The keys to success are within you. Discover your strengths and potential by preparing thoroughly, mentally and emotionally. Study, review, practice test-taking strategies, and learn how to reduce personal tension. The rewards begin with your license to practice as a professional nurse. You are needed in the health care field of the 1990s, and are welcomed as a care giver and a colleague!

Table 1.6 Keys to Success on the NCLEX-RN

Know the Test Format
- An integrated exam
- Pass/fail score
- Single response, multiple-choice items
- Based on measurement of safe nursing behaviors for common health problems

Review Concepts
- Growth and development
- Pharmacology and pathophysiology
- Effects of culture and nutrition on health
- The nursing process
- Categories of human needs

Where Should You Begin?
- Consider your strengths and your learning style.

How Should You Prepare?
- Review course notes and texts.
- Consider a review program.
- Use human resources and support services.

Strategies to Promote Success
- Begin with self-evaluation.
- Sharpen test-taking skills.
- Learn methods to reduce stress.
- Be self-confident.

Just Before the Exam
- Get a good night's rest.
- Avoid late cramming.
- Eat breakfast.

During the NCLEX-RN
- Be precise in marking answer spaces.
- Use time wisely.
- Be "test wise."
- Keep emotions under control.

References

Kane, M., Kinsgsbury, C., Colton, D. & Estes, C. (1986). *A study of nursing practice, role delineation and job analysis of entry-level performance for registered nurses*. Chicago: National Council of State Boards of Nursing.

McQuaid, E. & Kane, M. (1982). *The state board test pool examination for registered nurse licensure*. Chicago: Chicago Review Press.

National Council of State Boards of Nursing. (1982). *Test plan for the National Council licensure examination for registered nurses*. Chicago: National Council of State Boards of Nursing, Inc.

National Council of State Boards of Nursing. (1987). *Test plan for the National Council licensure examination for registered nurses*. Chicago: National Council of State Boards of Nursing, Inc.

Test wiseness—Test taking skills for the adult. (1978). New York: McGraw-Hill.

Young, M. & Kopala, B. (1981). Plan for success: Preparing for the 1982 state boards. *Imprint*, 28 (6), 50–51, 70–71, 85.

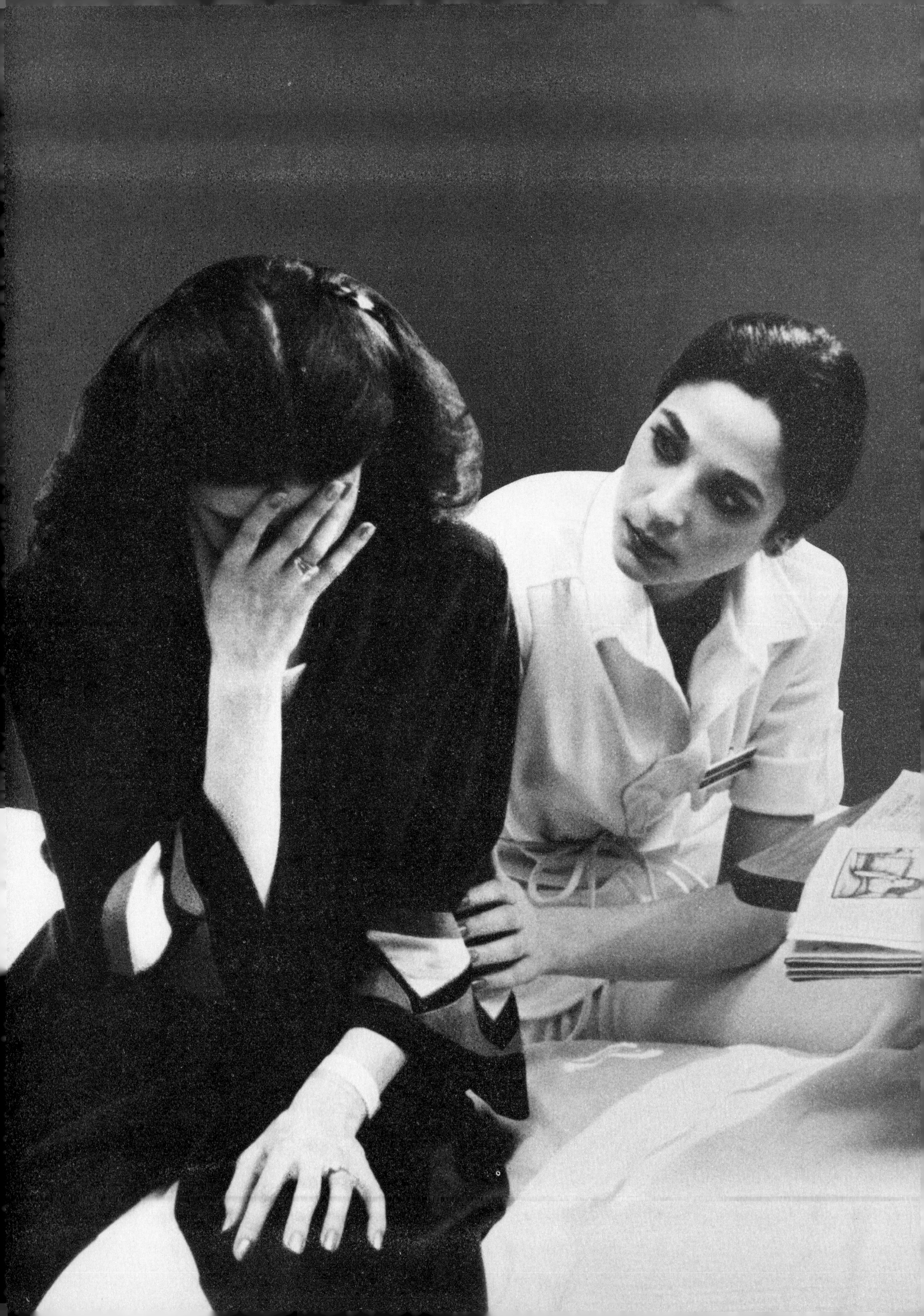

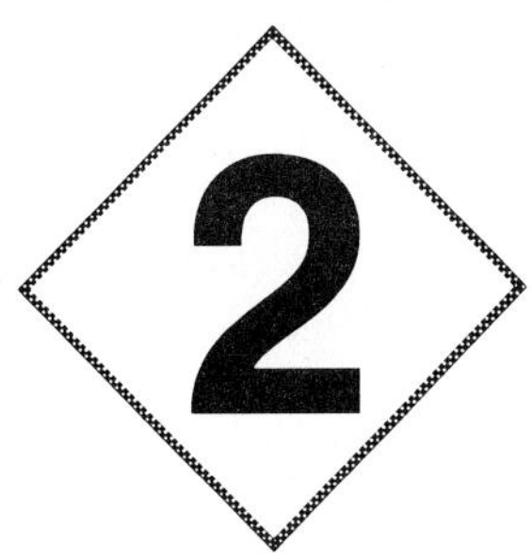

Nursing Care of the Client with Psychosocial, Mental Health/ Psychiatric Problems

Coordinator

Alene Harrison, EdD, RN

Contributors

Carolyn Billings, MSN, RN, CS
Sharon Golub, MN, RN
Ann L. Jessop, MSN, RN
Janet Elizabeth Bloomer Kristic, MSN, RN
Susan McCabe, MS, RN
Gail D. Wegner, MS, RN, CS
Janet Sullivan Wilson, MEd, RN

Section 2: Nursing Care of the Client with Psychosocial, Mental Health/ Psychiatric Problems

INTRODUCTION 15
Overview 15
Scope of the Profession 15
Interpersonal Relationships 15
Roles Assumed by the Nurse 16
Locations of Practice 16
Psychosocial Characteristics of the Healthy Client 16

THERAPEUTIC USE OF SELF 21
Theoretical Knowledge Base 21
Nurse-Client Relationship 22
Nursing Process 24
Interpersonal Treatment Modalities 25

LEGAL ASPECTS OF PSYCHIATRIC NURSING 28
Civil Procedures 28
Criminal Procedures 28
Recent Judicial Precedents 29
Role of the Nurse 29

LOSS, DEATH AND DYING 30
General Concepts 30
Overview 30
Application of the Nursing Process to the Client Experiencing a Loss 31
Selected Health Problems 31
Loss 31
Death and Dying 32

ANXIOUS BEHAVIOR 36
General Concepts 36
Overview 36
Application of the Nursing Process to the Client Experiencing Anxious Behavior 37
Selected Health Problems 40
Phobias 40
Dissociative Reactions 41
Obsessive-Compulsive Disorders 42
Anorexia Nervosa 43
Bulimia 43
Psychosomatic Disorders 44
Conversion Disorders 45
Post-Traumatic Stress Disorder 46

CONFUSED BEHAVIOR 48
General Concepts 48
Overview 48
Application of the Nursing Process to the Client Exhibiting Confused Behavior 48
Selected Health Problems 48
Chronic Confusion 48

ELATED-DEPRESSIVE BEHAVIOR 50
General Concepts 50
Overview 50
Application of the Nursing Process to the Client with an Affective Disorder 52
Selected Health Problems 53
Depression 53
Elation and Hyperactive Behavior 58

SOCIALLY MALADAPTIVE BEHAVIOR 62
General Concepts 62
Overview 62
Application of the Nursing Process to the Client Exhibiting Socially Maladaptive Behavior 62
Selected Health Problems 63
Violence in the Family 63
Hostile and Aggressive Behavior 66
Sexual Acting Out 67
Antisocial Behavior 68

SUSPICIOUS BEHAVIOR 70
General Concepts 70
Overview 70
Application of the Nursing Process to the Client Exhibiting Suspicious Behavior 70
Selected Health Problems 70
Paranoia 70

WITHDRAWN BEHAVIOR 72
General Concepts 72
Overview 72
Application of the Nursing Process to the Client Exhibiting Withdrawn Behavior 76
Selected Health Problems 80
Specific Schizophrenic Disorders 80

SUBSTANCE USE DISORDERS 81
General Concepts 81
Overview 81
Application of the Nursing Process to the Client with a Substance Use Disorder 82
Selected Health Problems 83
Alcohol 83
Drugs Other Than Alcohol 87

GLOSSARY 91

REPRINTS 95
Horsley, G. "Baggage from the Past" 97
Harris, E. "Lithium" 101
DiMotto, J. "Relaxation" 106
Harris, E. "Extrapyramidal Side Effects of Antipsychotic Medications" 111
Harris, E. "Antipsychotic Medications" 116
Harris, E. "Depression" 124
Campbell, E., Williams, M., & Mlynarczyk, S. "After the Fall—Confusion" 126
Harris, E. "Sedative-Hypnotic Drugs" 130
Hoff, L. & Resing, M. "Was This Suicide Preventable" 136
Acee, A. & Smith, P. "Crack" 142

TABLES
2.1 Life Cycle Stages 17
2.2 Theoretical Models 22
2.3 Social Determinants of Mental Health and Illness 23
2.4 Communication Skills in the Nurse-Client Relationship 24
2.5 Manifestations of Anxiety 37
2.6 Stress Management 39
2.7 Antianxiety Agents (Minor Tranquilizers) 41
2.8 Medications Used to Treat Affective Disorders 51
2.9 Suicide Methods 56
2.10 Major Tranquilizers (Neuroleptics) 75
2.11 Side Effects of Major Tranquilizers 76
2.12 Selected Problems Behaviors and Interventions 77
2.13 Types of Withdrawn Behavior (Schizophrenia) 80
2.14 Signs and Symptoms of Withdrawal and Overdose of Common Drugs of Abuse 89

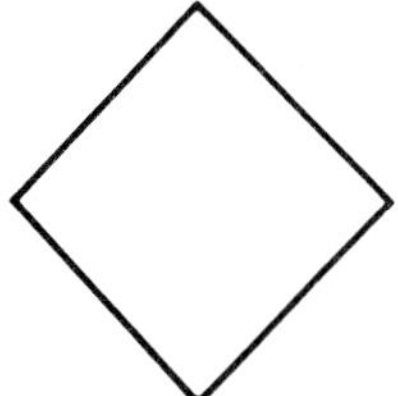

Introduction

Overview

1. This section reviews content that is general to all nursing—that is, communicating with clients and the nurse-client relationship—as well as content that is specific to psychiatric nursing. The NCLEX-RN examination will test your knowledge of communication and interpersonal relationships in *all* sections of the examination.
2. *DSM-III*-R: the sections in this book are organized in the format of client problem behaviors and the *Diagnostic and Statistical Manual of Mental Disorders*, 3rd Ed.-revised (American Psychiatric Association: 1980). The *DSM-III*-R categorizes and codes psychiatric diagnoses. These categories and codes are used by physicians and other health care providers to make diagnoses, to compile statistics, to apply for grants, and to report for third-party payment (insurance). Each diagnosis includes a description of diagnostic criteria. NCLEX will not ask you to diagnose the client's disorder.

Scope of the Profession

1. Psychiatric nursing is a specialized area of nursing that utilizes both science and art to provide nursing care to individuals and groups in a wide variety of settings. The nurse-client relationship is the vehicle through which the nurse fulfills both independent and dependent roles. Psychiatric/mental health nursing includes the promotion of mental health and prevention of mental illness. It includes the care and rehabilitation of the psychiatrically ill and the mental health care of the physically ill.
2. Scientific focus: on human behavior
   a. To understand biopsychosocial principles underlying emotional problems
   b. To be aware of safe and effective treatment measures such as psychotherapy, medications, ECT
3. Purposeful use of self
   a. To apply principles of the nurse-client relationship to all interactions
   b. To be aware of oneself as a principal in the relationship and countertransference issues
   c. To recognize and use one's own feelings and reactions as a guide to increasing empathy and trust, and understanding the client
   d. To act as an appropriate behavioral/social role model
4. Dependent practice involves implementation and coordination of physician's orders
   a. Know important aspects of each client problem in order to assess and report findings accurately
   b. Apply knowledge and use skills therapeutically in assessment and treatment
   c. Work collaboratively, sharing information about the client's progress
5. Independent practice involves utilization of the nursing process and development of individualized nursing care plans

Interpersonal Relationships

1. Therapeutic relationships
   a. Between nurse and individual client includes
      1) the initiation, development, and termination of a therapeutic relationship (objective, professional, empathic interactions)
      2) the nurse's role modeling appropriate behavior
      3) the nurse's treating the client as a unique individual worthy of respect, and not focusing solely on the client's symptoms
      4) the nurse's being consistent and reliable in increasing the client's trust and security, and decreasing defensive acting-out behavior
   b. In a group includes
      1) working with clients concerning the here-and-now living problems they confront
      2) providing information and role modeling
      3) clients getting feedback from other group members
2. Collaboration with other professionals
   a. Coordinating and planning holistic health care
   b. Sharing implementation of the care plan

according to skills needed, e.g., physical therapist, occupational therapist, rehabilitation counselor
    c. Working interdependently with other health professionals

Roles Assumed by the Nurse: nurses are involved directly in the care of the client and may assume many different, overlapping roles

1. Therapist
    a. Therapy focusing on problems of daily living may be done
        1) on a one-to-one basis (nurse-client communication); focus is on problem solving
        2) in groups such as assertiveness groups, grooming groups, adolescent groups; focus is on dealing with specific problems, providing emotional support and reality orientation, and increasing social skills and social acceptance
    b. Individual psychotherapy
        1) therapist and client meet regularly; the client learns to identify own problems and practices new ways of handling them
        2) the client has the opportunity to develop a close relationship with another person (the therapist), to grow from that experience, and to generalize new insights and behavior to other areas of life
    c. Group psychotherapy: nurse may be group leader or coleader
    d. Family therapy
        1) the therapist meets with the client and the family in various combinations
        2) family dynamics are stressed and scapegoating of the "identified patient" is decreased
    e. Sociotherapy: within the community mental health movement, psychiatric nurses provide services aimed at prevention of mental illness and reinforcement of healthy adaptation; specifically, this is done by teaching, by developing therapeutic relationships, and by recognizing early indications of problems and intervening appropriately
2. Surrogate parent: the nurse is perceived in the role of nurturer, authority figure, parent as part of therapy with adults and children
3. Teacher: the nurse educates the client regarding biopsychosocial health needs, medications, nutrition, and productive ways of interacting and coping with stress
4. Social agent: the nurse assists the client to utilize community agencies and social networks and helps people learn about mental health, mental illness, and the prevention of mental illness
5. Coordinator of client care
6. Patient advocate
7. Researcher
8. Administrator
9. Supervisor
10. Expanded and advanced roles as nurse clinical specialists

Locations of Practice: the role of the nurse is often dictated by the type of mental health facility

1. In hospitals: the type of involvement the nurse has in client care varies with the theoretical model in use at the individual facility; the nurse may
    a. Work under direction of psychiatrists
    b. Formulate care plans
    c. Observe, support, and listen to clients
    d. Assist clients in developing new behaviors
    e. Provide clients with an environment to try new behaviors
    f. Administer medicines and physical nursing care
2. In community mental health centers
    a. The nurse may
        1) provide outclient care using a variety of therapies
        2) do primary prevention in the community through
            a) classes designed to fulfill community needs
            b) crisis intervention
    b. There is a blurring of roles
        1) psychiatrists, psychologists, social workers, psychiatric nurses, and community mental health care workers work together in counseling, home visits, record keeping
        2) psychiatrists prescribe drugs; nurses administer medications; both may do physical exams

Psychosocial Characteristics of the Healthy Client

1. Infant through adolescent
    a. See Table 2.1 and *The Healthy Child*, page 577.
2. Young adult years (20–40)
    a. Cognitive development
        1) thinking and learning are problem centered
        2) thinks at an abstract level and compares ideas mentally or verbally with previous memories, knowledge, and experience

Table 2.1 Life-Cycle Stages

Common Name/Age	Freud	Erikson	Sullivan	Tasks
Infancy Birth–18 months	Oral • sexual gratification through mouth • dependent drives • pleasure of biting • aggressive drives and body image develop • differentiates self from mother	Trust vs Mistrust • exchanges with parents lay basis for trust or mistrust of others in later life	Development of a self-system Others gratify needs and satisfy wishes	Dependent drives Aggressive drive Differentiation from mother
Toddler 18 months–3 years	Anal • excretory control learned • concepts of cleanliness, punctuality, self-control, personal independence learned	Autonomy vs Shame and Doubt • self-control • personal independence and self-worth develop	Acculturation Delay gratification	Shame, disgust Control, cleanliness Punctuality Independence Self-worth
Preschool 3–6 years	Phallic/Oedipal • pleasure-genitals • attachment to parent of opposite sex • competition with parent of same sex • resolves by identifying with parent of same sex • develops sexual identity, guilt	Initiative vs Guilt • sharing, competing, self-motivation • learns to control jealousy, rage, envy, guilt	Playmates: forms satisfactory relationships with peers	Guilt, values Establishment of masculine or feminine role Sharing, competing Self-motivation
School-age 6–12 years	Latency • limited sexual image • socialization outside home • intellectual and social growth • friends • control over aggressive, destructive impulses	Industry vs Inferiority • skill mastery • work and play in groups • intellectual growth	Chums: relates to friend of same sex	Intellectual and social growth Mastery of skills Establishment of friendships Group work and play Control over aggressive, destructive impulses
Adolescence 12–20 years	Genital • sexuality focuses on genitals • establishes identity • learns independance from parents, responsibility for self, intimacy with one of opposite sex	Identity vs Role Diffusion • sense of self and identity apart from parents	Early: satisfactory relationships with members of opposite sex Late: intimate relationship with member of opposite sex	Independence from parents Responsibility for self Independent identity Acceptance of sexual and peer relationships
Young adult 20–40 years		Intimacy vs Isolation • learns to establish relationship with partner, gratifying social relationships		Establish intimate relationship with partner Gratifying social relationships Work adjustment
Middle age 40–60 years		Generativity vs Stagnation • productivity at home, work, community • child rearing		Productivity at home, work, community Can include reproduction, child rearing

(*continued*)

Table 2.1 Continued

Common Name/Age	Freud	Erikson	Sullivan	Tasks
Older adult 60 years–death		Integrity vs Despair • views past and remaining life as meaningful whole		Fulfillment Increased dependence Death of spouse, friends, self

3) learns formally and informally by emphasizing principles and concepts
4) objective, realistic

b. Emotional development
1) sexuality is a powerful determinant
2) expected to be responsible, have good impulse control
3) Erikson's task: intimacy vs self-isolation or self-absorption

c. Moral/religious development
1) challenges values, principles defined by parents and identifies those to be retained or modified
2) values become individualized, integrated, and provide basis for future ethical decision-making

d. Body-image development
1) body image is flexible, subject to constant revision, may not reflect actual body structure
2) a social creation
3) close interdependence between body image and personality, self-concept, and identity; may be altered by illness, injury, disability

e. Life-style options
1) separates from parents in 20s and develops peer relationships
2) makes decisions regarding types of relationships to form (marriage, child rearing, communal, homosexual)
3) settles into career
4) establishes leisure activities

f. Developmental tasks
1) accepts self: stabilizing self-concept and body image
2) establishes independence
3) establishes a vocation to make worthwhile contributions
4) learns to appraise and express love responsibly
5) establishes intimate bond with another
6) establishes and manages residence
7) finds congenial social group
8) decides on option of a family
9) formulates philosophy of life
10) establishes role in community

3. Middle adult years (40–65)

a. Cognitive development
1) goal oriented
2) enhanced by experiences, motivation
3) decreased memory functioning
4) less retained from oral information
5) continued learning emphasized
6) emphasis on realistic thinking
7) problem-centered thinking
8) attitudes may be less flexible

b. Emotional development
1) transitional, self-assessment period
2) channels emotional drives without losing initiative and vigor
3) masters environment
4) controls emotional responses
5) values age and life experiences
6) Erikson's task: generativity vs self-absorption and stagnation

c. Moral/religious development
1) integrates new concepts from wider sources
2) beliefs are less dogmatic
3) personal philosophy offers comfort, happiness

d. Body-image development
1) adapts to climacteric; changes accepted as part of maturity
2) reinforces positive self-concept
3) prefers experiences, insights, values of current age

e. Life-style options
1) reflects work ethic
2) increasing leisure time
3) differentiates compulsive work and play from healthy work and play
4) recognizes self-creativity
5) increases preparation for retirement

f. Developmental tasks
1) develops new satisfaction as a mate; supportive to mate; develops sense of unity with mate

2) assists offspring to become happy, responsible adults
3) takes pride in accomplishments of self and spouse
4) balances work with other roles
5) assists aging parents
6) achieves social and civic responsibility
7) maintains active organizational membership
8) accepts physical changes of middle age
9) makes an art of friendship
10) balances leisure with service pursuits
11) develops more depth of personal philosophy by reevaluating values and examining assets

4. Elderly (over 65)
a. Cognitive development
1) may decrease as a result of physiologic deterioration
2) environmental events may affect cognition
a) loss of self-esteem
b) isolation
3) must deal with a will, financial status, and property

b. Emotional development
1) reflects on meaningfulness of life, puts success and failure into perspective
2) sense of wisdom, knowledge, and self-reliance, of being able to cope with whatever comes along
3) Erikson's task: integrity vs despair

c. Moral/religious development
1) may become more spiritually oriented
2) value system changes from a material orientation to a more value-oriented outlook

d. Body-image development
1) must integrate continued physiologic changes
2) may see body as less dependable, therefore less desirable

e. Life-style options
1) may depend on finances, family situation, state of health
2) increased leisure time upon retirement
3) adjusting to fixed income
4) developing new hobbies and friends

f. Developmental tasks
1) continued self-development (recognizing positive experience of aging)
2) adapting to family responsibilities
3) maintaining self-worth, pride, and usefulness
4) dealing with loss of spouse, friends, upcoming end to life

5. Sexuality and cultural components related to the healthy client
a. Sexuality
1) an intrinsic part of each human
a) biologic, sociocultural, psychologic, and ethical components
b) significant part of Maslow's higher-order needs
c) integral part of Erikson's task for early adulthood: intimacy vs isolation
2) definitions
a) *gender*: internal sense of masculinity or femininity
b) *sexual role behavior*: all we do to disclose ourselves as male or female to others
c) *self-concept/self-esteem*: the perceptions each individual has of self
d) *body image*: a person's opinion of the appearance, function, and separateness of one's own body; a component of self-concept
3) sexual role dissatisfaction can occur with a wide variety of problems/disease states
a) common physical problems
- spinal cord injuries, neuromuscular disease
- cancer of reproductive organs, genitals
- diabetes mellitus
- hypertensive drug regimens
- cardiac problems (fear)
- advancing age, menopause
- colostomy
- obesity
- venereal diseases
- infertility
- endocrine disorders
- chronic illness
- rectal, prostate carcinoma

b) common biopsychosocial problems
- disturbances in body image, self-concept
- transvestitism, transexualism
- orgasmic or erectile dysfunction
- post-traumatic stress disorder

c) drugs that adversely affect sexuality
- alcohol
- antipsychotic tranquilizers, antidepressants, MAO inhibitors
- antihypertensives
- chemotherapeutic agents
- hormones and hormone antagonists

4) sexual functioning is multidimensional and influenced by a large number of variables;

it is relative to each individual, the individual's life-style, culture, values, and choice of love object (e.g., heterosexuality, homosexuality, bisexuality)

5) a critical part of nursing care of the client with respect to sexuality is that the nurse understand his/her own thoughts, feelings, beliefs, and misconceptions about this sensitive area

6) psychosocial counseling with client and significant others includes
- **a)** verbalizing feelings/concerns/fears
- **b)** encouraging client to maximize unaltered sexual characteristics
- **c)** realizing and verbalizing other characteristics that are part of clients' individuality

b. Cultural variables

1) definition: culture is the organized system of behavior or way of life for an identified social group. It includes knowledge, art, beliefs, morals, laws, customs, and values that are transmitted from one generation to another.

2) psychosocial support for client and significant others includes
- **a)** awareness of the components of a cultural orientation
  - ■ social institutions: family, religion, education, economics, politics
  - ■ communication systems
- **b)** identifying client's specific, culturally related nursing care needs
- **c)** tailoring interventions to be consistent with cultural practices of client

References

Beck, C., Rawlins, M., & Williams, S. (1988). *Mental health-psychiatric nursing: A holistic life-cycle approach*. St. Louis: Mosby.

Haber, J., Hoskins, P., Leach, A., & Sidelau, B. (1987). *Comprehensive psychiatric nursing* (3rd ed.). New York: McGraw-Hill.

Stuart, G., & Sundeen, S. (1986). *Principles and practice of psychiatric nursing* (3rd ed.). St. Louis: Mosby.

Wilson, H., & Kneisl, C. (1987). *Psychiatric nursing* (3rd ed.). Menlo Park, CA: Addison-Wesley.

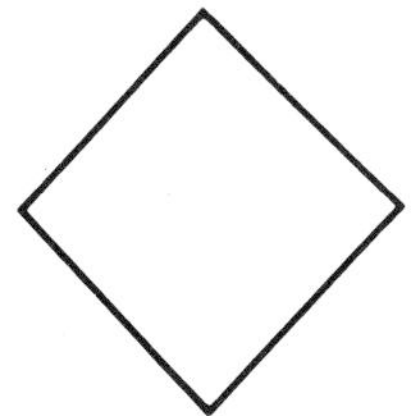

Therapeutic Use of Self

Theoretical Knowledge of Base

1. Theories of behavior
   Nursing interventions in the realm of human behavior are based on a variety of theories; see Table 2.2
2. Life-cycle stages (refer to Table 2.1)
   a. Freud: each stage must be negotiated successfully to avoid arrest at any one stage
   b. Erikson: focuses on psychosocial crises and developmental tasks. Each crisis must be successfully resolved so the individual will be able to meet subsequent crises
   c. Sullivan: focuses on social and environmental factors. A healthy personality develops through meaningful, gratifying interpersonal experiences with others in the environment
3. Defense mechanisms (Freud)
   a. Psychologic techniques the personality develops to manage anxiety, aggressive impulses, hostilities, resentments, frustrations, and conflicts between the id (pleasure-seeking impulses) and the superego (inhibiting)
   b. Used by both mentally healthy and mentally ill persons
   c. Measure of mental health is determined by the degree that defense mechanisms
      1) distort the personality
      2) dominate behavior
      3) disturb adjustment with others
   d. Specific defense mechanisms
      1) *suppression**: the conscious, deliberate forgetting of unacceptable or painful thoughts, impulses, feelings, or acts
      2) *repression**: unconscious, involuntary forgetting of unacceptable or painful thoughts, impulses, feelings, or acts
      3) *isolation*: separating thought and affect, allowing only the former to come to consciousness; it is a compromise mechanism
      4) *dissociation*: walling off certain areas of the personality from consciousness
      5) *denial**: treating obvious reality factors as though they do not exist, because they are consciously intolerable
      6) *rationalization**: attempting to justify feelings, behavior, and motives that would otherwise be intolerable, by offering a socially acceptable, intellectual, and apparently logical explanation for an act or decision
      7) *symbolization*: using an object or idea as a substitute or to represent some other object or idea
      8) *idealization*: conscious or unconscious overestimation of another's attributes, e.g., hero worship
      9) *identification*: attaching to one's self certain qualities associated with others; it operates unconsciously and is a significant mechanism in superego development
      10) *introjection*: incorporating the traits of others, internalizing feelings toward others
      11) *conversion*: the unconscious expression of mental conflict by means of a physical symptom
      12) *compensation**: putting forth extra effort to achieve in one area to offset real or imagined deficiencies in another area
      13) *substitution*: unconsciously replacing an unobtainable or unacceptable goal with a goal that is more acceptable or obtainable; the process is more direct and less subtle than sublimation
      14) *sublimation**: directing energy from unacceptable drives into socially acceptable behavior
      15) *reaction formation**: expressing unacceptable wishes or behavior by opposite overt behavior
      16) *undoing**: thinking or doing one thing for the purpose of neutralizing something objectionable that was thought or done before
      17) *displacement*: transferring unacceptable feelings aroused by one object or situation to a more acceptable substitute

*Most commonly referred to in psychiatric conditions.

Table 2.2 Theoretical Models

Models/Proponents	Assumptions	Treatment
Medical-Biologic	Emotional disturbance is an illness or defect. Illness is located in body or is biochemical. Disease entities can be diagnosed, classified, and labeled.	Physical/somatic: surgery, ECT, chemotherapy Therapists: physicians, others treating under MD's orders
Psychoanalytic (Freud, Erikson)	Emotional disturbance stems from emotionally painful experiences. Feelings are repressed. Unresolved, unconscious conflicts remain in the mind. Symptoms and defense mechanisms develop.	Therapy uncovers roots of conflicts through interviews within long-term therapy. Therapists: psychoanalysts, usually MDs
Social-Interpersonal (Sullivan, Peplau)	Emotional disturbance results from problematic interpersonal interaction. Client is seen as a subsystem of larger systems (e.g., family and community).	Client is approached in a holistic way. Intervention includes health promotion/illness prevention and alteration of harmful environments. Constructive interpersonal relationship is developed with therapist. Therapists: physician or nurse
Behavioral (Pavlov, Skinner, Wolpe)	Behavior can be modified by operant conditioning. • behavior that is reinforced tends to be repeated • behavior that is ignored tends to be eliminated Knowing the cause of the behavior is not helpful in treating deviant behavior.	Treatment aims at eliminating unwanted behavior by ignoring it and reinforcing wanted behavior. Response to behavior by therapists must be consistent. Therapists: physicians, nurses, psychologists, trained assistants.
Community Mental Health	When stresses and supports are in balance, the individual is socially competent. Emotional disturbance results from imbalance between stresses and supports (see Table 2.3). • too much stress and not enough support leads to social disorientation and disintegration • too much support and too little stress leads to social dependence, immobility, regression.	Treatment is aimed at maintaining or restoring balance between stresses and supports. Levels of prevention of mental illness • *primary*: promotion of mental health and disease prevention (anticipatory guidance, education, community organization, crisis prevention) • *secondary*: early treatment to prevent long-term illness (screening, early diagnosis, case finding, brief hospitalization, crisis intervention) • *tertiary*: treatment of chronic, long-term problems (halfway houses, partial hospitalization, day hospitals) Therapists: physicians, nurses, social workers, psychologists, other trained mental health workers

18) *projection**: unconsciously attributing one's own unacceptable qualities and emotions to others

19) *ideas of reference*: believing that one is the object of special and ill-disposed attention by others

20) *fantasy*: satisfying needs by daydreaming

21) *regression**: going back to an earlier level of emotional development and organization

22) *fixation*: never advancing the level of emotional development beyond that in which one feels comfortable

23) *withdrawal*: separating oneself from interpersonal relationships in order to avoid emotional expression or responsiveness

Nurse-Client Relationship

1. Purpose: to provide counseling, crisis intervention, or individual therapy

2. Characteristics

   a. Mutually defined relationship

   b. Mutually collaborative

Table 2.3 Social Determinants of Mental Health and Illness

Stress	Individual	Support
Social • poverty • poor housing • unemployment • crowding • high rate of mobility	Genetic information Constitutional traits Developmental traits • coping mechanism • ego strength	Social • churches and synagogues • schools • social welfare agencies
Personal • maturational – adolescence – aging • role changes • situational – loss – divorce – separation – illness		Personal • family network • friends • clergy • bartender • hairdresser

   c. Goal directed
   d. Interpersonal techniques facilitate communication
   e. Development of therapeutic relationship fostered
   f. Relationship differs from friendship
      1) specific boundaries established
      2) purpose, time, and place of interaction are specific
      3) professional demeanor and objectivity maintained
   g. Nurse assists client with problem resolution
   h. Successful relationship leads to mutual growth for client and nurse
3. Facts to remember
   a. It is not a friendship
   b. Its main benefit is to the client
   c. It presents an opportunity to the client to deal with the problems brought to treatment
   d. The nurse's approach to the relationship is crucial to the client's being able to express feelings
   e. Increased experience and education allow the nurse to have more discretion in relating to clients, but new practitioners should "go by the book"
4. Therapeutic communication
   a. Interpersonal techniques that facilitate communication
   b. Factors that influence the nurse's response
      1) client's stage of growth and development
      2) stage of the nurse-client relationship
      3) client's level of readiness
      4) goals of the interaction/priorities of care
   c. General guidelines: the best responses focus on
      1) actual client behaviors and nursing observations rather than inferences
      2) the here and now rather than the past
      3) description rather than judging
      4) sharing information and exploring alternatives rather than giving advice/solutions
      5) how/what rather than why
      6) orientation and presentation of reality (particularly for confused, disoriented clients)
   d. See Table 2.4 Communication Skills in the Nurse-Client Relationship
5. Phases of the nurse-client relationship
   a. *Initiating or orientating phase*: establishes boundaries
      1) when, how long, how often nurse will meet with client
      2) focus of relationship spelled out to client
      3) usually time of anxiety for client and nurse
         a) client may come late to or miss meetings; test boundaries
         b) client may exhibit nervous mannerisms
         c) client may sit silently, hallucinate, or exhibit delusions
         d) nurse may be more likely to use responses that block communication, because of own anxiety
      4) preparation for termination begins at this stage
   b. *Working phase*: exhibits reduction of anxiety in both client and nurse
      1) client accepts boundaries of relationship
      2) nurse uses interpersonal skills that foster communication
      3) client confronts problems and feelings
      4) client develops insights, learns methods of coping and problem solving
         a) begins to come to meetings on time
         b) uses the time with nurse as a "working" time
      5) nurse and client see each other as unique people
   c. *Terminating phase*: begins when work of relationship is over and builds on preparation made during orientation phase
      1) client and nurse summarize and evaluate work of relationship
      2) both express thoughts and feelings about termination

Table 2.4 Communication Skills in the Nurse-Client Relationship

Therapeutic Interpersonal Techniques

Technique	***Example***
Attending: indicating awareness of what is going on in interaction; includes giving feedback/recognition	Yes. Nodding. You're wearing a different blouse.
Encouraging Verbalization: promoting continued client verbalization	Um-hmm. And then? Go on.
Verbalization Observations: commenting on what nurse has perceived	You sound frustrated. I notice that you're biting your nails.
Reflecting Feelings: verbalizing either stated or implied client feelings	You're feeling anxious. You feel that no one cares about you.
Paraphrasing: restating the content of the message	Client: The doctor said I could go home tomorrow but I'm still having a lot of trouble walking. Nurse: You're wondering if you're ready to go home.
Questioning	
• Open Question: promotes freedom of response	What would you like to talk about today? What happens when you feel angry?
• Closed Question: limits freedom of response to short answer or yes/no	Have you ever been hospitalized before? Did you eat breakfast?
Giving Information: providing factual data	My name is . . . Lunch is at 12 noon. Visiting hours are from 2–8 P.M.
Clarifying: promotes understanding of what is unclear	I'm not sure I understand what you are saying.
Validating: checking perception of client verbalization	This is what I heard you say . . . Let me know if this is how you see it.
Focusing: directing flow of interaction	You were saying . . .
Requesting Description/Comparison: asking client to verbalize perceptions/similarities/differences	Describe how you are feeling now. Tell me when you feel angry. How does this compare with what happened when. . . .? What other times have you felt this way?
Summarizing: pulling together the salient points of an interaction	Today we have discussed three alternatives for . . . Last time we talked you were going to . . .

Blocks to Therapeutic Communication

Block	***Example***
False assurance	Everything will be all right. You don't need to worry. You're doing fine.
Giving advice	What you should do is . . . Why don't you . . . ?
Giving approval	That's the right attitude. That's the thing to do.
Requesting an explanation	Why are ypu upset? Why did you do that?
Agreeing with the client	I agree with you. You must be right.
Expressing disapproval	You should stop worrying like this. You shouldn't do that.
Belittling the client's feelings	I know just how you feel. Everyone gets depressed at times.
Disagreeing with the client	You're wrong. That's not true. No, it isn't.
Defending	Your doctor is quite capable. This hospital is well equipped. She's a very good nurse.

3) client may respond to termination similarly as to previous losses
4) client may have high anxiety in this stage, exhibited as
   a) hostility
   b) disparagement of relationship
   c) hallucinations, delusions
   d) regressive behaviors
5) initial boundaries of relationship should be maintained during termination
6) termination can be difficult for both client and nurse

Nursing Process: elicit client participation in each stage as appropriate

1. Assessment: Collecting and organizing data about the client by observation, interview, and examination; strengths and problem areas are identified
   a. Observation: note the ABCs (appearance, behavior, communication)
   b. Interview
      1) informal
      2) nursing history

c. Examination
   1) psychosocial assessment
      a) general appearance and behavior: age, grooming, dress, posture, body movements, eye contact, speech, affect, mood, attitude during interview
      b) thought processes, sensation, perception: logical, circumstantial, perseveration, flight of ideas, delusions, hallucinations, illusions
      c) cognitive functions: orientation, memory, attention and concentration, intellect, judgment, insight, communication, abstract thinking
      d) social processes: self-concept, interpersonal relations (family, peers, community), activities of daily living (ADL), leisure activities
   2) physical: complete review of systems, growth and development history, diet, exercise, rest, tobacco/drug/alcohol use, body image

2. Analysis: evaluating information gathered during assessment and making nursing diagnosis
3. Planning: developing client goals and nursing interventions to meet them
   a. Develop long- and short-term client goals
   b. Goals should be behaviorally stated
   c. Specify nursing interventions that will meet each goal
   d. Include nursing actions such as setting limits on unacceptable behavior without rejecting the client as a person, increasing or decreasing environmental stimuli, and providing individually appropriate activities
4. Implementation: carrying out the nursing care plan
   a. Carry out plan
   b. Establish a suitable environment for implementation (i.e., therapeutic milieu)
5. Evaluation: appraising client's response to nursing interventions and modifying the plan as necessary
   a. Appraise client response to nursing intervention based on the effect of the intervention on the client's behavior, client's concerns, and achievement of short-term goals
   b. Carried out by the individual nurse as well as by the total staff involved in the care
   c. Revise nursing care plan as necessary

Interpersonal Treatment Modalities

1. Psychotherapy
   a. Definition: goal-oriented, corrective emotional experience with a therapist in order to effect behavioral change, which may include
      1) increased well-being
      2) improved psychologic performance
      3) improved social performance
   b. Length of treatment
      1) may be long term, to allow client to gain insight and slowly take on new coping mechanisms
      2) may be short term, such as crisis intervention
2. Crisis intervention
   a. Definition: a time-limited (approximately 6 weeks), directive approach to help a client cope with a crisis
      1) person is in crisis when traditional methods of coping are not effective
      2) crises tend to resolve after several weeks; however, if the present one is ineffectively resolved, the person may have lost some ability to cope with future crises
   b. Therapy
      1) includes helping an individual or family cope with an immediate problem
      2) does not go into cause
      3) does not require insight as does traditional therapy
      4) deals directly and briefly with the individual's present situation
         a) clarifies situation and identifies problem
         b) teaches client new coping skills
         c) identifies and mobilizes external and internal resources
      5) attempts to return client to at least the previous level of coping
      6) helps persons in crisis become amenable to change because the crisis is intolerable (this is the motivation-of-crisis work)
      7) helps the client learn to problem solve and thus client may grow because of the intervention
      8) is the kind of intervention that may prevent maladaptation into more serious psychiatric symptoms
   c. The process of therapy includes
      1) establishing a nurse-client relationship
      2) being as active and directive as necessary to help client deal with crisis
      3) helping the client to establish therapeutic goals
      4) reinforcing that the relationship is time limited and therefore it is necessary to establish a termination date
      5) actively encouraging the client to express feelings and emotions regarding the crisis situation

6) assisting the client to develop new and more effective coping mechanisms
7) the client taking more responsiblity in subsequent sessions (if there is more than one)
8) a time-limited span: may take from one to several sessions, but is not a long-term process

3. Behavior modification
   a. Definition: altering undesirable behavior by systematically changing its consequences
      1) operates on the principle that behavior is determined by consequences
      2) changes in consequences result in change in behavior
      3) does not deal with cause of behavior
   b. Process of treatment
      1) identify the behavior to be changed (e.g., child throws temper tantrum when told it is time for bed)
      2) obtain baseline data re the behavior (e.g., frequency)
      3) identify the conditions and reinforcers that promote the behavior (e.g., child allowed to stay up late [rewarded] to stop temper tantrum)
      4) identify the conditions and reinforcers that will change or eliminate the behavior
   c. Techniques: systematic desensitization, ignoring the behavior, time out, token economy, aversion
   d. Positive reinforcers (rewards) are much preferable to aversion techniques
4. Milieu therapy: stresses the development of interpersonal and personal skills in a conducive environment
   a. Activities: include client government, occupational and recreational therapy
   b. Requirements: close collaboration between staff and clients toward mutually defined goals
   c. Heavy emphasis on maintaining independence of clients
   d. Clients are responsible for their own behavior
5. Therapeutic groups: more closely resemble real-life situations than one-to-one therapy
   a. Leading these groups requires training beyond basic nursing education
   b. Beginning nurse may colead a group
   c. Group members provide feedback for each other
   d. Variety of responses and reactions available for behavior displayed in group setting
   e. Three stages of development
      1) group orientation and development of identity
      2) group interaction and observation of dynamics
      3) resolution of dynamics and production of insights
   f. Members may examine patterns of relating to each other and authority figures in supportive atmosphere
   g. Group therapy more economical than one-to-one therapy; there are usually two therapists and 7–10 clients
   h. The goals and purposes are essentially the same as in one-to-one therapy
6. Family therapy: focuses on the family rather than on the individual
   a. Major problem: intolerance of differences
      1) healthy family can tolerate differences
      2) maladjusted family experiences differences as threats to individual identity and family unity; conflicts lead to splits, coalitions, scapegoating
   b. Major objective: to reestablish rational communication between family members
      1) family can reassess and recognize alliances
      2) family can resolve to accept differences between members
   c. Important difference between family therapy and group therapy
      1) in family therapy, the participants enter therapy with a long-standing system of roles and interactions, which the nurse-therapist must learn
      2) in group therapy, the relationship between participants begins with the first session; they have no history of a relationship
7. Self-help groups: use persons who have themselves surmounted problems. Nurses may serve as consultants/resource persons.
   a. Recovery, Inc.
      1) a consumer-funded group consisting of former mental clients and persons with nervous disorders
      2) focus is on the use of will power in avoiding deviant behavior
   b. Other self-help groups
      1) Parents without Partners
      2) groups for colostomy clients
      3) parents whose children have terminal diseases
      4) Overeaters Anonymous
      5) Reach for Recovery
      6) Alcoholics Anonymous (see page 85)
      7) Narcotics Anonymous

References

Beck, C., Rawlins, M., & Williams, S. (1988). *Mental health-psychiatric nursing: A holistic life-cycle approach* (2nd ed.). St. Louis: Mosby.

Burgess, A. (1984). *Psychiatric nursing in the hospital and the community* (4th ed.). Englewood Cliffs, NJ: Prentice-Hall.

Haber, J., Hoskins, P., Leach, A., & Sidelau, B. (1987). *Comprehensive psychiatric nursing* (3rd ed.). New York: McGraw-Hill.

Janosik, E., & Davies, J. (1986). *Psychiatric mental health nursing*. Boston: Jones and Bartlett.

Johnson, B. (1986). *Psychiatric-mental health nursing: Adaptation and growth*. Philadelphia: Lippincott.

Peterson, M. (1972). Understanding defense mechanisms (programmed instruction). *American Journal of Nursing*, *72*(9)(Supp.), 1–24.

Stuart, G., & Sundeen, S. (1986). *Principles and practice of psychiatric nursing* (3rd ed.). St. Louis: Mosby.

Wilson, H., & Kneisl, C. (1987). *Psychiatric nursing* (3rd ed.). Menlo Park, CA: Addison-Wesley.

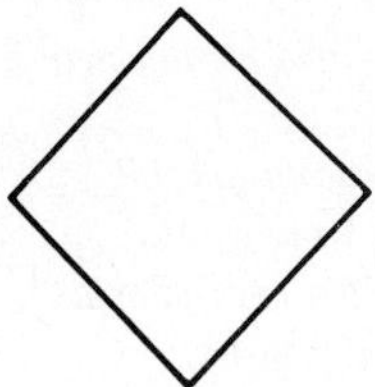

Legal Aspects of Psychiatric Nursing

Civil Procedures: the court protects the rights of psychiatric clients utilizing civil procedures. Many individuals are referred to psychiatric services through the courts. Psychiatric expert testimony is used by the courts when a person uses insanity or inability to stand trial as a defense.

1. Civil admission procedures
   a. General information
      1) the Mental Health Systems Act (1980) provided states with a Recommended Bill of Rights for mentally ill clients
      2) each state has its own mental health code determined by the legislature; it provides guidelines for admission procedures of the mentally ill to hospitals for treatment of mental illness
      3) there is disparity among states in legal commitment procedures
   b. Voluntary admission: any legal adult can apply for admission to an institution for the treatment of mental illness
      1) admission implies that the individual agrees to accept treatment and abide by hospital rules
      2) many states require that client give written notice to the hospital if requesting early discharge
      3) if physician believes this release to be dangerous to client or others, involuntary admission must be arranged through the court
      4) in most states a child under the age of 16 may be admitted if the parents sign the required application form
      5) in some states the minor has the right to protest admission by parents and petition the court for dismissal
      6) clients retain all rights with voluntary admission
   c. Involuntary admission: application for admission is initiated by someone other than the client
      1) requires certification by one or two physicians that person is a danger to self and/or to others
      2) the person has a right to a legal hearing within a certain number of hours or days
      3) commitment or discharge may be determined by the judge or jury
      4) most states limit commitment to 90 days
      5) extended commitment is usually for no longer than 12 months
      6) in most states, client retains the right to consult a lawyer at any time
   d. Emergency admission: any adult may execute an application for emergency detention of another. If a physician is not available, a magistrate must certify that the person is in risk of harming self or others. Medical or judicial approval is required to detain the person beyond 24 hours.
      1) a person who is hospitalized against his will may force court action for release through a procedure called habeas corpus
      2) the court will determine the sanity and alleged unlawful restraint of the person
2. Competency hearings: different and separate from admission hearings
   a. Admission to mental hospital does not mean a person is incompetent to manage own affairs
   b. Legally, *incompetency* indicates the person is no longer able to make responsible decisions for himself, his dependents, or his property
   c. Person declared incompetent has legal status of a minor, i.e., cannot
      1) vote
      2) make contracts or wills
      3) manage personal property
      4) drive a car
      5) sue or be sued
      6) hold a professional license
   d. A guardian is appointed for the incompetent person, and has the power of consent
   e. Procedure can be instituted by state or family

Criminal Procedures: many persons are referred to psychiatric services through the court system; psychiatric expert testimony is used by the courts when a person uses insanity or inability to stand trial as a defense

1. *Insanity*: a legal, not psychiatric, term meaning that because of mental illness the accused did not realize the extent or consequences of his actions, did not know right from wrong, or had impaired ability to resist "wrong," and thus is *not criminally responsible* for the unlawful act
   a. Sanity is determined by jury, based on psychiatric expert testimony
   b. The person accused of a crime will stand trial and plead not guilty by reason of insanity
      1) persons found guilty can be sentenced to prison
      2) persons found not guilty are committed to a mental hospital until judged sane by staff
      3) when released, person who was found not guilty by reason of insanity usually is free and has no legal ruling against self
2. *Inability to stand trial*: a person accused of committing a crime is not mentally responsible at time of trial
   a. The person is currently unfit to stand trial if he cannot understand the charge against him, or is incapable of cooperating with his own defense
   b. If found unfit to stand trial, must be sent to a psychiatric unit until legally determined to be competent for trial
   c. Once mentally fit, must stand trial and serve sentence, if then actually convicted

Recent Judicial Precedents

1. Give clients the right to treatment
2. Require institutions to devise specific plans of treatment for their individual clients
3. Require plans of treatment be the least restrictive of clients' liberty considering the individual's condition
4. Protect civil rights
5. Support confidentiality
6. Give client right to refuse treatment

Role of the Nurse

1. Functions as advocate for client
2. Gives care that reflects knowledge of client's legal rights as determined by the mental health code of the state in which the nurse practices
3. Implements nursing care that meets ANA Standards of Psychiatric-Mental Health Nursing Practice
4. Charts both legible and accurate *subjective* client data as well as *objective* observations and interventions in accordance with accepted nursing practice
5. Maintains confidentiality of client information
6. Consults a lawyer when clarification is needed
7. Knows difference between acts of omission and commission
   a. Omission: failing to do what should have been done
   b. Commission: doing what should not have been done
8. Ascertains client's understanding of consent
9. Provides necessary information at client's level of understanding
10. Monitors nursing actions relative to client protection to prevent assault or battery
    a. Assault: words or actions that produce genuine belief that action will occur without consent
    b. Battery: unconsented touching or restraining of a person without legitimate rationale

References

Cushing, M. (1986). The legal side: how the courts look at nursing practice acts. *American Journal of Nursing, 86*, 131–132.

Mittleman, R., Goldberg, H., & Waksman, D. (1983). Preserving evidence in the emergency department. *American Journal of Nursing, 83*, 1652–1656.

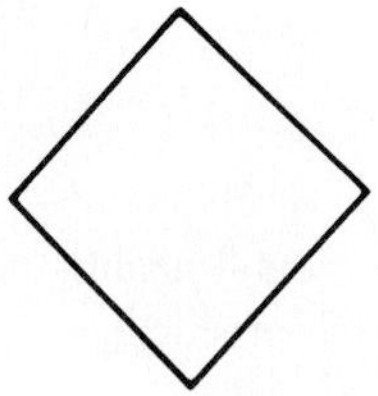

Loss, Death and Dying

General Concepts

Overview

1. Every human being experiences several losses during a lifetime, e.g., loss of a relationship or health, loss of a loved one, change in life-style. People deal with loss by grieving and integrating the subsequent changes into their life.
   a. Responses to loss vary greatly depending upon the individual's personality, previous experience with losses, and value of the person or thing lost.
   b. Behavior during normal grieving is similar to that seen in a depressed person, e.g., crying, fatigue, feelings of emptiness. Unlike grief, depression is a chronic state characterized by low self-esteem.
   c. People who are dying experience fear (e.g., pain, loneliness, meaninglessness).
2. Definitions
   a. *Loss*: the anticipated or actual removal of something or someone of value to a person
   b. *Grief*: the normal emotional responses to a loss, which subside after a reasonable time
   c. *Unresolved grief*: failure to complete the grieving process and cope successfully with the loss because of social and psychologic factors. Some circumstances that increase the likelihood of unresolved grief responses include:
      1) socially unspeakable loss, e.g., suicide
      2) uncertainty over loss, e.g., person missing in action
      3) need to be strong and in control
      4) ambivalence over lost object or person
      5) overwhelmed by multiple losses
      6) reawakens an old, unresolved loss
   d. *Mourning*: the expression of sorrow with outward signs of grief as a result of a perceived or threatened loss
   e. *Grief and mourning process*: the process a person goes through in adapting to a loss; this process is triggered by an *actual* or a *threatened* loss
3. The grief and mourning process, according to Engel
   a. Three stages
      1) *shock and disbelief*: usually lasts 1–7 days
      2) *developing awareness* of the loss: lasts several weeks to months
      3) *restitution*: takes a year or more
   b. Adaptive responses to a loss are
      1) first stage: crying, screaming, denial
      2) second stage: blaming self or bargaining; alternating between first-stage behaviors and asking questions about living with the loss
      3) third stage: making plans for the immediate future, speaking comfortably about loss
   c. Maladaptive responses to a loss are
      1) first stage: absence of crying or verbal expression of loss
      2) second stage: persistent guilt and low self-esteem
      3) third stage: isolation of self, lack of interest in living
      4) any time: any kind of destructive behavior
4. According to Kübler-Ross (the theorist most often associated with death and dying), there are five stages in the grief and mourning process of the dying person (these stages can be applied in evaluating other losses).
   a. *Denial*: may last from a few minutes at one extreme to the remainder of the time the person lives; it allows the person to mobilize defenses to cope with the terminal process; unconscious avoidance
   b. *Anger*: is expressed when the person begins to realize what is happening and that it can no longer be denied; can be overt or covert; manifested in affect, speech, behavior
   c. *Bargaining*: is usually done with God (e.g., an effort to get more time in exchange for church participation); an attempt to change the reality of the illness
   d. *Depression*: results from loss of function and also the anticipated loss of everything and

everyone of value; sadness and sometimes despair predominate

e. *Acceptance*: is almost devoid of feelings about the loss; the dying person has resolved feelings about death and found some peace and often wishes to be left alone or to associate with only one or two persons

5. A child's understanding and responses to death depend on
   a. Age
      1) preschooler can't differentiate between death and absence
      2) from 5–6 years old, they see death as something others experience, begin to accept death as a fact, believe death is reversible, not final
      3) from 6–9 years old, children associate death with injury; personify death (someone bad carries them away) or death is "old people"
      4) from 9–10 years old, they recognize everyone must die
      5) early adolescents understand permanency of death; difficult to see self dying before having a chance to live; may experience resentment, withdrawal, see self as different from others; also concerned about possible different reaction of others (e.g., withdrawal of friends); fantasies of rebirth, reunion, and reincarnation result
      6) all ages: underlying fear is of separation and pain, rather than fear of death itself
   b. Previous experience with death: relatives, friends, pets, family responses to death
   c. Knowledge of what is happening
   d. Other influences
      1) whether child is hospitalized; staff behavior
      2) parents' anxieties
      3) reaction of other family members, siblings
6. Children will convey their feelings and level of understanding of their impending death through symbols (drawings, stories, play with toys and other children) and behaviors such as anger, fear, hostility, withdrawal, bodily distress.

Application of the Nursing Process to the Client Experiencing a Loss

1. **Assessment**
   a. Current behavior
      1) stage of grief and mourning
      2) adaptive or maladaptive
   b. Previous losses
   c. Support system
2. **Analysis**
   a. Safe, effective care environment
      1) potential for violence: self-directed or directed at others
      2) knowledge deficit
      3) sensory—perceptual alteration (visual, auditory, kinesthetic, gustatory, tactile, olfactory)
   b. Physiological integrity
      1) potential activity intolerance
      2) pain
      3) impaired verbal communication
   c. Psychological integrity
      1) body image disturbance, personal identity disturbance, self-esteem disturbance
      2) anticipatory grieving
      3) dysfunctional grieving
   d. Health promotion/maintenance
      1) altered family processes
      2) altered growth and development
      3) altered health maintenance
3. **General Nursing Plan/Implementation and Evaluation**

Goal: Client will receive reinforcement for adaptive behaviors; will move through the grief and mourning process within an acceptable time frame.

Plan/Implementation

- Allow the client to utilize own method of coping as long as s/he is not physically destructive.
- Reinforce adaptive behavior; remember that suicidal ideation is not adaptive in any stage.
- Tell client that it is normal and expected to grieve over a loss.
- Help client to express feelings ("You look sad. What are you feeling right now?"); listen attentively and with empathy.
- Be alert to indications that client is moving into next stage of grieving.
- Recognize impact of previous losses, help client resolve past and present loss (see reprint page 97).

Evaluation: Client responds adaptively to the loss (e.g., talks about the specific loss; asks questions about the future).

Selected Health Problems

☐ Loss (Other Than Death and Dying)

1. **General Information:** types of loss
   a. Physical losses include loss of

2) usual function of a body part, e.g., paralysis of a limb
3) a valued object, e.g., a house
4) economic changes
5) loss of youth, beauty, health
6) a significant other, either through loss of a relationship or through death

b. Psychologic losses include losses/changes in
1) meaning in life, beliefs, and values
2) status, recognition, prestige
3) meaningful work, creative abilities
4) self-esteem and self-worth
5) nurturance and sense of belonging
6) loss of expected outcome, e.g., stillborn infant
7) changes in role identity, self-concept

2. Nursing Process

a. Assessment/Analysis (refer to page 31)

1) specific loss
2) meaning of loss to client
3) support system

b. Plans, Implementation, and Evaluation

Goal 1: Client will respond adaptively to the loss.

Plan/Implementation
- Allow client to cry, express anger, or exhibit other adaptive responses to the loss.
- Provide support for adaptive behavior (e.g., "It must be very difficult for you right now.").
- Help client to express feelings (e.g., "Other clients in your situation often feel sad or angry. How do you feel?").

Evaluation: Client exhibits adaptive behaviors (e.g., cries, feels sad).

Goal 2: Client completes all stages of the grief and mourning process.

Plan/Implementation
- Continue to help client to express feelings.
- When client asks questions about living with loss, tell the client only what s/he wants to know at this time (in-depth teaching can be done later when client is ready).
- Reinforce all adaptive behaviors.
- Expect that client will alternate between behaviors of stages.

Evaluation: Client asks questions about adapting to the loss; cries less frequently.

☐ Death and Dying

1. General Information

a. Responses to the dying process are highly individualized and may be greatly influenced by the client's physical status as well as his own personality. The interaction of client and family will have a strong bearing on the client's healthy progression through the process.

b. Nurse's responses
1) in order to be effective in helping the dying person, the nurse must focus on own beliefs, feelings, and behaviors in regard to death
2) the nurse who does not become aware of own feelings, fears, and beliefs about death may unwittingly inhibit client's expression of feelings; nurse's own feelings will become more powerful and decrease ability to help
3) nurses who understand their own feelings are better able to empathize with others' feelings
4) by looking at own beliefs about death and how people should respond to death, nurse can be aware of expecting others to respond in accordance with nurse's belief system

c. Establishing priorities
1) priorities may be determined by the client's psychologic and physical status
   a) at some point, pain or fatigue may demand more attention than the psychologic factors
   b) a client who cannot keep any food down or cannot feel relief from pain needs the nurse to respond to those factors immediately
2) the next most important action is to assist the client to deal with the manifestations of whatever stage client is in
3) assist the family to interact in healthy ways with client by healthy role-modeling, discussing illness and death with the client and family

d. DSM III-R Classification: uncomplicated bereavement

2. Nursing Process: Adult

a. Assessment/Analysis

1) physical condition and relationship to psychologic stimulus
2) knowledge of and response to diagnosis; people respond to dying similarly to the way they have responded to other major crises
3) stage in dying process: the stage can fluctuate, or client/family may be in more than one stage at a given time

a) current behavior
b) current affect and feelings expressed

4) support from significant others
5) expectations and resources
6) feelings about being in hospital or elsewhere
7) family assessment
   a) perception of diagnosis and prognosis; stage of loss
   b) feelings and their influence on client
   c) communication patterns
   d) needs and resources
   e) response to dying person and impact on client

b. Plans, Implementation, and Evaluation

Goal 1: (Stage 1) Client will begin to cope with the impending death by using denial.

Plan/Implementation

- Plan several brief interactions with client each shift (client may try to protect others by being "brave" and perhaps not seek out help and support from others).
- Teach client that some isolation and denial are normal responses.
- Allow use of denial until client has mobilized other defenses to deal with the impact of diagnosis and prognosis.
- Be honest when answering the client's questions about life, death, and treatment; do not be too harsh in your honesty, but do not minimize client's concerns; allow client to maintain hope.
- Do not reinforce client's denial of the condition. (E.g., if client says, "I can't believe it! It's not happening," nurse might say, "It must seem a bit unreal to you." Thus nurse neither reinforces nor rejects the client's denial, but accepts the need for denial.)
- Support client in dealing with denial expressed by family and friends.

Evaluation: Client initially denies and then begins to acknowledge the reality of the impending death.

Goal 2: (Stage 2) Client will verbalize anger about impending death.

Plan/Implementation

- Permit and encourage the verbal expression of anger (often the anger is displaced onto the nurse); remember that fear underlies anger; do not take the anger as a personal attack and react defensively.
- Know that anger may be turned inward and be manifested as guilt, (about not seeking medical attention earlier or other actions), allow expression of guilt feelings, but help client move away from self-blame.
- Listen to client's expressions of anger without offering any judgment; help client deal with anger arising from distancing behaviors of relatives and friends.
- Discuss possible alternative treatment and life-style changes introduced by the client; offer clear, factual information about any alternatives to assist client to make choices.

Evaluation: Client verbalizes anger about impending death.

Goal 3: (Stage 3) Client will use bargaining in an attempt to prolong life.

Plan/Implementation

- Permit client to cope by bargaining; client may say things like, "If only . . ." or "Maybe I could . . ."; know that this characteristic "magical thinking" allows client to feel some control.
- Assist client to make amends for past failures or grievances (perceived or real); help client to find meaning in life by reminiscing.
- Discuss importance of what is being bargained for using a sensitive, accepting approach.
- Allow client to make appropriate decisions (e.g., timing of, intervals between, or lack of interventions); explore risks and possible consequences, but allow client to make the decisions.

Evaluation: Client continues progress through the grief and mourning process by bargaining.

Goal 4: (Stage 4) Client will verbalize recognition of the inevitable and allow self to feel sadness and depression.

Plan/Implementation

- Understand that the client may express sadness by crying, talking, or withdrawing into silence; avoid trying to "cheer" client.
- Answer questions such as, "Am I going to die?" with a response such as "Do you feel you are going to die?"; support and discuss client's responses.
- Provide opportunities for client to express feelings about the impending loss of everything known and loved, changes in body image and self-esteem; accept sadness as grieving behavior, not as self-pity.
- Remind client that sadness is normal; explore

the difference that coping with the impending death rather than giving up can make.
- Help client to focus on the present and to make the most of each day.

Evaluation: Client verbalizes sad, depressed feelings; begins to talk about own death.

Goal 5: (Stage 5) Client will achieve acceptance of the inevitability of impending death.

Plan/Implementation
- Assist client to take care of personal and family matters as desired.
- Continue to allow discussion of the impending death but realize that full acceptance may not be achievable (rather, the client becomes resigned to the situation); do not try to force acceptance.
- Allow client to continue to participate in making decisions about care as desired.
- Allow client to decide when and if to spend some time alone; allow client to restrict visitors to short periods of time as desired.
- Promote a peaceful conclusion of the dying process by offering comfort and security measures as necessary.
- Know that the family may not be at the same level of coping as the client
  - assess the potential disruption the death will have on the family
  - use clear and factual terminology and information when speaking with them
  - remain as calm and unreactive as possible so as not to further stress the family with your own emotions and needs
  - use family rituals and customs whenever possible
  - spend time with them discussing their feelings
  - know that families respond to the dying member much as they handled other major crisis situations
  - family's greatest needs may be competent physical care for the ill member and empathy for the difficulty of their situation
  - they appreciate the nurse who helps them with packing, arranges a comfortable place to sleep in the hospital that night, or lets them call at any time to find out how their ill relative is or when they can visit

Evaluation: Client moves through the 5th stage of loss at own rhythm to a comfortable and dignified death; expresses feelings and concerns about impending death; participates in decision making for own activities of daily living (ADL) for as long as is possible; the family or significant other discuss feelings and concerns about death of loved one.

3. Nursing Process: Child

a. Assessment/Analysis

1) child's level of understanding and reaction/feelings about situation; ability to express self with symbols (e.g., play, stories, drawings)
2) parents' level of understanding and reaction/feelings about situation; parents' strengths and needs; support systems
3) child's physical condition (e.g., vital signs, pain, hydration, needs for range-of-motion exercises [ROM], skin care, comfort or security measures)
4) staff members' feelings and concerns, need for support
5) siblings' level of understanding; their responses to behavior and health changes in ill sibling, separation from hospitalized ill sibling

b. Plans, Implementation, and Evaluation

Goal 1: Child/family will express feelings, fears, anxieties, guilt they may be experiencing; will verbalize their understanding of the physical health status and the terminal process.

Plan/Implementation
- Determine what the child knows.
- Work through own feelings with other staff members.
- Allow and encourage the parents to express their feelings and accept those expressions in a nonjudgmental manner.
- Stress nurse's continuing availability.
- Permit child to express anger and hostility, but at the same time, do not be totally permissive regarding unacceptable behavior (child may perceive this permissiveness as total hopelessness and abandonment).
- Encourage child to draw or play with toys to express feelings
  - draw own body
  - draw a feeling
  - draw family
  - play doctor/nurse and act out feelings, including angry feelings; let nurse be the client
- Acknowledge the variety of family responses
  - shock, denial, guilt, bodily distress, anxiety
  - acceptance, belief in God

- overprotection, overindulgence
- encourage interaction/involvement of ill child and siblings
- stress on marriage: assist with marital stress by encouraging couple to spend an evening away from the hospital and to call when they feel concerned about their child

■ Help siblings to express their feelings, use drawing, storytelling, play therapy
- help parents understand that siblings' perceptions/interpretations/reactions may not be as intense as parents'
- "favorite child" angers other siblings; stress is also on siblings who need a chance to discuss feelings; they, too, may feel they did something to cause sibling to become ill

■ Refer family to self-help groups in community.

Evaluation: Child/family expresses some degree of awareness of the terminal process; verbalizes some feelings associated with grief and mourning.

Goal 2: Child will maintain as much independence as possible in ADL; will have minimal pain and discomfort; will ingest adequate food and fluid to meet body needs.

Plan/Implementation

■ Encourage child's participation in ADL as long as energy levels are not depleted.

■ Ensure adequate fluid and food; use supplements when necessary and allow child choice of food if possible

■ Preserve skin integrity by massage, lotions, sheepskin, water mattress.

■ Provide pain medication and comfort measures prn.

■ Use passive and active ROM.

■ Permit toys, music, and special objects to be with child.

■ Allow parents to participate in care; explain procedures to parents/child.

Evaluation: Child maintains independence in ADL (e.g., feeds self, ambulates to bathroom alone); has minimal pain and discomfort; ingests food and fluid to meet body needs.

References

Beck, C., Rawlins, M., & Williams, S. (1988). *Mental health—psychiatric nursing: A holistic life-cycle approach*. St. Louis, MO: Mosby.

Collison, C. & Miller, S. (1987). Using images of the future in grief work. *Image 19*(1):9.

Corr, C. & MacNeil, J. (1986). *Adolescence and death*. New York: Springer Verlag.

Lego, S. (1984). *The American handbook of psychiatric nursing*. Philadelphia: Lippincott.

Plaum, M. (1986). Understanding the final messages of the dying. *Nursing86*, *16*(6), 26–29.

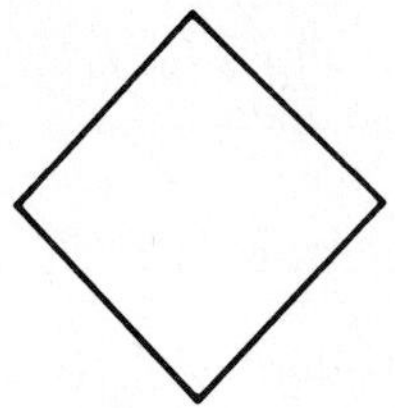

Anxious Behavior

General Concepts

Overview

1. Anxiety can be a problem in and of itself, but is also an aspect of other psychosocial problems. Anxiety is a subjective feeling brought on by a nonspecific threat to self. In mild degrees, it is a normal experience that motivates a person to take constructive action in a situation. As anxiety becomes more severe, it can interfere with perception, judgment, and behavior, and requires outside intervention to help the person to function constructively. Its prominence as a human occurrence makes it one of the most common concerns in psychosocial nursing. Recognition of anxious behaviors and the appropriate use of helping interventions are essential nursing skills in any health care setting.
2. Anticipatory anxiety, anxiety, and fear are all accepted official nursing diagnoses with established defining characteristics.
   - **a.** *Anticipatory anxiety*: an increased level of arousal associated with a perceived *future* threat to the self
   - **b.** *Anxiety*: a generalized feeling of dread and apprehension, which is a subjectively painful warning of a threat to the self or to significant relationships
   - **c.** *Fear*: a feeling of dread related to an *identifiable* source that is perceived as a threat or danger to the self or significant relationships
   - **d.** *Anxious behavior*: a manifestation of a subjective feeling resulting from the experience of anxiety, conflict, fear, or stress. Such response ranges from mild to severe, and represents a usual human reaction to a sense of threat.
3. General causes
   - **a.** A threat to biologic integrity
   - **b.** A threat to security of self; anxiety is a warning signal stimulating the organism to act against the threat
   - **c.** A person's own defenses/coping mechanisms are not working as well as they usually do
   - **d.** An unconscious conflict brought on by a nonspecific threat to self (psychoanalytic theory)
4. Four levels of anxiety: on a continuum from mild to panic, which primarily involves sensory perception and level of functioning
   - **a.** *Mild anxiety*: characteristics
     - 1) more alert than usual, increased questioning
     - 2) heightened capacity to deal with perception of impending danger
     - 3) focus of attention on immediate events
     - 4) person experiences mild discomfort, restlessness
     - 5) may be a useful motivating force; e.g., if a person experiences mild anxiety during NCLEX-RN, this may help to increase ability to answer questions
   - **b.** *Moderate anxiety*: characteristics
     - 1) narrowed perception
     - 2) reduced ability to listen and comprehend
     - 3) selective inattention, focus on one specific thing; "tunnel vision" develops
     - 4) increased tension; increased discomfort; verbalization about expected danger
     - 5) decreased ability to function
     - 6) physical symptoms, e.g., pacing, hand tremors, diaphoresis, increased heart rate, sleep and/or eating disturbances
   - **c.** *Severe anxiety*: characteristics
     - 1) greatly reduced perception; difficulty attending to, understanding, and processing information
     - 2) sense of impending doom
     - 3) increased physical symptoms, e.g., diaphoresis, dizziness, increased muscle tension, pallor
     - 4) survival response (fight or flight)
   - **d.** *Panic*: characteristics
     - 1) altered perception of and focus on reality
     - 2) helpless, fearful, panicky feelings
     - 3) physical symptoms, e.g., tachycardia, hyperventilation

4) extreme discomfort; extreme measures to decrease anxiety
5) feeling of personal disintegration
6) severe hyperactivity, loss of control

5. Diagnosis of anxiety: inferred from three kinds of data: physiologic changes, psychologic changes (see Table 2.5), and use of coping or defense mechanisms
   a. Physiologic changes
      1) involve primarily the autonomic nervous system
      2) physiologic operations tend to be speeded up by mild and moderate anxieties
      3) functioning tends to be slowed down by severe panic; can result in complete functional paralysis and death (in prolonged panic)
      4) knowledge of physical manifestations allows the nurse to intervene prior to the panic stage
      5) during panic, when the physical symptoms are severe, immediate intervention is imperative
   b. Psychologic changes
      1) psychologic manifestations accelerate as anxiety level increases and can become extremely uncomfortable to the person
      2) maladaptive behaviors are mechanisms used to avoid acceleration of anxiety to the panic state (e.g., rumination, rituals, compulsivity)
   c. Coping mechanisms: may be a defense mechanism or any means used to resolve, or at least delay, the conflict
      1) constructive: client, alerted by warning signal that something is not going as expected, resolves the conflict
      2) destructive or disturbed: client tries to protect self from anxiety without resolving the conflict, which can be expressed in maladaptive or dysfunctional behavior

Table 2.5 Manifestations of Anxiety

Physiologic	Psychologic
Tachycardia	Tension
Palpitations	Nervousness
Excessive perspiration	Apprehension
Dry mouth	Irritability
Cold, clammy, pale skin	Indecisiveness
Urinary frequency	Oversensitivity
Diarrhea	Tearfulness
Muscle tension	Agitation
Tremors	Dread
Narrowing of focus	Horror
	Panic

Application of the Nursing Process to the Client Exhibiting Anxious Behavior

NOTE: The same nursing process is utilized with all anxiety-related behaviors regardless of whether they are functional or dysfunctional

1. **Assessment**
   a. Level of anxiety (signs and behavior)
   b. Physiologic and psychologic signs and symptoms
   c. Cause, if known
   d. Coping mechanisms (constructive and/or destructive)
   e. Problem behavior (e.g., weekly episodes of gastritis indicating moderate anxiety related to work conflict)
   f. Support systems and their involvement with client
2. **Analysis**
   a. Safe, effective care environment
      1) impaired home maintenance management
      2) potential for trauma
      3) knowledge deficit
   b. Physiological integrity
      1) impaired verbal communication
      2) altered nutrition: less/more than body requirements
      3) sleep pattern disturbance
   c. Psychological integrity
      1) anxiety
      2) ineffective individual coping
      3) disturbed self-esteem/body image/and personal identity disturbance
      4) post-trauma response
   d. Health promotion/maintenance
      1) impaired adjustment
      2) altered family processes
      3) altered health maintenance
      4) self-care deficit (specify)
3. **General Nursing Plans/Implementation and Evaluation**

Goal 1: Client will develop an open, trusting relationship with the nurse.

Plan/Implementation

- Approach client in unhurried way and actively listen to concerns and feelings.
- Encourage client to express feelings and concerns about unmet needs or stressful situation.

- Be aware of feelings and behavior and their impact upon client.

Evaluation: Client expresses concerns and unmet needs to the nurse (e.g., concern about failure or rejection).

Goal 2: Client will use anxiety as a motivation for change.

Plan/Implementation

- Help client express feelings about stressful situations, unmet needs
  - assist client to acknowledge or name the feelings being experienced
  - express genuine attitude of interest and concern
- Be nonjudgmental and offer unconditional acceptance.
- Offer reassurance by giving appropriate information, correcting misinformation; repeat the process if necessary as client may have reduced hearing perception; use short, concise statements.
- Work with client to identify anxiety-causing situations that can be avoided.
- Teach client to recognize how client is manifesting anxiety in behavior.
- Help client identify situations that trigger anxiety.
- Assist client to use stress-reduction techniques (e.g., biofeedback, visualization, talking it out) to cope with anxiety; refer to Table 2.6.
- Be aware that client and nurse have reciprocal influence on each other
  - anxiety is contagious
  - find constructive ways to control own anxiety, frustration, or anger
- Prevent mild anxiety from escalating by intervening early, whenever possible.
- Provide physical care as needed to severely anxious client.

Evaluation: Client expresses feelings; identifies situations that cause anxiety; incorporates at least one stress-reduction technique into daily routine; experiences no more than moderate anxiety.

Goal 3: Client will recognize own behaviors of anxiety and gain insight into cause of problems.

Plan/Implementation

- Assist client to recognize anxiety by exploring the feelings that precede anxious behavior.
- Help the client to distinguish between thoughts, feelings, and behaviors.
- Utilize the nurse-client relationship to increase the client's ability to gain insight into the cause of problems.
- Provide a new perspective on the situation, i.e., help client "redefine" the problem.
- Utilize biofeedback learning to help client to recognize own tensions.
- Teach client to evaluate the threat, expectations, or unmet needs and to assess own capabilities realistically.

Evaluation: Client identifies own behaviors that are linked to current anxiety; tells nurse when feeling increasingly anxious; can state cause(s) of current anxiety.

Goal 4: Client will learn and demonstrate alternative methods of coping with anxiety.

Plan/Implementation

- Examine client's patterns of coping with anxiety.
- Reinforce effective and constructive coping mechanisms.
- Teach client alternative methods of coping, e.g., visual imagery, relaxation, talking it out.
- Know that the client with mild-moderate anxiety is generally not hospitalized for treatment depending upon
  - severity of the symptoms
  - incapacity of function
  - threat to self or others
  - nature of the home environment
- Observe physical status and intervene directly as necessary for client's well-being

Evaluation: Client learns two new coping mechanisms (e.g., talking about feelings, guided imagery; experiences more control over anxiety).

Goal 5: Client will be able to cope with severe to panic anxiety and reduce anxiety at least one level.

Plan/Implementation

- Understand that a severely anxious client may neglect physical needs, exhaust self, or actually injure self; give physical care and protection as indicated.
- Remove client from other clients if anxiety is increasing.
- Anticipate and prevent mild disturbances from developing into severe or panic stage by identifying with client early signs of disturbance.
- Allow client to determine what stresses client can handle.
- Know that coping mechanisms keep the anxiety within tolerable limits.

Table 2.6 Stress Management

Stress is a generalized, nonspecific response of the body to any demand, change, or perceived threat, whether positive or negative. *Stressors* are the circumstances or events that elicit this response and may be real or anticipated. *Distress* is damaging or unpleasant stress.

Signs of Distress

- accident proneness
- alcohol and drug abuse
- chronic fatigue
- decrease or increase of appetite
- diarrhea or constipation
- emotional instability
- emotional tension
- frequent urination
- grinding of teeth
- headache
- impulsive behavior
- inability to concentrate
- increased smoking
- insomnia
- irritability
- neck or back pain
- neurotic or psychotic behavior
- nightmares
- sexual problems
- stuttering
- sweating

GOAL

The patient will maintain homeostatic or optimal adaptive coping by preventing, or recognizing promptly, excessive levels of stress; the patient will utilize effective measures to manage stress by describing a plan to cope with stress in an adaptive way that includes exercise, relaxation, creative problem solving, and sharing feelings and concerns with a significant other.

Stress Reduction Techniques	Nursing Implications
Identify stressors (e.g., work, relationships, environmental, health, aging, financial, spiritual, emotional)	Have patient examine how s/he reacts to life occurrences (e.g., frustration, knot in stomach, loss of control). Discern between positive and negative stressors; explain that stress is unavoidable and can be useful to motivate.
Modify or eliminate stressors	Review possibilities for simple and major changes. Discuss alternatives, advantages and disadvantages of reducing stressors.
Develop effective coping mechanisms	
• daily exercise	Suggest methods to reduce stress through exercise (e.g., walking, running, dancing, swimming, gardening, participating in sports, body movement exercises, yoga). Assist in developing a plan of regular activity. Refer to community gyms, health clubs, and YMCAs. Advise consultation with personal physician for contraindications to exercise program.
• develop alternative ways to relax (e.g., drawing, pottery, carpentry, writing, music, photography, reading, watching the sunset, taking a bubble bath)	Review with patient activities enjoyed and suggest s/he devote at least an hour/day to an activity. Refer to recreation departments, adult education programs, community colleges.

Stress Reduction Techniques	Nursing Implications
• relaxation techniques –progressive relaxation –autogenic training –guided imagery	Guide patient through a relaxation exercise to experience its usefulness. Begin relaxation with deep breathing. Use guided imagery to induce relaxation (e.g., "Take another deep breath and let all the tension release. With each breath you become more relaxed. Now, imagine yourself in a peaceful, quiet setting [garden, beach, etc."]). Refer to cassettes, books, and classes on learning and practicing relaxation techniques.
• diaphragmatic breathing; periodic deep breathing	Practice diaphragmatic breathing with patient • sit or recline in a comfortable position with legs uncrossed • place one hand on the chest and the other hand on the diaphragm, approximately 2 inches below the bottom center of the breastbone • inhale so the diaphragm expands and the hand covering the diaphragm moves out while the other hand remains almost still • as you exhale, the diaphragm relaxes and the hand covering it moves inward

(continued)

Table 2.6 Continued

Stress Reduction Techniques	Nursing Implications	Stress Reduction Techniques	Nursing Implications
• positive affirmations creating positive, active, new beliefs about oneself and immersing them into the subconscious mind by repeating them frequently	Teach to • write out the statements and place them on mirror, steering wheel, refrigerator, desk, etc. • repeat the statements several times daily • be specific, positive, and brief (e.g., "I am relaxed," not "I am not tense.") • use the present tense, "I am," not "I will." (e.g., "I am learning to express my feelings. I am expressing anger in a positive way. I am loveable.")	• improve self-care	Discuss personal habits that contribute to distress • self-medication • poor nutrition • neglecting early warning signs of tension • nonassertiveness • drinking, smoking Demonstrate positive ways to express and become more aware of feelings. Teach creative problem solving; brainstorm alternatives and other possibilities. Discuss importance of setting priorities, taking one thing at a time.
• balance work and recreation	Teach importance of • seeking work that one enjoys and is capable of doing or learning • learning to take relaxation breaks • taking regularly scheduled vacations • taking a "mental health" day away from work in lieu of a sick day		

Note: from *Nursing care planning guides for adults* by R. Caine & P. Bufalino, 1987, Baltimore, Williams & Wilkins. Used with permission.

- Do not attempt to argue, ridicule, or reason with a client regarding defense mechanisms.
- Help client to adopt and develop effective, positive coping mechanisms.
- When tranquilizing agents are prescribed
  - refer to Table 2.7
  - administer as ordered to provide symptomatic relief of anxiety and tensions and to create stability so client may be more able to participate in process of therapy
  - know that drugs have potential for addiction and should be prescribed for only short periods of time; drugs may also rob client of motivation for change
  - teach client that minor tranquilizers should not be taken with alcohol, as each affects the CNS and enhances the effect of the other
  - teach the client actions and side effects of drugs (a common side effect of tranquilizers is drowsiness; therefore persons taking these drugs should avoid driving or involvement in any potentially dangerous activity)
- When client's anxiety has decreased, negotiate reasonable limits on anxious behavior.
- Do not reinforce phobias, rituals, or physical complaints by giving them undue attention.
- Provide physical protection from repetitive acts; some ritualistic behaviors can cause physical discomfort, e.g., compulsive hand washing.
- Know that client may not be able to sit and may need to keep moving; if so, nurse should walk with him.

Evaluation: Client reduces anxiety to at least a moderate level; does not injure self or others; has a constructive, effective coping mechanism (e.g., talking about feelings, utilizing relaxation techniques, punching bag).

Selected Health Problems

□ Phobias

1. General Information

a. Definition: intense, irrational, fearful reactions to objects or situations, which may interfere with normal function of the person

b. Common phobias

1) agoraphobia: marked fear and avoidance of being alone or in public places from which escape would be difficult

2) social phobia: persistent fear and compelling desire to avoid situations in which the person is exposed to scrutiny of

Table 2.7 Antianxiety Agents (Minor Tranquilizers)

Drug	Action	Side Effects	Nursing Implications
Benzodiazepine derivatives (Atavan, Librium, Serax, Tranzene, Valium, Xanax)	Act on limbic, thalamic and hypothalamic levels of CNS; produces hypnotic, sedative, anxiolytic, skeletal muscle relaxant, and anticonvulsant effects. Range of CNS depression from mild sedation to coma	Hypotension, drowsiness, dizziness, ataxia, lethargy, headache, dry mouth, constipation, urinary retention, changes in libido, paradoxical excitement. Psychic and physical dependence.	Caution client to avoid potentially hazardous activities because of drowsiness. Warn client of danger of concurrent use of alcohol or other CNS depressants. Be aware that these drugs may potentiate suicidal tendencies. Monitor vital signs. Report paradoxic excitement. Avoid abrupt withdrawal (may produce reactions).
Meprobamate (Equanil, Miltown)	CNS depressant similar to barbiturates; acts on multiple CNS sites: hypothalmus, thalmus, limbic, and spinal cord	Drowsiness, ataxia, dizziness, vertigo, slurred speech, headache, skin rash, weakness. Psychic and physical dependence.	Know that meprobamate is highly lethal in overdose; consider possibility of suicide attempts and take precautions. Caution client regarding the concurrent use of alcohol or other CNS depressants. Avoid rapid withdrawal (convulsions and death can result). Caution client to avoid potentially hazardous activities due to drowsiness.
Antihistamines (Vistaril, Atarax)	Central cholinergic effect and CNS properties; used for sedative effects as nighttime sleep aid	Drowziness, dry mouth, headache.	Caution client to avoid potentially hazardous activities due to drowsiness. Warn client of additive effects with alcohol and other drugs.

others for fear of being humiliated or embarrassed

3) simple phobia: persistent fear and desire to avoid an object or situation (other than agoraphobia or social phobia)
   a) claustrophobia: fear of closed places
   b) acrophobia: fear of heights
   c) zoophobia: fear of animals

c. Ego defense mechanism utilized is displacement

d. General treatment measures include individual or group psychotherapy, progressive relaxation and desensitization, behavior modification, and reciprocal inhibition

e. *DSM-III*-R classification: panic disorder (with or without agoraphobia), social phobia, simple phobia

2. Nursing Process

a. Assessment/Analysis: refer to Anxiety, page 37

b. Plan, Implementation, and Evaluation

Goal 1: Client will identify and discuss fear.

Plan/Implementation

- See General Nursing Plans 1–4 page 37.
- Carefully explore the fear with client helping to specify the fearful experience.
- Positively encourage client's participation in treatment (e.g., desensitization, behavior modification, individual and group therapy) to reduce phobic responses.

Evaluation: Client can state situation that caused the fear and talk about the associated feelings.

☐ Dissociative Reactions

1. General Information

a. Definition: hysterical reactions characterized by bizarre behavior in which the individual splits off one portion of the conscious mind from the total when that portion represents some major, otherwise unresolvable, conflict

b. Precipitating event: catastrophic event; characterized by memory loss of the event when person returns to "normal state"

c. *DSM-III*-R classifications
   1) *psychogenic amnesia*: sudden, extensive inability to recall important personal information
   2) *psychogenic fugue*: sudden, unexpected travel away from home or customary workplace with assumption of new identity and inability to recall one's past identity
   3) *multiple personality disorder*: existence in an individual of two or more distinct personalities, each of which is dominant at specific times
   4) *depersonalization disorder*: loss of sense of one's own reality in the absence of psychosis (e.g., self-estrangement, feeling of unreality)

d. Ego defense mechanism utilized in repression; example
   1) person may not remember a certain, anxiety-provoking period of life
   2) these clients can be admitted to a psychiatric unit not remembering who they are and where they are from; these are termed "John Doe" admissions
   3) dynamics: in using the mechanism of repression, the person removes from consciousness own identity and the situation that caused the overwhelming anxiety

e. Treatment: hypnosis, group or individual psychotherapy

2. Nursing Process

a. Assessment/Analysis
   1) careful observation and assessment of client's physical condition to help rule out organic causes such as brain tumor
   2) note patterns of dissociative behavior, including
      a) preceding events, duration, frequency
      b) client's reaction to milieu, persons, events

b. Plans, Implementation, and Evaluation

Refer to General Nursing Plans 1–4, page 37.

☐ Obsessive-Compulsive Disorders

1. General Information

a. Definition: presence of obsession (uncontrollable, recurring thoughts) or compulsion (a ritualistic act done in an attempt to relieve the anxiety related to the thoughts or to make the thoughts go away); considered to be a psychologic conversion reaction to anxiety

b. Ego defense mechanisms utilized are displacement and undoing; the person attempts to displace unconscious, hostile, aggressive impulse into unrelated acts (e.g., hand washing); in so doing, the person attempts to undo or negate the unacceptable impulse

c. Signs and symptoms: may include ritualistic behaviors, e.g., compulsive hand washing or cleanliness or habitual responses such as extreme thrift, neatness, or insistence on same daily routine, with panic or bizarre behavior if usual routine is broken

d. Treatment: individual, family, or group psychotherapy; desensitization; behavior modification; antidepressants

e. *DSM-III*-R classification: obsessive-compulsive disorder

2. Nursing Process

a. Assessment/Analysis
   1) note patterns of compulsive behaviors including preceding events, and client's reactions to specific situations and persons
   2) listen for description of obsessions

b. Plan, Implementation, and Evaluation

Goal: Client will accept limits on repetitive acts and participate in alternative adaptive activities.

Plan/Implementation

- Give client a schedule to follow so that ritualistic/repetitive behaviors are *limited*, but not prohibited.
- Allow client to have choices in schedule and participate in decisions as to how time and energy will be used.
- Do not abruptly interrupt the repetitive act, as it is allaying anxiety; interruption allows the anxiety to break through and can cause panic.
- Set reasonable limits on repetitive behavior; give the client adequate warning that at a certain time another activity will begin.
- Engage in alternative activities with client; do not expect the client to proceed in another activity alone.
- Provide physical protection from repetitive acts; some ritualistic behaviors can cause physical discomfort, e.g., compulsive hand washing.
- As ritualistic/repetitive behaviors decrease, assist client to express feelings and concerns in socially acceptable ways.

Evaluation: Client washes hands (or other compulsive act) fewer times/day compared with admission; begins to participate in other activities.

☐ Anorexia Nervosa

1. General Information

a. Definition: a symptom complex with compulsive resistance to eating and maintaining body weight; intense fear of becoming obese; loss of weight in excess of 15% of recommended body weight with no known physical illness to account for weight loss; body image disturbance (feel fat when thin and emaciated); in females, absence of at least 3 consecutive menstrual periods

b. Onset: usually 12–18 years of age

c. Etiology (several causes hypothesized): primary hypothalmic disorder; atypical affective disorder; phobic avoidance of adulthood; control of one's identity; disturbance in family relationships especially with mother; societal demands for perfection and control; ambivalence toward mother and independence

d. Prevalence reported in 12–18-year-old females ranges from 1 in 100 to 1 in 800

e. Prognosis: reports of up to 21% die from malnutrition, intercurrent infection, or other physical problems; 17%–77% recover

f. *DSM-III*-R classification: listed with other eating disorders of childhood and adolescence, e.g., bulimia and pica (craving unnatural foods such as plaster from walls, dirt, clay)

g. Complications: metabolic abnormalities, muscle wasting, weakness, fatigue, bradycardia, orthostasis, decreased systolic BP, body below 36°C.

h. Treatment: bedrest, hospitalization for intravenous or oral feedings to restore electrolyte and nutritional balance, psychotherapy, behavior modification, family therapy, pharmacotherapy (tricyclics, Periactin with caution)

2. Nursing Process

a. Assessment/Analysis

1) weight and percentage of normal body weight lost
2) eating patterns (amount and types of foods taken, time)
3) vomiting after eating, or if food is forced
4) anemia, hypotension, amenorrhea
5) relationships and interactions with parents, friends, staff, other clients
6) feelings about eating, body image, self
7) positive coping mechanisms, strengths, interests
8) family history of anorexia or bulemia
9) fluid/electrolyte balance
10) dental erosion, oral hygiene
11) vital signs

b. Plans, Implementation, and Evaluation

Goal 1: Client will regain/maintain fluid and electrolyte balance and have adequate nutrition for growth and development.

Plan/Implementation

- Avoid threats, pleas, and health advice.
- Keep accurate I&O; observe amounts and types of food eaten.
- Observe for 2 hours after eating, to prevent vomiting/regurgitation.
- Administer tube feedings/intravenous feedings as ordered.
- Provide positive reinforcement for weight gain rather than amount of food eaten.

Evaluation: Client regains/maintains fluid and electrolyte balance and has adequate nutrition for growth and development.

Goal 2: Client will express feelings and concerns about self and treatment plan; will participate in treatment plan.

Plan/Implementation

- Provide opportunities for choice and decision making in treatment plan and ADL, e.g., time of meal, type of food to be eaten, hygiene, exercise, leisure activities.
- Know that control issues are important dynamic; client needs to accept responsibility for self without guilt or ambivalence. Set and maintain firm limits; be clear about limits and consistent with treatment plan.
- Provide opportunities for staff to meet to ventilate feelings about manipulative and self-destructive behavior.

Evaluation: Client expresses feelings and concerns about self/treatment plan; participates in treatment plan (e.g., makes decisions about schedule and activities).

☐ Bulimia

1. General Information

a. Definition: syndrome characterized by recurrent binge eating with lack of control (average of 2 binge episodes per week for 3 months), regular self-induced vomiting, use of laxatives or diuretics, dieting/fasting, vigorous exercise to prevent weight gain, overconcern with weight and body shape; usually maintain normal weight and appear healthy.

b. Onset: adolescence or early adulthood (17–23 years of age)

c. Prevalence: reports of 1%–4.5% of women affected, 0.4% men

d. Etiology: same as anorexia

e. Prognosis: good if identified early; tends to be episodic with remissions and relapses

f. Complications (usually result of vomiting and laxative abuse): callous formation on back of hand due to trauma from teeth while stimulating gag reflex; dental erosions and cavities; Mallory-Weiss tears resulting in bloody vomitus and blood loss; acid-base changes, especially hypokalemia; ipecac toxicity; hyperactivity; depression/suicide attempts

g. Treatment: psychotherapy, family therapy, behavioral therapy, hospitalization, outpatient treatment, pharmacotherapy (tricyclic antidepressants and MAO inhibitors), diet therapy, restoration of normal fluid/electrolyte balance

2. Nursing Process

See assessment, plans/implementation, and evaluation for anorexia page 43.

☐ Psychosomatic Disorders

1. General Information

a. Definition: psychologically meaningful environmental stimuli are temporarily related to the initiation or exacerbation of a physical condition with demonstrable organic origin or known pathophysiologic process

b. Psychosomatic disorders are sometimes confused with hypochondriasis; the latter is an exaggerated concern with one's physical health and there is no associated organic pathologic condition

c. Reactions: include eczema (skin), migraine headaches (cardiovascular system), backaches (musculoskeletal system), gastrointestinal and respiratory disorders, and psychogenic pain

d. Ego defense mechanism utilized is repression: emotional tension is unconsciously channeled through visceral organs

e. Occurrence: often seen in medical settings and becomes a psychiatric problem when anxiety escalates in spite of physical disorder

f. Possible secondary characteristics

1) *dependence*: a person may manifest normal or abnormal dependency needs
   - a) difficulty in making decisions
   - b) extreme lack of confidence
   - c) a need for more help in meeting problem situations
   - d) anxious persons often lack the confidence and living skill to set up a beneficial living situation
2) *secondary gain*: describes an experience of the person resulting from the primary symptom that may be advantageous and/or satisfying to that person
   - a) this can be a severe problem, because if the secondary gain is great, recovery may not be chosen by the client; recovery is delayed or prevented
   - b) this is an unhealthy way of controlling one's environment rather than doing so in a more socially acceptable way
3) *controlling behavior*: refers to a situation in which a person attempts to exercise a dominating influence over another person
   - a) the controlling person feels helpless because of a lack of control over matters pertaining to own self and welfare
   - b) fear of this loss generates anxiety and often provokes aggressive, manipulative behaviors
   - c) controlling behavior includes manipulative techniques to get other persons to do things they would not choose to do (e.g., stay with ill person, feel sorry for person) and generally provokes anger in the manipulated person
4) *self-centeredness*: sometimes referred to as narcissism
   - a) the self-centered person uses others to satisfy excessive needs, usually irritates others, and is isolated from the comfort and help of good relationships with others
   - b) often believes that any other type of relationship cannot be achieved
   - c) low self-esteem leads to belief that needs can be met only through excessive self-attention
   - d) *DSM-III*-R classification: psychological factors affecting physical condition

2. Nursing Process

a. Assessment/Analysis: see Assessment, page 37

b. Plan, Implementation, and Evaluation

Goal: Client will express feelings, perceptions, and concerns about symptom and treatment plan; client will participate in treatment plan.

Plan/Implementation

- Know that physical symptoms are real.
- Verbally recognize and reinforce authentic communication of feelings, concerns, and perceptions.
- Give appropriate information about medications and treatment.
- Negotiate areas of self-care and independent activity.
- Understand unconscious motivation of the behavior and differentiate it from malingering (a deliberate effort to use an illness to avoid an uncomfortable situation).
- Focus intervention on understanding and alleviation of primary symptoms.
- Encourage exploration with you of the motivation for client's behavior.
- Explore alternatives to the primary symptom for handling anxiety (e.g., talking directly about the concern, asking for help and support, setting limits with others, saying "no" appropriately).
- Recognize person's means of attempting to gain control (negativism, obstinacy, silence, avoidance, increased chatter, crying).
- Set limits on controlling/manipulative behaviors; state time limits; make expectations clear; do not impose unnecessary controls.
- Utilize alternative approaches that allow attainment of the therapeutic goal while permitting the client to retain feeling of control; avoid a battle of wills.
- Be consistent and support other staff to be consistent.
- When manipulative behaviors occur, provide opportunities for staff meetings to ventilate feelings and coordinate care.

Evaluation: Client accepts limits on controlling/manipulative behaviors; develops alternative coping mechanisms; participates in self-care.

☐ Conversion Disorders

1. General Information

a. Definition: hysterical reactions that are manifested by the dysfunction of an organ of special meaning to the person

b. *DSM-III*-R classification: a sub-classification of somatiform disorder, conversion disorder

c. Conversion disorders differ from hypochondriasis in that in hypochondriasis there is no loss of function. They differ from psychosomatic disorders in that in psychosomatic disorders there is a demonstrable organic origin or known pathophysiologic process; in conversion disorders there is not.

d. Characteristics include
   1) symbolic expression of anxiety (e.g., anxiety about seeing something is controlled by becoming blind, a teacher loses voice)
   2) there is no demonstrable physical lesion
   3) symptoms do not follow motor-nerve paths
   4) the person shows little concern about the incapacity caused by the symptoms ("*la belle indifférence*")

e. Defense mechanisms utilized are repression and displacement
   1) primary gain: repression keeps anxiety or need out of client's awareness
   2) may have secondary gain of attention; does not have to do work, take care of self

2. Nursing Process

a. Assessment/Analysis
   1) symptoms of physical disorder and vital signs
   2) client's perceptions of symptoms: "*la belle indifférence*"

b. Plan, Implementation, and Evaluation

Goal: Client will obtain symptomatic relief from anxiety and physical symptoms; will participate in self-care and therapy process.

Plan/Implementation

- Observe and record behavior and physical condition and assist with lab tests, x-ray procedures, etc., to help rule out organic basis for symptoms.
- Do not focus on physical symptoms; assist client to change focus to healthy interests (music, exercise, friends, plans).
- Engage in alternative activities with client; do not expect client to proceed in another activity alone—share it with the client.
- Monitor responses to drug therapy.

Evaluation: Client is relieved of physical symptoms and experiences decreased anxiety; participates in self-care and therapy process.

☐ Post-Traumatic Stress Disorder

1. General Information

a. Definition: anxiety neurosis resulting from severe external stress that is beyond what is usual or tolerable for most people

b. Stressors: rape, military combat, natural disasters (e.g., earthquakes), physical accidents involving loss of life of another or loss of body part or its functions (e.g., post-accident permanent paralysis), accidental disasters caused by people (e.g., crashes, fires), intentional disasters (e.g., bombing, torture), victims of criminal assaults (e.g., robbery)

c. Characteristics
- **1)** re-experiencing trauma in at least one of the following ways
  - **a)** recurrent/intrusive recollections of event
  - **b)** recurrent dreams of event
  - **c)** sudden acting out or feeling as if traumatic event were recurring, owing to environmental or ideational stimulus
- **2)** numbing of responsiveness to or decreased involvement with external world after the trauma
  - **a)** markedly diminished interest in one or more significant activities
  - **b)** feeling of detachment or estrangement from others
  - **c)** constricted affect
- **3)** at least two of the following symptoms, which were not present before the trauma
  - **a)** hyperalertness or exaggerated startle response
  - **b)** sleep disturbance
  - **c)** guilt about surviving or about behavior required for survival
  - **d)** memory impairment or trouble concentrating
  - **e)** avoidance of activities that arouse recollection of traumatic event
  - **f)** intensification of symptoms by exposure to events that symbolize or resemble traumatic event

d. Related factors
- **1)** physical injury may be present because of the nature of the trauma
- **2)** depression and anxiety are usually present

e. Dynamics: loss of self-esteem and loss of control in the traumatic situation have led to the behavior and feelings described above

f. *DSM-III*-R classification: Post-traumatic stress disorder

2. Nursing Process

a. Assessment/Analysis
- **1)** nature of the traumatic event
- **2)** duration of disorder
- **3)** degree of impairment
- **4)** preexistence of problems that may complicate situation (e.g., anxiety, depression)
- **5)** presence and degree of symptoms
- **6)** positive support system available

b. Plans, Implementation, and Evaluation

Goal 1: Client will recount the traumatic event and cope with feelings related to it.

Plan/Implementation
- Support client through process of recounting the event and venting feelings.
- Acknowledge significance of the traumatic event and the appropriateness of client's feelings.
- If there is a need to return to the scene of the trauma, help the client to select supportive resources to accompany him/her.
- Review goals and plans for crisis intervention (page 37), depression, rape and loss (page 31).
- Involve client in a recovering group of people with similar problems (e.g., Victims for Victims).

Evaluation: Client describes the event and discusses feelings related to it (e.g., sadness, anger).

Goal 2: Client will resume involvement in external world.

Plan/Implementation
- Take measures to prevent the client from becoming isolated.
- Gradually increase reinvolvement in pretrauma activities.
- Discuss feelings about activities.
- Reinforce client's involvement in activities.
- Give information about social, financial, or health resources.

Evaluation: Client gradually resumes involvement in activities of importance to client.

References

Barry, P. (1984). *Psychosocial nursing assessment and intervention*. Philadelphia: Lippincott.

Griffin, M. (1986). In the mind's eye. *American Journal of Nursing*, *86*, 804–806.

Haber, J., Hoskins, P., Leach, A., & Sidelau, B. (1987). *Comprehensive psychiatric nursing*. New York: McGraw-Hill.

Lego, S. (ed.) (1984). *The American handbook of psychiatric nursing*. Philadelphia: Lippincott.

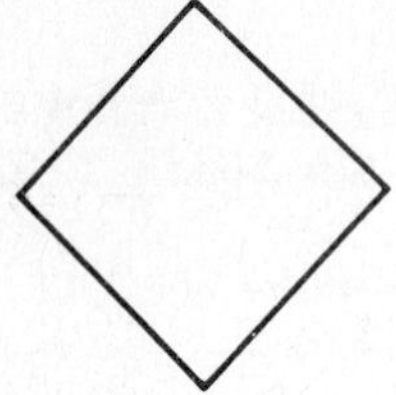

Confused Behavior

General Concepts

Overview: Confusion can be related to physiologic or psychologic disturbances and seen on a continuum from mild to severe; acute, temporary, or chronic. It is a biopsychosocial disorder involving the inability to comprehend and/or integrate words, relationships, or events.

Confusion can be a symptom of physical disturbances such as respiratory abnormalities, electrolyte imbalance, infection, biochemical or nutritional imbalances, cerebral disease or destruction, and physical or psychologic trauma. It may also be seen in functional psychotic disorders, severe depression, acute psychologic crises, and substance abuse.

Application of the Nursing Process to the Client Exhibiting Confused Behavior

Certain physiologic and environmentally induced confused behaviors are short-lived and directly associated with factors that can be controlled, changed, or improved. When the causative factors create permanent or progressive changes, the confusion becomes a chronic state—the selected health problem outlined below.

Selected Health Problem

☐ Chronic Confusion

1. Definition

- **a.** A mental dysfunction related to the response of the brain to disease, damage, or an aging process; a persistent clinical syndrome
- **b.** Specific syndromes
  - **1)** Alzheimer's disease: degeneration of the cortex and atrophy of cerebrum; usually begins in persons in their early 60s, death 1–10 years post onset
  - **2)** Korsakoff's syndrome: associated with chronic alcoholism
  - **3)** trauma-induced confusion, e.g., stroke, residual problems related to neurosurgery
- **c.** Confusion of varying degree and influence is noted in chronic organic brain syndromes
- **d.** *DSM-III*-R classification: organic mental syndromes: delirium and dementia, amnestic syndrome, organic mental syndrome not otherwise specified, primary degenerative dementia of the Alzheimer type, multi-infarct dementia, senile dementia not otherwise specified, presenile dementia not otherwise specified, dementia associated with alcoholism

2. Nursing Process

- **a. Assessment/Analysis**
  - **1)** onset history
  - **2)** orientation to person, time, and place
  - **3)** problems with cognition; decreased attention, comprehension, abstract thinking, and calculation
  - **4)** memory: impairment of recent or remote memory; may use confabulation to cover memory loss
  - **5)** judgment and decision making
  - **6)** speech patterns
  - **7)** paranoid ideation
  - **8)** self-care abilities
  - **9)** previous coping mechanisms
  - **10)** personality and affectual changes
  - **11)** social interaction
  - **12)** feelings and concerns about treatment, impairment
  - **13)** family involvement
  - **14)** physiologic problems: respiratory, skin, cardiac, nutrition, rest and activity
- **b. Analysis**
  - **1)** safe, effective care environment
    - ■ potential for trauma
    - ■ sensory-perceptual alteration (specify)
    - ■ knowledge deficit
  - **2)** physiological integrity
    - ■ activity intolerance
    - ■ sleep pattern disturbance
    - ■ altered nutrition: less than body requirements
  - **3)** psychological integrity
    - ■ altered role performance
    - ■ social isolation
    - ■ personal identity disturbance
  - **4)** health promotion/maintenance
    - ■ self-care deficit

- ineffective family coping
- impaired adjustment

c. Plans/Implementation, and Evaluation

Goal 1: Client will maintain or improve self-care activities to maintain optimal physiologic functioning.

Plan/Implementation

- Arrange for client to have needed eyeglasses, hearing aid, false teeth, and other assistive devices for activities of daily living (ADL).
- Plan ADL schedule based on client's established patterns; allow client to make schedule and activities decisions as appropriate.
- Give client specific, simple directions for ADL; provide assistance only if client cannot function alone; allow sufficient time for activities and give advance notice.
- Provide range-of-motion (ROM) exercises at least once daily; assist with ambulation as necessary.
- Schedule rest periods during the day as needed.
- Follow client's established bedtime routine; avoid use of sedatives, which may *increase* confusion.
- Offer and encourage nutritionally balanced foods and fluids.
- Keep skin clean, dry, and free from surface irritants or pressure that impedes circulation
- Assist client in maintaining neat, appropriate, attractive appearance.
- Supervise medication consumption (kind, time, amount); know side effects of drugs given and carefully observe and record client responses to all medications and treatments.
- Record vital signs and I&O daily.

Evaluation: Client performs ADL; attains and maintains ambulation; sleeps sufficient hours to obtain optimal rest; maintains adequate nutritional intake; maintains skin integrity; receives assistance only as required.

Goal 2: Client will regain and maintain contact with reality.

Plan/Implementation

- Establish routine; avoid changes in routine or environment.
- Provide hourly orientation to time/place/person using clocks, calendars, signs, pictures, and written reminders.
- Put client's picture and name (big letters) on room door and the bed.
- Use concrete symbols, photographs of client's past to strengthen sense of continuity.
- Answer questions as often as needed, using short, simple sentences; demonstrate acceptance nonverbally to reinforce verbal communications; build on the reality-based statements of the client to strengthen conversation; talk about familiar subjects; establish eye contact, face directly when addressing client.
- Assist client to use previously successful coping mechanisms.
- Provide adequate sensory stimulation, avoiding both sensory deprivation and overload.
- Utilize touch: back rub, skin care, hold hands if you/client are comfortable doing so.
- Respect client's privacy, space, time, and possessions.
- Avoid physical restraints or environmental confinement, which increase helplessness; assign staff to wandering clients for short time periods.
- Obtain necessary orders and administer appropriate symptomatic chemotherapy; observe and record behavioral changes.
- Educate and relate to the family and friends, so they will not withdraw from the client
  - discuss client's behavior, memory loss, and confusion; recognize and help them to work through their own feelings of helplessness, anger, depression, love, and guilt; discuss importance of continued interaction for client and significant others
  - help them prepare for client's continuing care by raising questions, exploring alternatives, and deciding on a goal and plan of action that meets their needs as well as the client's
  - refer to Alzheimer's support group

Evaluation: Client is oriented to person, time, and place; interacts with others appropriately; family and friends maintain interaction with client; client and family make reasonable plans for client's continuing care.

References

†Blakeslee, J. (1988). Untie the elderly. *American Journal of Nursing*, *88*, 833–834.

Campbell, E., Williams, M., & Meynarczyk, S. (1986). After the fall—confusion. *American Journal of Nursing*, *86*, 151–154.

Harp, A. & Borger, F. (1985). A test in time. *American Journal of Nursing*, *85*, 1107–1111.

Pajk, M. (1984). Alzheimer's disease: Inpatient care. *American Journal of Nursing*, *84*, 215–222.

Shapira, J., Schesinger, R., & Cummings, J. (1986). Distinguishing dementias. *American Journal of Nursing*, *86*, 698–702.

†Highly recommended.

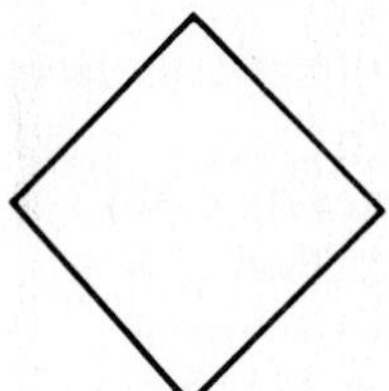

Elated-Depressive Behavior

General Concepts

Overview

1. Affective disorders are a variety of states and syndromes. They include extremes in mood and affect such as depressive or manic behavior and unresolved grief.
2. Affective states may be viewed as a mood state or a clinical syndrome. For example, the mood state of depression may occur in a normal person, in a client with a psychiatric syndrome, or in a medical client.
3. Management modalities (treatment): depends on the severity of the symptoms and includes psychotherapy, chemotherapy, convulsive therapy (electroshock), and milieu therapy in a hospital setting or on an ambulatory basis.
   a. Chemotherapy consists of antidepressant drugs (see Table 2.8, reprints)
   b. Psychotherapy is aimed toward achieving insight into the underlying depression, acknowledging feelings of worthlessness, and increasing self-esteem
   c. Milieu therapy in hospital offers client a safe emotional and physical environment
      1) requirements for treating elation or depression in hospital include
         a) protection from self-harm
         b) removal from unbearable pressures encountered outside the hospital
         c) need for problem solving in a sheltered, supportive environment with access to other therapies, reliable atmosphere
         d) staff attitudes that demonstrate interest and a desire to offer the help needed
      2) staff reaction to elated or depressed clients is often characterized by a feeling of ineffectiveness
         a) this can lead to avoidance of client, request for assignment change
         b) engenders further feelings of worthlessness in client, creating further withdrawal
         c) the feelings must be dealt with to ensure a therapeutic milieu
         d) staff must recognize potential for this rejection cycle and avoid it; the staff can support each other in treating client
         e) avoid becoming defensive with manic clients
            - clients have uncanny sensitivity to others' weaknesses and inadequacies; they constantly point these out
            - staff must tolerate criticisms without becoming defensive
            - defensiveness fuels attack and is counterproductive
   d. Electroconvulsive therapy (ECT)
      1) only form of shock (convulsive) therapy still in use
      2) one of the chief benefits is that it often makes a client more accessible to psychotherapy
      3) electric shock is delivered to brain through electrodes on one or both temples
         a) produces immediate unconsciousness
         b) produces a cerebral seizure
         c) effective in remission of symptoms
      4) Usually given every other day, 3 times a week for 10–12 treatments
      5) Candidates for ECT
         - severely depressed elderly with chronic disease that precludes use of antidepressants
         - severely depressed, suicidal patients who do not respond to antidepressants or psychotherapy
         - inpatients when tricyclic and tetracyclic antidepressants are contraindicated (e.g., cardiac patients, pregnant women)
      6) side effects: temporary confusion, amnesia

Table 2.8 Medications Used to Treat Affective Disorders

Name and Dosage	Action	Side Effects	Nursing Implications
Tricyclic Antidepressants			
Amitriptline HCl (Elavil) 75–100 mg/day (initial) adjusted to 300 mg/day Impiramine HCl (Tofranil) 75–100 mg/day (initial) up to 300 mg/day Doxepin HCl (Adapin, Sinequan) 30–150 mg/day up to 300 mg/day for therapeutic effect Combination Clordiazepozide-Amitriptyline (Limbitrol) 75–100 mg/day up to 300 mg/day	Blocks reuptake of neurotransmitters at neuronal membrane; effects of norepinephrine and serotonin may be potentiated resulting in antidepressant effect; strong anticholinergic activity	All tricyclics and tetracyclics: Dizziness, nausea, excitement, blurred vision, constipation, dry mouth, anorexia, insomnia, drowsiness, excessive perspiration, gynecomastia, skin rash, hypotension	Assess suicide potential. Observe side effects and treat symptomatically. Do not give with or immediately following treatment with MAO inhibitors. Monitor blood pressure. Teach client • avoid alcohol • check with MD before taking over-the-counter meds • ways to avoid problems with orthostatic hypotension • importance of oral hygiene • take with meals to avoid gastic irritation.
Tetracyclic Antidepressants			
Maprotiline HCl (Ludiomil) 75–150 mg/day Zimelidine (Zelmid) 100–300 mg/day	Similar to the tricyclics but does not appear to influence reuptake of serotonin		Institute seizure precautions.
Other Antidepressants			
Fluoxetine hydrochloride (Prozac) 20 mg/day initially, may be increased to 80 mg/day	Inhibition of CNS neuronal uptake of serotonin	Rash, anxiety, nervousness, insomnia, drowsiness, fatigue or asthenia, tremor, sweating, anorexia, nausea, diarrhea, weight loss, dizziness, lightheadedness; may activate mania	Assess suicide potential. Observe for mania, side effects. Teach client • avoid alcohol • avoid driving car or operating heavy machinery until response is determined • check with MD before taking other prescribed medications or over-the-counter meds • notify MD if client becomes pregnant
Mono-Amine-Oxidase (MAO) Inhibitors			
Isocarboxazid (Marplan) Initially 30 mg/day then 10–30 mg/day	Inhibition of monoamine oxidase, enzyme mainly in nerve tissue, liver and lungs, increases concentration of amines (epinephrine, norepinephrine, dopamine, serotonin) causing an antidepressant effect	Headache, dizziness, dry mouth, blurred vision, postural hypotension, increased appetite, dermatitis, hepatitis, euphoria, activates latent schizophrenia	Potentiates action of narcotics, barbiturates, sedatives, topine derviatives. May cause severe headaches, hypertension with natural foods (e.g., aged cheese) and alcoholic beverages (beer and wine). Teach client dietary restrictions.
Lithium			
Lithium carbonate (Eskalith, Lithane) Dosage determined by blood level and by behavior	Monovalent cation that competes with potassium, sodium, calcium, and	GI discomfort (nausea, vomiting, stomach pain, diarrhea), thirst, dazed feeling, drowsiness, hand	Remind client to take medicine. Assess drug level every 3–4 days.

(continued)

Table 2.8 *Continued*

Name and Dosage	Action	Side Effects	Nursing Implications
• blood level: 0.6–1.5 mEq/liter • maintenance level: 0.5–1.3 mEq/liter (300 mg/day tid) • toxic level: 2.0 mEq/liter or above • acute mania: 1–1.4 mEq/liter (20–30 mg/kg/day in 2–3 doses)	magnesium at cellular sites; interferes with reuptake of central monoamine neurotransmitters	tremor, tinnitus, blurred vision	Teach importance of regular medication schedule and blood work. Assess suicide potential. Monitor salt and fluid intake. Teach client • salt and fluid intake • avoid caffeine • take with meals

Application of the Nursing Process to the Client with an Affective Disorder

1. **Assessment**
   a. Affect
      1) powerlessness, worthlessness
      2) helplessness
      3) fears and crying
      4) anger, hostility (directed inwardly in depression, outward in elation)
      5) elation, exaltation
      6) anxiety
      7) depression related to guilt and repressed hostility; leads to self-condemnation and punishment
   b. Cognition
      1) narrowed perception and interests
      2) impaired concentration
      3) delusional thinking
      4) loquaciousness, flight of ideas in elated stage

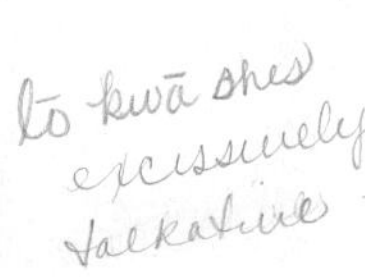

   c. Behavior
      1) decreased motor activity or agitation/hyperactivity
      2) decreased or increased communications
      3) changes in social interactions
      4) inappropriate dress
   d. Physical changes
      1) eating disorders (excessive or insufficient eating)
      2) sleep disturbances (too much or too little)
      3) interest in sex (increase or decrease)
      4) weakness, fatigue
      5) constipation/diarrhea
   e. Strengths and capabilities
      1) usual coping strategies
      2) family and peer relationships
      3) hobbies and pastimes (often very limited in depression)
2. **Analysis**
   a. safe, effective care environment
      1) impaired home maintenance management
      2) potential for violence: self-directed
      3) knowledge deficit
   b. physiological integrity
      1) altered bowel elimination
      2) altered nutrition: less/more than body requirements
      3) sleep pattern disturbance
      4) sexual dysfunction
   c. psychological integrity
      1) hopelessness
      2) chronic/situational low self esteem
      3) social isolation
   d. health promotion/maintenance
      1) impaired adjustment
      2) altered family processes
      3) altered health maintenance
      4) self-care deficit (specify)
3. **General Nursing Plans, Implementation, and Evaluation**

Goal 1: The elated or depressed client will demonstrate increased ability to cope with feelings by sharing feelings with others.

Plan/Implementation

- Spend time with client at least twice daily; start with 5–10 minutes, increase time as you and client can tolerate it; encourage client to identify and verbalize feelings, accept what is said; use silence when appropriate—the presence of a caring person is helpful when learning to cope with painful feelings; *avoid* false reassurance, overcheerfulness.
- Focus on client's feelings; allow ventilation in ways that seem comfortable to the client; share with client that the only way to get through

feelings is to stay with them and experience them.
- Help client explore meaning of loss, somatic symptoms, feelings tone, "It seems like it just isn't worth it." "You've had a hard time lately, and you're learning to deal with your feelings." "You've lost someone you loved, and you're going through grief and mourning." "Sounds like you remember the good parts and the rough parts of this relationship, and you're beginning to be ready to risk again."

Evaluation: Client discusses feelings with nurse and others; shares feelings of sadness and of wanting to cry.

Goal 2: The elated or depressed client will use acceptable expressions of anger.

Plan/Implementation
- Assist client to identify angry feelings.
- Explore sources of anger and help client to express anger verbally.
- Avoid arguments, involvement in client's set of rules, and avoid discussions that involve moral values.
- Prevent punishment that extends to self-mutilation (remove sharp objects, matches, cigarettes).
- Involve client in minimal tasks and activities.
- Help client explore ways to cope with anger; talk about alternate ways to express anger (handball, racquetball, hitting a punching bag or mattress, shouting, singing, confronting with words, swearing, using batacus, tearing up phone books, throwing sponges or bean bags).

Evaluation: Client shoots baskets in the gym; tells staff "it feels good to let off steam."

Goal 3: The elated or depressed client will identify feelings of guilt.

Plan/Implementation
- Acknowledge client's view of guilt but show that this is client's view, not nurse's.
- Assist client to express guilt: explore situation and persons with whom the client experiences guilt, "I feel guilty when I . . ."; have client try to replace the word "guilt" with "resentment"; explore feelings about this; most situations that involve guilt also involve feelings of anger and resentment; work on these feelings with client.
- Give positive reinforcement to reality-oriented behavior and realistic expectations.

Evaluation: Client acknowledges guilty feelings; discusses reasonableness of feelings.

Goal 4: The elated or depressed client will improve interpersonal relationships.

Plan/Implementation
- Explore the identity of persons in client's life with whom feelings can be shared; if there is no one, explore how this came about, feelings about this situation, and ways to change situations; use role-playing or psychodrama to try alternative ways to initiate sharing of feelings.
- Explore client's feelings about listening to others' feelings; often people who have problems tolerating their own feelings feel overwhelmed with others' feelings; practice sharing feelings and setting limits on listening to problems; practice reciprocal sharing of feelings in role playing; discuss how to set limits and keep relationship.
- Discuss effect of irrational demands and negativity on relationships. Support self-direction and decision making. Role play interpersonal relationships, decision making. Assertiveness training. Explore needs met by dependency, helplessness; discuss what client would lose if behavior changed.
- Explore expectations of self and others in relationships; discuss consequences of unrealistic expectations; realistically assess expectations, strengths in relationships.

Evaluation: Client reinstates relationships with family and friends; initiates contact with a significant person at least once a week; follows through with social engagements as feasible.

Selected Health Problems

☐ Depression

1. General Information

a. Definitions

1) a disorder of mood or affect characterized by feelings of dejection, sadness, and hopelessness

2) operational definition: gratification is received from a love object; loss of love object leads to frustration, anxiety, grief, guilt, and hostility; this results in loss of self-esteem and depression

b. Precipitating factors

1) loss of a loved one through separation or death is the most common precipitant; the loss must be significant to the person

2) threats to self-esteem: disruption in the interpersonal and intrapersonal input of love, respect, and approval results in decreased self-esteem

3) success: paradoxically, one may become depressed upon achieving success; this is due to the anticipation of loss of self-esteem if one does not live up to the expectations implied by the success
4) physical illness: depression is interrelated with many physical illnesses because of real or anticipated loss of function, independence, role of well person
5) self-image: changes in perception of self as a result of physical, emotional, or life-style changes including role changes, body changes

c. States of depression: depression may be felt to some degree by anyone; in terms of severity of disruption, there are four kinds of depression
   1) *transitory depression*
      a) seldom seen as presenting problem
      b) may be related to environmental or physiologic stress
      c) symptoms
         - affect: quiet, unhappy, helplessness or hopelessness
         - cognition: difficulty making decisions, self-deprecation, feelings of inadequacy, focus on personal problems
         - behavior: decreased activity, restrained, inhibited
         - physical changes: mild physical discomforts
      d) short-lived; person institutes own cure
   2) *reactive depression* (exogenous)
      a) *DSM-III*-R classification: uncomplicated bereavement
      b) related to precipitating environmental or physiologic stress or personal loss (e.g., death of someone close)
      c) responses follow stages of grief and mourning process (refer to Loss, Death and Dying, page 30).
      d) symptoms
         - affect: withdrawn, apathetic, anger
         - cognition: personal derogation, suicidal thoughts, preoccupation with loss or stress
         - behavior: serious impairment of activity, domestic disturbances
         - physical changes: mild changes, weight loss or gain of less than 10 lbs, feels worse as day progresses
      e) the crisis period takes about 6 weeks; complete resolution is usually achieved in 6–12 months; grief is normal reactive depression
   3) *neurotic depression*
      a) *DSM-III*-R classification: dysthymic disorder
      b) cognitive changes much greater and may be long-standing based on inability to get love from others and lack of supportive experiences
      c) symptoms
         - affect: powerlessness, helplessness, anxiety, hostility, anger, fear, crying
         - cognition: cognitive triad present—negative self image, negative view of world, negative expectations for future; indecisive, self-blame, decreased concentration and memory, suicidal ideation
         - behavior: psychomotor retardation, decreased grooming and self-care, constant repetition of a life experience or regret, decreased social interaction but maintains ability to work, etc.
         - physical changes: weakness, fatigue, somatic preoccupation, eating changes, sleep changes, decreased sexual interest
   4) *psychotic depression* (endogenous)
      a) *DSM-III*-R classification
         - major depressive episode with psychotic features including severe impairment of reality testing and physiologic disturbances
         - manic episode with psychotic features
      b) depression brought on by severe environmental blows to security; mobilization of extreme guilt; may have biochemical/genetic causes
      c) symptoms
         - affect: despondent, despairing, little feeling tone, helplessness, worthlessness, emptiness
         - cognition: delusional thinking, cognitive triad present and marked; thought pattern more despondent in morning, lifts as day progresses
         - behavior: markedly depressed (vegetative) or agitated depending on type
            - *agitated depression*: anxious, tense, extremely restless; pacing,

hand wringing, skin picking, poor eating and sleeping
- *retarded depression*: general physical and cognitive slowness, sitting idly, hanging head, looking haggard; indecisive and uncooperative
- *bipolar depression (manic-depression)*: episodes of well-defined, self-limiting mania or depression, usually in repeating cycles, with or without an interval of normalcy
  * person usually recovers completely from both phases, but there is a tendency for recurrence
  * may experience only the depressive phase, only the manic phase, or both at different times in life

■ physical changes
- vegetative signs: anorexia, weight loss of more than 10 lbs, constipation, insomnia, amenorrhea/impotence
- insomnia, early morning awakening
- lack of self-care

5) *seasonal affective disorder*

a) cyclical major depressive disorder that is affected by changes in day length occurring in the fall-winter months

b) symptoms (appear as the days shorten during winter months)
- ■ sadness, irritability, anxiety during depressed periods
- ■ overeating
- ■ carbohydrate craving, weight gain
- ■ sleep duration increases
- ■ quality of sleep decreases
- ■ drowsiness during daytime, fatigue
- ■ difficulties at work, in interpersonal relationships

c) symptoms may be mediated by the secretion of melatonin, a substance thought to mediate seasonal behavior, and affected by day–night rhythms

d) treatment: studies have shown good results with bright light application in the morning or evening hours every day (reverses the depressive changes by extending the photoperiod by 4–6 hours); clients respond to treatment after 2–4 days.

e) *DSM-III*-R classification: recurrent major depression, seasonal pattern

2. Nursing Process

a. Assessment/Analysis

1) signs and symptoms (refer to "States of Depression" page 54)

a) affect

b) degree of cognitive change: cognitive triad (i.e., emotional, physical, and behavioral changes), unlike other symptoms, occurs only in depression; the more severe the cognitive triad, the more debilitating the depression

c) behavior

d) physical changes

e) morning-evening mood variation
- ■ reactive depression: fatigue level affects depression; feel more depressed when tired
- ■ neurotic depression: more depressed in morning; mood improves as day progresses
- ■ psychotic depression: feel more depressed in morning; mood improves as day progresses

2) severity and level of depression (refer to "States of Depression" page 54)

3) priorities for care

a) safety

b) physical needs

c) self-esteem

4) suicide potential

a) suicidal risk: persons at high risk for suicide include
- ■ adolescents and people over 50 years old
- ■ single males
- ■ black males
- ■ alcoholics, isolated and unhappy persons
- ■ police, physicians
- ■ depressed persons
- ■ hallucinating persons responding to voice commands
- ■ those with a history of family suicide
- ■ persons experiencing a maturational or situational crisis or a chronic or painful illness
- ■ previous attempters

b) suicidal plan
- ■ method—assess degree of lethality (margin for error); see Table 2.9

Table 2.9 Suicide Methods

Lower Lethality	Higher Lethality
Cutting wrists	Slashing jugular
Tranquilizers	Barbiturates/sedatives
Inhaling gas	Carbon monoxide
Swallowing caustic substances	Aspirin
	Medications combined with alcohol
	Jumping
	Drowning
	Hanging
	Setting self on fire
	Explosives
	Automobile crash
	Shooting self

- availability (the more available, the higher the risk)
- specificity of plan

c) change in behavior, e.g., calmness: may mean person has worked out a plan; as depression lifts, client may have energy to carry out plan

d) giving away valued things: saying good-bye, making amends, asking medical questions

e) ambivalent feelings
- coexistence of opposing emotions in client (e.g., wants to live/die, experiences love and hate toward deceased or absent person)
- inability to express anger and hostility toward another person, turns hate and aggression inward toward self, leading to self-destructive thoughts/actions
- feelings of ambivalence are common in severely depressed clients, particularly when the depression is related to the loss of a person important to them

f) changes in activities of daily living
- sleep patterns
- work habits
- eating patterns (refer also to reprint "Was This Suicide Preventable?", page 136)

b. Plans, Implementation, and Evaluation

Goal 1: Client will be protected from suicidal gestures.

Plan/Implementation

- Assume responsibility for safety of client; inspect unit for dangerous items such as sharp items (scissors, nail files, razor blades), pills; remove from client area.
- Restrict client to observable areas; observe closely for suicidal ideation/gestures.
- Utilize open questioning about suicidal plans and ideas.
- Set limits on repetition of story of suicidal feelings or gesture.
- Establish nurse-client relationship that shows nurse as respectful, knowledgeable, able to help solve problems; nurse's attitude should reflect firmness and confidence.
- Allow client to express feelings.
- Involve client in activities that ensure success, e.g., attaining small goals in activities of daily living (ADL), exercise.
- Provide realistic reassurance; convey attitude that client will succeed.
- Assess client's abilities realistically and provide only the help needed; irrational demands should be discussed openly and refused.
- Stress client's capabilities/strengths.
- Work with client to prepare list of problems and corresponding solutions; use all resources available, including family and community resources; give client sense that problems are manageable.
- Know that suicidal client behavior may cause nurse to feel anger, guilt, or to experience rescue fantasies; staff need to meet daily for mutual support, planning, and reality testing.
- Do not withdraw when ambivalence is directed toward nursing staff; continue to offer listening and socialization.
- Utilize emergency methods to counteract suicidal attempts (e.g., lavage, one-to-one observation).
- If suicide attempt occurs, assist client/family to share and work through feelings and concerns.
- Acknowledge the coexistence of opposing (ambivalent) emotions in the client and family.
- Review and evaluate interventions.

Evaluation: Client makes no gestures of physical harm; gives all potentially dangerous materials to staff; receives frequent safety checks.

Goal 2: Client will meet physical care needs independently.

Plan/Implementation

Food and Fluid Intake

- Find acceptable eating pattern based on client's

likes, dislikes, and usual eating habits. If client is anorexic and apathetic to food, provide frequent, small meals and snacks of easy foods to eat; leave a thermos of hot chocolate, oatmeal cookies, crackers and cheese, 7-Up, etc., at bedside for small snacks at night or during day. Monitor food and fluid intake.

- Weigh weekly (continued loss of weight may indicate deepening depression; weight gain may indicate decreased depression).

Sleep/Rest

- Help client follow usual bedtime routine. If client sleeps continuously during the day and does not rest at night, work with client to maintain schedule of activity and rest during daytime. Recognize that insomnia increases fatigue and fatigue increases depression. Sedatives are generally ineffective; therefore, use other nursing measures (e.g., warm milk, snacks, back rub, warm bath).

Elimination

- Maintain adequate fluid intake.
- Provide adequate fiber in diet.
- Monitor elimination.

Grooming and Hygiene

- Help client establish routine and schedule for bathing, care of hair, skin, nails, clothes. If client is unable to initiate self-care, approach in matter-of-fact manner, e.g.,"It's time to bathe, Mr. Watkins." Convey expectation that client can perform self-care. Give positive reinforcement to any care of self.

Activity

- Consider personal preferences and needs; help client do things for self (many depressed clients become dependent on others, but activity usually helps them to feel better).
- Assign daily responsibility for ward-maintenance to help renew sense of self-worth and purposefulness. Simple tasks (emptying ashtrays, straightening chairs, putting away cards, games, or crafts equipment) with supervision may be appropriate for deeply depressed clients; more difficult tasks can be gradually assigned as client tolerates. Assignments should not be demeaning or demanding.
- Assess previous hobbies and pastimes. Assist with simple crafts that can be finished in one sitting to increase sense of accomplishment; encourage group singing, poetry reading, painting, working with clay, to assist client to become more comfortable in groups and to establish community and group socialization; client may need nurse's presence to tolerate group activities at first; simple exercises, walks, may progress to group sports; avoid competitive activities.
- Plan activity schedule based on client's morning-evening mood variation; teach client about variation
  - reactive depression: plan group and other activities in morning and following afternoon rest period
  - endogenous: do not plan therapy sessions or demanding activities early in day.

Medications

- Discuss rationale for medication as client can tolerate and assimilate teaching.
- Teach side effects, administration (see Table 2.8).

Evaluation: Client ingests adequate food and fluids; achieves adequate sleep-activity pattern; has adequate elimination; dresses and grooms self daily; participates in activities.

Goal 3: Client receiving ECT will be free from preventable injury.

Plan/Implementation

- Prep client as if going to OR.
- Explain procedure thoroughly and answer client questions, concerns.
- Ensure consent form is in chart.
- Arrange for spine x-ray, if required.
- Keep client NPO.
- Remove dentures, hairpins, etc.
- Give medications as ordered: muscle relaxant (e.g., succinylcholine) to reduce tonic/clonic movements; atropine sulfate to dry secretions and prevent bradycardia and asystole; short-acting barbiturate (e.g., pentothal) for sedation.
- Sit with client before treatment to provide support.
- After treatment, check client's pulse and respirations; observe reaction upon awakening.
- Orient client to time and place and to the fact that treatment has been administered (temporary memory loss and confusion are the most distressing side-effects following ECT).
- Stay with client a minimum of one hour after ECT; check vital signs; monitor confusion.

Evaluation: Client recovers from ECT safely; is oriented to time, place, and person.

Goal 4: Client will increase interactions with staff, other clients, and family.

Plan/Implementation

- Assist client to identify, define, and problem solve difficult areas in social relationships (e.g., client who is hypercritical of self and others can discuss and practice a softer, more accepting approach).
- Help client to look at situations where client may push others away out of fear of rejection (i.e., reject them before being rejected).
- Practice social skills, use role playing.
- Go with client to group activities, choosing short, simple group activities that client identifies as least threatening (exercise, sports, music).
- Involve client in activity that provides chance for success (e.g., simple occupational therapy activities).
- Refer to page 57.

Evaluation: Client spends increasing time with staff, other clients, and family; identifies problems in relationships; practices new social skills with staff and other clients.

Goal 5: Client will discuss feelings about self and situation.

Refer to General Nursing Goals 1, 2, and 3, page 52.

Goal 6: Client will increase independent decision making.

Plan/Implementation

- Assess areas in which client is making own decisions and give positive reinforcement to self-enhancing ones.
- Assist with decision making when client is profoundly depressed.
- Expect client to make own decisions, with support as depression lifts.

Evaluation: Client participates in planning own activities and schedule.

Goal 7: Family members will maintain relationship with client.

Plan/Implementation

- Provide family members opportunity to discuss their feelings of anger, guilt, inability to help client.
- Help family understand client's anger, dependency, negativism.
- Discuss ways family can respond to excessive demands and dependency.
- Review expectations and goals for family and individual family members; explore alternatives for unrealistic expectations.

Evaluation: Family members discuss feelings, expectations, and goals with appropriate staff; maintain interaction with client by letter, phone, or visit; bring client home when appropriate and assist with recreation and socialization.

□ Elation and Hyperactive Behavior

1. General Information

a. Definition: elation is a seemingly pleasurable affect that is characterized by an air of happiness and self-confidence as well as extreme motor activity

b. Precipitating factors

- **1)** results from a real or threatened loss of self-esteem
- **2)** massive denial of depression
- **3)** may develop from early childhood
  - **a)** child first begins to be independent of mother
  - **b)** mother is threatened by this; responds as if this independence is bad
  - **c)** child fears loss of mother's love
  - **d)** child attempts to meet expectations for compliance

c. Types

- **1)** *mild*: euphoric state of mind, mild exhilaration
  - **a)** happy, unconcerned, uninhibited, expansive, "life-of-the-party" mood
  - **b)** mood can change rapidly to irritability and anger; irritability is expression of anxiety and hostile impulses
  - **c)** very active, but activity is sometimes inappropriate for age and place
  - **d)** relationships are superficial
  - **e)** *DSM-III*-R classification: hypomanic episode
- **2)** *acute*: moderate degree of mania called hypomania
  - **a)** extreme emotional lability ranging from wild euphoria to fury; readily provoked by harmless remarks, seems to forgive and forget
  - **b)** thought disorders: flight of ideas, delusions of grandeur, short attention span, pressure of speech
  - **c)** little sleep, fatigue, very uninhibited, possibly sexually indiscreet
  - **d)** psychomotor activity is extremely exaggerated
  - **e)** often requires hospitalization
  - **f)** *DSM-III*-R classification: manic episode, moderate or severe without psychotic features

3) *delirium* or *delirious mania*: maximum intensity of reaction
   a) disorganized, seriously delusional
   b) disoriented, incoherent, agitated
   c) prone to self-injury, burn-out, and dehydration
   d) immediate intervention is necessary to meet physical needs
   e) *DSM-III*-R classification: manic episode, severe with psychotic features
4) may *alternate* between *manic and depressive phases*
   a) usually hospitalized first for manic episode
   b) may have rapid cycling (manic and depressive) phases succeed each other without a period of remission; *DSM-III*-R classification: bipolar disorder, manic
   c) may have numerous hypomanic and mild depressive episodes; *DSM-III*-R classification: cyclothymia

d. Prognosis: good, even without treatment, provided that the person does not suffer from complete physical exhaustion in manic phase or commit suicide in depressed phase

2. Nursing Process

a. Assessment/Analysis

1) physical needs
   a) nutrition: decreased appetite or unwillingness to stop activity to eat may lead to weight loss
   b) hydration
   c) sleep/rest: activity pattern and insomnia may lead to exhaustion
   d) elimination: may be incontinent; constipation
   e) may ignore injuries or symptoms of physical illness
   f) hygiene and grooming: inappropriate dress, excessive makeup; diaphoresis
2) affect
   a) degree of euphoria
   b) lability: rapid mood change from happy to sad without apparent provocation
   c) anger
   d) anxiety
3) cognition
   a) feelings of worthlessness, loneliness are masked by elation
   b) flight of ideas
   c) delusions of grandeur and/or persecution
   d) inadequacy, low self-esteem
   e) short attention span
4) behavior
   a) degree and appropriateness of activity
   b) aggression, manipulation, acting out
   c) demanding, verbally hostile
   d) pressured speech (loquaciousness)
   e) impulsivity
   f) decreased inhibitions leading to profanity, sexually indiscreet acts
   g) pseudoindependence (false independence and confidence)
   h) superficial relationships

b. Plans, Implementation, and Evaluation

Goal 1: Client will meet physical needs independently.

Plan/Implementation

Food and Fluid Intake

- Nutrition: provide high-calorie finger foods that can be eaten on the run; note amount of food ingested; monitor weight.
- Hydration: provide fluids at frequent intervals; fluid intake of 2,000 ml/day.

Sleep/Rest

- Provide medication to induce sleep and rest; provide opportunities for frequent short naps.
- Reduce stimuli in environment to help calm client; use soft lighting, low noise level, simple room decorations; quiet room if necessary.

Elimination

- Monitor elimination, maintain fluid intake, establish toileting schedule if necessary.

Hygiene and Grooming

- Provide flexible schedule for showering and changing clothing; provide loose, comfortable clothing; limit access to clothing if necessary to maintain appropriate dress or decrease frequency of changes; assist with hygiene.

Safety

- Watch for physical symptoms.

Medications

- Administer lithium and other medications as ordered (see Table 2.8); observe for side and/or toxic effects; teach client and family about lithium therapy.

Evaluation: Client receives adequate sleep and rest; ingests appropriate amounts of food and fluids; maintains hygiene and grooming; remains free from injury and verbalizes knowledge of medication regimen.

Goal 2: Client will cope adaptively with hostility and aggression.

Plan/Implementation
- Assist client to understand purpose that hostility and aggression serve.
- Ignore or respond minimally to hostile behavior which is not destructive to avoid positive reinforcement.
- Do not react defensively to criticism or profanity client directs to you or other staff.
- Set limits on behavior; "I cannot allow you to hurt people. You'll have to go to the quiet room for half an hour." Be consistent in expectations and limits; collaborate with other staff members to set, enforce and evaluate limits; enforce limits in clear, firm manner.
- After hostile or aggressive episode, discuss feelings before, during, and after the episode. Explore effect of client's behavior on self and others; explore alternative behavior.
- Reduce stimuli; use solitary time for hygiene, laundry, etc.
- Develop behavioral contract.
- Do not hurry manic clients; hurrying them will result in more anger and hostility.
- Utilize measures to prevent overt aggression, e.g., distraction, reduction of environmental stimuli; avoid competitive games; use large motor skill activities that are not highly structured or confining (e.g., walks, exercise, dance, painting).
- Utilizing quiet persuasion is most effective.

Evaluation: Client discusses feelings related to hostility and aggression; engages in appropriate physical activities to relieve tension.

Goal 3: Client will demonstrate realistic independence; will develop ability to problem solve, make requests appropriately, and negotiate.

Plan/Implementation
- Do not discuss grandiose ideas/plans.
- Assess client's abilities realistically.
- Give help only when client is incapable.
- Discuss capabilities calmly with client; reinforce client's self-esteem; convey expectation that client can function independently.
- Involve client in planning ADL.
- Inform client that staff will not comply with unreasonable demands while conveying acceptance of client.
- Give client feedback about effects of dependency and demands: "I become annoyed when you repeatedly ask me to do things for you that we decided you would do."
- Assist client to identify feelings, needs, means of seeking gratification.
- Assist client in developing decision-making skills; explore possible consequences of decisions/behavior.
- Assist to develop alternate behavior; teach client to use assertion, problem solving, negotiation.

Evaluation: Client makes decisions and takes actions independently; makes requests in a quiet voice, and sets limits on own demanding behavior.

Goal 4: Client will recognize and set limits on own manipulative, acting-out behaviors and impulsivity.

Plan/Implementation
- Avoid impatience and anger if client is manipulative or acts out.
- Inform client of behaviors expected in short, clear sentences.
- Set firm, definite limits on client's behavior; consistently enforce limits.
- Teach client that it is the manipulative behavior that is being rejected, not client.
- Avoid arguments or displaying disapproval of vulgarity, profanity, or overt sexual behavior resulting from extreme euphoria.
- Remove client from public places when this behavior could embarrass client or family.
- Protect other clients from sexual overtures.
- Use chemical or physical restraints as necessary to prevent leaving hospital or injuring self or others.

Evaluation: Client displays manipulative, acting-out behaviors and impulsivity less frequently than on admission.

Goal 5: Family will recognize indications that client needs treatment.

Plan/Implementation
- Discuss expectations of family and client.
- Explore need for and ways of setting limits.
- Teach family criteria for seeking treatment
  - noncompliance with lithium regimen
  - anorexia, weight loss, insomnia
  - hyperactivity, excessive spending
  - increased use of alcohol
  - delusions of grandeur or persecution
  - sexual impulsivity
  - aggressive, demanding, acting-out behavior
  - rapid mood changes

Evaluation: Family lists indications of need for treatment.

References

[†]Brenners, D., Harris, B., & Weston, P. (1987). Managing manic behavior. *American Journal of Nursing*, *87*, 620–623.

Campbell, L. (1986). Depression: Acute care in the hospital. *American Journal of Nursing*, *86*, 288–291.

Crockett, M. (1986). Depression: A case of anger and alienation. *American Journal of Nursing*, *86*, 294–298.

Valente, S. (1985). The suicidal teenager. *Nursing85*, *15*(12), 47–49.

Wilson, J. (1987). Unmasking depression. *Nursing Life*, *7*(6), 57–64.

[†]Highly recommended.

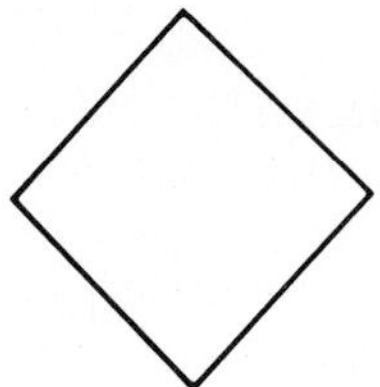

Socially Maladaptive Behavior

General Concepts

Overview: Socially maladaptive or acting-out behavior includes a great many different problem behaviors and conditions. All human beings live within a social system and each social system has values and rules by which to live with other human beings. When an individual copes with tension and anxiety by acting out against the social system's values and rules, society considers the individual to be socially maladapted.

Societies utilize many different ways to deal with socially maladaptive/acting-out behavior. Courts, jails, and prisons may be used if laws are broken. Psychotherapy may be used; it facilitates the reentry into society of such persons and helps them to change maladaptive behaviors to adaptive, healthy behaviors.

A society will provide social structure, which minimizes stress, social disorder, and upheaval through promotion of a healthy environment and through the provision of services essential to physical and mental health. These services include health care, schools, religious institutions, the justice system, recreational facilities, and welfare services.

When the structure and expectations of society are stable forces, the family and individual will decrease acting-out behavior. Social unrest, economic stress, health care inequities, moral decay, or dysfunctional families may precipitate or perpetuate stress and anger.

Application of the Nursing Process to the Client Exhibiting Socially Maladaptive Behavior

1. **Assessment**
   - **a.** Immediate events that precipitated socially maladaptive/acting-out behavior: characteristics and frequency
   - **b.** Physiologic changes that accompany angry feelings
   - **c.** Coping behavior that client uses to handle stress and anger: adaptive and maladaptive
   - **d.** Defense mechanisms used to cope with angry feelings
   - **e.** *DSM-III*-R classifications: antisocial or borderline personality disorders; conduct disorder; intermittent explosive disorder; passive–aggressive personality disorder
2. **Analysis**
   - **a.** Safe, effective care environment
     - **1)** potential for violence: self-directed or directed at others
     - **2)** potential for injury
   - **b.** Psychological integrity
     - **1)** ineffective individual coping
     - **2)** self esteem disturbance, personal identity disturbance
     - **3)** impaired social interaction
     - **4)** rape trauma syndrome
     - **5)** altered patterns of sexuality
   - **c.** Health promotion/maintenance
     - **1)** noncompliance
     - **2)** ineffective, disabling family coping
     - **3)** altered family processes
3. **General Nursing Plan, Implementation, and Evaluation**

Goal: The socially maladaptive client will decrease unacceptable behavior; will utilize assertive behaviors as a means of expressing independence and control.

Plan/Implementation

- Provide structure and set limits on behavior that is physically destructive to others or the environment.
- Consistently enforce limits (inconsistent limit setting increases the client's belief that manipulative behavior is productive).
- Be aware of own nonverbal messages to client; avoid acting defensively or aggressively.
- Stress to staff the importance of not chastising client or rejecting client's efforts to cope by using aggressive behavior.
- Teach client the difference between assertiveness (asking for what one wants, standing up for rights) and aggression (getting what one wants at the expense of others).

- Recognize and point out manipulative behaviors in a nonjudgmental way; do not allow client to manipulate staff or other clients; discuss effect of manipulation on relationships.
- Reinforce positive (assertive) approaches ("I would like . . ." versus "Do this . . .").
- Discuss consequences of impulsive actions; help client develop problem-solving skills.
- Increase self-esteem by supporting strengths.
- Teach stress-reduction techniques (e.g., imagery, relaxation).
- Praise efforts of family/significant others as they attempt to assist the client in coping.

Evaluation: Client reduces frequency of unacceptable behavior; can describe the difference between assertion and aggression; can demonstrate at least one assertive behavior; uses positive coping mechanisms to handle stress (e.g., relaxation).

Selected Health Problems

☐ Violence in the Family

1. General Information

a. Definitions
  1) violence is the expression of the aggressive drive, normally present, in a destructive manner
  2) a learned behavior, learned either through exposure and imitation or indirectly when an individual is unable to channel aggressive impulses constructively.

b. Some violent persons feel guilty about their behavior, and others do not. Behaving violently, either with or without feeling guilty, can cause a mental health problem for the person or those dependent upon him.

c. Victims of abuse generally are persons who are dependent on others for their physical, financial, and emotional care; their abuser is often their caretaker. Victims can include
  1) children
  2) spouses
  3) elderly parents or other adults
  4) children or adults in long-term care settings

d. Characteristics of abuse (violence) in the family
  1) victims have little capacity to defend themselves; may be weaker or younger (child, weak woman or man)
  2) the abuser is physically stronger than the abused
  3) the dynamics of abuse need to be viewed in terms of the following aspects
    a) intrapersonal: internal psychodynamics of those involved
    b) interpersonal: socializing framework of beliefs and values and interaction of individual with others
    c) sociocultural: power structure and belief system of the family or institution
  4) the victims of abuse (child or adult) often believe that they have done something to warrant the abuse; they have low self-esteem; they may feel a need for punishment
  5) abused adults (e.g., battered women) often believe they could not survive outside the home setting without the abusing person and thus are emotionally, if not physically, trapped
  6) abused persons fear the consequences of telling someone outside the family of their treatment; they also feel ashamed and for that reason may not tell health care personnel
  7) abused persons often include the elderly who are physically, financially, and emotionally dependent on family or other adults

e. Multidisciplinary treatment
  1) case finding: health care personnel are often the ones who have the opportunity to assess children and adults for possible abuse, especially when they are seen for injuries
    a) be alert for abuse cases, especially in emergency rooms, pediatrics, ambulatory clinics
    b) carefully document bruises, cuts, etc., size, and location; also document interaction patterns of client and significant other; these become evidence
    c) all suspected child abuse cases must be reported and will be investigated by the state child welfare agency; in some states elder abuse is also reportable
    d) medical personnel cannot be charged with defamation of character if they report an abuse that does not check out as such
    e) assess both the abuser and abused; documentation of behaviors, symptoms, is important for legal aspects

- **f)** help both to receive emotional treatment if they are willing
- **2)** community services: numerous branches of the health care system respond to client abuse situations
  - **a)** treatment and intervention by child welfare agencies may include alternative living situations for the abused
  - **b)** various community agencies provide classes on parenting, dealing with older parents, problem-solving skills, and appropriate expression of emotion, e.g., Parents Anonymous (a self-help group for actual or potential child abusers)

2. Nursing Process

a. Assessment/Analysis

- **1)** the victim: assess for
  - **a)** presence of injuries that do not fit the description of the accident
  - **b)** evidence of multiple bruises, chipped front teeth, or burns, particularly of the type inflicted by a cigarette
  - **c)** x-ray reports that indicate old healed fractures
  - **d)** retarded growth and/or development of the child with no history of pathologic conditions (e.g., walks late, cannot feed self, underweight)
  - **e)** child's clothing inappropriate in relation to weather conditions
  - **f)** evidence of poor hygiene
  - **g)** no immunization appropriate to the child's age
  - **h)** child wary of adults or caretaker from the referring facility
  - **i)** child adapts to hospital unit quickly
  - **j)** child does not seek out parents for comfort or affection
  - **k)** child does not cry when parents leave
  - **l)** grabbing behavior/lap hunger exhibited by the young child
  - **m)** child shows provocative behavior that generates anger in others
  - **n)** delinquent or runaway behavior; teenage pregnancy
  - **o)** adult victim reluctant to talk about injuries, particularly if spouse, parent, adult child, or caretaker from the referring facility is present
- **2)** the abuser: assess for
  - **a)** denial of abuse; an abuser may or may not see self as such
  - **b)** history of child abuse in family; abusive parents themselves were often abused as children and have learned that pattern of expressing anger
  - **c)** perception of victim; abusers may view the victim as "bad," as someone who tries to make them angry and does things on purpose to irritate or upset them; they view the victim this way regardless of developmental or social inabilities of the victim (e.g., a one-year-old child is viewed as breaking something on purpose to upset them)
  - **d)** knowledge of normal growth and development; abusers often have unrealistic expectations for child's age
  - **e)** guilt or remorse may be absent or abuser may feel guilt or remorse but be unable to stop; abusers who cannot stop—without remorse—include alcoholic or drug abusers as well as other persons
  - **f)** evidence of dysfunctional attachment process in new parent; withdrawal from the child; expresses fears that he will hurt the child
  - **g)** extreme overprotectiveness
  - **h)** defensiveness about behavior with child
  - **i)** evidence of psychosis
  - **j)** alcohol and/or drug abuse
  - **k)** low self-esteem; low self-acceptance
  - **l)** hostility, depression
  - **m)** hypochondriacal complaints
  - **n)** impulsiveness in decision making
  - **o)** seductive behavior toward child
  - **p)** explains need for physical punishment due to "badness" in victim
- **3)** family or caretaker dynamics: assess for
  - **a)** behavior expected of abused child is not appropriate to child's age
  - **b)** describes abused child as "difficult" or "hateful"
  - **c)** ascribes a special, negatively perceived characteristic to the abused person
  - **d)** lack of knowledge of normal growth and development, including the aging process
  - **e)** divorce, separation, abandonment, death of spouse
  - **f)** financial, housing, or personal crisis; severe stress
  - **g)** behavior toward crying/injured child is aloof, not comforting or affectionate

i) family refuses to allow diagnostic procedures
j) parents withdraw from hospitalized child
k) parents or caretaker complains of difficulty in coping with the abused person and/or own life
l) impaired communications, low self-image
m) evidence of misuse of defense mechanisms, e.g., projection, scapegoating, denial
n) emotionally cut off from families of origin
o) parents or caretaker gives history of being physically abused as child
p) family or caretaker has been experiencing chronic sustained anxiety or recent loss

b. Plans, Implementation, and Evaluation

Goal 1: The abuser will discuss feelings and needs related to violence openly and honestly with nurse.

Plan/Implementation
- Acknowledge own feelings about abuser and abused; recognize the needs of both (nurse may feel angry with abuser and sympathetic with victim); be aware of impact of own feelings on client care.
- Treat abuser with respect; know that the abuser may not view own actions as abusive, may be unable to stop the behavior, or may have low self-esteem and need assistance in developing positive self-regard.
- Assist abuser or caretakers to recognize importance of meeting own needs for affection, belonging, and self-esteem.
- Discuss appropriate ways to express and meet need.
- Discuss expectations for need fulfillment by those in abuser's care.
- Explore expectations related to meeting abuser's needs and needs of those in abuser's care.
- Assist client to identify events that trigger anger and violence.
- Teach stress-reduction skills.

Evaluation: Abuser begins to talk about feelings, anxieties, and frustrations rather than acting out violently.

Goal 2: Victim will manage psychological and physical trauma related to violence.

Plan/Implementation
- Encourage expression of feelings in both adult and child victims; provide child with drawing materials and dolls to act out feelings.
- Discuss adult victim's strengths, coping abilities, ability to function independently.
- Attend to physical needs caused by specific trauma (e.g., burns, fractures).
- Provide physical and emotional comfort (e.g., analgesics, therapeutic use of touch: stroking, holding).
- Refer to in-hospital support services and community services (e.g., mental health center, crisis intervention hot-line, individual and group counseling).
- Discuss use of support services if violence reoccurs.
- If unsafe to return home, contact social service or child/adult protective services for placement.

Evaluation: Victim expresses feelings; has physical needs met; identifies available support services; verbalizes plan of escape if violence reoccurs.

Goal 3: Abuser will learn ways to relate to victim without the use of violent behavior.

Plan/Implementation
- Practice open, direct communication that does not attack listener.
- Assist abuser to acknowledge emotional problems when they occur, explore childhood experiences with violence (some were abused as children, thus need to learn new ways of handling conflicts).
- Explore alternative ways of expressing anger (e.g., physical activities, discussion, relaxation).
- Teach effective problem-solving skills.
- Teach parents normal growth and development and realistic expectations of children at various ages; discuss appropriate methods of limit-setting and discipline as opposed to physical use of force.
- Reinforce positive parenting strategies.
- Assist in incorporating older parent into family home and life-style while maintaining independence for all family members.
- Identify resources in community to assist family in managing situation: day/home care agencies to provide partial relief from total care for elderly, Parents Anonymous to help discuss

feelings and problems and share solutions, mental health center for counseling.

Evaluation: Abuser identifies appropriate alternatives to handle feelings, seeks referral for counseling; attends peer support groups.

☐ Hostile and Aggressive Behavior

1. General information

a. Definitions

1) aggression: forceful goal-directed action that may be verbal or physical; the motor counterpart of the affect of rage, anger, and hostility

- **a)** defensive response to anxiety and loss of self-esteem and power
- **b)** constructive when it is problem-solving and appropriate as a defense against realistic attack
- **c)** can become healthy when channeled into appropriate expression, e.g., assertiveness
- **d)** pathological when it is unrealistic, self-destructive, not problem-solving, and is the outcome of unresolved emotional conflict
- **e)** unhealthy when out of person's control and results in physical or emotional harm to others.

2) *passive-aggressive behavior*: resistance to demands for adequate performance in both occupational and social functioning are met by timidity, sullenness, stubbornness, forgetfulness, and obstruction

- **a)** if the behavior is characteristic of the person, it may be considered a personality disorder (*DSM-III*-R classification)
- **b)** the person is acting out anger in very indirect ways, e.g., always late, forgetting to do things that are important to another person
- **c)** the anger of the other person provides the passive-aggressive person with attention and release for anger

b. Dynamics

1) behavior is a response to a perceived threat

2) feelings of anxiety occur, accompanied by helplessness

3) judgment and reasoning decrease as anxiety increases

4) verbal or physical aggression occurs as an attempt to alleviate anxiety

2. Nursing Process

a. Assessment/Analysis

1) refer to assessment page 37

2) aggressive behaviors

- **a)** increase in motor agitation
- **b)** verbal threats/abusive language
- **c)** tense and angry affect
- **d)** demanding
- **e)** self-directed anger
- **f)** manipulative
- **g)** noncompliant

3) level of control

- **a)** ability to listen and follow directions
- **b)** ability to identify source of anger and verbalize feelings appropriately
- **c)** ability to explore alternative ways of expressing anger

4) nurse's perception of impending violence

b. Plans, Implementation, and Evaluation

Goal 1: Client will increase control and decrease aggressive behavior.

Plan/Implementation

- Refer to General Nursing Plan page 37.
- Encourage verbal identification of source of angry feelings.
- Explore alternative ways of dealing with anger.
- Avoid power struggles
  - allow flexibility in decision-making as long as it is within safe parameters
  - if decision poses risks to self, other patients, or staff, explain why you cannot go along with it and do not give in.
  - set limits on disruptive behavior; apply limits consistently.
- At signs of increased loss of control
  - reduce stimuli; remove objects or persons that agitate client; move client to area with few people and minimal noise, light, activity, etc.
  - explain what is happening, tell client that s/he will be safe, and ask whether s/he has any questions; express an attitude of calm and helpfulness
  - if client expresses fear of hurting self or others, initiate steps to avert it; remove weapons or objects that could be used destructively
  - explain to client that the behavior can be controlled externally if s/he cannot regain self-control
  - offer medication, explaining that s/he is unable to control the behavior voluntarily

and if s/he refuses to take the medication, s/he will be restrained

Evaluation: Client decreases aggressive behavior, calms self, begins to verbalize feelings.

Goal 2: Client will be safely restrained to restore control and prevent injury to self and others.

Plan/Implementation

- Be aware of state laws governing use of restraints and care of client in restraints.
- Follow agency's policy and procedure in the application of and subsequent care and documentation of care of client in restraints.
  - have sufficient number of staff members available to apply restraints
  - give range-of-motion exercises for each extremity and check for full circulation at periodic intervals
  - remove each restraint at specified intervals
  - monitor client in restraints continually and document behavior and care at regular intervals
  - never leave client in restraints alone
- Remove physical restraints when medication takes effect.
- Explain use of restraints to any other clients who observed episode; encourage discussion of fears of loss of control and availability of help.
- Explain that restraints were used to help client regain control and prevent injury to self and others.

Evaluation: Client is free of restraint-related injury; staff applies restraints uneventfully.

☐ Sexual Acting Out

1. General Information

a. Definitions

1) includes sex acts with partners who are legally unable to consent, such as children (pedophilia), with persons who choose not to consent, sex acts accompanied by force or violence (rape), and invasion of other people's privacy without their knowledge (e.g., voyeurism)

2) voyeurism: the person repeatedly observes other people's naked bodies without their knowledge or consent in order to obtain sexual gratification

3) exhibitionism: a person exposes sexual organs when it is socially inappropriate

4) sadomasochism: obtaining sexual pleasure from having pain inflicted upon oneself or others; may be part of a rape incident or may also be part of other sexual encounter

5) rape: legal definitions of rape vary from state to state, but most include sexual intercourse without the consent of the other person; statutory rape is the seduction of a minor, even though the minor consented

b. Profile of a rapist

1) rape is an aggressive sexual act and a crime of violence and power

2) rapists act for the purpose of venting anger and hostility and exercising control and power

3) many rapes are planned

4) the majority of rapists are male, and in the case of child victims, usually someone the child knows; acquaintance rape is also a possibility with an adult victim

c. Responses to rape

1) Victim can be any age; majority are female but men can be victimized (usually by other men)

2) because of shame and embarrassment, most crimes are not reported

3) common reactions of the victim are shame, guilt, embarrassment, self-blame, anger; fears of injury, mutilation, sexually-transmitted diseases and pregnancy; fear of how significant others will react to incident

4) the victim's response varies from expressing feelings through talking or behavioral manifestations (e.g., crying, trembling, agitation)

5) the significant other's reactions to the rape are similar to the victim's and also vary (e.g., anger, support, isolation)

6) the psychological effect of rape may be long-lasting affecting interpersonal relationships with significant others, impairing sexual functioning, and creating feelings of helplessness, anxiety, and depression

7) self-awareness of one's own reaction to rape is imperative to deal therapeutically with the victim and significant others

2. Nursing Process

a. Assessment/Analysis

1) victim's perception of incident

2) victim's coping ability

3) anxiety level

4) signs of physical trauma (e.g., bruises, scratches)

5) availability of significant others, support network

6) impact of rape incident on significant others
7) victim's immediate concerns (e.g., emotional control, legal information or assistance, physical care, pregnancy or venereal disease protection/information)

b. Plans/Implementation and Evaluation

Goal 1: Victim will return to pre-rape level of functioning; immediate physical and psychological needs met by staff.

Plan/Implementation

- Provide a private location for interview, examination, and crisis intervention.
- Document client's perception of incident, physical trauma, psychological status, coping ability, and physical assessment findings; assist in collection of physical evidence.
- Use empathetic, nonjudgmental approach; do not give advice; be sensitive to victim's feelings while gathering information and physical evidence; avoid asking for unnecessary repetition of events by client.
- Encourage verbalization of rape; incident; if client is unable to talk about incident, acknowledge difficulty and traumatizing experience; allow immediate use of denial; explain that anger, sadness may occur later.
- Encourage client to ventilate present feelings about incident; do not dwell on actual sexual act unless client needs to discuss this; allow expression of anger (may be directed at staff).
- Help client assess present coping ability.
- Explain common behavior and feeling responses that may occur.
- Encourage client to actively problem-solve, prioritize concerns, and make decisions (e.g., who to tell, legal recourse, physical care, pregnancy prevention).
- Explore feelings of guilt or self-blame; reinforce responsibility of rapist, not of victim, for the act; inform client that whatever s/he did (either fighting or submitting) were necessary for self-protection.
- If victim is child
  - use drawing, play to assist child to ventilate feelings
  - use calm approach, be aware of own nonverbal communications that may convey anger to child
  - reinforce that child has done nothing wrong and will not be punished
  - explain all procedures thoroughly
- Give victim/significant others information about community resources (e.g., rape trauma group, legal aid, rape crisis center, counseling)
- Refer for follow-up to crisis counseling, marital and sexual functioning counseling.

Evaluation: Victim verbalizes need for intervention, complies with intervention, and verbalizes willingness to seek referral.

Goal 2: Significant others will verbalize feelings and give victim support.

Plan/Implementation

- Assess significant other's reaction (self-blame or victim-blame are common) and present coping ability.
- Reinforce rapist's responsibility for act and necessity of victim's actions for self-preservation.
- Provide teaching about typical reaction of victim and significant others to rape trauma (increased anxiety and fear within 48 hours followed by adjustment; reappearance of anxiety later).
- Explain how significant other can be supportive to victim
  - encourage victim to ventilate but do not force discussion of rape
  - assist victim to resume daily activities
  - support victim's decision for follow-up care, litigation, etc.
  - do not withold emotional and physical comfort, (e.g., touching, holding, stroking)
  - avoid overprotection or isolation
  - provide safety/protection measures victim needs to feel safe (e.g., new locks, escort at night)
- Talk with family away from victim; encourage verbalization of anger to nurse rather than to victim
- If victim is child
  - help parents recognize that victim is still child and has age-related needs for physical comfort and reassurance and protection
  - help family plan ways to return to usual family activities as soon as possible.
- Provide referral to community resources for additional support and assistance

Evaluation: Significant others discuss traumatic experience and give support to victim.

☐ Antisocial Behavior

1. General Information

a. Definition: disorder manifested by persistent pattern of consistent violation of the rights of others; pattern of life-long maladaptive behaviors.

b. *DSM-III*-R classification: personality disorder
c. Characteristics
   1) easily frustrated
   2) persistent pattern of self-defeat and failure to follow any life plan
   3) absence of anxiety
   4) reluctance to accept rules and regulations
   5) poor judgment and failure to learn by experience
   6) poor interpersonal relations
   7) minimal insight and poor impulse control
   8) absence of guilt
   9) suspiciousness, emotional lability, rigidity
   10) inability to feel or express emotion
   11) poor concentration and motivation
   12) behaviors differ from psychotics in that these clients do not exhibit ego disintegration, impaired thought processes, or poor reality testing
   13) behaviors differ from neurotics in that these clients do not have fixed and exaggerated psychological defenses
   14) behaviors differ from borderline personality disorders in that these clients do not exhibit unpredictability, self-destructiveness self-mutilation, or identity confusion
d. Treatment: apply external controls to limit the acting-out behavior
   1) these behavior patterns are difficult to change; respond poorly to treatment
   2) long-term psychotherapy is of some success, but relatively few clients remain in psychotherapy because of expense, time involved, poor motivation, and lack of insight
   3) self-help groups have had some success

2. Nursing Process

a. Assessment/Analysis

1) characteristics of personality disorders
2) behavior: manipulation, impulsiveness, narcissism, seductiveness, demanding, histrionics, acting out, violence

b. Plans, Implementation, and Evaluation

Goal 1: Client will interact with peers and staff within socially accepted norms; will follow treatment program.

Plan/Implementation

- Refer to General Nursing Plan, page 62
- Set firm and consistent limits to be consistently applied by all staff.
- Call staff conferences to discuss behavior and plans for setting limits and dealing with behavior; write limits on care plans so all staff can follow intervention.
- Communicate verbally and give written information to client on units rules and routines; explain consequences if expectations are violated; avoid lengthy or complex discussions of rules or limits.
- Be aware of manipulative behavior: setting up staff, playing one staff member against the other, using other clients.
- Do not make agreements with client without checking all other staff members about what has been told to the client.
- Confront client in a matter-of-fact way when behavior is not acceptable (e.g., manipulating).
- Encourage development of positive goals for change.
- Give positive feedback when client is conforming to socially accepted norms.
- Explore social relationships and problem areas; role-play social situations; use group therapy to point out problem behaviors.

Evaluation: Client increasingly complies with rules of the treatment program; interacts acceptably with others.

References

Campbell, J., & Humphries, J. (1984). *Nursing care of victims of family violence*. Reston, VA: Reston.

[†]Curry, L., Colvin, L., & Lancaster, J. (1988). Breaking the cycle of family abuse. *American Journal of Nursing, 88*, 1188–1190.

Fontaine, K., (1987). Violence. In J. Cook & K. Fontaine (Eds.), *Essentials of mental health nursing*. Menlo Park, CA: Addison-Wesley.

Leach, A.N. (1987). Rape. In J. Haber, P. Hoskins, A. Leach, B. Sideleau (Eds.), *Comprehensive psychiatric nursing* (3rd ed.). New York: McGraw-Hill.

[†]Morton, P. (1986). Managing assault. *American Journal of Nursing, 86*, 1114–1116.

Neal, M., Cohen, P., & Reighley, J. (1983). *Nursing care planning guides, set 4* (2nd ed.). Baltimore: Williams & Wilkins.

[†]Palmer, M. & Deck, E. (1987). Teaching your patients to assert their rights. *American Journal of Nursing, 87*, 650–654.

Sennhauser S. (1987). Personality Disorders. In J. Cook & K. Fontaine (Eds.), *Essentials of mental health nursing*. Menlo Park, CA: Addison-Wesley.

Sidelau, B. (1987). Patterns of Abuse. In J. Haber, P. Hoskins, A. Leach, B. Sidelau (Eds.), *Comprehensive psychiatric nursing* (3rd ed.). New York: McGraw-Hill.

[†]Highly recommended.

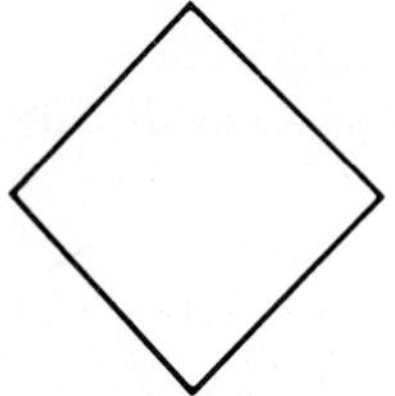

Suspicious Behavior

General Concepts

Overview: Suspicious behavior occurs when a person is hypersensitive to, and preoccupied with, the behavior and motivations of others. In mild forms, such behavior may include taking normal protective precautions to avoid becoming the victim of a truly dangerous person. In severe forms, such behavior results from abnormal and unwarranted distrust of others and results in extreme, unwarranted, and inappropriate efforts to protect self.

Suspicious behavior may be part of an organic mental disorder or schizophrenic disorder, may be the predominant problem as in paranoid disorders or paranoid personality disorders of a nonpsychotic type, or may occur with substance abuse.

Application of the Nursing Process to the Client Exhibiting Suspicious Behavior

All adults have some level of sensitivity and preoccupation with the behavior and motivation of others. When this behavior becomes exaggerated, it is paranoia, the selected health problem discussed below.

Selected Health Problems

☐ Paranoia

1. General Information

- **a.** Definition: behavior characterized by hostility and mistrust of others resulting from grandiose and/or persecutory delusions
- **b.** Types
  - **1)** paranoia: an insidious development with permanent well-organized, well-defined, unshakable delusional system that is contradicted by social reality; chronic; seen less frequently than paranoid schizophrenia
  - **2)** acute paranoid disorder: this is the sudden onset in individuals who have experienced drastic environmental changes (e.g., immigrants, boot camp POWs); rarely becomes chronic
- **c.** Characteristics
  - **1)** suspiciousness
  - **2)** grandiose, persecutory, jealous, or erotic delusions
  - **3)** usually no hallucinations
  - **4)** haughty, superior manner
  - **5)** constant vigilance
  - **6)** tendency toward hostility, anger, and aggression; projected outward
  - **7)** usually no impairment of intellectual or occupational functioning; distrust may be in only one area of life, with others relatively untouched
  - **8)** often severe impairment of social and marital functioning with progressive estrangement from others as client "gathers evidence" to support delusion
  - **9)** duration of at least one week
  - **10)** rarely seek help themselves; client sees nothing unusual about delusions; brought in by associates or relatives for help
  - **11)** client tends to stimulate avoidance and dislike in others
- **d.** Dynamics
  - **1)** lack of trust
  - **2)** low self-esteem
  - **3)** increased anxiety level
  - **4)** denial
  - **5)** projection resulting in delusions
  - **6)** decreased repression
  - **7)** poor reality testing in area related to delusions
- **e.** *DSM-III*-R classification: paranoid disorder

2. Nursing Process

- **a. Assessment**
  - **1)** duration: at least 1 week; chronic if over 6 months; acute if less than 6 months
  - **2)** delusions
  - **3)** anxiety level
  - **4)** problem behavior
    - **a)** superiority

b) expression of hostility, anger, or aggression
c) social and/or marital impairment
5) self-esteem

b. **Analysis**

1) safe, effective care environment
   a) potential for violence: self-directed or directed at others
   b) knowledge deficit
   c) sensory-perceptual alteration (specify)
2) physiological integrity
   a) altered nutrition: less than body requirements
   b) sleep pattern disturbance
3) psychological integrity
   a) anxiety
   b) social isolation
   c) altered thought processes
4) health promotion/maintenance
   a) noncompliance
   b) self care deficit (specify)
   c) diversional activity deficit

c. **Plans/Implementation and Evaluation**

Goal 1: Client will develop a trusting relationship with a staff member.

Plan/Implementation

- Establish regular times and places for meetings; keep appointments or notify in advance of cancellation.
- Be honest, accurate, and matter of fact in communication.
- Make mutual expectations and promises clear and abide by them.
- Be accepting and nonjudgmental.

Evaluation: Client develops a trusting relationship with a staff member as evidenced by a willingness to cooperate with and confide in staff member.

Goal 2: Client will learn to define and test reality regarding the delusional system.

Plan/Implementation

- Help client to recognize delusions as signs of anxiety and poor self-esteem.
- Do not argue about content of delusions, but focus on reality (arguing results in client defending the delusions).
- Limit discussion of delusions.
- Acknowledge client's feelings and beliefs, but point out that these are not shared; appear quizzical and express some doubt about delusions.
- Be honest and reliable.
- Focus on the here and now.

Evaluation: Client gives up delusion; verbally expresses feelings of anxiety.

Goal 3: Client will demonstrate improved self-esteem.

Plan/Implementation

- Identify strengths: encourage client to focus on them.
- Assist client in developing a relationship with another client.
- Assist client in gradually developing relationships within groups.
- Assist client in gaining insight into underlying dynamics of behavior.
- Intervene with problem behavior (e.g., superiority, hostility and anger, aggression; refer to those behaviors in *Socially Maladaptive Behavior*).

Evaluation: Client is able to begin an appropriate relationship with other clients and groups; controls problem behavior.

Goal 4: Client will improve social and marital functioning.

Plan/Implementation

- Encourage client to discontinue behavior that disrupts social and marital relationships (e.g., spying, accusations, letter writing, threats).
- Identify feelings that lead to problem behavior.
- Encourage client to express anxiety, tension, anger, and fears verbally.
- Find constructive outlets for the feelings (e.g., relaxation techniques, physical exercise, public service); avoid overly aggressive, competitive activities.
- Help client to establish or reestablish trusting, supporting relationship with family members (e.g., promote open, direct communication and involvement in mutually agreed-upon activities).
- Assist family to explore their feelings about client's behavior; provide information about client's status; help family to examine ways to respond to client.

Evaluation: Client improves social and marital relationships; communicates feelings, needs, and wants to family; family members state they feel comfortable around client.

References

Stuart, G., & Sundeen, S. (1986). *Principles and practices of psychiatric nursing* (3rd ed.). St. Louis: Mosby.

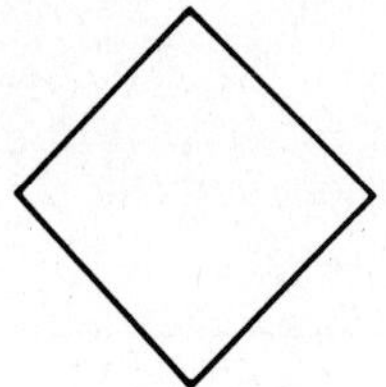

Withdrawn Behavior

General Concepts

Overview

1. Definition: an individual responds to stress by retreating from interactions with people and environment. In extreme situations, the person withdraws from reality.
2. Behavioral continuum
   - **a.** Healthy; temporary pulling back from a stressful situation and focusing psychic energy internally
     - **1)** to remove self from stressful situations, to think, and to take a temporary retreat is a healthy and sometimes necessary response
     - **2)** the individual who plunges forward without thinking can cause undue pain to self and others; each person needs solitary time to think, to plan, to reflect, and to regroup before acting
   - **b.** Unhealthy: isolating oneself from others and the world to the extent that relationships and the ability to function in society are seriously impaired
     - **1)** may retreat to avoid facing important social situations; social skills are not learned and a cyclical pattern of withdrawal results
     - **2)** examples of unhealthy uses of withdrawal include
       - **a)** excessive fantasizing that keeps the person from having to deal with day-to-day problems of living
       - **b)** excessive TV watching or involvement in only solitary activities to avoid social encounters
     - **3)** schizophrenia is the most severe form of withdrawal; the person's thought patterns, communications, and relationships with others prevent functioning in a productive manner
3. Withdrawn behaviors: though withdrawn behaviors occur on a continuum, this section focuses primarily on the most severe form of withdrawal, i.e., schizophrenic disorder
   - **a.** Etiologic factors: no consensus about cause; various theories
     - **1)** biologic: genetic or physical defect is the cause
     - **2)** psychologic: internal dynamics related to difficulties in thought process, affect, and behavior are the cause
     - **3)** sociologic: family relationships and rigid social expectations are the cause; schizophrenic behavior is learned, i.e., communication patterns, response to double-bind communication are learned from parents
   - **b.** Dynamics: the person views the world as so threatening that withdrawal from interpersonal relationships, social situations, and reality are seen unconsciously as the only alternative
   - **c.** Behavioral, psychologic, and sociologic manifestations (Bleuler's 4 "As": affect, autism, associative looseness, and ambivalence; fifth "A" usually present is auditory hallucinations)
     - **1)** behavioral manifestations: the behaviors of schizophrenic withdrawal are manifested in varying ways and degrees of severity
       - **a)** *affect* (feeling tone or mood) of the withdrawn client is often diagnostic of the status of illness
         - ■ a specific criterion in judgment is the appropriateness of the affect; that is, the degree to which it is in keeping with the situation at hand, both quantitatively and qualitatively
         - ■ responses may be excessive, or they may be inappropriately minimal, often referred to as "flat." A flat affect is demonstrated by a blunt or dull emotional tone of expression; it is a generalized impoverishment of emotional reactivity
         - ■ inappropriate affect is that which is incongruent with the situation or the content of thought
       - **b)** *behavior disorganization*, in which the client reacts to stress in an

unpredictable or bizarre manner (e.g., pacing, rigid posturing)

c) *disregard of hygiene and grooming* can range from looking unkempt to bizarre clothing and makeup or disregard for bodily care

d) *disregard of physical safety* includes not being concerned about placing self in dangerous situations, such as walking in a busy street or causing self-inflicted wounds; these persons need close observation

e) *nutrition deficits* because of poor eating habits

f) *regression*, in which the client returns to behavior patterns exhibited at an earlier stage of development (e.g., thumb sucking, baby talk, fetal position)

- main defense mechanism used in schizophrenia
- allows the person to be dependent and to return to the predictable behavior experienced in childhood

2) psychologic manifestations: these refer to the interpersonal dynamics of the person

a) *autism*: extreme withdrawal from real world and preoccupation with idiosyncratic thoughts and fantasies

- a common characteristic of schizophrenic behavior
- this persistent tendency to withdraw from involvement with the external world and to become preoccupied with ideas and fantasies that are egocentric and illogical causes autistic clients to be unresponsive
- it is difficult to establish communication with them; they may be mute; their conversations may be irrelevant or lack coherence

b) *hallucinations*: a sensory perception that occurs without an external stimulus

- can be auditory, visual, or tactile, olfactory, or gustatory
- usually occurs in psychotic disorders but can occur in both chronic and acute organic brain disorders
- auditory hallucinations are the most common form occurring in clients with schizophrenia, although visual, tactile, olfactory, and gustatory hallucinations may be experienced
  - some clients describe the experience as very definite; others describe it with an element of vagueness
  - the auditory hallucinations are often threatening and aggressive, and the client's response to them may account for acts of violence
  - hallucinations temporarily lessen anxiety, because they offer a substitute for interaction with real persons whom the client fears; such experiences are therefore counterproductive and conducive to further withdrawal from reality; when the client becomes aware that others see that s/he is hallucinating and becomes ashamed and embarrassed, and this increases anxiety and loneliness

c) *delusion*: a false belief or opinion that is unreasonable and causes distortion in judgment

- delusion of grandeur is a false, grandiose, or expansive belief that one is a very important or powerful person or entity (e.g., sees self as royalty or as Jesus)
- delusion of persecution is a false belief that one is victim of others' hostility and aggressiveness (e.g., "The FBI is after me.")
- although delusions represent a withdrawal from reality into fantasy, their function is to secure the client's identity
- this function makes these belief systems rigid and inaccessible to reason, permitting no modification; any attempt to correct the client's beliefs makes the nurse seem as an enemy
- trying to reason the client out of false beliefs will make client work harder to improve the delusion, thus reinforcing it and making it more entrenched

d) *depersonalization*: feelings of unreality or strangeness concerning either the environment or the self, or both

- a common phenomenon in the schizophrenic process resulting from the client's poor self-concept
- client treats self as an object
- client seems to have resigned not

only from the world of reality but also from self; this leads to extreme social isolation

e) *associative looseness*: one experience or idea reminds the client of a completely different experience, which is interpreted in an autistic manner
- the thought process loses its continuity so that thinking and expression become confused, bizarre, incorrect, and abrupt
- communication is disconnected, follows no logical sequence, and is confusing to the listener

f) *ambivalence*
- occurs normally, from time to time, in all persons and is popularly known as "mixed feelings"
- classic behavior in schizophrenia; characterizes the stormy, chaotic relationships the schizophrenic has with relatives, friends, and associates
- because of the ambivalence, minor difficulties can lead to disruption of relationships with significant others

3) sociologic manifestations

a) poor social skills: difficulty with conversation and even physical closeness

b) retreat from social situations

c) few or no friends: often has no friends, or relationships are considered to be friendships in spite of minimal contact

d) pathologic family relationships: often severe communication problems

e) erratic employment history

f) difficulty maintaining an independent living situation: unable to care for self, will not pay rent regularly or take care of physical needs; some can do the caretaking tasks but tend to isolate themselves

d. Management: long-term management with continuing follow-up is frequently necessary

1) medications: major tranquilizers (see Table 2.10)

a) actions: modify intense anxiety, tension, and psychomotor excitement; alleviate delusions and hallucinations

b) benefits: allow the client to participate in other forms of therapy

c) side effects: not addictive but do have troublesome, sometimes irreversible, and occasionally dangerous side effects; see Table 2.11)

d) nursing role
- administer the medications, observe client response, intervene to prevent complications related to drug side effects, and teach client and family about the drug, e.g., action, side effects, and need to take on long-term basis
- record and report side effects or problems

2) milieu therapy

a) utilized to increase the effectiveness of other psychiatric treatment methods

b) promotes a positive living environment for each client

c) uses the interactions within the social context as an opportunity to assess client and implement treatment

d) uses the inpatient hospital setting as a therapeutic environment

e) milieu therapy manipulates both physical and emotional properties of the hospital ward, taking into account the specific needs of individual clients and groups of clients in an effort to promote a positive living experience for each client and the maximum of positive, behavioral change

f) the therapeutic milieu takes into account the stimuli in the environment (it can be increased or decreased), limit setting, protection, and activities

g) nurses—on the unit at all times—are in a position to make the greatest contribution to milieu therapy; they can
- provide a positive role model of care and concern for others
- note and report the kinds of interactions among clients, clients and staff
- provide the flexibility to promote opportunity for the client's behavioral experimentation and growth

h) planned interactions designed to promote independence and develop social skills:
- *government*: clients elect officers to run meetings, negotiate with staff, and administer the various unit activities (e.g., kitchen cleanup, dayroom cleanup); clients report to

Table 2.10 Major Tranquilizers (Neuroleptics)

Generic Name (Trade Name)	Dosage	Action	Nursing Implications for all Major Tranquilizers
Phenothiazines			
Chlorpromazine (Thorazine)	100–1,000 mg/day	Phenothiazines block dopamine-mediated transmission, depress lower levels of central nervous system, antipsychotic activity, decrease psychomotor activity; in combination with piperazine stimulate withdrawn client to increasing socialization and communication	Check BP prior to administration; observe for orthostatic hypotension; teach client to rise slowly from sitting or lying position; have client remain in lying position 30–60 minutes after IM dose.
Acetophenazine (Tindal)	6–120 mg/day		
Carphenazine (Proketazine)	75–400 mg/day		
Perphenazine (Trilafon)	6–64 mg/day		Monitor periodic liver function tests, blood counts.
Trifloperazine (Stelazine)	4–10 mg; may be slowly increased to 15–20 mg		Notify physician of complaints of sore throat, nose blood, rash, fever or other infections.
Fluophenazine HCl, decanoate or enanthate (Prolixin, Permitil)	0.5–1.0 mg PO daily, not to exceed 20 mg; 12.5–25 mg q2wk IM		Observe for early signs of pseudoparkinsonism; if it occurs, explain to client and administer prescribed antiparkinsonian drug.
Thioridazine HCl (Mellaril)	20–800 mg/day		Observe for warning signs of tardive depkinesia (tongue-like movements) and report.
Butyrophenones			
Haloperidol (Haldol)	1.5–6 mg/day; 6–15 mg, up to 100 mg to achieve control	Butyrophenones and thioxanthenes similar to the phenothiazines; more potent dopaminergic effects	Warn client that drowsiness may occur until tolerance is developed; avoid driving a car or operating machinery until tolerant.
Thioxanthenes			
Chloroprothixene (Taractan)	100–600 mg		Observe for dryness of mouth, visual or retinal changes, rash, gastric irritation, constipation. May be administered with food, water or milk to reduce gastric irritation.
Thiothixene (Navane)	6 mg daily, slowly increase to 20–30 mg; rarely exceeds 60 mg		Maintain fluid intake to decrease mouth irritation and constipation.
Dihydroindolones			
Molindone HCl (Moban)	25–225 mg	Dihydroindolones as per phenothiazines; suppress aggressive behavior	Do not administer antacids within 1 hour of these medications given orally.
Dibenzoxanzephines			
Loxapine HCl (Loxitance C)	25–250 mg	Dibezoxanzephines act on ascending reticular activating system; activate withdrawn client	Teach client • avoid alcohol • consult MD before taking other meds • report sore throat in absence of other cold symptoms • appropriate diet and exercise to avoid weight gain • precautions to avoid skin damage due to photosensitivity • side effects • high fiber diet, fluids, exercise to prevent constipation
Loxapine Succinate (Loxitane)	25–250 mg		

the president of the government

- *self-care*: clients may be required to change their own bed linen, do their own laundry, and keep their rooms clean; these activities help clients to maintain or learn independence even while hospitalized
- *assessment of group skills*: several

Table 2.11 Side Effects of Major Tranquilizers

Parkinsonian-type
- pseudoparkinsonism
- dystonia
- akathisia

Hypotension
Photosensitivity
Anticholinergic effects (blurred vision, dry mouth, constipation, difficulty starting urination)
Agranulocytosis (rare)
Jaundice (rare)
Increased restlessness
Drowsiness
Weight gain
Skin rashes
Amenorrhea with false-positive pregancy test, galactorrhea
Ejaculation difficulties, gynecomastia
Decreased libido

activities are done in groups; clients attend and participate according to their ability

- *occupational therapy*
  - generally carried on in a room off the nursing unit, assigned for that special purpose
  - although nurses are sometimes involved in the activities of that department, generally registered occupational therapists and student occupational therapists plan and conduct the program for the clients in accordance with specific orders of the psychiatrists
  - gives the client an opportunity to
    * keep occupied
    * express self nonverbally if communication is a problem
    * follow activities prescribed to achieve specific psychologic results
- *activity therapy*: includes art, music, and recreation as a planned, therapeutically designed activity
  - the activities may be carried out by regular unit personnel or by specially trained therapists
  - nurses are often involved and assume some of the functions of the activity therapists

3) nurse-client relationship

a) purpose: to assist the client to function as independently as possible, to deal with problems and to complement the medical treatment

b) development of trust
- focuses on development of trust that will stand as a model for relationships with others, in contrast with those client has experienced thus far
- schizophrenics develop relationships slowly, if at all, and use their ambivalence to push others away; therefore, the orientation phase of the relationship is the most difficult for them

c) *DSM-III*-R classification: schizophrenia

Application of the Nursing Process to a Client Exhibiting Withdrawn Behavior

1. Assessment

a. Suicide potential
  1) autistic thinking; aggressive/hostile voices; a confused, depressed mood, low self-esteem increase suicide risk
  2) refer to *Elated-Depressive Behavior* page 50

b. Behavioral, psychologic, and sociologic manifestations (refer to page 72)

2. Analysis

a. safe, effective care environment
  1) potential for violence: self-directed or directed at others
  2) sensory-perceptual alteration (visual, auditory)
  3) impaired home maintenance management

b. physiological integrity
  1) impaired verbal communication
  2) sleep pattern disturbance
  3) altered nutrition: less than body requirements

c. psychological integrity
  1) ineffective individual coping
  2) chronic low self-esteem
  3) altered thought processes
  4) impaired social interaction

d. health promotion/maintenance
  1) impaired adjustment
  2) ineffective family coping: compromised
  3) noncompliance

3. General Nursing Plans/Implementation and Evaluation (see Table 2.12)

Goal 1: Client will remain physically safe.

Table 2.12 Selected Problem Behaviors and Interventions

Behavior	Interventions
Aggression	Prevention—early recognition of increased excitement. Encourage verbal expression of feelings surrounding behavior. Reduce stimuli. Avoid reinforcement, e.g., competitive games. Provide distraction. Set limits. Protect other clients.
Anger	Acknowledge or name feeling. Explore sources. Encourage to express verbally. Explore appropriate outlets. Avoid arguing.
Anxiousness	Acknowledge or name the behavior or feeling. Explore sources. Encourage appropriate expression. Give reassurance. Recognize that anxiety in nurse increases client's anxiety.
Associative looseness (thought disorder)	Relate in a concrete manner. Focus on immediate situation. Point out reality. Clarify verbalizations that are not understood.
Autism	Accept at stage client is in; do not push. Give ample time for responses. Do not reinforce dependency. Use silence appropriately.
Controlling behavior	Recognize means of controlling: negativism, obstruction, silence, avoidance, insults, yelling, increased chatter, crying. Do not impose unnecessary controls. Allow client some control. Develop trust: security in giving up control.
Delusions	Avoid arguing. Avoid arousing suspicion. Be honest and reliable. Be consistent. Acknowledge client's feelings. Point out reality: client's beliefs are not shared.
Dependence	Assess abilities and capabilities. Provide only help needed. Encourage to solve problems and make decisions. Display attitude of firmness and confidence. Discourage reliance beyond actual need. Encourage successful participation.
Hallucinations	Help to recognize as manifestation of anxiety. Encourage to give up hallucinations. Help to relate with real persons. Do not give attention to content.
Hopelessness, helplessness	Structure small successes. Give encouragement. Exhibit expectation that client will succeed. Encourage identification of strengths.
Hostility	Avoid arguing with the client. Acknowledge and name feelings. Explore the source of hostility with client. Encourage to express hostility verbally, rather than resort to physical aggression. Explore appropriate outlets for hostility (e.g., physical activities).
Low self-esteem, feeling worthless	Prevent isolation. Acknowledge client's view. Avoid system of shoulds and should nots and discussions regarding moral judgments. Avoid power struggles. Give minimal tasks and grade them to manageable size. Prevent self-mutilation.
Manipulation/acting out	Spell out acceptable and unacceptable behavior. Set firm and definite limits. Consistently enforce limits. Avoid involvement in intellectualization; i.e., responsibility for behavior rests with client. Treat infractions with withdrawal of privileges. Ensure that staff is united, firm, and consistent. Maintain sense of authority.
Ritualistic behaviors	Do not interrupt repetitive act: could lead to panic. Set limits on repetitive behavior. Engage in alternative activities with client. Provide physical protection from repetitive acts.
Secondary gain	Understand unconscious motivation of the behavior and differentiate it from malingering. Understand and alleviate primary symptoms. Encourage client to explore the motivation of the behavior. Explore alternatives to the primary symptom for handling anxiety.
Somatic behaviors	Do not focus on physical symptoms. Give appropriate information regarding somatic complaints. Point out reality, i.e., correct misinformation.
Superiority	Suggest solitary activities for client. Put client in charge of things, not people. Give client activities at which client can succeed.

Plan/Implementation

- Keep harmful objects away from impulsive clients.
- Observe client at frequent intervals.
- Observe for physical problems (e.g., infection, constipation) that may be outside client's awareness.
- Observe for side effects of drugs; (see reprint section page 111).
- Monitor rest and sleep; use comfort measures such as pillows, snacks, warm baths to induce sleep.

Evaluation: Client does not injure self; experiences only minimal side effects of drugs; has adequate rest and sleep.

Goal 2: Client maintains adequate nutrition and fluid and electrolyte balance.

Plan/Implementation

- Observe for signs of dehydration (e.g., dry skin, lips); encourage to drink fluids.
- If client is not eating, assess the reasons (e.g., delusions about food being poisoned, too agitated to sit for meals, unaware of poor eating habits).
- Assist client to find methods to ensure adequate food intake (e.g., permit food from home if client fears hospital food is poisoned; provide finger foods client can eat while walking).
- Provide positive reinforcement for good eating habits.
- Teach about nutrition as needed.

Evaluation: Client maintains adequate food and fluid intake; skin is hydrated.

Goal 3: Client demonstrates improved hygiene and grooming.

Plan/Implementation

- Identify specific client needs for assistance (e.g., with severe withdrawal, client may need nurse to provide care; client with poor reality orientation or attention span may need assistance; more self-sufficient client may only need encouragement).
- Use gentle firmness and consistent interest in client's needs.
- Provide matter-of-fact positive reinforcement for appropriate grooming and cleanliness.
- Be sure equipment for physical care is available to client.

Evaluation: Client does self-care for hygiene (hair, nails, clothing, bathing).

Goal 4: Client will develop a trusting relationship with staff member; will demonstrate increased ability in social interaction.

Plan/Implementation

- Know that staff reactions can be the crucial element negating or facilitating attainment of the therapeutic goal for the client
  - staff members may find themselves withdrawing from the client because this disorder is often chronic, the prognosis is pessimistic, and client's behavior provokes feelings of frustration, helplessness, and incompetence
  - withdrawal on the part of the staff reinforces the client's past experiences of rejection and feelings of low self-esteem
  - in own defense, the client will withdraw further into world of fantasy, negating progress towards the therapeutic goal planned
  - in addition, the client may test staff involvement by trying to push staff away
  - offer support and encouragement to other staff members; meet regularly to provide support
- Use consistent, predictable behavior with client.
- Persevere even though client may be unreliable or rejecting.
- Meet for short intervals at regularly scheduled times to increase trust.
- Use silence; share that you are willing to spend time without talking if client so chooses.
- Allow ample time for response if client very regressed; use general comments that do not push client for answer.
- Allow client to set the pace of the relationship.
- Accept where the client is in his/her illness; if communication is to be restored, the nurse must understand that client is frightened and both wants and fears contact from others, makes responses slowly, and needs ample time to trust nurse's sincerity and interest.
- Listen in nonjudgmental way to client's thoughts/feelings.
- Know that autistic clients are extremely sensitive to the feeling tones of others; they pick up negative clues from the nurse, who may be unaware of them.
- Role model socially appropriate behavior.
- As client begins to accept the nurse, client may become very dependent; a therapeutic goal requires that the nurse maintain contact on a professional level and not reinforce the dependency.
- Observe verbal and nonverbal behaviors that may indicate any interest in activities; give support to any expression of interest.

Evaluation: Client develops a relationship with one staff member; begins to interact with other clients.

Goal 5: Client will define and test reality; will dismiss internal voices/hallucinations, delusions.

Plan/Implementation

- Recognize disorientation as manifestation of severe withdrawal related to anxiety and frustration.
- Be meticulously honest and reliable, especially with the suspicious client.
- Do not give attention to content of hallucinations or delusions (gives them legitimacy): avoid arguing about content.

- Acknowledge client's feelings and beliefs; point out that these are not shared.
- Relate to client in a realistic and concrete manner, focusing on the immediate situation; it is helpful for the nurse to point out reality to the client by saying that s/he doesn't understand and asking for clarification as needed.
- Encourage to give up hallucinations or delusions; help to recognize hallucinations or delusions as sign of anxiety.
- Reassure that hallucinations and delusions do go away and can be dismissed as client focuses on real people and situations.
- Help client to relate with real persons.
- Assist client who has depersonalization to discuss feelings of estrangement with trusted individuals
  - first with a nurse in whom client has developed a trusting relationship
  - as client's condition permits, in group therapy sessions or similar groups involving other persons who may recount similar experiences
- Focus on reality of the client's body and environment during these discussions.

Evaluation: Client dismisses internal voices/hallucinations/delusions; increases ability to relate to real persons and situations.

Goal 6: Client increases communication with family members.

Plan/Implementation

- Accept client's feelings and thoughts and help client do the same.
- Explore present family patterns with client; family assessment and intervention during the client's hospitalization may be done.
- Help client identify feelings associated with family interactions.
- Help client view self as unique person with values and beliefs that are sometimes different from family's.
- Practice social skills to use with family members; use role playing, assertion techniques.
- Provide opportunity for family members to talk about the client's illness and treatment to decrease hostility and withdrawal from client; help family explore social resources.

Evaluation: Client increases adaptive communication with family members.

Goal 7: Client will increase successful decision-making skills.

Plan/Implementation

- Relate in a concrete manner; focus on the immediate situation.
- Encourage decision making at level of client's ability; use therapeutic milieu as tolerated by client.
- Increase complexity of decisions as tolerated.
- Provide with tasks of increasing complexity.
- Do not reinforce unneeded dependency.

Evaluation: Client increases ability to make decisions.

Goal 8: Client will demonstrate social skills in individual and group settings.

Plan/Implementation

- Role model appropriate social interaction.
- Role play social situation with client.
- Assist client to develop a relationship with one other client.
- Encourage client to relate to others during activities.
- Do not push client beyond present abilities; may need encouragement to begin developing social skills.
- Help client to relate to others in more complex situations, slowly as tolerated.

Evaluation: Client behaves appropriately in individual and group settings; interacts with other clients; demonstrates fewer problem behaviors.

Goal 9: Client will develop ability to be as self-supporting as possible.

Plan/Implementation

- Support client in finding a healthy living situation; may be at home, a halfway house, or in own apartment depending on client's social skills and ability to be self-motivating.
- Support client in finding employment as appropriate; employment history and assessment of skills in occupational therapy can help in developing employment plan.
- Allow family to discuss feelings about plans for client's living and employment plans; help them evaluate their expectations and role in supporting client in living and employment settings.

Evaluation: Client finds healthy living situation; develops a plan to be self-supporting.

Selected Health Problems

☐ Specific Schizophrenic Disorders

Characterized by withdrawal, all are distinguished by other characteristic behaviors. General Nursing Plans and Evaluations, page 76, are used in addition to care specific to the distinguishing characteristics, see Table 2.13.

References

Beck, C., Rawlins, R., & Williams, S. (1988). *Mental health—psychiatric nursing: A holistic life-cycle approach* (2nd ed.). St. Louis: Mosby.

Mathewson, M. (1986). *Pharmacotherapeutics: A nursing process approach*. Philadelphia: Davis.

Stuart, G., & Sundeen, S. (1986). *Principles and practices of psychiatric nursing* (3rd ed.). St. Louis: Mosby.

Table 2.13 Types of Withdrawn Behavior (Schizophrenia)

Type	Characteristics	Additional Nursing Care
Paranoid	Delusions of persecution/grandeur Hallucinations Ideas of reference Hostility/aggression Superiority	Interventions specific to delusions (see "Suspicious Behavior," page 70), hostility, superiority, and aggression (see "Socially Maladaptive Behavior," page 62)
Catatonic	Severe withdrawal, regression Catatonic stupor, waxy flexibility, muteness or Catatonic excitement, severe agitation, grimacing, bizarre gestures/posturing	Prevent complications of immobility: infection, skin breakdown, urinary and fecal incontinence, constipation.
Undifferentiated	Mixed schizophrenic symptoms over long time period	See General Nursing Plans page 76.
Childhood	Onset in early childhood Withdrawal, impaired relationships, disturbed affect Ritualism Self-mutilation Increased or decreased sensitivity to sensory stimuli *No* hallucinations or delusions	Prevent self-mutilation Behavior modification
Other psychotic disorders • schizophreniform disorders • brief reactive psychosis • schizoaffective disorder • atypical psychosis	Sudden onset Last less than 6 months No prior history of disturbed interpersonal relationships Minimal residual defects	See General Nursing Plans page 76.

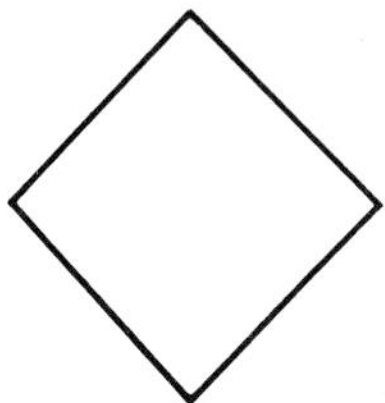

Substance Use Disorders

General Concepts

Overview

1. Definitions
   a. Substance use disorder: ". . . maladaptive behavior associated with more or less regular use of the substances." (*DSM-III*-R)
   b. Polydrug abuse: mixing drugs and alcohol in varying degrees (particularly dangerous because of potentiating and toxic interactions of drugs and alcohol)
2. Etiology: not known, but thought to be an interplay of physiologic, psychologic, and sociocultural factors
3. Interaction variables
   a. The person
      1) no specific personality type identified
      2) most frequently, the person shows signs of immaturity, low tolerance for frustration, low self-esteem, environmental deprivation, conflicts over parental upbringing, and conflict between values and behavior
      3) it is not known if substance abuse fosters development of these characteristics or if the characteristics trigger the abuse
      4) major psychiatric disorders generally associated with substance abuse are antisocial personality and affective disorders
   b. The family: substance abuse may relate to overall anxiety level in family as well as in individual
   c. The environment: social aspects and peer pressure may lead the person into drug culture and antisocial acts
   d. The substance: which substance the person uses depends on the cultural group, availability, costs, and federal regulation of the item (alcohol and/or drug substances other than alcohol)
4. Substance abuse is associated with behavior changes related to more or less regular use of a substance that affects the central nervous system acutely or chronically. Three criteria distinguish substance *abuse* from substance *use*
   a. Pattern of Pathologic Use: depending on the substance, client manifests inability to cut down or stop use despite physical problems; needs daily use for adequate functioning; intoxication throughout the day; episodes of a complication of substance intoxication, e.g., alcoholic blackouts
   b. Impairment of Social or Occupational Functions: legal and economic difficulties because of cost, procurement, or complications of intoxication, e.g., auto accident
   c. Duration of Abuse: disturbance of at least a month
5. Substance Dependence
   a. Definition: a more severe form of substance use disorder than substance abuse
   b. Manifestations
      1) a physiologic need for a substance evidenced by withdrawal or tolerance
      2) almost always, a pathologic use pattern occurs that causes impairment in social or occupational functioning
      3) rarely, manifestations are limited to physiologic dependence
      4) alcohol or cannabis dependence requires evidence of occupational or social impairment; diagnosis of other substance-dependence categories requires only evidence of withdrawal or tolerance
   c. Length of dependence: regular maladaptive use for over six months qualifies as "continuous dependence"
   d. Social implications: although accessibility, chance, peer pressure, and curiosity play a part in who will ingest a drug and who will not, they do not account for the fact that one person becomes addicted and another does not
   e. Concepts
      1) physiologic dependence: an altered physiologic state produced by the repeated administration of the drug, which necessitates its continued administration to

prevent a withdrawal syndrome
2) addiction: the compulsive use of a chemical substance with physiologic and psychologic dependence
3) habituation: repeated use of a substance that results in psychologic dependence
4) tolerance: markedly increased amounts of the substance are required to achieve the desired effect, or there is a markedly diminished effect with regular use of the same dose
5) withdrawal: a substance-specific syndrome following cessation or reduction of intake
6) lethality: the amount of a substance that constitutes a fatal dose
7) potentiation: two or more substances combined have a greater effect than simple summation (1 + 1 = 3)

6. Substance use disorders by health professionals is a serious problem
   a. Narcotic addiction by physicians estimated at 1%–2%, or 30 times greater than in general population
   b. Estimated 40,000 alcoholic nurses in US
   c. Problems with impaired health professionals' job performance result in danger to clients and the professionals themselves and compromise teamwork
   d. It is the responsibility of health professionals to report concerns about a colleague to supervisor, and for supervisor to take appropriate actions
   e. Professionals are helping, not harming, a substance-abusing colleague by bringing problems to attention of someone qualified to help.

Application of the Nursing Process to a Client with a Substance Use Disorder

1. **Assessment**
   a. Substance use history (substance abusers are well-known for denying use or seriously understating extent of use. To increase likelihood of accurate history, ask questions in a logical and nonthreatening manner. Family and friends may provide more accurate information or use denial.)
      1) history of recent prescription and nonprescription drug use
      2) drugs client has prescribed for self, e.g., nicotine, alcohol, cocaine, marijuana
   b. Work performance
      1) excessive use of sick time
      2) decreasing productivity or "job shrinkage"
      3) decreasing ability to meet schedules and deadlines
      4) sloppy or illogical work
      5) frequent errors in judgment; in drug-addicted nurses, medication errors, incorrect controlled-drug wastage, or incorrect narcotic counts
   c. Blood levels of suspected substance of abuse
   d. Level of consciousness, reality orientation, mental status exam
   e. Family history of substance abuse

2. **Analysis**
   a. Safe, effective care environment
      1) potential for injury
      2) sensory-perceptual alteration: visual, auditory, kinesthetic, gustatory, tactile, olfactory
      3) potential for violence: self-directed or directed at others
   b. Physiological integrity
      1) altered nutrition: less than body requirements
      2) impaired physical mobility
      3) sleep pattern disturbance
   c. Psychological integrity
      1) anxiety
      2) ineffective individual coping
      3) chronic low self esteem
   d. Health promotion/maintenance
      1) ineffective family coping: compromised
      2) altered family processes
      3) noncompliance

3. **General Nursing Plans/Implementation and Evaluation**

Goal 1: Client will withdraw from substance that is abused or creating dependency.

Plans/Implementation

- It is important *not* to do any of the following
  - scold, argue, moralize, blame, or threaten
  - lose one's temper
  - enable person to cover up consequences of actions
  - be overly sympathetic
  - put off facing problem
- Control symptoms via prn medication; take vital signs q2h and report elevations to physician.
- Assess potential for violence.
- If client is agitated, confused, assaultive, belligerent, stay with client; reassure that current symptoms are only the result of body's

responding to the abused substance, and that they are temporary; reassure that client will regain control; use restraints only if necessary for safety (follow hospital policy carefully).

- Deal with hallucinations by reinforcing reality; speak to client slowly in a calm voice; provide a quiet environment; stay with client until the frightening symptoms have decreased.
- Provide physical care advocated for additional diseases/conditions that client may have.
- Keep client ambulatory as much as possible; if necessary, walk with client several times a day.

Evaluation: Client withdraws from abused substance, free from complications.

Goal 2: Client will obtain treatment necessary to abstain from substance abuse or dependence.

Plans/Implementation

- Sit and talk with client at least twice daily; your presence will say client is not being rejected; be aware of your own nonverbal distancing maneuvers; establish good eye contact.
- Do not punish or reprimand client for failures or nonresponse to your suggestions/ interventions (punishment serves only to give client fuel for continuing to deal with failure or rejection by drinking or taking drugs); ignore it, but do praise *any* positive responses.
- Have client make decisions about daily care in hospital; involve in some type of occupational therapy, anything in which client can achieve some measure of success (helps increase self-confidence and self-esteem).
- Provide opportunities to decrease social isolation and improve social skills (mealtimes, groups, recreation periods); calmly, gently, point out unacceptable behavior such as manipulative acts; reinforce positive social behaviors (e.g., initiating friendly conversations); praise all efforts at participation in activities.

Evaluation: Client participates in prescribed treatment.

Goal 3: Client will develop a positive life-style that is free from substance use, abuse, or dependence.

Plan/Implementation

- Help the client to gradually become aware of the denial by poking holes in denial process; encourage client's assessment of how denial serves client, including delineation of the self-defeating aspects.
- Help client look at alternative coping methods and deal with abstinence one day (or one morning, one evening) at a time.
- Work with client to develop sound discharge planning regarding employment counseling, ongoing support via outpatient counseling, or long-term inpatient treatment.
- Arrange for client and family to attend group counseling sessions, if available in hospital, to discuss feelings, problems, changing behaviors, pressures, sources of support, etc.
- Provide information about other types of therapy available, e.g., stress-reduction programs, employee assistance, aftercare programs, and local mental health clinics, self-help groups.

Evaluation: Client's approach to daily living is positive and free from substance abuse or dependence.

Selected Health Problems

☐ Alcohol

1. General Information

a. Definitions

1) *alcohol* is a mind- and mood-altering substance classified as a central nervous system depressant

2) *alcoholism (alcohol dependence)*

a) no precise agreement on definition, but most refer to these clinical features: chronicity; preoccupation with drinking; loss of control over drinking; damage to health, relationships, and/or work; using alcohol as a solution to most problems

b) the World Health Organization defines alcoholism as a chronic disease or disorder of behavior characterized by alcohol consumption that exceeds customary use and interferes with the drinker's health, interpersonal relations, or economic functioning

c) in some settings may be further defined as alcoholism with no evidence of any preexisting major psychiatric problem (primary alcoholism) or alcoholism occuring after the onset of a major psychiatric disorder (secondary alcoholism)

b. Effects

1) at low levels of consumption, there is little apparent effect on the drinker; moderate

levels may produce euphoria; and in large amounts, alcohol acts as a sedative
2) alcohol depresses higher cortical functions, acts as a disinhibitor and tranquilizer, and serves to reduce anxiety rapidly (excessive drinking is often the way a person copes with anxiety)

c. Scope of alcohol abuse and dependence
1) estimates
a) one third of general hospital clients, but these clients are rarely admitted with alcoholism diagnosis
b) one out of 10 Americans who drinks is an alcoholic
c) 6.6 million adults in US are alcoholic
d) one in 10 alcoholics is diagnosed and treated
2) occurrence: alcoholism and related problems are widespread among
a) city residents
b) minorities
c) poor men under 25 years of age
d) persons who have experienced childhood disruptions, e.g., broken homes, alcoholic parents
e) rural or small-town persons who have moved to urban areas
f) people of Swedish, Polish, Irish, northern French, and Russian origin

d. Characteristics: common but not exclusive to alcoholics are
1) low self-esteem
2) feelings of isolation, depression
3) emotional immaturity and excessive dependence
4) anger and hostility
5) highly anxious in interpersonal relationships
6) inability to express emotions adequately
7) ambivalence toward authority
8) grandiosity
9) compulsiveness, perfectionism
10) sexual-role confusion
11) excessive use of denial, projection, rationalization

e. Withdrawal from alcohol and detoxification
1) symptoms develop when there is a physiologic dependence and the intake of alcohol is interrupted or decreased without substitution of other sedation
2) complete cessation of use of alcohol is not necessary for the development of withdrawal symptoms; the beginning of withdrawal can be a reflection of diminished use in those who have developed a marked tolerance and physical dependence
3) monitored detoxification for withdrawal is the top priority need of the alcoholic client
4) withdrawal syndrome has four major manifestations: tremulousness, hallucinations, convulsive seizures, and delirium tremens; this is a progressive process and involves four stages
- *stage 1*: 8 hours plus after cessation: symptoms include mild tremors, nausea, nervousness, tachycardia, increased blood pressure, diaphoresis
- *stage 2*: symptoms include profound confusion, gross tremors, nervousness and hyperactivity, insomnia, anorexia, general weakness, disorientation, illusions, nightmares; auditory and visual hallucinations begin
- *stage 3*: 12–48 hours after cessation: symptoms include all those of stages 1 and 2, as well as severe hallucinations and grand mal seizures (''rum'' fits)
- *stage 4*: occurs 3–5 days after cessation: symptoms include initial and continuing delirium tremens (DTs), which are characterized by confusion, severe psychomotor activity, agitation, sleeplessness, hallucinations, and at onset, uncontrolled and unexplained tachycardia; DTs are a medical emergency (fatality rate is 20% even with treatment)

f. Prognosis: motivation and recognition of the problem are necessary for the elimination of alcohol use; the person experiences fluctuations of sobriety, during which acknowledgment of illness and movement toward a new way of life are punctuated by relapse, shock, and denial; alcoholics are considered as recovering, not cured

g. Treatment: approaches used in all alcohol treatment models
1) general measures include vitamin and nutritional therapy, sedatives, tranquilizers, and/or disulfiram (Antabuse); avoid drugs containing alcohol, e.g., elixirs, cough syrups, mouth washes
2) detoxification: the acute phase of treatment
a) involves close observation and safety measures to prevent severe reaction while withdrawing from alcohol
b) magnesium sulfate 50% solution and high doses of chlordiazepoxide

(Librium) are used to prevent seizures and hallucinations

c) thiamine 50–100 mg IM to treat malnutrition

d) education and group process are frequently used after detoxification when client is able to understand instructions

3) rehabilitation

a) aim is to build treatment motivation and overcome denial in clients and significant others

b) the alcoholic has to learn to give up alcohol forever

c) the person is helped to learn new ways of problem solving and living a satisfying life without alcohol; this is enhanced by a therapeutic relationship that increases the alcoholic's self-confidence, feelings of self-worth, and attempts to become more independent

4) major models of treatment

a) chronic disease model

- views alcoholism as a primary, physiologic, incurable disease
- views psychosocial problems as result of drinking
- includes a maintenance program of recovery
- emphasis is on self-diagnosis by the alcoholic

b) psychiatric model

- focus on unique needs as defined by psychiatric perspective
- varying psychotherapeutic treatment regimen depends on individual

c) family systems model

- views family relationships as a contributing factor; chemical dependency is viewed as a family illness
- examines childhood development of alcoholic, such as drinking patterns of parents, ethnic attitudes, and socialization process regarding drinking behaviors
- looks at family roles, communication patterns, family rules, and power structure in the family
- identifies how present family relations recreate old patterns of avoidance or dependence
- utilizes family commitment and caring to promote recovery
- integrates recovering alcoholic into revised family structure

5) Alcoholics Anonymous (AA) is a self-help group of recovering alcoholics

a) 12-step program to achieve sobriety, which members do at their own pace

b) run entirely by sober alcoholics

c) requires members to devote themselves completely to mutual help

d) remarkable success with chronic alcoholism

e) has member groups for families of alcoholics who themselves suffer from codependency (i.e., dependency on the alcoholic)

- Al-Anon is an organization of friends and family
- Alateen is an organization of teenagers affected by alcoholism
- AC-A is an Al-Anon organization for adult children of alcoholics
- the emphasis is on changing oneself to make the most of one's life, education, guidance in relating to the alcoholic family member, the sharing of problems and experiences, and support based on a 12-step program

6) long-term treatment may also take place in the controlled environment of a private or public facility and in an outpatient setting

a) depending on particular model used, emphasis varies among group process, education, psychotherapy, family therapy, and AA

b) AA is the backbone to maintain sobriety; some clients attend daily

h. Preventive measures: include helping the client learn to

1) tolerate psychologic stress

2) do advance planning for anticipated painful events (surgery, separation from a loved one)

3) reduce social isolation

4) communicate honestly

i. *DSM-III*-R classifications: Alcohol intoxication, uncomplicated alcohol withdrawal, alcohol withdrawal delirium, alcohol hallucinosis, alcohol dependence abuse

2. Nursing Process

a. Assessment/Analysis

1) physical assessment/history

a) skin: spider angiomata, jaundice, acne rosacea, multiple bruises, age of bruises (purple, yellow), mahogany finger stains, "dirty tan," flushed ruddy complexion
b) orthopedic system: vaguely explained fractures, moderate muscle wasting of proximal muscle groups of lower and upper extremities
c) cardiovascular system: a first episode of paroxysmal atrial tachycardia as adult, ventricular premature contractions, paroxysmal atrial fibrillation, erratic hypertensive course (alcohol elevates bood pressure)
d) gastrointestinal system: early tooth losses, esophagitis, gastritis, pancreatitis, palpable liver, peptic ulcer, epistaxis, anorexia, weight loss, jaundice, cirrhosis
e) neurologic system: tremors that worsen with movement, vertigo and nystagmus that clear during the day, vaguely described memory lapses (blackouts), insomnia, seizures, peripheral neuropathy, hallucinations
f) genitourinary system: mild proteinuria, orgasmic/erectile dysfunction; prostatitis
g) indications of fluid and electrolyte imbalance
h) respiratory system: repeated upper respiratory infections

2) psychologic assessment
   a) suicide potential
   b) extent of cognitive disturbance
   c) mental status exam
   d) occurrence of signs and symptoms related to major psychiatric disorders
3) other: although not diagnostic in themselves, the following raise possibilities and should be explored further
   a) numerous transient medical symptoms in various organ systems without mention of drinking
   b) unwarranted complaints and signing out against medical advice (hospitalized clients)
   c) functioning at lower job level than intelligence and education would indicate; changing jobs frequently
   d) alcoholism in close relatives (parental alcoholism increases likelihood fivefold)
   e) child or spouse abuse
4) stage of alcoholism and related symptoms (dependent on amount of consumption and the physical makeup of the person)
   a) *early*: 5–10 years of controlled social drinking with some tolerance symptoms
      - signs: dependence on alcohol; without it the person is irritable, has insomnia and tremors; has need for a morning drink; is defensive and tries to conceal drinking problem
   b) *middle*: symptomatic; dependence increases and tolerance decreases
      - signs and symptoms: blackouts, periods of amnesia; life centered on drinking; social, recreational, and occupational activities affected
      - physical changes: chronic gastritis, fatty infiltration of the liver; all organs can be affected
   c) *late or chronic*: damage to the central nervous system
      - signs: organic brain syndrome, Wernicke's syndrome, Korsakoff's syndrome, pancreatitis, cirrhosis of the liver, nutritional deficiencies
      - withdrawal signs (usually occur 72–96 hours after alcohol stopped)
        - minor: flushed face, sweating, bloodshot eyes, anorexia, nausea/vomiting, tachycardia
        - alcohol withdrawal delirium (delirium tremens): coarse tremors, slurred speech, vivid hallucinations, unpredictable acts, confusion, disorientation, seizures, high blood pressure, 9%–15% mortality rate
5) strengths and stressors, coping mechanisms
6) beliefs, attitudes, feelings, concerns about alcohol consumption
7) codependency behaviors in family and friends: enabling behaviors that perpetuate the drinking behaviors, dependence on alcoholic, super-responsibility in children, denial and poor coping, signs of chronic stress
8) prescription- or street-drug use

b. Plans/Implementation and Evaluation

Goal 1: Client will withdraw from alcohol free from systemic complications.

Plan/Implementation

- Observe for withdrawal symptoms (anxiety, anorexia, insomnia, tremor, disorientation leading to delirium, tachycardia, hallucinations) beginning shortly after last drink and lasting 5–7 days.
- Monitor for delirium tremens (severe withdrawal behaviors) beginning 2–3 days after cessation of alcohol ingestion and lasting 48–72 hours.
- Give anti-anxiety drugs as ordered.
- Institute seizure precautions.
- Monitor I&O, administer 2,500 cc/day; avoid caffeinated drinks.
- Weigh daily to monitor fluid retention.
- Monitor electrolytes; report abnormalities.
- Give vitamin/mineral supplements, especially B vitamins.

Evaluation: Client withdraws from alcohol without evidence of nutritional imbalance, seizures, fluid and electrolyte imbalances; remains safe during episodes of disorientation, hallucinations.

Goal 2: Client will develop healthier coping mechanisms to deal with the stress of life.

Plan/Implementation

- Express concern for client's situations and confidence in ability to recover.
- Intervene to decrease denial and manipulative behavior.
- Discuss your observations of client's behavior with him/her, being as frank as possible; help client relate this behavior to alcohol intake.
- Deal with angry behavior resulting from confrontation; know that although the anger may be directed at staff it may stem from emerging insight into the problems; direct anger into nondestructive outlets (e.g., exercise, art or music).
- Intervene in withdrawal behavior that may result from grieving process and result in relapse; express confidence in client's ability to recover.
- Discuss drinking pattern with client to identify triggers, cues, "slippery places"; talk about what a life-style without alcohol would be like.
- If on Antabuse therapy to control impulsive drinking; explain symptoms if alcohol is ingested (headache, severe GI distress, tachycardia, hypotension).
- Discuss possibilities of continuing psychotherapy, a 12-step program (AA, Alanon, Alateen), or a transitional living program; arrange for a referral if patient is receptive.
- Initiate frequent staff conferences to share ideas of therapy, insights, and ventilate responses to client's manipulative or angry behavior.
- Develop a mutually agreed-upon "contract" for behavior change.

Evaluation: Client practices new coping behaviors; increases self-esteem, social skills; explores group support; initiates insight or behavioral therapy.

Goal 3: Client and family will accept the support of concerned others; will establish a life-style without alcohol.

Plan/Implementation

- Involve client in assertion therapy; involve in group therapy to help client recognize the impact of behavior on others.
- Reinforce contacts with 12-step programs and psychotherapy.
- Encourage new relationships that do not involve alcohol; be supportive during loss of old relationships.
- Permit family to express anger regarding patient's behavior; help them see their roles as enablers.
- Help family and staff understand that relapse is a strong possibility but does not mean failure or futility.
- Know that alcohol-dependent persons are susceptible to the adoption of other dependencies and developing "cross addictions."

Evaluation: Client and family attend therapy and support groups; client engages in and practices behaviors that decrease social isolation and strengthen new behaviors; family recognizes and decreases "enabling" behaviors.

☐ Drugs Other Than Alcohol

1. General Information

a. Opiates and opiate derivatives, synthetic opiates (e.g., morphine, Demerol, dilaudid, codeine, heroin): chronic abuse results in tolerance, physical dependence, habituation, and addiction

1) psychologically, most opiate addicts show a similarity to alcoholics in some aspects of their personality; they are emotionally immature, dependent, hostile, aggressive; and they take drugs to relieve inner tensions

2) opiate addicts sometimes differ from alcoholics in that they handle feelings passively, by avoidance rather than by acting out; choosing drugs (opiates) seems to suppress these inner tensions
3) availability (abuse may begin following surgery or illness), curiosity, and peer pressure play a role in the use of opiates; social factors, such as urban versus rural differences and social class, also play a role
4) cultural values regarding the use of opiates may play a role in the rates of addiction
   a) Asian countries in which opiate addiction has been tolerated have a high rate
   b) Western European counties, where opiate addiction is treated as a medical rather than a legal problem, have low rates
5) may be in methadone maintenance program as part of treatment and continue to misuse drugs

b. Barbiturates and other sedative drugs (e.g., Equanil, Librium, Doriden, Placidyl, Valium); if compulsively and chronically abused, cause tolerance, habituation, addiction, and physical dependence
1) there is a general, depressant, withdrawal syndrome associated with all of these drugs
2) many users of the sedative drugs began with a physician's prescription; prescription drugs are considered socially acceptable in western society for the relief of tension and insomnia
3) persons who become chronic and compulsive users of these drugs have a variety of underlying psychologic difficulties; they may be
   a) anxious or insecure
   b) trying to relieve hostile and aggressive impulses
   c) trying to escape tension through the drug's intoxicating effect
4) withdrawal must be managed gradually due to danger of seizures

c. Amphetamines and cocaine (see also reprint, page 142): have a stimulating effect upon the user
1) when these drugs are chronically and compulsively abused, they result in tolerance and habituation
2) when the drug is withdrawn, general fatigue and depression occur along with changes in sleep EEG; these symptoms are not considered a clinical withdrawal syndrome, and physical dependence is not associated with the abuse of these drugs
3) chronic use can result also in a toxic psychosis, characterized by vivid hallucinations and persecutory delusions
4) social, cultural, and psychologic factors have all been cited as causative: family history of alcoholism and psychopathology, availability, peer pressure, curiosity, and physician prescription; the use of these drugs by persons who are overweight or depressed is more socially acceptable than by those who take them for thrills
5) many amphetamine or cocaine addicts are also compulsive users of barbiturates, alcohol, or morphine

d. Hallucinogens (e.g., lysergic acid diethylamide [LSD], mescaline, PCP [angel dust], STP): produce tolerance, and in some persons, habituation
1) these agents do not produce physical dependence with its concomitant withdrawal syndrome or addiction
2) may produce acute panic and anxiety states and toxic psychosis, characterized by hallucinations and persecutory delusions
3) historically, these drugs were used in connection with religious practices of American and Mexican Indians
4) recently they have been used by persons who wish to explore their feelings in altered states of drug-induced intoxication
5) persons who abuse these drugs are thought to be psychologically insecure, dependent, hostile, and immature
6) social class seems to be a factor in the use of hallucinogens, with those in the middle or upper class being more frequent users

e. *DSM-III*-R classification: drug intoxication, drug withdrawal, personality disorder, drug dependence abuse

2. Nursing Process

a. Assessment/Analysis

1) physiologic problems: respiratory, circulatory, neurologic problems associated with withdrawal (priority); see Table 2.14
2) after emergency treatment, assess for problems arising from
   a) consequences of drugs

Table 2.14 Signs and Symptoms of Withdrawal and Overdose of Common Drugs of Abuse

Drugs	Overdose	Withdrawal
Narcotics		
Codeine	Shallow, slow breathing	Watery eyes, runny nose
Morphine	Clammy skin	Yawning
Meperidine	Pinpoint pupils	Anorexia
Heroin	Convulsions	Irritability, tremors, panic, insomnia
Methadone	Coma	Chills, sweating, gooseflesh
Hydromorphone	Death	Abdominal pain, nausea
Opium		
Stimulants		
Amphetamines	Agitation, panic	Apathy
Cocaine	Increase in body temperature	Fatigue, long periods of sleep
Preludin	Hallucinations, paranoia, violence	Irritability
Ritalin	Convulsions	Depression, suicidal
	Death	Disorientation
Depressants		
Barbiturates (Seconal, Tuinal, Nembutal, Phenobarbital)	Shallow breathing	Anxiety
	Cold, clammy skin	Insomnia
Methaqualone (Quaalude)	Dilated pupils	Tremors
Chloral hydrate	Weak, rapid pulse	Delirium
Doriden	Coma, death	Convulsions
Benzodiapines (Equinil, Librium,	Sedation	Death
Miltown, Valium, Serax, Tranxene)	Potentiates barbiturates and alcohol	Anxiety
		Poor muscle coordination, dizziness
Hallucinogenics and Cannabinoids		
PCP	Longer, more intense "bad trips"	No clinically significant effects
LSD	Psychosis, violence	Insomnia
Mescaline	Death	Hyperactivity
Marijuana	Fatigue	Decreased appetite
	Paranoia, confusion	
	Psychosis, depersonalization	

References: *Professional Guide to Drugs*, 1982.
Clinical Pharmacology and Nursing Management, 1983.
For further information: National Clearinghouse for Drug Abuse Information, P.O. Box 416, Kensington, MD 20795 (301) 443-6500.

From: Neal, M., Cohen, P., Reighley, J. *Nursing care planning guides, set 6*. Baltimore, Williams & Wilkins, 1986. Used with permission.

- nasal septum erosion (cocaine)
- potential seizures (cocaine, barbiturate withdrawal)
- tolerance

b) sepsis associated with drug injection
- abscesses of skin and subcutaneous fat deposits
- hepatitis
- septicemia

c) neglect of nutritional needs
- malnutrition
- loss of teeth, dental caries
- respiratory infections

3) behavior problems
a) denial and/or underreporting of use
b) somatic complaints
c) blaming others
d) anger, hostility, self-pity, mistrust
e) family, social employment, and financial problems
f) low frustration tolerance
g) criminal or "antisocial" behavior
h) grandiosity
i) high dependency needs
j) violence
k) suicidal attempts

4) pattern of drug use, family problems

b. Plans/Implementation and Evaluation

Goal 1: Client will withdraw from drug, free from respiratory failure, shock, toxic psychosis.

Plan/Implementation
- Intervene in respiratory failure: maintain a patent airway, give oxygen, administer naloxone hydrochloride (Narcan).
- Administer IV fluids for shock, as ordered.
- Assess the level of coma or stupor.
- Administer drugs, as ordered to suppress withdrawal or to counter a toxic psychosis.

- Give antibiotics as ordered.
- Restrain client as necessary for safety.

Evaluation: Client withdraws from drug; has patent airway; is free from signs of shock or toxic psychosis.

Goal 2: Client will decrease purposive drug-seeking, manipulative- and acting-out behavior.

Plan/Implementation

- Set firm and consistent limits.
- Clearly define acceptable and unacceptable behavior.
- Know that the client often will complain that a nurse who does not cooperate lacks trust.
- Be aware that the client may plead, cry, ask for money, steal, simulate drug withdrawal syndrome to obtain drugs.
- Have entire staff adopt consistent approach to client's behavior.

Evaluation: Client decreases purposeful drug-seeking and manipulative/acting-out behavior; accepts limits of unit.

Goal 3: Client will decrease intellectualization; will focus on problem solving and activities of daily living (ADL).

Plan/Implementation

- Know that client may exhibit dependency behaviors, blame parents, society, world conditions for drug-taking behaviors; be aware that client may try to involve nurse in intellectual discussion about the above, but do not discuss these with client.
- Keep focus on client's responsibility for own behavior; do not plead or exhort.
- Focus on problems in ADL and possible solutions.

Evaluation: Client discusses living problems and develops some solutions.

Goal 4: Client decreases denial and superficiality; explores alternative coping mechanisms; verbalizes some awareness of consequences of own actions.

Plan/Implementation

- Confront the client face to face with facts about self that client attempts to avoid; use only after foundation of trust and acceptance has been laid or when group relationship is cohesive.
- Avoid discussions of "why" client abuses drugs.
- Avoid nagging client to promise total rehabilitation; realistic approach to possibilities of success must be taken.
- Know that 90% of drug abusers relapse
  - the most effective treatment to date has been that given by former abusers (e.g., Narcotics Anonymous); having been in the situation, these persons are familiar with the demanding behaviors, manipulations, rationalizations, intellectualizations, and denial of drug abusers, and are able to handle them with firmness and with supportive concern; clients are less likely to "put one over" on them.
- Do not make moral judgments.
- Be aware of own rescue, angry or hostile feelings toward drug abusers; try to control your reactivity in client's presence.

Evaluation: Client decreases use of denial; begins to explore alternative coping; visits postdischarge treatment facility; decreases number and frequency of drug-abuse incidents.

References

Jacobs, P., & Stringer, G. (1983). The person who abuses substances. In R. Murray & M. Huelskvetter (Eds.), *Psychiatric nursing, mental health*. Englewood Cliffs, NJ: Prentice Hall.

†Powell, A. & Minick, M. (1988). Alcohol withdrawal syndrome. *American Journal of Nursing*, *88*, 312–315.

†Highly recommended.

Glossary

Terms Common to Psychiatric Nursing

Addiction: The compulsive use and procurement of chemical substances on which the individual has become dependent; has a high tendency to relapse after withdrawal.

Affect: The mood or emotion an individual shows in response to a given situation. Affect can be described, according to its expression, as appropriate, blunted, blocked, flat, inappropriate, or displaced.

Akathesia: A side effect of some antipsychotic drugs; motor restlessness, feeling of inner disquiet, inability to sit or lie quietly.

Ambivalence: The coexistence of two opposing feelings toward another person, object, or idea (examples: love-hate, pleasure-pain, like-dislike).

Anxiety: Apprehension, tension, or uneasiness that stems from the anticipation of danger, the source of which is largely unknown or unrecognized. Primarily of intrapsychic origin. May be pathologic when it interferes with effectiveness in living, achievement of desired goals or satisfactions, or reasonable emotional comfort.

Autism: Extreme withdrawal from the real world and preoccupation with idiosyncratic thoughts and fantasies.

Commitment Procedure: The legal procedure for admission to a psychiatric hospital. This procedure can be involuntary, compulsory, or emergency.

Confabulation: Defensive attempts to fill in details about the past that the client cannot recall because of memory loss. Imaginary experiences are often related in a detailed and plausible fashion.

Conflict: A psychoanalytic term describing the mental struggle that occurs when there are opposing impulses, drives, and demands of the id, ego, and superego.

Confusion: A cluster of behaviors related to cognitive impairment and characterized by inattention, disorientation, memory loss, loss of social skills, disruptive behaviors, noncompliance, and problems with self-care.

Countertransference: Arousal in the therapist of reactions toward the client based on unconscious feelings and attitudes.

Covert: Secret or hidden reasons for conscious actions or behavior.

Crisis Intervention Therapy: Brief psychiatric treatment in which individuals (and/or families) are assisted in their efforts to cope and problem solve in crisis situations. The treatment approach is immediate, supportive, and direct.

Delirium Tremens (DTs): A withdrawal syndrome precipitated in chronic alcoholics deprived of alcohol; associated with metabolic and nutritional disturbances. Early signs include restlessness, irritability, fear, and apprehension. Progression is to confusion, disorientation, illusions, hallucinations, and convulsions.

Delusion: A false belief or opinion that is unreasonable and causes distortion in judgment

a. delusion of grandeur: a false, grandiose, or expansive belief that one is a very important or powerful person or entity;

b. delusion of persecution: a false belief that one is victim of others' hostility and aggressiveness.

Depersonalization: Feelings of unreality or strangeness concerning either the environment or the self or both.

Double Bind: Interaction, generally associated with schizophrenic families, in which a message contains mutually contradictory signals. Best characterized by the ''damned if you do, damned if you don't'' situation.

Dystonia: May occur during first few days of antipsychotic drug therapy; acute tonic muscle spasms, most frequently involving tongue, jaw, eyes, and neck, but may involve whole body.

Ego: The part of the personality, according to Freudian theory, that mediates between the primitive, pleasure-seeking instinctual drives of the id and the self-critical, prohibitive, restraining forces of the superego. Functions to resolve intrapsychic conflict by keeping thoughts, interpretations, judgments, and behavior practical and efficient. The ego, directed by the reality principle, is the contact with the real world.

Extrapyramidal Reaction: The usually reversible side effect of some major psychotropic drugs on the extrapyramidal system of the CNS. Characterized by a variety of physical signs and symptoms (similar to those seen in clients with Parkinson's disease) including muscular rigidity, tremors, drooling, restlessness, shuffling gait, blurred vision, and other neurologic disturbances.

Family Therapy: Treatment of more than one member of the family simultaneously in the same session. The treatment may be supportive, directive, or interpretive. The assumption is that a mental disorder in one member of a family may be a manifestation of a disorder in other members and in their interrelationships and functioning as a total group.

Flight of Ideas: A disturbance in the progression of thought characterized by an increased associative activity, a rapid digression from one idea to another with no progress toward the goal idea.

Group Therapy: Application of psychotherapeutic techniques by one or more therapists to a group of persons who have similar problems and are in reasonably good contact with reality. The optimal size of a group is 6–10 members.

Hallucination: A sensory perception that occurs without an external stimulus. It can be associated with any of the five senses although auditory, visual, or tactile are most common. Usually occurs in psychotic disorders but can occur in both chronic and acute organic brain disorders.

Id: In Freudian theory, the id is the reservoir of psychic energy. It is guided by the pleasure principle, curbed by the ego, and is unconscious. The id wants what it wants when it wants it.

Ideas of Reference: False interpretation of external events and incidents as having direct reference to the self.

Illusion: A misinterpretation of the sensory stimuli, usually auditory or visual, or a real experience.

Incompetence: A legal decision that the client cannot successfully manage aspects of own daily living; results in loss of many civil rights; reversible only by another court hearing.

Insight: The ability of a person to understand self and the basis for emotions, attitudes, and behavior.

Interpersonal: All that occurs between persons, e.g., spoken words, gestures, looks, changes in body positions, expressions of emotion such as laughing, crying, etc.

Intrapsychic: All that takes place within the mind (psyche).

Lability: Unpredictable, frequent mood changes.

Latent: Feelings, drives, and emotions that influence behavior but remain repressed, outside of conscious thought or action.

Limit Setting: A clear enunciation of the rules of behavior and social relationships and the point beyond which going is forbidden, and a consistent enforcement of the rules.

Loose associations: Communication that does not have clear connections between thoughts.

Manipulation: A skillful handling, control, or management of others' behavior or of a situation for one's own purposes.

Mental status examination: A structured assessment of all aspects of an individual's mental functioning; includes physical, emotional, cognitive, and social functioning.

Milieu: The immediate environment, both physical and social.

Narcissism: Self-love; excessive interest in one's own appearance, comfort, importance, abilities, etc. In Freudian theory, arrest at the first stage of development in which the self is the object of all attention and pleasure.

Neologism: A new word that is invented or made up by condensing other words into a new one; used by patient typically in schizophrenia.

Neurosis: An impairment of personality development and growth characterized by excessive use of energy for unproductive purposes. The chief symptom is anxiety, which is either felt directly or controlled by various psychologic mechanisms to produce other, subjectively distressing symptoms. Although in some of its forms and degrees it is incapacitating, it does not interfere with the person's contact with reality.

Orientation: Ability to correctly identify and relate self to time, place, and person.

Overt: Open, conscious, and unhidden actions, behavior, and emotions.

Paranoid: Unwarranted suspiciousness and distrust of others.

Personality: The characteristic way in which a person behaves; the deeply ingrained pattern of behavior that each person evolves, both consciously and unconsciously, as a style of life or way of being in adapting to the environment.

Phobia: An irrational, persistent, obsessive, intense fear of an object or situation, which results in increased anxiety and tension and interference with the person's normal functioning.

Psychoanalysis: A form of psychotherapy developed by Freud, based on his theories of personality development and disorder. Involves an examination of the free associations of a client and the interpretation of client's dreams, emotions, and behavior. Its focus is mainly on the way the ego handles the id tensions. Psychoanalysis is a lengthy treatment concerned only with the intrapsychic processes of the individual. Success is measured by the degree of insight the client is able to gain into the unconscious motivations of his or her behavior.

Psychodrama: A form of group psychotherapy, developed by Moreno, in which clients dramatize their emotional problems. By assuming roles in order to act out their conflicts, they reveal repressed feelings that have been disturbing to them.

Psychodynamics: The usually unconscious forces that are presumed to be at work in a person that result in particular behaviors.

Psychogenic: Implies the causative factors of a symptom or illness are mental rather than organic.

Psychosis: A major mental illness characterized by any of the following symptoms: loss of contact with or a denial of reality, bizarre thinking and behavior, delusions, hallucinations, regression, and disorientation. Intrapsychically, it results from the unconscious becoming conscious and taking over control of the person. In psychosis, the ego is overwhelmed by the id and the superego.

Psychotherapy: The treatment of mental disorders or psychosomatic conditions by psychologic methods using a variety of approaches including psychoanalysis, group therapy, family therapy, psychodrama, hypnotism, simple counseling, and suggestion.

Reality: The way things acutally are.

Schizophrenogenic: The object or situation that is thought to be causative in the development of schizophrenia.

Significant Others: The meaningful persons in one's life, usually parents and siblings, spouse, guardians, extended family, close friends.

Stressor: Any stimulus that produces a state of tension and is perceived by the person as being challenging, harmful, or threatening.

Superego: In Freudian personality theory, the part of the psyche that guides and restrains, criticizes and punishes, just as the parents did when the individual was a child. It is unconscious and it is learned. Like the id, the superego also wants it own way. It has a conscious component called the conscience.

Tardive dyskinesia: Choreiform or athetoid movements resulting from long-term use of antipsychotic drugs; typical movements are tongue writhing or protrusion, chewing, lip puckering, toe and ankle movements, leg jiggling, and movements of neck, trunk, and pelvis.

Therapist: A person who, by reasons of training and experience and knowledge, is able and willing to use skills to assist clients in the recovery and maintenance of health.

Transference: In Freudian theory, a carrying over and attaching to the therapist unconscious feelings and attitudes that the client has toward family or significant others.

Unconscious: The repository of those mental processes of which the individual is unaware. The repressed feelings and their energy are stored in the unconscious and directly influence the individual's behavior.

Word Salad: A jumbled mixture of words and phrases that have no meaning and are illogical in their sequence. Seen most often in schizophrenia, e.g., "backter dyce tonked up snorfel blend."

References

American Psychiatric Association. (1985). *A psychiatric glossary*. Washington, DC: Author.

Beck, C.K., Rawlins, R.P., & Williams, S.R. (1988). *Mental-health psychiatric nursing: A holistic life-cycle approach*. St. Louis: Mosby.

Stuart, G.W., & Sundeen, S.J. (1987). *Principles and practices of psychiatric nursing*. St. Louis: Mosby.

Bibliography

*Acee, A.M., & Smith, D. (1987). Crack. *American Journal of Nursing*, *87*, 614–617.

Barry, P. (1984). *Psychosocial nursing assessment and intervention*. Philadelphia: Lippincott.

Burgess, A. (1984). *Psychiatric nursing in the hospital and the community* (4th ed.) Englewood Cliffs, NJ: Prentice-Hall.

*Campbell, E., Williams, M.L., & Meynarczyk, S. (1986). After the fall—confusion. *American Journal of Nursing*, *86*, 151–154.

Campbell, J., & Humphries, J. (1984). *Nursing care of victims of family violence*. Reston, VA: Reston.

Campbell, L. (1986). Depression: Acute care in the hospital. *American Journal of Nursing*, *86*, 288–291.

Carpenito, L. (1983). *Nursing diagnosis: Application to clinical practice*. Philadelphia: Lippincott.

Cook, J., & Fontaine, K. (Eds.). *Essentials of mental health nursing*. Menlo Park, CA: Addison-Wesley.

Crockett, M. (1986). Depression: A case of anger and alienation. *American Journal of Nursing*, *86*, 294–298.

Cushing, M. (1986). The legal side: how the courts look at nursing practice acts. *American Journal of Nursing*, *86*, 131–132.

Davis, M., Eshelman, R., & McKay, M. (1980). *The relaxation and stress reduction workbook*. Richmond, CA: New Harbinger.

Dawson, P. et al. (1986). Preventing excess disability in patients with Alzheimer's disease. *Geriatric Nursing*, *7*, 298–301.

*DeGennaro, M., et al. (1980). Antidepressant drug therapy. *American Journal of Nursing*, *80*, 1304–1310.

*DiMotto, J. (1984). Relaxation. *American Journal of Nursing*, *84*, 754–758.

DiNitto, D., et al. (1986). After rape: Who should examine rape survivors. *American Journal of Nursing*, *86*, 538–540.

Ebersole, P. & Hess, P. (1985). Toward healthy aging: Human needs and nursing responses. St. Louis: Mosby.

Griffin, M. (1986). In the mind's eye. *American Journal of Nursing*, *86*, 804–806.

*Harris, E. (1981). Antipsychotic medications. *American Journal of Nursing*, *81*, 1316–1323.

*——. (1981). Lithium. *American Journal of Nursing*, *81*, 1310–1315.

*——. (1981). Extrapyramidal side effects of antipsychotic medications. *American Journal of Nursing*, *81*, 1324–1328.

*——. (1981). Sedative-hypnotic drugs. *American Journal of Nursing*, *81*, 1329–1334.

*——. (1986). Drugs and depression. *American Journal of Nursing*, *86*, 292–293.

Hays, A. & Borger, F. (1985). A test in time. *American Journal of Nursing*, *85*, 1107–1111.

*Horsley, G.C. Baggage from the past. *American Journal of Nursing*, *88*, 60–63.

Janosik, E.H., & Davies, J.L. (1986). *Psychiatric mental health nursing*. Monterey, CA: Jones and Bartlett.

Johnson, B. (1986). *Psychiatric-mental health nursing: Adaptation and growth*. Philadelphia: Lippincott.

Kendrick, D.W. & Wilber, G. (1986). When in seclusion. . . . *American Journal of Nursing*, *86*, 1117.

Lessing, D.Z. (1987). Home care for psychiatric problems. *American Journal of Nursing*, *87*, 1317–1320.

Mathewson, M. (1986). *Pharmacotherapeutics: A nursing process approach*. Philadelphia: Davis.

Mittleman, R., Goldberg, H., & Waksman, D. (1983). Preserving evidence in the emergency department. *American Journal of Nursing*, *83*, 1652–1656.

Murray, R., & Huelskoetter, M. (1983). *Psychiatric/mental health nursing: Giving emotional care*. Englewood Cliffs, NJ: Prentice-Hall.

Neal, M., Cohen, P., & Cooper, P. (1980). *Nursing care planning guides, set 1* (2nd ed.). Baltimore: Williams & Wilkins.

——. (1980). *Nursing care planning guides, set 2* (2nd ed.). Baltimore: Williams & Wilkins.

Neal, M., Cohen, P., & Reighley, J. (1983). *Nursing care planning guides, set 3* (2nd ed.). Baltimore: Williams & Wilkins.

——. (1983). *Nursing care planning guides, set 4* (2nd ed.). Baltimore: Williams & Wilkins.

Neal, M., Cohen, P. & Reighley, J. (1986). *Nursing care planning guides, set 6*. Baltimore: Williams & Wilkins.

Pajik, M. (1984). Alzheimer's disease: Inpatient care. *American Journal of Nursing*, *84*, 215–222.

Pasquali, E., Alesi, E., Arnold, H., & De Basio, N. (1985). *Mental health nursing: A bio-psycho-cultural approach* (2nd ed.). St. Louis: Mosby.

Peterson, M. (1972). Understanding defense mechanisms (programmed instruction). *American Journal of Nursing*, *72* (9)(Supp), 1–24.

Plaum, M. (1986). Understanding the final message of the dying. *Nursing 86*, *16* (6), 26–29.

Potts, N. (1984). Eating disorders: The secret pattern of binge/purge. *American Journal of Nursing*, *84*, 33–35.

Ronsman, K. (1988). Pseudodementia. *Geriatric Nursing*, 50–52.

Shapira, J., Schesinger, R., & Cummings, J. (1986). Distinguishing dementias. *American Journal of Nursing*, *86*, 698–702.

Sanger, E., & Cassino, T. (1984). Eating disorders: avoiding the power struggle. *American Journal of Nursing*, *84*, 30–33.

Wilson, H., & Kneisl, C. (1987). *Psychiatric nursing* (3rd ed). Menlo Park, CA: Addison–Wesley.

*See Reprint section

Reprints
Nursing Care of the Client with Psychosocial, Mental Health/Psychiatric Problems

Horsley, G. "Baggage from the Past"
Harris, E. "Lithium"
DeMotto, J. "Relaxation"
Harris, E. "Extrapyramidal Side Effects of Antipsychotic Medications"
Harris, E. "Antipsychotic Medications"
Harris, E. "Drugs and Depression"
Campbell, E., William, M., & Mlymarcyk, S. "After the Fall—Confusion"
Harris, E. "Sedative-Hypnotic Drugs"
Hoff, L. & Resing, M. "Was This Suicide Preventable"
Acee, A. & Smith, P. "Crack"

BAGGAGE FROM THE PAST

BY GLORIA C. HORSLEY

One in five of your patients may suffer from unresolved grief. Here's how a psych nurse consult can help.

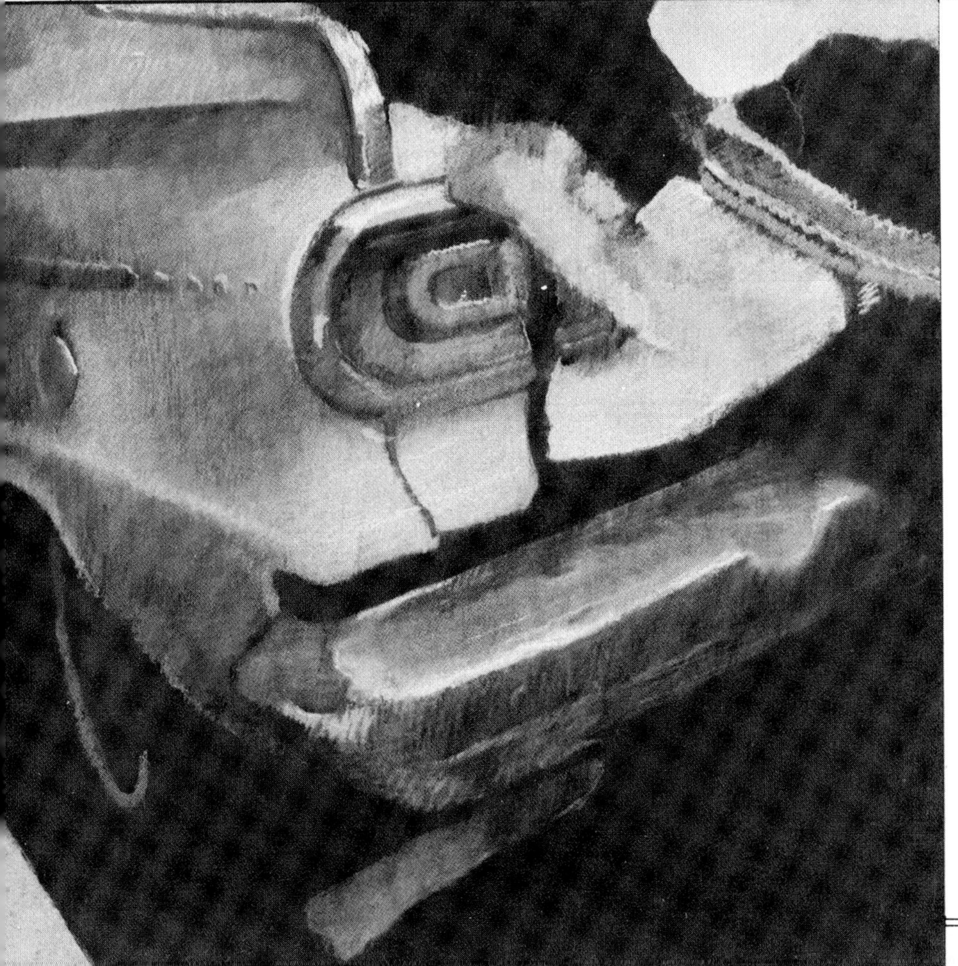

We all carry it around, but when a patient checks into the hospital with baggage from the past, his reaction to the smallest problem can be unexpectedly intense—and can threaten recovery.

In two years as the psychiatric liaison nurse for a 200-bed surgical service, I received 175 requests for consultation from staff nurses. Often, the reason prompting the request was a patient's demanding behavior—"always on the call button"—or oversensitivity to apparently insignificant events. But, for one of every five patients, the real problem was a compound crisis: the present trauma had crashed into some past, unresolved loss.

For the hospitalized person still grieving over past losses, the bur-

Gloria C. Horsley, RN, MS, is a family therapist in private practice in Pittsford, NY, and a PhD candidate in child and family studies at Syracuse (NY) University.

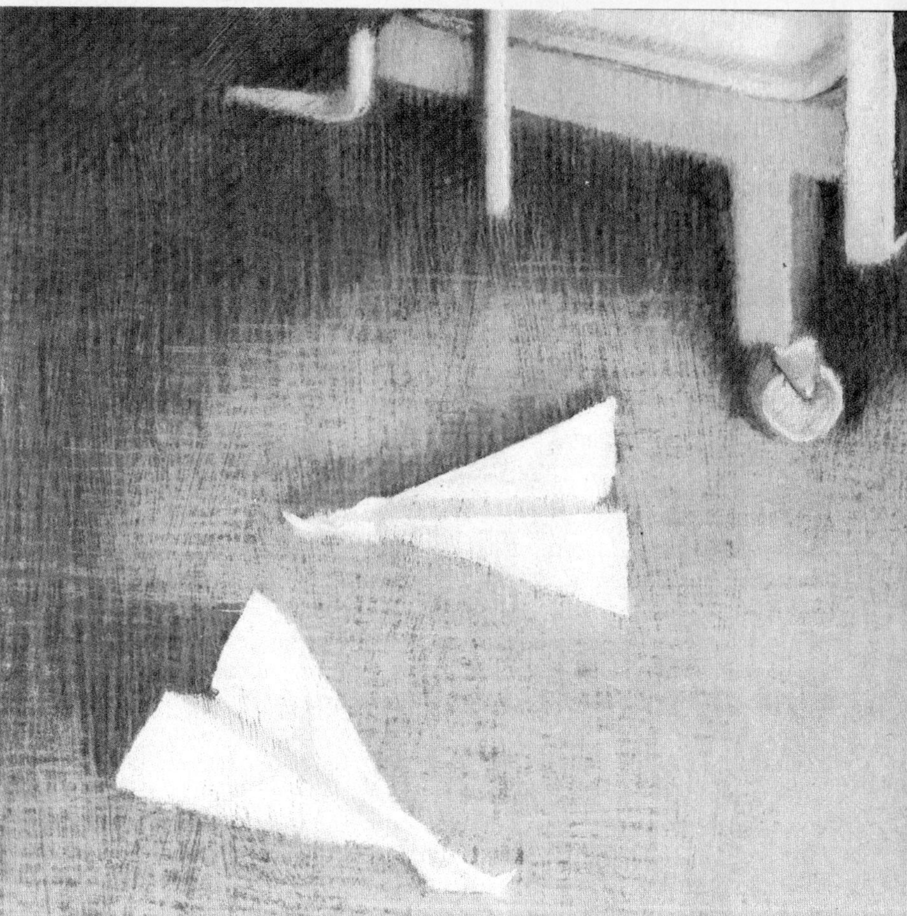

den of the current crisis drains the energy needed for recuperation. Physical pain, fear, and medication all can weaken the psychological defenses, allowing feelings about an earlier loss to surface(1). The grieving person may express these feelings indirectly, through fragmented sleep and disturbing dreams, or directly, by constant demands for attention and complaints that his needs are not met promptly. A grieving patient can be quick to anger and can have spells of crying or depression.

"NOT JUST *THIS* CAR ACCIDENT"

Ms. D, for instance, a 26-year-old orthopaedic patient, was "crying a good part of the day," said the nurses who requested a psychiatric nursing consultation.

Seven days before the consultation, she had had surgery for internal injuries sustained in a car accident. Her pain was only partially relieved by meperidine (Demerol). My first thought was that Ms. D might have caused the accident, but she denied this and said she was hit by a drunken driver.

I asked Ms. D to review the accident with me. In our discussion Ms. D said that, when she was 11, her mother had been killed when her car was hit by a truck. As she spoke of her mother's death she wept, and said that, as in her own accident, the driver hadn't even tried to avoid hitting them.

I encouraged her to identify the similarities in her feelings after the two accidents. We discussed her anger with the drivers and her anger toward her father for putting her into a foster home.

At the time of her mother's death, her grandmother told her that as the eldest of three children she must be strong and not cry. Ms. D was not allowed then to grieve openly for the loss of her mother and her home.

Ms. D described recurrent dreams since childhood of her mother trapped in the car, of looking through the window at her mother's bleeding body, and of being unable to open the car door or scream for help. We worked on *reality testing* around this dream. In doing this, we discussed the actual details Ms. D remembered and compared them to her dream. Ms. D said she felt guilty and helpless in her present circumstances, as she had when she was a child.

Before her injury, Ms. D was a responsible person who held a full-time job and handled the family's financial problems. Her husband, who managed a small grocery store, seemed angry and helpless when he visited her. He made heavy demands, asking Ms. D to make financial decisions. He was frustrated and confused by her childlike behavior. When Mr. D asked for some decision, Ms. D would say, "I can't think now." She whined constantly about the pain, folded her arms, put her legs over the side of the bed, and rocked back and forth.

To intervene, the staff and I told Ms. D that she need not be as strong as she had been after her mother's accident. We agreed to reassure and to comfort her when she expressed frustration over her situation.

In response to this supportive approach, Ms. D regained some of her ego defenses and became slightly less agitated. By the time I had my third session with her, Ms. D asked that we deal with her present crisis, because this now seemed more important.

During my subsequent visits to the unit, Ms. D and the staff were working together in an increasingly productive manner. She was requiring less pain medicine and the staff supported her emotional needs. Because she still had many issues to resolve, I suggested that she consider seeking further professional help after discharge. She agreed to do so.

"I WON'T BE NURSED BY A MAN"

Mr. J, 69, was depressed and anxious, according to the ICU staff. His refusal to be nursed by a man also was a problem.

Mr. J had had a coronary bypass. One week after surgery, complications developed that required surgical debridement of his sternum.

Two weeks after the debridement, when I visited, Mr. J was in severe pain and had difficulty breathing. Nevertheless, he was bright and cheerful for a man in extreme distress and talked will-

STEPHEN JOHNSON

ingly about his career in banking.

When asked why he had refused care from a man, Mr. J's voice flattened and tears welled in his eyes. He said the nurse reminded him of his son. Further questioning revealed that two of his three sons had died in separate airplane crashes in the past 10 years.

He was feeling special guilt over the son who died when he was 17, who was killed while flying with a group of exchange students. Against his wife's wishes, Mr. J had urged his son to go on this trip. Mr. J recalled how he and his wife had heard of the fatal crash on the evening news.

The other son died at the age of 24, several years after the first accident. He went down in a small plane and was lost for three days.

Mr. J's brother was with the search party that found the body. The following year, Mr. J's brother died of cancer. "I never thanked my brother for finding Ned and bringing his body home," the patient cried bitterly.

Mr. J had never talked to anyone about these three deaths. He saw himself as a strong, silent man who should not exhibit grief.

Now his coping mechanisms were seriously compromised by fear of death and by weakness from anemia and dyspnea. (I have often found that patients who have low hematocrits sometimes think they are on the brink of losing control.) Thoughts of his sons were emerging into his consciousness—why now, Mr. J wondered.

I suggested that the presence of the nurse, a young man, triggered these thoughts. When I pointed out that Mr. J's emotional reactions were understandable in view of his pain, low oxygen level, and two surgeries—and that this was a *temporary* loss of control—Mr. J was greatly relieved.

After Mr. J identified the connection between his past losses and present anxiety, he began dealing with some of his pain at the loss of his sons and brother. Encouraged to explore his feelings, Mr. J developed a more tolerable level of recall and expressed sorrow and a sense of loss.

Several days after this one visit, Mr. J left the ICU. He was much less anxious, said he was sleeping better, and looked forward to returning home. The staff confirmed his more rested and relaxed state.

Several men nursed Mr. J after he left the ICU. His last nurse before discharge had the same name as Mr. J's deceased youngest son. Mr. J was able to point out the fact without becoming upset. Two weeks after the ICU consultation, Mr. J went home. He seemed willing to seek follow-up with a therapist to continue to work through his grief and loss.

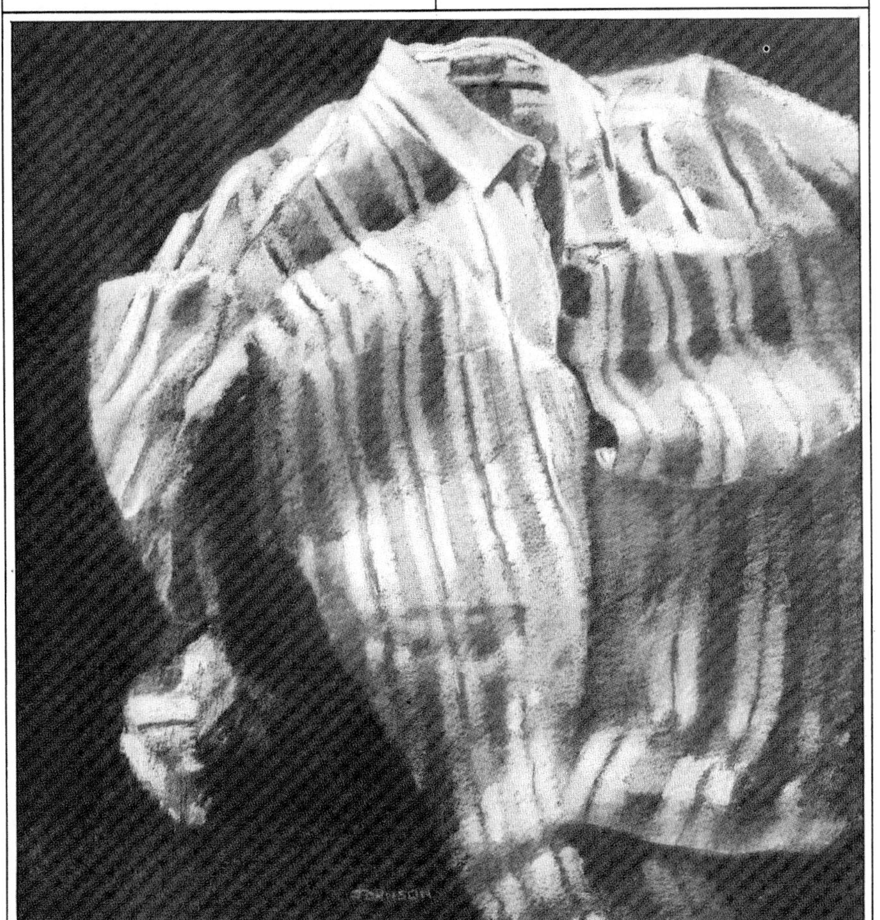

"CAN I SAVE MYSELF?"

Mr. T was described as a "frightened, depressed 23-year-old" by the staff who requested psychiatric nursing consultation.

Shot in the stomach two weeks earlier by the ex-husband of his girlfriend, Mr. T twice underwent surgery to control bleeding. He was in pain and frightened that he would bleed again and that the assailant would come to the hospital to kill him. His girlfriend spent most days with him, but they hardly talked. Mr. T had one dream over and over, he said. He couldn't get it out of his mind and was having trouble sleeping. The dream was about trying—unsuccessfully—to save a dying man.

I asked Mr. T whether his current emotional state might be connected to any past trauma. He said that when he was 16, he was walking home from school and saw a group of children by a pond. The children said a man had fallen into the water, so Mr. T quickly took off his shirt and shoes, dove in, pulled the man out, and started mouth-to-mouth resuscitation. The man did not respond.

Mr. T said he would never forget the terrible feeling of realizing that

A FRAMEWORK FOR HANDLING PAST GRIEF

The phenomenon of present grief complicated by unresolved grief is not new. When dealing with reactive conflicts that center on delayed grief, the Lindemann, Worden, and Caplan models of grief resolution can be useful(3-5). These specify that the patient must share the grief, verbalize feelings of guilt, accept the pain of bereavement, experience fear of insanity and change in feelings, express sorrow and a sense of loss, find an acceptable level of recall, and formulate a future relationship to the deceased.

Lindemann described typical behaviors of patients whose present grief stems from an earlier loss:

- ☐ Intense, fresh grief provoked by any mention of the loss.
- ☐ Minor events triggering intense grief.
- ☐ Unwillingness to move material possessions of the deceased person.
- ☐ Physical symptoms like those of the deceased occurring at the anniversary of the death.
- ☐ Depression, sadness, fixation on illness.
- ☐ Radical changes in life-style, usually within the first year or two(3).

Patients grieving only for present losses—the loss of a limb, sight, or hearing, or changes in body image, body function, or family relationships—tend to show many of the same signs as those with unresolved grief. A careful assessment of past history, however, usually will reveal no significant early death of family members or friends or traumatic events. When early losses have occurred these patients are able to discuss them with an appropriate range of emotions.

Patients dealing only with immediate loss tend to think of the future and to be extremely anxious about such issues as independent living. Patients with unresolved grief, on the other hand, are unable to work through the past losses and may show signs of depression or of giving up.

The thought or feeling (precipitant) aroused by the current trauma somehow evokes a past conflict or loss. To identify these and explore psychodynamic issues, the Burgess and Baldwin model is useful(1). Using this model, the patient can be encouraged to examine the crisis to look for clues to the precipitant. You can search with the patient for similarities between the past and present experiences. Find out which old memories, feelings, or thoughts might have emerged, unexplained, into consciousness.

To assess present coping responses and precrisis functioning, identify with the patient and family his past emotional style, support systems, and communication skills.

Finally, offer recommendations for interventions that are time-limited and directed toward restoring the patient to healthy emotional functioning. Keep the focus on the stressor rather than on the patient.

---

the man was his next-door neighbor and that he was dead. Mr. T discussed the recent fears of his own death, as well as his revulsion and despair at having given mouth-to-mouth resuscitation to a corpse. He voiced anger, fear, and frustration at his inability to save the neighbor, and could identify these same feelings about his present situation—he feared he would be unable to save himself from being shot again.

It took only one interview for Mr. T to see how his past trauma was interfering with his present ability to cope. He quickly lost his discomfort about the drowning and focused on the current crisis.

Mr. T's quick resolution of his past grief points out how the length and intensity of grief work is influenced by the patient's relationship to the deceased(2). The neighbor was not highly significant in Mr. T's life. He needed to resolve the event rather than to find an acceptable level of recall.

Having dealt with the event, Mr. T reestablished his usual coping mechanisms and focused his energy on current problems.

He asked that I see him at a time when his girlfriend would not be present. At this visit, he discussed his fear of her ex-husband, who was free on bail. Mr. T felt greatly relieved when staff suggested taking his name off the room door and telling the admitting desk not to give out his room number.

On future visits, I found Mr. T increasingly open and verbal. By the time of discharge, three weeks later, Mr. T had decided to end his relationship with his girlfriend because he believed that as long as he maintained it his life would be in danger. He planned to move to his parents' home until he was well enough to get an apartment. Encouraged by his improving health, he was eager to return to work.

All patients in crisis do not respond as constructively as these patients did. In general, however, I have found that the grieving hospitalized patient can begin to deal with past losses in even one to three sessions lasting 20 minutes to an hour. As his defenses recover, the patient is able to summon the energy to begin coping with the present crisis.

Crisis intervention takes time, which busy staff often lack. And the interviewing and psychotherapeutic skills to render effective therapy require training. To attempt crisis intervention without adequate training can harm the patient by stimulating feelings of guilt or personal invasion.

It is best for staff nurses to collaborate closely with a psychiatric nurse specialist when encouraging patients to vent feelings. Nurse-to-nurse consultation often can improve the care of these patients and help them resolve their grief.

REFERENCES

1. Burgess, A. W., and Baldwin, B. *Crisis Intervention Theory and Practice: A Clinical Handbook.* Englewood Cliffs, NJ, Prentice-Hall, 1981.
2. Engel, G. L. Grief and grieving. *Am.J.Nurs.* 64:93-98, Sept. 1964.
3. Lindemann, E. Symptomatology and management of acute grief. *Am.J.Psychiatry* 101:141-148, Sept. 1944.
4. Worden, W. J. *Grief Counseling and Grief Therapy: A Handbook for the Mental Health Practitioner.* New York, Springer Publishing Co., 1982.
5. Caplan, G. *Principles of Preventive Psychiatry.* New York, Basic Books, 1964.

Lithium

Reprinted from American Journal of Nursing, July 1981

By Elizabeth Harris

Lithium is the treatment of choice for the short-term management of the manic phase of bipolar disorder (DSM III terminology for what was formerly called manic-depressive illness), and for long-term prophylaxis for bipolar disorder. Lithium is approved by the FDA for only these two uses.

The drug is dramatically effective when it works, and does not produce the sedation or "chemical straitjacket" effect of the antipsychotics. In addition, it causes no known long-range harm as do the antipsychotics.

Lithium is the lightest known solid element. It exists in its natural form as a salt and is also manufactured for patient use as a salt. It is easily absorbed after oral administration, reaching peak serum levels in one to three hours. The body does not metabolize lithium: it exists in the body as an ion and is distributed evenly throughout the total body water compartment. It is not bound to protein. Lithium is excreted by the kidneys, where it competes with sodium for reabsorption in the proximal tubules. The mechanism of therapeutic action is, as yet, unknown, but there are many theories currently under investigation.

In patients with bipolar disorder, lithium is 80 percent effective in treating the manic phase. When used prophylactically, it decreases the frequency or diminishes the intensity of the manic relapses. It is slightly less effective in preventing depressive relapses, so that often tricyclic or MAO inhibitor antidepressants must be added to the patient's regimen. Patients who have rapid cycling (four or more episodes per year) are less likely to respond favorably to lithium.

For patients who have recurrent episodes of depression without intervening episodes of mania or hypomania (unipolar depressed patients), the treatments of choice are antidepressants or ECT. But, from recent studies, statistics show that lithium may be equally effective. Depressed patients with the following characteristics are thought to be as likely to respond to lithium as to antidepressants or ECT:

- history of mild hypomania
- family history of bipolar disorder
- cyclothymic personality (a chronic mood disturbance with numerous periods of mild depression and hypomania)
- history of postpartal depression
- hypersomnia or hyperphagia
- early age of onset of illness with recurrent cyclical depressions that are not related to environmental events
- endogenous symptom patterns associated with one or more of the above.

Schizoaffective disorder is a nonspecific DSM III term for conditions with some features of schizophrenia and some features of affective illness. Patients with this diagnosis do less well with lithium than patients with a clear-cut bipolar disorder, but enough respond that these patients are often given a trial with lithium.

Studies with alcoholic patients have shown lithium to be useful in some who are primarily depressed and may drink to alleviate their depression. Lithium, however, has not been shown to be useful in alcoholic patients who are not primarily depressed.

Several investigators have reported that violent acting-out behavior decreases significantly when patients who exhibit these behavioral disorders receive lithium. These studies suggest that lithium maintenance may help certain nonpsychotic patients with the following characteristics:

- extreme, rapid reactions to slight provocation with anger or violence
- inability to reflect on actions before acting
- inability to control rage once it has erupted.

In 1972, Rifkin reported that patients with emotionally unstable character disorder respond to lithium maintenance. These are adolescent patients with chronic maladaptive behavior patterns, such as poor acceptance of reasonable authority, truancy, poor work history, and manipulativeness. The core problem seems to be brief mood swings from depression to hypomania that last hours to days. These mood swings are not usually related to environmental or interpersonal events, but seem to occur on their own schedule. In these patients, lithium is thought to stabilize mood and, therefore, decrease the need for maladaptive behavior in response to the mood swings.

Guidelines for Use

Because of its narrow therapeutic index, lithium is considered a potentially dangerous drug. The amount of drug that is therapeutic is only slightly less than the amount that produces toxicity. This is compounded by the fact that no two patients respond alike to lithium or absorb or excrete it at exactly the same rate. The dose requirement for one patient may be two times the lethal dose for another. The dosage is adjusted by measuring serum levels and by observing for clinical signs of toxicity. Before a patient receives lithium, he should have baseline studies of renal, thyroid, cardiac, and electrolyte status.

Lithium is available in the United States as tablets or capsules of 300 mg. of lithium carbonate (Lithane, Lithonate, Lithotabs, Eskalith). It is also available in liquid form as lithium citrate. In this form, 5 cc. equals 8 mEq., which is the equivalent of 300 mg. of lithium carbonate. This form is useful for patients who cannot swallow tablets or capsules. There is no parenteral form.

Because lithium is rapidly absorbed, with peak effects in one to three hours and a narrow therapeutic index, it must be given in at least two divided doses daily. There are some long-acting or slow-release forms available, but so far these have been shown to offer no advantage over the short-acting forms(1).

Patients are usually started on

Side Effects and Toxicity of Lithium

Level	Symptoms
Mild below 1.5 mEq./1.	metallic taste in the mouth fine hand tremor (resting) nausea polyuria polydipsia diarrhea or loose stools muscular weakness or fatigue
Moderate 1.5-2.5 mEq./1.	severe diarrhea nausea and vomiting mild to moderate ataxia incoordination dizziness, sluggishness, giddiness, vertigo slurred speech tinnitus blurred vision increasing tremor muscle irritability or twitching asymmetrical deep tendon reflexes increased muscle tone
Toxicity 2.5-7.0 mEq./1.	nystagmus coarse tremor dysarthria fasciculations visual or tactile hallucinations oliguria, anuria confusion impaired consciousness dyskinesias—chorea, athetoid movements grand mal convulsions coma death

900 to 1,200 mg. per day in divided doses. Geriatric patients receive lower doses. Dosages are raised slowly in increments of 300 mg. until symptoms remit or toxicity occurs. During this time, serum lithium levels are tested two or three times a week until the blood level is stable. Patients' symptoms usually respond at levels of 0.8 mEq./l. to 1.5 mEq./l. (toward the high end of the range in mania), though this is quite variable. Some patients have responded best at 0.4 mEq./l., while others do not respond until they are over 1.5 mEq./l.

Blood for serum levels is always drawn in the morning, 10 to 14 hours after the last dose of lithium, to standardize measurement. If blood is drawn at any other time, or if the patient mistakenly takes his morning dose before his blood is drawn, the level will be erroneous and must be reported as such.

Once a therapeutic serum level is attained, it takes 7 to 10 days for a clinical response. If the patient is unmanageable during this lag period, it is usual practice to treat the patient with an antipsychotic drug until the lithium begins to take effect. After the initial clinical response, it takes another week or two for the patient to return to his normal mood state. If the manic patient shows no clinical response to the lithium after three weeks with adequate blood levels, he is then considered to be refractory to lithium.

Once the patient's symptoms are in control and he has returned to a normal mood state, he may be continued on lithium maintenance. Patients with bipolar or unipolar disorder are usually not maintained unless they have had at least two major affective episodes. It is only patients with recurrent, disruptive, cyclical relapses who should be subjected to the cost, inconvenience, and risks of long-term chemotherapy. If the decision is made to maintain a patient, his serum level is usually dropped to somewhere between 0.7 and 1.0 mEq./l. (approximately 600 to 1,500 mg of lithium carbonate), where his psychiatric symptoms are controlled, and few side effects are present.

Manic patients usually require a considerably lower dose once their mania is controlled. If the dose is not reduced as soon as the symptoms remit, the patient will often begin to show signs of toxicity, as his lithium level rises in response to his decreasing tolerance for it. Once the patient is on a stable maintenance dose, serum levels are tested less frequently, and finally tested every three months. Some patients maintained on lithium continue to have episodes of depression or, less often, of mania, but the episodes are less frequent and less intense. Only 20 percent of compliant patients show no change in severity over time. Patients who do respond will find that their response is better the longer they take lithium. Relapses become very infrequent or cease altogether.

There are no clear guidelines about how long to continue maintenance treatment, but some clinicians suggest that a patient who remains symptom free for three to five years should be given a trial off lithium.

Side Effects and Toxicity

Most patients will experience side effects. They include a fine resting tremor of the hands; nausea or slight abdominal discomfort; polyuria; thirst; mild diarrhea; muscle weakness or fatigue; and edema of the feet, hands, abdominal wall, or face. These may begin as early as two hours after the first dose and usually occur as isolated symptoms. Most side effects occur at therapeutic serum levels, and most subside in the first few weeks of treatment; some will resolve only to recur periodically throughout the course of treatment.

All side effects are reversible and fairly innocuous, though they may be quite distressing to the patient. Most of these effects are best treated with the reassurance that they will probably stop after a few weeks. If the effects persist, they can be treated by decreasing the lithium dose, by omitting several doses, or by temporarily discontinuing the drug. If nausea is the main problem, it can usually be treated by giving the drug with meals. If the polyuria is severe, but less than three liters per day, it should be considered within normal limits. If the tremors persist, and the patient must have fine motor coordination for his work, he may respond to propranolol (Inderal), 20 to 120 mg./day in divided doses.

If the patient's side effects begin to occur in clusters or gradually progress, this may be a sign of developing toxicity. Fortunately, when toxicity occurs, it usually occurs in a progressive fashion, so that it can often be detected before it becomes harmful to the patient (see table, at left). Certainly, if the patient complains of one or more of these symptoms, it is wise to inquire about them and examine the patient for the full range of symptoms.

Toxicity can occur for many reasons. An increased intake of lithium by a medication error on the part of the patient or staff or by an intentional overdose will cause toxicity. Hemoconcentration, caused by fever, dehydration, excess sweating, diarrhea, or vomiting, can raise the lithium level to a toxic degree. Diminished excretion of lithium secondary to renal disease or a low-salt diet can also raise serum levels.

When toxicity is suspected, it is wise to rely on clinical judgment rather than serum levels. The most recent serum level may not reflect a more recent change in clinical status, and it may be impossible to get a stat sample that is accurate, that is, after a 10-to 14-hour lithium fast. If, upon questioning and examination, the patient shows signs of toxicity, withhold the lithium and inform the patient's physician. For mild or moderate toxicity, the lithium dose is usually lowered or held until the patient's symptoms remit and an accurate level can be drawn. Lithium has an average serum half-life of 24 hours; serum will gradually clear if no more lithium is given.

In more severe toxicity, the lithium is discontinued and the patient is given supportive care and monitored until the lithium is cleared from his body. Blood pressure and intake and output are monitored, and fluid and electrolytes are replaced as necessary. Stronger measures can include osmotic diuresis with mannitol or urea or diuresis with I.V. theophylline. If the lithium level exceeds 3.0 mEq./l., many clinicians suggest starting hemodialysis or, when unavailable, peritoneal dialysis.

Most patients recover gradually as their serum lithium level decreases. Those patients who have died had serum levels above 5 mEq./l.(2). Death is usually caused by complications of coma, such as pneumonia, or by shock or cardiac arrest. If the patient survives after reaching a serum level greater than 5.0 mEq./l., there may be such permanent aftereffects as dementia or cerebellar ataxia.

Long-Term Effects

Now that a number of patients have been receiving lithium maintenance for over 10 years, some long-term effects are being seen. These are, for the most part, innocuous and reversible.

The effect that has received the most attention is renal toxicity. There were some initial reports of structural kidney damage that raised quite a stir. The current thought is that data collected until now indicate that 10 to 15 years of continuous lithium treatment does not lead to marked progressive impairment of glomerular filtration rate with risk of terminal azotemia. In a certain proportion of patients, the treatment leads to impairment of renal concentrating ability, which may be fully reversible, partially reversible, and perhaps in some patients, irreversible(3). The latter problem, the progressive inability to concentrate urine due to a suppression of ADH, can progress in a minority of patients to a nephrogenic diabetes insipidus. A basic rule is that if a patient's 24-hour urine volume is more than three l./day, more specific tests of urine concentrating ability should be performed. If present, diabetes insipidus will sometimes respond to a thiazide diuretic.

Some elderly patients develop organic brain syndrome (OBS) without other signs of toxicity after several years of maintenance. If the OBS is attributable to the lithium, it will reverse when the lithium is discontinued. Some patients develop goiters or chemical hypothyroidism after several years. If the lithium is discontinued, the patient becomes euthyroid in approximately six weeks. If it is essential that the patient continue to receive lithium, the hypothyroidism can be treated with thyroxine (Synthroid). It is extremely rare for patients to develop clinical symptoms of hypothyroidism or myxedema.

Two other long-term side effects reported are weight gain and, less frequently, cogwheel rigidity. In order to evaluate these long-term side effects, periodic laboratory and physical examinations should be performed.

Drug Interactions

Lithium is often used in combination with other drugs. Some combinations have been found to be safe, while others are potentially harmful.

Antipsychotics. Lithium is most often used in combination with an antipsychotic for treatment of acute manic episodes. Lithium is clearly the treatment of choice for acute mania, but there is a lag period between initial administration of lithium and symptom reduction. During this time the patient may be acutely and floridly manic to the point of being dangerous to himself or others and unmanageable even in an inpatient psychiatric setting. In these circumstances, an antipsychotic will dampen the patient's behavior. Below the surface, the mania will continue until the lithium takes effect, but the patient's behavior will be more manageable. Antipsychotics most often used in this way are chlorpromazine (Thorazine) and haloperidol (Haldol). Often, very high doses are needed. Once the mania is under control with lithium, the antipsychotic can be tapered and discontinued. It is worth bearing in mind that the antiemetic properties of the antipsychotics will mask nausea and vomiting as signs of lithium toxicity. There are no other precautions with this drug combination.

Antidepressants. These are also commonly used in combination with lithium. Patients on lithium maintenance are more likely to have depressive relapses than manic relapses. Patients who do continue to suffer depressive relapses may be treated with a combination of lithium plus a tricyclic or MAO inhibitor antidepressant. Either class of antidepressant combines safely with lithium.

Diuretics. Any class of diuretics may decrease lithium excretion. If diuretics are administered, monitor lithium levels and clinical status more frequently.

Nephrotoxins. Lithium toxicity has been precipitated by the tetracyclines and by spectinomycin (Trobicin).

Antiinflamatory agents. Lithium retention and toxicity have been reported with indomethacin (Indocin) and phenylbutazone (Butazolidin).

Antihypertensives. When first started, these can cause a transient decrease in renal function that can lead to lithium retention.

Digoxin. Lithium can potentiate digoxin toxicity by decreasing intracellular potassium. The combination can cause severe nodal bradycardia and slow atrial fibrillation. The combination of lithium, digoxin, and a thiazide diuretic is especially dangerous.

Psychostimulants. Lithium can antagonize the highs of cocaine and amphetamines.

Alcohol. Alcohol intoxication with lithium can cause clouding of consciousness, ataxia, tremor, and incoordination. Lithium can be given safely in combination with disulfiram (Antabuse).

Analgesics. Lithium may potentiate the effects of morphine.

Muscle relaxants and anesthetics. Lithium can prolong neuromuscular blockade of succinylcholine (Anectine) and pancuronium (Pavulon). For patients having surgery, lithium should be discontinued 48 to 72 hours before surgery and restarted on the postoperative return of bowel sounds. Patients having ECT should be monitored closely postanesthetic. Because of reports of neurotoxicity in patients taking lithium and having ECT, these two treatments should probably not be combined(4).

Contraindications

Absolute Contraindications	
Renal failure **Renal tubular disease**	Since Lithium (Li) is excreted via the kidneys, these conditions make treatment difficult or hazardous; these patients should be treated only in the hospital.
Acute MI	Li toxicity can cause arrhythmias and cardiac failure in patients with preexisting heart disease.
Myasthenia gravis	Symptoms are aggravated by Li. Li interferes with the release of acetylcholine and with depolarization and repolarization of motor endplates.
First trimester pregnancy	Studies have shown an increased incidence of cardiac defects in the fetus.
Breast-feeding	Human breast milk has 30-100% the Li serum concentration of the mother; it can cause Li toxicity or hypothyroidism in the infant.
Myeloid leukemia	Li causes reversible leukocytosis at therapeutic serum levels in most patients.
Children under 12 years	FDA recommendation.
Relative Contraindications	
Organic brain syndrome or dementia	Li can exacerbate preexisting OBS or dementia.
Seizure disorders	Li therapy can worsen preexisting complex partial seizures; it can be used in other forms of epilepsy with EEG and clinical monitoring.
Cardiac conduction defects	Even at therapeutic levels, Li can aggravate preexisting arrhythmias and conduction defects; these patients should be treated only in the hospital with ECG monitoring.

Patient Teaching

All patients should have knowledge of their disease, the alternatives of treatment for their condition, and the risks and benefits of all the treatment alternatives. For patients receiving lithium, this includes teaching about lithium's risks and benefits.

Patients on maintenance will be required to see their health care provider for periodic physicals and lab exams. They will need to obtain and self-administer lithium at least twice daily for at least several years. They may have to tolerate some uncomfortable side effects, and not a day will go by that they will not be reminded that they have a chronic illness. Some patients whose hypomanic periods were pleasurable or even profitable in some business or personal way may miss their "up" periods. In many ways, patients on lithium maintenance have the same problems as other patients with chronic diseases. They have a great many adjustments to make.

The nurse can help these patients by discussing the chronic nature of their problem and the adjustments they must make to it. She can help by fully exploring the risk-benefit ratio so that the patient can better decide about his treatment. It is often helpful to introduce the patient to another patient on lithi-

he Use of Lithium

Parkinson's disease	Li can aggravate preexisting Parkinson's disease.
2nd and 3rd trimester pregnancy	If it is necessary to treat pregnant patients, keep the dose as low as possible and divide doses throughout the day.
Delivery	Li renal clearance drops 50% after delivery; discontinue Li 2 weeks before delivery and resume ½ the former dose after delivery.
Controlled cardiac failure	Li can accumulate with fluid and increase the risk of toxicity.
Tardive dyskinesia	This syndrome is reported to be either improved or aggravated by Li.
Cerebellar disorders	These disorders can mask the symptoms of toxicity.
Diabetes mellitus	Li can increase or decrease glucose tolerance; watch for signs either way.
Ulcerative colitis; ileostomy	GI disease may be aggravated, since Li can cause diarrhea.
Psoriasis; acne	These skin conditions are frequently aggravated by use of Li.
Senile cataracts	Li may increase the speed of development of cataracts.
Electrolyte imbalance; dehydration	Li increases the risk of toxicity.
Acute neurological disorders	These disorders can mask the symptoms of toxicity.
Goiter or hypothyroidism	These conditions can be aggravated by the use of Li; when they occur during Li treatment, they respond to the use of thyroxine.
Low-salt diet	Li is more likely to reach toxic levels.
Suicidal or impulsive patients	Li overdose can be fatal.

um with whom he can share information and problems.

The patient and his family will need to be able to list the side effects and signs of toxicity and should know how to contact their health care provider in the event that toxicity develops. The patient and his family should be able to recognize the signs of recurrence of mania, including euphoria, decreased sleep, increased talkativeness, increased motor activity, grandiosity, and upsurge of sexual interest, distractability, spending sprees, or racing thoughts. These are signs of relapse and should be reported immediately. They should also recognize and report such symptoms of depression as anhedonia, psychomotor retardation, loss of appetite, crying, and hopelessness. It is especially important to teach the patient's family and/or friends, since the manic patient may lack the good judgment to report his symptoms, and a depressed patient may not have the energy.

Women of childbearing age should practice effective birth control. If the patient is considering having children, she and her mate should be advised about the risks to the fetus of her continuing lithium versus the risks to her and her family of discontinuing it.

The patient will need to know his schedule for follow-up. He will need a clear schedule for administering lithium. It may increase compliance to link the taking of doses with mealtimes and bedtime. Reinforce the need for divided doses. If a patient forgets one dose, tell him to skip it rather than double up on the next dose. Doubling up on a dose may cause a brief toxic reaction. Advise the patient to tell other health care providers that he is taking lithium and to keep the physician prescribing his lithium abreast of any other health problems. Advise him of the possible precipitants of toxic reactions: fever, weight-loss diets, profuse sweating, decreased fluid or salt intake, loss of appetite, vomiting, and diarrhea. Advise that he limit alcohol consumption to one drink per day. If your patient has polydipsia, advise against quenching his thirst with high-calorie drinks that might cause weight gain.

Most importantly, give your patient a realistic picture of what lithium can and cannot do. Some patients feel lithium will take away all their problems. It clearly will not do that. What it may do is take away the extreme mood states of depression and mania. To some patients this may make life seem dull and colorless, but it probably will also make it less disrupted by severe episodes of illness and hospitalization. Patients also may need encouragement not to despair if they continue to have minor relapses. In fact, there are only a small number of bipolar patients who remain without relapses from the beginning of treatment. Most have recurrences that stop in the first few months or year of treatment. These are considered good responders. Some have recurrences beyond the first year, but the episodes are shorter and less disruptive. And, some 20 percent, the lithium nonresponders, continue to suffer recurrences of undiminished severity.

References

1. Klein, D. F., and others. *Diagnosis and Drug Treatment of Psychiatric Disorders: Adults and Children*. 2d ed. Baltimore, Md., Williams & Wilkins Co., 1980, p. 426.
2. Shou, M. The recognition and management of lithium toxicity. IN *Handbook of Lithium Therapy*, ed. by F. N. Johnson. Baltimore, Md., University Park Press, 1980, p. 399.
3. Vestergaard, Per. Renal side effects of lithium. IN *Handbook of Lithium Therapy*, ed. by F. N. Johnson. Baltimore, Md., University Park Press, 1980, p. 354.
4. Tyrer, Stephen, and Shopsin, Baron. Neural and neuromuscular side effects of lithium. IN *Handbook of Lithium Therapy*, ed. by F. N. Johnson. Baltimore, Md., University Park Press, 1980, p. 297.

RELAX

Six techniques you can teach to patients, incorporate into your care, and use yourself—even when you just have ten seconds to spare.

Relaxation, an effective adjunct to the treatment of a variety of ailments, can be achieved through simple techniques that can easily be taught to patients. Patients requiring minor invasive procedures—such as the drawing of blood, or insertion of intravenous catheters—can reduce their anxiety levels by following any one of a number of routes to relaxation. Those with asthma can learn to use these techniques when they anticipate attacks. Relaxation can relieve headaches and menstrual cramps and reduce both acute and chronic pain by alleviating tension in rigidly held muscles surrounding painful areas.

Several characteristics are common to all relaxation methods:

Rhythmic breathing. Most relaxation techniques start with slow deep breathing. As a person becomes relaxed, he consumes less oxygen; so breathing becomes slower and shallower. Although the rate and depth of breathing changes, the rhythm becomes constant. Thus, rhythmicity itself characterizes relaxation. (See chart, next page, for other physiologic changes brought about by relaxation.)

Reduced muscle tension. Some people relax so thoroughly that they can't move their arms or legs. Whether or not such profound relaxation is attained, almost any relaxation method will significantly ease muscle tension.

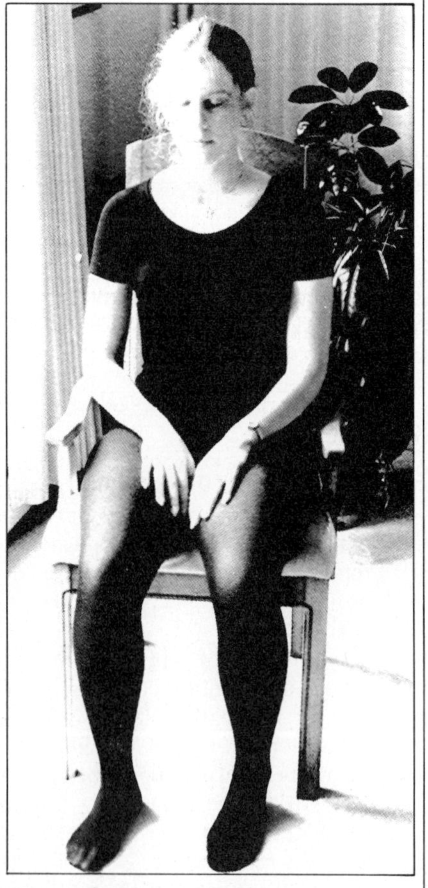

An altered state of consciousness. Your state of consciousness corresponds to your brain waves. The waking, alert state is called beta. During relaxation, you move to a level of consciousness called alpha(1). In the alpha state, which falls between full consciousness and unconsciousness, thought processes become less logical and more associative and creative. Your sense of time and body may be distorted: A 15-minute relaxation exercise may seem to last two minutes or two hours; your body might feel very large or very small; you might feel a heavy, or a light, floating feeling; or, you might experience your body as boundless, at one with the surrounding environment(2).

You have a heightened ability to focus on one idea or image. Focus may be on breathing, sensory experiences, or tension(3). Or, you might concentrate on a particular image, thought, or problem. Alpha state and focused mental activity are the major reasons why mental imagery is so effectively paired with relaxation. Although clients are seldom aware of moving from the beta to the alpha state, when relaxation is finished and they return to the beta level of consciousness they are aware of feeling more alert.

Clinical experience suggests there are individual differences in people's experiences of relaxation. Not everyone will demonstrate all characteristics of a relaxed psychophysiologic state.

RELAXATION TECHNIQUES

Full-body relaxation. A common type of relaxation, this 15-minute method—involves paying attention to different parts of your body, noting any ten-

Jean Wouters DiMotto, RN, MSN, is a psychophysiologist and educator. She is currently completing law school at Marquette Univerity, Milwaukee, WI.

ATION

BY JEAN WOUTERS DiMOTTO

Reprinted from American Journal of Nursing, June 1984

sion, and replacing it with warmth and relaxation.

If the patient is willing, this is a good relaxation technique to use while giving a bed bath. While preparing the patient for her bath, give the breathing instructions (see chart, p. 758). As you wash each part of her body, ask her to notice any tension in that part. For example, you could say, "As I wash your arm, notice any tightness or tension in it." As you rinse her arm say, "Breathe in warmth and relaxation to this arm and exhale the tension." Dry her arm with slower motions than you used to wash or rinse, saying, "Notice the warmth and relaxation you now feel in this arm." Repeat these instructions as you wash each body part, dealing with her hands independently of her arms, her arms separately from her shoulders, her neck from her face, and her feet from her calves. The bath is likely to take about 20 to 30 minutes, so keep the water warm; cold water inhibits relaxation.

As is true of most relaxation exercises, it is fairly easy for patients to do the exercise themselves once you have done it with them a few times.

Modified autogenic relaxation. This method can be useful in the treatment of asthma, hyperventilation, high blood pressure, cold hands or feet, headache, and ulcers(4). Relaxation is attained through a series of statements—or autosuggestions—about various bodily functions. After assuming a relaxing position, breathe in slowly and deeply, then slowly exhale, repeating to yourself the phrases shown in the chart on p. 0000. Inhale as you identify the parts of your body and exhale as you describe how relaxed you feel.

People enjoy this method and use it because the calming results are so obvious. After a while, subsequent use relaxes them more thoroughly and quickly. For some, just thinking the first statement produces relaxation.

Sensory pacing. While your uncon-

WHAT HAPPENS WHEN WE RELAX?

Physiologic manifestations	Cognitive manifestations	Behavioral manifestations
decreased pulse decreased blood pressure decreased respirations decreased oxygen consumption decreased carbon dioxide production and elimination decreased muscle tension decreased metabolic rate pupil constriction peripheral vasodilation increased peripheral temperature	altered state of consciousness, usually alpha level heightened concentration on single mental image or idea receptivity to positive suggestion	lack of attention to and concern for environmental stimuli no verbal interaction no voluntary change of position passive movement easy

Adapted from: Graves, H.H., & Thompson, E.A., "Anxiety: A Mental Health Vital Sign." In: Longo, D.C. and Williams, R.A. (Eds.), Clinical Practice in Psychosocial Nursing: Assessment and Intervention, *N.Y., Appleton-Century-Crofts, 1978.*

BODY POSTURES FOR RELAXATION

Sitting, reclining, or lying down are all postures conducive to relaxing. In each of these positions, the body should be well supported by a chair, bed, or couch. It is important that your primary position be balanced. Crossing your legs, dropping your head to one side, or leaning your upper body over a table will strain the affected muscles after ten to twenty minutes. Not only will these muscles remain tense, the discomfort will interfere with your attaining or remaining in alpha-level consciousness(5).

Sitting. Sit all the way back resting against the entire back of the chair. Place your feet flat on the floor. (If you're wearing high heels, remove your shoes.) Separate your legs so they're not touching each other. You can hang your arms by your sides or rest them on chair arms. Or, you can place each of your hands flat on each of your thighs. A fourth possibility is to rest your palms on your thighs, letting your fingers hang loosely between your legs.

Align your head with your spine. You can hold it comfortably straight, tilt it slightly forward, or rest your chin on your upper chest. If you choose to hold your head straight, you may unknowingly drop it forward as you relax. This is fine, since your head remains aligned with your spine.

You are now in a balanced, sitting position. Complete your preparation by loosening any tight clothing and making sure you are moderately warm.

Reclining and lying down. Many of the positioning principles for sitting apply. Separate your legs and point your toes slightly outward. Rest your arms at your sides without touching your sides. Keep your head aligned with your spine. You can lie flat or place a small, thin pillow under your head. Thick, large pillows will cause neck and back strain.

You will be able to maintain these postures for as long as you choose, without straining any muscle group. The only problem with reclining or lying down is that it's easy to fall asleep in these positions. In a recent study showing that relaxation training produces prolonged reduction of blood pressure, the author noted that the individual needs to remain awake to obtain maximum benefit from relaxation training(6). If, on the other hand, your purpose for relaxing is to induce sleep, then of course, reclining or lying down are the preferred positions.

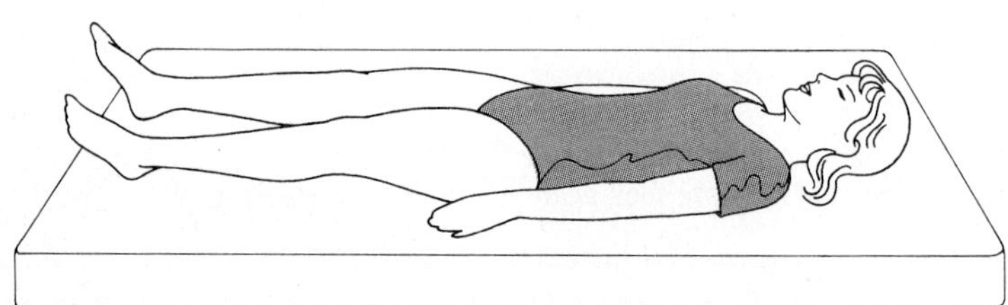

correct

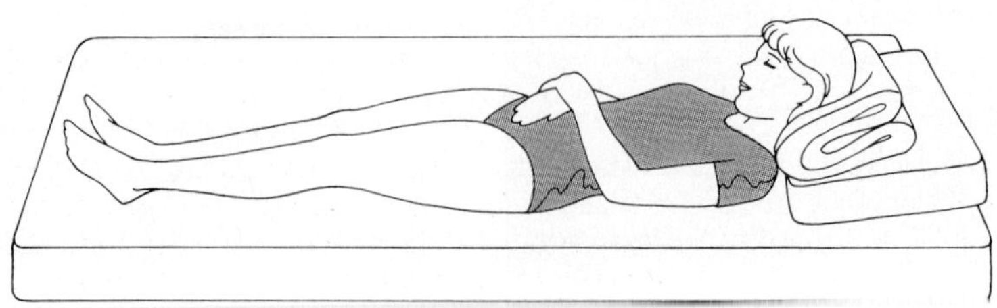

incorrect

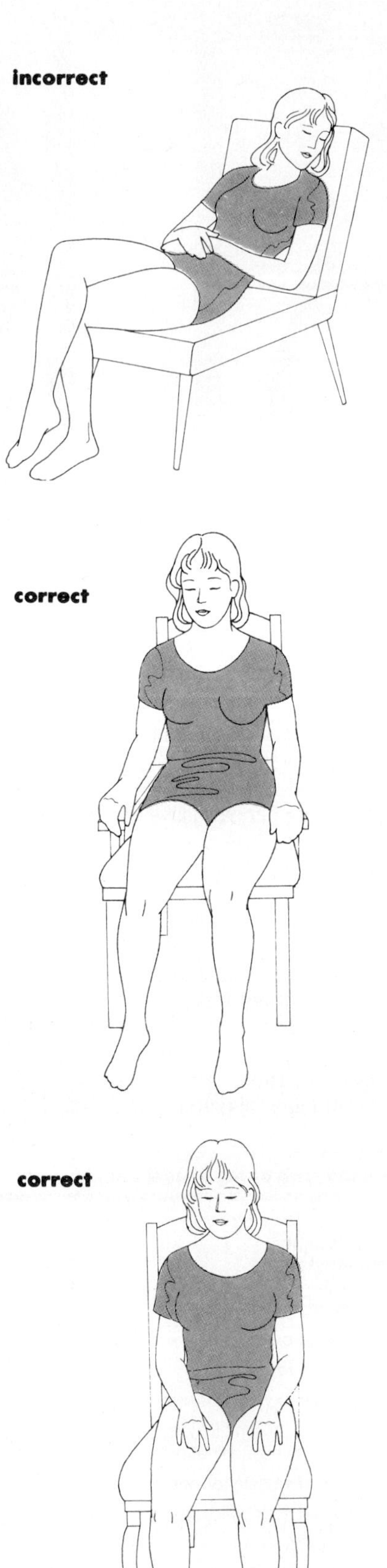

scious mind constantly takes in information from all five senses, your conscious mind is seldom aware of input from more than one or two senses at any moment. By consciously calling attention to the sensory experience you are having at a particular instant, you synchronize, or pace, your conscious and unconscious minds. If your body is motionless in one of the relaxed postures and you continue pacing for two to four minutes, you will attain relaxation (see chart, next page).

The method is simple and effective, particularly for patients in units where there are a lot of environmental stimuli, such as critical care units and outpatient departments. It is also good for people who have trouble concentrating on different parts of their bodies.

If a patient is having difficulty with the exercise, repeat the first part of each sentence (as listed in the chart) and have the patient finish the sentence with what he is aware of at that moment. If at the end the patient doesn't feel relaxed, repeat the pacing.

Color exchange. This method uses two senses—kinesthetic and visual. Sensations of tension or pain are converted to colors, then exhaled. The exhaled color is replaced with white light that is inhaled (see chart, next page). The concept of white light—healing, peaceful energy—has been used by Eastern people for centuries.

Color exchange is especially effective in the late afternoon and early evening, a time when people who have worked all day feel fatigued, and when patients who spend most of their day in bed feel restless and uncomfortable. Using this method will reduce the day's tension, replenish energy, and relieve pain. It is also a good way to end a back rub.

Music. Any restful music is appropriate, but classical music is most conducive to relaxation because its rhythms and harmonic structures are often perceived as soothing. As people listen to classical music, they tend to let their thoughts wander, either away from their present concerns to more pleasant topics, or to creative perspectives on problems with which they are struggling.

A number of classical selections can be used. Pachelbel's Canon in D Major, Mozart's Piano Concerto No. 21 in C Major, and much of Vivaldi's and Bach's music are apt. Particularly, good selections from Vivaldi include *The Four Seasons,* the concerti for mandolin, the baroque guitar concerti, and the six flute concerti (Opus 10). Relaxing selections from Bach include the *Goldberg Variations,* and the six concerti after Vivaldi.

The adagio, larghetto, and largo movements of Vivaldi and Bach have rhythms similar to the human heartbeat. When they listen to these movements, people's pulse rates and other biological rhythms tend to synchronize themselves with the beat of the music. This is particularly true with the largo movement's slow, stately, restful rhythm. The result is deeper, more efficient relaxation(7).

Another excellent choice is Halpern's *Soundscapes.* These are meditative collections of sounds without any familiar rhythm that are designed to relax, balance, and attune the listener(8). Similar selections include Horn's *Inside* albums, Andrew's *Kuthumi* and *The Violet Flame,* and Scott's and Yuize's *Music for Zen Meditations.*

> Postop patients who use relaxing techniques feel less pain and tension, and use fewer narcotics.

Music can also serve as background accompaniment while using other relaxation methods. Recordings or tapes of environmental sounds (i.e., streams of water, soft rain, wind) are particularly helpful. You can create relaxation tapes for yourself or your patients.

Ten-second relaxation techniques. Even a short exercise can lower pulse and respiration rates, although using stimulants such as caffeine shortly before relaxing interferes with a person's ability to slow physiologic processes.

Two relaxation techniques take only 10 seconds. Both are useful when, for example, postoperative patients begin to feel incisional pain and become tense, as when ambulating or changing positions.

You yourself can use these techniques during a busy day when there is no opportunity to take a break. While walking to a patient's room, taking an elevator, using the restroom, or sitting down to chart, you can lower your tension level with a 10-second exercise: Eyes open, let your lower jaw drop as if you were starting to yawn. Rest your tongue on the bottom of your mouth behind your lower teeth. Breathe slowly and rhythmically through your mouth: inhale, exhale, then rest. Do not form or even think words.

Research on patients who used this technique showed they felt significantly less incisional pain and bodily tension than those who didn't use the technique, and that they used fewer narcotics in the first 24 hours after surgery(9).

The second technique is done while sitting or standing. Close your eyes. Focus on a tiny imaginary star one inch in front of the tip of your nose. Take four deep breaths slowly through your mouth while continuing to focus on the star. This brief exercise requires intense concentration, and is especially helpful when you want to clear your mind as well as relax.

Ending relaxation techniques. The simplest and most comfortable way to end an exercise is to gradually open your eyes and stretch as though you were coming out of a deep sleep. Stretching helps move you from the alpha level of consciousness to the beta level of alert wakefulness. Although some people advocate jerking or contracting an arm or leg, it is more abrupt and less comfortable than stretching. After stretching, get up and move about a bit to become fully alert, especially if you are going to drive or operate medical machinery.

The more often you relax, the easier and faster you relax; relaxation becomes a conditioned response. Simply slowing your breathing, or performing a 10-second relaxation technique, or thinking of a phrase such as "relax," or "down you go," will trigger relaxation.

Relaxing regularly does not necessarily mean relaxing daily. Once a week is probably enough to establish a conditioned response. It is not necessary to use the same relaxation method each time in order to condition yourself; which relaxation method you choose is a matter of personal preference. Patients will also have preferences, so it is usually a good idea to teach them at least two methods.

USING RELAXATION TECHNIQUES

Relaxation by Sensory Pacing

Assume a relaxing position and slowly repeat and finish each of the following sentences, either in a low voice or to yourself.
Now I am aware of seeing . . .
Now I am aware of feeling . . .
Now I am aware of hearing . . .

Start with your eyes open, allowing them to close when they feel heavy. Begin by repeating and finishing each sentence four times. Then repeat and finish each sentence three times, then two times, then one time. Once your eyes are closed, what you see will be in your mind's eye.

Reference: Carter, P. and Gilligan, S. Personal Communication, 1980.

Full Body Relaxation

Assume a relaxing position. Note your breathing. Is it fast, slow, even or uneven, deep or shallow? Now, change your breathing to slow, abdominal breathing, breathing all the way in, down to your navel. Count to 4, inhaling on 1 and 2, exhaling on 3 and 4. Continue this.

Become aware of your face, your jaws, and your neck. Notice any tightness or tension in these parts. Breathe in warmth and relaxation. Exhale the tension.

Become aware of your shoulders, your arms, your hands and fingers. Notice any tightness or tension. Again, breathe in warmth and relaxation. Exhale the tension.

Become aware of your back—from your shoulders to your tailbone. Notice tightness or tension anywhere in your back. Breathe in, relaxing your back. Exhale the tension.

If you're feeling warm, you're relaxing.

Move to your chest and abdomen. Relax your abdominal muscles. Notice any tightness or tension. Breathe in warmth and relaxation. Exhale the tension.

You may notice that some parts of your body are tingling. It means you're relaxing.

Now move to your pelvic area and buttocks. Notice any tightness or tension in these parts. Breathe in warmth and relaxation to these areas and exhale the tension.

You may feel very heavy, as though you could sink deeply into your chair or bed. Or, you may feel light enough to float on a cloud or sit on a flower. Either way is fine. It means you're relaxing.

Move to your thighs. Notice any tightness or tension in those muscles. Breathe in warmth and exhale tension.

Move to your knees, then your calves, ankles, and feet. Notice any tightness or tension. Breathe in, relaxing all the way down to the tips of your toes. Exhale the tension.

Take time now to enjoy the peace you feel. When you're ready to end the relaxation period, count to ten, slowly open your eyes, wriggle your fingers and toes, and stretch as if you are just waking up.

Modified Autogenic Relaxation

Assume a relaxing position.

Slowly take in a very deep breath. Exhale very slowly.

Repeat each of the following phrases to yourself four times. Say the first part of the phrase as you breathe in for 2 to 3 seconds. Hold your breath in for 2 to 3 seconds. Then say the last part of the phrase as you breathe out for 2 to 3 seconds. Hold your breath out for 2 to 3 seconds.

Breathe in	Breathe out
1. I am	relaxed.
2. My arms and legs	are heavy and warm.
3. My heartbeat	is calm and regular.
4. My breathing	is free and easy.
5. My abdomen	is loose and warm.
6. My forehead	is cool.
7. My mind	is quiet and still.

References: Bauman, Edward, and others. The Holistic Health Handbook. *Berkeley, And/Or Press, 1978.*
Pelletier, Kenneth R. Mind as Healer, Mind as Slayer. *New York, Dell, 1977.*

Relaxation by Color Exchange

Assume a relaxing position. Concentrate on your breathing as you slowly take four deep breaths.

Notice any body tension, tightness, aches, or pains. Give the tension or discomfort a color, the first color you think of.

Now breathe in pure white light from the universe. Send the light to the tight or painful place in your body. Surround the color of your discomfort with the white light.

Exhale the color of your discomfort and inhale white light to take its place. Continue breathing in white light and exhaling the color of your discomfort.

Now, continue breathing in white light until your entire body is filled with the light and you have a sense of peace, well being, and energy.

Reference: Radtke, Dawn, D. Personal communication, 1980.

You may find that the more often you teach relaxation techniques to patients, the faster and more deeply you relax when you do an exercise yourself—one way the caregiver benefits directly from the care given.

For years, women preparing for childbirth have learned various breathing patterns and relaxation techniques in order to give birth without tranquilizers or analgesics. New mothers breastfeeding their babies can relax before feeding to increase the flow of milk. They are also more likely to feel at ease and to enjoy the experience.

Relaxation is useful preoperatively not only to help people sleep but to reduce their anxiety about upcoming surgery. Postoperatively, relaxation can be used to relieve pain. And, people can use relaxation to reduce the stress in their lives and to achieve even better health. In whatever nursing setting you choose to practice, there will be numerous indications for teaching relaxation to your patients.

REFERENCES

1. Wallace, R. K., and others. A wakeful hypometabolic physiologic state. *Am.J.Physiol.* 221:795-799, Sept. 1971.
2. Trygstad, Louise. Simple new ways to help anxious patients. *RN* 43:28-32, Dec. 1980.
3. McCaffery, Margo. *Nursing Management of the Patient with Pain.* 2nd ed. Philadelphia, J.B. Lippincott Co., 1979.
4. Davis, Martha, and others. *The Relaxation and Stress Reduction Workbook.* 2nd ed. Richmond, CA, New Harbinger, 1982.
5. Guyton, A. C. *Textbook of Medical Physiology.* 5th ed. Philadelphia, W.B. Saunders Co., 1976.
6. Agras, W.S. Relaxation therapy in hypertension. *Hosp. Prac.* May 1983, p. 134.
7. Ostrander, Sheila, and others. *Superlearning.* New York, Delacorte Press, 1979.
8. Halpern, Steven. *Tuning the Human Instrument.* Belmont, CA, Spectrum Research Institute, 1978.
9. Flaherty, G. G., and Fitzpatrick, J. J. Relaxation technique to increase comfort level of postoperative patients: a preliminary study. *Nurs.Res.* 27:352-355, Nov.-Dec. 1978.

Extrapyramidal Side Effects of Antipsychotic Medications

Reprinted from American Journal of Nursing, July 1981

By Elizabeth Harris

The extrapyramidal side effects of antipsychotic drugs are often confusing, frightening, uncomfortable, and embarrassing for patients. About one-third of all patients taking antipsychotic medications will experience EPS(1). While these side effects are difficult to prevent, they are fairly easily controlled when accurately diagnosed and treated.

Untreated EPS can be so distressing that patients will stop taking their medications in order to alleviate the symptoms. Van Puten found that most patients with schizophrenia who refuse to take their drugs upon discharge from the hospital do so because of discomfort from EPS(2).

Unless health care professionals are knowledgeable about antipsychotic drugs, the symptoms of EPS may be misdiagnosed as any of the following conditions: epilepsy, meningitis, encephalitis, poliomyelitis, tetanus, malingering, hysteria, stroke, joint dislocation, calcium deficiency, or depression. In fact, EPS have been improperly treated with such aggressive measures as hospitalization, lumbar puncture, and tracheotomy(3-5).

These are four general classes of EPS:

- parkinsonism
- dyskinesias and dystonias
- akathisia
- tardive dyskinesia.

Parkinsonism. Drug-induced parkinsonism is a syndrome similar in appearance to the naturally occurring Parkinson's disease. This syndrome is thought to be caused by the dopamine blockade created by the antipsychotics. The syndrome consists of akinesia, muscular rigidity, alterations of posture, tremor, masklike facies, shuffling gait, loss of associated movements, hypersalivation, and drooling.

The usual time of onset of this side effect is after the first week of treatment but before the end of the second month of treatment. Patients seem to accommodate to this effect, so that the symptoms fade over two or three months with or without treatment.

Akinesia is often experienced as fatigue, lack of interest, slowness, heaviness, lack of drive or ambition, or vague bodily discomforts. If severe, it can interfere with the patient's psychosocial and rehabilitative activities. Akinesia can often be confused with depression, demoralization, schizophrenic inertia, or negativism.

One patient I cared for who had chronic schizophrenia spent several weeks lying mute in bed. Her psychosis had been treated, but she seemed unable to mobilize herself to return to work. We incorrectly assumed that she was either severely depressed or negativistic, when, in fact, she was suffering from akinesia. Three days after treatment for akinesia was started, she returned to work.

Akinesia should be suspected when patients say they feel weak, less spontaneous, less interested in conversation, generally apathetic, and less inclined to initiate usual activities. To the observer, the patient seems anergic, with fewer gestures and diminished spontaneity. Test the patient's strength in both hands. The patient with akinesia will have decreased muscle strength. Ask the patient if he feels slowed down; the patient with akinesia will almost always answer yes.

Rigidity is a plastic hypertonicity that affects both axial and limb musculature; it is often mistaken for tension or anxiety. Rigidity is most easily tested for by holding a patient's elbow in the palm of your hand with your thumb positioned over the flexor tendons. Flex and extend the arm with your other hand, asking the patient to relax the arm and allow you to do the moving. You may find a smooth resistance to movement, known as "lead-pipe" rigidity, or a ratchet-like phenomenon, known as "cogwheel" rigidity. Either finding is evidence of drug-induced rigidity, rather than simple increased tension. Rigidity will most likely be seen three or four days to two weeks after therapy is started, with a peak incidence at two to four weeks.

Patients with drug-induced parkinsonism tend to have a stooping posture and a festinating, or shuffling and somewhat propulsive, gait. Their tremor is faster and more irregular than that seen in true Parkinson's disease and can be present during movement or at rest at speeds of about 5 cycles/second.

The tremor usually begins in one or both upper extremities and, when severe, involves the tongue, jaw, and lower extremities(6). This symptom is first seen at a half week, peaks at 2 to 6 weeks, and declines at 8 to 16 weeks. This symptom will be most difficult for patients whose work or hobby calls for fine motor coordination.

The masklike facies of parkinsonism can be mistaken for the flat affect of schizophrenia. The difference is that the patient with masklike facies will employ means other than facial gestures to indicate a wider range of affect.

The loss of associated movements is most easily seen in the decreased or absent arm swing. The patient with this symptom will often walk with the forearms perpendicular to the trunk. Patients frequently describe themselves as looking like a puppy begging for a bone, or like a kangaroo. Hypersalivation and drooling are present only in severe cases of parkinsonism.

Patients often describe their parkinsonian symptoms in graphic ways. One patient described her slowness (akinesia) as a feeling of being under water. Many describe the akinesia by saying they feel like robots or zombies. Patients who drool often say that they feel like babies.

When these parkinsonian symptoms become most severe, patients have been known to develop neuroleptic malignant syndrome. This syndrome has been reported only with high doses of potent neuroleptics like fluphenazine (Prolixin) and haloperidol (Haldol)(7-10). Neuroleptic malignant syndrome is gradual in onset, with milder parkinsonian symptoms progressing to mutism, posturing, waxy flexibility, incontinence, and sometimes fever and coma. Improvement follows slowly after decreasing the dose of neuroleptic or adding an anticholinergic drug. One study showed a more rapid relief of symptoms when patients were treated with amantadine (Symmetrel)(7).

This syndrome can easily be confused with worsening of schizophrenic symptoms, but, unlike a worsening of schizophrenia, the syndrome does not respond to an increased dose of antipsychotics. Higher doses of antipsychotic drugs only make the patient appear more deeply catatonic, while decreasing the dose will ameliorate the catatonialike symptoms. One patient with this reaction to haloperidol was transferred to the neurology service to rule out encephalitis. Her symptoms resolved gradually when all her antipsychotic medications were discontinued.

Neuroleptic-induced parkinsonism is easily controlled. Some of the symptoms can usually be eliminated by decreasing the dose of neuroleptic or by changing to another drug with a lesser incidence of this syndrome. If these measures are ineffective or if they are impractical for clinical reasons, the antiparkinsonian agents are commonly administered. (See chart, next page.)
If one of these drugs is unsuccessful, another agent should be tried. Sometimes, if side effects do not respond to one medication, they will respond to another.

Amantadine (Symmetrel) and benztropine mesylate (Cogentin) have long serum half-lives and, therefore, can be given on a once- or twice-a-day schedule. These drugs are, however, slightly more expensive than the others. The other antiparkinsonian drugs have shorter half-lives and should be given in divided doses throughout the day.

Amantadine's effectiveness may diminish over time, necessitating a change to another antiparkinsonian drug.

Since drug-induced parkinsonism usually abates in a month or two, with or without treatment, the dose of antiparkinsonian medications should be reduced gradually over two or three months and then discontinued. There is often no recurrence of parkinsonism.

Dyskinesias and dystonias. Dyskinesias are coordinated, involuntary, stereotyped, rhythmic movements of the limbs and trunk that are seen more commonly in males(11).

The dystonias are uncoordinated, bizarre, jerking or spastic movements of the neck, face, eyes, tongue, torso, arm, or leg muscles; backward rolling of the eyes in the sockets (oculogyric crisis); sideways twisting of the neck (torticollis); protrusion of the tongue; or spasms of the back muscles (opisthotonus). These symptoms occur suddenly and dramatically. They are extremely frightening to patients and staff and are often painful as well.

These symptoms are sometimes so severe as to lead to respiratory distress or difficulty talking or swallowing. In fact, the nurse will sometimes become aware of an acute dystonic reaction when a patient approaches with a look of terror, pointing to his sharply twisted jaw, but unable to speak, even to ask for help. Some patients first become aware of this symptom when they find it difficult to chew or swallow food. Other patients will present with a complaint that their eyes keep rolling up in their heads against their will. What at first sounds like it may be a delusion turns out to be an oculogyric crisis. If untreated, these symptoms wax and wane and remit spontaneously in about a week(12). If treated, they remit almost immediately and usually do not recur.

Dystonias may be seen anytime after administration of the first dose of an antipsychotic agent. The incidence peaks in a week and declines in two weeks. The duration of an episode ranges from a few minutes to several hours. Dystonias are twice as common in males and occur more often in younger people(11-13). Patients usually welcome treatment for these painful and frightening symptoms.

Severe, acute dystonic reactions can be treated with parenteral diphenhydramine (Benadryl). Doses of 25 to 100 mg., given intravenously, should be effective in one minute. The same dosage given IM should work in 15 minutes, and an oral dose should work in one hour. Another useful drug is benztropine (Cogentin) 2 mg. I.V. or IM(6). Any of the antiparkinsonian drugs can be administered orally, but the oral route is painfully slow for a patient in an acute crisis. After the acute symptoms have subsided, it is common to give a maintenance dose of antiparkinsonian medications for two or three months to prevent a recurrence.

It is important to treat these reactions quickly because they are so frightening to patients. Reassure the patient that he is experiencing a common side effect of his medication. Tell him how you will be treating the symptoms, and depending on the drug and route used, tell him how long he can expect to wait before feeling relief. It is a good safeguard when a patient is begun on an antipsychotic medication to request that the physician also write a PRN order to give IM diphenhydramine or benztropine in the event of an acute dystonic reaction.

Akathisia. Akathisia is the symptom that most often leads to noncompliance(2). Akathisia is a very discomforting feeling of restlessness and agitation. One patient called it the "walkies and the talkies." The patient finds he is unable to lie down, to sleep, or to sit still. If forced to sit, the patient often shifts his posture, taps his feet, or squirms and fidgets in the chair. Often he cannot resist the compulsion to stand up and walk around. In a situation where a long period of sitting is required, such as in a movie or a therapy session, the patient will sit and stand repeatedly with an obvious inability to stop himself. He thus finds it difficult to perform such activities as reading books, watching television, sewing, or knitting. When standing still, the patient often rocks and shifts his weight. The more severe the akathisia, the more desperate the patient becomes. Occasionally, he experiences the feeling as sexual excitement. More often, the affects he experiences are terror, fright, anger, or rage. In desperation, the patient

Drugs Used as Antiparkinsonian Agents

Generic name	Trade name	Usual daily dose (mg.)
Anticholinergics		
benztropine mesylate	Cogentin	1-6
trihexyphenidyl hydrochloride	Artane (and others)	2-15
procyclidine hydrochloride	Kemadrin	5-20
cycrimine hydrochloride	Pagitane	3.75-15.0
biperiden hydrochloride	Akineton	2-6
ethopropazine hydrochloride	Parsidol	50-600
Antihistamines		
diphenhydramine hydrochloride	Benadryl (and others)	25-200
chlorphenoxamine hydrochloride	Phenoxene	150-400
orphenadrine hydrochloride	Disipal	50-250
Others		
amantadine hydrochloride	Symmetrel	100-300

may become suicidal, violent, or homicidal.

Akathisia is often mistaken for psychomotor agitation. If it is treated with an increase in the dose of the antipsychotic medication, the akathisia becomes worse. In contrast, one or two doses of an antiparkinsonian medication will sometimes relieve it.

Likewise, the patient often erroneously attributes akathisia to a psychological cause. It is important that we clearly explain that the restlessness the patient is experiencing is a side effect of the medication rather than an emotional state.

To differentiate akathisia from anxiety or agitation, several questions can be asked. Ask if the patient ever felt like this before taking his medication. A no answer suggests akathisia. Ask, "Do you feel restless inside? Do you feel more comfortable standing up or walking around than you do sitting or lying down?" If the answers are yes, the patient is likely to be suffering from akathisia. In addition, the patient almost always experiences the symptoms as ego-alien and may feel it is more difficult to endure the akathisia than his original symptoms.

Akathisia is first seen after two weeks of drug treatment. The peak incidence is at 6 to 10 weeks, with a decline at 12 to 16 weeks. It is more common in women and in middle age. The symptoms tend to appear and disappear spontaneously, but accommodation does not develop as it does with parkinsonism. Over half of patients with akathisia also have other extrapyramidal side effects (7,11,12,14).

Akathisia is the EPS most refractory to treatment with antiparkinsonian medications. The first attempt at treatment of akathisia is to reduce the dose of antipsychotic or to change to a drug with a lower incidence of akathisia (see chart at left). If neither of these measures are successful, an antiparkinsonian agent can be tried. If the first trial is unsuccessful, a second trial with another antiparkinsonian drug may succeed. If all else fails, akathisia can be treated with diazepam (Valium). The symptoms should subside in three days if the diazepam is effective(15).

Tardive dyskinesia. If detected early, this syndrome is frequently reversible. Symptoms consist of coordinated, rhythmic, stereotyped, abnormal, involuntary sucking, chewing, licking, and pursing movements of the tongue and mouth. Sometimes, choreiform movements of the extremities are seen. Grimacing, blinking, and frowning are common. Also seen are tongue protrusion and rocking. The symptoms may occur after long-term use of high doses of antipsychotic drugs, often first appearing after the dosage is decreased or the medication discontinued. More recently, cases have been reported following short-term use of moderate doses.

Two of the earliest signs of tardive dyskinesia (TD) are excessive blinking and fine, vermiform movements of the tongue. The symptoms then progress with a fluctuating course until, finally, they interfere with activities of daily living, such as bathing, dressing, or even eating. The symptoms can be suppressed by intense, voluntary effort and are absent during sleep. They are embarrassing to most patients.

It is reported by the APA task force on late neurological effects of antipsychotic drugs that 10 to 20 percent of patients receiving antipsychotic drugs for a year or more develop tardive dyskinesia. Possible predisposing factors are age, being female, presence of organic brain disease, use of antiparkinsonian drugs, use of high-potency neuroleptics, presence of dementia, history of ECT or leucotomy, or a history of tricyclic antidepressant use(16).

Much research is being done to find a cure for tardive dyskinesia. So far, none has been found. There are, however, some guidelines for prevention. Antipsychotics should be used for as short a time as possible, always taking into consideration the balance between the need for the antipsychotic and the risk of tardive dyskinesia. One study showed that only 40 percent of patients, when taken off antipsychotics after six months, require reinstitution of the drug because of exacerbation of symptoms(17). Antiparkinsonian agents should be used only when indicated and, when possible, should be discontinued no later than three months after institution of treatment.

All patients on antipsychotics should be screened for tardive dyskinesia at least every three months. A common tool for this purpose is the AIMS test (Abnormal Involuntary Movement Scale). If any symptoms of tardive dyskinesia are noted, the antipsychotic should be discontinued if clinically possible. In some cases, ECT is then used to treat the patient's acute psychotic symptoms. In the difficult situation where there is no satisfactory alternative to continuing antipsychotic medication, the patient and family should be advised of the patient's condition and of the risks involved in further treatment with antipsychotics. Only if the patient understands the risks involved and is willing to proceed, should antipsychotics be continued. Some institutions require the patient's written consent.

Principles of Treating EPS

The most obvious way to prevent EPS is to use the least amount of antipsychotic medications for the shortest time possible. One study suggests that all patients should have a drug-free trial after six months of treatment, with reinstitution of medications only if there is an exacerbation of symptoms. Fully half of such patients should be able to function well without reinstitution of chemotherapy(17). Others suggest a drug-free trial for all patients at 6 to 12 months after institution of drug treatment(15).

When antipsychotics are used, they are best used initially in divided doses to increase the sedative, hypnotic, and motor-inhibiting properties during the patient's acute psychosis. After a few days, when control is satisfactory, the patient should be put on a once- or twice-a-day schedule. Clinical benefit from the antipsychotic is the same, but on a less frequent dosage schedule, the patient will experience fewer side effects(17). The usual practice is to schedule a single dose for bedtime or arrange a BID schedule, with the larger portion of the total dose at bedtime. It is important to remember that many EPS can be treated by decreasing the dose of the antipsychotic or by changing antipsychotics.

Basically, all antipsychotic drugs produce equal improvement, yet, at times, some will work when others fail. All produce the same range of side effects, though one drug may produce more of one side effect and less of others. For example, high-potency drugs, such as haloperiold (Haldol), trifluoperazine (Stelazine), fluphenazine (Prolixin), and perphenazine (Trilafon), have the greatest incidence of parkinsonism, dystonias, and akathisia. Thioridazine (Mellaril) has the least incidence of EPS, but it has the disadvantages of creating ejaculatory disturbances in a small percentage of males and of having an upper dosage limit of 800 mg. Chlorpromazine and thioridazine commonly cause sedation and orthostatic hypotension. The long-acting injectables, fluphenazine decanoate and enanthate, cause EPS more quickly than other dose forms—within 12 hours to 5 days of injection.

Because EPS are so uncomfortable and frightening to patients and because they often lead to drug resistance, some clinicians believe it is best to treat all patients on antipsychotics with prophylactic doses of antiparkinsonian medications. This would seem to be a very sensible approach. Yet, there are some very good reasons why prophylactic use of antiparkinsonian (AP) drugs is unwise. They include the following:

- Prophylactic AP medications have not been shown to prevent all EPS.
- Not all patients develop EPS.
- Excess doses of AP drugs can cause atropine psychosis.
- Use of AP medications may decrease the blood level of antipsychotics by interfering with absorption.
- AP medications may worsen the symptoms of TD or may add to the risk of developing TD.
- AP medications have their own side effects.
- AP medications add to the patient's expense.

When administering AP medications, watch for the following side effects: paralysis of bladder or bowel; confusion; burred vision; dry mouth; lethargy; dizziness; GI disturbance; dry, flushed skin; and dilated pupils. These are more likely to occur with high doses in young or middle-aged patients or with moderate or low doses in elderly patients.

Nursing Implications

The nurse's approach to extrapyramidal side effects and to their treatment is also important for the patient. When patients are begun on antipsychotic medications, they and their friends or family should be taught about the side effects that may be dangerous.

When a patient experiences EPS, he often attributes his discomfort to emotional distress, to some fault of his own, or to a sinister outside force. Explain to the patient that he is having a side effect of his medication. Validate for the patient that other people with the same symptom find it uncomfortable, unpleasant, or even painful. Tell him that the side effect is usually treatable and that everything possible will be done to treat it quickly. Inform the patient's physician of your findings and discuss the appropriate treatment.

After treatment begins, it is important to monitor the course of the symptoms to evaluate any necessary changes in treatment. It seems to be a great relief to our patients when they see we are familiar with their distress and know how to help them with it.

There is a misconception that there is a relationship between EPS and drug efficacy. There have been no conclusive studies that show antipsychotic drugs to be more effective when the patient experiences EPS. When a patient is stiff or drooling, you know that he has swallowed and absorbed some of his medication, but this does not increase the likelihood that the medication will work to treat his psychosis.

A second common misconception is that EPS are constant in strength and appearance. A nurse who observes that a patient's symptoms occur only in the presence of other people or that they disappear when a patient is alone, will sometimes conclude that the patient is malingering or manipulating. Similarly, a patient whose drug-induced restlessness interferes with sitting still more in group therapy than during a card game will often be accused of copping out. On the contrary, EPS are known to wax and wane over time or with the patient's affective state and level of anxiety(6). The nurse should expect to see EPS occur more often or to be more pronounced in stressful situations.

References

1. Newton, M., and others. How you can improve the effectiveness of psychotropic drug therapy. *Nurs. '78* 8:46-55, July 1978.
2. Van Putten, T. Why do schizophrenic patients refuse to take their drugs? *Arch.Gen.Psychiatry* 31:67-72, July 1974.
3. Mills, J. Dystonic reactions to phenothiazines. *JEN* 4:43-46, Nov.-Dec. 1978.
4. Cavenar, J. O., Jr., and others. Misdiagnosis of severe dystonia. *Psychosomatics* 20:209-210, Mar. 1979.
5. Baldessarini, R. J. *Chemotherapy in Psychiatry.* Cambridge, Mass., Harvard University Press, 1977, p. 41.
6. Lipton, M. A., and others. *Psychopharmacology: A Generation of Progress.* New York, Raven Press, 1978, p. 1021.
7. Baldessarini, *op. cit.*, p. 36.
8. Grunhaus, L., and others. Neuroleptic malignant syndrome due to depot fluphenazine. *J.Clin.Psychiatry* 40:99-100, Feb. 1979.
9. Baldessarini, R. J. The "neuroleptic" antipsychotic drugs. Part 2. Neurologic side effects. *Postgrad.Med.* 65:123-128, Apr. 1979.
10. Gelenberg, A. J., and Mandel, M. R. Catatonic reactions to high-potency neuroleptic drugs. *Arch.Gen.Psychiatry* 34:947-950, Aug. 1977.
11. Klein, D. F., and Davis, J. M. *Diagnosis and Drug Treatment of Psychiatric Disorders.* Baltimore, Williams & Wilkins Co., 1969, p. 98.
12. Murphy, J. E., and Stewart, R. B. Efficacy of antiparkinson agents in preventing antipsychotic-induced extrapyramidal symptoms. *Am.J.Hosp.Pharm.* 36:641-644, May 1979.
13. Shader, R. L., and DiMascio, Albert. *Psychotropic Drug Side Effects: Clinical and Theoretical Perspectives.* Baltimore, Williams & Wilkins Co., 1970, p. 93.
14. Van Putten, T. The many faces of akathisia. *Compr.Psychiatry* 16:43-47, Jan.-Feb. 1975.
15. Gelenberg, A. J. Treating the outpatient schizophrenic. *Postgrad.Med.* 64:48-56, Nov. 1978.
16. Schwartz, H. J. Tardive dyskinesia and the long-term patient. *Hosp.Community Psychiatry* 30:465-467, July 1979.
17. Gardos, G., and Cole, J. O. Maintenance antipsychotic therapy: is the cure worse than the disease? *Am.J.Psychiatry* 133:32-36, Jan. 1976.
18. McAfee, H. A. Tardive dyskinesia. *Am.J.Nurs.* 78:359-367, Mar. 1978.

Reprinted from American Journal of Nursing, July 1981

Antipsychotic Medications

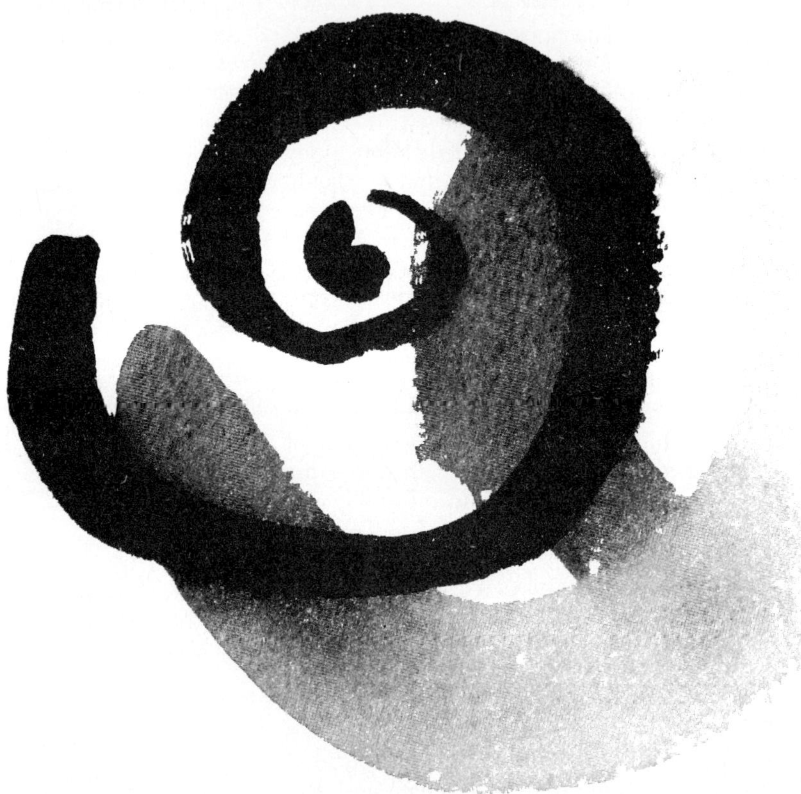

By Elizabeth Harris

Many people mistakenly believe that only patients with schizophrenia take antipsychotic medications (also called neuroleptics, or major tranquilizers). This, however, is not the case.

The antipsychotics are used in the treatment of psychotic conditions that may be caused by schizophrenia, mania, agitated psychotic depression, paranoid disorders, involutional or senile psychosis, a psychotic reaction to amphetamines, organic dementia, and acute brain syndromes(1). Antipsychotics are used to treat the acute psychotic symptoms of these conditions. They are also used prophylactically to prevent psychotic relapse in patients with schizophrenia.

There is also some confusion as to which symptoms these drugs alleviate and which symptoms they do not. The symptoms that respond to antipsychotics are agitation, rage, overreactivity to sensory stimuli, hallucinations, delusions, paranoia, combativeness, insomnia (when this is a symptom of the psychosis), hostility, negativism, and thought disorder. These drugs, however, do not correct poor judgment, poor insight, or social and interpersonal disabilities; they also cannot change an individual's personality(2).

The antipsychotics are also used in treating disorders other than psychosis. They have antiemetic properties and can be used specifically for this purpose(3). Antipsychotics have also been used to treat intractable hiccoughs(4). Haloperidol is used to treat Gilles de la Tourette syndrome(5). Finally, these drugs have been used in combination with other drugs for pain control(3-6).

There are six major classes of antipsychotics grouped according to their chemical structure. The phenothiazine class is further divided into three subclasses (see chart, page 1319). The phenothiazines, the first widely used antipsychotics, were first used in this country in the mid-

1950s. Chlorpromazine was the first phenothiazine and is the prototype of this class.

Another commonly used method of classifying these drugs divides the antipsychotics into two classes—high potency and low potency. The high-potency drugs, such as haloperidol and fluphenazine, are given in low milligram doses and exert a greater antipsychotic effect per milligram. The low-potency drugs, such as chlorpromazine and thioridazine, have higher milligram doses and exert a lesser antipsychotic effect per milligram. This classification scheme is used primarily to discuss side effects, since the low-potency drugs have side effects that differ from those of the high-potency drugs.

All antipsychotics are thought to exert their effect by blocking the dopamine receptors in the brain(7). This is the mechanism of action for both their antipsychotic action and also their neurological side effects. These drugs also have anticholinergic properties that are not thought to contribute to their antipsychotic effect, but which are responsible for some of their side effects.

General Properties

The antipsychotics are rapidly absorbed after oral or intramuscular administration. After oral administration, clinical effects are apparent in 30 to 60 minutes. Following IM administration, effects are seen in about 10 minutes. Antipsychotics are highly lipophilic, so that most of the drug that is absorbed is bound to proteins or membranes(8). The remaining free or unbound drug is available to the central nervous system and, thus, active.

Metabolism of the antipsychotics occurs largely through oxidation by the hepatic microsomal enzymes(9). The serum half-life is fairly short (about 24 hours), yet varying amounts of the drug will linger in the body for weeks or even months after a drug is discontinued.

The antipsychotics and their metabolites begin to accumulate in body tissues, particularly in fatty tissues, from the first dose. As the patient continues to receive these drugs, the tissues take on greater amounts until a saturation point is reached. When the drug is discontinued, the body tissues slowly release their accumulation back into the bloodstream where it can be metabolized and excreted. Therefore, patients who stop their medications after a course of treatment often stay protected from relapse for some time, as their body continues to free small amounts of the medication. For this same reason, patients may experience side effects for weeks after receiving their last dose. Traces of drugs or their metabolites have been found in urine two or three months after discontinuation of the drug(10).

Antipsychotics have a high therapeutic index; they can be given at very high doses with minimal risk. They are not addicting, do not produce euphoria, and there is no tolerance to their antipsychotic effects. However, patients show considerable accommodation to many of their side effects(11). The antipsychotic effect occurs anywhere from several hours to three weeks after the first dose. After the initial antipsychotic effects are seen, it can take anywhere from weeks to months for full improvement to be apparent(12). It is important to make patients aware of this lag period to prevent discouragement when there is no immediate favorable response.

Selection of a Drug

All six classes of antipsychotics have the same antipsychotic effect. None of the newer drugs have been found to be more effective than chlorpromazine(13).

The choice of a drug for a specific patient depends on several factors. If a patient or one of his relatives has responded favorably in the past to one particular drug, then the chances are greater that he will respond well to that same drug. In patients (or relatives) who have had a severe unfavorable reaction, that particular drug is best avoided. For a patient who is acutely disturbed and requires parenteral medication, the choice is limited to the drugs that have injectable forms. For a patient who will need high doses of medication, it would be best to avoid thioridazine, which is the only antipsychotic that has an absolute upper limit to the dose range (800 mg.). For some patients, cost of the drug may be a factor. Some newer drugs are several times more expensive than the older ones.

After all these considerations are taken into account, the choice of drug will depend largely on the different side effects of each drug. For example, the low-potency drugs, such as chlorpromazine and thioridazine, have a higher incidence of the side effects of hypotension and sedation but fewer extrapyramidal symptoms (EPS).

On the other hand, the high-potency drugs, such as fluphenazine, haloperidol, and trifluoperazine, have a low incidence of sedation and hypotension but a high incidence of EPS because they are potent dopamine blockers. Clinicians often choose a drug based on which side effect they believe will be more easily tolerated by the patient. Two long-acting, injectable drugs are available for use in patients who have a history of noncompliance with medication: fluphenazine enanthate and fluphenazine decanoate. Both are long-acting depot injections with a slow, even absorption. The enanthate form can be given in dosages of 12.5 mg. to 50 mg. every 3 to 14 days. The decanoate is given in the same dosages every two to four weeks. The differences between the two forms are in length of action and side effects. The decanoate has been reported to have somewhat fewer side effects(14).

When these medications were first developed, they were thought to provide the answer to the problem of noncompliance and subsequent relapse. Obviously, it seems to be easier to ensure patient compliance when a professional administers the drug by injection every two weeks or so than when the patient is relied on to take oral doses once a day or more often without supervision.

Unfortunately, the early promise of these drugs to greatly reduce relapse in schizophrenia has not proven itself. The use of these drugs has been somewhat limited by the incidence of EPS. Like other piperazine phenothiazines, depot fluphenazines often induce EPS. In addition, there have been disappointing findings regarding their ability to prevent relapse. Results of the recent National Institute of Mental Health Collaborative Fluphenazine Study show that depot fluphenazine markedly improves compliance by 20 to 50 percent over the use of oral fluphenazine. But, despite this increased compliance, the relapse rate after 12 months is equal to that of the oral drugs. This raises doubt about any real advantage of these drugs (15). Nonetheless, these drugs are an important part of the armamentarium and preferred by some patients who do not want the responsibility for taking oral medications on a daily basis.

There is considerable evidence against using more than one antipsychotic at a time. This is reasonable, considering that each has equal antipsychotic effect, and all have the same mechanism of action. Another reason to avoid using more than one antipsychotic is that if the patient responds, it will be unclear to which drug he responded. Likewise, if he has severe side effects, it would be impossible to know which drug caused them.

Contraindications

Antipsychotic drugs should never be used in treating patients who have severe CNS depression or who are in coma as a result of alcohol or barbiturate use or from excessive use of narcotics. These patients are at risk for a synergistic effect that can lead to respiratory paralysis or circulatory collapse. Patients in coma or with severe CNS depression from brain damage or trauma are also at risk for respiratory paralysis.

There are a number of relative contraindications to the use of antipsychotics. Patients who have a known sensitivity or severe allergic response to one of these drugs are at risk for another allergic response if treated with the same drug. If these patients are given a drug from another class of antipsychotic, they should be carefully observed for a sensitivity reaction(16). Patients who have Parkinson's disease may have a recrudescence of symptoms when treated with these drugs due to increased dopamine blockade. This may occur whether or not the patient is being treated pharmacologically for the Parkinson's disease(17).

Patients with a history of a blood dyscrasia are more likely to develop a dyscrasia as a side effect to these drugs than will someone with no such history. Those with a history of liver damage or dysfunction may be more at risk to develop obstructive jaundice when treated with antipsychotics, and those with severe liver damage may not be able to detoxify and inactivate these drugs adequately(18). The anticholinergic properties of the drugs may result in increased intraocular pressure in patients with acute narrow angle glaucoma. Patients with chronic wide angle glaucoma can usually be safely treated with these drugs if the glaucoma is treated with cholinergic eyedrops throughout the course of treatment with antipsychotics(19). Men who have prostatic hypertrophy are more at risk for urinary hesitancy or retention when they are treated with these drugs because of their anticholinergic properties.

Pregnant women should be treated with these drugs only when necessary, especially during the first trimester of pregnancy. Antipsychotics have not conclusively been shown to be teratogenic, but they do pass the blood-placenta barrier and can cause extrapyramidal symptoms or a postnatal depression syndrome, followed by agitation, in newborns delivered from mothers treated with antipsychotics. Antipsychotics are also secreted in human milk in small quantities, and should probably be avoided by nursing mothers.

When a pregnant woman is in need of these drugs, it is necessary to weigh the risks to mother and child of allowing the psychotic symptoms to continue untreated, versus the risks of possible, but unproven, risks to the fetus. In some cases it is a greater risk to allow psychotic symptoms to go untreated(20).

Guidelines for Use

There is wide variation in the way antipsychotics are instituted, the doses used, and the length of the course of treatment. All these factors depend on the patient's age, size, and weight and his history, symptoms, and behavior.

The dosage ranges are wide because of the high therapeutic index. In general, there does seem to be a low limit of effectiveness, below which there is no appreciable antipsychotic effect. This level is 300 mg. of chlorpromazine or its equivalent for any other drug(21). Above this minimum level, there is tremendous variability in the effective dose. Several studies have shown that most patients do as well at doses of less than 1,500 mg. of chlorpromazine or its equivalent than they do at a higher dose(22). However, some patients who do not respond at lower doses do respond at very high doses. Studies report the use of up to 7,000 mg. of chlorpromazine, 1,500 mg. fluphenazine, 1,000 mg. haloperidol, or 600 mg. trifluoperazine(23). At these doses, there are few reports of side effects that are any more intense than those reported at lower doses. Since few patients seem to need such high doses, most patients receive daily doses of somewhere between 300 and 1,600 mg. of chlorpromazine or its equivalent. In the last several years, serum level assays of antipsychotics have become available, but they are of little value in judging when a dose is adequate, since serum levels have not been correlated with antipsychotic effect.

Antipsychotics are usually prescribed as follows: The patient is first given a small test dose to rule out severe hypotension, sedation, or severe allergic response. This test dose is usually about 50 mg. of chlorpromazine or its equivalent. If the patient has no untoward reaction, he is usually started on a schedule of small, daily, divided doses in the range of 600 to 1,200 mg. of chlorpromazine or its equivalent. In patients who are over 40 years of age or who are less acutely ill, the dosage range is 300 to 600 mg. of chlorpromazine or its equivalent. Doses are gradually increased until a dose is reached at which the side effects are unacceptable, or at which clinical improvement occurs(24). At this point, the dose is reduced carefully to the highest

The Antipsychotics			
Generic name	Trade name	Approximate potency relative to chlorpromazine	IM Form
Phenothiazines			
Aliphatics			
chlorpromazine	Thorazine	100 mg.	yes
triflupromazine	Vesprin	25-50 mg.	yes
Piperidines			
thioridazine	Mellaril	100 mg.	no
mesoridazine	Serentil	25-50 mg.	yes
piperacetazine	Quide	10-15 mg.	no
Piperazines			
trifluoperazine	Stelazine	5 mg.	yes
acetophenazine	Tindal	20 mg.	no
fluphenazine	Prolixin	1-4 mg.	yes
fluphenazine enanthate	Prolixin Enanthate	no reliable correlation	yes
fluphenazine decanoate	Prolixin Decanoate	no reliable correlation	yes
perphenazine	Trilafon	8-12 mg.	yes
prochlorperazine	Compazine	15-50 mg.	yes
butaperazine	Repoise	10-15 mg.	no
carphenazine	Proketazine	25-50 mg.	no
Thioxanthenes			
chlorprothixene	Taractan	50-100 mg.	yes
thiothixene	Navane	2-10 mg.	yes
Butyrophenones			
haloperidol	Haldol	1.6-2 mg.	yes
Dihydroindolones			
molindone	Lidone Moban	10-15 mg.	no
Dibenzoxapines			
loxapine	Loxitane Daxolin	10-20 mg.	no
Diphenylbutyl piperidines			
penfluridol pimozide	both are experimental		

dose at which there is clinical improvement of symptoms with minimal side effects.

After 5 or 10 days, when the patient's symptoms are in control and tolerance has developed to the acute side effects, the patient can have his dosage schedule rearranged so he gets the same total dose but divided into one or two doses instead of three or four(25). Patients tend to prefer one dose at bedtime, as it is easier to carry out a simple regimen that does not call for carrying medication during the day. If there are side effects, they will be more likely to occur at night when the patient is asleep. It is also less expensive to buy fewer tablets or capsules of larger doses than to buy more of the smaller dose tablets or capsules.

The patient continues on his dose for a full drug trial of three to six weeks(26). If at that time there has been no improvement, one must question if the patient is actually taking his medicine. Often, lack of response is a result of noncompliance. If the patient continues to be symptomatic and you are fairly certain he is taking his medication, he may require a drug from a different class or subclass.

Even after a full trial of a second drug, there will be some patients who do not respond. There are several alternatives. They can be given a trial of a third antipsychotic, or these patients can be given intramuscular medications with the hope that their nonresponse is due to inadequate absorption in the gut. Occasionally, a nonresponder to oral medications will respond to an IM dose(27). Another alternative for the nonresponder (this comprises 10 to 20 percent of patients with schizophrenia) is electroconvulsive treatment (ECT)(28).

Once the acute phase of the illness is past (usually in 4 to 12 weeks), the dose can be very slowly lowered to a maintenance dose that is often one-half to one-fifth the highest dose used to control the psychotic symptoms(29).

How long a patient remains on maintenance medication will depend on the likelihood that he will have a recurrence of symptoms. A patient having a first psychotic episode, unless it was so severe that it was life threatening, will not require long-term maintenance. Even after a second psychotic episode, there is no need for maintenance medication if the episodes are mild or separated in time by several years. Long-term maintenance is used for patients who have a history of recurring psychotic episodes (usually patients with schizophrenia) where there is a high probability of future relapse. Patients who are continued on long-term maintenance run a risk of developing tardive dyskinesia (see the next article).

Whenever antipsychotics are discontinued, they should be gradually tapered. If chlorpromazine or thioridazine is abruptly withdrawn, the patient may experience such symptoms as nausea, vomiting, and diarrhea within 48 hours of withdrawal. With abrupt discontinuation of high doses of high-potency drugs, there may be withdrawal dyskinesias that should diminish over time(30,31).

Rapid Neuroleptization

There are times when the usual method of treating patients with these drugs is inadequate. When a patient is acutely psychotic and in severe psychic pain, or when he is combative or assaultive or in imminent danger of harming himself or others, rapid neuroleptization may be required.

Before proceeding to medicate such an acutely disturbed patient, it is important to perform a brief physical exam first. This may be difficult because of the patient's inability to cooperate. However, it is imperative to at least check the patient's neurological and cardiovascular status to rule out intracranial tumor, hypertension, hypotension, head injury, or toxic delirium. A brief history, particularly for drug use in the preceding week, is important.

Once the patient has been examined and the above conditions ruled out, antipsychotics are begun orally or intramuscularly. (See table above). The patient is given an initial dose. Then, depending on his response, the same dose is repeated every 30 to 60 minutes until the patient is sedated or falls asleep or until the acute psychotic symptoms (severe anxiety, hallucinations, delusions, suspiciousness, aggressiveness, grandiosity) abate. Before each dose, the patient should have his blood pressure and pulse taken, lying down and standing, to test for orthostatic hypotension, and a brief mental status examination should be performed.

Drugs Used for Rapid Neuroleptization

Drug	Dose range for single dose IM
loxapine	5-10 mg.
perphenazine	4-30 mg.
trifluoperazine	1-10 mg.
fluphenazine	1-25 mg.
haloperidol	1-10 mg.
thiothixene	4-30 mg.
chlorpromazine	25-100 mg.

High-potency drugs may reduce the risk of sedation, hypotension, and cardiovascular side effects. However, in practice, some clinicians prefer chlorpromazine because of its sedating properties(32,33).

Most patients will respond favorably to such a regimen after 2 to 10 consecutive doses. When a response occurs, the patient can be changed to a daily oral dose equal to one to one and one-half times the effective IM dose required in the first 24 hours.

As a general rule, geriatric patients have diminished absorption, distribution, metabolism, and excretion of all drugs. Antipsychotics are no exception. Because the elderly are more sensitive to the anticholinergic effects of the antipsychotics, these patients are more likely to experience side effects at a lower dose and can more quickly develop toxic reactions with symptoms of confusion, disorientation, lethargy, restlessness, delirium, or agitation. Elderly patients may experience severe orthostatic hypotension that can result in falls and trauma. They are also more prone to the sedative effects of chlorpromazine and thioridazine, which have the greatest anticholinergic activity. Elderly men with prostate enlargement are more likely to develop urinary hesitancy or retention, and older patients of both sexes are more prone to constipation and bowel obstruction as side effects.

Because they are the least anticholinergic and, thus, have a lesser incidence of sedation and hypotension, such high-potency drugs as haloperidol are recommended for elderly patients(34). Doses of antipsychotics for the elderly are often one-third to one-half those of younger adults, but usually not below the minimum effective dose of 300 mg. of chlorpromazine or its equivalent(35). Doses are raised slowly with careful monitoring of side effects.

Antipsychotic medications are used in children for the same indications as in adults. Smaller doses are often used because of the smaller body size. Doses are 20 to 50 percent of adult doses(36).

Side Effects

Although some side effects are fairly common with these drugs, they are usually not severe or dangerous. They are, however, uncomfortable and sometimes frightening to many patients. When they are recognized and dealt with appropriately, the patient can have a significantly more comfortable course of treatment.

Many of the side effects will diminish after several days or weeks of therapy. Many side effects, however, can be treated by a reduction in dose, and all side effects are reversible, with the exception of some cases of tardive dyskinesia (see the article beginning on page 1324).

Some drugs have a greater in-

Drug Interactions with the Antipsychotics

Agent	Effect
Alcohol and/or barbiturates	Speeds the action of liver microsomal enzymes so antipsychotic is metabolized more quickly; potentiates CNS depressant effect
Tricyclic antidepressants	Can lead to severe anticholinergic side effects; antipsychotics can raise the plasma level of the antidepressant, probably by inhibiting metabolism of the antidepressant
Hydrochlorthiazide and hydralazine	Can produce severe hypotension
Guanethidine	Antihypertensive effect is blocked by chlorpromazine, haloperidol, and thiothixene
Cigarettes	Heavy consumption requires larger doses of antipsychotic
Meperidine	Respiratory depression is enhanced by chlorpromazine
Anticonvulsants	Seizure threshold may be lowered by antipsychotic requiring adjustment of anticonvulsant
Levodopa	Antiparkinsonian effect may be inhibited by antipsychotics
General anesthesia	Antipsychotic may potentiate effect of anesthetic

cidence of certain specific side effects. In general, it is true that any side effect can occur with any of these drugs. No two patients will have exactly the same side effects with the same drug, and often a patient who experiences a particular side effect on one drug will not experience the same symptoms with another drug.

Sedation. This effect is most common with chlorpromazine, but it can occur with the other drugs. Accommodation to this side effect usually occurs a week or two after the dose has been stabilized. If the sedation is severe, a reduction in the dose should alleviate the symptom. If sedation is mild, it can be treated by encouraging the patient to get up in the morning and get moving in an effort to fight the sedation. Reassure the patient that the symptom will pass with time. For patients with sleep disturbance, sedation will afford the patient a good night's sleep.

Orthostatic hypotension. This effect results from alpha-adrenergic blockade and is more common with low-potency antipsychotics, though it can occur with high-potency drugs as well. Orthostatic hypotension usually occurs early in the course of treatment and usually disappears one or two weeks after the dose is stabilized. The patient experiences this side effect as dizziness or light-headedness, especially in the morning when getting out of bed. The patient often reports accompanying tachycardia or palpitations as his heart rate increases to compensate for the hypotension. To validate these symptoms, the patient's blood pressure and pulse should be taken lying and standing. A fall in systolic blood pressure of 30 mm. Hg or greater is significant.

When this side effect is mild, reassure the patient that the symptom will pass in a week or two. Advise him to get out of bed slowly in the morning, sitting at the side of the bed for a full minute before standing. Likewise, throughout the day, he should rise from sitting positions slowly. Surgical elastic stockings can help in mild cases to prevent venous pooling. When more severe, especially in elderly patients, orthostatic hypotension can result in falls that can lead to fractures or other injuries. If severe, it can be treated by reducing the dosage or by changing to a high-potency drug with a lower incidence of this side effect. Occasionally, the orthostatic drop can be so severe that it can cause fatal cardiac arrest(37).

Alterations in sexual functioning. All antipsychotics can diminish sex drive. This can be beneficial for patients who are hypersexual. For others, this side effect can be distressing. When a patient reports this as a problem, bear in mind that a reduced sex drive can have any number of causes other than medication. It may result from the patient's illness or from current conflicts with the sexual partner(s).

Thioridazine has caused ejaculatory difficulty in males. Patients with this side effect can achieve erection, but they are either unable to ejaculate or they have retrograde ejaculations(38).

Depression of hypothalamic functions. This can lead to a variety of symptoms. Appetite can be increased, leading to weight gain. This is fairly common, particularly for patients taking chlorpromazine, and it is best treated with diet and exercise. Molindone, however, is purported to prevent weight gain and even cause weight loss in obese patients(39).

Occasionally, women will become amenorrheic. When this occurs, bear in mind that the cause of the amenorrhea may be pregnancy or simply the stresses concomitant with the patient's illness. Occasionally, women may also develop galactorrhea. When mild, patients will often tolerate this side effect and wear small breast pads in their bra. When severe, it is best treated by reducing the dose of drug or changing to another drug. Women can have false-positive pregnancy tests while taking antipsychotics.

Male patients can develop gynecomastia. This is usually intolerable to the patient and calls for a change in the drug.

Seizures. All the antipsychotic medications lower the seizure threshold. Patients with a preexisting seizure disorder may need an increase in prophylactic antiepileptic medication. Patients with no history of seizure disorder may have grand mal seizures if given high doses of antipsychotics or if given rapidly increasing doses. This, however, is a rare occurrence. Such patients are not protected from further seizures by the addition of an antiepileptic drug and are best treated by reducing the dose of the antipsychotic(40).

Decreased tolerance to alcohol. Warn patients who plan to drink alcoholic beverages to take a smaller amount than usual and observe their response before proceeding. They may feel intoxicated by a much smaller amount of alcohol than they are accustomed to.

Anticholinergic side effects. These symptoms include nasal congestion, dry mouth, blurred near vision, constipation, and urinary hesitancy or retention. Chlorpromazine and thioridazine are the most anticholinergic of these drugs, and haloperidol and the piperazine phenothiazines are the least(41). Nasal congestion can be relieved temporarily by nasal decongestants but probably is best tolerated until the body adjusts. Dry mouth is best relieved by frequent rinsing or sucking on hard candies or chewing gum. Sugarless gum and candies are preferred, since the sugar in regular candies can foster monilial infections.

Blurred near vision usually abates in a week or two after the dose of medication is adjusted. Patients should be discouraged from getting new glasses unless the blurring continues for more than two weeks after the dose is stabilized.

Constipation, when mild, can be treated by encouraging the patient to increase his intake of bran, fluids, and fresh fruits and vegetables. A mild laxative will also help. When severe, constipation has been known to cause intestinal obstruction.

Urinary hesitancy can lead to urinary retention. This can be treated acutely with catheterization and with the addition of a cholinergic medication such as bethanechol(42). A reduction in antipsychotic dose will also help, or the offending medication can be discontinued and replaced with one that is less anticholinergic.

When antipsychotics are used in combination with other drugs that have anticholinergic properties, such as antiparkinsonian drugs or tricyclic antidepressants, the risk of severe anticholinergic side effects is increased. Some patients, commonly the elderly or those taking several drugs with anticholinergic properties, can develop a psychotic picture with the following symptoms: purposeless overactivity; agitation; confusion; disorientation; dry, flushed skin; tachycardia; sluggish, dilated pupils; bowel hypomotility; dysarthria; and memory impairment. The treatment of this syndrome, often called "atropine psychosis," is discontinuation of the medication(s). IM or I.V. physostigmine may be used in severe cases (43).

Allergic symptoms. The most common allergic response is a pruritic maculopapular rash. It usually appears on the face, neck, and chest about 2 to 10 weeks after the drug is first administered(44). This side effect is most common with chlorpromazine. If the rash is mild, it needs no treatment and will often clear on its own. If it is severe, the medication can be discontinued until the rash clears. A second trial on the same drug may not cause another rash(45). If the patient is acutely disturbed and cannot do without medication, a different drug can be started immediately. Those administering these drugs can develop contact dermatitis from contact with the liquid concentrate or tablets.

Phototoxicity. This is most common with chlorpromazine and rare with high-potency drugs(46). It consists of an extreme sensitivity of the skin to sunlight, such that brief exposure can cause sunburn. Patients should be advised to test for this reaction with a brief exposure to the sun. If they are sensitive, they can wear protective clothing or use a sunscreening lotion containing para-amino benzoic acid.

Cholestatic jaundice. This is a rare side effect of the phenothiazines(47). Early symptoms include malaise, fever, nausea, and abdominal pain. In another week after these symptoms appear, the patient develops itching and jaundice. This side effect is reversible and is usually benign and self-limiting. It is treated by discontinuing the drug, bed rest, and a high-protein, high-carbohydrate diet. It is most common with chlorpromazine and usually occurs in the first month of treatment. If a patient is acutely psychotic, he can be immediately started on a different antipsychotic(48).

Agranulocytosis. This is another rare side effect that occurs in the first eight weeks of treatment. It is most common in older women and most often occurs with low-potency phenothiazines and thioxanthenes(49). It develops abruptly with sore throat, fever, malaise, and sores in the mouth. If these symptoms develop in a patient started on antipsychotics in the past two months, a complete blood count should be drawn immediately, as leukopenia confirms the diagnosis. This should be considered to be an extreme emergency, and is treated by stopping the drug and initiating reverse isolation. If the initial phase of the illness is not fatal, the leukocyte count will return to normal in 7 to 10 days, with rapid recovery. Other blood dyscrasias reported include eosinophilia, thrombocytopenia, anemia, aplastic anemia, and pancytopenia.

Pigmentation of the skin and eyes. This can occur with long-term treatment with low-potency phenothiazines or with thioxanthenes (50). Pigmentation begins as a golden brown coloration, which can progress to slate gray, metallic blue, or purple. It occurs in skin surfaces often exposed to sunlight and is caused by deposition of pigment granules similar to melanin. Pigment can also be deposited in the conjunctiva, sclera, lens, and cornea. These eye changes are usually of no functional significance and do not impair vision(51). The pigment is reabsorbed after the drugs are discontinued.

Pigmentary retinopathy. This has been reported in patients taking thioridazine in doses higher than 800 mg. a day(51). It can cause blindness. Thus, thioridazine is never prescribed in amounts greater than 800 mg. per day.

Hypothalamic crisis. This is a rare but serious side effect(52). Some patients have only one symptom—hyperpyrexia. Other patients have additional symptoms of diaphoresis, drooling, tachycardia, dyspnea, seizures, and unstable blood pressure. This side effect is treated by stopping the drug and treating the individual symptoms.

Hyperglycemia. Occasionally, the side effect of hyperglycemia will unmask a previously undiagnosed case of mild diabetes mellitus. Patients previously diagnosed as having diabetes may need some alteration in insulin dose or diet to compensate(53).

Cardiac changes. These are usually mild and result from the anticholinergic action of the antipsychotics. They consist of mild ECG changes that are due to altered repolarization rather than to myocardial damage(54). In patients with preexisting cardiovascular disease, an ECG should be done before starting antipsychotic medications, and a cardiology consult should be obtained. The best drugs for patients with cardiac disease are those with low anticholinergic effects, such as haloperidol and the piperazine phenothiazines(55).

Gastrointestinal distress. Although many antipsychotics have antiemetic properties, heartburn or nausea can occur. Patients who have gastrointestinal distress usually respond to taking their medications at mealtimes or with a glass of milk.

This comprehensive list of side effects may seem overwhelming; however, in practice, side effects are usually mild. Even so, they can be annoying to the patient and should be recognized and treated. We should encourage patients to continue their medications despite the discomforts of the mild side effects until the maximum therapeutic effect is obtained. Only at that point can the patient decide whether the favorable effects of the drug outweigh whatever discomforts it brings.

Patients and their families often have a variety of misconceptions and fears about antipsychotic drugs. Many believe that these drugs are addictive. This is clearly not true, and the belief should be immediately dispelled. Many people argue against taking their drugs because they feel they are unnatural. The truth is that they are no more unnatural than the psychosis they are designed to treat. What these drugs do, when they are effective, is to return a very disturbed person to his more "natural" or usual state of mind.

Another common misconception is that patients who take high doses are "crazier" than patients who take low doses. Nurses often overhear patients comparing their dosage levels. Explain to patients with this fear that the dose depends on a number of individual factors, such as age, weight, and metabolism, and there is no relationship between number of milligrams and severity of illness.

When patients are started on these drugs, it is important that they be told what the drug will do and what it will not do. For example, a socially isolated, unemployed woman with auditory hallucinations and disorganized thinking can be told that the drug will help stop the hallucinations and help clear up her thinking but will not get her a job and find her friends. It is important that patients have a realistic notion of what to expect. Many hold the mistaken belief that antipsychotics will solve all their problems. In fact, they will only treat the psychosis and thereby free the patient to work on his other problems.

When patients are started on these medications, they should also be given a clear idea of what their course of treatment will be—low doses at first, then gradually increasing doses until the drug takes effect. The patient should be informed that it often takes several days, weeks, or even months to see a complete response. He should be informed of the most common early side effects, such as dystonias, parkinsonism, and sedation and be asked to inform the staff of any unusual symptoms. Patients who will be on maintenance for some months should be told about the risk of tardive dyskinesia and should be taught the early symptoms and the importance of early detection.

Patients leaving the hospital and all outpatients, as well as their families, should know the name of the drug being taken and the exact dose, the number of tablets or capsules, and the exact dose schedule. They should be taught that failure to continue medications when they are prescribed for long-term maintenance has been proven to increase greatly the risk of relapse. And, patients and their families should be taught to recognize the symptoms of relapse and told to report to their health care provider immediately if these symptoms appear.

The symptoms of relapse are somewhat different in different patients, but can include difficulty concentrating, loss of appetite, trouble sleeping, restlessness, preoccupation with one or two thoughts, social withdrawal, paranoia, hallucinations, religious preoccupation, delusions, and many other symptoms. The patient and his family can usually tell you about the particular symptoms of relapse by thinking back to the time just before treatment began.

Outpatients should be told what to do if they forget or skip a dose. If the patient is taking divided doses, he should add the missed dose to the next dose. If he takes only one dose per day, he should skip the missed dose. Patients should be told that they may feel, at times, like stopping or changing the schedule for their medications but that they should check with their health care provider first. They should be warned of a possible decrease in tolerance to alcohol. If they are on a sedating drug, they should be warned about the danger of operating cars or dangerous machinery before their body has had time to adjust to the sedating properties.

When antipsychotic medications are used properly and patients are monitored carefully for side effects, the treatment of acute and painful psychotic episodes can be humane and expeditious.

References

1. Baldessarini, R J *Chemotherapy in Psychiatry* Cambridge, Mass., Harvard University Press, 1977, p 31
2. *Ibid*, p 32
3. Bergersen, B S *Pharmacology in Nursing* St Louis, C V Mosby Co, 1976, p 677
4. Appleton, W S, and Davis, J M *Practical Clinical Psychopharmacology* 2d ed Baltimore, Md, Williams & Wilkins, 1980, p 60
5. Gilman, A G, and others, eds Goodman and Gilman's *The Pharmacological Basis of Therapeutics* 6th ed New York, Macmillan Publishing Co, 1980, p 418
6. Irons, P D *Psychotropic Drugs and Nursing Intervention* New York, McGraw-Hill Book Co, 1978, p 15
7. Snyder, S H The dopamine hypothesis of schizophrenia focus on the dopamine receptor *Am J Psychiatry* 122 197-202, Feb 1976
8. Gilman, A G, and others, eds *Goodman and Gilman's The Pharmacological Basis of Therapeutics* 6th ed New York, Macmillan Publishing Co, 1980, p 404
9. *Ibid*, p 405
10. Baldessarini, *op cit*, p 23
11. *Ibid*, p 24
12. Appleton and Davis, *op cit*, p 30
13. Baldessarini, *op cit*, p 60
14. Klein, Donald F, and others *Diagnosis and Drug Treatment of Psychiatric Disorders Adults and Children* 2d ed Baltimore, Md, Williams & Wilkins Co, 1980, p 101
15. Schooler, N R, and others Depot fluphenazine in the prevention of relapse in schizophrenia *Psychopharmacol Bull* 15 44-47, Apr 1979
16. Klein and others, *op cit*, p 47
17. Gilman and others, *op cit*, p 481
18. *Ibid*, p 404
19. Baldessarini, *op cit*, p 50
20. Lipton, M A and others, eds *Psychopharmacology A Generation of Progress*, New York, Raven Press, 1978, p 1047
21. Baldessarini, *op cit*, p 28
22. Appleton and Davis, *op cit*, p 32
23. Aubree, J C, and Loder, M H High and very high dosage antipsychotics a critical review *J Clin Psychiatry* 41 341-350, Oct 1980
24. Shader, R I, and Jackson, A H Approaches to schizophrenia IN *Manual of Psychiatric Therapeutics*, ed by R I Shader Boston, Little, Brown & Co, 1975, p 87
25. *Ibid*, p 88
26. Gilman and others, *op cit*, p 415
27. Klein and others, *op cit*, p 109
28. Salzman, Carl Electroconvulsive therapy IN *Manual of Psychiatric Therapeutics*, ed by R I Shader Boston, Little, Brown & Co, 1975, p 116
29. Appleton and Davis, *op cit*, p 39
30. Appleton and Davis, *op cit*, p 61
31. Baldessarini, *op cit*, p 45
32. Appleton and Davis, *op cit*, p 29
33. Klein and others, *op cit*, p 92
34. Appleton and Davis, *op cit*, p 56
35. Salzman, Carl, and others Psychopharmacology and the geriatric patient IN *Manual of Psychiatric Therapeutics*, ed by R I Shader Boston, Little, Brown & Co, 1975, p 173
36. Baldessarini, *op cit*, p 40
37. Shader and Jackson, *op cit*, p 91
38. Appleton and Davis, *op cit*, p 66
39. Gardos, G, and Cole, J O Weight reduction in schizophrenics by molindone *Am J Psychiatry* 134 302-304, Mar 1977
40. Klein and others, *op cit*, p 198
41. Baldessarini, *op cit*, p 103
42. Appleton and Davis, *op cit*, p 74
43. Baldessarini, *op cit*, p 49
44. Appleton and Davis, *op cit*, p 67
45. Gilman and others, *op cit*, p 413
46. Klein and others, *op cit*, p 192
47. *Ibid*, p 195
48. *Ibid*, p 196
49. Baldessarini, *op cit*, p 53
50. *Ibid*, p 50
51. Klein and others, *op cit*, p 193
52. Baldessarini, *op cit*, pp 48-49
53. Appleton and Davis, *op cit*, p 69
54. Klein and others, *op cit*, p 184
55. Gilman and others, *op cit*, p 404

DRUGS AND DEPRESSION BY BETH HARRIS

Reprinted from American Journal of Nursing, March 1986

DEPRESSION

Tricyclic Antidepressant	Major depression Bipolar disorder, depressed Atypical depression Schizoaffective disorder Dysthymic disorder	Imipramine (Tofranil)	150–300 mg
		Desipramine (Norpramin)	100–300 mg
		Amitriptyline (Elavil)	150–300 mg
		Nortriptyline (Pamelor)	50–100 mg
		Doxepin (Sinequan)	75–300 mg
		Protriptyline (Vivactil)	15–60 mg
		Trimipramine (Surmontil)	50–200 mg

Sedation	Reassure patient that this is temporary. Evaluate degree of sedation. Possibly change time of drug administration.
Dry mouth	Usually temporary. Frequent sips of water or chewing unsweetened gum will help.
Blurred vision	Reassure patient that blurring is usually temporary.
Constipation	Encourage patient to increase fluid and fiber intake. Give stool softeners or laxatives if severe. In rare cases, intestinal obstruction may occur.
Urinary hesitance	Record output and palpate bladder if retention is suspected. Explain urinary retention and possible need for catheterization or the use of cholinergic agents. May require change of medicine.
Nasal congestion	Reassure patient that this is usually temporary. Use a room vaporizer or nasal sprays if severe.
Orthostatic hypotension with reflex tachycardia	Reassure patient that symptoms may be temporary. May cause falls in the elderly. Use fall prevention precautions. Encourage patient to rise slowly from a sitting or lying position. Record lying and standing BPs.
Tremor	Reassure patient that this is a benign side effect. Give beta-blockers if prescribed.
Problems with orgasm (either sex) or with erection (in men)	Reassure patient that problem may be caused by depression and, if so, will be relieved by the medicine. If caused by the medicine, the problem is almost always reversible.
Slowing of intracardiac conduction, quinidine-like effect	Monitor cardiac status of patients with preexisting heart disease. Check blood presure and pulse at least twice daily. Repeat EKGs 2–3 times a week until dose is adjusted.
Lowered seizure threshold	Initiate seizure precautions for patients with preexisting seizure disorders. Note in Kardex or by other method so that staff is alerted to the possibility of seizures.

Tetracyclic Antidepressant Other antidepressants	Same as the tricyclics	Maprotiline (Ludiomil)	125–225 mg
		Amoxapine (Asendin)	150–600 mg
		Trazodone (Desyrel)	150–600 mg
		Nomifensine (Merital)	100–300 mg

Maprotiline—Same as the tricyclics

Amoxapine—Same as the tricyclics and all antipsychotic side effects

Trazodone—Same as the tricyclics and cardiac irritability

Nomifensine—Same as the tricyclics

Monoamine Oxidase Inhibitor (MAOI) Antidepressant	Same as the tricyclics	Isocarboxazid (Marplan)	30–40 mg
		Phenelzine (Nardil)	60–90 mg
		Tranylcypromine (Parnate)	30–60 mg

Insomnia	Give all doses before 3 PM, e.g., 8–12–3 or 8–12.
Orthostatic hypotension with reflex tachycardia	See previous discussion of this problem.
Dry mouth	See previous discussion of this problem.
Hypertensive crisis	Occurs when patient fails to adhere to a low tyramine diet and/or to adhere to certain medicine restrictions. Teach patient foods and medicines to avoid. Give patient a list of restrictions to carry at all times. Explain symptoms of impending hypertensive crisis: stiff neck, headache, palpitations, chest pain, nausea. Can be fatal.
Weight gain	Teach patient to control with a moderately calorie-restricted diet.
Sedation	See previous discussion of this problem.
Headache	Conservative measures may or may not be effective. Patient should be kept quiet. Apply warm or cold compresses and give aspirin or acetaminophen as needed.
Excitement	Dosage or medicine may have to be changed if severe.
Constipation	See previous discussion of this problem.
Difficulty with orgasm	See previous discussion of this problem.
Blurred vision	See previous discussion of this problem.

Drug Class	Indications	Name of Drug	Usual Daily Dose
Antipsychotic	Major depression with psychotic features Bipolar disorder with psychotic features Schizoaffective disorder	Chlorpromazine (Thorazine)	300–1200 mg
		Thioridiazine (Mellaril)	300–800 mg
		Trifluoperazine (Stelazine)	15–60 mg
		Fluphenazine (Prolixin)	6–24 mg
		Perphenazine (Trilafon)	24–96 mg
		Thiothixene (Navane)	30–120 mg
		Haloperidol (Haldol)	6–24 mg
		Molindone (Moban)	30–120 mg
		Loxapine (Loxitane)	30–120 mg

Side Effects	Nursing Management
Parkinsonism (akinesia, stiffness, tremor, mask-like facies, shuffling or propulsive gait, loss of associated movements)	Administer antidyskinetic medicines such as diphenhydramine (Benadryl) or benztropine (Cogentin) if prescribed. Reassure patient that side effects are treatable.
Dystonia	Administer antidyskinetic medicines if prescribed, preferably in IM form. Reassure patient that side effect is treatable. Reduce sensory stimulation until symptoms subside.
Akathisia (restlessness)	Administer antidyskinetic medicines if prescribed, or other medicines used to treat akathisia, such as diazepam (Valium). Reassure patient that this is treatable.
Tardive dyskinesia	Teach patients taking antipsychotics about tardive dyskinesia: its definition, prevalence, early detection, possible irreversibility, and lack of definitive cure. Observe for early signs using the AIMS scale.
Sedation	See previous discussion.
Orthostatic hypotension with reflex tachycardia	See previous discussion.
Dry mouth	See previous discussion.
Blurred vision	See previous discussion.
Constipation	See previous discussion.
Urinary hesitance	See previous discussion
Nasal congestion	See previous discussion.
Problems with orgasm (either sex) or erection (in men)	See previous discussion.
Weight gain	See previous discussion.
Amenorrhea	Reassure patient that side effect is temporary and does not harm reproductive ability.
Decreased tolerance to alcohol, sedative-hypnotics and narcotics	Advise patient to limit alcohol to 1 to 2 drinks per day and to limit use of sedative-hypnotics and narcotics. Warn patient that these substances will have a much more powerful effect if patient is taking antipsychotics.
Rash	Reassure patient that rash is not harmful and is temporary.
Sensitivity to sunburn	Advise patient to use sunscreen lotion and to cover skin with clothing when outdoors for prolonged periods.
Cardiac arrhythmias	See previous discussion.
Lowered seizure threshold	See previous discussion.

Drug class	Indications	Name of Drug	Usual Daily Dose
Antimanic	Bipolar disorder Major depression, recurrent Schizoaffective disorder	Lithium carbonate (Lithonate, Eskalith, Lithobid, Lithane, Lithotabs) Lithium citrate	300–1500 mg

Side Effects	Nursing Management
Lithium toxicity	Results from an excessively high serum blood lithium level due to overdose, dehydration, fasting, a large drop in salt intake, or kidney dysfunction. When toxicity is suspected, hold the lithium and assess patient for toxic symptoms: nystagmus, coarse tremor, dysarthria, fasciculations, confusion, impaired consciousness, seizures, ataxia, severe diarrhea, vomiting, hyperreflexia, lack of coordination. For severe toxicity, diuresis or renal dialysis may be required. Lithium toxicity can be fatal. Periodic (every 2 mo.) serum lithium levels are necessary to keep within therapeutic range of approximately 0.5 to 1.5 meQ/liter. Advise patient not to take the morning dose of lithium on the day the level will be drawn.
Tremor	See previous discussion.
Nausea/abdominal discomfort	Reassure patient that discomfort is temporary and advise taking lithium with food or milk.
Polyuria/polydipsia	Encourage patient to increase fluid intake to quench thirst. Reassure patient that sign is not dangerous. If polyuria is severe, measure the 24-hour urine volume. If it is greater than 4 liters, a kidney workup may be in order. Encourage patient to maintain a stable fluid and salt intake. Carry out baseline and repeat kidney function studies on all patients taking lithium.
Mild diarrhea or increased number of bowel movements	Reassure patient that sign is usually temporary. If severe, reduced drug dosage may be required for 2 or 3 days.
Muscle weakness or fatigue	Explain to patient that these symptoms are often temporary, lasting only a few weeks, although they may persist as long as patient takes lithium. Encourage activity—walking, exercise.
Edema of the hands, face, or feet	Reassure patient that swelling is not dangerous and is not a sign of heart or lung disease.
Weight gain	See previous discussion.
Hypothyroidism	Carry out baseline and repeat thyroid function studies (every 6 mo.) on all patients taking lithium. Observe for signs of hypothyroidism—dry, coarse skin, facial or periorbital swelling, dull expression. Reassure patient that if this occurs, it is easily treated with thyroid replacement.
Worsening of dermatological conditions such as acne or psoriasis	Administer standard treatments, such as salves, antibiotics, or steroids, for these conditions.

AFTER THE FALL— CONFUSION

BY EMILY B. CAMPBELL/MARGARET A. WILLIAMS/SUSAN M. MLYNARCZYK

It's all too familiar: Independent elders, suddenly hospitalized, become confused. These nurses found out why.

Reprinted from American Journal of Nursing, February, 1986

Elvira Jones, age 78, was admitted to the orthopedic unit three hours after she fell at a church reception. She had fractured the neck of her right femur. On admission, she was alert and oriented. The day after the hip pinning, Ms. Jones became confused and stayed so for four days.

Here is an all-too-familiar case of an older person who had been functioning well but, when admitted suddenly to the hospital, developed episodes of confused behavior for no apparent reason. How extensive is the problem, and how can this confusion be prevented?

We decided to survey elderly patients hospitalized after surgical repair of a fractured hip.

We defined four behaviors as evidence of confusion: disorientation to time, place, or people in the environment; communication unusual for the person, such as yelling and calling out; unusual or inappropriate behavior, such as attempting to get out of bed or pulling off dressings; and evidence of illusions or hallucinations.

On orthopedic units in four hospitals, 170 hip fracture patients with an average age of 78 were monitored postoperatively for confusion. Every eight hours, nurses assessed patients for the four behaviors. If a behavior was not present, a score of 0 was assigned. If it was present at some time during the shift in mild form, the score was 1; if markedly present at some time during the shift, the score was 2. The highest possible confusion score for each shift was 8, for a total of 24 for each day.

Like Ms. Jones, none of the patients had a history of mental impairment, yet 52 percent became confused within five days after surgery(1). Of these, 36 percent were considered to have mild confusion (a 5-day confusion score of 1–15) and 16 percent were considered to have moderate/severe confusion (a score of more than 15).

Analysis of admission data for 21 possible risk factors as indicated through pilot studies and an extensive review of the literature showed that postoperative confusion was most likely in older patients who were not active before the injury and who did poorly on a simple 10-item mental status test. After admission, certain clinical factors—urinary problems, slow mobilization, and pain—were also associated with confusion. Having visitors, having personal possessions nearby, seeing time pieces, and using radio or television were associated with less confusion(1).

HOW NURSING CARE CAN REDUCE CONFUSION

Once we had identified the extent of the problem and risk factors, we were ready to move into the intervention phase—after which we concluded, "Yes, nursing care *can* reduce the incidence of confusion in patients like Ms. Jones." When specified measures were incorporated into nursing care of 57 similar patients on three of the four orthopedic units we studied, the incidence of confusion dropped from 52 to 44 percent. Tests controlling for risk factors among the two groups showed the reduction was not due to chance alone ($p < .02$)(2).

The chart on a following page summarizes the clinical interventions used in the four-year study(2).

The interventions were crafted from personal experiences, discussions with other nurses, and measures reported in

The authors are at the University of Wisconsin School of Nursing in Madison. Emily B. Campbell, RN, MS, and Margaret A. Williams, RN, PhD, are professors. Susan M. Mlynarczyk, RN, MS, is a social science research specialist. *The study on which this paper is based was supported by grant R01 NU00754 fron the Division of Nursing, Health Resources and Services Administration. The authors acknowledge the help of head nurses Susan Rosenbek, Agnes Trace, and Jane Masbruch who, with their staffs, made this study possible.*

Severe pain, inadequate pain relief, and slow postop mobilization were clear harbingers of confusion.

the literature(3-6). We also identified interventions based on risk factors documented in the initial survey of 170 patients. The three major risk factors, however, were those over which nurses have little control: increased age, low pre-injury activity level, and impaired mental status on admission. Risk factors that were found to be potentially amenable to nursing intervention included urinary problems, slow postoperative mobilization, and pain.

Some of the relationships among these risk factors were not always clear, however. For example, confusion and slow mobilization were often found in the same patients, but a cause-and-effect relationship in either direction was not documented.

It is important to note that, because aging reduces an individual's physiologic reserves, stress and insult may easily tip the balance and confusion may be the major—or only—manifestation of failure in one or more body systems. For example, drug toxicity, nutritional deficiencies, infections, metabolic disturbances, and impaired cerebral metabolism are but a few of the potential physiologic reasons for confusion(7,8). Others may be psychosensory problems such as stress, fear, anxiety, disruption in the pattern of life, and sensory deprivation(4,7,9).

We developed two protocols: One set to manage the six major factors thought to *contribute* to the development of confusion and the second to manage the four major behavior problems usually *associated with* acute confusion. Related goals for each problem were identified and a repertoire of nursing strategies was specified.

CONTRIBUTING FACTORS

Six major factors thought to contribute to confusion are:

Strange environment. Being uprooted from a familiar environment and confined in a hospital, regardless of the reason, can be stressful and frightening. Lack of regular contact with family and friends who would normally reconfirm one's sense of identity, unfamiliar routines and habits, restricted activity, and pain may predispose the patient to confusion. Being captive in a situation with limited opportunity to control what is happening can contribute to a profound sense of helplessness. Furthermore, when the environment is too fast-paced for the patient to understand what is happening, it can be frightening and overwhelming.

If we could see the hospital environment through the eyes of the older person, the appropriate interventions would become clearer. Routines, procedures and equipment can be described slowly and clarified frequently so that the person will have a better understanding of what is expected. For example, explain how to get help when meals are served, where the bathroom is, how to use the bedpan.

Most important, the older person can be helped to establish his identity with the staff. "Therapeutic socializing," encouraging reminiscence and life review, will help staff to see the person as an individual and reinforce the patient's sense of identity.

Altered sensory input. In the hospital, a patient may bounce between periods of overstimulation and understimulation. Staff often hurry in and out of rooms. Because older people need more time to process information, however, they may be overwhelmed when rushed into activities and may be befuddled by instructions given quickly. Being left alone, subject to sensory deprivation, is another hazard; if the patient is denied eyeglasses or hearing aid, the problem is compounded and the sense of isolation deepened.

Loss of control and independence can overwhelm anyone but is particularly threatening for the older person. The impact of sudden hospitalization, unanticipated surgery, prolonged recovery, and an uncertain future leave the person feeling completely out of control. Efforts must be made to enable the person to control the situation when possible. It helps to explore with the patient the impact the injury will have on his future. It may be necessary to discuss the advantages and disadvantages of temporary nursing home placement, of staying with a son or daughter, and other alternatives.

Disruption in life pattern. Sudden hospitalization disrupts the pattern and meaning of one's life and can lead to confusion. Calling a patient by the preferred name can comfort. Reminiscing and visits or calls from family and friends help link past and present and reinforce identity and feelings of competence.

Immobility and pain are, unfortunately, the common lot of patients with hip fractures. Even more distressing, older patients often are undermedicated for pain because staff hesitate to administer more than minimum doses of analgesic. In fact, in our preliminary survey, we found that a low level of narcotic administration, severe pain, and slow postoperative mobilization clearly were associated with development of confusion(1).

Physical activity, including range of motion, has both physiologic and psychologic benefits. Physiologically, it minimizes the deconditioning aspects of inactivity and immobility. Older people are particularly vulnerable to disuse atrophy. Because of the normal changes of aging, they do not have the reserves with which to "bounce back." Psychologically, movement, touch, change of position, and change of the visual field can relieve boredom and provide sensory stimulation.

Disrupted pattern of elimination. In the survey, in the intervention phases of this study, and in an earlier exploratory study we found a relationship between urinary elimination problems and confusion(1,2,10).

Hospitalization inevitably interrupts long-established elimination patterns. The problem may be circular: Worry and apprehension about the timing of, privacy for, and assistance with elimination may overwhelm the person and increase the potential for confusion;

STRATEGIES FOR MANAGING CONFUSION

MANIPULATING CONTRIBUTING FACTORS

Problem	Goal	Intervention
Strange environment	To establish meaning in environment	Provide normal living cues: curtains open during day, clock with large face where patient can see it (not obscured by glare or curtain), calendar within view, daily newspapers, hand mirror available. Ask patient how he or she wants the area organized. Encourage friends and family to bring in familiar objects. Encourage reminiscence. Ask the patient about the meaning of objects, such as pictures of relatives. Weave orienting material into conversation: *Good morning, Ms. Jones, it's already Friday, January 24. Does it seem like your operation was only three days ago?* Explain setting, routines, and role of personnel. Describe coming events such as meals, physical therapy, etc. Use frequent repetition.
Altered sensory input	To ease processing of environmental stimuli	Have eyeglasses (clean) and hearing aid (functional) in place when needed. Have adequate light, but avoid glare and lighting that produces sharp contrasts and shadows. Keep a night light on unless the person needs total darkness to sleep. Make eye contact at patient's level. Use touch as appropriate, for example, backrubs and handclasps. Turn patient and change position periodically. Try to pace activities to avoid rushing the patient. If a schedule cannot be adjusted, talk slowly while explaining the activity to give the person time to understand the information.
Loss of control and independence	To restore sense of control	Be sure patient has control over environment and care as far as possible. For example, even when a patient has no choice but to be out of bed, allow him or her to decide the time. Help patient discuss thoughts and feelings. Be nonjudgmental, accepting, and supportive. Build on patient's strengths and abilities. Help patient to understand procedures and treatments; re-clarify as necessary and encourage questions. Provide privacy.
Disrupted life pattern	To provide continuity with established life patterns	Limit the number of hospital staff who interact with patient. Call patient by preferred name. Encourage family to visit and call. Reassure family that they are not in the way. Help family to understand and help patient. Encourage patient to reminisce about life experiences. Phrases like "Remember when . . . ?" or "What was it like . . . ?" help to start the person talking. Integrate life-review interactions during care, e.g., during bathing and walking.
Immobility and pain	To reduce or relieve pain. To minimize effects of inactivity.	Anticipate and prevent pain. Involve patient in pain management and mobility. Ask what patient thinks will ease the pain or what position is most comfortable. Differentiate operative site pain from general discomfort, since the approach to relief differs. Encourage the patient to move as much and as often as possible, including bed exercises as prescribed. Focus on abilities, but deal realistically with disabilities. If patient tires quickly, allow rest periods but do not reduce activity.
Disrupted elimination patterns	To maintain or restore normal pattern	Assess usual habits and/or difficulties and plan accordingly. Explain how bedpans will be used. Provide for privacy. Actively involve patient in planning how best to meet elimination needs. If the person needs an indwelling catheter, explain how it feels. Respect the fear many patients have of having "an accident" and try to prevent it. In the case of incontinence, assess for cause (e.g., immobility or pain). Follow the simple routine of offering the bedpan at regular intervals.

CONTROLLING ASSOCIATED BEHAVIOR

Problem	Goal	Intervention
Confused behavior (e.g., disorientation, yelling, etc.)	To reduce or eliminate episodes of confusion	Describe the behaviors and the context. Assess for precipitating factors, both physiologic and environmental. Were there antecedent events? Is there a pattern? Possible physiologic factors are many: electrolyte imbalance, drugs, hypoxia, hypoxemia, hypotension, hypoglycemia, dehydration, pain. Use reality-orienting approaches, provide reassurance and the presence of a concerned person when possible.
Sundowning	To reduce or eliminate episodes of confusion	Review events at end of day to assess potential for sundowning: Ask open-ended questions, such as *Tell me how things went for you today* to uncover undue fatigue, unmet toilet needs, pain, unusual events, and the fear of being left alone—all associated with sundowning. Provide security; offer to check person at specific intervals. Relieve pain and discomfort. Continue reality-orienting approaches and provide reassurance. Again, the presence of a concerned person may help prevent sundowning.
Unsafe behavior and/or frightened behavior	To help patient regain control of situation	Control own agitation; be calm, matter-of-fact, don't raise voice. Patient is probably begging for control of the situation. Gently introduce a reality-based activity, e.g., offer a backrub or water or food. Try to reassure by use of gentle touch. Avoid confrontation or argument. Nurse's behavior should inspire sense of safety and security. Avoid use of restraints unless absolutely necessary. With guidance, help patient touch and "explore" tubes or intrusive equipment that may be frightening and confusing. Calmly sit at bedside to offer comfort. Talk quietly about how frightening it must seem, while carefully describing reality and demonstrating by your presence that you are there to help the person regain control.
Hallucinations or illusions	To clarify reality	Listen carefully to the patient's description, since there may be a basis in fact and the patient has simply misinterpreted the environment (illusion). Never support misperception. Calmly describe reality but don't argue. Reassure with comments such as *It may seem as if chickens are under your bed, but the sound you hear is the television in the next room. Remember you are in a hospital now and I am here to help you.* Such a statement acknowledges the worry without making the patient feel stupid, describes reality by explaining the possible sources of the noise, reminds the person that he/she is in the hospital, and gives assurance that someone is there to help. If possible, rearrange environment to preclude more error.

Primary nursing is ideal, but if not possible, consistent assignments at least lessen the demands placed on patients.

then confusion may diminish the ability to deal with elimination needs.

Questions about how to manage elimination needs may be embarrassing and go unanswered unless the nurse brings them up. For instance, has the patient experienced frequency? Urgency? Dribbling? How were these managed at home?

ASSOCIATED FACTORS

Sometimes, even when we have done all we can to compensate for the contributing factors, confusion still occurs. Here are our thoughts behind the protocols for factors associated with confusion:

Behavior suggestive of confusion. Usually, the first signs of acute confusion are disorientation to time, followed by place, then person. Disorientation to person generally means that the patient does not recognize others. Unlike the patient in a severe psychotic state or later stages of dementia, the confused patient seldom fails to know who *he* is. Other early signs of confusion can be shortened attention span, marked restlessness, purposeless activity, and anxiety. Without intervention, the patient may withdraw, show signs of suspicious thoughts, become very talkative, hostile, or abusive. Confabulation, illusions and hallucinations may be present in severe confusion.

If confusion develops or is suspected, assessment of the situation as well as the behavior is critical to prevent misinterpreting and mislabeling. In fact, confusion has been described as "a highly subjective state recognized by the observer as behaviors that do not make sense in this context"(4). The behavior, however, may make sense given the *patient's* perception of the situation. In that case, interventions need to be directed toward altering the perceptual problem rather than attempting to control the behavior.

Illusions, for example, may disappear when the object that is misperceived is accurately described and labeled, or handled or seen by the patient. Noise, glare, and shadows may contribute to misperceptions. Identification of the many people, often similarly clad, in the hospital environment can be difficult even for someone in good health. Complete orientation to time and place can be difficult for anyone in the absence of orienting cues, as anyone who has vacationed abroad can attest.

Sundowning, a well-known phenomenon, is confusion that sets in as night falls. Factors thought to be associated with sundowning include fatigue at the end of the day, pain, elimination discomfort, lower light, fewer and different staff on the evening shift, and the end of visiting hours. Such factors can give the person an overwhelming sense of being left alone. Fear can build to the point where reality is distorted and confusion begins. The presence of family or other supportive people during the evening hours may reduce sundowning.

Frightened behavior, in severe confusion, may threaten the patient's own safety. Pulling out IVs or indwelling catheters, getting out of bed when contraindicated, combativeness, anger, agitation, and screaming are usually frightened attempts to regain control.

The person's fear, not the behavior, must be the focus of the intervention. Can the fear or threat be identified? It is essential that the nurse be calm and controlled, instilling a sense of comfort and security by tone of voice, by the use of touch, and by the gentle introduction of reality-based activities such as a backrub or offering a drink of juice or some food.

Hallucinations or illusions that signal confusion can be aggravated by diffuse lighting, exaggerated shadows, and unfamiliar sounds and tactile sensations. Patients who are having hallucinations need calm and constant reminders of reality: "It may seem as if snakes are in your bed, but you are seeing the folds in your bed linen. See what happens when I straighten the covers. Remember, you are in the hospital now and I am here to help you." Such an explanation supports the patient in several ways: It acknowledges the worry or fear that there may be snakes on the bed without making the person feel stupid, helps the person remember that he is in the hospital, and clarifies the fact that the person is not alone and that someone is there to help. If the snakes are an illusion, not a hallucination, the explanation should describe reality by explaining the visual distortion.

Some aspects of hospitalization are difficult to change. Nurses in the study, for example, found it difficult to do anything about the number of people who interact with the patient. Yet care can be taken in assigning nursing personnel to patients. Primary nursing is ideal, but if this is not possible, at least attempting to maintain consistent assignments will limit some of the demands placed on patients. Continuity of care was significantly greater during the intervention phase of our study, and we believe that it contributed to the reduced incidence of confusion.

REFERENCES

1. Williams, M. A. and others. Predictors of acute confusional states in hospitalized elderly patients. *Res.Nurs.Health* 8:31-40, Mar. 1985.
2. _____ . Reducing acute confusional states in elderly patients with hip fractures. *Res.Nurs.Health* 8:329-337, Dec. 1985.
3. Chatman, M. A. The effect of family involvement on patients' manifestations of postcardiotomy psychosis. *Heart Lung* 7:995-999, Nov.-Dec. 1978.
4. Wolanin, M. O., and Phillips, L. R. *Confusion: Prevention and Care.* St. Louis, The C.V. Mosby Co., 1981.
5. Hahn, Karen. Using 24-hour reality orientation. *J.Gerontol.Nurs.* 6:130-135, Mar. 1980.
6. Nowakowski, Loretta. Disorientation—signal or diagnosis. *J.Gerontol.Nurs.* 6:197-202, Apr. 1980.
7. Ahronheim, J. C. Acute confusional states in the elderly. *Semin.Fam.Med.* 3:20-25, Feb. 1982.
8. National Institute on Aging Task Force. Senility reconsidered: treatment possibilities for mental impairment in the elderly. *JAMA* 244:259-263, July 18, 1980.
9. Trockman, G. Caring for the confused or delirious patient. *Am.J.Nurs.* 78:1495-1499, Sept. 1978.
10. Williams, M. A., and others. Nursing activities and acute confusional states in elderly hip-fractured patients. *Nurs.Res.* 28:25-35, Jan.-Feb. 1979.

Sedative-Hypnotic Drugs

Reprinted from American Journal of Nursing, July 1981

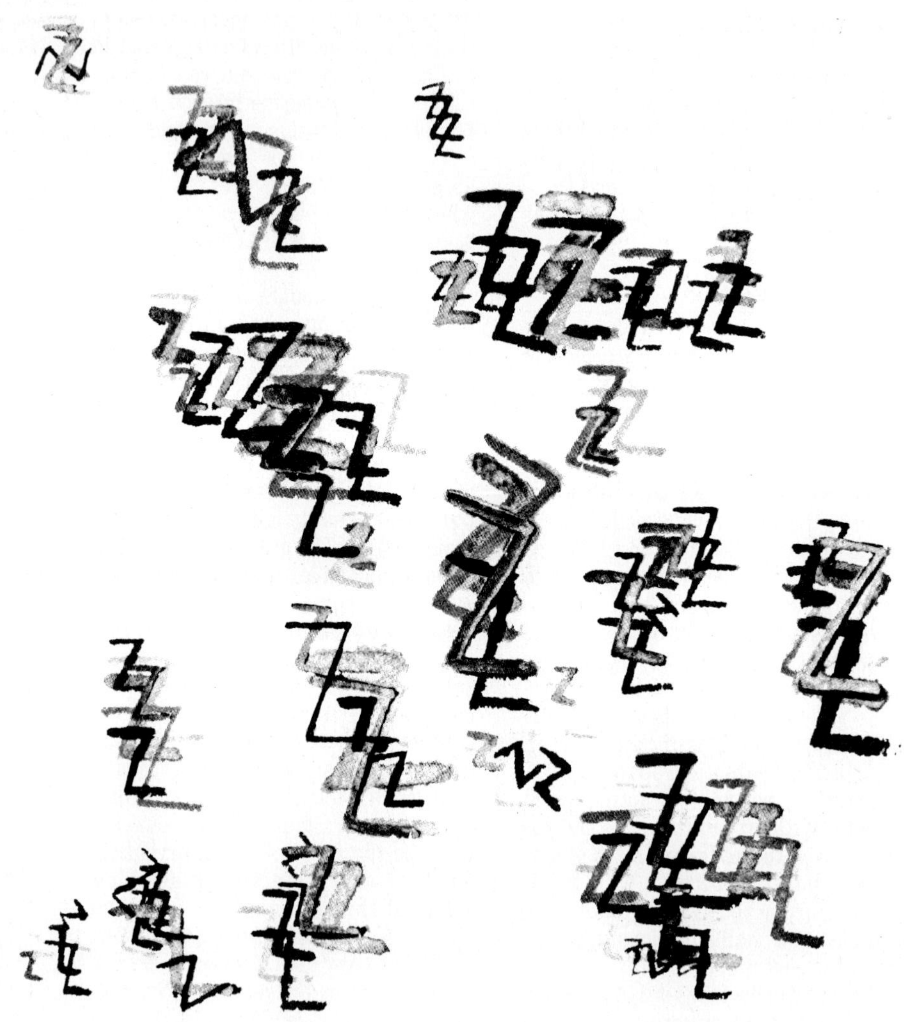

By Elizabeth Harris

The sedative-hypnotics are among the most widely used drugs. But, many authorities maintain, these drugs also are the most widely misused.

Sedative-hypnotics are used to treat anxiety and sleep disturbances, which occur often in both sick and well individuals and can be attributed to a great many causes. They may be symptoms of other conditions. For example, sleep disturbance is a symptom of depression, and anxiety can be due to hyperthyroidism. If so, it is the underlying condition that needs to be treated. But, if the anxiety and sleeplessness are severe or intolerable to the patient, or if they adversely affect his health, and particularly when they seem to be temporary, the use of a sedative-hypnotic may be in order.

Each time a patient presents with anxiety or sleep disturbance, it is important to assess carefully the circumstances around the development of the symptom and to exam-

Classification of the Sedative-Hypnotics

I. Barbiturates

II. Nonbarbiturates
A. Benzodiazepines
B. Nonbenzodiazepines
1. Propanediols
2. Quinazolines
3. Acetylinic alcohols
4. Piperidinedione derivatives
5. Chloral derivatives
6. Monoureides

Classification of the Barbiturates

Short acting
secobarbital
pentobarbital

Intermediate acting
butabarbital
amobarbital

Long acting
phenobarbital

ine the patient to discover the cause. If a cause can be found and treated, there may be no need to treat the symptom alone.

It may be that these drugs are best used sporadically to treat a patient during the height of his symptoms. Administration of these drugs should be seen as an adjunctive, symptomatic treatment that is not curative, but only a means to alleviate distress, so that the underlying problem can be worked on more effectively.

The sedative-hypnotics, also referred to as anxiolytics, or minor tranquilizers, have been classified in two different ways. One scheme divides them into two classes: the sedatives produce a calming, quieting effect, and the hypnotics induce sleep. In practice, however, it is impossible to place these drugs with certainty into one or the other of these two classes. In fact, all of these drugs in small amounts will produce sedation and in large amounts will induce sleep. It is true that some drugs are preferred for one effect or the other; however, the sedative-hypnotic division is somewhat arbitrary.

A better system is to classify the drugs according to their chemical structure. (See chart, page 1333.) Two other classes of drugs are also used for their sedative-hypnotic effects: the antihistamines and the beta-adrenergic blockers. Because these drugs are so different from other sedative-hypnotics, they will be considered separately.

The sedative-hypnotics are central nervous system (CNS) depressants. In small doses (sedative doses), they create a calming, relaxing effect—an anxiolytic effect. In larger doses, the CNS depression is greater, and the patient will show signs of intoxication, similar to alcohol intoxication, including slurred speech, ataxia, silliness, dizziness, diplopia, and blurred vision. If the patient at this point is provided a quiet, comfortable environment, he will fall asleep—the hypnotic effect. Still larger doses can lead to coma or death.

Tolerance develops with all these drugs, usually within several days. The patient finds that a dose of the drug that relieved his symptoms a few days earlier no longer works as well. The patient may then resort to increasing doses of the drug to produce the desired effect. It is worth noting that a cross-tolerance also develops with all these drugs, so that switching periodically from one drug to another does not help (1,2).

All of these drugs, if taken in large enough doses or long enough, can lead to physical and emotional dependence. Once physical dependence has developed, there are characteristic signs of withdrawal if the drug is abruptly discontinued. Shortly after the last dose (about 24 hours to 2 weeks, depending on the half-life of the drug), the patient will exhibit some or all of the following signs: insomnia, weakness, muscle tremors, anxiety, irritability, sweating, anorexia, fever, nausea and vomiting, headache, incoordination, and restlessness. After a few days, if the patient continues to abstain from the drug, he may develop postural hypotension, tinnitis, incoherence, delirium, psychosis, convulsions, and, eventually, status epilepticus, cardiovascular collapse, or loss of the temperature-regulating mechanism.

The severity of the withdrawal syndrome will depend on the drug, its dose, and the duration of its administration(3,4). It is important to be aware of the symptoms of withdrawal and intoxication, since either may occur in a patient who takes these drugs.

The Barbiturates

The barbiturates are a large, fairly old and well-known group of drugs that are derived from barbituric acid. Phenobarbital is the barbiturate most commonly prescribed(5).

All barbiturates are metabolized into inactive metabolites by the hepatic microsomal enzymes. The inactive metabolites are then excreted in the urine. Phenobarbital is unusual in that 50 percent of the drug is excreted unchanged in the urine(6).

All the barbiturates are equally effective as sedative hypnotics. Traditionally, the choice of a particular compound depends on the duration of action required. For these purposes, barbiturates are divided according to their half-lives into the short, intermediate, and long-acting compounds. In practice, it has not yet been proven that there are noticeable clinical differences in onset of duration of action, but the system of classification persists(7). The only noticeable clinical difference based on duration of action is that phenobarbital, a long-acting barbiturate, can accumulate in the body to toxic levels if it used repeatedly in patients who have trouble metabolizing it.

All the barbiturates can be used either for daytime sedation or for sleep. The hypnotic dose is generally three or four times the sedative dose. When used as hypnotics, there is conclusive evidence that the barbiturates are useful for no longer than 7 to 14 consecutive nights (8,9).

One advantage of the barbiturates is that they are less expensive than the other sedative-hypnotics. However, their disadvantages far outweigh this advantage.

Disadvantages. When used as

hypnotics, all barbiturates suppress REM (rapid eye movement) or dreaming sleep. It is unclear what the clinical effects of REM suppression are, but what is clear is that after the barbiturate is discontinued the patient can have a rebound effect, with restless sleep, frequent and intense dreaming, or nightmares, for a number of nights or weeks(10).

When used as sedatives or anxiolytics, the barbiturates can cause daytime drowsiness and somnolence. After just a single dose, the patient can have a "hangover" the next day with irritability or excitement and impairment of judgment and fine motor skills(11).

Barbiturates have a narrow margin of safety, particularly as tolerance develops and the effective dose approaches the lethal dose. Barbiturates are often used successfully alone or in combination with other CNS depressants as instruments of suicide. Doses as low as 10 to 15 times the therapeutic dose have been lethal(12).

Tolerance occurs in 7 to 14 days, and there is a high potential for physical dependence with a month or more of use. The long-acting phenobarbital is the only barbiturate that is rarely abused because it has less tendency to produce intoxication or euphoria(13,14).

Barbiturates activate or induce the hepatic microsomal enzymes, which cause more rapid than usual metabolism of a number of drugs, including the barbiturates themselves (this is part of the explanation for tolerance), coumarin derivatives, MAO inhibitor antidepressants, tricyclic antidepressants, phenothiazines, phenytoin, systemic steroids including oral contraceptives, griseofulvin, and rifampicin (15).

Because of these serious drawbacks, barbiturates are seldom indicated for use as oral antianxiety agents and many authorities believe they should be used as hypnotics only for intractable insomnia(16).

The National Institute for Drug Abuse recommends only the following uses for barbiturates:

- thiopental as an anesthetic agent
- phenobarbital, because of its selective anticonvulsant effect, as a first-line drug for treatment of grand mal or cortical focal seizures; other barbiturates, including pentobarbital, amobarbital, or thiopental, given intravenously, are recommended for emergency treatment of seizures
- amobarbital, intravenously, for narcotherapy or intramuscularly, for rapid sedation in patients who are psychotic, manic, or enraged; when used in psychosis, amobarbital is combined with an antipsychotic.
- pentobarbital and secobarbital, as preoperative sedatives(17).

Some drugs, such as Tuinal, combine two barbiturates. Use of these combination drugs is strongly discouraged by most authorities because of the increased risk of abuse and dependence.

Benzodiazepines

The benzodiazepines, chlordiazepoxide (Librium) and diazepam (Valium), are among the most frequently prescribed drugs.

The benzodiazepines offer a number of advantages over the barbiturates. First, they produce less daytime sedation and mental cloudiness while still affording at least an equal antianxiety effect.

Second, they have a higher therapeutic index, so that they rarely are agents for successful suicide. Just as the therapeutic dose is far less, proportionally, than a toxic dose, so also is the difference between the sedative and hypnotic dose greater than for barbiturates (18).

Third, because the benzodiazepines do not activate the hepatic microsomal enzymes significantly, they do not interfere with the metabolism of other drugs.

Fourth, the risk of physical dependence is lower than for any of the other sedative-hypnotics.

Fifth, some studies report greater, more consistent efficacy than with barbiturates and a wider range of usefulness. Others report no significant difference in efficacy (19-21).

As a result of these five factors, it can be said that benzodiazepines may be somewhat more effective as sedative-anxiolytics or hypnotics, and that they are definitely safer than barbiturates. There is overwhelming support in the literature for the use of benzodiazepines in preference to barbiturates, except for the specific indications listed for the barbiturates.

The benzodiazepines also have several disadvantages. All, except the short-acting forms (lorazepam and oxazepam), are converted in the liver to active metabolites with long half-lives. These metabolites are eventually excreted in the urine. This means that the long-acting benzodiazepines can accumulate to a toxic level over several days of continuous use. This can be a particular hazard in the elderly or in patients with liver disease. Such patients are better treated with lorazepam or oxazepam, which have no active metabolites and are quickly excreted(22).

Another effect of the breakdown into active metabolites with long half-lives is that the withdrawal syndrome due to the long-acting benzodiazepines can be prolonged. In fact, the syndrome may not even appear until up to two weeks after the last dose is taken(23).

Tolerance to the benzodiazepines develops, but less quickly than with barbiturates. Dependence is a lesser risk, though there are recent reports that dependence and withdrawal can occur, even when the drugs are taken at therapeutic doses. Oxazepam appears to have the least potential for abuse(24,25).

Another disadvantage is that the intramuscular forms of diazepam and chlordiazepoxide are absorbed slowly, irregularly, and incompletely. Lorazepam, however, is available in an intramuscular form that is well absorbed. Although the benzodiazepines do suppress REM sleep in adequate dosage, there is no evidence of a rebound effect after the drug is discontinued(26).

The benzodiazepines are all equally effective as sedative-hypnotics and differ from each other only in duration of action and pharmacokinetics. They can be divided by duration of action: lorazepam and oxazepam are short acting, and the others are relatively long acting. One resulting consideration is that the short-acting agents must be given in divided doses, whereas the long-acting agents can be given once daily at bedtime after an initial week of divided doses.

There are some specific uses for benzodiazepines in addition to their general use as sedative-hypnotics. Flurazepam may have more potent hypnotic effects and is recommended for use as a hypnotic. As such, it is effective for up to 28 consecutive nights. Chlordiazepoxide and diazepam are often used to detoxify patients who are physically dependent on alcohol. This is possible because of the cross-tolerance that develops.

Benzodiazepines are particularly effective in treating anticipatory anxiety and have been shown to be effective in treating anxiety associated with physical illness. Klein favors using benzodiazepines with tricyclic antidepressants to treat panic disorders. The benzodiazepine treats the anticipatory anxiety (the anxiety of anticipating a panic attack) and the tricyclic treats the panic attacks themselves(27).

Baldessarini suggests using them for agitation during the lag period before antidepressants become effective, and Klein recommends their use in the residual phase of psychosis when the patient is anxious and demoralized and needs the help of an anxiolytic to engage in new activities that will help raise self-esteem(28,29).

Benzodiazepines are also used as preoperative medications. Diazepam is often prescribed as a muscle relaxant, although controlled studies show that it is no more effective than aspirin or placebo. In fact, all CNS depressants have some muscle relaxation effects. Diazepam is used intravenously for emergency treatment of status epilepticus, and clonazepam has been approved for use as an anticonvulsant(30,31). Chlordiazepoxide is the only benzodiazepine available generically at reduced cost.

Nonbarbiturate, Nonbenzodiazepine Compounds

This is another large group of fairly old drugs that are being prescribed less and less since the advent of the benzodiazepines. The National Institute of Drug Abuse reports that although these drugs are equally as effective as other sedative-hypnotics, they offer no advantage over barbiturates or benzodiazepines and may lead to serious toxicity. The disadvantages of this group are many. They present a high risk of abuse and physical dependence; they have a narrow margin of safety; they suppress REM sleep; and with the exception of chloral hydrate, they activate the hepatic microsomal enzymes. Shader argues against the use of meprobamate and other propanediols, but one propanediol, tybamate, produces few withdrawal symptoms and may, therefore, have an advantage(32,33). Chloral hydrate causes distressing GI side effects and can displace and therefore potentiate other protein-bound drugs(34). Methaqualone has been widely abused for years. Paraldehyde, once thought to be a very safe drug, has some major problems. It has a very low therapeutic index, a strong aromatic odor, and a burning, disagreeable taste. It also decomposes on exposure to light and air, and reacts rapidly with some plastics. When given IM it should be given in a glass syringe. Paraldehyde also causes aseptic necrosis when given IM and may cause pulmonary edema. Glutethimide, methyprylon, and ethchlorvynol have pronounced anticholinergic properties and are erratically absorbed from the GI tract. This makes management of overdoses of these drugs especially difficult.

Guidelines for Use

There is overwhelming agreement among psychopharmacologists that when any of these agents are used to treat anxiety or sleep disorder, the course of treatment should be brief and/or intermittent. None of these agents has been shown to be helpful as a hypnotic for any longer than 28 nights. Most are helpful only for 7 to 14 consecutive nights. When used as sedatives, the drugs produce tolerance fairly quickly, so that a higher dose is needed for a therapeutic effect. If this continues unabated, physical dependence develops. Yet, there are times of stress when these agents are indicated for severe anxiety or sleeplessness.

When a patient complains of anxiety or sleeplessness, and an underlying cause is not apparent, it would be wise to try such conservative measures as listening to the complaint, providing reassurance where appropriate, or teaching relaxation techniques, yoga, or meditation. Patients who suffer from sleep disturbance can be helped to create a relaxing routine before bedtime and to increase exercise and decrease caffeine intake during the day. These measures alone may be successful. If not, a sedative-hypnotic may provide the only humane treatment.

Side Effects

Daytime sedation is the most common side effect of sedative-hypnotics. It occurs slightly less with benzodiazepines than with other sedative-hypnotics(35). Paradoxical excitement can occur as a side effect of any of these drugs. This is similar to the disinhibition that can occur with alcohol and can appear as excitement, hostility, rage, confusion, depersonalization, or hyperactivity.

Other rare side effects include blood dyscrasias, rash, photosensitivity, nonthrombocytopenic purpura, menstrual irregularities, GI discomfort, nausea, and vomiting(36).

As is true with many other kinds of drugs, the elderly experience more side effects from the sedative-hypnotics. Elderly patients are more prone to daytime sedation and to the paradoxical excitement effect. Because they have a diminished capacity to metabolize and eliminate these drugs, older patients are more prone to toxic accumulation over time. For this reason, the shorter-acting drugs should be used.

Finally, because elderly patients are often on a variety of medications, special attention must be paid to possible drug interactions.

Contraindications

Absolute contraindications include severe respiratory compromise, known hypersensitivity to individual compounds, and acute intermittent porphyria(37,38).

These drugs should be avoided

The Sedative-Hypnotics

Generic name	Trade name	Hypnotic dose	Sedative dose (total daily dose)	Half-life (hr.)
Barbiturates				
secobarbital	Seconal	100-200 mg.	90-200 mg.	19-34
pentobarbital	Nembutal	100-200 mg.	60-80 mg.	15-48
amobarbital	Amytal	100-200 mg.	60-150 mg.	8-42
butabarbital	Butisol	100-200 mg.	20-200 mg.	34-42
phenobarbital	Luminal and others	100-200 mg.	30-90 mg.	24-140
thiopental	Pentothal	Used for anesthesia		
methohexital	Brevital	Used for anesthesia for ECT only		
Nonbarbiturates				
Benzodiazepines				
flurazepam	Dalmane	15-30 mg.		24-100
nitrazepam	Mogadon	5-10 mg.	Not available in U.S.	18-34
chlordiazepoxide	Librium and others	25	15-80 mg.	6-30
diazepam	Valium	10	6-40 mg.	20-90
oxazepam	Serax	10-30	30-60 mg.	3-21
clorazepate	Tranxene and others		15-60 mg.	40-200
prazepam	Verstran	10-20	20-60 mg.	24-200
lorazepam	Ativan	2-4	2-6 mg.	10-20
Nonbenzodiazepines				
Propanediols				
meprobamate	Equanil Miltown and others	800	0.4-1.2 gm.	10
tybamate	Solacen Tybatran		500-1,500 mg.	
Quinazolines				
methaqualone	Quaalude Parest Optimil Sopor and others	150-300 mg.	250-300 mg.	10-42
Acetylinic alcohols				
ethchlorvynol	Placidyl	0.5-1 gm.	200-600 mg.	10-25
Piperidinedione derivatives				
glutethimide	Doriden	250-500	125-750 mg.	5-22
methyprylon	Noludar	200-400 mg.	150-400 mg.	
Chloral derivatives				
chloral hydrate	Noctec Somnos and others	0.5-2 gm.		
chloral betaine	Beta-Chlor	870 mg.-1 gm.		
triclofos	Triclos	750 mg.-1.5 gm.		
Monoureides				
paraldehyde	Paral	3-8 gm.		

whenever possible in patients with a history of drug or alcohol abuse or suicide attempts by overdose because of the increased risk of abuse. Patients with a history of peptic ulcers should avoid chloral hydrate because of its irritation of the GI tract. In patients with uremia or hepatic insufficiency, hypnotics can precipitate coma due to inadequate metabolism and excretion of the drugs. Patients with renal or hepatic disease can be treated with smaller doses or short-acting compounds. Patients in pain should not receive these drugs unless their pain is controlled, or their discomfort will increase.

The safe use of these compounds in pregnancy and breast-feeding has not been established. There is some evidence of an increased incidence of cleft lip and palate after diazepam use in the first trimester, but there is no other evidence of sequelae of first trimester use(39). However, when barbiturates or benzodiazepines are used in the last trimester of pregnancy, there have been reports of physical dependence in the fetus or neonatal depression, accompanied by poor sucking, hypotonia, and hypothermia. In addition, barbiturates and benzodiazepines are excreted in small amounts in human breast milk and can cause lethargy and weight loss in the breast-fed infant. Most authorities agree that sedative-hyp-

Antihistamines

Generic name	Trade name	Average daily dose
diphenhydramine	Benadryl	25-100 mg.
hydroxyzine	Atarax Vistaril	25-200 mg.
promethazine	Phenergan	50-200 mg.

notics should be avoided whenever possible during pregnancy and breast-feeding (40,41).

As with any other drug, patients must be told the expected course of treatment, and the name, dose, and schedule of the drug. In addition patients using these drugs should be warned of the risk of tolerance and dependence and told how these risks will be minimized. They should be told not to increase their dosage without contacting the health care provider and not to take an extra tablet or more when their symptoms are not immediately ameliorated with the prescribed dose.

Patients should also be informed that these drugs will not treat the cause of the anxiety or sleeplessness but will only treat the symptoms.

Patients should be advised not to use alcohol or other CNS depressants while taking these medications because of the additive effect. They should be advised against operating cars or any dangerous machinery that requires muscular coordination and mental alertness.

Because of the possible drug interactions with many of these agents, patients should be asked to notify all health care providers when they are taking these drugs.

If the patient lives with children, he should be advised to keep the tablets or capsules in a safe place where children cannot find them and mistake them for candy.

Beta-blockers

The most commonly studied drug in the beta-blocker group is propranolol (Inderal). Propranolol is a beta-adrenergic blocking agent that is used primarily to treat cardiac arrhythmias, angina, and hypertension. Recently, it has also been used experimentally to treat such peripheral autonomic symptoms of anxiety as trembling, tachycardia, palpitations, diaphoresis, and hyperventilation.

The medication does not allay the inner feeling of anxiety; it only removes the outward manifestations. It seems particularly useful for patients whose anxiety appears in specific, highly stressful situations where the possible sedation and mental clouding of the sedative-hypnotics are undesirable—for example, public speaking, musical recitals, acting, or job interviews. Propranolol may also be helpful to patients who focus on the somatic symptoms of anxiety. It is not helpful, however, in treating anticipatory anxiety.

The mechanism of action is thought to be a peripheral beta-adrenergic blockade, although there may also be some central effects. Dosages recommended are 30 to 120 mg. per day in three or four divided doses.

There can be troubling side effects, such as insomnia, hallucinations, impairment of metabolism of other drugs, lethargy or depression, GI distress, or rash. Inderal is contraindicated in some cardiac and pulmonary diseases. The use of propranolol as an antianxiety agent is not FDA approved.

Antihistamines

These drugs can be prescribed to treat sleep disturbance or anxiety states, although these are not the primary uses of the antihistamines. They are less effective sedative-anxiolytics than the sedative-hypnotics and tend to create daytime sedation. When used as hypnotics, they are less powerful than the sedative-hypnotics and are often ineffective. In addition, they can create unwanted and sometimes dangerous anticholinergic side effects. Yet they are effective for some people and are fairly commonly used.

References

1. Baldessarini, R J *Chemotherapy in Psychiatry* Cambridge, Mass., Harvard University Press, 1977, p 132
2. U S National Institute of Drug Abuse *Sedative-Hypnotic Drugs, Risks and Benefits*, ed by J R Cooper Washington, D.C., U S Government Printing Office, 1977, p 15
3. *Ibid*, p 16
4. Gilman, A G, and others, eds *Goodman and Gilman's The Pharmacological Basis of Therapeutics* 6th ed New York, Macmillian Publishing Co, 1980, p 339-375
5. National Institute of Drug Abuse, *op cit*, p 60
6. Gilman and others, *op cit*, p 357
7. Greenblatt, D J, and Shader, R I Psychotropic drugs in the general hospital IN *Manual of Psychiatric Therapeutics* ed by R I Shader Boston, Little, Brown & Co, 1975, p 5
8. Gilman and others, *op cit*, p 353
9. National Institute of Drug Abuse, *op cit*, p 15
10. *Ibid*, p 6
11. Gilman and others, *op cit*, p 358
12. National Institute of Drug Abuse, *op cit*, p 9
13. Koch-Weser, J, and Greenblatt, D J The archaic barbiturate hypnotics *N Engl J Med* 291 790-791, Oct 10, 1974
14. Solomon, F, and others Sleeping pills, insomnia and medical practice *N Engl J Med* 300 803-808, Apr 5, 1979
15. Committee on the Review of Medicines Recommendations on barbiturate preparations *Br Med J* 2 719-720, Sept 22, 1979
16. *Ibid*
17. National Institute of Drug Abuse, *op cit*, p 106
18. Klein, D F, and others, eds *Diagnosis and Drug Treatment of Psychiatric Disorders: Adults and Children* 2d ed Baltimore, Md, Williams & Wilkins Co, 1980, p 547
19. Shader and Greenblatt, *op cit*, p 35
20. Klein and others, *op cit*, p 526
21. National Institute of Drug Abuse, *op cit*, p 8
22. Hoyumpa, A M Jr Disposition and elimination of minor tranquilizers in the aged and in patients with liver disease *South Med J* 71 (Suppl) 23-28, Aug 1978
23. Baldessarini, *op cit*, p 144
24. *FDA Bull* Prescribing of minor tranquilizers Feb, 1980
25. ______ Binding, A The abuse potential of benzodiazepines, with special attention to oxazepam *Acta Psychiatr Scand* 274 111-116, 1978
26. Feinberg, I, and others Flurazepam effects on sleep EEG *Arch Gen Psychiatry* 36 95-102, Jan 1979
27. Klein and others, *op cit*, p 564
28. Baldessarini, *op cit*, p 135
29. Klein and others, *op cit*, p 547
30. Gilman and others, *op cit*, p 466-467
31. Anderson, G D Benzodiazepines *Nurse Pract* 5 47, 50-51, 60, Jan-Feb 1980
32. Shader and Greenblatt, *op cit*, p 33
33. Klein and others, *op cit*, p 546
34. Greenblatt and Shader, *op cit*, p 4
35. Baldessarini, *op cit*, p 140
36. Appleton and Davis, *op cit*, p 158
37. National Institute of Drug Abuse, *op cit*, p 12
38. Gilman and others, *op cit*, p 358
39. Goldberg, H L, and DiMascio, A Psychotropic drugs in pregnancy IN *Psychopharmacology: A Generation of Progress*, ed by M A Morris and others New York, Raven Press, 1978, p 1051
40. Committee on the Review of Medicines, *op cit*
41. Goldberg and DiMascio, *op cit*

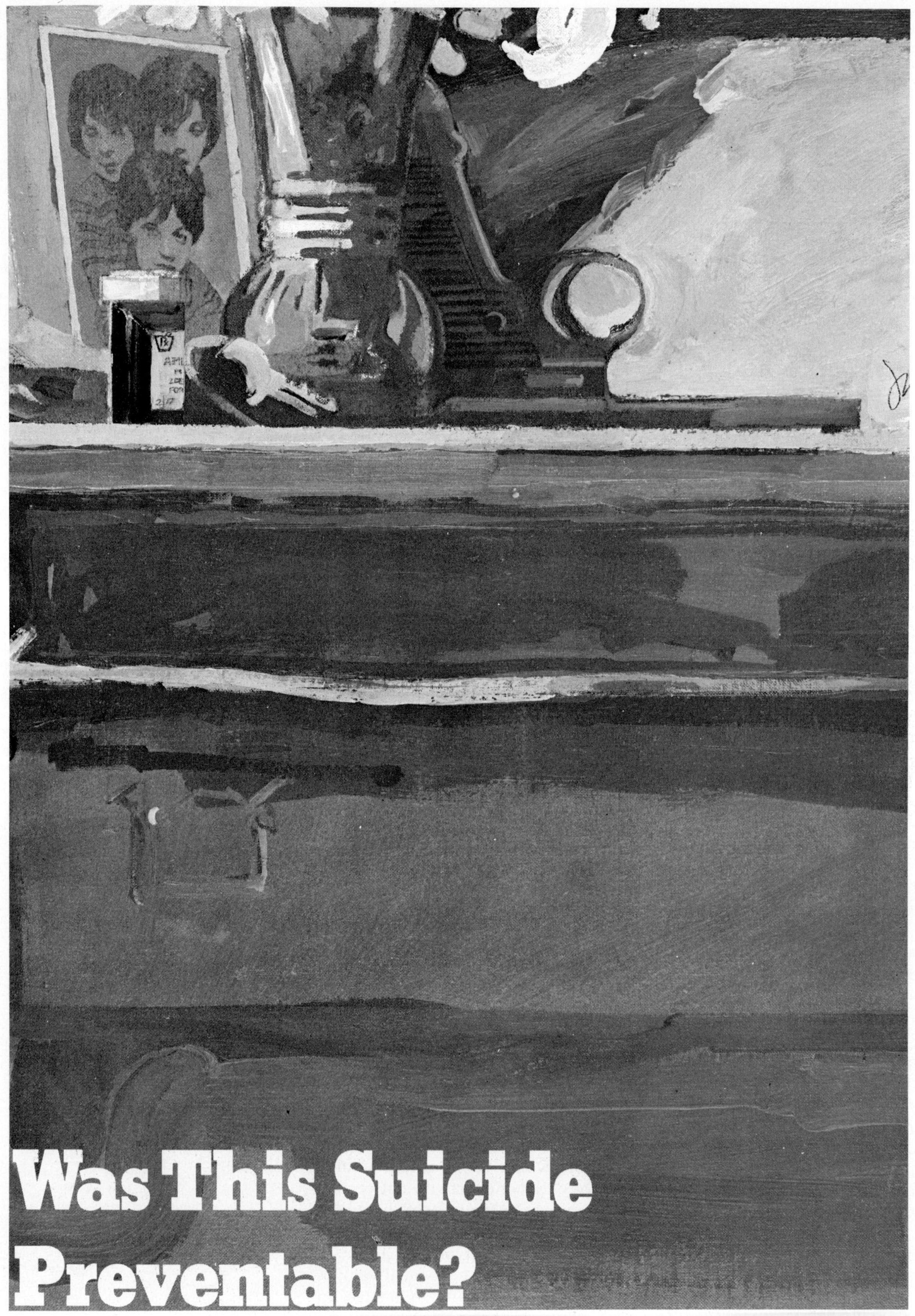

Was This Suicide Preventable?

Reprinted from American Journal of Nursing, July 1982

By Lee Ann Hoff
Marcia Resing

Mr. Smith killed himself only hours after being assessed by several mental health professionals. Judged to be nonsuicidal but in need of hospitalization, he was nevertheless sent home. The mental health facility serving him had no emergency holding service and made no effort to contact his family.

What went wrong? Was this an unnecessary death? What could have been done to prevent this suicide? What is the role of the nurse in preventing unnecessary death?

The Circumstances

Mr. Smith had sought help two years earlier, when his wife divorced him and obtained custody of their three children. At that time, he was severely depressed and unable to work, but psychotherapy, milieu therapy, and medication enabled him to return to his job. He functioned well until he married for a second time and experienced an increase in job responsibilities. When he reported feelings of paranoia at work, sexual inadequacy, and depression, he was treated with phenothiazines. The phenothiazines, however, caused him to fall asleep at work; and because being awake and alert was vital to his job, the medication resulted in increased stress. Taking vacation time, he sought psychiatric treatment at the day hospital. Sensing that hospitalization might be necessary, his therapist re-

LEE ANN HOFF, RN, MSN, MA, is a psychiatric nurse clinician with specialty training in suicidology and crisis intervention. The author of *People in Crisis* (Addison-Wesley, 1978), she is chief certification examiner of the American Association of Suicidology. She is teaching crisis intervention and doing research on violence against women.

MARCIA RESING, RN, MSN, recently completed a master's program in psychiatric nursing and is a head nurse in a psychiatric hospital.

Ms. Hoff and Ms. Resing worked in a supervisor-student relationship at the time of the suicide discussed in this article. The names of their university affiliations are withheld for purposes of privacy.

The authors thank Mary Correa, Marion Garey, Patricia Sparks, and Patricia Wahl for their thoughtful reviews of this paper.

How It Might Have Been

The following interview excerpt illustrates some recommended techniques for assessing lethality and establishing the basis of a service plan for a suicidal person. It is not a complete assessment interview, rather it focuses on critical lethality assessment techniques.

Principles and techniques	Interview
• problem identification	*Nurse:* Hello Mr. Smith, I'm Lois Haney. Can you tell me what's troubling you? *Mr. Smith:* Well, it seems like everything is going wrong.
• reflection	*Nurse:* Everything's going wrong? *Mr. Smith:* It sure is.
• focusing • identifying hazardous event	*Nurse:* What seems to be troubling you most? *Mr. Smith:* It's hard to say, because everything seems all mixed together in a big mess.
• empathy • focusing	*Nurse:* You sound really frustrated. . . . Why don't you start with what's been happening in just the last couple of days. *Mr. Smith:* Well, I've been off work on account of falling asleep on the job. . . . I've been trying to get things worked out with my wife (we just got married a few weeks ago), and my medication is bugging me. . . . I'm not sure I should be taking it anymore. Nothing seems to be working out right.
• empathy	*Nurse:* That's a lot of things to put up with.
• determining extent and boundary of problem	How long has this been going on? *Mr. Smith:* Oh, maybe the last 4 or 5 weeks or so. That's why I took some time off work.
• summarizing • identifying precipitating factor	*Nurse:* I see . . . so there's a problem with your wife, and you've got questions about your medicine, and you're having trouble staying awake at work. I think we need to talk about these things some more, but before we do, can you tell me what made you come in today, since these things have been going on for a while? *Mr. Smith:* Well, I'm supposed to go back to work tomorrow and I just can't face it.
• empathy	*Nurse:* You sound like you don't know which way to turn . . . really frustrated. *Mr. Smith:* Yes, I am. I just don't know how I can stand it anymore.
• clarification	*Nurse:* You mean you sort of feel like giving up? *Mr. Smith:* I sure do.
• reflection • empathy • assessing for suicidal ideation and possible plan	*Nurse:* Sounds to me like you're pretty desperate. Are you so discouraged that you've maybe thought about killing yourself? *Mr. Smith:* Well, yes, I've thought about it, but I don't think I could go through with it.

ferred him to the psychiatric evaluation clinic at the main hospital.

[*As a graduate student in this evaluation center, one of the authors—Marcia Resing—met Mr. Smith. She describes what happened.*]

"Mr. Smith presented as a casually dressed, clean-shaven, attractive man, but he appeared somewhat older than his 36 years. He walked slowly to the interview room, eyes downcast, and shoulders bent. I began by asking his reasons for coming to the evaluation center. He responded slowly, in an expressionless voice. He wasn't sure why he had come and could not state what he needed. It was difficult to get him to relate the events that led to his present difficulties. Throughout the interview his affect remained listless, his eye contact poor. At one point, though, I remember catching his eye and joking with him—and he lifted his head and smiled. I thought to myself: This man has life underneath that mask of depression. I wanted to help liberate that vitality, but how?

"I did a mental status examination and assessed Mr. Smith for suicidal tendencies. I asked him if he felt badly enough about his life to hurt himself. He half-smiled and said no, that he was afraid to really do anything. He said he had tried suicide before by wrecking his car. On another occasion he tried to poison himself by plugging up the car's exhaust system with a hose, but he said that the attempt was unsuccessful because the hose melted.

"After the interview I consulted with another staff member; we decided that Mr. Smith was probably too depressed to act on suicidal impulses. Still, we felt unsure about how to help him.

"I spent the rest of the afternoon consulting with the day-hospital therapist, the administrator of the clinic, and the psychiatric resident, and we agreed that Mr. Smith might need hospitalization. But since the psychiatric resident alone had the authority to admit a client to the inpatient unit, Mr. Smith would have to wait for several more hours to see the resident.

"I felt very uncomfortable with this plan. Mr. Smith had come to us early that morning requesting assistance, and since that time no one had taken direct responsibility for helping him. It appeared that all this agency could offer him was hospitalization, a disposition I was not convinced was proper. I decided, however, that all I could do was document my impressions and hope that this would help the psychiatrist formulate a treatment plan. I wrote, 'no suicidal ideation present.' I left feeling so frustrated that I did not even say good-bye to Mr. Smith.

"Four days later I returned to the clinic and learned that late in the afternoon on the day of the interview, after being seen by the psychiatrist, Mr. Smith had gone home. The next morning he shot himself. The records indicated that the psychiatrist had recommended hospitalization, but because no beds were available, Mr. Smith had been placed on the waiting list. The psychiatrist indicated in the records that Mr. Smith was not suicidal at the time of the interview.

"After hearing this shocking news, I informed my supervisor, cancelled my afternoon appointments, and went home. I was confused, frustrated, angry, and depressed. I did not understand what had gone wrong; I concluded that Mr. Smith's death was totally unnecessary. I wondered whether things might have been different had I told my supervisor about this client on the day I saw him. Still, many professionals had seen Mr. Smith. . . ."

Theory, Analysis, and Recommendations

The case of Mr. Smith is tragic. Yet, when we reflect on a suicide, it is important to avoid two common responses—blaming and excusing—and to focus instead on examining what went wrong and what might have prevented the death.

A tenet of crisis theory and suicidology is that the evaluation of a person in emotional distress is incomplete if it does not include direct assessment for suicide risk—a lethality assessment(1). Most mental health professionals seem to think that a lethality assessment is part of a general psychiatric examination of clients presenting with emotional or mental dysfunction. Evidence for this assumption is revealed during intake conferences by such statements as, "He does not appear to be suicidal," or "I do not believe that she is suicidal." Or the evidence of risk is presented in terms of depression, for example, "He is only mildly depressed," or "She is too seriously depressed to commit suicide." When questioned about the basis for these judgments the worker is often unable to produce facts.

One reason for this indirect approach to lethality assessment may be that some mental health workers deliberately refrain from asking about suicidal ideation out of the mistaken belief that bringing up the subject will put the idea into the client's head. Contrary to this popular myth, the fact is that the motivation to commit suicide is far too complex to be caused by the power of suggestion, particularly when questions are asked by someone intending to help—not harm—the client.

Some health workers believe that persons contemplating suicide won't reveal their plans anyway, so there is no point in asking a direct question. In fact, however, suicidal persons are more likely to conceal their intentions when they sense that the helper is avoiding the subject. By the same token, a worker who is confident and direct will usually convey to suicidal persons that they are talking with someone who can help them control frightening self-destructive tendencies. If the worker doesn't shy away from the issue, the sharing of suicidal plans is a more likely result.

Such data as the client's appearance, the worker's impressions, and the perceived degree of depression are unreliable as indicators of suicidal risk when considered apart from other signs. And direct communication is not only critical to the assessment process; it is a basic step in helping a suicidal person.

Suicide researchers propose that in considering signs that help predict suicide we must identify those signs that characterize people who actually kill themselves, and differentiate them from signs that are also present in the larger group of suicide attempters, as well as in the population at large(2,3,4). Even though health and mental health professionals have historically used depression as a major criterion for predicting suicide risk, studies of completed suicides show that depression *alone* is not an accurate predictor. A considerable number of people suffer from varying degrees of depression and may or may not be suicidal.

In assessing suicide risk, then, which signs are the most reliable? Some authorities suggest that workers should identify not only particular signs, but also the *patterning* of signs(4,5). In this context, assessing risk for suicide is aided by an understanding of two concepts central to the process of self-destruction—ambivalence and communication.

Ambivalence. People who kill themselves have invariably gone through a process of weighing the relative advantages of life and death, even though the process may not seem to outsiders to have been thorough or objective. In fact, a suicidal person's ambivalent state of mind (simultaneously desiring life and death) forms the very foundation for the possibility of intervention. Contrary to the popular belief that once a person has decided to commit suicide, there's nothing we can do to stop him or her, so long as a person has not in fact committed suicide, one can safely assume that he or she is still open to considering other responses to life's stresses and problems. Thus, the outcome of suicide is not inevitable.

Communication. People who engage in self-destructive behavior are sending cries for help to those around them. Some examples are: "I'm angry at my mother. . . . She'll really be sorry when I'm dead." "I can't take any more problems without some relief."

Unlike most people, who usually try to get what they need or want by simply asking for it, self-destructive people typically have a history of failed communication. They are either unable to express their needs directly, or their needs are insatiable and therefore impossible to fulfill. Failing to communicate their needs by ordinary means, self-destructive persons learn that self-injury is a powerful method of telling those around them that they are hurting and probably desperate.

• exploring ambivalence • direct questioning • determining suicidal method	*Nurse:* So you're thinking about suicide but aren't sure. . . . What have you thought about doing? *Mr. Smith:* I guess something better than last time.
• clarification	*Nurse:* Last time? *Mr. Smith:* That's right . . . when I tried to do it before.
• determining history of suicide attempts	*Nurse:* You mean you've tried to kill yourself before? *Mr. Smith:* Yes.
• determining specifics of previous attempts (time, method, outcome)	*Nurse:* When was that? *Mr. Smith:* Oh . . . not long ago, just about a year . . . I think it was April. *Nurse:* What did you do to yourself then. *Mr. Smith:* I tried to wreck my car by driving off the road. *Nurse:* What happened? *Mr. Smith:* I went off the road, but I didn't really get hurt. *Nurse:* When was that? *Mr. Smith:* A year ago, after my wife left me.
• determining history of communication patterns	*Nurse:* When that happened did you talk with anyone about your suicide attempt? *Mr. Smith:* No, I felt too foolish to talk to anyone about it.
• determining further history of suicide attempts	*Nurse:* Have you made other attempts to end your life besides that one? *Mr. Smith:* I tried to block the exhaust of my car once with a hose, but it melted. I did that about the same time last year. . . . That was the only other time.
• identifying ambivalence	*Nurse:* So you've tried twice before to kill yourself, and now you feel as badly as you did then . . . but you're not sure you could go through with it. *Mr. Smith:* (nods yes)
• determining method of current plan	*Nurse:* You mentioned that if you decide you want to end your life now you would choose a different method than before. *Mr. Smith:* I have guns at home.
• determining specificity of current plan • assessing for danger to others	*Nurse:* Are you thinking about shooting yourself or anyone else? *Mr. Smith:* Only myself.
• empathy	*Nurse:* It sounds like you're feeling very desperate. *Mr. Smith:* I guess I am.
• identifying social resources	*Nurse:* Is there someone at home now who can be with you? *Mr. Smith:* My wife.

For some, the message is, "I really want to die. . . . life is no longer worth living." Others are less certain: "I don't really want to die. . . . I just want someone to understand how miserable I am and that if things don't change I will, in fact, kill myself."

Thus, the helping person faces a double challenge: to discover the degree of ambivalence in the self-destructive person and to determine the essential message the person is trying to communicate.

There are numerous signs that can be used to predict whether or not a person is a high suicide risk:

Suicide plan. Studies reveal that the majority of persons who die by suicide have deliberately planned to do so by an available "high-lethal" method—a gun, sleeping pills, carbon monoxide poisoning. The risk of death is further increased if the attempter has full knowledge that the method is lethal and if no possibility of rescue is included in the plan.

History of suicide attempts. Among those who kill themselves, significant numbers have a history of other suicide attempts. Those who have made previous attempts with high-lethal methods or who have changed the method of self-injury from low- to high-lethal are at greater risk than those with a history of low-lethal attempts.

Resources and communication with significant others. Internal resources include emotional strength, problem-solving ability, and other personality factors that help in coping with difficulties and stress. External social resources consist of a network of persons on whom one can rely during times of stress and crisis.

Therefore, if a person has a *history of high-lethal suicide attempts, a specific plan for suicide, an available high-lethal method, and lacks both personal and social resources,* his or her immediate and long-range risk for probable suicide is very high.

There are other demographic and personal factors that increase risk: For example, the general ratio of male to female suicides in America is approximately 3 to 1. The rate among young urban black males between ages 25 and 40 is twice that for white males the same age(6).

Suicide risk is higher among those who have suffered a recent *loss,* whether through marital separation, death, or divorce. Other significant losses include job termination, a decline in social status, or financial disaster.

The presence of *physical illness, drug,* or *alcohol problems* also increases suicide risk. People who are suicidal are often physically isolated; such *isolation* exacerbates feelings of being cut off, socially and psychologically, from significant others. In cases of extreme isolation, hospitalization can be a life-saving measure if other high-risk signs are also present. Suicide risk can, however, be increased by hospitalization—well intended though it may be—if hospitalization results in the patient's feeling even more cut off from significant others.

How can we apply these indicators of suicidal danger to specific people like Mr. Smith, who are giving covert and overt signals of distress? First, it should be remembered that *all* self-destructive behavior is serious, indicating either a cry for help or a message of intent to die. Secondly, since self-destructive behavior is serious, the challenge lies in distinguishing self-destructive behavior that is an indication of intent to die from that which is a cry for help. A person who takes ten tranquilizers knowing death is not likely, but who hopes thereby to bring about some change to make life more bearable, is a low risk for suicide in the immediate sense, but may be a high risk in the future, depending on what happens as a result of the current attempt.

In Mr. Smith's case, hindsight tells us that he was in fact a high risk for suicide. We have seen how Mr. Smith was assessed in the psychiatric evaluation clinic. His denial was accompanied by a half-smile, the meaning of which was not pursued. Was Mr. Smith's half-smile related to the suicidal plan he was considering but which no one asked him about? And was he perhaps testing the interviewer to determine whether she could handle his scary ideas without panic or censure? We do not know. But we do know that these possibilities were not explored by direct, detailed questioning, and that Mr. Smith was judged to be nonsuicidal without data regarding his current plans.

Clearly, if the assessment team had judged Mr. Smith to be an immediate high risk for suicide, their response would have been different. However, many health and mental health workers apparently do not have up-to-date knowledge or training in the theory and techniques of lethality assessment. The standard assessment procedure in psychiatric practice—the mental status examination—reveals data about a client's cognition and judgment. This assessment technique, however, is *not* sufficient to determine suicidal danger(7).

The American Association of Suicidology (AAS)—the national standard-setting body for suicide prevention and crisis services—recommends that health and mental health workers receive a minimum of 40 hours of training in crisis intervention and suicide prevention(8). The nurse who interviewed Mr. Smith was in her second quarter of a master's program in psychiatric nursing and, at the time of the suicide, had not yet received the mere six hours of crisis content planned for her program. Because nurses, like police, pastors, and teachers, are front-line personnel in suicide prevention and crisis work, they frequently are the first contact for desperate people who use self-injury or suicide as solutions to critical life events.

One of the lessons to be learned from this tragic case is the great importance of assessment based on more than guesswork or vague generalizations. While there was an attempt to assess Mr. Smith for danger of suicide, what was lacking was the knowledge that a history of high-lethal suicide attempts is very significant. Because Mr. Smith had tried to kill himself by a car crash and with carbon monoxide poisoning a year earlier, he should have been asked in detail about his current plans for suicide.

Not only is such direct questioning a most valuable tool for assessment, but it can also be an essential link between life and death. It establishes direct communication between the suicidal person and a caring human being, and this can help to counteract the sense of isolation and despair the client is feeling.

Effective communication with potentially suicidal people does not require extensive training in psychotherapy or counseling, but can be carried out in the ordinary course of gathering information and expressing concern for a person who appears upset or depressed(9). (See the sample interview and discussion of how Mr. Smith's case might have been handled.)

While recognizing that crisis intervention is not a panacea, we hope that this analysis and sharing of our experience will be helpful in preventing unnecessary deaths as well as in preventing unnecessary pain for health and mental health workers. A suicide is always a painful message, but we believe that the guilt, scapegoating, and/or frustration so common to survivors can be minimized for workers with up-to-date knowledge and experience in assessing and helping people at risk for suicide.

References

1. Hoff, L. A. *People in Crisis*. Menlo Park, Calif., Addison-Wesley Publishing Co., 1978, Chap. 5.
2. Breed, Warren. Five components of a basic syndrome. *Life-Threatening Behav.* 2:3-18, Spring 1972.
3. Beck, A. T., and others, eds. *The Prediction of Suicide*. Bowie, Md., Charles Press, 1974, p. 194.
4. Brown, T. R., and Sheran, T. J. Suicide prediction: a review. *Life-Threatening Behav.* 2:67-98, Summer 1972.
5. Farberow, Norman, ed. *Suicide in Different Cultures*. Baltimore, University Park Press, 1975.
6. Hoff, *op. cit.*, pp. 122-130.
7. *Ibid.*, pp. 293-327.
8. *Hoff, L. A., and others, eds. *Certification Standard Manual for Suicide Prevention and Crisis Intervention Programs*. 2nd ed. Denver, American Association of Suicidology, 1981.
9. McGee, R. K. *Crisis Intervention in the Community*. Baltimore, University Park Press, 1974.
10. Langsley, D. G., and Kaplan, D. M. *Treatment of Families in Crisis*. New York, Grune & Stratton, 1968.
11. Polak, P. R., and Kirby, M. W. The crisis of admission. *Soc.Psychiatry* 2 (4): 150-157, 1967.
12. ______. Social systems intervention. *Arch.Gen.Psychiatry* 25:110-117, Aug. 1971.
13. ______. A model to replace psychiatric hospitals. *J.Nerv.Ment.Dis.* 162:13-22, Jan. 1976.
14. Harsell, Norris. *The Person in Distress*. New York, Human Services Press, 1976.

*This manual can be obtained from the AAS Central Office, 2459 South Ash, Denver, Colo. 80222.

• establishing links to social network	*Nurse:* I'm concerned about your returning home when you're feeling this way. I think you need to have some help right now. I would like to call your wife and have her come in so we can talk together. *Mr. Smith:* I guess it's OK.

At this point, the interview and assessment process might proceed in several directions. Mrs. Smith needs to be assessed as a potential social resource for Mr. Smith's protection from self-destruction. If it is found that, for the time being at least, she is part of the problem rather than a resource for crisis resolution, other resources such as hospitalization should be explored.

Let's assume, however, that the following additional data have been obtained from Mr. and Mrs. Smith: Mrs. Smith is upset about the possibility of Mr. Smith's not returning to work the next day. She is also concerned about his problem of impotence and has only vague knowledge of his previous suicide attempts. She agrees to remove the guns from the house and then come in to see the counselor with her husband. (Removal of lethal weapons is a crucial suicide prevention technique that should be carried out as soon as possible.) Both Mr. and Mrs. Smith are afraid that even though the guns are removed, if they have an argument he might try some other means of attempting suicide.

From the above interview data, then, what is Mr. Smith's risk for suicide, and how can possible suicide best be prevented? First, the data suggest that Mr. Smith is a high risk for suicide because he has a *specific plan, an available high-lethal method, a history of previous high-lethal suicide attempts, and is unable to communicate his desperate suicidal feelings to his significant others.*

Planning then, should be based on this assessment of suicide risk, with Mr. and Mrs. Smith actively involved in the planning process. Also, in crisis situations it is acceptable for the helper to assume a more active role in the helping process than would be appropriate in, say, psychotherapy. For example, the worker can suggest to Mr. and Mrs. Smith that the guns should be removed from the home. Once a self-destructive person like Mr. Smith trusts that the worker is willing and able to help protect him from his self-destructive impulses, he will feel more secure and will welcome such a safety measure as removal of the guns. Thus, he would probably agree to the worker's suggestion that his wife remove the guns before coming to the clinic.

A service plan for Mr. Smith might have included the following:

Crisis Intervention. 1. Have wife remove guns from home. 2. Arrange interview with Mrs. Smith individually and with her husband. 3. Arrange for Mr. Smith to stay in the hospital 24-hour emergency holding unit. This will provide immediate protection against suicide while further evaluation of Mr. Smith's home and marital situation, his medication regimen, and possible need for hospitalization are done. We recognize that such 24-hour emergency holding units are not a routine part of many emergency psychiatric programs. However, this does not detract from their need and usefulness, particularly if mental health and crisis workers subscribe to the philosophy that the majority of crises can be successfully managed in the community and that psychiatric hospitalization can as easily be the source of still another crisis as it can be the solution to the crisis initially presented(1,10–14). 4. Make appointment for Mr. and Mrs. Smith to be seen in crisis counseling sessions daily or every other day until the acute suicidal urges have subsided and other immediate problems have been resolved.

Follow-up Service. 1. Mr. Smith should have ongoing individual and/or group therapy for his depression. 2. His medication regimen should be re-evaluated on a regular basis. 3. Family/marital therapy may be indicated as the recent marriage was an identified stressor in Mr. Smith's current crisis.

Since Mr. Smith, in fact, killed himself, crisis intervention and follow-up efforts should have been focused on his wife and other survivors of the suicide.

While there are no absolutes in the challenging business of lethality assessment, suicide prevention, and crisis work, in certain cases suicide is definitely preventable. We think that Mr. Smith's was one such case.

CRACK

These potent cocaine crystals cause explosive highs and easy addiction. This detox program helps to break the cycle.

BY ANNA M. ACEE/DOROTHY SMITH

"Once you start using crack, you can't stop," observe those familiar with people trapped in the addiction.

Crack, a purified, free-base form of cocaine hydrochloride, acquired its name because of the sound made by crystals popping when it is heated. It is also called rock because of its appearance(1).

Crack differs from traditional cocaine powders—cocaine hydrochloride, cocaine sulfate, and cocaine base—in more than appearance. The powder is "snorted"—inhaled through the nose—or dissolved and taken intravenously. Unlike crack crystals, the powder is not smoked; in fact, smoking actually destroys powdered cocaine. Cocaine is somewhat self-limiting when it is inhaled. The inherent vasoconstrictive properties of cocaine actually diminish absorption through the nasal vasculature as the user continues to inhale the drug(2).

Anna M. Acee, RN, MA, is clinical specialist, psychiatric day treatment program, and Dorothy Smith, RN, MA, is assistant supervisor and clinical specialist, both at Bernstein Institute, Beth Israel Medical Center, New York, NY. Ms. Acee is also an adjunct clinical instructor, Lienhard School of Nursing, Pace University.

Crack, on the other hand, is always smoked: flakes are placed in a pipe or sprinkled on a tobacco or marijuana cigarette. The self limiting property of inhaled cocaine is lost when crack is smoked because the drug is directly absorbed into the lungs. Moreover, crack reaches the brain in a more concentrated form(1).

Crack also differs from other street cocaine by its purity. Cocaine is usually 15 to 25 percent pure. But crack may be as much as 90 percent pure(1). The danger of overdose and severe toxicity is therefore heightened. And the cocaine-induced psychological symptoms—psychosis, paranoia, hallucinations, and violence—are intensified when crack is used(3).

Why is crack so popular? The sense of superiority, power, and exhilaration that cocaine brings undoubtedly makes it seductive. Crack is still associated with glamour—the way inhaled cocaine and heroin were in the 1960s and 1970s.

Crack's short, intense high is produced in four to six seconds with the euphoria lasting five to seven minutes. In contrast, when cocaine is snorted, its effects occur in one to three minutes and last up to half an hour. Crack's fleeting high is followed by a period of deep depression that strongly reinforces addictive behavior patterns and guarantees almost continuous use of the drug(1).

Crack users describe five stages as they come down from the drug's high: worries about where they can get more crack, deep depression, loss of energy and appetite, difficulty sleeping, and feelings of revulsion about themselves. Heavy crack smokers can go through all five stages after a single binge, which can last as long as the user can afford the habit(1).

The administration route also contributes to the drug's popularity. Many people perceive smoking as being less dangerous and less invasive than other routes. It does not destroy the nasal membranes the way inhaling cocaine does, nor is there the threat of infectious disease associated with IV use(1).

GETTING OFF CRACK

Widespread cocaine abuse has changed the way we think about treating drug addiction. Today, we think in terms of the broad concept of chemical dependency: the pathological relationship of a person to a mind-altering chemical(4).

The pathological relationship is

PHOTOGRAPHY/SANDOR ACS

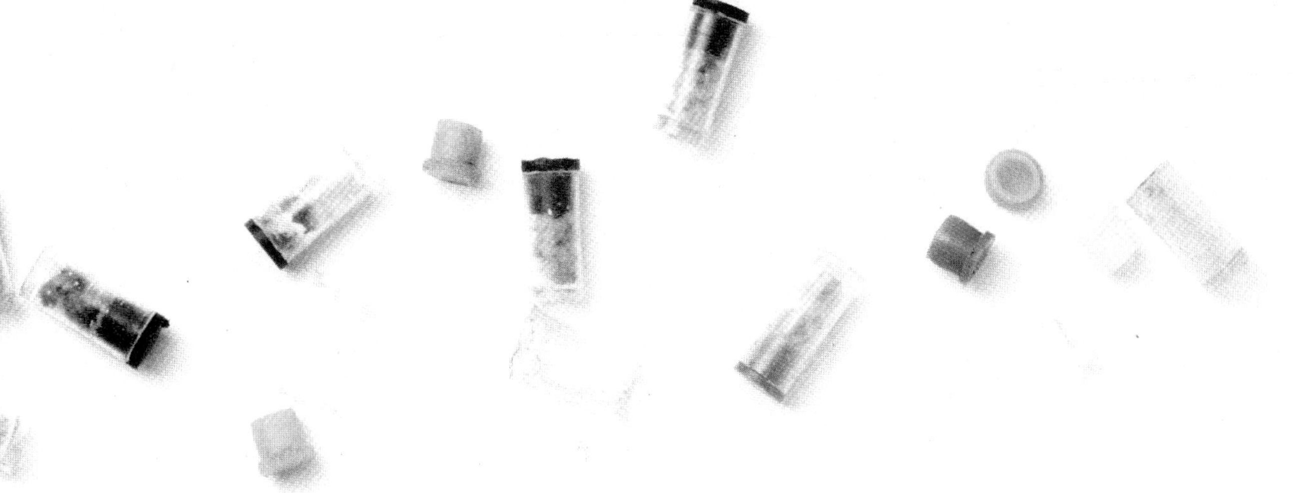

characterized by the addict's life revolving around obtaining the drug, by his inability to refuse the drug when it is offered, and by his continued use of the drug despite the hazards he experiences. The immediate goal of detoxification is to break the pattern of drug use.

Recreational users follow a different pattern: their involvement with a drug usually includes friends and is easily limited to when the drug is readily available. They can usually begin outpatient rehabilitation without the help of a detoxification unit.

Detoxification is only the first step in a substance abuser's rehabilitation. To be eligible for admission to our detox unit, patients must have used cocaine for at least four months. We also require referral from a long-term treatment facility, an employee assistance program, or a methadone maintenance program. The patient must demonstrate motivation toward making the essential long-term commitment for rehabilitation and recovery and follow-up care after discharge.

For those who cannot afford a 28-day inpatient rehabilitation program, whether due to financial or time constraints, the 7- to 10-day detoxification program serves as an orientation and preparation for outpatient rehabilitation programs.

When a patient is admitted, we note any signs and symptoms of withdrawal, oversedation, or acute intoxication (see box). Because of crack's short-lived effect, however, we rarely see intoxication symptoms when patients come to the detoxification unit.

In the first 12 hours, patients are often restless. Hypersomnia and overeating are also frequent. The paranoia and depression experienced when coming down from crack and other forms of cocaine are relatively short-lived and abate during the first 72 hours after the last drug dose.

We avoid antidepressants and anxiolytic agents. Instead we support clients through this period by assuring them that they will experience relief shortly. Meanwhile, we never minimize their discomfort.

SUBSTANCE HIGHS AND LOWS

	INTOXICATION	WITHDRAWAL
COCAINE	Elevated blood pressure, tachycardia, diaphoresis, tremors, pressured speech, euphoria, increased energy, alertness, insomnia, dilated pupils.	Lack of energy, depression, oversleeping, overeating, inability to concentrate, irritability, restlessness.
HEROIN	Respiratory depression, constricted pupils, lethargy, drowsiness, confusion, euphoria.	*Mild:* Lacrimation, rhinorrhea, gooseflesh, sneezing, sniffling, yawning. *Severe:* Extreme agitation, generalized body aches, nausea, vomiting.
BARBITURATES	Respiratory depression, slowed mental and physical activity, relaxation, drowsiness, slurred speech, ataxia. Loss of impulse control, resulting in mood swings, release of sexual and aggressive impulses; occasionally, combativeness.	Tremulousness, weakness, insomnia, diaphoresis, nausea, vomiting, loss of appetite, headache, malaise. Can progress to include suicidal thinking, grand mal seizures and status epilepticus, hallucinations, delirium, even death.
ALCOHOL	Basically the same as with barbiturate abuse. Smell of alcohol on breath.	Same as with barbiturates.

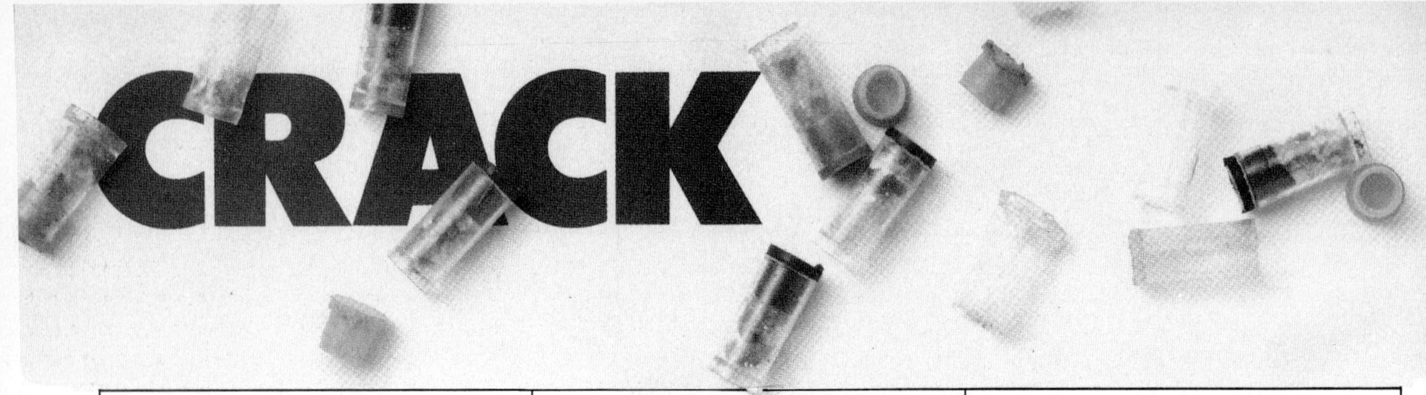

Abnormal vital signs may indicate anxiety or infection. Cocaine-induced skin lesions may cause a negative self-image that influences interaction with staff and peers.

Cocaine abusers commonly complain of anxiety, impaired memory, and depression. Sometimes anxiety and depression are related to patients' concerns about their situations and their feelings of powerlessness to effect appropriate changes. Symptoms may also be due to psychosis that existed before their drug abuse.

To help patients whose memories are impaired, we give each patient written schedules of unit activities and we post daily schedules on the bulletin board.

An important assessment goal is to determine how drug abuse has eroded not only physical health (see box), but also familial, educational, social, and employment activities.

In both group sessions and individual counseling we encourage patients to discuss their feelings to help them gain perspective. Knowing that others experience similar feelings of guilt, doubt, or isolation can alleviate these feelings. Reality-testing can make such feelings less overwhelming.

Observing interactions among patients and between patients and staff is the primary way we assess motivation.

Surreptitious behavior suggests an attempt to obtain contraband drugs. For example, a patient may make frequent phone calls, then seek an excuse to leave the locked unit. To deter drug-seeking, we keep the unit locked and do not allow visitors. Of course, family members do come in to plan subsequent care together with the patient and counselor.

PHYSICAL EFFECTS OF COCAINE USE

While the exact physical effects of long-term crack use are unknown, long-term cocaine users lose weight, develop skin problems (such as facial dermatitis and perioral dryness and peeling), experience convulsions, have difficulty breathing, and spit up black phlegm. The source of the black phlegm is uncertain. Because crack is inhaled directly into the lungs, long-term crack users can also develop intermittent abnormal pulmonary gas exchange that subsides without treatment(2).

Cocaine slows digestion, masks hunger, stimulates the central nervous system, and induces agitation, restlessness, apprehensiveness, and sexual arousal. Cocaine also elevates blood pressure, temperature, pulse, and blood sugar. Cardiovascular problems, such as hypertension, tachyarrhythmias, myocardial infarction, cerebral hemorrhage, and even death, can result. IV users frequently develop cellulitis from using contaminated needles and syringes. Dental problems are common due to neglect and poor nutrition(2,6,7).

When we observe surreptitious behavior, we confront the person and point out how his actions inhibit his attaining or maintaining sobriety. Frequently, however, patients are very supportive with one another, extending encouragement and sympathy to someone experiencing discomfort. In fact, peer support is a key part of many rehabilitation programs: recovered users become mentors.

A daily meeting gives our multidisciplinary staff a chance to validate observations and correct possible misconceptions. It also allows us to examine a problem from each other's perspectives—sometimes perspectives that have not yet been considered regarding a given client.

Daily staff discussions also counter manipulative behavior that can promote staff dissension. A client may, for example, seek sympathy from one staff member by complaining about another. Another tactic is to misquote staff members so that it appears they are contradicting, or even demeaning, each other.

Motivations for treatment. A crack addict, like other chemically dependent people, uses both denial and compliance as major defense mechanisms.

We often see career addicts with dual addictions. Their motivation for treatment frequently centers on staying out of jail, obtaining welfare benefits, or retaining custody of their children.

For example, a 25-year-old woman had been attending a methadone maintenance treatment program for six years. She had been a model patient until she began snorting cocaine and smoking free-base five months before admission. She admitted that she came in to detoxify so that she could get a letter from her counselor to get her children back. They had been taken to a temporary shelter when she left them alone overnight while she was at a "crack house."

A crack user may experience severe difficulty sooner than users of other drugs. But since his relationship with the drug is not so long-standing, the seriousness of the crack addiction can be masked by the patient's denial. One 22-year-old man, for instance, maintained that he came in to detoxify only to satisfy his mother who, he said, overreacted when she found a marijuana cigarette in his room.

At first we were inclined to discharge this first-time client and

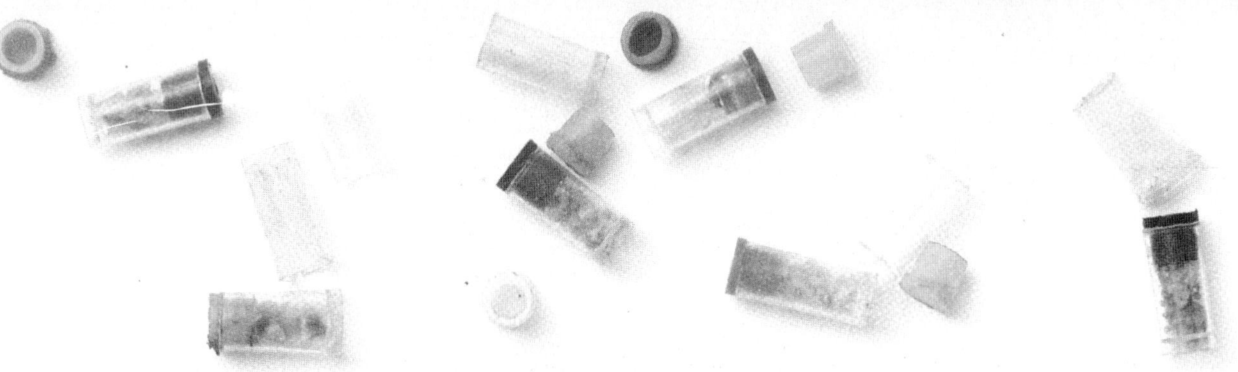

recommend outpatient treatment. When he then reassured his mother, "See, I don't have a drug problem," she called and told us that she and her husband had become alarmed when they had begun to miss sums of money and jewelry from their home. They had given their son an ultimatum to seek help or to move out of the house.

When we reviewed the conflicting stories at the staff meeting, we realized that, although he had appeared to comply with the unit's program, he had been simply going through the motions.

In fact, he was not acknowledging the extent of his addiction. He had been using crack for about a year. Already he was spending up to $1,500 a week on the drug—not only stealing but selling drugs to continue the habit.

He had experienced a seizure a month before admission during one of his heavier binges. During his last week's binge, which ended about three days before admission, he had lost at least 20 pounds.

Interactions with staff that focus on somatic complaints are another form of denial. We respond by helping the patient see how his physical problems are linked to his drug use.

The detoxification process provides an atmosphere that enables the patient to recognize the need for long-term treatment. To accomplish this, we use health teaching with peer-support and counseling groups to explain the nature of chemical dependency. Attendance at group sessions is mandatory: failure to comply is grounds for administrative discharge.

Despite emphasis on the group milieu, one-to-one staff-patient interaction is equally important. Individual counseling provides the chance to reflect on personal life direction and to synthesize the information that has been presented. We expect that the patients will understand:

☐ Chemical dependency is a progressively deteriorating disease if left unchecked.

☐ Individuals are not responsible for their disease, but they are responsible for their recovery.

☐ They cannot blame people, places, or things for their dependency. They must face their problems and their feelings.

☐ Rehabilitation and recovery are lifelong enterprises that begin with a commitment to a long-term treatment effort.

The value of detoxification by itself is limited. We now recognize that successful long-term treatment must address more than the psychodynamics related to addictive behavior. The focus must be on the entrenched cycle of euphoria, abstinence, dysphoria, and continued abuse that gives detoxification its revolving door(5).

Rehabilitation must center on abstinence. Our program emphasizes self-help, supported through groups such as Cocaine Anonymous. Like Alcoholics Anonymous, the chemically dependent help each other in these groups without medical, political, or religious supervision. The career addict will need a more structured discharge plan, perhaps including escorted transportation to a halfway house or residential treatment facility.

During detoxification, we help patients take the first step: to admit they have become powerless in relation to the drug. For the chemically dependent, taking this first step—recognizing that the drug has made life unmanageable—is a step toward survival.

WHO USES CRACK?

A random survey of 458 people who called the 1-800-COCAINE national hotline during May 1986 found that 33 percent used crack. The majority of crack users were males (72%), 20 to 29 years old (94%), earned more than $10,000 a year (57%), and spent more than $100 a week on the drug (75%)(3,8).

Eighty-one percent had switched to crack from occasionally snorting cocaine powder. Eighty-two percent reported a compulsion to use the drug again as soon as the brief high wore off; 78 percent reported the onset of compulsive use and significant drug-related problems within two months of first use.

Drug-related physical complaints reported by the callers included chest congestion (64%), chronic cough (40%), and convulsions with loss of consciousness (7%). Psychiatric complaints included severe depression (85%), loss of sexual desire (58%), memory lapses (40%), violent behavior (31%), and suicide attempts (18%)(8).

REFERENCES

1. New York State Division of Substance Abuse Services. *Report on Crack.* Albany, The Division, 1986, p. 2.
2. New York Department of Health, Poison Control Center, City Health Information. *Crack: Cocaine Repackaged.* The Department, New York City, 1986, Vol. 5, No. 10.
3. Gold, M. S. *800-COCAINE* New York: Bantam Books, 1984.
4. Peterson, R. M. *Hooked on a Line.* Palm Beach, FL, Palm Beach Institute Foundation, 1983.
5. Drakis, C. Brain mechanisms and pharmacologic treatment of cocaine abuse. Presented at *Cocaine: The Clinical Challenge* the first national conference on cocaine, sponsored by U.S. Journal Training, Inc., Nov. 17-19, 1985.
6. Mittelman, H. S., and others. Cocaine. *Am.J.Nurs.* 84:1092-1095, Sept. 1984.
7. Cregler, L. L., and Mark, H. Medical complications of cocaine abuse. *N.Engl.J.Med.* 315:1495-1500, Dec. 4, 1986.
8. Washton, A. M., and others. Survey of 500 callers to a national cocaine helpline. *Psychosomatics* 25:771-775, Oct. 1984.

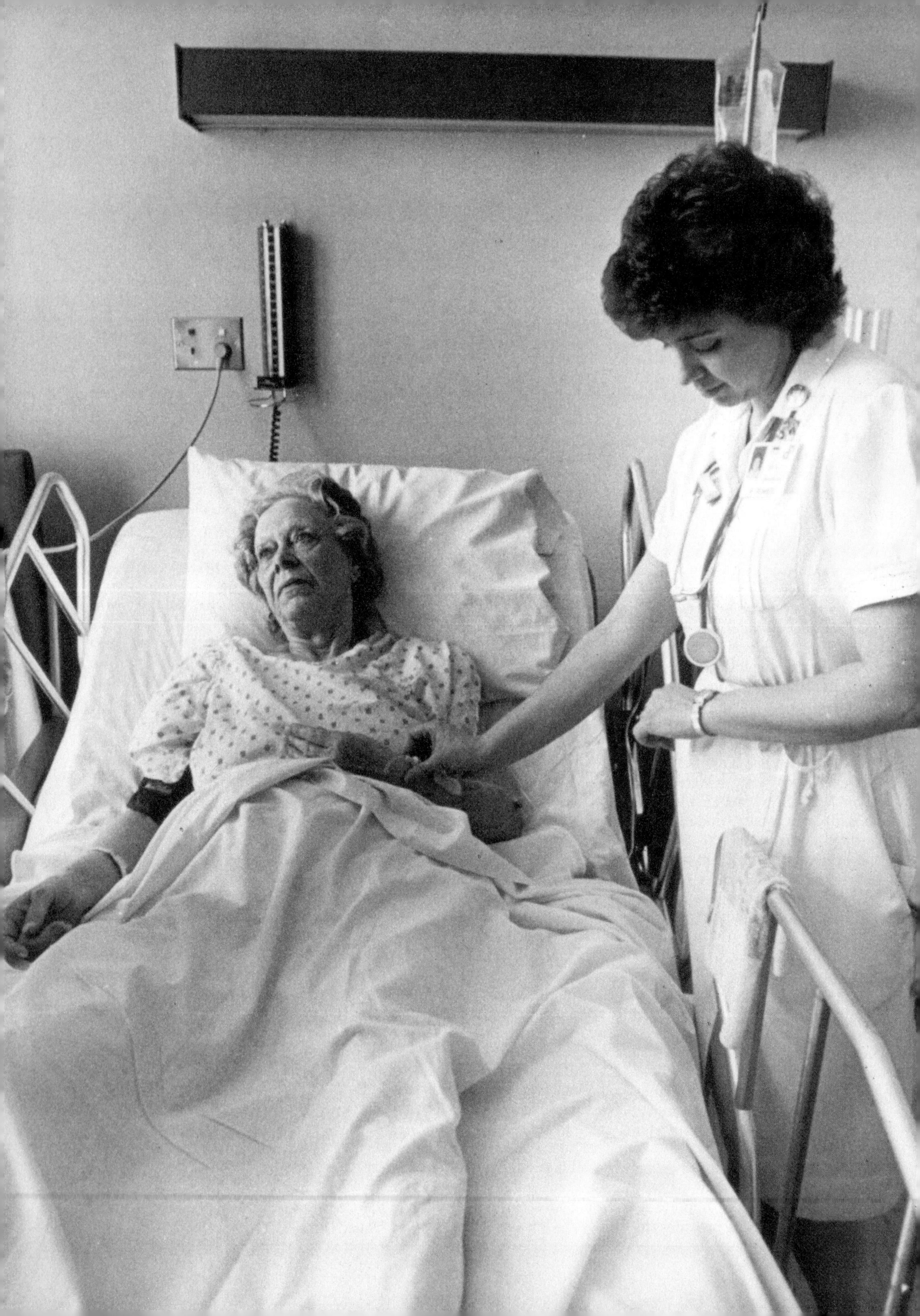

Nursing Care of the Adult

Coordinators

Patricia E. Downing, MN, RN
Paulette D. Rollant, MSN, RN, CCRN

Contributors

Suzette Cardin, MS, RN, CCRN
Virginia L. Cassmeyer, PhD, MSN, RN
Robin Donohoe Dennison, MSN, RN, CS
Deborah Ennis, MSN, RN, CCRN
Alma J. Labunski, MSN, RN, Doctoral Cand.
Esther Matassarin-Jacobs, PhD, RN
Kathleen Deska Pagano, PhD, RN
Judith K. Sands, EdD, RN

Section 3: Nursing Care of the Adult

THE HEALTHY ADULT 151
Characteristics of the Healthy Young and Middle-Aged Adult 151
Characteristics of the Elderly Healthy Adult 153
Application of the Nursing Process to the Healthy Adult 154

SURGERY 157
Overview/Physiology 157
Perioperative Period 157
Discharge 160

OXYGENATION 162
General Concepts 162
Overview/Physiology 162
Application of the Nursing Process to the Client with Oxygenation Problems 164
Selected Health Problems Resulting in Interference with Cardiac Functioning 169
Cardiopulmonary Arrest 169
Shock 170
Angina Pectoris 171
Myocardial Infarction 173
Pacemaker 177
Congestive Heart Failure (CHF) 178
Hypertension 182
Circulatory Problems 183
Selected Health Problems Resulting in Interference with Respiration 185
Chronic Obstructive Pulmonary Disease 185
Pneumonia 188
Tuberculosis 190
Pulmonary Embolus 192
Chest Tubes and Chest Surgery 193
Cancer of the Lung 195
Cancer of the Larynx 196

NUTRITION AND METABOLISM 199

THE DIGESTIVE TRACT 199
General Concepts 199
Overview/Physiology 199
Application of the Nursing Process to the Client with Digestive Tract Problems 201
Selected Health Problems Resulting in Problems with Digestion 205
Hiatal Hernia 205
Gastritis 205
Peptic Ulcer Disease 206
Diverticulosis/Diverticulitis 209
Cholecystitis with Cholelithiasis 210
Pancreatitis 211
Hepatitis 212
Cirrhosis 213
Complications of Liver Disease: Esophageal Varices, Ascites, Hepatic Encephalopathy 214

THE ENDOCRINE SYSTEM 216
General Concepts 216
Overview/Physiology 216
Application of the Nursing Process to the Client with Endocrine System Problems 218
Selected Health Problems 219
Hyperpituitarism 219
Hypopituitarism 220
Hyperthyroidism 220
Hypothyroidism 222
Hyperparathyroidism 222
Hypoparathyroidism 223
Hyperfunction of the Adrenal Glands 223
Hyposecretion of the Adrenal Glands 225
Hypofunction of the Pancreas: Diabetes Mellitus 225

ELIMINATION 232

THE KIDNEYS 232
General Concepts 232
Overview/Physiology 232
Application of the Nursing Process to the Client with Kidney Problems 236
Selected Health Problems Resulting in Alteration in Urinary Elimination 242
Cystitis/Pyelonephritis 242
Urinary Calculi 243
Cancer of the Bladder 244
Acute Renal Failure 245
Chronic Renal Failure 247
Dialysis 249
Kidney Transplantation 252
Benign Prostatic Hypertrophy 254
Cancer of the Prostate 256

THE LARGE BOWEL 257
General Concepts 257
Overview/Physiology 257
Application of the Nursing Process to the Client with Large Bowel Problems 258
Selected Health Problems Resulting in Alteration in Large Bowel Elimination 259
Alteration in Normal Bowel Evacuation 259
Inflammatory Bowel Disease (Regional Enteritis, Ulcerative Colitis) 261
Total Colectomy with Ileostomy 263
Mechanical Obstruction of the Colon 264
Cancer of the Colon 265
Hemorrhoids or Anal Fissure 266

SAFETY AND SECURITY 268
General Concepts 268
Overview/Physiology 268
Application of the Nursing Process to the Client with Problems of Safety and Security 270
Selected Health Problems Resulting in an Interference with Sensation and Perception 275
Acute Head Injury 275
Intracranial Surgery 276
Cerebrovascular Accident 277
Spinal Cord Injuries 279
Parkinson's Syndrome 281
Multiple Sclerosis 283
Amyotrophic Lateral Sclerosis 284
Myasthenia Gravis 285
Cataracts 286
Retinal Detachment 289
Glaucoma 290
Nasal Problems Requiring Surgery 291
Epistaxis 291

ACTIVITY AND REST 293
General Concepts 293
Overview/Physiology 293
Application of the Nursing Process to the Client with Activity and Rest Problems 293
Selected Health Problems Resulting in an Interference with Activity and Rest 295
Fractures 295
Fractured Hip 297
Amputation 299
Arthritis 300
Collagen Disease 302
Herniated Nucleus Pulposus 302

CELLULAR ABERRATION 306
General Concepts 306
Overview/Physiology 306
Application of the Nursing Process to the Client with Cancer 307
Selected Health Problems 311
Hodgkin's Disease 311
Cancer of the Cervix 312
Cancer of the Endometrium of the Uterus 313

Cancer of the Breast 313
Acquired Immune Deficiency Syndrome 315

REPRINTS 317

Section 3: Tables

3.1 Basic Four Food Groups 152
3.2 US Recommended Daily Nutrition for an Average Healthy Adult 153
3.3 Stages of General Anesthesia 159
3.4 General Points Regarding Anesthetic Agents 160
3.5 Calculating IV Rates 160
3.6 Postoperative Diet Modifications 160
3.7 Classes of Analgesics 161
3.8 Emergency Drugs 170
3.9 Angina Pectoris Drugs 173
3.10 Blood Tests for Myocardial Infarction 175
3.11 Anticoagulant and Thrombolytic Drugs 176
3.12 Approximate Sodium Content in Selected Food Items 177
3.13 Cholesterol and Saturated Fat Content in Selected Items 177
3.14 Congestive Heart Failure 179
3.15 Cardiac Glycoside Drugs 179
3.16 Antihypertensive Drugs 180
3.17 Foods High in Potassium 182
3.18 Bronchodilator Drugs 187
3.19 Cough Medications 187
3.20 Antibiotics 189
3.21 Antituberculosis Drugs 191
3.22 Gastrointestinal Hormones 200
3.23 Digestive Enzymes 200
3.24 Drugs Used to Treat Peptic Ulcer Disease 207
3.25 High Fiber/Roughage Diet 210
3.26 Principles of a Low-Fat Diet 210
3.27 Hormones 217
3.28 Steroid Drugs 226
3.29 Hypoglycemic Agents 227
3.30 Diabetic Meal Planning with Exchange Lists 229
3.31 Differentiating Hypoglycemia from Ketoacidosis (Hyperglycemia) 230
3.32 Fluid Imbalance 234
3.33 Electrolyte Imbalances 235
3.34 Acid-Base Imbalance 237
3.35 Laboratory Tests Used to Evaluate Renal Function 238
3.36 Drugs Used to Treat Urinary Tract Infections 241
3.37 Diuretic Drugs 246
3.38 Low-protein Diet Sample Menu 247
3.39 Immunosuppressive Drugs 253
3.40 Prostatectomies 255
3.41 Antidiarrheal and Laxative Drugs 260
3.42 Comparison of Crohn's Disease and Ulcerative Colitis 262
3.43 Foods to be *Avoided* on a Low Residue Diet 263
3.44 Cranial Nerves 269
3.45 Parasympathetic and Sympathetic Effects 269
3.46 Spinal Cord 280
3.47 Drugs Used to Treat Parkinsonism 282
3.48 Drugs Used to Treat Myasthenia Gravis 286
3.49 Eye Medications 287
3.50 Anti-inflammatory Drugs 301
3.51 Anti-gout Medications 303
3.52 Antiemetic Drugs 310
3.53 Staging of Hodgkin's Disease 312

Section 3: Figures

3.1 The Normal Heart 163
3.2 Pressures in the Systemic Circulation of the Vascular System 164
3.3 Areas of Auscultation of Heart Valves 165
3.4 Pulmonary Volumes and Capacities of an Adult 166
3.5 Components of a Normal Electrocardiogram 167
3.6 Distribution of Typical Angina Pain 172
3.7 Coronary Blood Supply 174
3.8 Myocardial Infarction 174
3.9 Typical Enzyme Patterns after Acute Myocardial Infarction 175
3.10 Pattern for Rotating Tourniquets 181
3.11 Common Manifestations of Chronic Arterial and Venous Peripheral Vascular Disease 184
3.12 Water-Seal Chest Drainage 194
3.13 Pleur-evac System 195
3.14 Components of the Kidney 233
3.15 Components and Functions of the Nephron 233
3.16 Schematic Representation of Dialysis 249
3.17 Normal Male Anatomy 254
3.18 Types of Prostatectomies 256
3.19 The Eye 270
3.20 Decorticate Posturing 272
3.21 Decerebrate Posturing 273
3.22 Areas of the Brain that Control Certain Motor and Sensory Functions 278

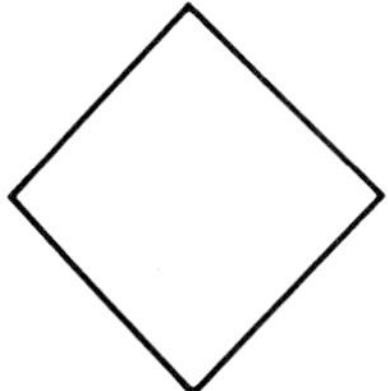

The Healthy Adult

Health

1. Definition
   a. No universally accepted definition
   b. Defined by the World Health organization in 1946 as "state of complete physical, mental, and social well being and not just absence of disease or infirmity . . . fundamental right of every human being."
   c. Defined by the American Nurses Association (ANA) in 1980 as "a dynamic state of being in which the developmental and behavorial potential of an individual is realized to the fullest extent possible. Each human being possesses various strengths and limitations, resulting from the interaction of hereditary and environmental factors. The relative dominance of the strengths and limitations determines an individual's place on the health continuum; it determines the person's biological and behavioral integrity, his wholeness."
2. Characteristics
   a. Dynamic state, dependent upon individual's ability to adapt continually to changing internal and external environment
   b. Continuous spectrum, extending from obvious disease, through absence of discernible disease, to state of optimal functioning
   c. Involves physical and psychosocial aspects
   d. Norms change with age
3. Duration of life
   a. Life span
      1) constant, genetically determined
      2) average appears fixed at 85 years old, with maximum of 115
   b. Life expectancy (United States)
      1) changes with advances in disease control and treatment
      2) born in 1900: 47 years; born in 1989: 75.0 years
4. Levels of health promotion
   a. Primary: prevention of disease; promotion of health
   b. Secondary: early diagnosis; prompt treatment
   c. Tertiary: prevention of complications of disease

☐ Characteristics of the Healthy Young and Middle-Aged Adult (20–65 years)

1. Physiologic characteristics
   a. General
      1) growth and development appropriate for age
      2) symmetrical body
      3) no pain
      4) balanced sleep pattern
   b. Integument
      1) skin
         a) clean, intact, smooth, warm, dry
         b) normal turgor and texture
         c) odorless
         d) no lesions
         e) normal color (e.g., no jaundice, cyanosis)
      2) mucous membranes
         a) pink, intact, hydrated
         b) no lesions
      3) hair
         a) normal distribution and amount
         b) normal texture
         c) no dandruff, scales
      4) nails
         a) pink nail beds
         b) rapid capillary filling of nail beds after compression
         c) no clubbing of fingers
   c. Neck
      1) trachea in midline
      2) no masses
   d. Eyes
      1) symmetrical placement
      2) white sclera
      3) pink conjunctiva
      4) PERRLA (*p*upils *e*qual, *r*ound, *r*eact to *l*ight and *a*ccommodation)
      5) visual acuity 20/20 without or with correction
   e. Ears
      1) symmetrical placement

2) auditory acuity (hearing) normal (i.e., can distinguish whispered words at 20 feet)
3) no drainage from external auditory canal
4) equilibrium maintained (no vertigo)

f. Thorax and lungs
1) open, unobstructed airway
2) respirations (eupneic)
 a) effortless, noiseless, odorless
 b) rhythmical, normal depth
 c) rate: 12–20/minute at rest
3) normal breath sounds: tracheobronchial, bronchovesicular, vesicular (no adventitious sounds)
4) resonant on percussion (no dullness)
5) no cough or sputum
6) thorax: normal anterior-posterior diameter (i.e., AP diameter less than lateral to lateral diameter)

g. Cardiovascular
1) normal sinus rhythm (NSR)
2) rate: 60–80/minute at rest
3) blood pressure approximately 120/80 at rest
4) no chest pain
5) no palpitations
6) normal palpable arterial pulses in the extremities (radial, brachial, femoral, popliteal, tibial, dorsalis pedis)
7) normal skin color and temperature (e.g., no cyanosis, pigmentation)
8) no peripheral edema
9) no varicosities/ulcerations of extremities

h. Abdomen
1) soft, nontender
2) flat, no distension
3) normal, active bowel sounds
4) no palpable organomegaly or masses

i. Gastrointestinal/nutrition
1) normal weight for height
2) normal appetite
3) balanced, adequate diet; see Tables 3.1, 3.2 (see also Tables 4.7 and 4.8)
4) normal digestion (e.g., no food intolerance, indigestion)
5) well nourished
6) teeth present, in good repair
7) normal mastication (i.e., no difficulty or pain with chewing)
8) no difficulty swallowing
9) regular bowel habits, stools brown and formed

j. Musculoskeletal
1) good posture and body alignment
2) body movements coordinated (no tremors or involuntary movements)
3) muscles: firm, symmetrical, strong, normal tone (no spasms, contractures, weakness, atrophy, or paralysis)
4) normal gait (foot strikes heel to toe, normal base of support, arms swing in coordination with leg movements)
5) joints
 a) full, unimpaired range of motion
 b) no deformities
 c) nontender, nonswollen, no crepitation

k. Neurologic
1) mental status/cognitive functioning
 a) oriented to person, place, time
 b) alert, conscious
 c) memory intact: short- and long-term
 d) capable of abstract thinking
 e) articulates without difficulty

Table 3.1 Basic Four Food Groups

Milk Group	Fruit/Vegetable Group
Calcium Protein Riboflavin	Vitamins A and C Carbohydrate
3 or more glasses daily—Children 4 or more glasses daily—Teens 2 or more glasses daily—Adults	4 or more servings daily
Milk, cheese and other milk products	Dark green or yellow vegetables; citrus fruit or tomatoes

Meat Group	Grain Group
Protein, Niacin Thiamin, Iron	Carbohydrate, Niacin Thiamin, Iron
2 or more servings daily	4 or more servings daily
Meats, fish, poultry, eggs or cheese—with dry beans, peas, nuts as alternates	Whole grain or enriched breads, cereals, pastas, and rice

Source: Dairy Nutrition Council Inc, Chicago, IL. Used with permission.

Table 3.2 US Recommended Daily Nutrition for an Average Healthy Adult (23–50 years old)

	Women	Men
	120 lb (55kg) 64 in (163cm)	154 lb (70kg) 70 in (178cm)
Calories	2,000 kcal	2,700 kcal
Protein[1]	44 G (176 kcal)	56 G (224 kcal)
Fat[2]	66 G (594 kcal)	90 G (810 kcal)
Carbohydrate[3]	285 G (1,140 kcal)	383 G (1,532 kcal)
Cholesterol	300 mg	300 mg
Sodium	1,100–3,300 mg	1,100–3,300 mg
Calcium	800 mg	800 mg
Iron	18 mg	10 mg
Fluids	1,500 ml	1,500 ml

[1]8%–12% of total calories; 0.8g/kg
[2]30% of total calories (10% saturated fat & 20% from poly- or monosaturated fat)
[3]58% of total calories (48% complex carbohydrate, 10% simple sugar)

Source: *Recommended Daily Allowances* (RDA), National Research Council. Daily Goals for the US, US Senate Select Committee on Nutrition & Human Needs. American Heart Association.

f) dress/behavior/mood appropriate (no excessive aggression, violence, withdrawal, depression)

2) sensory
   a) pain perception intact
   b) light touch, pressure, and vibration perception intact
   c) temperature perception intact
   d) sight, hearing, taste and smell perception intact
   e) proprioception (sense of body position) perception intact
3) motor (see also *Musculoskeletal*, page 154)
   a) coordinated movement
   b) normal gait
   c) no tremors or involuntary movements
   d) no atrophy, weakness, or paralysis of muscles
   e) reflexes intact and normal (including deep tendon reflexes)

l. Genitourinary
1) normal sexual function for age and sex
2) genitals
   a) good hygiene
   b) no lesions or abnormal discharge
3) breasts
   a) symmetrical size and placement
   b) no masses
   c) no abnormal discharge from nipples
4) micturition (urination)
   a) nonpainful
   b) voluntary control
   c) no difficulty controlling stream
   d) no frequency or urgency
   e) bladder empty after voiding
   f) approximately 300 ml/voiding
   g) urine: amber, clear, specific gravity 1.001–1.020

2. Psychosocial characteristics (see *Nursing Care of the Client with Psychosocial, Mental Health/ Psychiatric Problems* page 16)

☐ Characteristics of the Elderly Healthy Adult (over 65 years)

1. Physiologic characteristics

a. Norms: normal physiologic changes (vs abnormal pathologic changes) have not been completely identified.

b. General changes
1) general tissue desiccation and slowed cell division
2) slowed, weakened speed of response to stimuli
3) slowed rate of tissue repair
4) decreased metabolism
5) mechanisms of homeostasis less rapid and less efficient
6) rate of change is individual, influenced by factors such as heredity and stress
7) high incidence of health problems (e.g., CHF, osteoporosis, cataracts)

c. Integument
1) skin
   a) dry, wrinkled, loss of elasticity
   b) decreased perspiration and sebum
   c) fragile, easily injured
   d) decreased subcutaneous tissue
   e) decreased skin turgor
   f) increased sensitivity to cold
2) hair
   a) decreased number of hair follicles, generalized loss
   b) scant, fine, greying
   c) hirsutism (female)
   d) possible hereditary baldness
3) nails
   a) dry
   b) thick
   c) brittle

d. Eyes
1) slowed accommodation to light
2) decreased visual acuity

a) far sightedness due to slow lens accomodation (presbyopia)
b) narrowed field of vision (tunnel)

e. Ears
1) decreased acuity
2) sensorineural hearing deficit (presbycusis): gradual loss of high-frequency tones

f. Thorax and lungs
1) decreased lung capacity
2) decreased elasticity of tissue
3) increased AP diameter of thorax

g. Cardiovascular
1) decreased vascular elasticity
2) increased systolic BP
3) decreased cardiac output
4) less tolerance to position change

h. Gastrointestinal/nutrition
1) slowed digestion; increased food intolerances
2) decreased metabolism: caloric requirement, approximately 1,000 calories/day
3) redistribution of body fat: increased fat in trunk, especially in the abdomen
4) teeth and gum problems common
5) atonic constipation common

i. Musculoskeletal
1) tire easily, less stamina
2) symmetrical decrease in muscle bulk
3) decreased muscle strength and tone
4) impaired range of motion resulting from stiff joints
5) generalized loss of from 6–10 cm in stature resulting from
a) flexion of knee and hip joints
b) narrowing of intervertebral discs
6) body takes on bony, angular appearance
7) osteoporosis common (especially in vertebral bodies and neck of femur)

j. Neurologic
1) general
a) slowed speed of impulse transmission
b) progressive decrease in number of functioning neurons in CNS and sense organs
c) normal neurologic functioning possible because of tremendous reserve of numbers of neurons
2) mental/cognitive function
a) altered capacity to retain new information and learn new tasks
b) some impaired memory and mental endurance
3) sensory
a) some impaired sensory perception (hearing, smell, sight, taste, touch, temperature, pain)
b) gradual decrease of visual and auditory acuity
4) motor
a) slowed reaction to stimuli; lengthening of reaction time
b) decreased coordination and balance

k. Genitourinary
1) decreased renal capacity to concentrate urine at night
2) nocturia
3) ability to function sexually may continue well into older years

2. Psychosocial Characteristics (see *Nursing Care of the Client with Psychosocial, Mental Health/ Psychiatric Problems* page 15 and Table 2.1)

☐ Application of the Nursing Process to the Healthy Adult

1. Assessment

a. Health history
1) usual health status
2) present health status
3) family history (e.g., familial cancer, heart disease)
4) previous illness
5) immunization status
6) allergies
7) psychosocial
a) age, sex, race, marital status
b) role in family
c) cultural heritage
d) language
e) education
f) economic status
g) occupation
h) housing
i) religious practices
j) recreational/social activities
k) personal habits: tobacco, alcohol
8) physical
a) personal hygiene habits/practices
b) eating habits/patterns
c) dental history
d) bowel and bladder habits
e) sleep and rest habits
f) activity level
g) work habits
h) sexual habits

b. Physical exam
1) methods
a) inspection: looking, observing
b) auscultation: listening

c) palpation: feeling, touching, pressing
d) percussion: tapping

2) head-to-toe appraisal (see physiologic characteristics of the young, middle aged, and elderly adult pages 151–154)

2. Analysis

a. Safe, effective care environment
1) knowledge deficit
2) potential for injury
3) sensory-perceptual alteration (specify)

b. Physiological integrity
1) altered growth and development
2) altered nutrition: more/less than body requirements
3) potential activity intolerance

c. Psychological integrity
1) self esteem disturbance
2) spiritual distress
3) altered patterns of sexuality

d. Health promotion/maintenance
1) knowledge deficit
2) health-seeking behaviors
3) altered health maintainance

3. General Nursing Plans, Implementation, and Evaluation

Goal 1: Adult individual will use health practices that promote optimal health.

Plan/Implementation

- Teach, support and act as role model as necessary to assist the individual to
  - maintain personal hygiene
  - maintain nutrition
    - * eat sensible, well-balanced diet (see Tables 3.1, 3.2, 4.7, 4.8)
    - * avoid foods high in saturated fat, cholesterol, and simple sugars
    - * eat adequate fiber
    - * limit alcohol use
  - maintain proper body weight
  - exercise regularly
  - obtain adequate rest and sleep
  - avoid tobacco use
  - avoid prolonged sun exposure

Evaluation: Individual maintains normal weight for height.

Goal 2: Adult individual will experience safe environment; will be free from accidental injury.

Plan/Implementation

- Teach as necessary to ensure that individual
  - has safe home (e.g., fire alarms, ample lighting)
  - has safe working conditions (e.g., safety devices, no toxic material)
  - travels safely (e.g., automobile seat belts)
  - recreates safely (e.g., no diving in shallow water)

Evaluation: Individual is free from serious accidents.

Goal 3: Adult individual will undergo routine health exams.

Plan/Implementation

- Recommend and help schedule as necessary annual physical exam
  - routine dentist/dental hygienist visits
  - attendance at screening clinics (e.g., hypertension, glaucoma, diabetes)
- Teach guidelines for early detection of cancer; see *Cellular Aberration*, General Nursing Plan 1 page 309.

Evaluation: Individual has dental exam/check every 6 months, yearly physical exam.

References

Bates, B. (1987). *A guide to physical examination*. (4th ed). Philadelphia: Lippincott.

Berliner, H. (1986). Aging skin. *American Journal of Nursing*, *86*, 1138–1141.

Berliner, H. (1986). Aging skin: Part 2. *American Journal of Nursing*, *86*, 1259–1261.

Burggraf, V., & Donlon, B. (1985). Assessing the elderly: System by system, part 1 (programmed instruction). *American Journal of Nursing*, *85*, 974–984.

Carnevali, F. & Patrick, M. (Eds.). (1986). *Nursing management for the elderly* (2nd ed.). Philadelphia: Lippincott.

Dychtwald, D. (Ed.). (1986). *Wellness and health promotion for the elderly*. Rockville, MD: Aspen.

Ellis, F. & Nowlis, E. (1985). *Nursing: A human needs approach*. Boston: Houghton-Mifflin.

Henderson, M. (1985). Assessing the elderly: Altered presentations, part 2 (programmed instruction). *American Journal of Nursing*, *85*, 1103–1106.

Krause, M. & Mahan, L. (1984). *Food, nutrition and diet therapy*. Philadelphia: Saunders.

Lewis, S. & Collier, I. (1987). *Medical-surgical nursing*. New York: McGraw-Hill.

Moore, P., & Williamson, G. (1984). Health promotion: Evolution of a concept. *Nursing Clinics of North America*, *19*, 195–206.

New longevity record in the United States. *Statistical Bulletin*, *69*(3), 10–15.

Phipps, W. Long, B. & Woods, N. (Eds.). (1987). *Medical surgical nursing: Concepts and clinical practice* (3rd ed.). St. Louis: Mosby.

Porter-O'Grady, T. (1985). Health vs illness, nurses can chart the course of the future. *Nursing and Health Care*, *6*(6), 319–321.

†Sensory changes in the elderly (programmed instruction). (1981). *American Journal of Nursing*, *81*, 1851–1880.

Shaver, J. (1985). A biopsychological view of human health. *Nursing Outlook*, *33*(4), 186–191.

Shine, M. (Ed.). (1983). Symposium on gerontologic nursing in acute care. *Nursing Clinics of North America*, *18*, 355–421.

Steffl, B. (Ed.). (1984). *Handbook of gerontological nursing*. New York: Van Nostrand Reinhold.

†Highly recommended

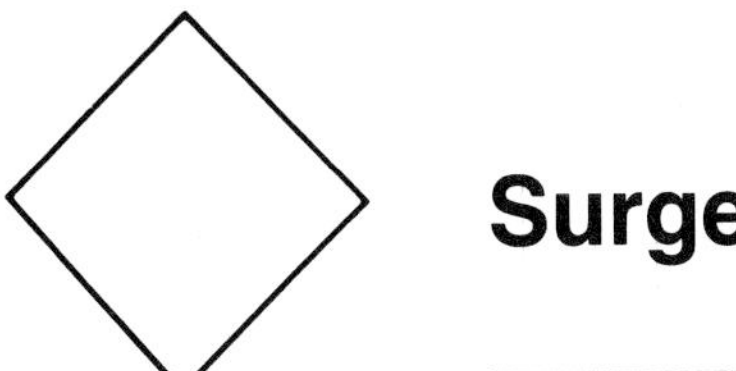

Surgery

(The nursing care presented in this unit concerns problems in the care of clients undergoing surgery.)

General Concepts

Overview/Physiology

1. Surgery is a stressful event
2. General considerations
   - a. Dangers are always present for all surgery clients
   - b. One complication usually leads to another
   - c. Close monitoring is needed throughout the perioperative period
3. Most common types of complications
   - a. Respiratory
     - 1) atelectasis (air blockage by mucus plugs to portion of lung leading to collapse)
     - 2) hypostatic pneumonia
   - b. Circulatory
     - 1) thrombophlebitis and phlebothrombosis (refer to "Circulatory Problems" page 183)
     - 2) shock; volume depletion (refer to "Shock" page 170)
   - c. Wound
     - 1) hemorrhage
     - 2) infection
     - 3) dehiscence (wound separation)
     - 4) evisceration (separation with protrusion of contents through incision)
   - d. Urinary
     - 1) retention
     - 2) oliguria
   - e. Gastrointestinal
     - 1) paralytic ileus (neurogenic disruption of intestine often related to hypokalemia, decreased autonomic innervation, absent peristalsis)
     - 2) singultus (hiccoughs)
   - f. Negative nitrogen balance: greater nitrogen excretion than amount ingested
4. Factors affecting client's response to surgery and development of complications
   - a. Age: very old and very young are less able to tolerate stress of surgery
   - b. Nutritional status: malnutrition and/or obesity increase risk of poor wound healing
   - c. Presence of other chronic illnesses
     - 1) COPD increases risk of pulmonary problems
     - 2) cardiovascular disease decreases ability to deal with stress of surgery
     - 3) renal disease increases risk of fluid and electrolyte problems
     - 4) diabetes mellitus increases risk of poor wound healing
     - 5) chronic glucocorticoid therapy increases risk of fluid and electrolyte problems, poor wound healing
   - d. Prolonged immobility after surgery increases risk of thrombophlebitis, abdominal distension, urinary retention, and pulmonary complications
   - e. Type of operation: some operations are more frequently associated with complications (e.g., atelectasis after gallbladder surgery)
5. Each institution has basic admission, preoperative, intraoperative, and postoperative routines. The following content emphasizes general principles of care that apply to all situations.

☐ Perioperative Period

1. General Information

- a. Pre-op care may need to be completed within 1 or 2 hours in an emergency or day surgery situation, or may be given over a longer period for elective surgery.
- b. Post-op care may be given in recovery room, ICU, or on general floor.
- c. Adequate physiologic and psychologic preparation and care are extremely important to the client's successful recovery.
- d. For day surgery clients: Many procedures are now performed in ambulatory surgery or day surgery settings. These persons need the same care as that required by inpatients. Diagnostic tests are usually done as an outpatient during

the week prior to surgery. The client may see the anesthesiologist, sign consents, and receive some preoperative teaching at this time. Postoperatively, a time and place must be provided to instruct the client/family about diet, fluids, activity, care of wounds, medications, and what to expect re returning to work, comfort, and nausea and vomiting. Clients need someone to help them get to and from the hospital if they receive a general anesthetic.

2. Nursing Process

a. Assessment

1) total health status of the client and activities of daily living (ADL) preoperatively
2) general physical exam preoperatively as described for the healthy adult (if time is limited, focus on cardiovascular, pulmonary, neurologic, renal)
3) post-op assessment focuses on systems affected by potential complications and surgery
4) for day surgery clients: ability to get home, do care at home
5) diagnostic tests
   a) every client
      - CBC
      - electrolytes
      - urinalysis
      - ECG
   b) special considerations
      - type and crossmatch (as necessary)
      - prothrombin time, partial thromboplastin time (PTT), bleeding time and/or clotting time
        - underlying bleeding or coagulation problem
        - receiving anticoagulants or to receive anticoagulants during surgery
        - liver problems or jaundice
      - blood gases and pulmonary function tests (if pulmonary problem is present or pulmonary-cardiovascular surgery is planned)
6) diagnostic tests (post-op) will vary with type of surgery

b. Analysis

1) safe, effective care environment
   a) knowledge deficit (pre-op)
   b) potential for injury (intra-op)
   c) potential for infection (post-op)
2) physiological integrity
   a) ineffective breathing pattern, potential ineffective airway clearance (intra-, post-op)
   b) potential decreased cardiac output (intra-, post-op)
   c) urinary retention (post-op)
   d) pain (post-op)
   e) potential altered nutrition: less than body requirements (post-op)
3) psychological integrity
   a) anxiety (pre-op)
   b) fear (pre-op)
   c) body image disturbance (post-op)
4) health promotion/maintenance
   a) self care deficit (specify) (post-op)
   b) knowledge deficit (post-op)
   c) altered health maintenance (post-op)

c. Plans, Implementation, and Evaluation

Goal 1: Client and significant others will be prepared for surgery.

Plan/Implementation

Day before surgery

- Assess learning needs and expectations of surgery.
- Clarify expectations of surgery.
- Explain pre-op procedures, post-op routine to client and significant others.
- Ensure diagnostic tests completed.
- Evaluate nutritional status.
- Do bowel prep if required.
- Ensure adequate rest the night before surgery; sedate prn.

Day of surgery

- Monitor vital signs and report immediately if different from admission vital signs.
- Have client shower.
- Remove hairpins, jewelry, medals to avoid loss, injury.
- Remove prosthetic devices (i.e., dentures, artificial body parts).
- Apply antiembolic stockings as ordered.
- Have client void immediately before the administration of premedications.
- Premedicate as ordered (not used as frequently as in the past).
- Put side rails up following premedication.
- Provide quiet environment.

Evaluation: Client and significant other explain surgery and post-op routine; client demonstrates coughing, rests well before surgery; completes all diagnostic tests.

Goal 2: Client will experience a safe environment in the operating room.

Plan/Implementation

- Prepare skin as appropriate.
- Maintain sterility of equipment and operating team.
- Prevent static electricity by proper attire, safety of electrical equipment, proper grounding.
- Position client appropriately.
- Maintain contact with client during induction of general anesthesia (see Table 3.3)
- Assist with monitoring for potential complications of anesthetic agents (see Table 3.4).
- Attend to client during intubation and extubation; be prepared to assist as necessary.
- Promote hemostasis and have appropriate equipment, supplies available (hemostats, ligatures, electrocoagulation, bone wax, styptics, gelatin sponges, cryoprobe, laser beam, saline packs).
- Monitor sponge usage; weigh sponges for blood loss as indicated.
- Measure content of suction bottles; subtract irrigation fluid to approximate blood loss.

Evaluation: Client is positioned appropriately; enters operative stage of anesthesia without difficulty; remains stable throughout surgical procedure; is transported to recovery room in stable condition; does not develop any disturbance in circulation (e.g., excess blood loss, signs of shock).

Table 3.3 Stages of General Anesthesia

Stage	Duration	Manifestations
I	Beginning of induction to loss of consciousness	Loss of judgment powers Hearing acute
II	Loss of consciousness to loss of eyelid reflex	Cerebral or voluntary control lost Hypersensitive to incoming impulses Hearing acute
III	Extends from loss of eye reflex to cessation of respiratory effort; surgery performed in this stage; reflexes absent and muscles relaxed	Functions of medulla retained
IV		Respiratory paralysis Cardiac failure Death

Goal 3: Postoperatively, client's respiratory, circulatory, fluid and electrolyte, and neurologic status will be optimal.

Plan/Implementation

- Monitor vital signs, I&O, IV infusion, electrolytes, drainage tubes, neurologic status, and surgical wound dressing.
- Report changes to physician.
- Begin turning, coughing, deep-breathing exercises qh after airway is removed.
- Monitor respiratory rate, character with vital signs.
- Suction nasopharynx as needed.
- Administer respiratory-assistance drugs as ordered.
- Use inspiratory spirometer as indicated.
- Give IV therapy, drugs as ordered (see Table 3.5 for calculating IV rates).
- Use voiding-inducement techniques as necessary.
- Start oral fluids when appropriate (see Table 3.6).
- Keep side rails up until client's neurologic status is normal.
- Use restraints as necessary.

Evaluation: Cleint's breath sounds are clear; client coughs well; BP remains stable; skin is warm and dry; nail beds blanch briskly; I&O is in balance; IV is infusing appropriately; client responds appropriately; has dry and intact surgical dressing.

Goal 4: Client will be free from discomfort during the post-op period.

Plan/Implementation

- See reprint on pain, page 320.
- Position comfortably; turn q2h; begin ROM exercise as appropriate; ambulate to prevent abdominal distension and other complications of immobility as appropriate.
- Assess pain
  - source of discomfort
  - location, character, intensity, and duration of pain
  - level of anxiety
  - factors that intensify or decrease discomfort
  - type of anesthetic administered
  - vital signs before and after administration of medication
- Give analgesics as appropriate (see Table 3.7 for common analgesics).
- Utilize comfort measures, relaxation, distraction.
- Observe client's response to pain-relief

Table 3.4 General Points Regarding Anesthetic Agents

Type	Definition	Major Complications
General inhalation	Gases and vapors administered via mask or ET tube; blocks pathways to brain and renders patient unconscious; used for major operations of thorax, abdomen, head, and neck.	Cardiac dysfunction (dysrrhythmias, arrest) Respiratory dysfunction (broncho- and laryngospasms, aspiration failure) Cardiovascular dysfunction (shock, hypotension) Neurologic complications (convulsions, CVA) Others (renal and liver problems, malignant hyperthermia)
Intravenous	Drugs given directly into vein; used for induction and as adjunct to inhalation agents. Do not abolish all pain reflexes.	Respiratory dysfunction (arrest, bronchospasm, laryngospasms) Cardiac and cardiovascular dysfunction (hypotension, depression) Neurologic dysfunction (convulsions)
Regional	Drugs injected into nerve track/endings to block selected fibers; may be given topically, locally, spinal, epidural, etc. Do not decrease anxiety, fear; must have a cooperative patient.	Hypotension, anaphylactic shock Respiratory paralysis can occur with spinal Headache

Table 3.5 Calculating IV Rates

$$\frac{\text{amount of IV fluid (ml)}}{\text{time to infuse (min)}} \times \text{drip factor (gtt/ml)} = \text{IV rate (gtt/min)}$$

Example: The order is for 1,000 ml D_5W to run for 10 hours. The drip factor is 15 gtt/ml.

$$\frac{1{,}000 \text{ ml}}{\underset{(60 \times 10)}{600 \text{ min}}} \times \frac{15 \text{ gtt}}{1 \text{ ml}} = \text{IV rate of 25 gtt/min}$$

measures (e.g., amount, onset, duration of relief).

- Prevent nausea and vomiting
  - assess rationale for occurrence (e.g., type of anesthesia, surgery)
  - give antiemetics prn as ordered
  - give frequent oral hygiene

Evaluation: Client's pain is relieved; offers no complaints of nausea.

Table 3.6 Postoperative Diet Modifications

Diet	Foods Allowed	Comments
Clear liquids	Tea, Jell-O, broth, strained juices	Provides liquids, but inadequate calories and nutrients
Full liquids	Soups, milk, unstrained juices, ice cream, custards, pudding	Provides more calories and nutrients. If selected carefully can meet many nutritional needs.

☐ Discharge

1. General Information: discharge planning starts at admission

2. Nursing Process

a. Assessment/Analysis

1) client's ability to do self-care at home
2) significant others
3) home situation

b. Plan, Implementation, and Evaluation

Goal: Client and significant others are prepared for client's discharge.

Plan/Implementation

- Determine discharge date with consultation with physician.
- Teach client and significant other as appropriate re: medications, return appointment, treatments, activity, diet.
- Refer to appropriate community health agency.

Evaluation: Client states time of return appointment; lists medicines to take and how.

Table 3.7 Classes of Analgesics

Morphine-like Agonists
codeine
morphine
hydromorphone (Dilaudid)
methadone (Dolophine)
levorphanol (Levo-Dromoran)
oxycodone
oxymorphone (Numorphan)
meperidine (Demerol)
Partial Agonist
buprenorphine (Buprenex)
Mixed Agonist-Antagonists
pentazocine (Talwin)
nalbuphine (Nubain)
butorphanol (Stadol)
Non-narcotics
aspirin
acetominophen
ibuprofen (Motrin)
fenoprofen (Nalfon)
diflunisal (Dolobid)
naproxen (Naprosyn)

Note: See reprint "Relieving Pain," page 320, for more information.

References

*American Pain Society. (1988). CE: Relieving pain: An analgesic guide. *American Journal of Nursing*, *88*, 816–826.

Brozenec, S. (1985). Caring for the postoperative patient with an abdominal drain. *Nursing85*, *15*(4), 55–57.

Kleiman, R., Lipman, A., Hare, B., & MacDonald, S. (1987). PCA versus regular IM injections for severe post-op pain. *American Journal of Nursing*, *87*, 1491–1492.

Luce, F. (1984). Clinical risk factors for postoperative pulmonary complications. *Respiratory Care*, *29*, 484–495.

McCaffrey, M. (1987). Equigesic doses. *Nursing87*, *17*(8), 56–57.

McConnell, E. (1983). After surgery: How can you avoid the obvious and not so obvious hazards. *Nursing83*, *16*(2), 74–84.

McConnell, E. (1987). *Clinical considerations in perioperative nursing*. Philadelphia: Lippincott.

Montanari, J. (1986). Action STAT: Wound dehiscence. *Nursing86*, *16*(2), 33–36.

Montanari, J. (1985). Documenting your post-op assessment findings. *Nursing85*, *15*(8), 31–35.

Norheim, C. (1985). Spinal anesthesia; As bad as it sounds. *Nursing85*, *15*(4), 42–44.

Phipps, W., Long, B., & Woods, N. (Eds.). (1987). *Medical-surgical nursing: Concepts and clinical practice* (3rd ed.). St. Louis: Mosby.

Smith, C. (1985). Detecting acute abdominal distension. *Nursing85*, *15*(9), 56–57.

*See reprint section

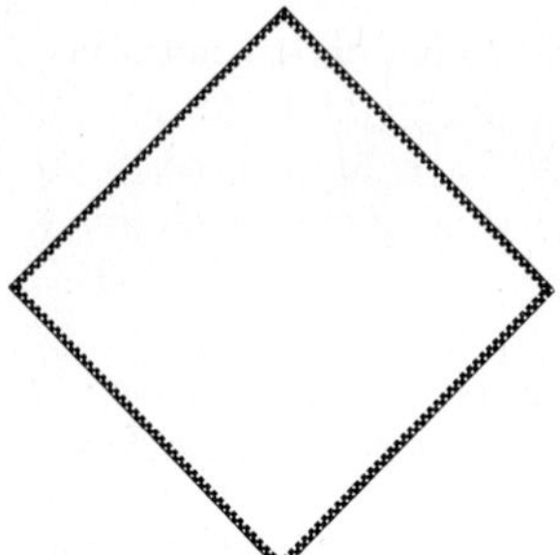

Oxygenation

(The nursing care presented in this unit concerns selected health problems related to disturbances in the cardiovascular and respiratory systems.)

General Concepts

Overview/Physiology

1. The cardinal purpose of the cardiovascular and respiratory systems is to provide adequate oxygenation to the body as a whole
   a. Respiratory system: responsible for the intake of oxygen (O_2), elimination of carbon dioxide (CO_2); plays a major role in maintaining acid-base balance
   b. Cardiovascular system: responsible for the transport of O_2, CO_2, nutrients, and waste products
2. The heart is a high-energy pump that forcefully ejects blood with enough pressure to perfuse the pulmonary and systemic circulatory systems.
3. Flow of blood through the heart: inferior and superior vena cava → right atrium → tricuspid valve → right ventricle → pulmonary valve → pulmonary arteries → lungs → pulmonary veins → left atrium → mitral valve → left ventricle → aortic valve → aorta → systemic circulation (see Figure 3.1)
4. Blood returning to the right side of the heart is unoxygenated, venous blood. Blood ejected from the left side of the heart into the systemic circulation is oxygenated, arterial blood.
5. The heart is surrounded by a sac of fibrous tissue known as the pericardium. Between the pericardium and epicardium there is a small space that contains a few drops of fluid that lubricate the heart surface.
6. The heart itself is composed of three layers
   a. Epicardium: outer layer; coronary arteries lie on this surface (this layer is structurally the same as the visceral pericardium)
   b. Myocardium: middle layer; cardiac muscle activity originates here
   c. Endocardium: inner layer; lines the valves, chordae tendineae, and papillary muscles
7. The cardiac impulse originates automatically in the sinoatrial (SA) node, travels to the right and left atria → atria contract. Then the impulse reaches the atrioventricular (AV) node, accelerates through the bundle of His, bundle branches, and Purkinje's fibers, and is distributed rapidly and evenly over the ventricles → ventricles contract. The conduction process is regulated by the autonomic nervous system
   a. Sympathetic stimulation increases the heart rate
   b. Parasympathetic or vagal stimulation decreases the heart rate
8. Mean arterial pressure = cardiac output × total peripheral resistance; cardiac output = stroke volume (amount of blood ejected/beat) × heart rate. Arterial pressure can be increased by increasing cardiac output (either stroke volume, heart rate, or both), or by increasing total peripheral resistance. Both cardiac output and total peripheral resistance are influenced by a variety of factors, particularly the autonomic nervous system. Stimulation of the sympathetic nervous system increases heart rate, stroke volume, and total peripheral resistance.
9. Blood pressure varies throughout circulation: greatest in the arterial system; lowest in the venous portion (see Figure 3.2).
   Central venous pressure (CVP) is the pressure within the right atrium; normal = 4–10 cm H_2O (0–5 mm Hg).
10. The respiratory system is composed of upper and lower airway structures
   a. Upper airway: nose and nasopharynx, mouth, oropharynx, and larynx
   b. Lower airway: trachea, mainstem bronchi, bronchioles, alveolar ducts, and alveoli
   c. Airways provide a passageway for air and also filter, warm, and humidify inspired air
11. The lungs lie in and are protected by the thoracic cavity. This bony cage is composed of the sternum and ribs anteriorly and the ribs, scapulae, and vertebral column posteriorly. The thoracic cavity is lined with a serous membrane,

Figure 3.1 The Normal Heart

a. Superior vena cava **b.** Inferior vena cava **c.** Right atrium **d.** Tricuspid valve **e.** Right ventricle **f.** Pulmonary valve **g.** Pulmonary artery **h.** Right pulmonary veins **i.** Left pulmonary veins **j.** Left atrium **k.** Mitral valve **l.** Left ventricle **m.** Aortic valve **n.** Aorta

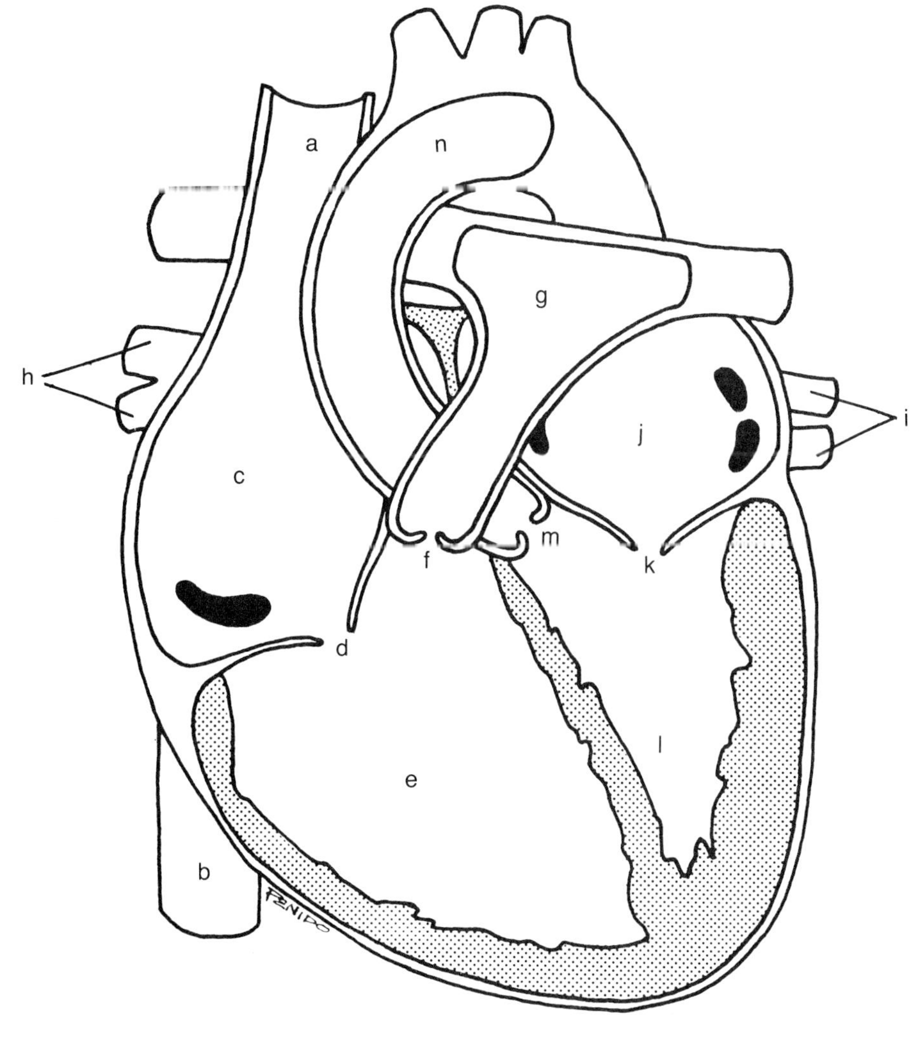

the pleura; one surface of the pleura lines the inside of the rib cage (parietal pleura), the other covers the lungs (visceral pleura). The pleural space (which is really a potential space) exists between the surfaces of the two pleurae. Substmospheric pressure in the pleural space is responsible for the continued expansion of the lungs.

12. The basic gas-exchange unit of the respiratory system is the alveolus. Pulmonary capillaries lie adjacent to each alveolus; O_2 and CO_2 are exchanged across the alveolar-capillary membrane by the process of diffusion.

13. The neural control of respirations is located in the medulla. Under normal conditions, this center is stimulated directly or reflexly by the concentration of CO_2 in the blood (pCO_2). Chemoreceptors located in the carotid arteries and aortic arch also stimulate the respiratory center of the medulla and respond primarily to hypoxia in the blood (reduced pO_2).

14. The rhythmic breathing pattern is dependent on

Figure 3.2 Pressures in the Systemic Circulation of the Vascular System

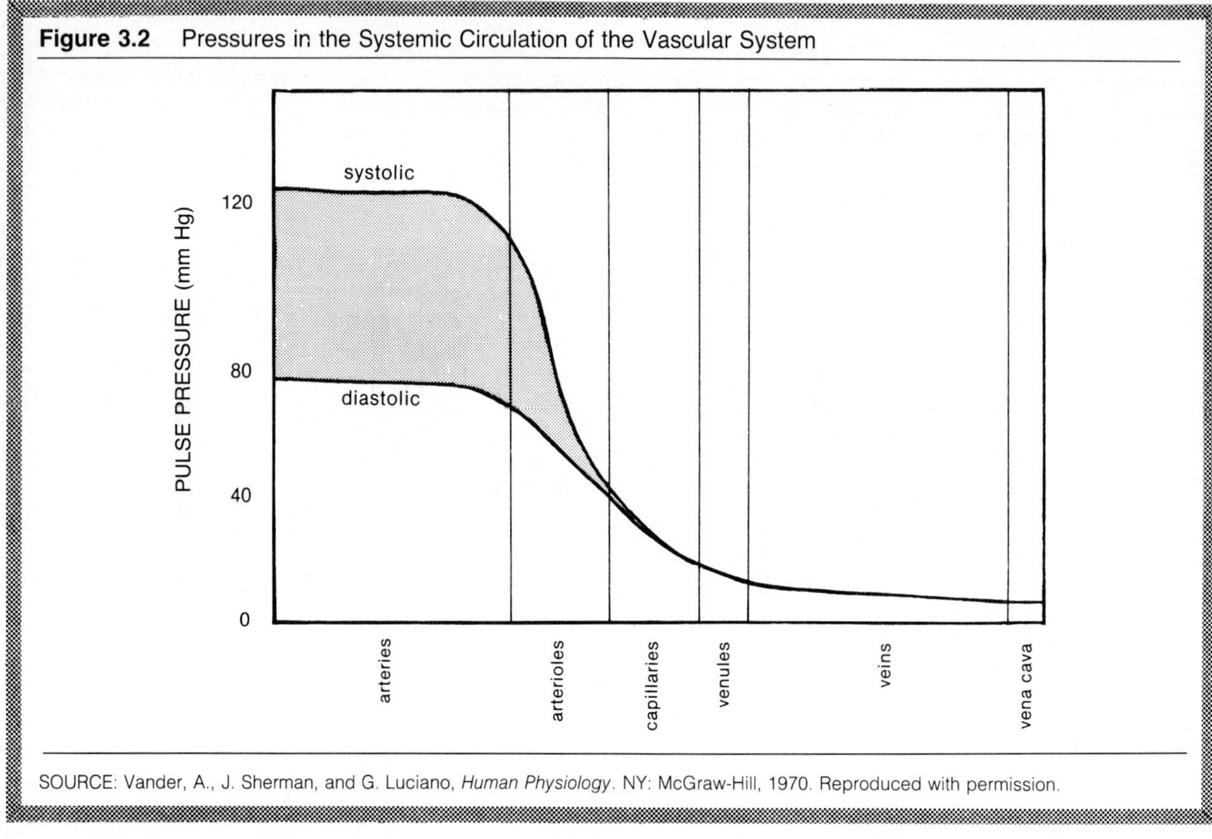

SOURCE: Vander, A., J. Sherman, and G. Luciano, *Human Physiology*. NY: McGraw-Hill, 1970. Reproduced with permission.

the cyclical excitation of the respiratory muscles by the phrenic nerve (to the diaphragm) and the intercostal nerves (to the intercostal muscles).

15. Blood is the fluid that circulates through the cardiovascular system
   a. Composition
      1) cells: RBCs, WBCs, platelets
      2) plasma: water, protein, electrolytes, and various organic constituents
   b. Functions
      1) RBC (hemoglobin): carry O_2 from the lungs to tissue and CO_2 from tissue to lungs
      2) WBC: defense against microbial invasion
      3) platelets: hemostasis
   c. Volume: approximately 5,000 ml

16. The major steps of clot formation are thromboplastin → prothrombin → thrombin → fibrinogen → fibrin (clot).

Application of the Nursing Process to the Client with Oxygenation Problems

1. Assessment
   a. Health history
      1) dyspnea or chest pain/discomfort
         a) when (e.g., rest, activity)
         b) relieved by what
      2) cough
         a) when
         b) productive/nonproductive; character and amount of sputum, if productive
      3) smoking
         a) type, pack/years (number of packs per day × number of years)
         b) when stopped, duration
      4) allergies
         a) to what?
         b) symptoms
         c) relieved by what
      5) orthopnea or paraoxysmal nocturnal dyspnea (PND)
         a) when
         b) relieved by what (e.g., number of pillows, rest)
      6) edema, syncope, dizziness, or headache
         a) when
         b) relieved by what
      7) fatigue or weakness
         a) when
         b) relieved by what
         c) compare with client's normal level of exercise
      8) changes in life-style
         a) ADL
         b) work

c) leisure
9) diet (have the client describe previous 24-hour intake)
a) restrictions (e.g., sodium, cholesterol)
b) difficulties complying with prescribed diet
c) alcohol intake
d) food preferences/intolerances
e) who shops/prepares meals
10) medications (prescription and nonprescription)
a) dose
b) side effects
c) effectiveness
11) personal or family history
a) pulmonary problems (e.g., tuberculosis, pneumonia, asthma)
b) cardiac problems (e.g., angina, myocardial infarction, hypertension)

b. Physical examination
1) vital signs
a) blood pressure: lying/sitting/standing, and in both arms
b) pulse: rate and rhythm
c) respirations: rate, depth, effort
d) temperature
2) inspection of chest
a) use of accessory muscles
b) presence of retraction
c) degree of excursion
d) chest deformity
3) palpation of chest
a) areas of pain/tenderness
b) presence of carotid thrills, atypical pulsation
c) change in tactile fremitus
d) anatomical landmarks: aortic, pulmonic, tricuspid, and mitral area correspond to where value closing is the loudest (see Figure 3.3)
- aortic: 2nd intercostal space to the right of the sternum
- pulmonic: 2nd intercostal space to the left of the sternum
- tricuspid: 4th–5th intercostal space to the left of the sternum
- mitral: 5th intercostal space in the midclavicular line

e) point of maximal impulse (PMI); for most clients apical pulse is their PMI
4) percussion of chest
a) resonance = air
b) dullness = fluid and/or consolidation
5) auscultation of the lungs
a) normal vesicular breath sounds

Figure 3.3 Areas of Auscultation of Heart Valves

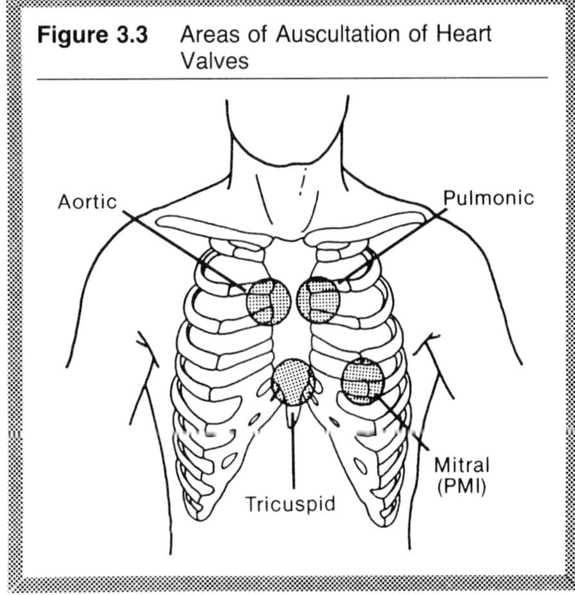

b) adventitious breath sounds
- rales
  - high-pitched crackling
  - caused by air passing through abnormal secretions in alveoli
- rhonchi
  - loud, coarse gurgling
  - caused by air passing through abnormal secretions in bronchi
- wheezing
  - high-pitched whistling
  - caused by air passing through narrowed bronchi

6) auscultation of the heart
a) apical pulse (see Figure 3.3)
- rate and rhythm
- pulse deficit = apical minus radial pulse (*NOTE*: The two pulses must be taken at the same time by *two* practitioners)

b) normal heart sounds
- S_1 (lub)
  - closing of mitral and tricuspid valves
  - at onset of ventricular systole
- S_2 (dub)
  - closing of aortic and pulmonary valves
  - at onset of ventricular diastole

c) extra heart sounds
- S_3, S_4
  - abnormal in adults
  - sometimes normal in children and young adults

- murmurs: caused by turbulent blood flow

7) skin and extremities
   a) skin color (e.g., pallor, cyanosis, rubor)
   b) skin temperature
   c) edema
   d) peripheral pulses: presence, strength, equality

c. Diagnostic tests
   1) pulmonary function tests: the direct or indirect measurement of various lung volumes; done to assess lung function; see Figure 3.4
      a) *tidal volume* (TV): volume of gas inspired and expired with a quiet normal breath (500 cc)
      b) *inspiratory reserve volume* (IRV): maximal volume that can be inspired at the end of a normal inspiration (3,100 cc)
      c) *expiratory reserve volume* (ERV): maximal volume that can be forcefully exhaled after a normal expiration (1,200 cc)
      d) *residual volume* (RV): volume of gas left in lung after maximal expiration (1,200 cc)
      e) *minute volume* (MV): volume of gas inspired and expired in 1 minute of normal breathing (6 liters/minute)
      f) *vital capacity* (VC): maximal amount of air that can be expired after a maximal inspiration (TV + IRV + ERV) (4,800 cc)
   2) sputum specimens
      a) examinations
         - culture and sensitivity
         - cytology
      b) nursing care
         - collect specimen in morning
         - collect sterile specimen
         - collect sputum, not saliva
   3) chest x-rays/tomograms
   4) lung scan: following injection of radioactive material, lung is scanned for presence of obstruction or areas that are poorly perfused
   5) bronchoscopy
      a) insertion of a rigid or flexible

Figure 3.4 Pulmonary Volumes and Capacities of an Adult (Values Vary with Age, Sex, Weight, and Height)

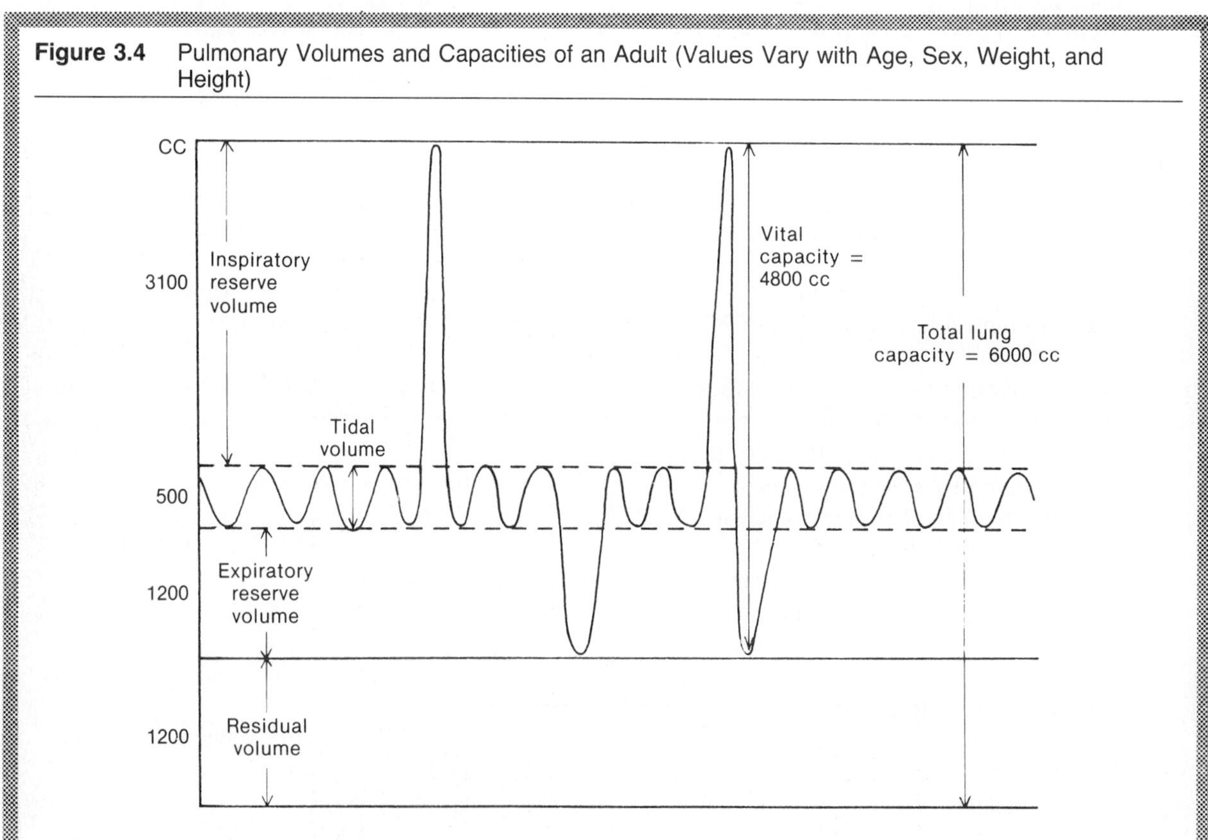

SOURCE: Adapted by P. Downing from Burrell, Z. and Burrell, L. *Critical Care*. St. Louis: Mosby, 1977. Used with permission.

fiberoptic bronchoscope through the oral cavity into the bronchus in order to visualize the area; bronchial brushing, biopsy, or bronchogram may be done during the procedure

b) nursing care: preparation
- explain procedure
- NPO 6–12 hours
- oral hygiene
- remove dentures
- premedicate

c) nursing care: postprocedure
- NPO until gag reflex returns
- observe respirations
- observe hoarseness, dysphagia
- observe for subcutaneous emphysema (crackling under the skin when pressed, caused by air from perforated airway)
- bloody sputum normal after biopsy

6) ECG

a) monitor (see Figure 3.5)

b) resting 12-lead

c) exercise (stress test)
- treadmill or bicycle
- ECG shows cardiac function during exercise

7) myocardial scan: following injection of radioactive thallium, heart is scanned to detect areas of poorly perfused myocardium

8) echocardiography: cardiac wall motion is visualized by ultrasound

9) cardiac catheterization/angiography

a) under local anesthesia and fluoroscopy, a catheter is inserted into the femoral or brachial artery (left heart catheterization) or an antecubital vein (right heart catheterization). The injection of radiopaque dye permits visualization of the heart vessels, chambers, and valves and measurement of pressures and oxygen concentrations

b) preparation
- explain procedure

Figure 3.5 Components of a Normal Electrocardiogram

The P wave represents atrial depolarization; the P-R segment, atrial depolarization and transmission of the cardiac impulse through the AV node. The QRS complex represents ventricular depolarization; the ST segment, the refractory period of the ventricular muscle. The T wave represents ventricular repolarization. The U wave may not be present.

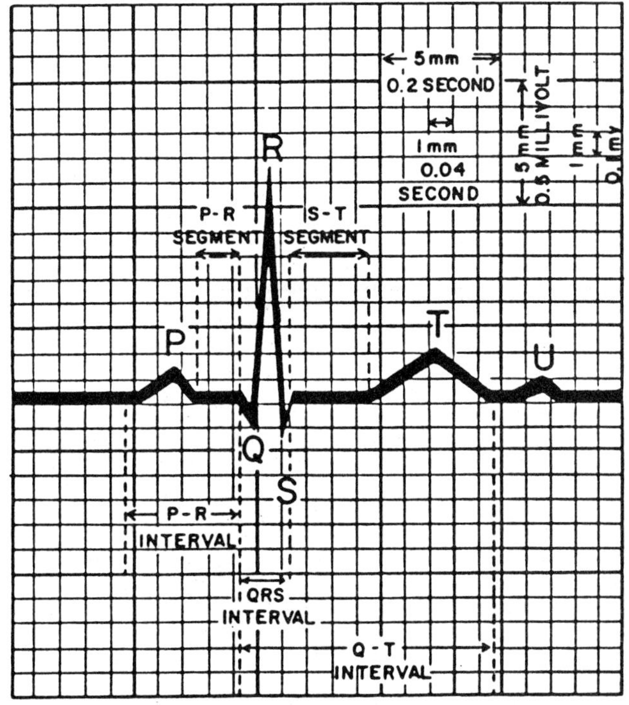

- NPO 6–12 hours
- take and record pulses/temperature of all extremities
- check for allergy to iodine

c) nursing care: postprocedure
- monitor vital signs
- monitor pulse/temperature in area distal to arterial puncture site (spasms/emboli can cause these to diminish or disappear); emboli formation requires immediate intervention)
- prevent stress on incision line (e.g., no bending of affected limb, no ambulation for 12–24 hours if femoral site)
- use pressure dressing at puncture site

10) hematologic studies (normal values will vary slightly from laboratory to laboratory)

a) arterial blood gases (ABG)
- test of arterial blood to assess oxygenation, ventilation, and acid-base status
- normal values
  - pH: 7.35–7.45
  - pO_2: 75–100 mm Hg
  - pCO_2: 35–45 mm Hg
  - % Hgb saturation: 96%–100%

b) CBC
- WBC: 5,000–10,000/mm^3
- RBC: 4.2–6.2 million/mm^3
- Hgb
  - men: 14–18 gm/dl
  - women: 12–16 gm/dl
- Hct
  - men: 42%–54%
  - women: 38%–46%

c) electrolytes
- sodium: 135–145 mEq/liter
- potassium: 3.5–5.0 mEq/liter
- chlorides: 100–106 mEq/liter

d) lipids
- cholesterol: 120–200 mg/dl
- triglycerides: 40–150 mg/dl

2. Analysis

a. Safe, effective care environment
1) potential for injury
2) knowledge deficit
3) potential for infection

b. Physiological integrity
1) decreased cardiac output
2) impaired gas exchange
3) activity intolerance

c. Psychological integrity
1) ineffective individual coping
2) anxiety
3) body image disturbance

d. Health promotion/maintenance
1) impaired adjustment
2) health-seeking behaviors
3) noncompliance

3. General Nursing Plans, Implementation, and Evaluation

Goal 1: Client will maintain patent airway and adequate oxygenation.

Plan/Implementation
- Monitor respiratory status (e.g., vital signs, breath sounds, skin color).
- Reduce anxiety.
- Limit/space activities to decrease O_2 need.
- Turn frequently if on bedrest.
- Place in Fowler's position to increase air exchange.
- Humidify air.
- Administer O_2 as needed.
- Cough and deep breathe frequently.
- Avoid sedatives that depress respirations and cough reflex (e.g., narcotics).
- Force fluids to liquefy bronchial secretions.
- Suction as needed; provide hyperventilation before and after suctioning to decrease chances of hypoxia.
- Carry out postural drainage if needed
  - give humidified air or bronchodilators 10–15 minutes before
  - no longer than 15 minutes at one time
  - clapping/vibration can be done with postural drainage
  - avoid clapping/vibrating over sternum, breast tissue, below ribs
  - follow with coughing to be effective

Evaluation: Client is well oxygenated (pO_2 greater than 60 mm Hg).

Goal 2: Client's cardiac work load will be decreased.

Plan/Implementation
- Monitor cardiovascular status (e.g., vital signs, pulse deficit, skin color).
- Limit activity to decrease O_2 need.
- Promote rest.
- Administer O_2 as needed.
- Monitor I&O of fluids to prevent circulatory overload.
- Give diuretics as ordered to reduce circulating blood volume (see Table 3.16).
- Prevent constipation (e.g., use stool softeners).

■ Reduce anxiety.
Evaluation: Client's cardiac workload is decreased; pulse decreases from 100 to 84.

Goal 3: Client will remain free from the hazards of immobility.

Plan/Implementation
■ Turn frequently.
■ Deep breathe and cough as needed.
■ Provide passive ROM exercises as needed.
■ Teach client ankle flexion exercises.
■ Give good back care.
■ Apply antiembolic hose.
■ Give anticoagulants if ordered (see Table 3.11).
Evaluation: Client remains free from thrombophlebitis, decubitus ulcers, pulmonary consolidation.

Selected Health Problems Resulting in Interference with Cardiac Functioning

☐ Cardiopulmonary Arrest

1. General Information
a. Definition: complete failure of the heart to perfuse adequately and the lungs to ventilate adequately
b. Classification: medical emergency

2. Nursing Process
a. Assessment/Analysis
1) *A*-airway
2) *B*-breathing
■ determine breathlessness
■ look for chest to rise and fall
■ feel for flow of air
3) *C*-circulation
■ determine pulselessness
■ check carotid pulse

b. Plans, Implementation, and Evaluation

Goal 1: Client will have an open airway and receive adequate ventilation.

Plan/Implementation
■ Place client in supine position on a flat, firm surface.
■ Assume rescuer position: kneel at level of client's shoulders.
■ Clear airway of foreign matter if present.
■ Open airway by head-tilt/chin-lift maneuver.
■ Watch for breathing.
■ Ventilate mouth to mouth if no breathing.
■ Give two full breaths of 1–1½ seconds each.
■ Use Heimlich's maneuver (subdiaphragmatic abdominal thrust) to clear airway, if unable to ventilate.
■ Watch for breathing.
■ Continue mouth-to-mouth ventilation, if no breathing but pulse is present, at a rate of 12/minute (once every 5 seconds)
■ If available
– use airway and Ambu bag
– administer 100% O_2
Evaluation: Client is well ventilated (e.g., chest rises and falls with rescue breathing).

Goal 2: Client will circulate adequately oxygenated blood.

Plan/Implementation
■ Check carotid pulse
■ Begin external chest compression after initial two breaths if carotid pulse absent
– assume rescuer position: arms straight, elbows locked, shoulders directly over hands
– locate proper hand position: hands one over other, long axis of heel over long axis of *lower half* of sternum, fingers *off* chest
■ Depress lower half sternum 1½–2 inches at a rate of 80–100/minute.
■ One rescuer: give 15 compressions/2 ventilations.
■ Two rescuers: give 5 compressions/1 ventilation with a pause for ventilation (1–1½ seconds).
■ Continue CPR until spontaneous respirations and pulse return.
■ If available
– monitor ECG
– defibrillate
Evaluation: Client has carotid pulsation with each compression; maintains BP of 100 systolic.

Goal 3: Client will receive appropriate emergency drugs.

Plan/Implementation
■ Obtain cart with emergency drugs.
■ Start IV for drug administration.
■ Administer emergency drugs as needed (see Table 3.8).
■ Record accurately all drugs given.
Evaluation: Client receives appropriate doses of ordered drugs; client's heart resumes normal sinus rhythm.

☐ Shock

1. General Information

a. Definition: a syndrome associated with abnormal cellular metabolism; the pathology common to all shock is inadequate tissue perfusion

b. Causes
- **1)** hemodynamic disturbances of the
  - **a)** heart
  - **b)** blood vessels
  - **c)** blood volume
- **2)** disturbances within cells

c. Etiologic classification
- **1)** hypovolemic (decreased volume)
- **2)** cardiogenic (inadequate pump)
- **3)** neurogenic (pooling due to vasodilation)
- **4)** septic (caused by bacterial endotoxins; characterized by fever, early vasodilation, increased capillary permeability, and shift of fluid to interstitial space)
- **5)** anaphylactic (massive capillary vasodilation due to release of histamine and related substances)

d. Precipitating factors
- **1)** allergic reactions
- **2)** infections, particularly gram negative
- **3)** spinal anesthesia
- **4)** spinal cord trauma
- **5)** myocardial infarction
- **6)** pulmonary emboli
- **7)** dysrhythmias
- **8)** hemorrhage
- **9)** burns
- **10)** GI loss of fluid and electrolytes

e. Body's response to shock
- **1)** stimulation of the adrenal medulla by the sympathetic nervous system
  - **a)** tachycardia
  - **b)** tachypnea
  - **c)** vasoconstriction
  - **d)** redistribution of blood
  - **e)** cool, clammy skin; oliguria; decreased bowel sounds
- **2)** stimulation of renin-angiotensin-aldosterone system and ADH
  - **a)** thirst
  - **b)** decrease urine volume
  - **c)** increased concentration of urine
- **3)** stimulation of cortisol and growth hormone secretion
  - **a)** increased glucose metabolism
  - **b)** increased fat mobilization

2. Nursing Process

a. Assessment/Analysis
- **1)** identify high-risk client (e.g., clients with severe dysrhythmias, adrenocortical problems, severe GI fluid loss, hemorrhage, burns, allergic reactions, massive infections)
- **2)** vital signs: tachycardia, tachypnea; early BP may be normal due to compensatory mechanisms but will decrease later
- **3)** mental status: restless, early increased alertness, but as hypoxia occurs → decreased alertness → lethargy, coma

Table 3.8 Emergency Drugs*

Name	Indications
Atropine sulfate	Bradycardia
Bretylium tosylate (Bretylol)	Ventricular dysrhythmias unresponsive to lidocaine
Calcium chloride	Not recommended for cardiac arrest except when hyperkalemia, hypocalcemia, or calcium channel block toxicity is present
Dobutamine HCl (Dobutrex)	To increase cardiac contractility
Dopamine HCl (Intropin)	To increase BP and cardiac contractility; in small doses improves renal perfusion
Epinephrine	Asystole and ventricular fibrillation; to increase heart rate, cardiac output, and BP (beta- and alpha-receptor stimulant)
Lidocaine HCl (Xylocaine)	PVCs and ventricular tachycardia
Procainamide HCl (Pronestyl)	PVCs and ventricular fibrillation when lidocaine is not effective
Sodium bicarbonate	*Not recommended* routinely for metabolic acidosis during cardiac arrest; may be given in response to arterial blood gases
Verapamil (Calan)	Paroxysmal supraventricular tachydysrhythmias

*Drugs that should be readily available for all cardiac emergencies; recommended by American Heart Association.

4) skin changes
   a) pale, cool, clammy skin (hypovolemic and cardiogenic shock)
   b) flushed, cool if vasodilation present (neurogenic shock)
   c) flushed, warm early, then → cool, clammy (septic shock)
5) fluid status: check skin turgor, I&O, urine specific gravity, CVP

b. Plans, Implementation, and Evaluation

Goal 1: Client will remain free from any undetected change in cellular perfusion.

Plan/Implementation (high-risk client)
- Assess vital signs q4h; more frequently if unstable.
- Measure I&O at least q8h; qh if unstable.
- Note skin turgor, temperature, color q8h.
- Monitor ECG if dysrhythmias present.
- Obtain blood work as appropriate (CBC, electrolytes, BUN, creatinine, blood gases).

Evaluation: Client maintains stable vital signs, fluid balance; has no signs of impending shock.

Goal 2: Client will have adequate perfusion.

Plan/Implementation
- Monitor blood pressure (mean should be at least 80), pulse, respiration.
- Note and report dysrhythmias.
- Monitor CVP (normal = 4–10 cm H_2O); measure the same way each time.
- Maintain urine output of at least 30 ml/hour and equal to intake.
- Monitor mental status.
- Monitor GI function.
- Administer fluids as ordered: blood, colloid fluids, or electrolyte solutions as necessary (until CVP = 6–10 cm H_2O).
- Administer drugs only after circulating volume has returned to normal (Table 3.8).
  - adrenergic stimulants (epinephrine, dopamine, dobutamine, norepinephrine [Levophed], isoproterenol [Isuprel]) cause increase in contractility and heart rate to increase perfusion; some may also cause vasoconstriction
    * administer with a controlled-volume regulator
    * monitor BP q15min continually
    * wean off drugs as soon as possible
    * know that some of these drugs cause severe vasoconstriction and can worsen organ damage (renal failure, hepatic failure)
    * watch for extravasation of vasopressors (if norepinephrine or dopamine extravasates, infiltrate around area with regitine)
    * titrate drug infusion to keep BP at a mean of 80, or as ordered
  - vasodilators (nitroprusside, hydralazine) may be used to decrease cardiac workload
  - when using adrenergic stimulants and vasodilators together
    * if BP drops, decrease vasodilator first; then increase adrenergic stimulant
    * if BP increases, decrease adrenergic stimulant and then increase vasodilator
  - administer other drugs as ordered (e.g., cardiac glycosides to enhance cardiac contractility); see Table 3.15
- Position in modified Trendelenburg's (feet up 45° and head flat)

Evaluation: Client's BP is maintained at a mean of 80 mm Hg.

Goal 3: Client will have adequate O_2/CO_2 levels.

Plan/Implementation
- See General Nursing Plans page 168.
- Provide comfort measures (*NOTE*: If giving pain medications, do not use IM or subcutaneous route since medications may accumulate and not be absorbed; when perfusion improves, client may get overdose).
- Keep client warm, not hot or cold (heat causes sweating; cold causes shivering).

Evaluation: Client is well oxygenated (pO_2 greater than 60 mm Hg; no air hunger or cyanosis).

Goal 4: Client will be protected from injury, complications.

Plan/Implementation
- Keep side rails up; if client confused, watch carefully, avoid restraints.
- Apply antiembolic stockings to prevent venous stasis.
- Turn frequently to prevent decubitus ulcers, pulmonary problems.
- Use sterile technique with all procedures (e.g., changing IVs, suctioning) since client has decreased resistance to infection.

Evaluation: Client is free from preventable complications (e.g., falls, infections).

☐ Angina Pectoris

1. General Information

a. Definitions

1) atherosclerosis: fatty plaque deposited on the intima of the artery
2) arteriosclerosis: calcium deposits in the media of the artery
3) angina pectoris: chest pain caused by temporary ischemia of the myocardium; usually caused by atherosclerosis, arteriosclerosis, thrombus, or coronary artery spasm

b. Risk factors (coronary artery disease)
1) risk factors that cannot be controlled
   a) age
   b) sex
   c) family history
2) risk factors that can be controlled with medical supervision
   a) hypertension
   b) hyperlipidemia
   c) diabetes
3) risk factors that can be controlled by the person at risk
   a) smoking
   b) high stress
   c) sedentary life-style
   d) obesity

c. Precipitating factors (immediate): five "E"s
1) *e*xercise
2) *e*xertion: arteries are able to provide blood to myocardium at rest, but an increased demand on coronary circulation cannot be met temporarily
3) *e*motions: stimulation of sympathetic nervous system → increased demand on heart
4) *e*ating a heavy meal: increased perfusion of the gastrointestinal tract for digestion; pressure from full stomach against diaphragm
5) *e*xposure to cold

2. Nursing Process

a. Assessment/Analysis

1) precipitating factor(s)
2) pain
   a) pattern varies with each individual, but is usually the same for a specific person
   b) usually retrosternal
   c) tends to radiate into neck, jaw, shoulder, and down inner aspect of left arm (see Figure 3.6)
   d) short duration

Figure 3.6 Distribution of Typical Angina Pain

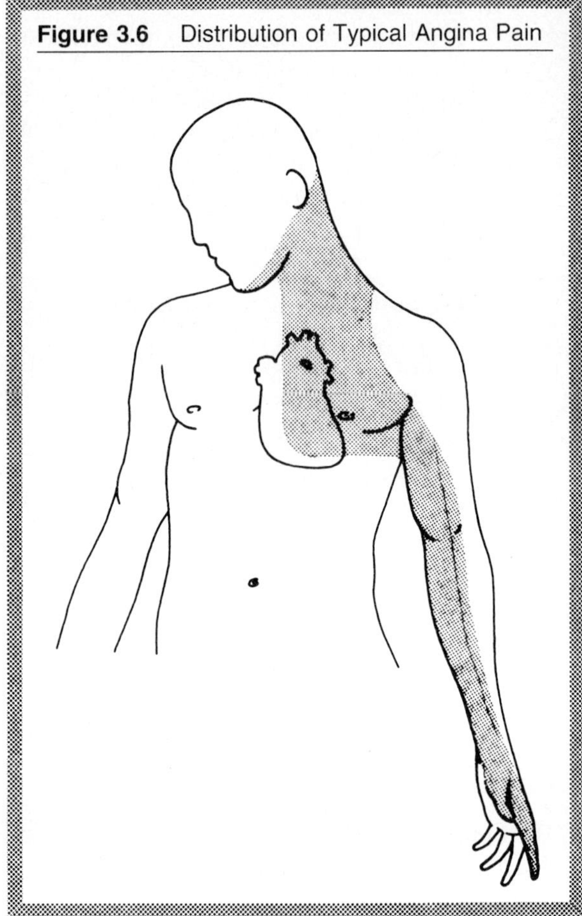

   e) usually relieved by rest and nitroglycerin
3) ECG changes (if any) are not permanent

b. Plans, Implementation, and Evaluation

Goal 1: Client will have improved perfusion of the myocardium.

Plan/Implementation
- Give vasodilating and beta-blocking drugs (see Table 3.9).
- Know action and side effects of these drugs.

Evaluation: Client performs daily activities without pain by spacing activities or by taking a nitroglycerin tablet prior to bathing, eating, or taking daily walks.

Goal 2: Client will learn methods to prevent attacks.

Plan/Implementation
- Teach client
  - to recognize symptoms
  - to take medications and cope with side effects
  - when to take medications (e.g., before

Table 3.9 Angina Pectoris Drugs

Name	Action	Side Effects	Nursing Implications
Nitrates			
Nitroglycerin (Nitro-Bid)	Generalized vasodilatation. Oxygen consumption and demand on myocardium are decreased.	Pounding headache, flushing, tachycardia, dizziness, orthostatic hypotension	Taken sublingually usually. Take at pain onset; repeat in 5 min × 2; if no pain relief, go to nearest ER. Also taken prophylactically before pain onset.
Nitroglycerin ointment (Nitrol) Nitroglycerin disc (Transderm-Nitro)	Absorbed through skin; long-acting vasodilatation	Relatively safe (same as nitroglycerin sublingual)	Applied to intact, hairless skin. Rotate sites.
Erythrityl tetranitrate (Cardilate) Isosorbide dinitrate (Isordil, Sorbitrate) Pentaerythritol tetranitrate (Peritrate, Pentafin, and Pentritol)	Long-acting vasodilatation	Less acute vasodilatation effect due to slower absorption. Can cause gastric irritation, nausea, vomiting.	
Calcium Channel Blockers			
Nifedipine (Procardia) Verapamil (Calan) Diltiazem (Cardizem)	Coronary artery spasm is inhibited. Oxygen consumption of myocardium is decreased.	Fatigue, headache, transient hypotension, nausea	
Beta Adrenergic Blockers			
Propranolol (Inderal)	Heart rate, cardiac contractility, cardiac output, and BP are reduced. Oxygen consumption of myocardium is decreased.	Fatigue, bradycardia, postural, hypotension, nausea, vomiting, diarrhea, bronchospasm.	Heart rate must be 50 or more before the drug is administered.

activity)
- to avoid precipitating factors if possible
- to decrease risk factors (e.g., quit smoking, control hypertension)
- to reduce dietary cholesterol and saturated fat to prevent further atherosclerosis (see Table 3.11)

■ Define activity level: space and eliminate activities that might precipitate angina (e.g., mowing grass, shoveling snow).

Evaluation: Client is able to explain medications, dosage, time schedule, side effects; has a tentative schedule for rest and activities.

Goal 3: Client will be able to state what to do if symptoms change.

Plan/Implementation

■ Teach client to identify own pain pattern and to recognize change in pain.

■ Instruct client to notify physician of change.

Evaluation: Client explains ways of dealing with a change in anginal pain.

☐ Myocardial Infarction

1. General Information

a. Definition: occlusion of one or more coronary arteries causing death of a portion of the myocardial tissue (infarct); see Figures 3.7 and 3.8

b. Incidence

1) leading cause of death in the United States

2) more common in men; rate in women rises after menopause

c. Risk factors (see risk factors for coronary artery disease page 172)

2. Nursing Process

a. Assessment/Analysis

1) chest pain

a) intense, crushing, substernal

b) not relieved by rest or nitroglycerin

2) ECG changes: elevation or depression of ST segment; T wave inversion; Q wave changes

Figure 3.7 Coronary Blood Supply

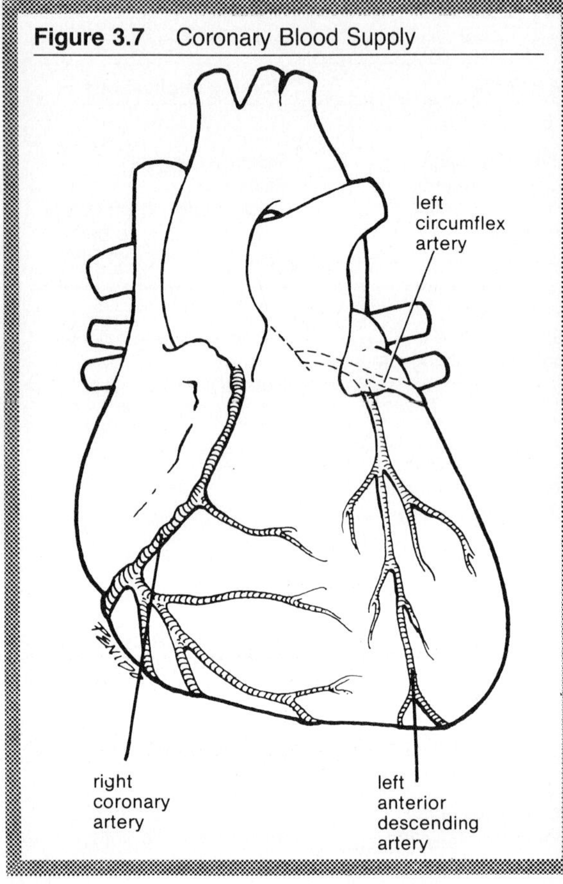

Figure 3.8 Myocardial Infarction

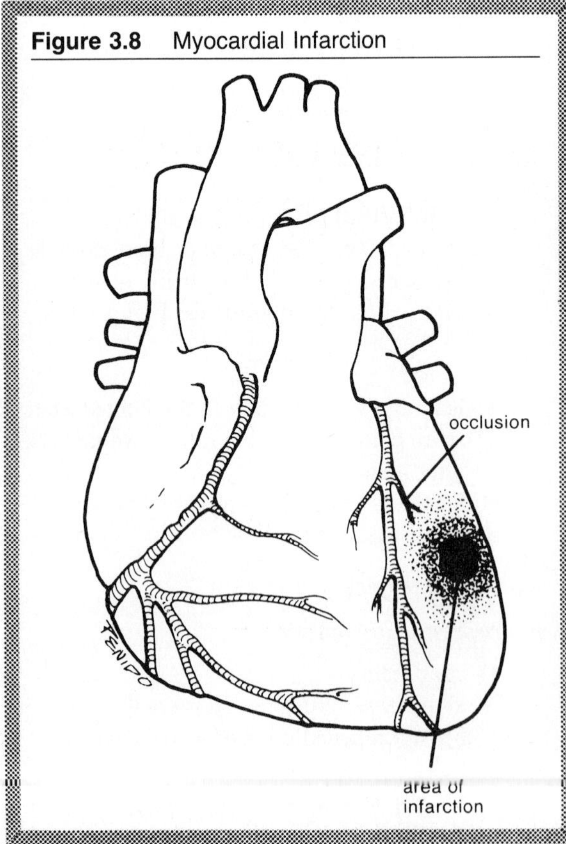

3) blood tests (see Table 3.10 and Figure 3.9)

b. Plans, Implementation and Evaluation

Goal 1: Client's chest pain will be controlled.

Plan/Implementation
- Give analgesics (e.g., IV morphine sulfate) until pain is relieved.
- Administer O_2 (4–6 liters/minute).
- Give sedatives prn to promote rest.

Evaluation: Client states pain was relieved.

Goal 2: Client's coronary blood flow will be increased or reestablished.

Plan/Implementation
- Administer thrombolytics as ordered (see Table 3.11).
- Provide post-procedure care after percutaneous transluminal coronary angioplasty
  - monitor arterial puncture site
  - keep head of bed elevated less than 30 degrees for 12 hours
  - monitor pulses distal to puncture site
- Monitor cardiac rhythm for reperfusion dysrhythmias.

Evaluation: Following angioplasty, client reports decreased chest pain; is free from dysrhythmias.

Goal 3: Client's cardiac workload will be decreased.

Plan/Implementation
- See General Nursing Goal 2
- Teach client to avoid Valsalva's maneuver (increases intrathoracic pressure and causes sudden temporary increase in work load).

Evaluation: Client's heart rate is decreased from 88 to 72.

Goal 4: Client will remain free from new blood vessel occlusions.

Plan/Implementation
- Administer anticoagulants as ordered (see Table 3.11).
- Know action, side effects, and antidotes of anticoagulants.
- Apply antiembolic hose.
- Teach client ankle flexion/extension exercises.

Evaluation: Client's condition remains stable; has no signs of further occlusions.

Goal 5: Client will remain free from complications.

Table 3.10 Blood Tests for Myocardial Infarction

Test	Abbreviation	Normal Values	Myocardial Infarction
Creatine phosphokinase	CPK	men: 17–148 units/L women: 10–79 units/L	elevated
Serum glutamic-oxaloacetic transaminase	SGOT	7–27 units/L	elevated
Lactic dehydrogenase	LDH	45–90 units/L	elevated
Erthrocyte sedimentation rate	ESR	men: 0–10 mm/hour women: 0–20 mm/hour	elevated
Leukocyte count	WBC	5,000–10,000 m^3/liter	elevated

Note: Normal values will vary somewhat depending on the laboratory doing the tests.

Plan/Implementation

- Monitor ECG for dysrhythmias.
- Monitor lab reports (enzymes and electrolytes); see Table 3.10 and Figure 3.9.
- Monitor for symptoms of cardiogenic shock (see page 170).
- Monitor for symptoms of congestive heart failure (see page 178).
- Monitor for symptoms of thrombophlebitis (see Fig. 3.11).

Evaluation: Client gradually improves without complications.

Goal 6: Client and significant others will be able to explain care during acute and recovery phase, and care that will follow discharge.

Plan/Implementation

- Teach
  - level of activity
  - diet
    - * calories reduced if client is obese
    - * sodium restricted (see Table 3.12)
    - * cholesterol and saturated fat restricted (see Table 3.13)
    - * high potassium if necessary (see Table 3.17)
  - medications
    - * administration
    - * schedule
    - * side effects
  - sexual activity: may resume sexual intercourse in 6–8 weeks following an *uncomplicated* MI

Figure 3.9 Typical Enzyme Patterns after an Acute Myocardial Infarction

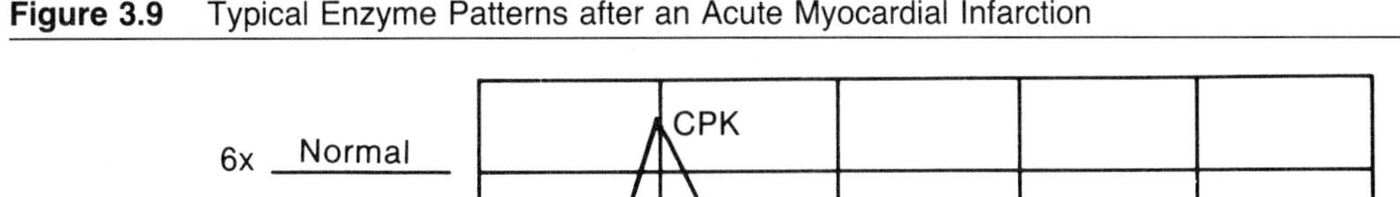

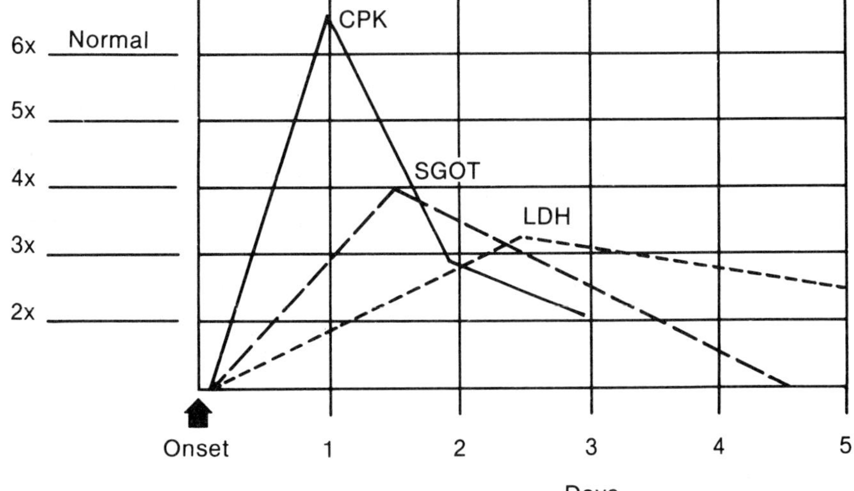

SOURCE: Burrell, Z. and Burrell, L. *Critical Care*. 4th Ed. St. Louis: Mosby, 1982. Used with permission.

Table 3.11 Anticoagulant and Thrombolytic Drugs

Name	Action	Side Effects	Nursing Implications
Heparin sodium	Prolongs clotting. Prevents formation of thrombin from prothrombin. Onset almost immediate. Lasts 4 hours. No effects on existing thrombi.	Hemorrhage epistaxis, hematuria, melena, ecchymosis, bleeding gums, transient alopecia	Parenteral: IV or subcutaneous. Monitor partial thromboplastin time (PTT). PTT maintained at 1½–2 times normal (normal = 30–40 seconds). Discontinue heparin if there is evidence of bleeding or if the PTT is overly prolonged. ANTIDOTE: Protamine sulfate. Use bleeding precautions (e.g., soft toothbrush, electric razor).
Bishydroxycoumarin (Dicumarol)	Prolongs clotting. Inhibits synthesis of prothrombin and other vitamin K dependent clotting factors. Slow onset (2–3 days). Lasts up to 9 days after last dose. No effect on existing thrombi.	Hemorrhage epistaxis, hematuria, melena, ecchymosis, bleeding gums. GI disturbances: diarrhea, vomiting, anorexia. INTERACTION: Salicylates *increase* anticoagulant effect.	Oral. Monitor prothrombin time (PT). PT maintained at 1½–2 times normal (normal = 12–15 seconds). Discontinue Dicumarol or Coumadin if the PT is overly prolonged or if bleeding occurs. No aspirin. ANTIDOTE: Vitamin K (AquaMEPHYTON). Use bleeding precautions as above.
Warfarin sodium (Coumadin)	Same as Dicumarol. Onset occurs within 18–24 hours. Cumulative effect lasts up to 7 days.	Same as Dicumarol.	Same as Dicumarol.
Streptokinase (Streptase)	Activates plasminogen and converts it to plasmin, which degrades fibrin clots. Immediate onset; residual effects last up to 12 hours after infusion.	Hemorrhage, oozing at site of puncture, incision, or cut; fever, allergic reaction, reperfusion dysrhythmias.	Parenteral: IV. Monitor, PT, PTT, and thrombin time. Monitor for hemorrhage. Maintain bleeding precautions. Start heparin before streptokinase is discontinued. Solu-Cortef frequently given before infusion to prevent allergic reaction. Administer all drugs through preexisting IV lines, by mouth, or by NG tube while streptokinase is infusing. Monitor cardiac rhythm for reperfusion dysrhythmias. No true antidote.
Tissue Plasminogen Activator (t-PA) (Activase)	Converts plasminogen to plasmin at fibrin surface; is more clot specific than streptokinase. Immediate onset; action lasts approximately 10 minutes.	Hemorrhage, oozing at site of puncture, incision, or cut; reperfusion dysrhythmias	Parenteral: IV bolus followed by 3–4 hour infusion. Monitor PT, PTT, and thrombin time. Monitor for hemorrhage. Maintain bleeding precautions. Start heparin before t-PA is discontinued. Administer all drugs through preexisting IV lines, by mouth, or by NG tube while streptokinase is infusing. Monitor cardiac rhythm for reperfusion dysrhythmias.

Table 3.12 Approximate Sodium Content in Selected Food Items*

Food Items	Portion	Sodium Content (mg)
Breads and Cereals		
White bread	1 slice	200
Regular Corn Flakes	1 oz	260
Dairy Products		
Milk	8 oz	130
American cheese	1 slice	238
Cottage cheese, low fat	4 oz	435
Fish and Shellfish		
Flounder, broiled filet	2 oz	355
Scallops	3½ oz	265
Fruits and Vegetables		
Tomato juice	6 oz	275
Peas, canned	5¼ oz	349
Meats and Poultry		
Chicken, roasted	2 pieces	57
Bacon	1 slice	101
Bologna	1 slice	226
Beef	3 oz	381
Miscellaneous Food Items		
Olives	1	130
Catsup	1 tbsp	154
Peanut butter	1 tbsp	167
Potato chips	14 chips	191
Italian salad dressing	1 tbsp	315
Chocolate pudding, instant	½ cup	404
Dill pickle	1 large	1,137
Beef broth	1 cube	1,152
Salt	1 tsp	2,400

*Exact amount of sodium varies with brands of food items.

Teaching Guidelines for Sodium-restricted Diets.

a. Discuss salt and other sodium-containing compounds.
b. Explain relationship of sodium to high blood pressure, rationale for eliminating sodium from diet.
c. Stress avoidance of foods and medications that contain multiple sodium compounds; read labels carefully.
d. Eat 3 well-balanced meals a day with foods naturally low in sodium.
e. Add no salt while preparing food and add no salt at table.
f. If sodium intake is limited to only 2 gm, food can be salted lightly during preparation, but no additional salt added at table.
g. Season food with non-sodium flavorings.
h. Seek advice from physician concerning salt substitutes.

- Identify symptoms to report to physician immediately
  - chest pain
  - dyspnea

Table 3.13 Cholesterol and Saturated Fat Content in Selected Items*

Food Items	Serving	Cholesterol (mg)	Saturated Fat (gm)
Dairy Products			
Milk, skim	8 oz	0	0
Yogurt, low fat	8 oz	11	1.8
American cheese	1 oz	27	5.6
Butter	1 tbs	31	7.1
Milk, whole	8 oz	33	5.1
Ice Cream	8 oz	59	8.9
Fish and Shellfish			
Clams	3 oz	50	0.4
Fish, lean	3 oz	59	0.3
Shrimp	3 oz	126	0.5
Meats and Poultry			
Beef liver	3 oz	372	2.5
Egg	1 whole	213	1.7
Beef, lean	3 oz	56	2.4
Chicken breast	3 oz	63	1.3
Fruits and Vegetables			
All fruits All vegetables	No cholesterol and generally no saturated fats (see vegetable oils below for two exceptions)		
Vegetable Oils			
Coconut oil	1 tbs	0	11.8
Palm oil	1 tbs	0	6.7
Olive oil	1 tbs	0	1.8
Corn oil	1 tbs	0	1.7
Safflower oil	1 tbs	0	1.2

*Exact amount of cholesterol and saturated fat varies with brands of food items.

  - fluid retention

Evaluation: Client explains own activity; plans menu for a sodium-restricted diet; knows what symptoms to report to physician immediately.

□ Pacemaker

1. General Information

a. Definition: An electronic device that delivers an electrical stimulus to the heart through electrodes sewn directly on the epicardium or placed in contact with the endocardium; may be temporary or permanent.

1) fixed rate: continuously fires at preset rate

2) demand rate: fires only if heart rate drops below given rate

2. Nursing Process

a. Assessment

1) rate, rhythm, and quality of all pulses

2) ECG: alterations in P wave, PR interval, QRS, and T waves

3) laboratory tests: electrolytes, serum digoxin levels

b. Plan, Implementation, and Evaluation

Goal: Client will undergo pacemaker implantation free from preventable complications.

Plan/Implementation

- Postprocedure
  - monitor for changes in pulse rate and rhythm
  - keep insertion site clean; inspect for signs of infection
  - monitor for temperature elevation
  - support extremity on which pacemaker attached (external pacemaker)
- Teach client with permanent pacemaker
  - level of activity
  - take own pulse daily
  - symptoms of pacemaker failure: vertigo, syncope, palpitations, hiccoughs, bradycardia
  - avoid improperly grounded electrical appliances (e.g., some power tools)
  - avoid sources of high frequency signals (e.g., radio towers)
  - schedule for battery replacement
  - carry identification card
  - importance of follow-up care

Evaluation: Client maintains a regular, normal heart rate postimplantation.

☐ Congestive Heart Failure (CHF)

1. General Information

a. Definition: state in which cardiac output is indaequate to meet the metabolic needs of the body; characterized by circulatory congestion.

b. Etiology: one or more of the following
  1) inflow of blood to heart greatly increased (e.g., excessive IV fluids, sodium and water retention)
  2) outflow of blood from heart obstructed (e.g., damaged valves, narrowed arteries)
  3) functional capacity of myocardium decreased; (e.g., myocardial infarction, dysrhythmias)
  4) metabolic needs of body accelerated (e.g., fever, pregnancy)

c. cardiac compensation
  1) mechanisms
    a) *tachycardia*: increases cardiac output
    b) *ventricular dilation*: increases volume of chambers
    c) *myocardial hypertrophy*: fibers of myocardium increase in length and diameter; heart contracts more forcibly
  2) terminology
    a) *compensated CHF*: compensatory changes maintain adequate cardiac output
    b) *decompensated CHF*: compensatory changes unable to maintain adequate cardiac output; CHF becomes symptomatic

d. Left-sided congestive heart failure: left ventricle cannot eject all blood from left atrium; therefore left atrium cannot accept all blood from pulmonary bed
  1) etiology
    a) hypertension
    b) mitral and/or aortic valvular disease
    c) ischemic heart disease: damage or infarction of the myocardium of the left ventricle
  2) pathophysiology: blood backs up in *pulmonary bed* (see Table 3.14 for results and symptoms)

e. Right-sided congestive heart failure: right ventricle cannot eject all blood from right atrium, therefore right atrium cannot accept all blood from systemic circulation
  1) etiology
    a) pulmonary disease
    b) tricuspid and pulmonic valvular disease
    c) ischemic heart disease: damage or infarction of the myocardium of the right ventricle
  2) pathophysiology: blood backs up in systemic circulation (see Table 3.14 for results and symptoms)

2. Nursing Process

a. Assessment/Analysis
  1) left-sided CHF
    a) dyspnea
    b) abnormal breath sounds (i.e., rales)
    c) abnormal heart sounds (i.e., S_3)
    d) arterial blood gas studies showing decreased pO_2 (i.e., less than 80 mm Hg)
  2) right-sided CHF
    a) elevated central venous pressure
    b) distended neck veins
    c) hepatomegaly (enlargement of the liver)
    d) abnormal liver function (hepatic congestion)
    e) peripheral edema

Table 3.14 Congestive Heart Failure

Results	Symptoms
Left-sided Pathophysiology: Blood backs up from left ventricle to *pulmonary* bed.	
Pulmonary congestion	Dyspnea, orthopnea, rales, paroxysmal nocturnal dyspnea
Pulmonary edema	(PND), decreased vital capacity, cyanosis
Cerebral anoxia	Irritability, restlessness, confusion
Decreased O_2 to cells	Extreme weakness, fatigue, oliguria
Right-sided Pathophysiology: Blood back up from right ventricle to *systemic* circulation.	
Increased hydrostatic pressure in systemic circulation	Peripheral edema, dependent edema: sacrum, ankles
Elevated venous pressure	Distended neck veins
Congestion in kidneys, retention of sodium	Oliguria
Venous congestion in extremities	Cool and cyanotic legs
Congestion in GI tract	Anorexia, nausea, bloating

3) both right- and left-sided congestive heart failure (CHF)
   a) cardiomegaly; PMI displacement
   b) oliguria
   c) weight gain
   d) tachycardia

b. Plans, Implementation, and Evaluation

Goal 1: Client will experience increased force and strength of contraction of the ventricles.

Plan/Implementation
- Administer cardiac glycosides as ordered (see Table 3.15).
- Monitor vital signs closely.

Evaluation: Client's heart rate is stable at 80 beats/minute.

Goal 2: Client will eliminate excess fluid.

Plan/Implementation
- Give diuretics as ordered (see Tables 3.16 and 3.37).
- Keep accurate I&O.
- Weigh daily.
- Restrict sodium intake.

Evaluation: Client's weight decreases to pre-CHF level.

Goal 3: See General Nursing Goal 2 (cardiac workload) page 168.

Goal 4: See General Nursing Goal 3 (immobility) page 168.

Goal 5: Client will remain free from pulmonary edema.

Plan/Implementation
- Monitor closely for symptoms
  - severe dyspnea
  - audible rales
  - frothy, blood-tinged sputum
  - extreme anxiety
- institute therapy *immediately* if pulmonary edema develops
  - place in Fowler's position
  - give O_2 by positive pressure if available (increases O_2 and helps to push fluid from alveolar space)

Table 3.15 Cardiac Glycoside Drugs

Name	Action	Side Effects	Nursing Implications
Digitalis leaf Digitoxin (Crystodigin, Purodigin) Digoxin (Lanoxin) Lanatoside C injection (Cedilanid)	Increases strength of myocardial contraction. Cardiac output is increased. Decreases heart rate. Promotes diuresis.	GI upset, visual disturbances, dysrythmias, heart block Hypokalemia potentiates digitalis action.	Take pulse before administration: if above 120 or below 60, hold medication and notify MD. Monitor serum K. High-potassium diet as needed.

Table 3.16 Antihypertensive Drugs

Name	Action	Side Effects	Nursing Implications
Diuretic Agents			
Thiazide diuretics			
Benzthiazide (Exna) Chlorothiazide (Diuril) Hydrochlorothiazide (Oretic, Hydrodiuril, Esidrix)	Increases sodium and chloride excretion by inhibiting renal reabsorption. Enhances potassium excretion. Relaxes peripheral arteriolar smooth muscles.	*Hypokalemia*: weakness, paresthesias, muscle cramps, nausea, paralytic ileus, cardiac disturbances *Hyponatremia*: thirst, diminished sweating, fever, weakness, confusion *Hyperuricemia*: usually asymptomatic; can cause gouty arthritis *Hyperglycemia*: usually asymptomatic; can cause nausea, vomiting, polydipsia, polyphagia, weight loss, dehydration; sensitivity reactions, GI disturbances	Monitor I&O, BP, weight, serum electrolytes. Modify dietary sodium and potassium as needed.
Potent, rapid-acting diuretics			
Ethacrynic acid (Edecrin) Furosemide (Lasix)	Increases sodium and chloride excretion by inhibiting renal reabsorption. Enhances potassium excretion.		
Potassium-conserving diuretics			
Spironolactone (Aldactone)	Increases sodium and chloride excretion, and decreases potassium excretion by blocking aldesterone (adrenal cortex mineralcorticoid).	*Hyperkalemia*: weakness, paresthesias, cardiac disturbances *Hyponatremia*: GI disturbances, sensitivity reactions	
Sympathetic Inhibiting Agents			
Reserpine (Serpasil, Reserpoid, Sandril, Rau-sed)	Acts by various complex mechanisms to inhibit synthesis, storage, and/or transport of norepinephrine, thereby depressing sympathetic nerve activity—as a result, cardiac output and/or peripheral vascular resistance are decreased. Reserpine and methyldopa also have central depressant effects.	Depression, nightmares, suicidal ideas, drowsiness, bradycardia, GI disturbances, dry mouth, increased appetite, excessive gastric secretion, nasal congestion	Monitor BP, P, weight. Teach importance of compliance. Advise hard candy for dry mouth. Instruct to rise and change position slowly.
Methyldopa (Aldomet)		Depression (less than reserpine), drowsiness (tends to subside with continued use), decreased mental acuity, GI disturbances, sodium and water retention, and loss of libido, sexual impotence and postural hypotension: less than guanethidine	
Guanethidine (Ismelin)		Postural hypotension, generalized muscle weakness especially on arising, diarrhea and other GI disturbances, sodium and fluid retention, failure to ejaculate, sensitivity to sympathomimetics found in some cold remedies (can result in hypertensive crisis)	
Propranolol (Inderal)	See Table 3.9		
Vasodilating Agent			
Hydralazine (Apresoline)	Acts directly on vascular	Headache, flushing,	Monitor: BP, P, weight.

(continued)

Table 3.16 Continued

Nitroprusside (Nipride) injection	smooth muscle to decrease peripheral resistance—relaxant effect more marked on arterioles than veins. Increases cardiac output, renal blood flow, and plasma renin activity.	tachycardia, palpitation, angina, GI disturbances, lupus-like syndrome (especially long-term administration with high doses), sodium and fluid retention	Teach importance of compliance. Instruct to rise and change position slowly.

Note: From "Hypertension—what patients need to know" by M. Long, E. Winslow, M. Scheuhing, & J. Callahan, 1976, *American Journal of Nursing*, *76*, pp. 765–780.

- apply rotating tourniquets (see Figure 3.10) to reduce circulating blood volume by obstructing *venous* flow in 3 extremities
  - * rotate one tourniquet every 15 minutes in *one* direction
  - * remove one at a time when edema is controlled
- give morphine sulfate IV (relieves anxiety and dilates pulmonary vascular bed)
- administer cardiac glycosides (see Table 3.15) as ordered
- give diuretic as ordered (e.g., furosemide); see Tables 3.16 and 3.37
- give aminophylline IV (see Table 3.18)

Evaluation: Client's respirations are 16/minute; lung fields are clear on auscultation.

Goal 6: Client and significant others will be able to explain need for care after discharge.

Plan/Implementation

■ Teach
- level of activity, balance between activity and rest
- sodium-restricted diet (see Table 3.12), high potassium as necessary (see Table 3.17)

Figure 3.10 Pattern for Rotating Tourniquets

Rotate *one* tourniquet every 15 min. in the *same* direction.

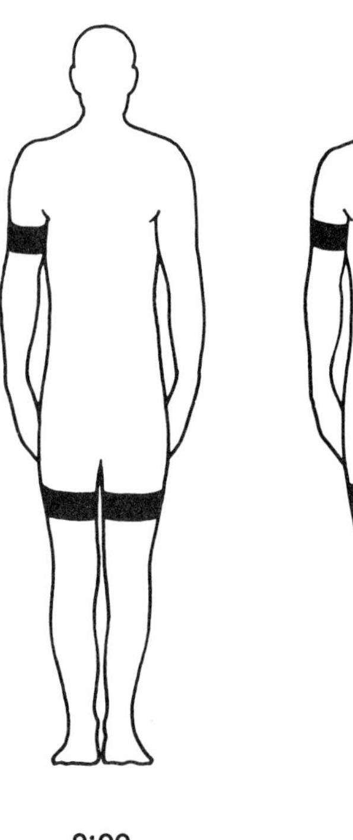
9:00

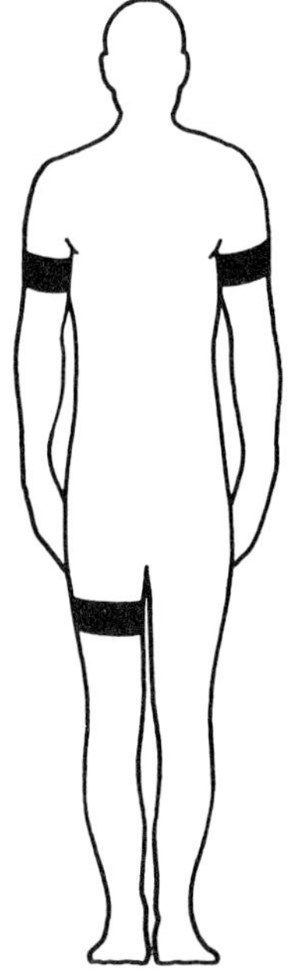
9:15

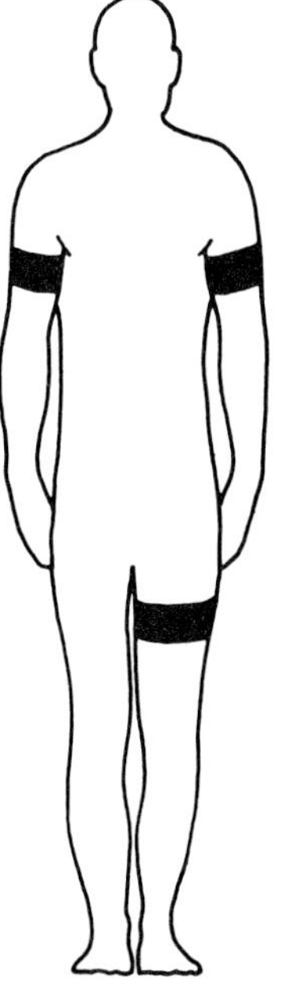
9:30

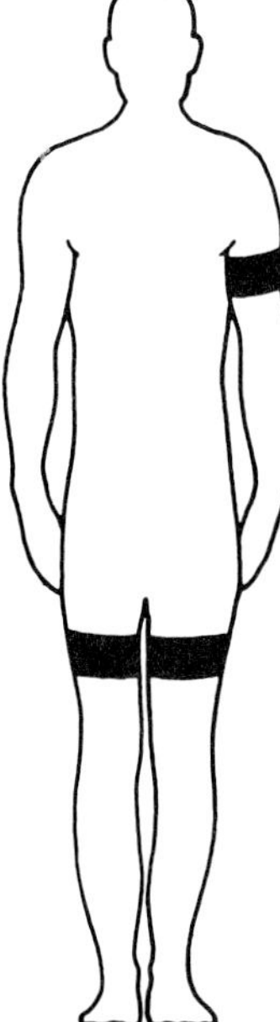
9:45

Table 3.17 Foods High in Potassium

Food	Portion	Potassium (mEq)
Whole milk	1 cup	9.0
Broiled meat	3 oz	9.6
Apricots (canned)	4 halves	7.9
Banana	1 small	9.5
Honeydew melon	⅛ medium	9.6
Fresh orange	1 medium	9.5
Dried prunes	4 large	12.0
Watermelon	² slice (1″ thick)	15.3
Baked potato	1 medium	12.9
Dried lima beans	½ cup cooked	14.5
Soybeans	½ cup cooked	13.8
Winter squash	½ cup cooked	10.0
Dried white beans	½ cup cooked	10.6

- medication administration, schedule, side effects
- application of antiembolic hose

■ Instruct client to weigh daily to monitor fluid balance.

Evaluation: Client correctly describes care needs for home (e.g., drug therapy, how to take own pulse).

□ Hypertension

1. General Information

a. Definition: a chronic elevation of systemic arterial BP in which the systolic pressure is *consistently* over 140 mm Hg and the diastolic is 90 mm Hg or higher

b. Incidence
   1) affects all age groups
   2) prevalence increases with age
   3) one of the major causes of illness and death in the United States

c. Blood pressure physiology
   1) determinants
      a) cardiac output
      b) total peripheral resistance
   2) regulation
      a) neural stimulation: autonomic nervous system
      b) humoral stimulation (e.g., catecholamines, aldosterone, angiotensin)

d. Pathophysiology
   1) no obvious early pathologic changes in blood vessels and organs
   2) large vessels (aorta, coronary arteries, basilar artery to brain, peripheral vessels in limbs) eventually become sclerosed and tortuous
   3) lumens narrow resulting in decreased blood flow to heart, brain, and lower extremities
   4) vessels become completely occluded, or rupture → hemorrhage
   5) damage to the intima of small vessels causes local edema and intravascular clotting
   6) decreased blood supply to tissues of heart, brain, kidneys causes dysfunction of these organs

e. Types
   1) primary (essential): approximately 90% of all cases; etiology unknown; types include
      a) *benign*: slowly progressive
      b) *malignant*: rapidly accelerating
   2) secondary: approximately 10%–15% of all cases; caused by an identifiable primary disease (e.g., pheochromocytoma, kidney disease)

f. Predisposing factors
   1) stress
   2) familial history
   3) obesity

2. Nursing Process

a. Assessment/Analysis
   1) BP elevated on at least three different occasions
   2) headache, change in vision (hemorrhages in retina, blurred vision)
   3) epistaxis
   4) personality change: forgetful and irritable

b. Plans, Implementation, and Evaluation

Goal 1: Client's BP will decrease to safe level and permanent damage will be prevented.

Plan/Implementation

■ monitor BP
■ modify life-style to reduce stress
■ modify diet
- calories reduced if client is obese
- sodium restricted (see Table 3.12)
- high potassium if needed (see Table 3.17)

■ exercise in a regular, planned program
■ avoid smoking
■ administer antihypertensive medications as ordered (see Table 3.16)

Evaluation: Client's blood pressure is reduced to 140/90.

Goal 2: Client will carry out self-care activities after discharge.

Plan/Implementation

- Teach client to
  - take own BP
  - modify life-style
  - institute exercise program
  - manage diet (sodium-restricted and low calorie, high potassium as necessary) (see Tables 3.12 and 3.17)
  - medications (see Table 3.16)
    - administration
    - schedule
    - side effects
    - importance of compliance
  - stop smoking
  - importance of follow-up care

Evaluation: Client lists all components of therapeutic regimen; keeps an appointment for return visit.

☐ Circulatory Problems

1. General Information

a. Definition: changes in blood vessels peripheral to the heart; types: arterial and venous

b. Types of arterial problems

1) *arteriosclerosis obliterans*: atherosclerotic plaque formation that involves arteries of lower extremities; occurs in men aged 50–70 and women after menopause
2) *Raynaud's disease*: intermittent constricting spasms of arteries of digits and extremities, resulting in pain and cyanosis
3) *Buerger's disease* (thromboangiitis obliterans): disease characterized by diffuse, inflammatory, proliferative changes in arteries and veins of extremities

c. Types of venous problems

1) *varicose veins*: dilated, tortuous superficial veins; incompetent valves cause dilation; increased pressure causes tortuosity; increased capillary pressure causes edema
2) *varicose ulcers*: ulcers resulting from circulatory insufficiency
3) *thrombophlebitis*: inflammation of vessel with thrombus formation
4) *phlebothrombosis*: thrombus formation in a vein without inflammation

2. Nursing Process: arterial problems

a. Assessment/Analysis: symptoms of impaired peripheral arterial circulation (see Figure 3.11)

b. Plans, Implementation, and Evaluation

Goal 1: Client will have adequate arterial blood flow to extremities.

Plan/Implementation

- Teach cleint to eliminate/avoid
  - tobacco
  - exposure to temperature extremes
  - trauma
    - tissue injury and infections
    - maintain good foot care
  - excessive exercise
  - vasospastic drugs (e.g., epinephrine)
  - constrictive clothing
- Modify diet
  - low cholesterol
  - moderate fat
  - reduced calories if client is obese
- Give thrombolytics or anticoagulants if ordered (see Table 3.11).

Evaluation: Client's extremities are warm; peripheral pulses are strong.

Goal 2: Client will have minimal discomfort.

Plan/Implementation

- Have client rest when pain occurs.
- Administer vasodilator adrenergic medications as ordered (e.g., isoxaprine HCl [Vasodilan]).

Evaluation: Client develops schedule of activities that keeps pain under control.

Goal 3: Client will be able to explain when surgery might be used; will be free from preventable complications.

Plan/Implementation

- Know that bypass surgery may be used if client has localized occlusion with arteriosclerosis obliterans; that infrequently sympathectomy may be used to treat Buerger's disease; that amputation is the treatment for gangrene.
- Provide post-op care: avoid strain on incision (do not bend joint over which graft passes), monitor for hemorrhage resulting from disruption of graft or occlusion of graft, administer anticoagulants as ordered (see Table 3.11).

Evaluation: Client explains the type of surgery that he may receive; is free from complications postoperatively (e.g., split incision, frank hemorrhage).

3. Nursing Process: venous problems

a. Assessment/Analysis: symptoms of impaired venous circulation (see Figure 3.11)

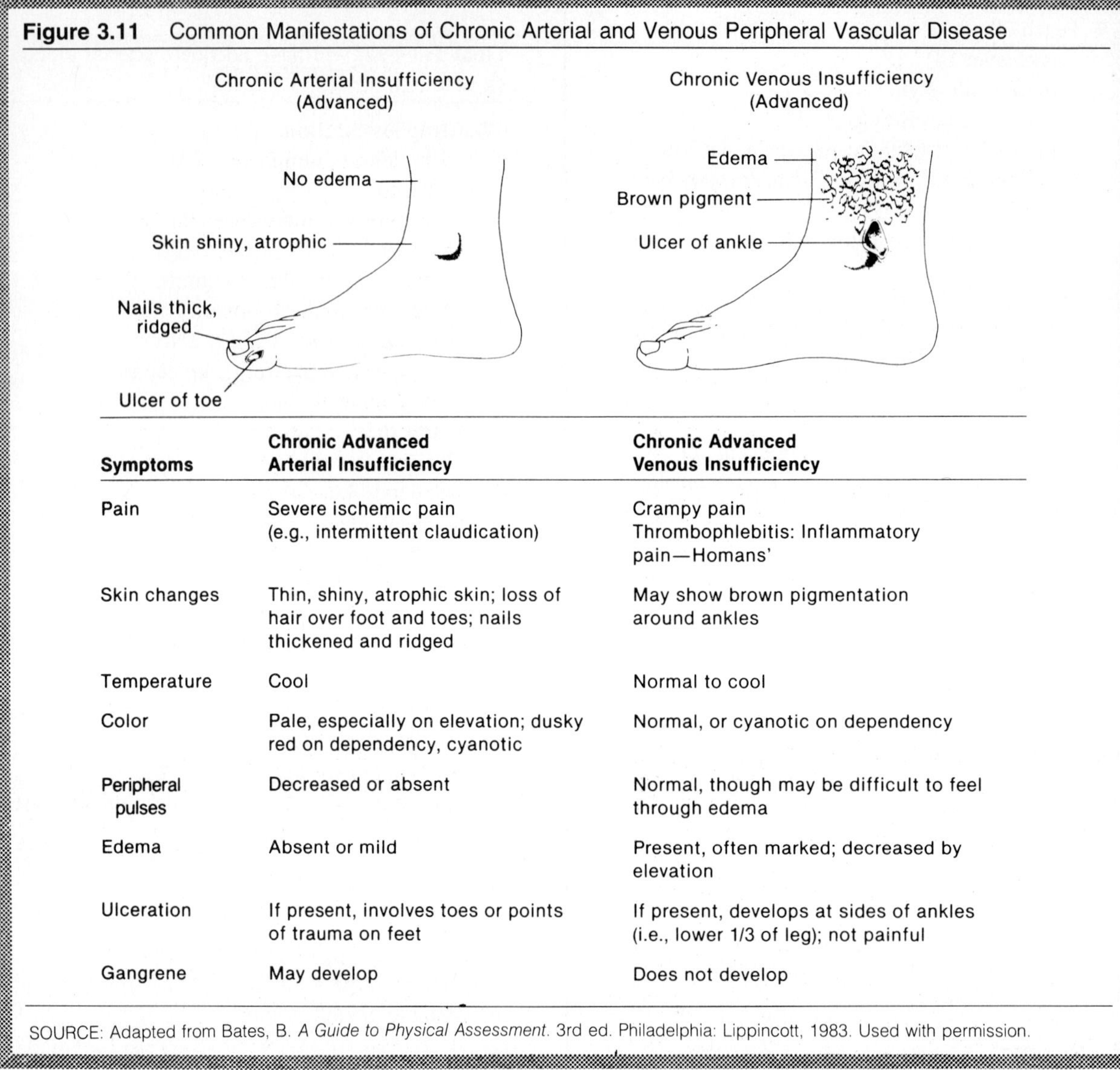

Figure 3.11 Common Manifestations of Chronic Arterial and Venous Peripheral Vascular Disease

Symptoms	Chronic Advanced Arterial Insufficiency	Chronic Advanced Venous Insufficiency
Pain	Severe ischemic pain (e.g., intermittent claudication)	Crampy pain Thrombophlebitis: Inflammatory pain—Homans'
Skin changes	Thin, shiny, atrophic skin; loss of hair over foot and toes; nails thickened and ridged	May show brown pigmentation around ankles
Temperature	Cool	Normal to cool
Color	Pale, especially on elevation; dusky red on dependency, cyanotic	Normal, or cyanotic on dependency
Peripheral pulses	Decreased or absent	Normal, though may be difficult to feel through edema
Edema	Absent or mild	Present, often marked; decreased by elevation
Ulceration	If present, involves toes or points of trauma on feet	If present, develops at sides of ankles (i.e., lower 1/3 of leg); not painful
Gangrene	May develop	Does not develop

SOURCE: Adapted from Bates, B. *A Guide to Physical Assessment*. 3rd ed. Philadelphia: Lippincott, 1983. Used with permission.

b. Plans, Implementation, and Evaluation

Goal 1: Client will have adequate venous blood flow from extremities.

Plan/Implementation

- Teach client to eliminate/avoid
  - tobacco
  - injury and infections
  - constrictive clothing (e.g., garters)
  - standing or sitting for long periods
  - crossing legs at knee
- Teach client to
  - wear antiembolic hose
  - elevate legs
  - do ankle push-ups when standing (promotes venous return)

Evaluation: Client's feet are warm; client is free from ankle edema.

Goal 2: Client with thrombophlebitis will be protected from dislodgment of thrombus.

Plan/Implementation

- Maintain bedrest 7–10 days.
- Prevent Valsalva maneuver.
- Elevate legs.
- Apply antiembolic hose.
- Apply warm, moist packs to involved site (prevent burns).
- Do not rub legs.
- Give anticoagulant therapy as ordered (see Table 3.11).

Evaluation: Client is free from any signs of an embolism.

Goal 3: Client's ulcers will heal.

Plan/Implementation

- Maintain bedrest with leg elevated when ulcer is acute.
- Monitor for signs of cellulitis and report immediately.
- Give antibiotics as ordered if infected.
- Know and inform client that skin grafting may be necessary.
- Explain the long-term nature of treatment to client.

Evaluation: Client's ulcer remains clean, uninfected; heals well.

Goal 4: Client with varicose veins will be able to describe surgical procedure and post-op care.

Plan/Implementation

- Elevate legs.
- Apply antiembolic hose.
- Teach client regarding planned surgical procedure.
- Monitor for bleeding, thrombosis postoperatively.

Evaluation: Client describes surgical procedure; applies antiembolic hose correctly.

Selected Health Problems Resulting in Interference with Respiration

☐ Chronic Obstructive Pulmonary Disease (COPD) or Chronic Obstructive Lung Disease (COLD)

1. General Information

- **a.** Definition: chronic respiratory disorders that involve a persistent obstruction of bronchial air flow
- **b.** Incidence
  - **1)** fastest growing cause of death in the US
  - **2)** occurs in adults and children
- **c.** Predisposing factors
  - **1)** smoking
  - **2)** environmental factors: smoke, coal, hay, asbestos, air pollution
  - **3)** allergic factors
  - **4)** chronic, recurrent respiratory infections
  - **5)** genetic factors (possibly)
- **d.** Pathophysiology
  - **1)** thoracic excursion is reduced due to bronchial obstruction, air trapping, and thoracic overdistension; possible inflammatory reaction in airways causes bronchial spasm and increased secretions
  - **2)** tidal volume, vital capacity, and inspiratory reserve necessary for effective coughing are decreased
  - **3)** person employs accessory muscles of respiration to facilitate breathing; purses lips to maintain open bronchioles with expiration
  - **4)** bronchial obstruction and air trapping lead to destruction of lung, permanently reduced alveolar ventilation, and CO_2 retention
  - **5)** decreased resistance increases susceptibility to respiratory infections (e.g., pneumonia)
  - **6)** respiratory acidosis (compensated) commonly occurs secondary to chronic CO_2 retention
- **e.** Hypoxemia
  - **1)** definition: deficient oxygenation of the blood
  - **2)** frequently chronic, possibly acute
  - **3)** characterized by
    - **a)** subtle changes in mentation such as restlessness, agitation, headache, drowsiness, and confusion (due to less O_2 to the brain and stimulation of the sympathetic nervous system)
    - **b)** tachycardia, hyperventilation will be seen early in hypoxia; possibly followed by bradycardia and hypoventilation
    - **c)** hypertension due to tachycardia may be present early with hypoxia
    - **d)** decreased pO_2 (less than 80 mm Hg)
- **f.** Hypercapnia
  - **1)** definition: excess of CO_2 in blood
  - **2)** can occur with hypoxemia; may be chronic or acute
  - **3)** characterized by
    - **a)** CNS depression: drowsiness, inability to concentrate, progressive loss of consciousness
    - **b)** early behavioral changes: irritability, inability to get along with others, discontentment with food, care, etc., inability to sleep
    - **c)** headache
    - **d)** tremors, dizziness, cardiac dysrhythmias
    - **e)** increased pCO_2 (greater than 45 mm Hg)
- **g.** Common examples of COPD

1) *bronchial asthma*: a chronic disease characterized by episodic attacks of respiratory distress due to constriction of the bronchi and bronchioles (refer to *Nursing Care of the Child* page 569)
2) *chronic bronchitis*
   a) definition: chronic inflammation of the bronchi with production of large amount of sputum that causes bronchial obstruction
   b) etiology and pathophysiology: air pollution or smoking cause inflammation of bronchial mucosa with resulting edema and copious production of mucus; also person is predisposed to recurrent respiratory infections by reduced ciliary motility in the bronchi
3) *emphysema*
   a) definition: chronic lung condition characterized by abnormal enlargement of alveoli and alveolar ducts with destruction of alveolar walls
   b) incidence: highest in men over age 50
   c) etiology: exact cause not identified
   d) pathophysiology: air trapped behind partially obstructed bronchioles produces overdistention and destruction of alveoli; loss of elastic recoil of lungs reduces respiratory flow; barrel chest develops

2. Nursing Process

a. Assessment/Analysis

1) respiratory distress (dyspnea on exertion progressing to dyspnea at rest)
2) apprehension
3) cough (productive)
4) lethargy (results from hypoxemia)
5) use of accessary muscles
6) abnormal breath sounds (rales, rhonchi, wheezing, decreased breath sounds)
7) weight loss
8) skin color
   a) flushed (hypercapnia)
   b) cyanosis (hypoxemia)
9) abnormal pulmonary function tests (e.g., decreased expiratory and inspiratory volumes, increased residual volume)
10) blood gases
    a) pO_2 decreased only with activity at first, then decreased continuously
    b) pCO_2 increases as disease worsens
11) respiratory acidosis, compensated (from chronic CO_2 retention)
12) frequent respiratory infections (decreased resistance)

b. Plans, Implementation, and Evaluation

Goal 1: Client will maintain a pO_2 of at least 60 mm Hg; airway will be clear, sputum will be thin and clear.

Plan/Implementation

- See General Nursing Goal 1 page 168.
- Administer bronchodilators as ordered (see Table 3.18).
- Administer expectorants (see Table 3.19) as ordered.
- Administer nebulizer as ordered
  - bronchodilators (see Table 3.18)
  - mucolytics (see Table 3.19)
- Teach relaxation techniques and breathing exercises (e.g., pursed-lip breathing).
- Administer low concentrations of humidified O_2 (1–2 liters/minute); *CAUTION*: high O_2 flow may precipitate respiratory failure in presence of hypercapnia and hypoxia.
- Encourage activity to tolerance.
- If client must be confined to bed for any period of time (usually infection or asthma attack)
  - semi-Fowler's or Fowler's position
  - turn frequently
  - encourage to take frequent deep breaths and to breathe out slowly and completely
  - active ROM exercises (passive if client too weak to do active exercises)
  - employ diversional activities to avoid napping during the day so as to prevent insomnia and nocturnal restlessness
  - *NOTE: avoid bedrest if at all possible to prevent hypoventilation, stasis of secretions, weakened ventilatory muscles, weakness of other muscles, and decreased cough reflex*
- Give diet as tolerated (e.g., small amounts of soft food 4–5 times/day).

Evaluation: Client's pO_2 remains greater than 60 mm Hg; pH remains between 7.35–7.45; sputum is clear and thin.

Goal 2: Client will be protected from any injuries.

Plan/Implementation

- Know that if client has hypoxia, hypercapnia, or uncompensated respiratory acidosis, may be lethargic, confused, or in coma.
- Use side rails, pad if necessary.
- Keep bed low to floor.
- Avoid restraints, sedatives, or tranquilizers.

Table 3.18 Bronchodilator Drugs*

Name	Action	Side Effects	Nursing Implications
Adrenergic Agents			
Epinephrine (Adrenalin) Ephedrine	Stimulates alpha- and beta-adrenergic receptors of sympathetic nervous system. alpha: peripheral vasoconstriction, increased BP beta: bronchodilation, increased cardiac irritability, increased heart rate	Nervousness, tremors, headache, palpitation, tachycardia, dysrhythmias	Monitor BP, pulse. Use cautiously with hypertension and coronary insufficiency.
Isoproterenol (Isuprel)	Stimulates beta adrenergic receptors of sympathetic nervous system: relaxes bronchioles, stimulates heart.	Similar to epinephrine	
Xanthine Compounds			
Aminophylline Theophylline	Relaxes smooth muscle of bronchial airway and blood vessels. Also has diuretic effect. Acts synergistically with adrenergic bronchodilators.	Dizziness, hypotension, restlessness, dysrhythmias, GI irritation (oral), cardiac stimulation	Monitor BP; observe for hypotension. Give oral preparations with food.

*See also Table 5.18

- If client is confused, have someone stay with client.
- Maintain quiet environment.
- Speak in low, calm, soothing tone.

Evaluation: Client is free from injury.

Goal 3: Client will be protected from CO_2 narcosis.

Plan/Implementation

- Know that uncontrolled O_2 delivery will eliminate hypoxic drive of respirations.
- Administer O_2 at *low* concentrations (1–2 liters/minute).
- Observe for symptoms of narcosis with O_2 therapy
  - decreased respiratory rate and depth
  - headache
  - skin changes (flushing)
  - behavioral changes: confusion → coma
  - blood gases
    * increased pCO_2
    * *increased* pO_2

Table 3.19 Cough Medications*

Name	Action	Side Effects	Nursing Implications
Expectorants			
Ammonium chloride Guaifenesin (Robitussin) Potassium iodide (SSKI)	Increases bronchial mucus secretion. Facilitates the expulsion of viscid, tenacious sputum.	Nausea, vomiting Drowsiness Gastric irritation	Force fluids: 6–8 glasses/day. Water alone may be the most effective expectorant.
Mucolytic			
Acetylcysteine (Mucomyst, Airbron)	Inhalant; liquefies respiratory mucus.	Bronchospasm (especially asthmatics); nausea, vomiting, rhinitis, stomatitis	Use cautiously with asthma.

*See also Table 5.18

- respiratory failure
- ■ Assist ventilation when needed.

Evaluation: Client maintains spontaneous respirations.

Goal 4: Client will live as actively as possible within the limitations of the disease.

Plan/Implementation

- ■ Teach client
  - level of activity: balance of activity and rest
  - breathing/relaxation exercises
  - effective coughing
  - postural drainage
  - diet
    - * small, frequent high-carbohydrate meals
    - * adequate fluids
  - medications
    - * administration
    - * schedule
    - * side effects
  - use of O_2 equipment
  - preventive health habits
    - * stop smoking
    - * avoid respiratory infections
    - * seek treatment for respiratory infections *early*
    - * avoid factors that precipitate bronchospasms (e.g., pollens, air pollutants)

Evaluation: Client develops a schedule that allows activities of daily living, work obligations, and social activities.

☐ Pneumonia

1. General Information

a. Definition: acute inflammation of the alveolar spaces of the lung

b. Etiology

1) microorganisms

- **a)** bacteria
- **b)** viruses
- **c)** fungi

2) chemicals

- **a)** inhalation (e.g., smoke)
- **b)** aspiration (e.g., vomitus)

c. Predisposing factors

1) decreased immunity (e.g., COPD)
2) debility (e.g., malnutrition)
3) immobility (e.g., postsurgery)

d. Pathophysiology

1) causative agent is inhaled
2) alveoli become inflamed and edematous
3) alveolar spaces fill with exudate
4) diffusion of O_2 and CO_2 is obstructed
5) involved lung tissue becomes consolidated

2. Nursing Process

a. Assessment/Analysis

1) chills, fever, malaise
2) chest pain (limits chest excursion)
3) respirations: rapid, shallow, dyspneic
4) tachycardia
5) productive cough
6) sputum

- **a)** viscid, tenacious
- **b)** rusty → yellow
- **c)** culture positive for causative microorganism

7) breath sounds (diminished over involved areas, rales, and pleural friction rub)
8) percussed dullness over involved area
9) leukocytosis
10) cyanosis with advanced hypoxia

b. Plans, Implementation, and Evaluation

Goal 1: Client's pulmonary ventilation will improve.

Plan/Implementation

- ■ See General Nursing Goal 1 page 168.
- ■ Administer organism-specific antibiotics (see Table 3.20).
- ■ Administer expectorants prn (see Table 3.19).
- ■ Discourage antitussives.
- ■ Care for tracheostomy if present (see tracheostomy care page 197).
- ■ Administer analgesics for chest pain.
- ■ Provide good oral hygiene.

Evaluation: Client has decreased dyspnea.

Goal 2: Client will remain free from atelectasis.

Plan/Implementation

- ■ Assess client status q2–4h for atelectasis (area of lung that is collapsed and airless).
- ■ Position client on unaffected side.
- ■ Check pulse rate.
- ■ See General Nursing Goal 1 page 168.

Evaluation: Client has clear lungs on auscultation; breathes easily.

Goal 3: Client will be able to care for self after discharge.

Plan/Implementation

- ■ Teach
  - activity level
  - avoid overfatigue
  - medications
    - * administration

Table 3.20 Antibiotics

Name	Action	Side Effects	Nursing Implications
			All antibiotics: • take culture if ordered *before* starting antibiotic • instruct client to take *entire* prescription
Penicillin			
Penicillin G crystalline (Crystapen) IV or IM procaine (Wycillin) IM only benzathine (Dicillin) IM only Penicillin V (PenVee K) oral	Bactericidal (interferes with cell wall synthesis) Effective against numerous gram-positive cocci, spirochetes, actinomycetes, and some gram-negative organisms.	Hypersensitivity (rash, urticaria, anaphylaxis); GI disturbance (oral); superinfection	Check allergy history before giving. Observe for hypersensitivity.
Penicillin-resistant penicillin oxacillin (Prostaphlin) methicillin (Staphcillin) nafcillin (Unipen)	Semisynthetic penicillin; effective against penicillin-resistant organisms such as *S. aureus*	Same as Penicillin G and V	Same as Penicillin G and V
Broad-spectrum penicillin ampicillin (Polycillin) amoxicillin (Amoxil)	Semisynthetic penicillin; effective against many gram-positive and gram-negative organisms.	Same as Penicillin G and V	Same as Penicillin G and V
Cephalosporins			
Cephalothin (Keflin) Cephalexin (Keflex)	Bactericidal (inhibits cell wall synthesis); effective against most gram-positive cocci, and many strains of gram-negative bacilli (similar to penicillin).	GI disturbance, hypersensitivity (rash), nephrotoxicity, cross sensitivity to penicillin (but anaphylaxis rare)	Monitor renal function. Check for history of allergy to penicillin.
Tetracyclines			
Tetracycline[1] (Achromycine) Minocycline (Minocin)	Bacteriostatic (inhibits protein synthesis); effective against wide variety of gram-positive and gram-negative organisms, rickettsiae, chlamydia, trophozite forms of amebae, and actino mycetes.	GI disturbance; hypersensitivity (rash, urticaria); photosensitivity; superinfection; permanent discoloration during tooth development	Do not give with milk, food, or antacids. Avoid sun exposure. Do not administer to pregnant women or children under 8 years.
Aminoglycosides			
Neomycin[1] Gentamincin (Geramycin) Kanamycin (Kantrex) Streptomycin[2]	Bactericidal (inhibits protein synthesis); effective against a wide range of gram-positive and gram-negative organisms and mycobacteria.	Ototoxicity Nephrotoxicity	Monitor hearing function. Monitor renal function.
Polypeptides			
Bacitracin[1]	Bactericidal (hinders cell wall synthesis); effective against most gram-positive organisms.	Nephrotoxicity	Used primarily as topical agent because of its nephrotoxicity.
Polymixins[1] Polymixin B (Aerosporin) Colistin (Coly-Mycin)	Bactericidal (hinders cell wall synthesis); effective against nearly all gram-negative organisms, except the proteus group.	Nephrotoxicity Neuromuscular blockade	Used topically. Use parenterally with caution. Parenteral: monitor renal function; use cautiously with respiratory insufficiency.

[1]See also Table 3.49.
[2]See also Table 3.21.

  * schedule
  * side effects
- breathing exercises

Evaluation: Client develops a plan for balanced rest and activity; knows actions and side effects of all prescribed medications.

☐ Tuberculosis

1. General Information

a. Definition: a reportable, communicable disease usually affecting the respiratory system

b. Incidence: 9.3 cases/100,000 US population; higher in nonwhites; an opportunistic disease in clients with AIDS

c. Etiology: *Mycobacterium tuberculosis*, an acid-fast bacillus

d. Predisposing factors

- **1)** lowered resistance caused by
  - **a)** overcrowding
  - **b)** poor sanitation
  - **c)** poor nutrition
  - **d)** poorly ventilated living conditions
  - **e)** debilitating diseases
  - **f)** immunosuppressive conditions
- **2)** virulence of organism
- **3)** length of exposure

e. Pathophysiology: tuberculosis bacillus is usually inhaled; transmitted by droplet produced by individual with active disease

- **1)** most common site of implantation is on alveolar surface of lung parenchyma
- **2)** induces hypersensitivity reaction in host
- **3)** inflammation occurs, then acute pneumonia develops
- **4)** caseous nodule (tubercle) is formed around organism
- **5)** organism never completely disappears but is walled off in lungs
- **6)** may remain quiescent for long time, but physical and emotional stress can cause organism to become active and multiply (reactivation process)
- **7)** inflammation can occur and tuberculous process begins again
- **8)** disease may also spread through lymphatics and vascular system (miliary tuberculosis)
- **9)** if medical therapy fails, surgical resection of one or more lobes may be advised

2. Nursing Process

a. Assessment/Analysis

- **1)** dyspnea
- **2)** pleuritic pain
- **3)** rales
- **4)** fatigue
- **5)** night sweats
- **6)** low-grade fever in afternoon
- **7)** weight loss
- **8)** anorexia
- **9)** hemoptysis (late symptom)
- **10)** abnormal chest x-ray
- **11)** sputum culture positive for *Mycobacterium tuberculosis* (*NOTE*: May take 3–12 weeks to obtain positive result)
- **12)** positive skin testing
  - **a)** OT (old tuberculin) (Mantoux)
  - **b)** PPD (purified protein derivative) is most reliable
    - ■ intradermal injection on inner aspect of forearm
    - ■ negative reaction: absence of erythema and/or induration after 48 hours
    - ■ positive reaction: 8–10 mm *induration* in 48 hours
      - indicates contact with tuberculosis bacillus but not necessarily an active infection
      - do chest x-ray and sputum cultures if positive
      - do not repeat skin testing in future (screen with a chest x- ray)
      - prophylactic chemotherapy may be indicated

b. Plans, Implementation, and Evaluation

Goal 1: Client's active tuberculosis will be arrested.

Plan/Implementation

- ■ Administer antituberculosis drugs as ordered (see Table 3.21)
  - first line drugs
  - second line drugs
- ■ Provide adequate rest (*not* bedrest).
- ■ Institute adequate diet.

Evaluation: Client's sputum culture converts to negative after 2 weeks of medications.

Goal 2: Staff, client's family, and others will be protected from infection with tuberculosis.

Plan/Implementation

- ■ Maintain appropriate isolation
  - necessary while client has positive sputum smear and culture and/or is coughing
  - discontinue after symptoms disappear (often within 2 weeks after start of treatment)

Table 3.21 Antituberculosis Drugs

Name	Action	Side Effects	Nursing Implications
			All antituberculosis drugs: stress the importance of compliance.
First-line Drugs: Drugs used for primary therapy; often used in combination to potentiate effect (e.g., INH, rifampin, and ethambutol).			
Isoniazid (INH)	Bactericidal (interferes with synthesis of cell wall)	Peripheral neuritis, pyridoxine deficiency (vitamin B_6); hepatotoxicity, glossitis, GI disturbance, hypersensitivity: fever	Give pyridoxine. Monitor liver function.
Rifampin (Rifadin)	Bactericidal (inhibits RNA synthesis)	Hepatotoxicity, GI disturbance, hypersensitivity: rash. May color urine, tears orange.	Instruct to expect orange body fluids.
Ethambutol (Myambutol)	Bacteristatic (inhibits protein synthesis)	Optic neuritis: decreased acuity and loss of color discrimination; gout	Test vision frequently. Monitor serum uric acid.
Streptomycin	Bacteristatic and cidal (inhibits protein synthesis)	Ototoxicity (eighth cranial nerve) Nephrotoxicity	Monitor ear and kidney function.
Second-line Drugs: Therapy used when primary therapy cannot be used or has failed.			
Pyrazinamide			
Capreomycin (Cepastat)			
Cycloserine (Seromycin)			
Ethionamide (Trecator-C)			
Kanamycin (Kantriex)			
Para-aminosalicylic acid (PAS)			

- Prevent the transmission of droplets
  - cover mouth, nose when coughing, sneezing, laughing
  - dispose of tissue by burning
  - careful hand washing when handling sputum
  - adequate air circulation (air changes will dilute number of bacilli in air of isolated client's room)
  - bacilli are killed by direct sunlight in 1–2 hours; boiling temperature of water kills bacilli in 5 minutes
- Emphasize the importance of continuing prescribed medication.
- Report to public health department for case finding.

Evaluation: Client's family does not contract tuberculosis.

Goal 3: Client will be able to cope with disease.

Plan/Implementation

- Know there is a social stigma associated with tuberculosis.
- Encourage expression of fears, concerns, questions.
- Spend time talking with client (see Table 2.4).

Evaluation: Client verbalizes a desire to practice safe health measures.

Goal 4: Client will care for self at home and will practice health habits that prevent reactivation of infection.

Plan/Implementation

- Teach
  - medication administration, schedule, side effects, importance of compliance
  - importance of activity
  - nutritious diet
  - isolation technique if necessary
  - not to swallow sputum
  - importance of follow-up care
- Arrange public health follow-up.

Evaluation: Client complies with medication regimen.

☐ Pulmonary Embolus

1. General Information

a. Definition: Obstruction of the pulmonary vascular bed; typically caused by a dislodged thrombus

b. Etiology: Thrombus

c. Predisposing factors
   1) hypercoagulability (e.g., oral contraceptives, dehydration, aging)
   2) alterations in integrity of blood vessel (e.g., recent surgery, trauma to vessel wall, vasculitis)
   3) venous stasis (e.g., immobility, obesity, pregnancy, thrombus formation in heart, CHF)

d. Pathophysiology
   1) most emboli arise as detached portions of venous thrombi formed in the right side of the heart or in the deep veins of the legs or pelvic area
   2) dislodgement of thrombi is influenced by intravascular pressure changes, natural mechanism of clot dissolution
   3) acute pulmonary artery obstruction causes
      a) increased alveolar dead space, loss of surfactant, alveolar collapse, regional atelectasis
      b) increased resistance to pulmonary blood flow
      c) acute right ventricular failure

2. Nursing Process

a. Assessment/Analysis
   1) respirations: rapid, shallow, dyspneic
   2) tachycardia
   3) pleuritic chest pain
   4) cough, possibly hemoptysis
   5) anxiety, restlessness
   6) abnormal heart sounds (e.g., S_3, S_4)
   7) abnormal breath sounds (e.g., rales, pleural friction rub)
   8) fever, elevated WBC
   9) abnormal arterial blood gases: decreased pCO_2, pO_2
   10) abnormal chest x-ray and lung scan
   11) massive pulmonary embolism: sudden shock, cyanosis, tachypnea and respiratory distress, mental clouding and anxiety, feeling of impending doom

b. Plans, Implementation, and Evaluation

Goal 1: Client will be protected from development and dislodgement of thrombus.

Plan/Implementation
- Encourage ambulation unless contraindicated.
- Perform active and passive range of motion.
- Apply antiembolic stockings.
- Maintain adequate hydration, steady IV rates.
- Avoid strain, Valsalva maneuver.
- Turn, cough, deep breath every 2 hours.
- Administer low-dose heparin as ordered.

Evaluation: Client is free from signs and symptoms of respiratory difficulty.

Goal 2: Client's pulmonary perfusion and ventilation will improve.

Plan/Implementation
- Observe for signs/symptoms of hypoxia.
- Monitor respiratory rate and rhythm.
- Turn every 2 hours.
- Administer O_2 at prescribed concentrations.
- Administer thrombolytics or anticoagulants as ordered (see Table 3.11).

Evaluation: Client exhibits no respiratory distress; has pink nailbeds, normal skin and mucous membrane color.

Goal 3: Client will maintain adequate cardiac output.

Plan/Implementation
- Monitor for signs/symptoms of acute right ventricular heart failure.
- Measure CVP as ordered.
- Auscultate heart sounds.
- Monitor cardiac rhythm.
- Monitor I&O.
- Administer pulmonary vasodilators (e.g., aminophylline) as ordered (see Table 3.18).
- Administer diuretics (e.g., furosemide) (see Tables 3.16, 3.37).

Evaluation: Client has normal heart rate, rhythm; BP, urine output within normal limits.

Goal 4: Client will experience reduced apprehension, fear, anxiety.

Plan/Implementation
- Administer sedation as ordered.
- Provide a quiet, nonstimulating environment.
- Provide calm reassurance.
- Explain all procedures thoroughly.
- Stay with client during episode of severe dyspnea, chest pain.

Evaluation: Client appears calm; verbalizes reduction in antianxiety.

Goal 5: Client will remain free of recurrence of thrombus formation of pulmonary embolus.

Plan/Implementation

- Teach
  - methods to prevent venous stasis
  - medications
    - * avoidance of complications of hemorrhage (see Table 3.11)

Evaluation: Client wears antiembolic stockings, avoids sitting or remaining in bed for long periods of time; takes anticoagulant drugs correctly.

☐ Chest Tubes and Chest Surgery

1. General Information

a. Clients who experience open-chest injuries, are surgically treated for lung cancer, or have open-heart surgery require similar care because of the opening of the thoracic cavity and the subsequent use of chest tubes

b. Lung expansion: supported by
- **1)** visceral and parietal pleura
- **2)** pressure in pleural space
- **3)** sucking effect on lung

c. Causes of disruption of airtight thoracic cavity
- **1)** spontaneous pneumothorax
- **2)** stab wound
- **3)** bullet wound
- **4)** thoracotomy
- **5)** tear of pleura by fractured ribs

d. Tension pneumothorax
- **1)** cause: closed chest wound; air is unable to escape on expiration; lung collapses as intrathoracic tension increases
- **2)** emergency treatment: chest tube if available, otherwise insert a needle to allow air to escape

e. Chest tube drainage (see reprint page 331)
- **1)** chest tube to open drainage bottle will not function: atmospheric pressure is greater than intrathoracic pressure → collapsed lung
- **2)** purpose of water seal: to seal off the end of chest tube so it acts as a one-way valve (air and fluid travel down the tube but room air cannot travel up the tube)
- **3)** 1-, 2-, or 3-bottle system of Pleur-evac (see Figures 3.11 and 3.12)
- **4)** two chest tubes used for client with lobectomy, segmental resection, or hemothorax; one chest tube with pneumothorax, cardiac surgery
  - **a)** placement
    - anterior, upper thoracic area for air removal
    - 2nd tube, if required, in posterior, lower thoracic area for drainage (drainage is heavier than air)
  - **b)** purpose
    - to remove air and/or drainage from pleural space
    - to help reexpand remaining lung tissue
    - to prevent shifting of mediastinum and collapsed lung tissue by equalization of pressure
- **5)** no chest tubes used for client with pneumonectomy
  - **a)** no lung left to reexpand
  - **b)** increased danger of mediastinal shift
- **6)** application of suction
  - **a)** controlled suction: intermittent positive pressure is used to facilitate removal of secretions and aid in lung expansion
  - **b)** uncontrolled suction: suction control bottle controls the amount of suction

2. Nursing Process

a. Assessment/Analysis
- **1)** patient: breathing (rate, regularity, depth, ease, breath sounds), anxiety, chest discomfort, level of understanding
- **2)** entry site: dressing, drainage, subcutaneous emphysema
- **3)** tubing: tight, taped connections; no kinks, compressions, dependent loops
- **4)** bottles (see Figure 3.12)
  - **a)** water seal bottle: tube submerged or chamber filled to prescribed level (usually 2 cm), fluctuations with respirations, excessive bubbling indicates air leak or open air vent if not on suction
  - **b)** drainage collection bottle: volume, type, rate of drainage; bottle below chest level
  - **c)** suction control bottle: tube submerged or chamber filled to ordered depth (usually 20 cm), gentle, continuous bubbling, tube open to atmosphere
- **5)** Suction source
  - **a)** no control bottle: water level at ordered level
  - **b)** control bottle: suction set so gentle, continuous bubbling occurs

b. Plans, Implementation, and Evaluation

Goal 1: Client will remain safe from malfunctioning water-seal system.

Plan/Implementation

- Check functioning of system.

Figure 3.12 Water-Seal Chest Drainage

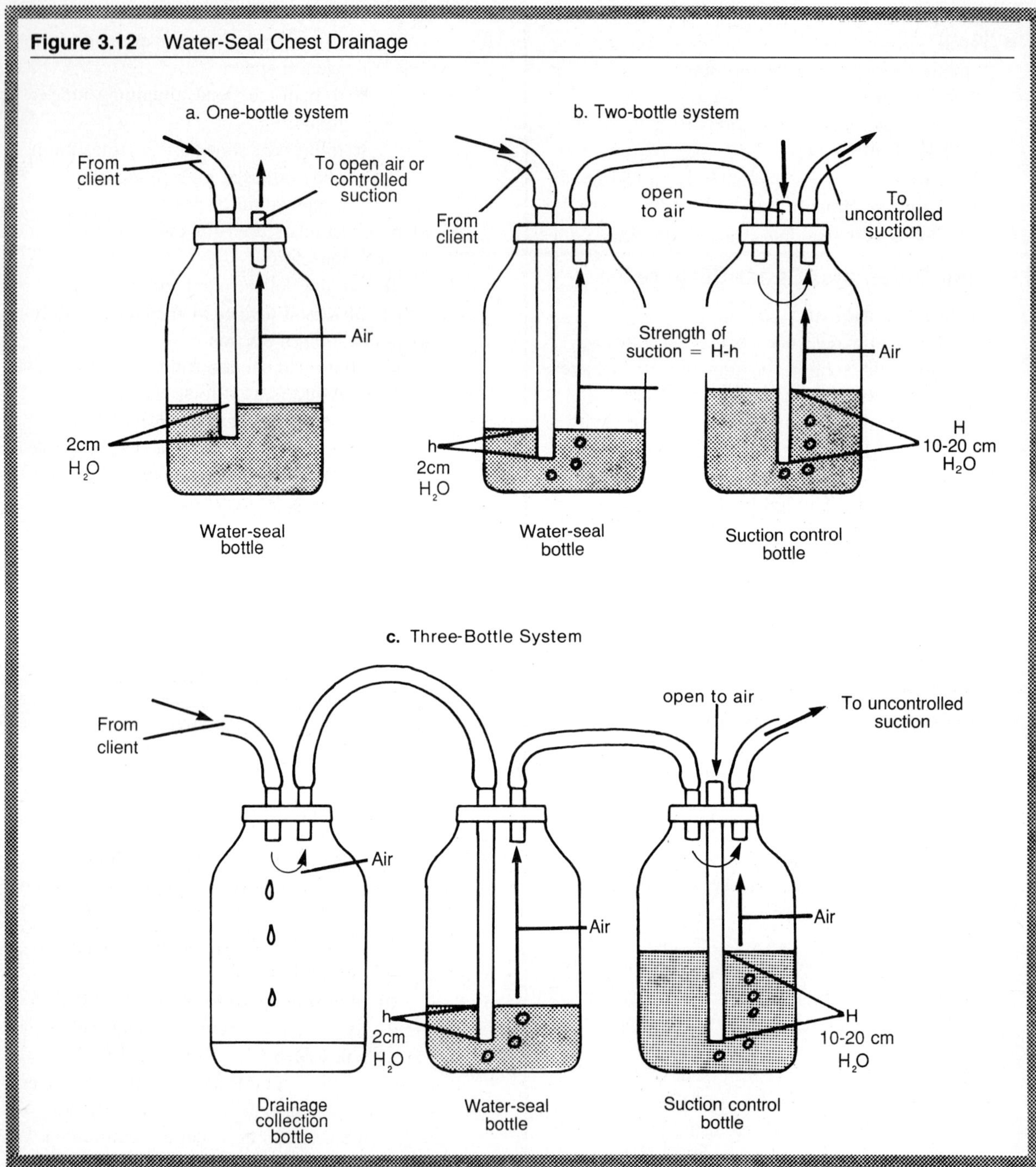

- Check that tube(s) is submerged at appropriate level or that water level(s) in Pleur-evac is correct.
- Tape all connectors.
- Know what to do if system breaks: have tube clamps at bedside and use clamps appropriately.

Evaluation: Client receives prompt and appropriate care if system breaks; water-seal drainage remains intact.

Goal 2: Client will have tube patency maintained.

Plan/Implementation
- Position tubes correctly; ensure that they are not kinked.
- Attach tube to bed linens to prevent it from falling over side and pulling at insertion site.
- Strip tubes as ordered.
- Check for fluctuation of drainage in tube of water-seal bottle.

Figure 3.13 Pleur-evac System

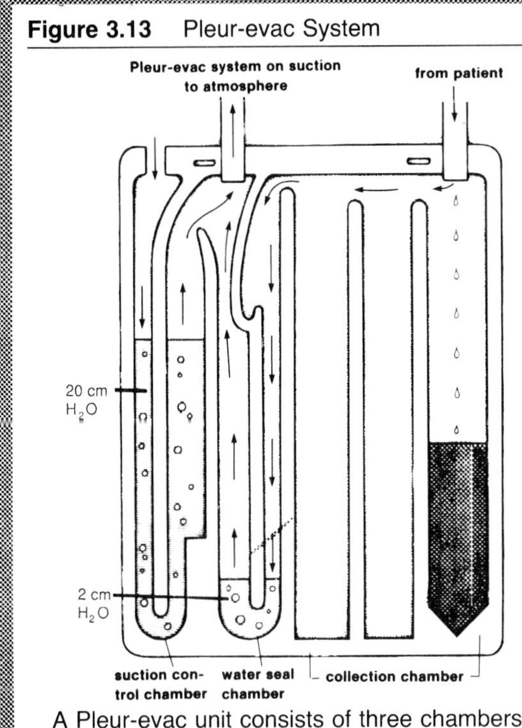

A Pleur-evac unit consists of three chambers comparable to a 3-bottle water-seal drainage system. The suction control chamber is equivalent to bottle #3—the breaker bottle. The water-seal chamber is equivalent to bottle #2—the water-seal bottle. The collection chamber corresponds to bottle #1—the drainage collection bottle.

Evaluation: Client has adequate air and fluid drainage (chest tubes remain patent).

Goal 3: Client will experience adequate lung reexpansion.

Plan/Implementation

- Assist with daily chest x-ray.
- Measure amount of drainage by marking bottle with tape and time of measurement (usual blood loss: 50–100 ml/hour 1st few hours post-op; then decreases to 10–20 ml/hour).
- Monitor for respiratory distress.
- Cough and deep breathe q2h, as needed.
- Provide comfort measures as needed; pain medications as ordered (Table 3.6).
- Position the client to ensure optimum lung expansion
  - pneumonectomy: lie on either affected side or back
  - all other thoracotomies: lie on unaffected side or back
- Assist with removal of tube
  - equipment needed: gauze sponges, tape, scissors to cut suture holding the tube
  - instruct client to exhale or inhale and hold breath
  - apply tight dressing of 4 × 4s over a piece of petrolatum gauze

Evaluation: Client has adequate lung reexpansion; breathes easily, has normal skin color.

□ Cancer of the Lung

1. General Information

a. Incidence

1) leading cause of cancer death in men and women; peaks in middle age

2) increasing in frequency, especially among women

b. Mortality rate is 20 times higher for those who smoke two or more packs daily

2. Nursing Process

a. Assessment/Analysis

1) cough: chronic, persistent

2) abnormal chest x-ray

3) positive sputum cytology

4) positive biopsy

5) hemoptysis, weakness, anorexia, weight loss, dyspnea, chest pain: symptoms of advanced disease

6) pleural effusion (peripheral tumors)

b. Plans, Implementation, and Evaluation

Goal 1: Client and significant others will be able to explain diagnostic tests and postprocedure care.

Plan/Implementation

- Assess level of knowledge of client/significant others.
- Explain procedures (e.g., bronchoscopy, sputum exams, page 166).

Evaluation: Client/significant others describe what to expect during and after procedures.

Goal 2: Client and significant others will be able to explain planned medical treatment.

Plan/Implementation

- Know that radiation therapy and/or chemotherapy are often given if surgery not possible or pre-op in conjunction with surgery.
- Prepare client and significant others for radiation and/or chemotherapy (see *Cellular Aberration* page 306).

Evaluation: Client describes expected actions and side effects of planned medical therapy.

Goal 3: Client and significant others will be able to explain preoperative care, postoperative needs, OR-RR-SICU environment and purpose of chest tubes.

Plan/Implementation
- Prepare client for surgery (see "Perioperative Period" page 157, *Cellular Aberration*, General Nursing Goal 2 page 309; and chest tube care page 193)
- Tour ICU.

Evaluation: Client demonstrates adequate coughing and deep breathing; describes ICU environment.

Goal 4: Postoperatively, client will have adequate respiratory function, stable cardiac function, and adequate pain control.

Plan/Implementation
- See "Perioperative Period" page 157.
- Monitor chest tubes; position appropriately for lung expansion (see chest tube care page 193).

Evaluation: Client remains free from post-op complications (breathes easily, has adequate I&O, experiences good control of pain).

Goal 5: Client and significant others will discuss fears and concerns.

Plan/Implementation
- Assess level of anxiety.
- Give emotional support/relieve anxiety (see Table 2.4).
- Maintain hope.
- Refer to appropriate support groups.

Evaluation: Client and significant others discuss fears, ask questions concerning diagnosis.

Goal 6: Client and significant others will be prepared for discharge.

Plan/Implementation
- Teach
  - levels of activity and rest
  - how to prevent respiratory infections (e.g., avoid crowds)
- Encourage client to stop smoking.
- Arrange follow-up appointment.

Evaluation: Client knows date for return appointment with physician; states a willingness to comply with restrictions.

☐ Cancer of the Larynx

1. General Information

a. Incidence: most common malignancy of upper respiratory tract

b. Risk factors
- **1)** irritants to mucous membranes (e.g., chemicals, allergens)
- **2)** smoking
- **3)** excessive alcohol intake
- **4)** familial predisposition
- **5)** chronic laryngitis
- **6)** voice abuse

c. Medical treatment
- **1)** surgical intervention
  - **a)** laryngectomy
  - **b)** laryngectomy with modified, radical neck dissection
- **2)** medical intervention
  - **a)** radiation therapy
  - **b)** chemotherapy not used

2. Nursing Process

a. Assessment/Analysis
- **1)** presistent hoarseness (early symptom)
- **2)** dysphagia, burning with hot liquids
- **3)** persistent sore throat
- **4)** pain in laryngeal prominence
- **5)** feeling that something is in throat
- **6)** swelling of the neck
- **7)** diagnostic tests: abnormal laryngoscopy, biopsy

b. Plans, Implementation, and Evaluation

Goal 1: Client and significant others will be able to explain planned medical treatment.

Plan/Implementation
- Know that radiation is often used as adjuvant therapy to surgery.
- Prepare client and significant others for radiation (see *Cellular Aberration* page 309).

Evaluation: Client describes expected actions and side effects of radiation therapy.

Goal 2: Client and significant others will be able to explain pre-op care, post-op needs, and the OR-RR environment.

Plan/Implementation
- Prepare client for surgery (see "Perioperative Period" page 157, and *Cellular Aberration* General Nursing Goal 2 page 309.
- Give frequent oral care.
- Advise no smoking, alcohol.
- Teach about post-op procedures
  - presence of drains/HemoVac
  - tracheostomy care and suctioning
  - breathing through tracheostomy tube, inhalation treatments

– possible IVs, tube feedings
- Discuss communication problems that will result.
- Determine methods of post-op communication (e.g., writing pad, picture board, call bell, magic slate, hand signals).

Evaluation: Client explains tracheostomy care; client, significant others, and nurse have plan for post-op communication.

Goal 3: Postoperatively, client will have adequate respiratory function.

Plan/Implementation

- See "Perioperative Period" page 157.
- Assess frequently
  - patency of airway
  - breath sounds, respiratory rate and depth
- Elevate head of bed 30°–45° (promotes drainage and facilitates respirations).
- Support head and neck.
- Administer humidified oxygen.
- Suction tracheostomy frequently
  - sterile suction setup
  - prepare equipment
  - hyperoxygenate client (suctioning can lower pO_2 10–30 mm Hg)
  - lubricate catheter (with H_2O-soluble lubricant) and insert catheter with suction turned off; advance catheter till client coughs
  - withdraw, rotating catheter and applying intermittent suction; suction no longer than 10–15 seconds at one time
  - hyperoxygenate client
  - repeat procedure allowing client to rest between suctionings
  - observe cardiac monitor if in use; if bradycardia or dysrhythmias occur, terminate suctioning immediately and hyperoxygenate client
  - if client has inflated endotracheal or tracheostomy tube in place and you must deflate cuff, use the following procedure
    * suction trachea via tube as outlined above
    * suction oro- and nasopharynx
    * open new sterile setup and then deflate cuff and suction through tube immediately
    * reinflate cuff just until air can no longer be heard, being careful not to overinflate the cuff
- Give laryngeal-tube care; clean tube at least q8h.
- Suction nasopharynx and tracheostomy using separate sterile catheters (or suction tracheostomy first, and nasopharynx second with same catheter).
- Give frequent oral hygiene.
- Check neck drains/HemoVac for drainage.

Evaluation: Client remains free from respiratory distress; has stable vital signs; rests comfortably.

Goal 4: Client will have satisfactory communication with staff and significant others postoperatively.

Plan/Implementation

- Use communication measures decided upon pre-op.
- Remain with client as often as possible.
- Explain to client how to summon nurse; respond promptly when called.
- Have significant others remain with client.

Evaluation: Client communicates needs effectively.

Goal 5: Client will receive adequate nutrition postoperatively.

Plan/Implementation

- Give IV therapy as ordered.
- Give NG tube feedings as ordered.
- Give vitamin supplements as ordered.
- Supervise 1st oral intake; know that aspiration is not possible unless a fistula has formed.
- Check skin turgor to monitor adequate hydration of tissues.
- Monitor I&O.

Evaluation: Client's weight remains stable; fluid intake approximates output.

Goal 6: Client will cope with change in body image.

Plan/Implementation

- See *Loss, Death and Dying* page 30.
- Enlist help of role models such as laryngectomees who have been rehabilitated.

Evaluation: Client's grooming and attitude demonstrate a positive self-concept.

Goal 7: Client and significant others will be prepared for discharge.

Plan/Implementation

- Teach
  - tube care
  - stoma care
  - proper clothing
  - diet
  - activity and recreation
  - bathing
  - oral hygiene
  - Medic Alert bracelet (neck breather)

- Refer to community health agency (e.g., Laryngectomee Club of American Cancer Society).
- Make referral to speech therapist.
- Arrange follow-up appointment.

Evaluation: Client explains care of tube and stoma.

References

Andreoli, K., et al. (Eds.). (1987). *Comprehensive cardiac care: A text for nurses, physicians, and other health personnel* (2nd ed.). St. Louis: Mosby.

Beavers, B. (1986). Health education and the patient with peripheral vascular disease. *Nursing Clinics of North America, 21*(2), 265–271.

Briody, M. (1984). The role of the nurse in modification of cardiac risk factors. *Nursing Clinics of North America, 19*(3), 387–396.

Cohen, S. (1981). New concepts in understanding congestive heart failure (programmed instruction), Part 1. *American Journal of Nursing, 81*, 119–139; Part 2. *American Journal of Nursing, 81*, 357–380.

Cornell, E. (1988). Tuberculosis in hospital employees. *American Journal of Nursing, 88*, 484–485.

Current care of the uncomplicated M.I. (1984). *American Journal of Nursing, 84*, 1410, 1439.

Davido, J. (1981). Pulmonary rehabilitation. *Nursing Clinics of North America, 16*(2), 275–283.

Do you remember how to interpret a T.B. skin test. (1984). *American Journal of Nursing, 84*, 1082.

Donner, C., & Cooper K. (1988). The critical difference: pulmonary edema. *American Journal of Nursing, 88*, 59.

Doyle, J. (1986). Treatment modalities in peripheral vascular disease. *Nursing Clinics of North America, 21*(2), 241–253.

Faulkenberry, J. (1985). Prevention and detection: Lung cancer. *Cancer Nursing, 8*(3), 185–194.

Filderman, A., & Matthay, R. (1985). Update on lung cancer. *Respiratory Therapy, 15*(6), 21–31.

Goodman, L., & Gilman, A. (Eds.). (1986). *Goodman & Gilman's the pharmacological basis of therapeutics*. New York: Macmillan.

Herman, J. (1986). Nursing assessment and nursing diagnosis in patients with peripheral vascular disease. *Nursing Clinics of North America, 21*(2), 219–231.

*†How to work with chest tubes (programmed instruction). (1980). *American Journal of Nursing, 80*, 685–712.

Jung, R. (1984). Current chemotherapy for tuberculosis. *Respiratory Therapy, 14*(2), 29–33.

Knudsen, N., Schulman, S., van den Hoek, J., & Fowler, R. (1985). Insights on how to quit smoking: A survey of patients with lung cancer. *Cancer Nursing, 8*(3), 145–150.

Lancaster, E. (1988). Tuberculosis on the rise. *American Journal of Nursing, 88*, 485.

Lung Cancer. (1987). *American Journal of Nursing, 87*, 1427–1446.

McCauley, K., & Weaver, T. (1983). Cardiac and pulmonary disease: Nutritional implications. *Nursing Clinics of North America, 18*(1), 81–96.

Moore, L., & Pulliam, C. (1986). An on the spot guide to antihypertensive drugs. *Nursing86, 16*(1), 54–57.

New CPR guidelines: Bicarbonate now a last resort. (1986). *American Journal of Nursing, 86*, 889.

†Nursing care of patients in shock. Part 1: Pharmacotherapy (programmed instruction). (1982). *American Journal of Nursing, 82*, 943–963.

Pagana, K. & Pagana, T. (1988). *Pocket nurse guide to laboratory and diagnostic tests*. St. Louis, MO: Mosby.

Peterson, F. (1983). Assessing peripheral vascular disease at the bedside. *American Journal of Nursing, 83*, 1549–1551.

Pinneo, R. (1984). Living with coronary artery disease. *Nursing Clinics of North America, 19*(3), 459–467.

Pinney, M. (1981). Pneumonia. *American Journal of Nursing, 81*, 517–518.

Price, S., & Wilson, L. (1982). *Pathophysiology, clinical concepts of disease processes*. New York: McGraw-Hill.

Purcell, J. et al. (1985). A pacemaker primer. *American Journal of Nursing, 85*, 553–568.

Purcell, J. (1982). Shock drugs: Standardized guidelines. *American Journal of Nursing, 82*, 965–974.

Rossi, L. et al. (1983). Calcium channel blockers, new treatment for cardiovascular disease, *American Journal of Nursing, 83*, 382–387.

Sheridan, E., Patterson, H., & Gustafson, E. (1986). *Falconer's the drug the nurse and the patient* (2nd ed.). Philadelphia: Saunders.

Sjoberg, E. (1983). Nursing diagnosis and the COPD patient. *American Journal of Nursing, 83*, 244–248.

Standards and guidelines for cardiopulmonary resuscitation (CPR) and emergency cardiac care (ECC). (1986). *Journal of the American Medical Association, 255*(21), 2905–2984, and *256*(13), 1727.

Turner, J. (1986). Nursing intervention in patients with peripheral vascular disease. *Nursing Clinics of North America, 21*(2), 233–240.

Wagner, M. (1986). Pathophysiology related to peripheral vascular disease. *Nursing Clinics of North America, 21*(2), 195–205.

Yes, reducing cholesterol does lower coronary heart disease incidence. (1984). *Ameican Journal of Nursing, 84*, 297–298.

†Highly recommended
*Reprint

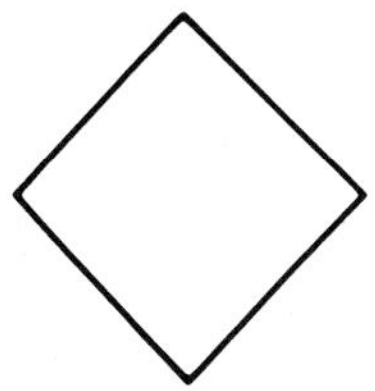

Nutrition and Metabolism

(The nursing care presented in this unit concerns selected health problems related to disturbances in the digestive tract and the endocrine system.)

The Digestive Tract

General Concepts

Overview/Physiology

1. Function: to transfer food and water from the external to the internal environment of the body and transform these substances into a form suitable for distribution to the cells via the circulatory system
2. Anatomy
   a. Upper gastrointestinal tract
      1) mouth, teeth, salivary glands
      2) esophagus
      3) stomach
   b. Lower gastrointestinal tract
      1) small bowel
      2) large bowel
      3) rectum
      4) anus
   c. Accessory organs of digestion
      1) liver
      2) gallbladder
      3) pancreas
3. Processes
   a. Digestion: the process of breaking down proteins, polysaccharides, and fat; accomplished by the action of acid and enzymes secreted into the GI tract
   b. Secretion: the process of elaborating a specific product as a result of glandular activity
      1) saliva (mouth): contains salivary amylase (hydrolyzes starch into maltase)
      2) gastric secretions
         a) mucus: lubricates stomach lining and content
         b) hydrochloric acid (HCl): essential to provide the acid medium necessary for the function of pepsin
         c) pepsin: breaks down proteins to polypeptides, proteoses, and peptones
         d) lipase (small amounts): digests butterfat
         e) gastrin: involved in stimulation and release of HCl
      3) small bowel secretions
         a) peptidases: split polypeptides into amino acids
         b) sucrase, maltase, isomaltase, lactase: split disaccharides into monosaccharides
         c) intestinal lipase splits fats into glycerol and fatty acids
         d) secretin and cholecystokinin-pancreozymin stimulate the pancreas and gallbladder
      4) pancreatic secretions
         a) trypsin, chymotrypsin, nucleases, carboxypeptidase, pancreatic lipase, and pancreatic amylase break down protein, fats, carbohydrates
         b) bicarbonate-rich isosmotic electrolyte solution
      5) gallbladder secretes bile
   c. Absorption: the process by which the small molecules that are the result of digestion cross cell membranes of the intestine and enter the blood and lymph
      1) carbohydrates and proteins are absorbed by active transport along with sodium
      2) fatty acids are absorbed by diffusion
      3) water and electrolytes are absorbed in the small and large intestines
      4) synthesis and absorption of vitamin K, thiamine, riboflavin, vitamin B_{12}, folic acid, biotin, and nicotinic acid take place in the large intestine as a result of bacterial activity, primarily *E. coli*
   d. Motility: the process by which contractions of the smooth muscle lining the walls of the GI tract produce movement of substances through the GI tract while digestion and absorption occur

Table 3.22 Gastrointestinal Hormones

Hormone	Source	How Stimulated	Action
Gastrin	Mucosa of stomach	Distention by food and vagal stimulation.	Stimulates secretion of hydrochloric acid.
Secretin	Duodenal mucosa	Gastric contents entering duodenum.	Stimulates secretion of pancreatic fluid.
Cholecystokinin	Duodenal mucosa	Fat in duodenum.	Contraction of gallbladder. Stimulates secretion of enzyme-rich pancreatic juice.

1) GI tract contains an intrinsic nerve supply that controls tone and peristaltic action
2) nerve fibers from both the sympathetic and parasympathetic branches of the autonomic nervous system supply the intestinal tract and interact with intrinsic nerve supply
3) the vagus nerve (the major autonomic nerve supplying the GI tract) is composed of motor parasympathetic fibers and many sensory fibers; parasympathetic stimulation *increases* motility and secretion; sympathetic stimulation *decreases* motility and secretion

e. Metabolism

1) all of the changes or body processes that take place in order to sustain life; the chemical changes that occur allow chemical energy to be changed to other forms of energy so that cellular functions can be maintained
2) intermediary metabolism includes all the cellular functions in the body's internal environment; this phase of metabolism begins after the ingestion and digestion of foodstuffs from the external environment
3) two-part process

Table 3.23 Digestive Enzymes

Enzymes that Digest	Source	Selected Action and Products
Carbohydrates		
Amylase	Parotid and submaxillary glands	Hydrolyzes starch to maltose.
Sucrase, maltase, isomaltase, lactase	Intestinal fluids	Split disaccharides into monosaccharides.
Pancreatic amylase	Pancreas	Splits starches into maltose and isomaltose.
Fats		
Gastric lipase	Gastric mucosa	Digests butterfat.
Intestinal lipase	Intestinal fluids	Splits fats into glycerol and fatty acids.
Pancreatic lipase	Pancreas	Hydrolyzes fat into glycerol and fatty acids.
Protein		
Pepsin	Gastric mucosa	Breaks down dietary protein into proteoses, peptones, and polypeptides.
Peptidases	Intestinal glands	Splits polypeptides into amino acids.
Trypsin	Pancreas	Splits proteins into peptide and amino acids.
Chymotrypsin	Pancreas	Splits proteins into polypeptides.
Carboxypeptidase	Pancreas	Splits polypeptides into smaller peptides.
Other		
Enterokinase	Duodenal mucosa	Activates trypsin.
Nucleases	Pancreas	Splits nucleic acids.

a) anabolism: the process of synthesis of smaller molecules to larger molecules; energy is saved
   - building process: proteins from amino acids, fats from fatty acids, polysaccharides from monosaccharides
   - increased during growth, pregnancy, recovery states, or times of increased intake

b) catabolism: the breaking down of larger molecules into smaller molecules
   - protein, fats, carbohydrates are broken down into units that can be used by the cells
   - excesses in catabolism are seen in starvation, illness, trauma
   - breakdown involves the release of CO_2, water, and urea with amino acid metabolism

4) adenosine triphosphate (ATP) is the high-energy phosphate that is the major source of energy for cellular function

5) adenosine diphosphate (ADP) is one of the end products released when energy is used and ATP is broken down

6) metabolic balance remains unless a change in the internal or external environment produces imbalances (for the balance to be maintained, the rate of catabolism must equal anabolism)

7) variances in metabolic rate occur with differences in sex, age, hormonal environment, seasonal and environmental temperature changes, culture, activity levels, ingestion of drugs (e.g., caffeine, nicotine, epinephrine)

8) materials needed for metabolism
   a) nutrients to supply energy and build tissue: glucose, glycerol, fatty acids, amino acids
   b) minerals, electrolytes
   c) materials (primarily proteins) to promote synthesis of enzymes and hormones
   d) vitamins that function as co-enzymes
   e) enzymes and hormones to function as organic cellular catalysts

9) metabolism governs the activities of muscle contraction, nerve impulse transmission, glandular secretion, absorption, and elimination

☐ Application of the Nursing Process to the Client with Digestive Tract Problems

1. Assessment

a. Health history
   1) normal dietary pattern: changes in appetite
   2) normal weight: changes in weight (how much, time period, planned vs. unplanned)
   3) change in energy level: weakness, fatigue, general malaise
   4) stool: changes in frequency, color, character
   5) urine: dark, orange or clear color, frequency
   6) indigestion or heartburn: pattern, frequency, drugs used, effectiveness
   7) difficulty in swallowing: dysphagia with onset by solids or liquids
   8) difficulty tolerating certain foods: allergies
   9) vomiting/nausea: character of vomitus; pattern of nausea; relationship to intake, other events
   10) abdominal pain: presence, location, character, pattern
   11) abdominal distention
   12) abdominal surgery
   13) skin: jaundice, bruising
   14) bleeding: onset, duration, extent
   15) alcohol habits

b. Physical examination of the abdomen (*NOTE*: Palpation is done last because it can stimulate bowel sounds)
   1) inspection
      a) skin characteristics: scars, striae, engorged veins, spider angiomata
      b) visible peristalsis, pulsations, masses
      c) contour: rounded, protuberant, concave, asymmetric
   2) auscultation: listen to all four quadrants
      a) bowel sounds: location, frequency (normally 8–20/minute in each quadrant), characteristics
         - normal: succession of clicks/gurgles
         - abnormal
           – hyperperistalsis: loud gurgles
           – paralytic ileus: absent or infrequent
           – intestinal obstruction: loud, rushing, high-pitched tinkling sounds proximal to the obstruction
           – air/fluid in stomach: succession of splashes
      b) bruits

3) percussion
   a) stomach (tympany normal)
   b) liver size (normally dull)
   c) gaseous distention
4) palpation
   a) pain
   b) masses, especially liver enlargement
   c) skin reflexes
   d) fluid waves

c. Diagnostic tests
1) hematologic studies: normal values will vary slightly from laboratory to laboratory
   a) general function
      - electrolytes
        - sodium: 135–145 mEq/liter
        - potassium: 3.5–5.0 mEq/liter
        - chlorides: 100–106 mEq/liter
      - CBC
        - WBC: 5,000–10,000/mm^3
        - RBC: 4.2–6.2 million/mm^3
        - Hgb
          * men: 14–18 gm/dl
          * women: 12–16 gm/dl
        - Hct
          * men: 42%–54%
          * women: 38%–46%
   b) liver function
      - serum glutamic-oxaloacetic transaminase (SGOT): 7–27 units/liter
      - serum glutamic-pyruvic transaminase (SGPT): 1–21 units/liter
      - bromsulphalein (BSP): less than 10% retention after 45 minutes
      - alkaline phosphatase: 13–39 units/liter
      - ammonia levels: less than 50 μg/dl
      - albumin: 3.5–5.0 gm/dl; globulin: 2.3–3.5 g/dl
      - bilirubin: less than 1 mg/dl
      - cholesterol: 120–200 mg/dl
      - hepatitis B surface antigen (HB_SAg) and hepatitis B surface antibody (anti HB_S): negative
      - prothrombin time: comparable to normal control
   c) GI function
      - gastrin: less than 300 pg/ml
   d) pancreatic function
      - glucose levels
        - glucose: 70–110 mg/dl
        - postprandial: less than 145 mg/dl
        - glucose tolerance: peak of 160–180 mg/dl
      - lipase: 2 units/ml or less
      - amylase: 4–25 units/ml
2) urine tests
   a) glucose, acetone
   b) urobilinogen
3) stool tests
   a) ova and parasites (stool must be warm)
   b) occult blood (guaiac)
   c) fecal fat (after a 72-hour collection)
   d) culture
4) radiographic studies
   a) flat plate of abdomen
   b) upper GI series (often with small bowel follow-through)
      - definition: x-ray of esophagus, stomach, duodenum following oral intake of contrast medium (barium)
      - nursing care pretest: keep NPO for 8 hours prior to test
      - nursing care post-test
        - give laxatives, force fluids to remove barium
        - encourage mobility to stimulate peristalsis
   c) lower GI, barium enema, refer to ''Large Bowel'' page 257
   c) cholecystogram
      - definition: x-ray visualization of gallbladder and biliary tract following oral ingestion of iodine dye
      - nursing care pretest
        - check for iodine allergies
        - administer dye (usually Telepaque in form of 6 tablets) given 12 hours before test (give with sufficient water 30 minutes apart since it may cause diarrhea)
        - give low fat evening meal the day prior
        - keep NPO for 8 hours prior to test
      - nursing care post-test: no special concerns
   e) cholangiogram (IV, via T-tube, or via common bile duct during surgery)
      - definition: x-ray visualization of gallbladder and biliary tract following injection of iodine dye
      - nursing care pretest
        - check for iodine allergies
        - keep NPO for 8 hours prior to test
        - ensure signed consent is on chart if applicable

- nursing care post-test: force fluids (dye acts as diuretic)

f) abdominal CAT scan: with or without contrast medium

5) endoscopy

a) definition: direct visualization of a part or parts of the GI tract through a lighted scope; may be a treatment modality as well (e.g., polypectomy, remove foreign objects, cauterize GI bleeding sites)

b) types

- esophagoscopy (esophagus)
- gastroscopy (stomach)
- duodenoscopy (duodenum)
- peritoneoscopy (liver, gallbladder, and mesentery)
- endoscopic retrograde cholangiography (ERCP) (pancreas and biliary tree)
- sigmoidoscopy (sigmoid colon)
- colonoscopy (entire colon)
- proctoscopy (rectosigmoid)

c) nursing care pretest

- keep NPO for 8 hours prior to test
- administer bowel prep for lower GI endoscopy
- ensure a signed consent is on the chart
- give pretest sedation as ordered

d) nursing care post-test

- check vital signs frequently the first 24 hours
- feed when gag reflex returns after upper GI endoscopy
- observe for bleeding (indicated by frequent swallowing/bloody emesis following exam of the upper GI system or bloody stools following exam of lower GI system), sharp pain (indicates perforation)
- force fluids as needed

6) hepatic angiography: liver, gallbladder, pancreas

a) nursing care pretest

- keep NPO 8 hours prior to test
- ensure a signed consent is on the chart

b) nursing care post-test

- observe for bleeding at puncture site
- apply sandbag or pressure dressing to site for 8–12 hours

7) abdominal ultrasound

a) definition: examination of the abdomen using sound waves

b) nursing care pretest

- give laxatives and cathartics the evening before
- keep NPO for 8 hours prior to test
- have client drink 6–8 glasses of water just prior to test and not void until test is over, or clamp Foley catheter (full bladder acts as a landmark)

c) nursing care post-test: no special concerns; if Foley is in place, check to ensure it has been unclamped

8) analytical studies

a) gastric analysis (with NG tube)

- definition: to determine amount/absence of digestive juices, bacteria, or parasites
- nursing care
  - keep NPO for 8 hours
  - insert nasogastric tube
  - collect fasting specimen
  - collect specimens after gastric secretions have been stimulated by food, alcohol, histamine, insulin, secretin
  - observe for vital-sign changes and anaphylaxsis when histamine, insulin are administered
  - have diphenhydramine (Benadryl) on hand for allergic reactions

b) gastric analysis (without NG tube)

- definition: analysis of stomach pH done with diagnex blue
- nursing care
  - keep NPO for 8 hours
  - have client empty bladder
  - give diagnex blue tablet
  - several hours later, have client empty bladder and send urine to lab (if gastric secretion has pH of 3 or less, the dye will have been excreted)

c) Schilling's test

- definition: assessing vitamin B_{12} absorption to differentiate between intrinsic factor deficiency and absorption problem
- nursing care
  - administer parenteral, saturating dose of nonradioactive B_{12} to a fasting client
  - 1–2 hours later, administer oral radioactive B_{12} test dose
  - start 24-hour urine specimen collection to assess levels of

radioactive B_{12} excreted (normal = 8%–40% of injected activity)

9) biopsies
   a) excisional
      - rectal (done at time of sigmoidoscopy)
      - gastric (done at time of gastroscopy)
   b) needle (percutaneous liver biopsy)
      - definition: a blind needle biopsy of liver tissue to establish a microscopic picture of the liver
      - nursing care pretest
        - ensure informed consent is on chart
        - check prothrombin time (if less than 40% test will not be done)
        - instruct client to hold breath while biopsy is being done and not to move during procedure
      - nursing care post-test
        - have client lie on right side with pillow or sand bag over the insertion point
        - take frequent vital signs the first 24 hours
        - assess for pain or respiratory difficulty

2. Analysis

a. Safe, effective care environment
   1) knowledge deficit
   2) potential for infection

b. Physiological integrity
   1) pain
   2) constipation or diarrhea
   3) altered nutrition: less than body requirements

c. Psychological integrity
   1) ineffective individual coping
   2) self-esteem disturbance

d. Health promotion/maintenance
   1) health-seeking behaviors
   2) noncompliance

3. General Nursing Plans, Implementation, and Evaluation

Goal 1: Client will ingest a diet that conforms to prescribed restrictions yet contains all needed nutrients.

Plan/Implementation

- Increase or decrease dietary nutrients as ordered.
- Teach client the rationale for dietary restrictions
- Assist clients to identify factors in their life-style which may interfere with compliance.
- Provide needed support and encouragement, involve family if possible.

Evaluation: Client selects appropriate diet from sample menus; verbalizes rationale for restrictions; expresses positive attitude toward diet alteration.

Goal 2: Client will be as comfortable and as pain free as possible.

Plan/Implementation

- Administer pain medications as appropriate.
- Use noninvasive pain-relieving techniques such as positioning, massage, distraction.
- Teach client and significant others about measures that will minimize pain when client is discharged (e.g., dietary regimen, medications).

Evaluation: Client states that s/he is pain free or experiencing only minimal pain; verbalizes measures to control pain after discharge.

Goal 3: Client's fluid and electrolyte balance will return to normal.

Plan/Implementation

- Institute replacement therapy or restrictions as ordered.
- Keep accurate I&O.
- Monitor daily weight.

Evaluation: Client's fluid and electrolyte levels are within normal limits.

Goal 4: Client will be knowledgeable about disease process, medications, and the prevention of complications.

Plan/Implementation

- Explain disease process.
- Discuss rationale for ordered treatment regimen.
- Provide information regarding the administration and side effects of all medications.
- Help client and significant other to identify factors that might trigger complications of the disease.

Evaluation: Client lists medications and describes the prevention of complications.

Selected Health Problems Resulting in Problems with Digestion

☐ Hiatal Hernia (Diaphragmatic Hernia)

1. General Information

a. Definition: a small opening in the diaphragm allows the esophagus and vagus nerve to pass through. When that opening is enlarged, stomach contents protrude into the thoracic cavity and regurgitation of stomach contents into the esophagus may occur.

b. Precipitating factors
   1) congenital or acquired weakness of the diaphragm
   2) obesity
   3) heavy lifting
   4) increased intra-abdominal pressure
   5) pregnancy

c. Medical treatment
   1) medical intervention: diet adjustment, change in eating pattern, medications
   2) surgical intervention: fundoplication and suturing of the stomach through the abdomen or thorax

2. Nursing Process

a. **Assessment/Analysis**
   1) heartburn, pain may radiate
   2) symptoms vary from mild to severe
   3) regurgitation of stomach contents, especially in recumbent position

b. **Plan, Implementation, and Evaluation**

Goal: Client will be free from pain/heartburn.

Plan/Implementation
- Follow high protein, low-fat diet
  - avoid caffeine, alcohol, and chocolate
  - take small, frequent meals; avoid hs meals
- Instruct client
  - to elevate the head of the bed at night 6–12 inches
  - to sit upright for at least 1 hour after meals
  - to avoid activities that increase intra-abdominal pressure (e.g., coughing, heavy lifting, tight belts, girdles)
- Take 30 ml antacids between meals, at bedtime, and PRN for discomfort; take other drugs as prescribed (e.g., Reglan, cimetidine).
- Avoid anticholinergic drugs.

☐ Gastritis

1. General Information

a. Definition: acute or chronic inflammation of the stomach

b. Predisposing factors
   1) dietary intolerances (commonly milk)
   2) alcohol
   3) drugs: aspirin, steroids, antibiotics (e.g, tetracycline)
   4) uremia
   5) certain systemic diseases: hepatitis, typhoid fever
   6) ingestion of strong acids or alkalis (corrosive gastritis)

c. Medical treatment
   1) diet adjustment; change in eating pattern; minimal alcohol intake
   2) use of antacids

2. Nursing Process

a. **Assessment/Analysis**
   1) nausea/vomiting
   2) indigestion
   3) hematemesis
   3) history of
      a) onset of pain
      b) ingested substances
      c) any systemic problems

b. **Plans, Implementation, and Evaluation**

Goal 1: Client will experience relief of nausea, vomiting, and hyperacidity.

Plan/Implementation
- Identify and remove cause if possible.
- Keep NPO until symptoms subside.
- Know IV fluids with electrolyte replacement may be given during acute phase.
- Give antacids as ordered.
- Introduce bland foods when client is able to take food; monitor tolerance.

Evaluation: Client regains adequate gastric functioning (e.g., no pain, eating well); tolerates foods (liquids).

Goal 2: Client will be free from complications.

Plan/Implementation
- Take emergency measures to prevent scarring/obstruction following ingestion of alkalis or acids; do not induce vomiting.
- Give bland diet, antacids as ordered.
- Know that vitamin B_{12} may be indicated for clients with chronic gastritis to prevent pernicious anemia.

Evaluation: Client regains adequate gastric functioning (e.g., no pain, eating well); tolerates foods (liquids).

☐ Peptic Ulcer Disease

1. General Information

a. Definition: sharply defined break in mucosa, which may involve the submucosa and muscular layers of the esophagus, stomach, and duodenum

b. Incidence (*NOTE*: references differ on incidence)
- **1)** gastric type: 2 times higher in men, usually over 50 years of age
- **2)** duodenal type: 4 times higher in men, 25–50 years age range; 80% of all ulcers of the GI tract

c. Predisposing factors
- **1)** cigarette smoking
- **2)** genetic predisposition
- **3)** chronic high-dose salicylate use
- **4)** severe physiological stress (gastric stress ulcers): severe burns, trauma, surgery
- **5)** ulcerogenic drugs (acute ulcers not chronic disease state): corticosteriods, anti-inflammatories, caffeine
- **6)** emotional stress (role unclear)
- **7)** presence of another chronic illness: arthritis, COPD

d. Pathophysiology
- **1)** gastric ulcers
  - **a)** decreased resistance of gastric mucosa to acid injury and back diffusion of gastric acid into mucosa. Barriers to back diffusion are broken down by alcohol, bile acids, and salicylates.
  - **b)** clients typically have normal rates of gastric emptying and normal gastric acid secretion.
- **2)** duodenal ulcers
  - **a)** increased gastric acid secretory rate
  - **b)** increased gastrin levels postprandially (gastrin is a potent stimulator of gastric acid secretion)
  - **c)** markedly increased rate of gastric emptying; more gastric acid propelled into duodenum

e. Diagnostic aids
- **1)** direct visualization (gastroscopy, duodenoscopy)
- **2)** upper GI
- **3)** gastric analysis (amount of HCl)
- **4)** stool exams (occult blood)

f. Complications of peptic ulcer disease requiring surgery
- **1)** hemorrhage
- **2)** perforation and peritonitis
- **3)** obstruction

g. Medical treatment
- **1)** medical intervention
  - **a)** drugs: histamine receptor antagonists, antacids (see Table 3.24), anticholinergics
  - **b)** rest
  - **c)** decreased stress
  - **d)** diet modification
- **2)** surgical intervention (for recurrent ulcers)
  - **a)** subtotal gastrectomy
    - ■ Billroth I: removal of part of stomach, anastomosis of remaining portion to duodenum
    - ■ Billroth II: resection of distal 2/3 of the stomach; anastomosis of jejunal loop to remaining portion with remaining duodenal stump sutured shut
    - ■ may result in pernicious anemia due to the removal of the parietal cells
  - **b)** vagotomy: severing of vagus nerve to eliminate acid-secreting stimulus to gastric cells
  - **c)** pyloroplasty: revision of passage between pyloric region and duodenum to enhance emptying in gastric atony associated with vagotomy

2. Nursing Process

a. Assessment/Analysis
- **1)** gastric
  - **a)** pain
    - ■ ½–1 hour after meals
    - ■ may be relieved by ingestion of food or liquid; if ulcer penetrates, food will aggravate pain
    - ■ described as burning or pressure in high epigastrium, may radiate
    - ■ may be asymptomatic
  - **b)** occasional nausea and vomiting
  - **c)** possible weight loss
  - **d)** hematemesis more common than melena
- **2)** duodenal
  - **a)** pain
    - ■ chronic and periodic (occurs 1–4 hours after eating and may occur in middle of night)

Table 3.24 Drug Therapy for Peptic Ulcer Disease

Generic Name (Trade Name)	Action	Use	Side Effects
Antacids			
Aluminum hydroxide (AlternaGel, Amphojel) Dried form (Alu-Cap)	Nonsystemic, works by neutralization.	Treat gastric/duodenal ulcers Management of phosphate stone formation	Constipation, phosphorus deficiency, intestinal obstruction
Basic aluminum carbonate (Basagel)	As with Amphogel.	As with Amphojel	Constipation
Calcium carbonate (Alka-2, Tums)	Rapid onset. High neutralizing capacity.	Peptic ulcers	Constipation, hypercalcemia, rebound hyperacidity
Magaldrate (Riopan)	Combination of aluminum and magnesium hydroxide. Nonsystemic neutralizing substance.	Antacid	Mild constipation or diarrhea Hypermagnesia in renal failure
Magnesium hydroxide (Milk of Magnesia)	Neutralizes HC1. Demulcent effect.	Antacid Laxative	Diarrhea, abdominal pain, nausea
Sodium bicarbonate	Systemic and local alkalizer.	Antacid	Acid rebound, systemic alkalosis
Antiflatulent			
Simethicone (Mylicon)	Decreases surface tension of gas bubbles. Prevents formation of mucus-surrounded gas bubbles.	Antiflatulent	None
Combination of Mixtures			
Aluminum and magnesium hydroxide (Maalox, Maalox #1, #2, Concentrate)	As above	Antacid	As above
Aluminum and magnesium hydroxide and Simethicone (Mylanta, Mylanta II, Maalox Plus)	As above	Antacid Antiflatulent	
Histamine Receptor Blocking Agent			
Cimetidine (Tagamet)	Inhibits release of HCl by occupying histamine receptors in gastric mucosa.	Duodenal ulcers Gastric hypersecretory states Prevent recurrent ulcers	Mild diarrhea, mental confusion, dizziness, gynecomastia
Ranitidine (Zantac)	As above. Greater reduction of acid secretion, longer duration of action.		As above but side effects are fewer; no gynecomastia or confusion.

- relieved by the ingestion of some types of food or by antacids
- located in epigastrium and may radiate around the costal border to the back
- described by the client as a gnawing, boring, or nagging sensation

b) melena or occult blood in stools

3) hemorrhage
- **a)** excessive hematemesis and/or melena
- **b)** signs and symptoms of shock

4) perforation/peritonitis: ulcer penetrates entire wall with leakage of GI contents, into abdominal cavity
- **a)** sudden onset of severe abdominal pain
- **b)** diffuse abdominal tenderness
- **c)** diminished bowel sounds

c) diminished bowel sounds
  - boardlike abdomen with diffuse distention
  - tachycardia, shallow respirations, diaphoresis

d) obstruction: can result from edema or scar tissue formation near the pylorus
  - fullness, nausea
  - profuse vomiting of undigested food

b. Plans, Implementation, and Evaluation

Goal 1: Client will be free from pain.

Plan/Implementation
- Give 30 ml antacid drugs 1–3 hours after meals, at bedtime, and PRN.
- Give histamine receptor antagonists as ordered with meals and at bedtime.
- Teach client to eliminate foods from diet that cause increased pain
  - try small frequent meals
  - avoid common stimulants of gastric acid secretion (e.g., caffeine, alcohol, spicy foods)
- Provide for increased rest; ensure a calm, peaceful environment.
- Assist client to stop smoking, if possible.

Evaluation: Client can tolerate diet without discomfort; states or institutes measures that decrease/prevent pain.

Goal 2: Client will identify and alleviate stressful factors in life-style.

Plan/Implementation
- Assist client/significant other to identify stressful factors in life/life-style.
- Encourage client to express emotions and needs.
- Teach client relaxation/stress-reduction techniques.
- Help client design a balanced work, play, rest schedule.

Evaluation: Client identifies stressors on the job and at home; begins to express emotions verbally; expresses a willingness to find an outlet to release stress; adheres to a mutually planned schedule of activities while in the hospital and at home.

Goal 3: Client will identify activities to prevent ulcer recurrence.

Plan/Implementation
- Teach client to avoid factors that tend to activate ulcer.
- Help client plan to balance work, play, rest.
- Clarify dietary restrictions, if any.
- Encourage reduction or elimination of smoking, alcohol, caffeine intake.
- Encourage follow-up health care.
- Teach regarding medications, side effects; time and method of administration; medications that irritate ulcer (e.g., ASA).

Evaluation: Client states measures that will reduce the chances of recurrence; follows prescribed diet; takes medication correctly; has a balanced activity schedule; stops or decreases smoking or alcohol ingestion.

Goal 4: Client will recover from GI hemorrhage or ulcer perforation with minimal complications; if surgery is performed the client will recover free from complications.

Plan/Implementation

Pre-op
- Institute measures to control bleeding as ordered
  - insert NG tube; irrigate stomach with cool saline until clear; connect to suction
  - give antacids/cimetidine (Tagamet) after acute bleeding has stopped
  - administer IV fluids; type and crossmatch client's blood in order to replace blood loss as ordered
  - offer emotional support
- Minimize consequences of perforation
  - give antibiotics as ordered
  - maintain client in Fowler's position to localize gastric contents to 1 area of peritoneum
- Do as much pre-op teaching as time allows; focus only on deep breathing; avoid turning and coughing (promote movement of intestinal contents).
- Include significant others in discussion of what the plan of care incorporates.

Post-op
- Provide standard post-op care, refer to *Surgery* page 157.
- Maintain client NPO for 5–7 days to allow incision to heal; progress to clear liquids and diet as tolerated.
- Maintain in semi-Fowler's position.
- Maintain NG tube to suction
  - do not irrigate or reposition unless ordered
  - record all NG drainage as output
  - observe color of drainage: should progress from bloody drainage → old blood → gastric secretions (greenish) within 24 hours.

Evaluation: Client is physically prepared for immediate surgery (e.g., NG tube in place; has vital signs and level of consciousness monitored at least q15 minutes); recovers from surgery free of respiratory complications, infection, or hemorrhage.

Goal 5: Client will recover from gastric surgery with minimal anemia.

Plan/Implementation

- Know that 20%–50% of clients will experience anemia postresection
  - vitamin B_{12} deficiency (pernicious anemia) if parietal cells of the stomach were removed
  - iron deficiency from blood loss
- Give dietary supplements as ordered.

Evaluation: Client recovers, is free from anemia; if anemic, accepts follow-up care.

Goal 6: Client will understand dumping syndrome and ways to control it.

Plan/Implementation

- Teach client
  - symptoms of dumping syndrome (following subtotal or total gastrectomy: food enters duodenum rapidly; hyperosmolarity of intestinal contents pulls H_2O from vascular bed and stimulates a neuroendocrine response)
    - * reaction occurs within *30 minutes* after eating
    - * client feels dizzy, weak
    - * pulse increased
    - * skin cool, clammy
  - prevention techniques
    - * eat small meals that are dry, contain moderate protein and fat and reduced carbohydrate (avoid refined sugars)
    - * drink liquids between meals only
    - * rest or lie down on left side for 30 minutes after meals if possible to slow gastric emptying
  - symptoms of postprandial hypoglycemia (rapid emptying of stomach contents into the intestine → rapid absorption of glucose → hyperglycemia → pancreas is stimulated to secrete excess of insulin → hypoglycemic reaction)
    - * occurs about *2 hours* after meal
    - * complaints of dizziness, weakness, restlessness
    - * pulse increased
    - * skin cool, clammy
    - * malabsorption results
  - prevention techniques
    - * same as dumping syndrome
    - * symptoms are quickly relieved by ingestion of sugared fluids or candy
- Know that if the above does not relieve the problem, surgical intervention may be necessary to narrow the opening between stomach and intestine.
- Know that for some clients dumping syndrome and subsequent malabsorption become chronic, unrelieved problems.

Evaluation: Client states symptoms of and methods to prevent dumping syndrome; identifies a plan for work and relaxation; selects appropriate foods from diet list.

☐ Diverticulosis/Diverticulitis

1. General Information

a. Definitions
  1) diverticulum: outpouching of the musculature of the colon
  2) diverticulosis: the condition of being afflicted with diverticulum
  3) diverticulitis: inflammation of the diverticulum
  4) fiber/roughage: plants or food stuffs not digested by the body
  5) residue: that part of food stuffs left after digestion and eventually winding up in the large intestine

b. Most common in the sigmoid colon

c. Risk factors
  1) diet low in fiber and high in refined and processed foods
  2) age (frequently over 40 years of age)
  3) chronic constipation

d. Medical treatment
  1) medical intervention:
    a) acute episodes: NPO, antibiotics, IV fluids; if eating a low fiber/roughage, low residue diet
    b) ongoing care: high fiber/roughage diet, high or low in residue (MD choice), bulk laxatives, antispasmodics
  2) surgical intervention: bowel resection with/without a temporary colostomy

2. Nursing Process

a. Assessment/Analysis
  1) diverticulosis is usually asymptomatic
  2) diverticulitis
    a) crampy, left lower quadrant pain
    b) constipation possibly alternating with diarrhea

c) fever and leukocytosis

b. Plans, Implementation, and Evaluation

Goal 1: Client's acute episode will subside without complications.

Plan/Implementation
- Keep client NPO until pain subsides, then advance to liquid diet.
- Give antibiotics, IV fluids, electrolytes as ordered.
- Keep on bedrest to decrease intestinal motility.
- Observe for complications of perforation/peritonitis.

Evaluation: Client remains free from pain and complications; has normal bowel function; tolerates diet.

Goal 2: Client will recover from any necessary surgery (e.g., bowel resection, colostomy) without complications. Refer to *Elimination* page 263.

Goal 3: Client will take measures to control diverticulosis.

Plan/Implementation
- Teach client
  - to eat a high-fiber/roughage diet (see Table 3.25 below)
  - to take bulk laxatives (e.g., psyllium hydrophilic [Metamucil]), as ordered
  - about use of ordered antispasmodics (e.g., propantheline [Pro-Banthine]), oxyphencyclimine [Daricon])
  - ways to decrease stress in life/life-style
  - to increase daily fluid intake
  - to avoid activities that increase intra-abdominal pressure
  - to avoid all nuts or fruits/vegatables with seeds to prevent the seeds from lodging in the intestinal pouches and causing infection

Table 3.25 High Fiber/Roughage Diet

Food Groups	Recommended Foods
Fruits	Fresh fruits with skin
Vegetables	Raw vegetables
Breads	Whole wheat and whole grain Bran-type cereals
Grains and flour	Wheat germ, cornmeal, rice, buckwheat
Protein substitutes	Legumes

Evaluation: Client remains free from symptoms of diverticulitis; tolerates high-fiber/roughage diet; decreases stress.

☐ Cholecystitis with Cholelithiasis

1. General Information

a. Definition: inflammation of the gallbladder caused by presence of stones (composed of bile pigment, cholesterol, calcium)

b. Incidence: higher in Caucasian women over age 40

c. Predisposing factors
- **1)** obesity
- **2)** middle age
- **3)** multiparity, use of birth control pills
- **4)** four times more common in women
- **5)** diabetes

d. Medical treatment
- **1)** medical intervention
  - **a)** low-fat diet (see Table 3.26 below)
  - **b)** weight reduction
  - **c)** drugs to dissolve stones
  - **d)** lithotripsy
- **2)** surgical intervention
  - **a)** cholecystectomy (removal of gallbladder and cystic duct): Penrose drain in gallbladder bed
  - **b)** choledocholithotomy (removal of stones in common bile duct): T-tube inserted into common bile duct
    - common duct exploration always requires T-tube insertion to prevent bile spillage into peritoneum and maintain ductal patency while healing takes place
    - crossbar of T-tube lies in common bile duct; long end is brought out through a stab wound in the abdomen and connected to receptacle for gravity drainage

Table 3.26 Principles of a Low-Fat Diet

Trim all visible fat from foods.
Use only lean meats; remove skin from poultry.
Restrict use of eggs.
Do not use fat for food preparation, no frying.
Use skim milk, low-fat cottage cheese.
Avoid use of sauces, gravies, and rich desserts.
Increase use of fish and seafood.

2. Nursing Process

a. Assessment/Analysis

1) abdominal pain, usually in the right upper quadrant; may radiate to back
2) fullness, eructation, dyspepsia following fat ingestion
3) nausea and vomiting (distention of bile duct initiates stimulation of vomiting center)
4) abnormal cholecystogram, ultrasound
5) signs of obstructed bile flow
   a) jaundice, pruritus
   b) clay-colored stools, dark amber urine

b. Plans, Implementation, and Evaluation

Goal 1: Client with an acute attack will be comfortable and relieved of symptoms.

Plan/Implementation

- Relieve pain with analgesics as ordered; meperidine (Demerol) is usually ordered since morphine causes spasms of bile ducts.
- Relieve reflex spasms with antispasmodics PRN as ordered; nitroglycerin may be used to relax smooth muscle.
- Relieve vomiting and decrease gastric stimulation with NG tube to suction.
- Give broad-spectrum antibiotics as ordered (ampicillin, tetracycline, cephalosporins are frequently used).
- Relieve pruritus: tepid cornstarch baths, cortisone ointments.

Evaluation: Client is pain free without itching, nausea, vomiting.

Goal 2: Client will recover from surgery without complications (refer to General Nursing Plans page 157).

Plan/Implementation

- Provide liberal pain medication (post-op pain is severe).
- Place in low to semi-Fowler's position; encourage frequent coughing and deep breathing to prevent atelectasis.
- Change dressings as needed (bile with a pH of 7.6–7.8 is very irritating to skin).
- Care for T-tube if present
  – avoid tension and obstruction of tubing
  – measure amount of drainage carefully, record as output (drainage will be 200–1,000 ml/day for 1st several days; continuing large amounts indicate obstruction)
  – clamp as ordered in 3–4 days before or after meals; assess tolerance
  – usually removed 10–12 days post-op following T-tube cholangiogram to determine status of duct
- Advance from clear liquids to diet as tolerated when ordered.

Evaluation: Client recovers from surgery free from skin irritation, diet intolerance, biliary tract complications; ambulates without difficulty.

☐ Pancreatitis

1. General Information

a. Definition: inflammation of the pancreas resulting in
   1) autodigestion by the trapped pancreatic enzymes
   2) obstruction and edema
   3) interstitial hemorrhage and tissue necrosis
b. Types
   1) acute: with or without hemorrhage; mortality rate is about 10%; pancreas returns to near normal following successful treatment
   2) chronic: organ destruction similar to acute, but normal tissue replaced by scar with tissue loss and ductal obstruction causing deficiencies in exocrine secretion
c. Risk factors
   1) alcohol abuse
   2) gallbladder disease
   3) abdominal trauma
   4) infections (especially viral)
   5) peptic ulcer disease
   6) many cases have no identifiable cause
d. Medical treatment: generally conservative: control pain, rest pancreas, support nutrition and hydration

2. Nursing Process

a. Assessment/Analysis

1) extreme epigastric pain extending to back
2) vomiting
3) abdominal distention
4) elevated serum amylase and lipase
5) elevated urinary amylase
6) low-grade fever
7) shock (kinin is a vasodilator activated by trypsin secretion)
8) jaundice
9) hyperglycemia

b. Plans, Implementation, and Evaluation

Goal 1: Client will be free from or have minimal pain.

Plan/Implementation
- Keep NPO until inflammation subsides.
- Know that meperidine (Demerol) is narcotic of choice; morphine is contraindicated since it causes spasm of the sphincter of Oddi.
- Give anticholinergics such as propantheline (Pro-Banthine) as ordered, to decrease secretions and relax the sphincter.
- Administer antacids frequently in mild cases.

Evaluation: Client states pain is subsiding.

Goal 2: Client will be free from shock in the acute phase (refer to "Shock" in *Oxygenation* page 170).

Goal 3: Client will maintain adequate nutrition.

Plan/Implementation
- Maintain NPO during acute phase, NG suctioning may be used. Specific mouth care orders.
- Administer total parenteral nutrition (TPN) as ordered if inflammation persists.
- Give clear liquids or elemental diet such as Vivonex after the inflammation subsides; progress to a low fat, bland diet.
- Teach to avoid stimulants, alcohol.
- Monitor blood sugar, urine sugar and acetone levels (PRN insulin may be necessary).
- Know that pancreatic enzymes may be given to aid fat digestion in chronic pancreatitis if attack is severe.

Evaluation: Client is free from nutritional deficiencies, digestive problems; ingests and tolerates prescribed diet; has no weight loss; chooses bland foods from diet menu.

Goal 4: Client will institute measures to prevent chronic pancreatitis.

Plan/Implementation
- Discuss with client ways to eliminate the underlying cause when possible.
- Suggest alcohol rehabilitation programs if indicated.

Evaluation: Client has no recurrences; joins and consistently attends Alcoholics Anonymous.

☐ Hepatitis

1. General Information

a. Definition: acute inflammatory disease of the liver caused by virus (most common), bacteria, and toxic or chemical injury.

b. Viral

1) type A

a) mode of transmission
- person-to-person via oral, fecal, or respiratory route
- contaminated food (particularly milk and shellfish), polluted water are commonly involved
- contaminated syringes and needles

b) incubation: 2–7 weeks

c) incidence
- worldwide
- higher during fall and winter months
- higher among children and young adults, those in institutional care

2) type B

a) mode of transmission
- parenteral route
- blood or blood component transfusions from an infected person
- contaminated needles and syringes
- mucosal transmission: dental instruments or venereal contact

b) incubation: 6 weeks to 6 months (average 2½–3 months)

c) incidence
- worldwide
- higher among recipients of blood and blood products (e.g., surgical, dialysis clients)
- users of illicit parenteral drugs

3) non-A/non-B: little is known; occurs in clients with multiple blood transfusions; treated similarly to hepatitis B

c. Pathophysiology

1) inflammatory infiltration of hepatic tissue

2) simultaneous inflammation, degeneration, and regeneration of cells

3) hyperplasia of Kupffer cells

d. Medical treatment

1) rest; nutritional support

2) interventions to minimize transmission

2. Nursing Process

a. Assessment/Analysis

1) jaundice

2) clay-colored stools

3) dark amber urine (bilirubin and urobilinogen excreted in urine)

4) pruritis (bile salts accumulate in skin)

5) right upper quadrant abdominal pain (stretching of liver capsule)

6) large tender liver

7) anorexia, nausea (visceral reflexes reduce peristalsis)

8) fatigue and weakness (reduced energy metabolism)

9) abnormal liver functions tests (increased bilirubin, SGOT, SGPT)
10) fever (inflammatory release of pyrogens)—rare in type B
11) bleeding tendencies in severe cases (reduced prothrombin synthesis)

b. Plans, Implementation, and Evaluation

Goal 1: Significant others and staff will be protected from the client's infection.

Plan/Implementation

- Know that if client has positive hepatitis antigen without signs of active disease, isolation is not needed except for precautions with syringes, needles, and blood products.

Hepatitis A

- Place client on enteric precautions.
- Use gown, gloves when in direct contact with client, blood, or excreta.
- Use disposable eating utensils and dishes.
- Use good handwashing techniques.
- Use hospital protocol and clearly label all linens.
- Provide gamma globulin to close household and sexual contacts.

Hepatitis B

- Place client on blood/body fluid precautions.
- Use gown, gloves when in direct contact with body fluids.
- Discard needles and syringes in appropriate containers; *do not recap needles.*
- Give hepatitis B immune globulin to exposed contacts.
- Advise hepatitis B vaccine for high risk persons (e.g., dialysis, critical care and emergency room, medical/dental personnel).

Evaluation: Staff members and client's significant others remain free from disease.

Goal 2: Client will have reduced metabolic demand on liver.

Plan/Implementation

- Place on bedrest; explain reason to client
  - limit activities until symptoms have subsided
  - provide environment for adequate rest
  - provide diversionary activities as needed
- Monitor liver function tests throughout care.
- Avoid administering drugs toxic to the liver; use sedatives and opiates with caution.
- Provide general comfort measures and interventions to control pruritis (refer to "Cholecystitis" Goal 1, page 211).

Evaluation: Client rests most of the day; sleeps throughout the night.

Goal 3: Client will have adequate nutrition.

Plan/Implementation

- Encourage well-balanced diet with adequate nutrients and calories; restrict fats if poorly tolerated; encourage fluids.
- Use mild antiemetics if needed prior to meals; offer small frequent meals.
- Know that good nutrition is hard to maintain because of anorexia and nausea.
- Have food available at client's bedside (e.g., hard candy).

Evaluation: Client's nutritional status appears adequate (no weight loss, intake equals output, normal energy level).

Goal 4: Client will remain free from reinfection.

Plan/Implementation

- Health teaching and preventive measures: type A
  - encourage optimal sanitation practices
  - instruct client in good personal hygiene
  - instruct client not to donate blood
- Health teaching and preventive measures: type B
  - instruct client not to donate blood
  - teach client to avoid sexual activity until liver function tests have returned to normal
  - test clients with history of drug abuse for hepatitis B antigen/antibody regularly

Evaluation: Client states methods to prevent transmission and recurrence.

☐ Cirrhosis

1. General Information

a. Definition: chronic disease with destruction of liver cells followed by cell regeneration and an increase in connective tissue; impaired function of liver and obstruction of venous and sinusoidal channels causing portal hypertension

b. Incidence: twice as common in men than women, higher in people 40–60 years old

c. Predisposing/precipitating factors
1) malnutrition
2) effects of alcohol abuse
3) chronic impairment of bile excretion
4) necrosis from hepatotoxins or viral hepatitis
5) chronic congestive heart failure

d. Pathophysiology
1) fatty infiltration of the liver
2) acute inflammation and tissue degeneration

3) obstruction of hepatic blood flow and elevation of venous pressure

e. Medical treatment

1) rest, nutritional and fluid support
2) prevent further liver damage

2. Nursing Process

a. Assessment/Analysis

1) early signs
   a) history of failing health
   b) anorexia, nausea, indigestion
   c) aching or heaviness in right upper quadrant
   d) fatigue
2) later signs
   a) abnormal liver function tests: elevated bilirubin, SGOT, SGPT, alkaline phosphatase
   b) intermittent jaundice
   c) edema and ascites, prominent abdominal wall veins, decreased serum albumin
   d) bleeding tendencies, prolonged prothrombin time, decreased platelet count
   e) anemia: folic acid deficiency, decreased RBC production, increased RBC destruction in spleen
   f) frequent infections, decreased WBC
   g) hormonal abnormalities, elevated estrogen levels
      - palmar erythema, vascular spiders
      - testicular atrophy, gynecomastia, amenorrhea

b. Plans, Implementation, and Evaluation

Goal 1: Client will have reduced metabolic demands on liver.

Plan/Implementation

- Provide bedrest during periods of acute malfunction.
- Have client rest before and between activities if anemia becomes worse.
- Eliminate ingestion of all substances toxic to liver: sedatives and opiates, alcohol.

Evaluation: Client rests quietly most of the day; keeps activities to a minimum; sleeps through the night.

Goal 2: Client will have adequate nutrition and hydration.

Plan/Implementation

- Give a high protein/carbohydrate/calorie (over 2,000), sodium-restricted diet.
- Plan small, frequent meals.
- Administer multiple-vitamin therapy as ordered (higher doses of thiamine and fat-soluble vitamins if there is deficient fat absorption).
- Restrict fluids and sodium intake if there is edema and/or ascites.
- Provide mouth care before meals (foul taste may be present).

Evaluation: Client eats prescribed diet; is adequately hydrated; maintains weight.

Goal 3: Client will be free from infection.

Plan/Implementation

- Encourage scrupulous personal hygiene.
- Know that reverse isolation may be necessary with extreme leukopenia.
- Assess for signs of urinary or respiratory infection.
- Turn frequently to prevent any skin breakdown.

Evaluation: Client has normal temperature; remains free from skin abrasions or inflammation.

Goal 4: Client will be protected from bleeding.

Plan/Implementation

- Monitor urine, stool, gums, skin for signs of bleeding or bruising.
- Avoid injections; apply pressure to venipuncture sites for at least 5 minutes.
- Monitor prothrombin time and PTT.
- Teach client to use soft toothbrush for oral care.
- Handle client gently and prevent scratching from pruritis.
- Administer vitamin K as ordered.

Evaluation: Client remains free of bleeding.

☐ Complications of Liver Disease: Esophageal Varices, Ascites, Hepatic Encephalopathy

1. General Information: Esophageal Varices

a. Definition: dilation of collateral veins that bypass a scarred liver to carry portal blood to vena cava; may occur in lower esophagus and stomach

b. Pathophysiology

1) as liver becomes increasingly cirrhotic, portal hypertension increases
2) collateral circulation in the esophagus develops in vessels that are weaker than normal vessels
3) as pressure in collateral vessels increases, they become overdistended and can rupture and bleed

c. Usually asymptomatic until the varices rupture
d. With hemorrhage mortality rate is greater than 50%
e. Treatment
   1) medical intervention: Sengstaken-Blakemore tube; vasopressin infusion
   2) surgical intervention: portacaval shunt (anastomosis between the portal vein and inferior vena cava [has a high mortality rate])

2. Nursing Process

a. Assessment/Analysis

1) abrupt active bleeding following
   a) increased abdominal pressure (physical exertion, Valsalva maneuver, coughing)
   b) mechanical trauma (abrasions from swallowing poorly chewed food)
   c) esophageal irritation by HCl, pepsin
2) hematemesis
3) signs of shock

b. Plan, Implementation, and Evaluation

Goal: Client will have esophageal bleeding effectively controlled.

Plan/Implementation
- If bleeding occurs perform gastric lavage with saline continuously until the returns are clear.
- Administer antacids as ordered.
- Monitor and treat client for shock as needed (see "Shock" in oxygenation, page 170)
  - administer blood transfusions as ordered
  - administer vitamin K to correct clotting problems
- Assist with insertion of Sengstaken-Blakemore tube
  - ensure balloon patency and accurate labeling of all ports prior to insertion
  - monitor balloon pressure frequently (at least q10)
  - assist client to expectorate secretions or gently suction oral cavity (client cannot swallow around tube)
  - monitor airway (danger of airway obstruction if tube moves)
  - provide comfort measures e.g., mouth and nasal care, positioning (esophageal balloon may be left inflated for up to 48 hours)
- Administer saline cathartics, lactulose, and enemas as ordered to reduce ammonia formation and possibility of hepatic coma.
- Give intestinal antimicrobials (e.g., neomycin) as ordered to decrease intestinal bacterial action.

Evaluation: Client's esophageal bleeding is promptly identified and controlled; condition remains stable.

3. General Information: Ascites

a. Definition: an abnormal intraperitoneal accumulation of watery fluid containing small amounts of protein
b. Pathophysiology
   1) portal hypertension
   2) decreased albumin production in liver; decreased colloidal osmotic pressure
   3) decreased removal of aldosterone by liver: sodium and water retention
c. Medical treatment
   1) medical intervention
      a) sodium-restricted diet
      b) diuretics
      c) paracentesis: removal of fluids from the peritoneal cavity; indicated if respiratory distress is present
   2) surgical intervention: LeVeen Shunt (placement of a catheter to shunt ascites from peritoneum to inferior vena cava)

4. Nursing Process

a. Assessment/Analysis

1) enlarged abdominal girth
2) fatigue
3) nutritional status: dehydration, malnutrition
4) abdominal pain, discomfort
5) respiratory difficulty
6) increased weight

b. Plan, Implementation, and Evaluation

Goal: Client will experience a reduction of ascites, and increased comfort.

Plan/Implementation
- Monitor fluid and electrolyte balance, I&O.
- Monitor daily weights.
- Measure abdominal girth at least every shift.
- Maintain high-Fowler's position for maximum respiratory effectiveness and comfort.
- Support abdomen with pillows.
- Maintain bedrest or restricted activity.
- Give sodium-restricted diet (usually no more than 1 gram daily).
- Administer diuretics as ordered (spironolactone [Aldactone] is drug of choice since it is potassium-sparing).
- Administer salt-poor albumin IV as ordered for

hypoalbuminemia; monitor carefully for signs of congestive heart failure, pulmonary edema.

- Assist with paracentesis if performed
  - have client void before the procedure
  - monitor client during and after the paracentesis for tachycardia, shock, dyspnea, and dizziness
  - observe puncture wound for leakage, signs of infection

Evaluation: Client is comfortable; undergoes paracentesis without complications; has ascites reduced; experiences a reduction in abdominal girth and respiratory distress.

5. General Information: Hepatic Encephalopathy

a. Definition: cerebral dysfunction associated with severe liver disease

b. Pathophysiology: inability of the liver to detoxify ammonia (convert ammonia to urea); cause is loss of functioning hepatic cells or no filtration of ammonia because blood bypasses liver

c. Higher incidence among clients who have had a portacaval shunt

6. Nursing Process

a. Assessment/Analysis

1) mental status, level of consciousness: lethargy → coma
- dullness, slurred speech
- behavioral changes, lack of interest in grooming or appearance

2) neurologic exam: twitching, muscular incoordination, asterixis (a flapping tremor)

3) elevated serum ammonia level

4) history of liver disease, portacaval shunt

b. Plans, Implementation, and Evaluation

Goal 1: Client will have decreased ammonia production.

Plan/Implementation

- Decrease ammonia formation in the intestine
  - prevent constipation
  - give laxatives, enemas as ordered
  - administer lactulose (Cephulac) and neomycin (oral or rectal) as ordered
- Reduce dietary protein to 20–40 gm/day (see Table 3.38); maintain adequate calories.

Evaluation: Client's serum ammonia level returns to normal limits; client tolerates a low protein diet.

Goal 2: Client will remain free from injury.

Plan/Implementation

- Perform general nursing measures for the unconscious client (refer to *Safety and Security* page 274).
- Assess mental status frequently.

Evaluation: Client regains consciousness free from injury.

Goal 3: Client and significant others will learn to prevent future episodes of encephalopathy.

Plan/Implementation

- Counsel client regarding low protein diet.
- Ensure client/family understand how to avoid and treat constipation.
- Ensure that client has an appointment for return follow-up care with physician.
- Teach family early signs of encephalopathy.

Evaluation: Client states measures to ensure proper bowel functioning; states principles of a low protein diet and planned rest periods.

The Endocrine System

General Concepts

Overview/Physiology

1. The endocrine system is a chemical communication system that functions together with the nervous system as the body's communication network

a. Endocrine glands synthesize and secrete chemical substnaces (hormones) that control and integrate body functions (see Table 3.27 on page 217)

1) secreted in minute amounts

2) circulated in the blood

3) regulated by

a) negative feedback systems

b) changes in the plasma concentration of specific substances

c) direct autonomic nervous system activity

d) circadian rhythms

4) action alters specific physiologic responses

a) growth and development

b) reproduction

c) metabolism

d) responses to stress and injury

b. Health problems involving the endocrine system result from hormone imbalances

1) primary problems: involvement of the

Table 3.27 Hormones

Gland	Hormone	Action
Hypothalamus	Releasing hormones	Stimulate relase of hormones from pituitary gland.
	Inhibiting hormones	Inhibit release of hormones from pituitary gland.
	ADH	See Pituitary, posterior lobe.
Pituitary, anterior lobe	Growth hormone (GH)	Acts directly on bones and other tissues to stimulate growth.
	Prolactin (LTH)	Stimulates development of mammary tissue and lactation.
	Thryotropic hormone (TSH)	Stimulates thyroid gland.
	Adrenocorticotropic hormone (ACTH)	Stimulates adrenal cortex.
	Melanocyte-stimulating hormone (MSH)	Stimulates darkening of the skin.
	Luteinizing hormone (LH)	Initiates ovulation and formation of corpus luteum.
	Follicle-stimulating hormone (FSH)	*Women*: stimulates ovarian development of graffian follicle. *Men*: maintains spermatogenesis.
Pituitary, posterior lobe	Antidiuretic hormone (ADH): produced in hypothalamus and stored in pituitary	Facilitates reabsorption of H_2O in the kidneys, vasoconstriction in arterioles.
	Oxytocin	Initiates expression of breast milk; stimulates uterine contractions at delivery.
Thyroid	Triiodothyronine (T_3) Thyroxine (T_4)	Control body metabolism and influence physical and mental growth; nervous system activity; protein, fat, carbohydrate metabolism; reproduction.
	Calcitonin	Lowers serum calcium levels, inhibits bone resorption.
Parathyroid	Parathormone (PTH)	Regulates calcium and phosphorus metabolism.
Pancreas	*Endocrine function* Insulin	Enables glucose to freely enter cells; helps muscle and tissue oxidation of glucose; promotes storage of glycogen.
	Glucagon	Increases gluconeogenesis in liver.
	Exocrine function (digestive enzymes)	
	Amylase	Aids carbohydrate digestion.
	Trypsin	Aids protein digestion.
	Lipase	Aids fat digestion.
Adrenal cortex	Glucocorticoids: cortisone, cortisol	Decrease protein synthesis; regulate serum glucose by increasing rate of gluconeogenesis; suppress the inflammatory and immune response; increase fat mobilization; support adaptation during stressful situations.
	Mineralocorticoids: aldosterone	Facilitate reabsorption of NA^+ and elimination of K^+.
	Sex hormones: primarily androgens	Responsible for development of secondary sex characteristics.
Adrenal medulla	Epinephrine	Initiates stress response.
	Norepinephrine	Causes vasoconstriction.
Ovaries	Estrogen	Responsible for secondary sex characteristics, mammary duct system, growth of graffian follicle in women.
	Progesterone	Prepares corpus luteum; maintains pregnancy.
Testes	Testosterone	Responsible for secondary sex characteristics, normal reproductive function in men.

target gland of the hormone

2) secondary problems: involvement of the primary gland of secretion (i.e., pituitary or hypothalamus)

2. Glands
   a. Pituitary
      1) anatomy
         a) lies in the sella tursica above the sphenoid at the base of the brain
         b) consists of two lobes connected by the hypothalamus
      2) functions (see Table 3.27)
         a) anterior lobe (adenohypophysis) secretes ACTH, MSH, TSH, FSH, GH, and prolactin
         b) posterior lobe (neurohypophysis) secretes ADH (vasopressin) and oxytocin
         c) regulates the function of the other endocrine glands through the stimulation of target organs
         d) controlled through the action of releasing and inhibiting factors from the hypothalamus
   b. Thyroid gland
      1) anatomy
         a) located at or below the cricoid cartilage in the neck, anterior to the trachea
         b) consists of two highly vascular lobes
      2) functions (see Table 3.27)
         a) controls the rate of body metabolism through the production of thyroxine (T_4) and triiodothyronine (T_3)
         b) produces calcitonin
   c. Parathyroid glands
      1) anatomy: four small glands located near or imbedded in the thyroid gland
      2) functions: secrete parathyroid hormone (PTH) and control calcium and phosphorus metabolism in the body
   d. Adrenal glands
      1) anatomy: two small glands lying in the retroperitoneal region, capping each kidney
      2) functions (see Table 3.27)
         a) adrenal cortex (outer capsule)
            - secretes the adrenocortical steroids (cortisol, cortisone, corticosterone)
            - secretes the mineralocorticoids (aldosterone)
            - secretes the adrenal sex hormones (androgen, estrogen, progesterone)
         b) adrenal medulla (inner parenchyma of gland)
            - stimulated by the sympathetic nervous system
            - secretes catecholamines (epinephrine and norepinephrine)
   e. Pancreas
      1) anatomy
         a) long, soft gland that lies retroperitoneally
         b) head of the gland is in the duodenal cavity and the tail lies against the spleen
      2) functions
         a) exocrine function to produce digestive enzymes
         b) endocrine function to control carbohydrate metabolism
            - glucagon secreted by alpha cells
            - insulin secreted by beta cells

Application of the Nursing Process to the Client with Endocrine System Problems

1. **Assessment**

   Hormones have very diverse systemic effects. Hypofunction or hyperfunction can result in dysfunction in a wide variety of organs and organ systems.
   a. Health history
      1) current symptoms
         a) change in client's energy level or stamina
         b) change in personal appearance
            - size of head, hands, or feet
            - weight, skin, or hair
            - secondary sex characteristics
         c) increased sympathetic nervous system activity
         d) change in alertness or personality
         e) change in sexual functioning
      2) past or family history
         a) abnormal progression in growth and development
         b) family history of diabetes, hypertension, infertility, mental illness
   b. Physical exam
      1) inspection: subtle or dramatic deviations from normal in body size, muscle tone, skin, hair, voice, and sexual characteristics
      2) palpation: limited to the thyroid gland
   c. Diagnostic tests
      1) measurement of the amounts of hormones present in serum or urine
      2) fluctuations in daily pattern of secretion means random specimens have limited value

d. Medical treatment
 1) medical intervention: replacement therapy, diet adjustment
 2) surgical intervention: partial or total gland removal

2. **Analysis**
 a. Safe, effective care environment
  1) knowledge deficit
  2) potential for injury
 b. Physiological integrity
  1) activity intolerance
  2) potential fluid volume deficit
  3) altered nutrition: more or less than body requirements
 c. Psychological integrity
  1) anxiety
  2) ineffective individual coping
  3) body image disturbance
 d. Health promotion/maintenance
  1) impaired adjustment
  2) noncompliance
  3) health-seeking behaviors

3. **General Nursing Plans, Implementation, and Evaluation** (refer to General Nursing Goals 1, 3, 4, for Digestive Tract Problems, page 204)

Goal 4: Client will adapt to changes in body image.

Plan/Implementation
- Assess client's perceptions of body.
- Encourage client to verbalize concerns.
- Provide client with correct information about the degree of symptom reversibility.

Evaluation: Client expresses self-acceptance and engages in usual social activities.

Selected Health Problems

☐ Hyperpituitarism

1. General Information

a. Definition: oversecretion of one or more hormones of the pituitary gland, frequently caused by tumors
 1) anterior pituitary → acromegaly or giantism
 2) posterior pituitary → syndrome of inappropriate secretion of ADH (SIADH)
b. Incidence
 1) acromegaly
  a) insidious onset in middle age
  b) more common in women than men
 2) SIADH
  a) may be triggered by malignancies or the stress of surgery and anesthesia
  b) syndrome is usually self-limiting
c. Diagnosis
 1) acromegaly
  a) thorough history and inspection
  b) plasma levels of GH
  c) skull x-rays, CAT scan
 2) SIADH
  a) clinical picture of sudden weight gain with decreasing urinary output
  b) serum sodium below 125 mEq/liter
  c) urine osmolality usually higher than plasma osmolality
d. Medical treatment
 1) acromegaly: surgical hypophysectomy by transsphenoidal approach if possible
 2) SIADH: strict fluid restriction to less than 1,000 ml/day

2. Nursing Process

a. **Assessment/Analysis**
 1) acromegaly
  a) increases in hat, shoe, and glove size
  b) protruding jaw, enlarged nose, jaw, hands, feet
  c) headache
 2) SIADH
  a) falling urine output
  b) sudden weight gain
  c) decreasing level of consciousness
  d) signs of sodium and potassium imbalance (see Table 3.33)

b. **Plans, Implementation, and Evaluation**

Goal 1: Client who has been treated by transsphenoidal hypophysectomy will be free from post-op complications.

Plan/Implementation
- Refer to "Intracranial Surgery" in *Safety and Security* page 276.
- Note any nasal leakage of cerebrospinal fluid.
- Prevent increased ICP.
- Monitor signs of diabetes insipidus or adrenal crisis.

Evaluation: Client remains free from post-op infection or alteration in mental status; maintains stable vital signs and fluid balance.

Goal 2: Client treated by hypophysectomy will be prepared for knowledgeable self-care (see General Nursing Goals 2 and 4 page 204).

Plan/Implementation

- Provide information about the importance of lifelong replacement therapy with regular medical supervision.

Evaluation: Client follows prescribed medication regimen, experiences minimal fluctuations in hormone levels, expresses self-acceptance.

Goal 3: Client with SIADH will reestablish normal fluid and electrolyte balance.

Plan/Implementation

- Restrict fluid intake as ordered (less than 1,000 ml/day).
- Maintain accurate I&O and daily weight records.
- Monitor for symptoms of sodium or potassium imbalance.
- Assess for signs of cerebral edema (refer to *Safety and Security* page 274).

Evaluation: Client's weight is stable; urinary output is within acceptable limits.

☐ Hypopituitarism

1. General Information

a. Definition: undersecretion of one or more of the hormones of the pituitary gland caused by disease, tumor, postpartum hemorrhage (Sheehan's syndrome), neurologic surgery, or trauma
   1) anterior pituitary → failure of GH secretion followed by failure of secretion of other hormones
   2) posterior pituitary → diabetes insipidus from failure of secretion of ADH

b. Diagnosis: see "Hyperpituitarism" page 219

c. Medical treatment: supplementary administration of the deficient pituitary hormones
   1) corticosteroids
   2) thyroid hormone
   3) growth hormone
   4) sex hormones
   5) vasopressin (pitressin)

2. Nursing Process

a. Assessment/Analysis

   1) anterior pituitary hypofunction
      a) dwarfism in children (GH)
      b) decreased stress tolerance (ACTH)
      c) decreased metabolism (TSH)
      d) menstrual irregularities, decreased or altered secondary sex characteristics (gonadotropin)
   2) posterior pituitary hypofunction: diabetes insipidus
      a) excessively high urinary output
      b) low urinary specific gravity
      c) elevated serum osmolality
      d) signs of dehydration and hypernatremia

b. Plans, Implementation, and Evaluation

Goal 1: Cient's hormone levels will be restored and maintained in the normal range.

Plan/Implementation

- Provide information about medications (i.e., name, dosage, side effects) and the importance of lifelong replacement with ongoing medical supervision.
- Teach client the effects of physical and psychologic stress on hormone needs.

Evaluation: Client follows prescribed medication regimen; adjusts life-style to maintain hormone balance.

Goal 2: Client with diabetes insipidus will reestablish and maintain normal fluid and electrolyte balance.

Plan/Implementation

- Administer replacement fluids as ordered.
- Keep accurate I&O; monitor daily weight, urine specific gravity.
- Monitor for signs of hypovolemic shock (refer to "Shock" in *Oxygenation* page 170).
- Administer vasopressin nasal spray or vasopressin (Pitressin) IM as ordered (usually every 36–72 hours).
- Teach client safe administration of nasal preparation.
- Teach signs and symptoms of fluid volume excess.

Evaluation: Client's fluid balance is within normal limits; client self-administers replacement medications safely.

☐ Hyperthyroidism (Graves' Disease)

1. General Information

a. Definition: oversecretion of the thyroid gland; second to diabetes in incidence; also called thyrotoxicosis
   1) a recurrent syndrome; may appear after emotional shock, stress, or infection
   2) occurs primarily in women 30–50 years of age
   3) a variety of causes have been identified including adenoma, goiter, viral

inflammation, and autoimmune glandular stimulation

b. Diagnosis
   1) elevated T_3, T_4, PBI, ^{131}I uptake values
   2) abnormal findings from thyroid scan

c. Complications
   1) cardiovascular disease
   2) exophthalmos owing to abnormal deposits of fat and fluid in the retro-ocular tissue
   3) thyroid storm or crisis: an extreme physiologic state of life-threatening hypermetabolism

d. Medical treatment
   1) medications
      a) propylthiouricil (PTU): antithyroid drug that depresses the synthesis of thyroid hormone; takes about three months to be completely effective
      b) iodine preparations (SSKI): decrease the size and vascularity of the gland (short-term use)
      c) propranolol (Inderal): adrenergic antagonist that relieves the adrenergic effects of excess thyroid hormone (e.g, sweating, tachycardia, tremors)
   2) radioactive iodine: limits the secretion of hormone by damaging or destroying thyroid tissue; treatment of choice for most adults
   3) surgical intervention (only performed when client is in a euthyroid state)
      a) subtotal thyroidectomy
      b) total thyroidectomy (if carcinoma present)

2. Nursing Process

a. Assessment/Analysis
   1) cardiovascular: elevated BP, bounding pulse, tachycardia, palpitations
   2) nutrition: weight loss, increased appetite, frequent stools
   3) integument: flushed, moist skin; heat intolerance
   4) musculoskeletal: fatigue, muscle weakness and wasting, fine tremors
   5) psychologic: anxiety, insomnia, mood swings, personality changes
   6) other: menstrual irregularities, change in libido
   7) exophthalmos

b. Plans, Implementation, and Evaluation

Goal 1: Client will return to and remain in euthyroid state.

Plan/Implementation
- Provide calm, restful physical environment with low levels of sensory stimulation
  - ensure physical comfort; comfortable environmental temperature
  - provide adequate rest
- Provide adequate nutrients
  - high-calorie (4,000–5,000), balanced diet
  - increased fluid intake
- Provide eye care if exophthalmos present
  - eye drops, dark glasses, patch eyes if necessary
  - elevate head of bed for sleep

Evaluation: Client enjoys restful sleep; verbalizes decreased discomfort and fatigue; maintains or increases body weight; is free from corneal damage.

Goal 2: Client undergoing thyroidectomy will be free from post-op complications.

Plan/Implementation
- Prepare client's room prior to return from OR with O_2, suction, tracheostomy set, and calcium gluconate at bedside.
- Monitor for signs of bleeding or excessive edema
  - elevate head of bed 30°; support head and neck
  - check dressings frequently, assess for constriction
  - check behind the neck for bleeding
- Assess for signs of respiratory distress, hoarseness (laryngeal damage is common)
- Be alert for the possibility of
  - tetany (owing to hypocalcemia caused by accidental removal of parathyroid glands)
  - thyroid storm: markedly increased temperature and pulse with increasing restlessness and agitation
- Administer food and fluid with care (dysphagia is common).

Evaluation: Client maintains normal vital signs; experiences no excessive bleeding or respiratory distress; supports head and neck during movement.

Goal 3: Client will maintain normal levels of thyroid hormone.

Plan/Implementation
- Provide client with information about prescribed medications (i.e., name, dosage, side effects) and the importance of ongoing medical supervision
  - total thyroidectomy necessitates lifelong

replacement medication
  - subtotal thyroidectomy necessitates careful monitoring of the return of thyroid function
- Teach client receiving radioactive iodine treatment symptoms of thyroid deficiency (hypothyroidism is common within 2–5 years).

Evaluation: Client follows prescribed medication regimen; is euthyroid.

☐ Hypothyroidism

1. General Information

a. Definitions: underactive state of the thyroid gland resulting in diminished secretion of thyroid hormone
  1) *cretinism*: deficiency occurring in infancy and childhood
  2) *myxedema*: deficiency occuring in adulthood, usually in the fifth to sixth decade; affects women five times more frequently than men

b. Diagnosis
  1) decreased T_3 and T_4
  2) elevated TSH and cholesterol

d. Complications
  1) cretinism: severe physical and mental retardation
  2) myxedema
    a) accelerated development of coronary artery disease
    b) organic psychosis
    c) myxedema coma: rapid development of impaired consciousness and suppression of vital functions

e. Medical treatment: thyroid replacement
  1) levothyroxine (Synthroid) is the drug of choice, if client does not have disabling cardiac involvement
  2) liothyronine (Cytomel) is useful in clients who experience allergic responses to other preparations

2. Nursing Process

a. Assessment/Analysis
  1) fatigue, weight gain, constipation
  2) dry skin, cold intolerance
  3) coarse, thinning hair
  4) mental sluggishness
  5) thick tongue, swollen lips
  6) menstrual irregularities, infertility
  7) extreme sensitivity to narcotics, barbiturates, anesthetics

b. Plan, Implementation, and Evaluation

Goal: Client will return to and remain in an euthyroid state.

Plan/Implementation
- Provide a warm environment conducive to rest.
- Avoid use of all sedatives.
- Assist client in choosing low calorie diet.
- Increase intake of fluid and roughage to relieve constipation.
- Increase physical activity and sensory stimulation gradually as condition improves.
- Monitor cardiovascular response to increased hormone levels carefully.
- Provide information about prescribed medication (i.e., name, dosage, side effects) and the importance of lifelong medical supervision.

Evaluation: Client follows prescribed medication regimen; loses weight; experiences increased activity tolerance and alertness

☐ Hyperparathyroidism

1. General Information

a. Definition: overactivity of one or more of the parathyroid glands
  1) primary: a problem within the gland itself; usually benign adenomas
  2) secondary: a compensatory response to other conditions that produce hypocalcemia (e.g., vitamin D deficiency, chronic renal disease, malabsorption)

b. Diagnosis
  1) elevated serum calcium, with low serum phosphate; elevated parathormone (PTH) levels
  2) x-rays show demineralization of bones, bone cysts, especially in hands

c. Complications
  1) renal stones/failure
  2) cardiac dysrhythmias
  3) bone fractures or collapse

d. Medical treatment
  1) medical intervention to lower calcium level
    a) hydration with normal saline, plus diuretics
    b) calcium-blocking agents
  2) surgical intervention: parathyroidectomy leaving any disease-free glands intact

2. Nursing Process

a. Assessment/Analysis (*NOTE*: Most clients are clinically asymptomatic.)

1) skeletal pain, weakness, fatigue, backache
2) vague abdominal pain, nausea and vomiting, constipation
3) depression, mental dullness
4) cardiac dysrhythmias
5) renal colic, stones

b. Plan, Implementation, and Evaluation

Goal: Client undergoing parathyroidectomy will be free from complications.

Plan/Implementation

- Provide low calcium diet pre-op; avoid milk and milk products.
- Encourage high fluid intake pre-op (at least 3,000 ml/day).
- Perform general post-op care as for thyroidectomy, and in addition
  - observe carefully for tetany
  - institute *high* calcium diet
- Encourage ambulation to stimulate bone recalcification.

Evaluation: Client maintains calcium values within normal range; experiences normal muscle functioning; follows prescribed diet.

☐ Hypoparathyroidism

1. General Information

a. Definition: Failure of the parathyroid glands to produce adequate amounts of PTH

b. Precipitating causes
1) usually surgically induced by thyroidectomy
2) idiopathic forms, possibly autoimmune in nature, are rare

c. Diagnosis
1) low serum calcium
2) elevated serum phosphate

d. Complications
1) cardiac dysrhythmias
2) premature cataract formation

e. Medical treatment
1) oral calcium preparations
2) high-dose vitamin D
3) aluminum hydroxide (Amphogel or Basalgel) to lower serum phosphate

2. Nursing Process

a. Assessment/Analysis

1) signs of tetany
   a) positive Chvostek's and Trousseau's signs
   b) muscle spasms
   c) tingling of fingers and around lips
2) cardiac dysrhythmias

b. Plan, Implementation, and Evaluation

Goal: Client will be free from the complications of prolonged calcium imbalance.

Plan/Implementation

- Acute stage
  - assess for symptoms of tetany frequently
  - keep calcium gluconate at bedside
- Chronic stage
  - provide high calcium, low phosphorus diet
  - provide information about prescribed medications (i.e., name, dosage, side effects)
- Teach client symptoms of calcium imbalance.

Evaluation: Client follows prescribed medication and diet regimen; is free from the symptoms of hypocalcemia.

☐ Hyperfunction of the Adrenal Glands

1. General Information

a. Definition: oversecretion of hormones from either the adrenal cortex or adrenal medulla
1) Cushing's syndrome: excessive secretion of glucocorticoids and possibly androgens from the adrenal cortex
2) pheochromocytoma: catecholamine-producing tumor of the adrenal medulla

b. Incidence
1) Cushing's syndrome
   a) true Cushing's syndrome is relatively rare, but occurs most frequently in women aged 20–60
   b) can result from adrenal tumors or excessive pituitary secretion of ACTH from any cause
   c) a common result of the chronic use of exogenous steroids
2) pheochromocytoma
   a) rare disorder; may occur in middle age in either sex
   b) has a familial tendency

c. Diagnosis
1) Cushing's syndrome
   a) increased plasma cortisol, blood glucose, urinary 17-hydroxysteroids and 17-ketosteroids; decreased potassium
2) pheochromocytoma
   a) elevated 24-hour urine vanillylmandelic acid (VMA) (*NOTE*: Client must avoid ingestion of fruits, coffee, vanilla, and chocolate prior to this test)
   b) elevated urine metanephrines

d. Complications
   1) Cushing's syndrome
      a) cardiac problems (e.g., CHF, hypertension)
      b) skeletal fractures
      c) opportunistic infections
   2) pheochromocytoma
      a) CVA
      b) renal damage
      c) blindness
e. Medical treatment
   1) Cushing's syndrome
      a) surgical adrenalectomy if tumor is present
      b) hypophysectomy for tumor of pituitary
      c) drug therapy with cortisol inhibitors
      d) alteration in exogenous steroid dose if possible
   2) pheochromocytoma
      a) surgical adrenalectomy
      b) pre-op drug therapy with alpha- and beta-blocking agents

2. Nursing Process

a. Assessment/Analysis

1) Cushing's syndrome
   a) abnormal fat distribution
      - weight gain, thick trunk, thin legs
      - moon face, buffalo hump (cervical dorsal fat pad)
   b) skin changes
      - thin fragile skin, red cheeks
      - purple striae (stretch marks)
      - bruises, acne
      - body hirsutism
   c) cardiovascular
      - hypertension
      - fluid overload, CHF
      - sodium and water retention, hypokalemia
   d) musculoskeletal
      - muscle weakness, decreased muscle mass, fatigue
      - osteoporosis, bone pain, fractures
   e) increased susceptibility to infection
   f) decreased resistance to stress
   g) increased secretion of pepsin and HCl acid
   h) hyperglycemia
   i) mental changes and mood swings
   j) changes in secondary sex characteristics, menstrual irregularities, amenorrhea
2) pheochromocytoma
   a) labile hypertension
   b) tachycardia, palpitations
   c) diaphoresis

b. Plans, Implementation, and Evaluation

Goal 1: Client with Cushing's syndrome will have fewer symptoms.

Plan/Implementation

- Provide diet low in calories and sodium, high in protein, potassium, and calcium
  - offer diet in small, frequent feedings
  - monitor for signs of hyperglycemia, GI bleeding
- Protect client from unnecessary exposure to infection
  - monitor vital signs regularly
  - use strict hygiene and asepsis
  - institute reverse isolation if needed
- Provide atmosphere conducive to rest; space activities and assist with care as needed.
- Observe for signs of CHF.
- Monitor daily weights, I&O, blood and urine glucose measurements.
- Offer needed support in dealing with changes in body image.

Evaluation: Client maintains or loses weight; experiences increased strength and stamina; is free from infection, accidental injury, or peptic ulceration; refers to self in a positive way.

Goal 2: Client treated with adrenalectomy will be free from complications.

Plan/Implementation

- Measure urine output accurately and frequently.
- Monitor vital signs frequently.
- Watch for signs of adrenal crisis; have IV fluids, pressor drugs, corticosteroids readily available.
- Minimize physiologic and psychological stress.
- Prevent thrombotic and respiratory problems.
- Monitor wound healing carefully.
- Teach regarding post-discharge self-care (e.g., diet, medications, activity level, follow-up care).

Evaluation: Client maintains stable vital signs, adequate urine output and respiratory gas exchange post-op; states self-care needs to expect after discharge.

Goal 3: Client with pheochromocytoma will have BP controlled prior to surgery.

Plan/Implementation

- Administer antihypertensives or blocking agents as ordered; monitor vital signs frequently.

- Provide rest and control anxiety.
- Provide sedation if needed.

Evaluation: Client's BP remains within prescribed parameters; client is free from palpitations or tachycardia.

☐ Hyposecretion of the Adrenal Glands

1. General Information

a. Definition: Addison's disease: insufficient secretion of glucocorticoids, mineralocorticoids, and possibly androgens from the adrenal cortex

b. Incidence
   1) rare disease occurring in 1 in 100,000; affects both sexes and usually occurs in middle age
   2) true Addison's is usually idiopathic but will occur after bilateral surgical removal of the adrenal glands

c. Diagnosis
   1) low serum cortisol levels
   2) low serum sodium and glucose
   3) elevated serum potassium

d. Complications: adrenal crisis: acute adrenal insufficiency with sudden, marked deprivation of adrenocortical hormones producing cardiovascular collapse

e. Medical intervention: steroid replacement maintained throughout life
   1) glucocorticoids
      a) cortisone usually given for maintenance
      b) hydrocortisone given in emergencies
      c) dose will need to be increased at any time of increased stress, including illness or surgery
   2) mineralocorticoids: fludrocortisone (Florinef) 0.05–0.2 mg daily (if more needed, long-acting preparation may be given)
   3) periodic testosterone injections to support protein anabolism

2. Nursing Process

a. **Assessment/Analysis** (*NOTE*: The clinical picture from the history and symptoms is often vague.)
   1) lethargy, apathy, loss of concentration
   2) gastrointestinal symptoms: anorexia, nausea, weight loss, abdominal pain
   3) bronzing of skin (from excess MSH production)
   4) muscle weakness and fatigue
   5) hypotension, fluid deficit
   6) hypoglycemia

b. **Plans, Implementation, and Evaluation**

Goal 1: Client will recover from an adrenal crisis.

Plan/Implementation
- Give large dose of glucocorticoids and vasopressors by IV infusion.
- Encourage complete bedrest; prevent physical activity and emotional stress.
- Monitor vital signs and fluid and electrolyte balance until condition stabilizes.

Evaluation: Client maintains vital signs within normal limits; exercises and returns to normal activity levels gradually.

Goal 2: Client will maintain normal hormonal balance.

Plan/Implementation
- Provide information about prescribed medications (i.e., name, dosage, side effects) and the importance of ongoing medical supervision.
- Teach to balance activity and rest, maintain a regular activity pattern.
- Promote good nutrition; monitor weight, fluid status, and I&O.
- Assist client to deal effectively with stress.
- Teach client the signs and symptoms of under- or overdose of medications, and conditions that will require dosage adjustments.

Evaluation: Client is asymptomatic; takes and adjusts medications as indicated; maintains ongoing medical care.

☐ Hypofunction of the Pancreas: Diabetes Mellitus

1. General Information

a. Definition: a chronic systemic disease producing disorders in carbohydrate, protein, and fat metabolism; results from disturbances in the production, action, or utilization of insulin; eventually produces destructive changes in a wide variety of organs and tissues. The insulin deficiency may be relative or absolute.

b. Incidence
   1) most common endocrine disorder; more than 10 million diabetics in the US
   2) diabetes and its complications are among the leading causes of death and disability in the US

Table 3.28 Steroid Drugs

Drugs	Action	Uses	Side Effects	Nursing Implications
Dexamethasone (Decadron) Hydrocortisone (Cortef, Solu-Cortef) Prednisone (Deltasone) Betamethasone Valerate (Valisone cream or ointment) Methylpredisolone Acetate (Medrol) Triamcinolone Acetate (Kenalog cream or ointment)	• Blocks inflammatory, allergic, & immune responses	• Replacement therapy • Inflammatory, allergic, & autoimmune responses	• Impaired wound healing • Salt & water retention • Leukopenia • GI ulceration (increased HCl secretion) • Hypertension • Diabetes • Cataracts • Osteoporosis • Hypokalemia • Sterility • Fatty redistribution • Protein catabolism • Hirsutism • Decreased growth in children	Teach: •• The need to avoid infections •• The need to increase steroids during times of physical & emotional stress •• Take with antacids •• Drugs cannot be abruptly stopped; tapering is needed •• Carry an ID stating steroid therapy is being used •• Side effects: body-image changes & how to minimize by a low salt & carbohydrate, high potassium diet •• Take in the morning to mimic normal release

c. Etiology
  1) basic etiology remains unknown
  2) considered to be a group of syndromes whose development is influenced by genetic factors, viruses, autoimmunity, and environmental factors such as stress and obesity

d. Types
  1) Type 1 (insulin dependent): results from destruction of the beta cells of the pancreas resulting in little or no insulin production; requires daily insulin administration
  2) Type 2 (non-insulin dependent): probably results from a disturbance in insulin reception in the cells; most common in middle aged, overweight adults

e. Pathophysiology: Type 1
  1) normally blood-glucose levels are maintained in the homeostatic range of 60–100 mg/100 ml by a series of feedback mechanisms
  2) in the absence of insulin, glucose accumulates in blood and urine leading to
    a) hyperglycemia
    b) glycosuria
  3) glucose is hypertonic and depletes the body of large amounts of water (from extracellular fluid) as it is excreted by the kidneys causing
    a) polyuria
    b) polydipsia
    c) loss of sodium and potassium
  4) glucose is then not available for cellular nutrition and this causes polyphagia
  5) fat and protein stores are broken down and used for energy; so utilization of these stores is not sufficient, causing
    a) ketoacidosis
    b) ketonuria
    c) weakness
  6) other metabolic effects
    a) micro- and macrocirculatory changes producing athero- and arteriosclerosis (e.g., coronary artery disease, peripheral vascular disease, retinal and kidney damage)
    b) alteration in immune and inflammatory response
      ■ glucose concentration in the skin creates an excellent medium for infection
      ■ glucose inhibits the phagocytic action of leukocytes → decreased resistance
    c) alterations in perception and coordination caused by developing neuropathies (a common complication the cause of which is poorly understood)

f. Pathophysiology: Type 2
- **1)** serum insulin level may be low, normal or even elevated
- **2)** pathology thought to be a combination of
  - **a)** slowed response in insulin release
  - **b)** reduced number of insulin receptors
  - **c)** receptor abnormality to insulin binding
  - **d)** peripheral resistance to insulin

g. Medical treatment
- **1)** drug therapy (see Table 3.29)
  - **a)** insulin: short-, intermediate-, and long-acting forms
  - **b)** oral hypoglycemic agents
- **2)** diet: individually planned regimens based on the client's age, sex, weight, and usual life-style (see Table 3.30)
  - **a)** diet is manipulated to distribute the nutrient intake appropriately over a 24-hour period
  - **b)** diet is planned using the American Diabetic Association's (ADA) exchange method of meal planning
  - **c)** diet is used to correct obesity when necessary
- **3)** exercise

2. Nursing Process

a. Assessment/Analysis
- **1)** type 1: initial symptoms
  - **a)** polyphagia, polyuria, polydipsia, weight loss
  - **b)** hyperglycemia, glycosuria, ketonuria
  - **c)** weakness, fatigue
- **2)** type 2: initial symptoms
  - **a)** may be asymptomatic
  - **b)** may have classic type 1 signs
  - **c)** weakness, fatigue, weight gain
  - **d)** hyperglycemia, glycosuria
- **3)** Glucose tolerance test is abnormal

Table 3.29 Hypoglycemic Agents

Description	Drugs that act to either stimulate the islet cells in the pancreas to secrete more insulin (oral) or act as insulin replacement when pancreatic function ceases (parenteral)
Uses	Treatment of diabetes mellitus
Side Effects	Hypoglycemic reactions, GI distress, neurologic symptoms, alcohol intolerance (oral preparations), allergic reactions
Nursing Implications	Know onset and duration of action for each agent and teach to client; monitor for and teach client to monitor for hypoglycemic reaction; stress compliance with total diabetic regimen; check for beef or pork allergy (insulin preparations); teach client self-administration of insulin including proper storage, care of equipment, site rotation, urine testing for sugar and acetone, and serum glucose checks (finger stick). Purified insulins are used infrequently as intermittent therapy or for patients with insulin allergy, lipodystrophy, gestational diabetes, or massive insulin resistance. They cannot be used interchangeably with standard purity insulin.

Types of Examples	Peak (hours)	Duration (hours)
Oral Agents		
Acetohexamide (Dymelor)		12–24
Chlorpropamide (Diabinese)	3–6	24
Tolbutamide (Orinase)	5–8	6–12
Tolazamide (Tolinase)	10	16
Glipizide (Glucotrol)	1–3	up to 24
Glyburide (Diabeta, Micronase)	2–8	24
Insulin (Usually are standard purity)		
Rapid acting (onset 1 hour)		
Crystalline zinc	2–4	5–8
Regular	2–4	4–6
Insulin zinc suspension prompt (Semilente)	6–10	12–16
Regular human (Humulin-R, Novolin-R)	1–3	3–5
Intermediate acting (onset 2–4 hours)		
Globin zinc (Iletin)	6–10	18–24
Isophane insulin suspension (NPH)	8–12	28–32
Insulin zinc suspension (Lente)	8–12	28–30
NPH human insulin isophane (Humulin-N, Novolin-N)	8–12	26–30
Long acting (onset 4–6 hours)		
Protamine zinc (PZI)	16–24	24–36
Insulin zinc suspension extended (Ultralente)	16–24	more than 36
Lente human insulin	16–24	24–30

b. Plans, Implementation, and Evaluation

Goal 1: Client will demonstrate knowledge of the principles of diet control.

Plan/Implementation

- Assess client's knowledge of a diabetic diet.
- Reinforce teaching of the dietician as needed.
- Encourage client to use the individualized meal plan.
- Reinforce the importance of not skipping meals.
- Measure foods accurately; do not estimate them.
- Discuss with client the diet modifications needed to compensate for changes in life-style or illness.
- Assist Type 2 client to lose weight as indicated.

Evaluation: Client makes appropriate selections from sample menus; maintains normal body weight; maintains fasting blood-sugar levels within normal ranges.

Goal 2: Client will correctly administer insulin, or other hypoglycemic agent as indicated.

Plan/Implementation

- Assess client's knowledge of hypoglycemics.
- Teach client preparation of injection, storage of insulin, and the principles of site rotation
  - insulin in current use may be stored at room temperature, all others in refrigerator or cool area
  - insulin must be at room temperature before administration
  - roll insulin to mix, double-check label concentration
  - if client mixes insulin, do so in same sequence each day; e.g., always draw up regular or shorter-acting insulin first followed by longer-acting preparations (i.e., clear to cloudy)
  - rotate sites so that no one site is used more frequently than once a month; know that switching from separate injections to a mixture of insulins in one injection may alter local response
  - inject at 45° or 90° angle
  - press, do not rub the site after injection
  - avoid smoking for 30 minutes after injection (cigarette smoking decreases absorption)
- Provide opportunities for multiple return demonstrations.
- Teach at least one family member to administer insulin.
- Teach client factors that influence the body's need for insulin
  - increased need: trauma, infection, fever, severe psychologic or physiologic stress, smoking marijuana
  - decreased need: active exercise

Evaluation: Client properly administers own insulin; shows no signs of lipodystrophy.

Goal 3: Client will monitor diabetic status regularly and correctly through the use of finger sticks or urine testing.

Plan/Implementation

- Assess client's knowledge of glucose monitoring.
- Teach client the principles of urine testing (used primarily for ketone monitoring)
  - consistent use of one product
  - test before meals and at bedtime using a fresh urine sample
  - record results in percentages
- Teach client about common medications that interfere with urine test results (e.g., vitamin C, cephalosporin antibiotics)
- Teach client proper technique for finger sticks
  - follow product guide carefully for timing results
  - use sides of fingers or earlobe
- Keep accurate date and time records for both urine and finger-stick testing.
- Teach client to notify physician if urine tests greater than 1% or finger-stick results are greater than the physician-specified limit.

Evaluation: Client demonstrates accurate urine testing and/or finger-stick glucose measurements; correctly interprets the results; maintains consistent, accurate records of the results; knows when to contact physician.

Goal 4: Client will establish and maintain a pattern of regular exercise.

Plan/Implementation

- Assess client's knowledge of the relationship between exercise and diabetes.
- Individualize exercise plan for each client; tell Type 2 client to have a cardiovascular evaluation before beginning an exercise program.
- Tell client to perform exercise after meals to ensure an adequate level of blood glucose
  - teach Type 1 client to carry a rapid-acting source of glucose
  - teach client that excessive or unplanned exercise may trigger hypoglycemia

Table 3.30 Diabetic Meal Planning with Exchange Lists[1]

% of Total Calories Food Exchange Group	12%–20% Protein in gm	+55%–60% CHO in gm	per serving	+20%–30% Fat in gm	= 100% Calories
Milk	8	12		trace	80
Vegetable (½ cup)[2]	2	5		–	25
Fruit	–	10		–	40
Bread	2	15		–	70
Meat	7	–		3	55
Fat	–	–		5	45

[1]Note: From *Exchange Lists for Meal Planning*, 1976, American Diabetes Association, Inc., American Dietetic Association.
[2]Some vegetables in the vegetable exchange can be used freely when raw. Starchy vegetables are listed in the bread exchange list.

Examples of Foods in Exchange Lists

Free Foods	List 1 Milk Exchanges	List 2 Vegetable Exchanges	List 3 Fruit Exchanges	List 4 Bread Exchanges	List 5 Meat Exchanges	List 6 Fat Exchanges
Coffee, tea Clear broth Gelatin (unsweetened) Pepper and other spices	Whole milk (omit 2 fat exchanges) Skim milk Buttermilk made with skim milk	Asparagus Beets Broccoli Cabbage Cauliflower Cucumbers Chard Collards Mushrooms Onions Tomatoes Turnips Raw vegetables (List 2) Chicory Chinese cabbage Endive Escarole Lettuce Parsley Radishes Watercress	Apple Applesauce Banana Strawberries Cantaloupe Cherries Grapefruit Orange juice Pear Pineapple Prunes, dried Watermelon	Bread Cereals Spaghetti, noodles Crackers Beans and peas (dried and cooked) Corn Potatoes	Meat and poultry Cold cuts Frankfurters Eggs Fish Shrimp Cheese: cheddar, cottage Peanut butter	Butter or margarine Bacon (crisp) Cream Mayonnaise Nuts Olives

General Rules (for all clients to know and follow carefully):

1. Eat all meals about the same time daily. Do not skip meals.
2. Eat only those foods, in the amount given, on the diet list.
3. Do not eat between meals UNLESS it is part of the dietary plan, unless replacing food not eaten at a previous meal, or unless an insulin reaction is "coming on."

Replacement Meals for Illness[3]

1. Drink liquids hourly to replace losses.
2. Carbohydrates are necessary to prevent ketosis; use simple sugars for easy digestion, 50–70 gms every 8 hours.

Standard Meal Plan	CHO Content	Replacements	CHO Content
3 meat exchanges	0	2 cups broth	0
2 bread exchanges	30	1 cup ginger ale	20
2 fat exchanges	0	½ cup jello	20
1 fruit exchange	15	⅓ cup grape juice	15
1 milk exchange	12	hot tea	0
	57 gm		55 gm

[3]From: G. Burtis, J. Davis, & S. Martin. *Applied Nutrition and Diet Therapy*. W.B. Saunders Co., 1988, used with permission.

Evaluation: Client engages in planned regular exercise without experiencing difficulties with hypoglycemia.

Goal 5: Client will practice good personal hygiene and positive health promotion to avoid diabetic complications.

Plan/Implementation

- Assess client's knowledge of health promotion/ complications.
- Teach client diabetic foot care
  - daily gentle cleansing and inspection
  - properly fitting shoes
  - use lanolin cream to prevent dryness and cracking of heels
  - avoid going barefoot
  - wear socks with shoes
  - visit a podiatrist regularly for care of nails, calluses, corns
- Teach client interventions to prevent peripheral vascular disease (refer to "Circulatory Problems" in *Oxygenation* page 183).
- Teach client the adjustments that must be made in the event of minor illness (e.g., colds, flu)
  - continue taking insulin or oral hypoglycemic regularly (infection increases the body's need for insulin)
  - maintain fluid intake, replace diet with appropriate liquids if unable to eat solid food (see Table 3.30)
  - increase the frequency of blood/ketone testing
  - contact physician if necessary
- Assist client to identify stressful situations in life-style that might interfere with good diabetic control.
- Encourage regular checkups by dentist and good daily hygiene.
- Advise regular eye exams.
- Teach aggressive care for minor skin cuts and abrasions; avoid clothing and activities that cause chafing and irritation.

Evaluation: Client maintains teeth and gums in good repair; maintains soft, intact skin; states adjustments that are to be made to maintain control during periods of minor illness.

Goal 6: Client will recognize the signs of hypoglycemia and ketoacidosis and take appropriate actions.

Table 3.31 Differentiating Hypoglycemia from Ketoacidosis (Hyperglycemia)

	Hypoglycemia (Insulin Reaction)	Ketoacidosis (Diabetic Coma)
Causes	Too much insulin, not enough food (delayed or missed meals), excessive exercise or work, diarrhea, vomiting	Too little insulin, too much or wrong kind of food, infection, illness, injuries, emotional stress
Onset	Sudden: regular insulin Gradual: modified insulin or oral hypoglycemic drugs	Gradual
Symptoms	Sweating, pallor, cold clammy skin, irritability, nervousness, tachycardia and palpitations, weakness and fatigue, headache, hunger, confusion, blurred vision; shallow, rapid respirations	Thirst, increased urination, nausea and vomiting, abdominal pain, headache, weakness and fatigue; late signs include symptoms of dehydration, Kussmaul respirations, fruity odor to breath, lethargy → coma
Urine	Negative for sugar and acetone	Positive for sugar and acetone
Blood Glucose	60 mg or less/100 ml	Greater than 400 mg/100 ml
Treatment	• Give about 10 gm carbohydrate – 4 oz fruit juice, or – 2 tsp corn syrup, or – 2 tsp honey, or – 5 Life Savers, or – 1 glass soft drink. • If client is unable to swallow, squeeze concentrated glucose between gums into mouth (Reactose, Glucose, Cake Mate, a decorating gel). • If necessary, 50% glucose IV may be given. • Obtain blood and urine specimens for lab testing. • Give complex carbohydrates from diet (e.g., crackers, milk) about 1 hour after treatment.	• Keep client flat in bed, and warm. • Have client, if conscious, drink liquids such as coffee, tea, broth, water, bouillon. • Record I&O • Obtain blood and urine specimens for lab testing. • Check and record vital signs and level of consciousness. • Administer parenteral fluids as ordered. • Administer regular insulin as ordered. • Connect to cardiac monitor and observe for potassium imbalance.

Plan/Implementation

- Assess client's knowledge about hypo-/hyperglycemia.
- Teach signs of hypoglycemia and the situations that may trigger it (see Table 3.31 for symptoms)
  - too much insulin or too little food
  - strenuous unplanned exercise
  - vomiting or diarrhea
  - emotional upsets
- Teach client to reverse hypoglycemia if possible with 10–15 gm of a rapid-acting carbohydrate.
- Teach client signs of ketoacidosis and situations that may trigger it (see Table 3.31 for symptoms)
  - failure to take insulin
  - too much food
  - episode of illness, infection, stress
- Teach client that development of ketoacidosis requires immediate transport to a health care facility
  - correct dehydration by administration of IV fluids
  - correct blood sugar level with administration of insulin (usually low-dose insulin infusion)
  - replace electrolytes as ordered
  - record I&O accurately (Foley catheter is usually necessary)
  - monitor ketones and blood glucose at frequent intervals
  - assess for decreasing LOC and declining cardiopulmonary status at frequent intervals
- Tell client to wear a diabetic alert bracelet or tag at all times.

Evaluation: Client lists the symptoms of hypoglycemia and ketoacidosis and states appropriate actions to take for each; wears a diabetic alert tag.

References

Adams, C. (1983). Pulling your patient through adrenal crisis. *RN*, *46*(10), 36–38.

Anderson, F. (1986). Portal systemic encephalopathy in the chronic alcoholic. *Critical Care Quarterly*, *8*(4), 40–52.

Atkins, J., & Oakley, C. (1986). A nurse's guide to TPN. *RN*, *49*(6), 20–24.

Baker, W. (1985). Hypophosphatemia. *American Journal of Nursing*, *85*, 99–1003.

Bryant, R. (1986). Diverticular disease. *Journal of Enterostomal therapy*, *13*(3), 114–117.

Buckingham, A. (1986). Arterial blood gases made simple, *Nursing Life*, *5*(6), 48–51.

Caine, R., & Bufalino, P. (1987). *Nursing care planning guides for adults*. Baltimore: Williams & Wilkins.

Dodd, R. (1984). Ascites: When the liver can't cope. *RN*, *47*(10), 26–30.

†Forbes, K. & Stokes, S. (1984). Saving the diabetic foot. *American Journal of Nursing*, *84*, 884–888.

Fredette, S. (1984). When the liver fails. *American Journal of Nursing*, *84*, 64–67.

Fredholm, N., Vignati, L., & Brown, S. (1984). Insulin pumps: The patients verdict. *American Journal of Nursing*, *84*, 36–38.

Gannon, R., & Pickett, K. (1983). Jaundice. *American Journal of Nursing*, *83*, 404–407.

Gavin, J. (1988). Diabetes and exercise. *American Journal of Nursing*, *88*, 178–181.

Gever, L. (1984). Anticholinergics. *Nursing84*, *14*(9), 64.

Gever, L. (1984). Ranitidine: New relief for peptic ulcers? *Nursing84*, *6*(6), 22.

†Graham, S. & Morley, M. (1984). What "foot care" really means. *American Journal of Nursing*, *84*, 889–891.

Green-Hernandez, C. (1987). Surgery and diabetes. *American Journal of Nursing*, *87*, 788–793.

Kirkman-Liff, B. & Dandoy, S. (1984). Hepatitis B: What price exposure? *American Journal of Nursing*, *84*, 988–990.

Larson, C. (1984). The critical path of adrenocortical insufficiency. *Nursing84*, *14*(10), 66–69.

Masoorli, S., & Piercy, S. (1984). A life saving guide to blood products. *RN*, *47*(5), 32–42.

McAdams, R., & Birmingham, D. (1986). When diabetes races out of control. *RN*, *49*(5), 46–53.

McCarthy, J. (1985). The continuum of diabetic coma. *American Journal of Nursing*, *85*, 878–882.

Moree, N., Huey, F., & Burk, J. (1984). Gallstone dissolving agents. How do the new drugs measure up? *American Journal of Nursing*, *84*, 907–908.

Neal, M., Cohen, P., & Reighley, J. (Eds.). (1983). *Nursing care planning guides, set 3* (2nd ed.). Baltimore: Williams & Wilkins.

Patras, A., Paice, J., & Lanigan, K. (1984). Managing GI bleeding; It takes a two tract mind. *Nursing84*, *14*(7), 26–33.

Patras, A., Paice, J., & Lanigan, K. (1984). Managing GI bleeding. *Nursing84*, *14*, 26–34.

Robertson, C. (1986). When an insulin dependent diabetic must be NPO. *Nursing86*, *16*(6), 30–31.

Salmon, M., & Mathos, E. (1984). New insulins. *Nursing84*, *14*(8), 65.

Stock, P. (1985). Action stat! Insulin shock. *Nursing85*, *15*(4), 53.

Strange, J. (1983). An expert's guide to tubes and drains. *RN*, *46*(4), 35–42.

Sweet, K. (1983). Hiatal hernia—What to guard against most in postop patients. *Nursing83*, *13*(12), 39–45.

Thatcher, G. (1985). Insulin injections: The case against random rotation. *American Journal of Nursing*, *85*, 690–692.

Wimpsett, J. (1984). Trace your patient's liver dysfunction. *Nursing84*, *14*(8), 56–57.

---

*See reprint section

†Highly recommended

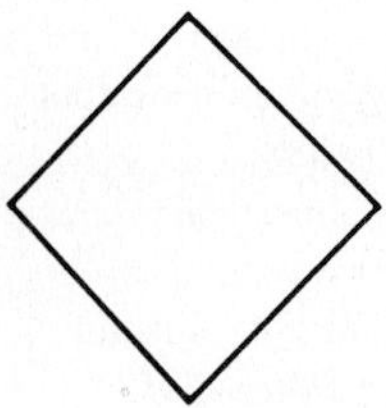

Elimination

(The nursing care presented in this unit concerns selected health problems related to disturbances in the kidneys and the large bowel.)

The Kidneys

General Concepts

Overview/Physiology

1. Kidneys
   - **a.** Location: paired organs that lie in the retroperitoneum at the costovertebral angle (CVA)
     - **1)** upper border: T-12
     - **2)** lower border: L-3
   - **b.** Size: 120–170 gm (4–6 oz) each
   - **c.** Regions (see Figure 3.14)
     - **1)** cortex
       - **a)** outer layer
       - **b)** contains glomeruli, proximal and distal tubules
     - **2)** medulla
       - **a)** middle layer
       - **b)** composed of 6–10 renal pyramids, formed by collecting ducts and tubules
       - **c)** deepest part of loop of Henle
     - **3)** pelvis
       - **a)** innermost layer
       - **b)** hollow collection area composed of calyces
       - **c)** papillae move urine into ureter by peristaltic action
   - **d.** Nephron (see Figure 3.15)
     - **1)** functional unit of kidney
     - **2)** one million nephrons in each kidney
     - **3)** composition
       - **a)** glomerulus
       - **b)** tubule
         - ■ Bowman's capsule
         - ■ proximal convoluted tubule
         - ■ loop of Henle
           - – descending limb
           - – ascending limb
         - ■ distal convoluted tubule
         - ■ collecting duct
     - **4)** action: all elements to be excreted or conserved are acted on in the nephron by the processes of filtration, concentration, reabsorption, or secretion
2. Ureters
   - **a.** Join with renal pelvis; distal end implanted in bladder
   - **b.** Composed of smooth muscles that have peristaltic action
   - **c.** Narrow at ureteropelvic junction, bifurcation of iliac vessels and join with bladder
3. Bladder
   - **a.** Stores urine until eliminated
   - **b.** Muscular organ (detrusor muscle)
4. Urethra
   - **a.** Passageway for urine during excretion
   - **b.** Surrounded by prostate gland in men
5. Functions of the kidney
   - **a.** Fluid and electrolyte balance
     - **1)** control of sodium balance
       - **a)** intake in normal diet is usually greater than needed
       - **b)** filtered by glomeruli
       - **c)** reabsorption in tubules is controlled by active and passive processes and by the renin-angiotensin-aldosterone system
     - **2)** control of chloride balance follows sodium
       - **a)** intake in normal diet is usually greater than needed
       - **b)** filtered by the glomeruli
       - **c)** actively transported out of the ascending loop of Henle
     - **3)** control of H_2O balance
       - **a)** intake controlled by social habits and thirst
       - **b)** reabsorption controlled by antidiuretic hormone (ADH) concentration in the collecting duct
     - **4)** control of potassium balance
       - **a)** intake adequate in normal diet
       - **b)** filtered by glomeruli

Figure 3.14 Components of the Kidney

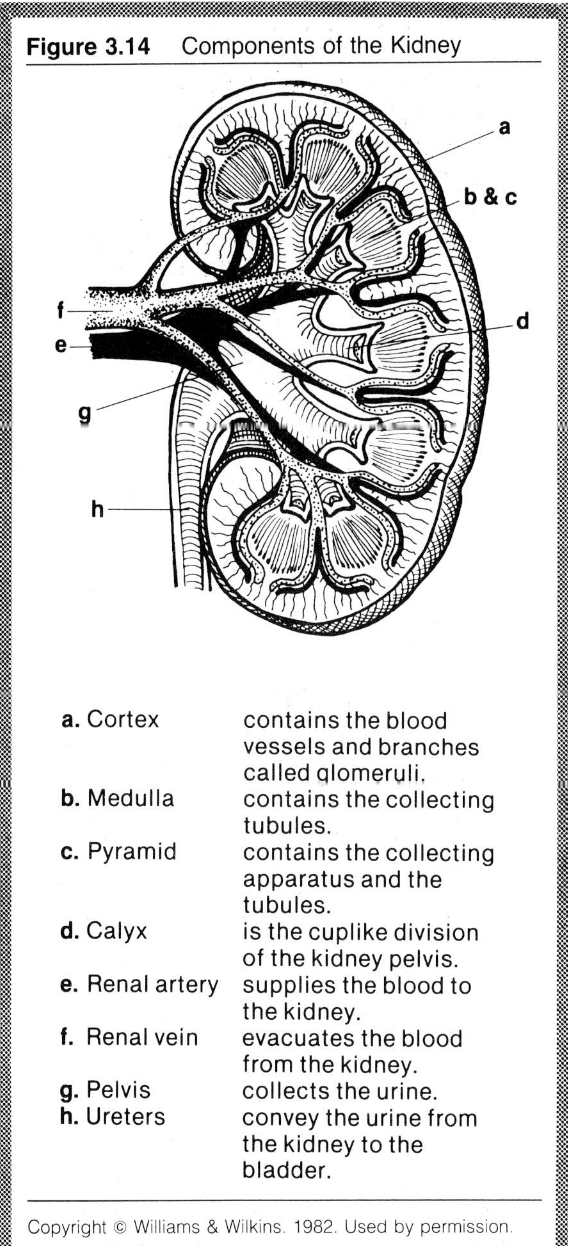

a. Cortex	contains the blood vessels and branches called glomeruli.
b. Medulla	contains the collecting tubules.
c. Pyramid	contains the collecting apparatus and the tubules.
d. Calyx	is the cuplike division of the kidney pelvis.
e. Renal artery	supplies the blood to the kidney.
f. Renal vein	evacuates the blood from the kidney.
g. Pelvis	collects the urine.
h. Ureters	convey the urine from the kidney to the bladder.

c) almost all filtered potassium is reabsorbed in proximal tubules

d) secreted into distal tubules and into distal ducts where there is selective secretion or reabsorption

e) dependent upon hormonal influence
- increase of aldosterone causes increased potassium secretion
- decrease of aldosterone causes decreased potassium secretion

f) potassium also lost through GI tract

b. Control of acid-base balance

1) excretion of organic acids

Figure 3.15 Components and Functions of the Nephron

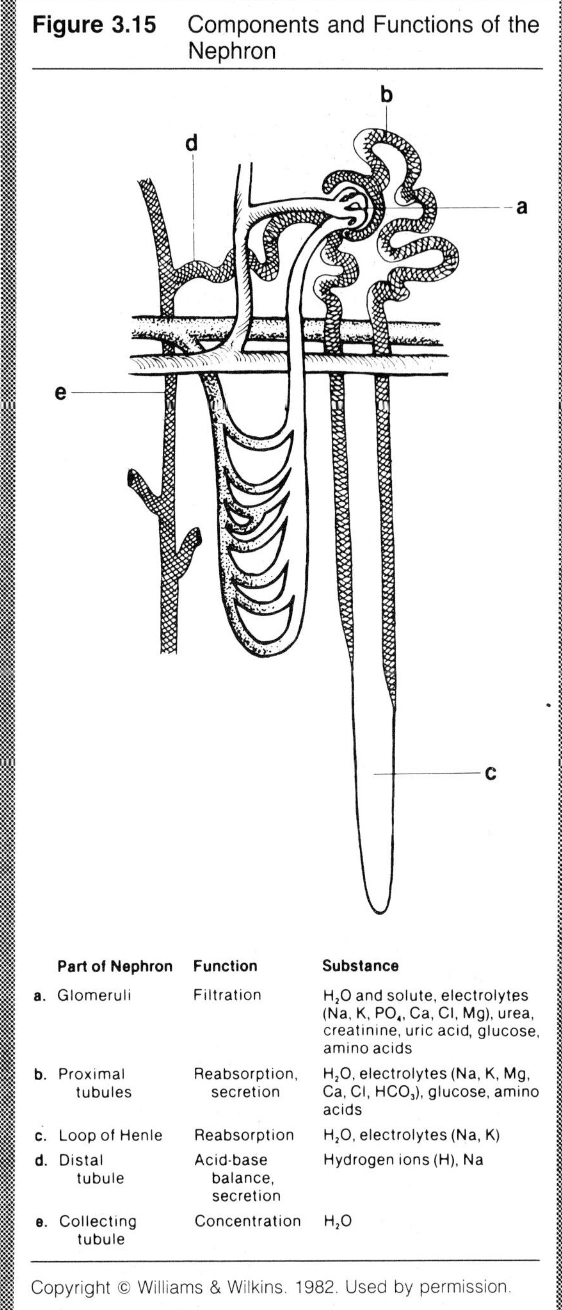

Part of Nephron	Function	Substance
a. Glomeruli	Filtration	H_2O and solute, electrolytes (Na, K, PO_4, Ca, Cl, Mg), urea, creatinine, uric acid, glucose, amino acids
b. Proximal tubules	Reabsorption, secretion	H_2O, electrolytes (Na, K, Mg, Ca, Cl, HCO_3), glucose, amino acids
c. Loop of Henle	Reabsorption	H_2O, electrolytes (Na, K)
d. Distal tubule	Acid-base balance, secretion	Hydrogen ions (H), Na
e. Collecting tubule	Concentration	H_2O

a) HPO_4 buffer system: $H + HPO_4 \rightarrow H_2PO_4$

b) NH_3 buffer system
- $NH_3 + H \rightarrow NH_4$
- $NH_4 + NaCl \rightarrow NH_4Cl + Na$

c) liberation of free hydrogen ions

2) conservation of bicarbonate

c. Excretion of waste products (primarily products of protein metabolism: urea and creatinine)

Table 3.32 Fluid Imbalance

Etiology	Assessment	Nursing Implications
Overhydration		
Renal failure Excessive fluid intake Excess IVs Water intoxication (GU irrigation with hypotonic fluids) Hypernatremia	Level of consciousness, vital signs, weight (increases), peripheral edema, venous pressure (increases), pulmonary edema, symptoms of CHF or increased intracranial pressure	*Prevention* • monitor IV fluids closely. • monitor urine output, I&O, weight. *Treatment* • reduce edema (e.g., positioning). • give diuretics as ordered. • limit intake. • maintain low sodium intake.
Dehydration		
Nausea and vomiting Increased urinary output Diuretics Insufficient intake (because of age, immobility, etc.) Inadequate replacement following excess fluid loss (diaphoresis, diarrhea)	Level of consciousness, vital signs, weight (may be decreased), skin turgor (poor), thirst, urine output	*Prevention* • monitor I&O. • replace lost fluids. • patient teaching re: excess perspiration. *Treatment* • replace fluids carefully. • monitor I&O, weight.

Table 3.33 Electrolyte Imbalances

	Problem	Etiology	Assessment	Nursing Implications
SODIUM	***Hypernatremia***			
	$Na^+ > 145$ mEq/L	*Hyperosmolar* Sodium increased in relation to water, water loss without sodium loss, dehydration	Increased hemoglobin, signs of dehydration, thirst, decreased BP, concentrated urine with high specific gravity	• Offer sodium-restricted diet, fluids. • Maintain strict I&O. • Prevent shock. • Maintain adequate urine output. • Monitor serum Na.
		Sodium excess Both sodium and water increased, renal failure, cirrhosis, steroid therapy, aldosterone excess	Edema, weight gain, hypertension, symptoms of fluid overload	• Offer low-sodium diet, water restriction. • Maintain strict I&O. • Monitor for signs of CHF or increased intracranial pressure. • Measure daily weight. • Administer diuretics (Na-wasting) as ordered.
	Hyponatremia			
	$Na^+ < 135$ mEq/L	*Hypo-osmolar or "dilutional"* Water increased in relation to sodium, water intoxication, exercise, IVs without NaCl, sodium-restricted diet	Fluid volume excess, increased urine output with low specific gravity, no thirst, nausea/vomiting, weakness/cerebral dysfunction	• Restrict water. • Monitor I&O, serum Na. • Watch for circulatory overload. • Replace Na carefully. • Give high Na diet.
		Sodium deficit Both sodium and water decreased, diuretics, GI losses, burns	Decreased BP, poor skin turgor, dehydration/shock, oliguria	• Monitor for shock. • Provide good skin care. • Give isotonic fluids. • Monitor I&O, serum Na.

(continued)

Table 3.33 Continued

	Problem	Etiology	Assessment	Nursing Implications
POTASSIUM	***Hyperkalemia***			
	$K^+ > 5.0$ mEq/L	Severe burns, crush injuries, Addison's disease, renal failure, acidosis, excessive K intake (oral or IV)	ECG changes (high T wave), skeletal muscle weakness, bradycardia, cardiac arrest, oliguria, intestinal colic and diarrhea	• Monitor cardiac function, serum K, neurologic signs. • Limit K intake. • Give D_{50} plus insulin as ordered. • Give exchange-resins (sodium polystyrene sulfonate [Kayexalate] PO or enemas) as ordered. • Give bicarbonate to correct acidosis. • Dialysis (renal/peritoneal).
	Hypokalemia			
	$K^+ < 3.5$ mEq/L	Diuretic therapy (thiazides), poor intake, GI loss, ulcerative colitis, Cushing's syndrome, alkalosis	Digitalis toxicity, muscle weakness and decreased reflexes, flaccid paralysis, paralytic ileus, CNS depression, lethargy, hypotension, anorexia, ECG changes (flattened T wave)	• Administer K slowly IV. • Monitor ECG. • Teach adequate K replacement when taking diuretics. • Administer PO K drugs/diet.
CALCIUM	***Hypercalcemia***			
	$Ca^{++} > 11$ mg	Immobility, hyperparathyroidism, bone metastasis, excess vitamin D intake, parathyroid tumor, osteoporosis, decreased renal excretion	Skeletal muscle weakness; bone pain; renal calculi; pathologic fractures; CNS depression, altered LOC; GI (constipation, nausea, vomiting, anorexia); decreased serum phosphorus	• Limit intake. • Patient teaching. • Prevent fractures. • Give phosphorus. • Maintain adequate I&O. • Monitor neurologic signs.
	Hypocalcemia			
	$Ca^{++} < 9$ mg	Hypoparathyroidism, low vitamin D in diet, parathyroidectomy, pregnancy and lactation, postthyroidectomy, rickets, renal disease	Tetany, tingling, paresthesias of fingers and around mouth/muscle twitching, cramps; positive Chvostek's and Trousseau's signs; laryngospasm; increased phosphorus	• Give Ca as needed. • Monitor for early muscle spasms, neurologic signs. • Monitor those at risk. • Give phosphate-binding antacids. • Monitor serum Ca.

(continued)

Table 3.33 Continued

	Problem	Etiology	Assessment	Nursing Implications
MAGNESIUM	***Hypermagnesemia***			
	$Mg^{++} > 2.8$ mEq/L	Renal insufficiency, diabetic ketoacidosis, excess Mg intake (antacids), dehydration	CNS and neuromuscular depression, hypotension, sedation, arrest	• Monitor replacement carefully. • Support respiration. • Teach client correct antacid intake. • Monitor neurologic signs.
	Hypomagnesemia			
	$Mg^{++} < 1.5$ mEq/L	Alcoholism, loss (GI diuresis), low intake, hypercalcemia, diabetes, toxemia, renal disease	Tremors and neuromuscular irritability, disorientation, positive Chvostek's and Trousseau's signs, convulsions	• Give Mg cautiously as ordered. • Monitor closely for Mg excess. • Teach adequate intake. • Monitor neurologic signs.

d. Production and secretion of erythropoietin in response to hypoxia (stimulates bone marrow to produce hemoglobin)

e. Manufacture and activation of vitamin D (plays a role in calcium metabolism: active form of vitamin D must be available for parathormone to work)

f. Regulation of arterial blood pressure: renin and aldosterone

- **1)** kidneys secrete an enzyme called renin, which acts on plasma protein to cause the release of angiotensin (a vasoconstricting substance)
- **2)** angiotensin increases total peripheral resistance leading to increased aldosterone secretion by adrenal cortex
- **3)** increased aldosterone stimulates increased sodium reabsorption
- **4)** increased sodium reabsorption leads to increased water retention and plasma volume, which increases arterial BP

Application of the Nursing Process to the Client with Kidney Problems

1. Assessment

a. Health history

- **1)** urinary retention, stasis (e.g., associated with pregnancy, neurogenic bladder, immobility, diabetes)
- **2)** bladder infections: caused by contamination from large intestine (especially young girls)
- **3)** intrusive procedures (e.g., catheterization, cystoscopy, coitus)
- **4)** bone demineralization
- **5)** metabolic disease
- **6)** changes in color (e.g., hematuria)
- **7)** changes in volume
  - **a)** polyuria: greater than 2,500 ml/day
  - **b)** oliguria: less than 400 ml/day
  - **c)** anuria: less than 100 ml/day
- **8)** changes in voiding pattern
  - **a)** nocturia
  - **b)** frequency
  - **c)** hesitancy
  - **d)** urgency
  - **e)** change in urinary stream
  - **f)** incontinence
    - ■ amount
    - ■ frequency of occurrence
    - ■ dribbling
- **9)** medications
  - **a)** diuretics
  - **b)** antibiotics
  - **c)** nephrotoxic agents: ASA, acetaminophen, mercaptomerin sodium, phenylbutazone, sulfonamides, gentamycin
  - **d)** cholinergics, anticholinergics

b. Physical examination

- **1)** inspection of genitals
- **2)** palpation of kidneys
- **3)** palpation of prostate
- **4)** pain
  - **a)** back
  - **b)** flank
  - **c)** CVA tenderness

c. Diagnostic tests (see Table 3.35)

- **1)** urine (visual inspection)

Table 3.34 Acid-Base Imbalance

Problem	Etiology	Assessment	Compensating Mechanisms	Nursing Implications
Respiratory Acidosis				
• pH < 7.35 • $pCO_2 > 45$ • HCO_3 normal	Hypoventilation • acute causes – respiratory infections – CNS depressant overdose – paralysis of respiratory muscles – atelectasis – brain damage – post-op abdominal distention • chronic causes – obesity – ascites – pregnancy.	Hypoventilation; tachycardia, irregular pulse; decreased chest excursion; headache, dizziness; cyanosis; drowsiness leading to coma.	Kidneys retain and manufacture more bicarbonate leading to • pH 7.4 • $pCO_2 > 45$ • $HCO_3 > 28$.	Turn, cough, and deep breathe qh. Suction prn. Monitor vital signs. Give respiratory stimulants as ordered. Give bronchodilators. Give O_2 cautiously to prevent CO_2 narcosis.
Respiratory Alkalosis				
• pH > 7.45 • $pCO_2 < 35$ • HCO_3 normal	Hyperventilation • emotions, hysteria • O_2 lack • fever • salicylate poisoning • CNS stimulation by drugs/disease.	Hyperventilation • light-headed • tingling of hands and face (tetany). Convulsions, diaphoresis, low serum K^+.	Kidneys excrete large amounts of bicarbonate leading to • pH 7.4 • $pCO_2 < 35$ • $HCO_3 < 23$.	Calm client. Slow the rate of ventilation. Use rebreather to increase pCO_2. Administer O_2 as needed.
Metabolic Acidosis				
• pH < 7.35 • pCO_2 normal • $HCO_3 < 23$	Bicarbonate loss • diarrhea • GI fistula. Acid gain • diabetic ketoacidosis • lactic acidosis • renal failure • salicylate intoxication • K^+ excess.	Headache, dizziness; Kussmaul's respiration; fruity breath odor; disoriented; coma; nausea/vomiting; high serum K^+.	Lungs hyperventilate to blow off CO_2 and reduce plasma carbonic acid content leading to • pH 7.4 • $pCO_2 < 35$ • $HCO_3 < 23$.	Administer sodium bicarbonate as ordered. Give insulin as ordered. Monitor I&O, vital signs. Support client.
Metabolic Alkalosis				
• pH > 7.45 • pCO_2 normal • $HCO_3 > 28$	Acid loss • vomiting or GI suction • steroid therapy • thiazide diuretics. Bicarbonate retention • excess use of bicarbonate (baking soda) as antacid • excess infusion of Ringer's lactate • citrated blood.	Headache, numbness and tingling leading to tetany and convulsions, hypoventilation, confusion and agitation, low serum K^+.	Lungs hypoventilate to retain CO_2 and increase plasma carbonic acid content leading to • pH 7.4 • $pCO_2 > 45$ • $HCO_3 > 28$.	Give IV ammonium chloride as ordered. Maintain K^+ level with diet or drugs. Teach client high K^+ diet if taking thiazide diuretics. Give acetazolamide (Diamox) as ordered. Maintain calm, quite environment.

a) color: pale to deep amber; changes with medication, food, or disease
b) volume: 30 ml or more/hour
c) appearance: clear
d) odor: strong ammonia after stored for a period of time

2) urinalysis

a) specific gravity: 1.015–1.025 (random samples)
- reflects concentrating ability of kidneys
- increases (greater than 1.035) with glucosuria, proteinuria, and dehydration

Table 3.35 Laboratory Tests Used to Evaluate Renal Function

Test	Normal Range	Usual Range in Renal Disease	What it Measures
Hemoglobin	12–18 gm/100 ml	Lowered	Formation of red blood cells
Blood urea nitrogen (BUN)	8–20 mg/100 ml	Elevated	Renal excretory function
Electrolytes Sodium	136–145 mEq/L	Elevated (not necessarily) or lowered	Fluid and electrolyte balance
Potassium	3.5–5 mEq/L	Elevated or lowered	Electrolyte balance
Chloride	90–102 mEq/L	Elevated (not necessarily) or lowered; has partnership with sodium	Fluid and electrolyte balance
Serum creatinine	0.4–1.2 mg/100 ml	Elevated	Renal function
Serum osmolarity	275–295 mOsm/L		Dissolved particles in the blood
Glucose	70–110 /100 ml	Slight hyperglycemia	
Blood pH Arterial Venous	 7.38–7.44 7.3–7.41	Usually lowered	Acidity vs. alkalinity of blood
Calcium	4–5 mEq/L	Usually lowered	Renal excretory function
Phosphorus	3.5–5.5 mEq/L	Elevated	Renal excretory function
Albumin	3.2–5.5 g/100 ml	Usually lowered	Albumin, (helps maintain blood's osmotic pressure)

Note: From "Renal Function Assessment," by E. Larson, 1982, in E. Larson, L. Lindbloom, & K. Davis, Eds. *Development of the clinical nephrology practitioner*. St. Louis: Mosby. Used with permission.

- decreases (less than 1.002) with distal renal tubular disease, endocrine disorders associated with insufficiency of ADH, and overhydration
- fixed (1.010) with glomerulonephritis

b) pH: 4.8–8.0
- reflects the acid-base balance
- greater than 8.0: alkaline; occurs with metabolic alkalosis, overuse of alkalizing medications, in presence of urinary tract infection (UTI)
- less than 4.8: acidic; occurs with metabolic acidosis, uncontrolled diabetes, some medications (e.g., ammonium chloride, high doses of vitamin C)

c) glucose
- normally not present
- may occur after heavy meal, emotional stress, or with infusion of glucose
- occurs abnormally with diabetes mellitus, pancreatic disorders, impaired reabsorption in the proximal tubules

d) ketones
- normally not present
- occur with uncontrolled diabetes, fasting, severe infections accompanied by nausea and vomiting

e) protein
- normally not present
- occurs with serious kidney or proximal tubular disorders, nephrotic syndrome, toxemia
- may occur after heavy protein meal, strenuous exercise, or prolonged standing

f) red blood cells
- normally 0–3/high power field
- increase with kidney malfunction or trauma to urinary tract or tumor or infection in urinary tract

g) white blood cells
- normally 0–4/high power field
- increase with infection within urinary tract system

h) hyaline casts
- normally not present
- indicate acute glomerulo- or

pyelonephritis, chronic renal disease, or renal calculi

i) granular casts
- normally not present
- indicates acute renal rejection (transplant), pyelonephritis, or chronic lead poisoning

3) urine culture and sensitivity
   a) voided specimen: bacterial count over 100,000 organisms/ml (if infection is cause)
   b) sterile, catheterized specimen: over 10,000 organisms/ml

4) tests of filtration function
   a) creatinine clearance (the most important test of kidney function)
   - amount of creatinine filtered by glomeruli (since creatinine is not reabsorbed and is only minimally secreted, this test is a measure of glomerular filtration rate)
   - determined by 24-hour urine specimen
   - normal values
     - 115 ± 20 ml/min
     - serum creatinine: 0.6–1.5 mg/100 ml
   - as glomerular filtration rate falls, serum creatinine rises and 24-hour urine creatinine decreases
   - advantage of serum creatinine: independent of protein metabolism

   b) blood urea nitrogen (BUN)
   - normal: 8–25 mg/100 ml
   - urea: end product of protein metabolism
   - increases with decrease in glomerular filtration
   - less reliable measure than serum creatinine because
     - after being filtered, urea is reabsorbed back into renal tubular cells
     - urea production varies according to the state of liver function, and protein intake and breakdown

5) radiologic tests
   a) KUB: kidney, ureters, bladder
   - simple x-ray without contrast medium
   - results indicate size, position, and any radiopaque calcifications

   b) tomography
   - x-ray at different angles: no contrast medium
   - useful for clear picture when colon and other organs block kidney
   - can distinguish solid tumors from cysts

   c) IVP: intravenous pyelogram (excretory urogram)
   - injection of contrast medium that is excreted by kidneys
   - allows visualization of kidneys, ureters, and bladder
   - used to diagnose masses, cysts, obstructions, renal trauma, bladder dysfunction
   - contraindicated in severe renal disease or dehydration and individuals allergic to shellfish or iodine
   - nursing care pretest
     - check for iodine allergies
     - ensure informed written consent is on the chart
     - tell client that a dye is injected and x-rays are taken at 2-, 5-, 10-, 15-, 20-, 30-, and 60-minute intervals
     - administer strong cathartic, enemas night before
     - NPO after midnight
     - have client void immediately prior to test
   - nursing care post-test: check for signs and symptoms of allergic reaction to dye and signs of acute renal failure

   d) nephrotomogram
   - techniques of tomography with IVP
   - provides a clearer visualization

   e) retrograde pyelogram
   - catheter is passed through urethra, urinary bladder, and into right or left ureter where contrast medium is injected
   - allows more detailed visualization of the urinary collecting system independent of the status of renal function
   - disadvantages: increased chances of trauma (catheter manipulation) and infection
   - nursing care pretest
     - check for iodine allergies
     - ensure informed written consent is on the chart
     - teach client concerning procedure

- administer cathartics, enemas evening before
- keep NPO after midnight

■ nursing care post-test
- observe amount of urine
- watch for hematuria
- watch for signs of urinary sepsis
- check for signs and symptoms of allergic reaction to dye

f) renal angiography, arteriography

■ catheter is introduced through the femoral artery to the renal artery

■ contrast medium is injected and 2–3 x-rays are taken at 2-second intervals

■ allows visualization of renal arteries, capillaries, and venous system

■ used to diagnose renal artery stenosis, renal masses, trauma, thrombosis, and obstructive uropathy

■ risks: bleeding, thrombosis, damage to vessels, allergic reaction

■ nursing care pretest
- check for iodine allergies
- ensure informed written consent is on the chart
- administer cathartics, enemas evening before
- ensure that chart contains hematologic evaluation
- have client void immediately prior to test

■ nursing care post-test
- maintain bedrest 12–24 hours; flat, no sitting
- check insertion site for hematoma formation
- check pressure dressing on insertion site
- monitor post-op vital signs
- check peripheral pulses distal to insertion site
- measure urine output

g) cystography

■ a flexible metal tube is inserted into the bladder and a dye is injected; x-rays are taken at 30-minute intervals

■ assesses bladder function and explores the possible presence of stones in the bladder

■ nursing care: same as retrograde pyelogram

h) cystoscopy

■ a cystoscope is inserted into bladder through the urethra

■ direct inspection of bladder to biopsy and resect tumors, to remove stones, cauterize bleeding areas, dilate ureters, and implant radium seeds

■ nursing care pretest
- ensure written informed consent is on the chart
- administer prep as ordered
- teach client about procedure (e.g., position [lithotomy], darkened room)
- keep NPO if general anesthesia will be used
- administer pre-op medication as ordered

■ nursing care post-test
- monitor urine output
- monitor urine color, blood-tinged is common
- provide comfort measures (back pain, bladder spasms, feeling of fullness are common), e.g., sitz baths and/or analgesics, e.g., belladonna and opium (B&O) suppository as ordered
- check temp and urine for signs of infection
- encourage increased fluid intake (unless contraindicated)

i) renal biopsy

■ a specially designed needle is inserted percutaneously to obtain sample of kidney tissue

■ determines histology of glomeruli and tubules

■ contraindications: a single, functioning kidney; infection; tumors; hydronephrosis; coagulation disorders; or uncooperative client

■ risks: uncontrolled bleeding, hematuria, loss of kidney function

■ nursing care pretest
- ensure written informed consent is on the chart
- check results of coagulation studies and hematocrit
- teach client to hold breath during procedure

■ nursing care post-test
- maintain bedrest for 24 hours with tight dressing or sandbag over insertion site

- force fluids
- monitor vital signs frequently
- monitor hematocrit frequently
- monitor urine
- teach to avoid strenuous activity for approximately 2 weeks

2. Analysis

a. Safe, effective care environment
  1) potential for infection
  2) knowledge deficit

b. Physiological integrity
  1) pain
  2) potential fluid volume deficit
  3) functional incontinence

c. Psychological integrity
  1) ineffective individual coping
  2) altered patterns of sexuality
  3) anxiety

d. Health promotion/maintenance
  1) impaired adjustment
  2) altered health maintenance
  3) knowledge deficit

3. General Nursing Plans, Implementation, and Evaluation

Goal 1: Client will be free from infection.

Plan/Implementation

- Collect necessary urine specimen for culture and sensitivity.
- Teach women proper perineal hygiene.
- Use and teach client good hand-washing techniques.
- Use strict sterile technique during catheterization procedures.
- Provide daily Foley catheter care using good techniques.
- Administer antibiotics as ordered, for full 10–14 days (see Table 3.36).
- Increase fluid intake to 3,000–5,000 ml/day,

Table 3.36 Drugs Used to Treat Urinary Tract Infections

Generic Name (Trade Name)	Action/Use	Side Effects	Nursing Implications
Urinary Analgesic			
Phenazopyridine HCl (Pyridium)	Exerts an anesthetic effect on the mucosa of the urinary tract as it is excreted in the urine. Used for relief of urinary tract pain.	Red-orange or rust discoloration of urine.	• Inform that urine will be orange colored. • Take drug with food. • Use Clinitest for urine testing.
Urinary Antiseptics			
Cinoxacin (Cinobac) Methanamine hippurate (Hiprex) Nitrofurantoin (Furadantin, Macrodantin)	Act as disinfectants within the urinary tract. Concentrated by the kidneys and reach therapeutic levels only within the urinary tract. Used to treat UTIs.	Nausea, vomiting, GI upset, diarrhea, hypersensitivity reaction, dizziness. Brown or rust discoloration of urine	• Keep urine acidic; give vitamin C (6–12 gm/day) or cranberry, plum, prune, or apple juice. • Give after meals to minimize GI upset. • Warn that urine may be brown or rust color. • Monitor I&O; maintain fluid intake of 1,500–2,000 ml/day.
Sulfonamides			
Co-trimoxazole (Bactrim, Septra) Sulfasalazine (Azulfidine) Sulfisoxazole (Gantrisin)	Bacteriostatic against gram-positive and gram-negative organisms. Excreted unchanged and dissolves well in urine. Used to treat UTIs, acute otitis media, inflammatory bowel disease, chronic bronchitis, parasitic infections, and for bowel sterilization pre-op.	GI disorders, hypersensitivity reactions, headache, peripheral hearing loss, crystaluria, hypoglycemia.	• Force fluids to 3,000–4,000 ml/day. • Keep urine alkaline. • Give with at least 8 oz of water 1 hour before or 2 hours after meals for maximum absorption. • Monitor I&O. • Monitor clients with potential renal or hepatic impairment closely. • Advise clients to complete drug course. • Warn about potential increased effect of oral hypoglycemics and false-positive Clinitest results when appropriate.

not contraindicated by renal or cardiovascular status.
- Acidify urine through acid-ash diet (e.g., meats, eggs, cheese, fish, fowl, whole grains, cranberries, plums, prunes) or by administration of methenamine hippurate (Hiprex) or vitamin C if compatible with antibiotic therapy.
- Teach good oral-hygiene techniques.
- Teach client signs and symptoms of upper respiratory infections (URI) and importance of seeking early treatment; screen client from staff or significant others with URIs; teach client to avoid exposure to persons with infections (strep infections can lead to glomerulonephritis).
- Monitor level of potentially nephrotoxic agents (i.e., gentamycin, tetracycline, tobramycin).
- Teach client potentially nephrotoxic agents.

Evaluation: Client is free from dysuria, frequency, fever and other signs of infection; states procedure for proper perineal hygiene; takes medications as prescribed; has I&O of at least 3,000–5,000 ml/day; lists signs and symptoms of URI and need for early treatment; states potentially nephrotoxic agents to avoid in the future.

Goal 2: Client will be free from discomfort.

Plan/Implementation
- Administer sitz baths to decrease urethral burning.
- Administer phenazopyridine HCl (Pyridium) or urinary antispasmodics if ordered (see Table 3.36 page 241).
- Apply hot water bottle or heating pad to suprapubic region.

Evaluation: Client is free from pain, discomfort; reports no burning with urination.

Goal 3: Client's normal urinary function will be maintained.

Plan/Implementation
- Measure urine output accurately.
- Collect urine specimens for routine urinalysis.
- Encourage adequate fluid intake.
- Observe for early signs of renal failure.

Evaluation: Client's urine output remains equal to or greater than 30 ml/hour; client remains free from symptoms of renal failure.

Goal 4: Client and significant others will receive emotional support.

Plan/Implementation
- See Table 2.4 on page 24.
- Provide encouragement when client becomes frustrated with treatment and progression of illness.
- Explain cause of disease and treatments to client/significant others as necessary.
- Allow client and significant others to express fears, feelings, and questions.
- Encourage discussion of diagnosis and ways to cope with problems (e.g., group session for families).
- Prepare the client for possibility of hemodialysis or peritoneal dialysis.
- Refer to social service or pastoral care as needed.

Evaluation: Client/significant others state necessity of treatments; show increasing acceptance of diagnosis and treatment; work through feelings and fears; discuss altered body image; have plans to alter life-style.

Selected Health Problems Resulting in Alteration in Urinary Elimination

☐ Cystitis/Pyelonephritis

1. General Information

a. Definitions
  1) *cystitis*: inflammation of the bladder wall
  2) *pyelonephritis*: inflammation of the kidney caused by a bacterial infection
    a) acute (short course): organisms gain access to the kidney by ascending from the lower urinary tract or via bloodstream; no permanent renal impairment
    b) chronic (slowly progressive): multiple, recurrent, acute attacks that scar the renal parenchyma, damaging tubules, vessels, glomeruli

b. Incidence: both more common in women

c. Risks/predisposing factors
  1) cystitis
    a) prostatic hypertrophy with urinary retention (men)
    b) contamination from large intestine (women)
    c) intrusive procedures: catheterization, cystoscopy
    d) coitus (women)
    e) atonic bladder (spinal cord injury)
    f) chronic disease (e.g., diabetes)
    g) pregnancy (because of pressure of uterus on bladder and urethra)
    h) chronic stasis (e.g., atonic bladder, immobility, and infrequent voiding)

2) pyelonephritis
   a) anomalies of the kidney
   b) pregnancy
   c) calculi
   d) diabetes mellitus
   e) neurogenic bladder
   f) instrumentation (i.e., procedures)
   g) bacterial infection elsewhere in the body

2. Nursing Process

a. Assessment/Analysis

1) cystitis (often asymptomatic)
   a) burning
   b) frequency
   c) urgency
   d) suprapubic pain
   e) slight hematuria
2) pyelonephritis
   a) symptoms of cystitis may or may not be present
   b) severe flank pain, CVA tenderness
   c) hematuria, pyuria
   d) fever
   e) chills
3) diagnostic tests
   a) urinalysis, urine C&S: midstream urine specimen for evaluation of bacterial content
   b) CBC: leukocytosis

b. Plans, Implementation, and Evaluation (refer to General Nursing Goals 1, 2, and 3 page 241)

☐ Urinary Calculi

1. General Information

a. Types
   1) calcium oxylate: hard, small; alkaline urine
   2) calcium phosphate: large, soft; alkaline urine
   3) cystine: metabolic, familial; acid urine
   4) uric acid: may be accompanied by gout; acid urinc
   5) struvite: large, soft; associated with urinary tract infections, alkaline urine

b. Incidence: can occur at any age

c. Locations
   1) bladder
   2) ureter (especially at narrow points)
   3) pelvis of the kidney

d. Risk factors
   1) supersaturation of urine with poorly soluble crystalloids (calcium, uric acid, cystine)
   2) infection: alkaline urine leads to precipitation of calcium and struvite
   3) increased concentration of urine
   4) stasis
   5) bone demineralization leading to increased calcium phosphate in serum and urine
   6) metabolic diseases (e.g., gout [increased uric acid])
   7) certain medications (e.g., corticosteroids, vitamin D [hypervitaminosis D])

e. Medical treatment
   1) medical interventions
      a) ambulation to increase the likelihood of passing the stone
      b) fluids to decrease the concentration of substances involved in stone formation, to promote passage of the stone, and to prevent infection
   2) surgical intervention
      a) *ureterolithotomy*: incision into ureter through an abdominal or flank excision to extract stones from the ureter
         - ureteral catheter is inserted to act as splint; ureter not sutured to avoid stricture; catheter is never irrigated to maintain patency
         - Penrose drain inserted around ureter to collect any extra drainage
      b) *pyelolithotomy*: removal of a stone from renal pelvis through a flank incision; Penrose drain inserted outside renal pelvis
      c) *nephrolithotomy*: parenchyma of kidney is cut and stone extracted through a flank incision
         - nephrostomy tube placed to divert urine and drain pelvis to allow kidney to heal; never irrigated unless specifically ordered
         - Penrose drain inserted
      d) *nephrectomy*: removal of kidney through a flank incision
         - may be needed if stone and infection have caused extensive damage to kidney parenchyma
         - Penrose drain inserted into renal bed

2. Nursing Process

a. Assessment/Analysis

1) pain
   a) renal colic: sudden, sharp, severe;

located in deep lumbar region; radiating to side
b) ureteral colic: same type pain radiating to genitalia and thigh
2) renointestinal reflex: nausea and vomiting, diarrhea, constipation
3) hematuria, frequency, altered pH of urine
4) increased WBC
5) fever, chills
6) signs of paralytic ileus with right-sided renal colic
7) if stone is formed in renal pelvis, may be asymptomatic for years until signs of infection occur
8) IVP results
9) urine for mineral precipitate
10) blood levels of uric acid, calcium, and phosphorus if metabolic problems suspected

b. Plans, Implementation, and Evaluation

Goal 1: Client will be free from pain.

Plan/Implementation
- Administer analgesics as ordered (often morphine is necessary because of severity of pain).
- Administer anticholinergics, propantheline (Pro-Banthine) as ordered, to relax smooth muscles.
- Encourage client to ambulate.
- Strain all urine for stones.

Evaluation: Client is free from discomfort; ambulates; strains all urine for stones.

Goal 2: Client will be free from infection leading to urinary calculi (refer to General Nursing Goal 1 page 241)

Goal 3: Client will decrease risk of stone formation.

Plan/Implementation
- Teach client importance of maintaining adequate fluid intake (3,000 ml/day).
- Teach client about medications and reason for prescription (e.g., to maintain recommended urinary pH).
- Teach client about any medication ordered to decrease levels of minerals (e.g., aluminum hydroxide + $PO_3 \rightarrow AlPO_3$, eliminated through the GI tract).
- Teach client how to measure urine pH.
- Assess diet for excess intake of substances that contribute to stone formation.
- Teach client about dietary restrictions.
- Explain advantages of regular exercise and voiding at least every 2 hours (e.g., to prevent stasis calculi).

Evaluation: Client states importance of maintaining large urine output; lists actions and need for medication to maintain recommended pH; demonstrates ability to monitor urinary pH; demonstrates adherence to dietary restrictions.

Goal 4: Client will be free from post-op complications.

Plan/Implementation
- Refer to *Surgery* page 159.
- Note urine: amount, color, specific gravity.
- Maintain adequate respiratory function following a flank incision.
- Encourage early ambulation.
- Monitor for
  - hypostatic pneumonia (client may be reluctant to deep breathe and cough because of discomfort)
  - hemorrhage
  - paralytic ileus (from reflex paralysis)
  - severe pain
  - urinary tract infection
- Give urinary antiseptics and anti-infectives as ordered (see Table 3.36 page 241).

Evaluation: Client rests comfortably; is free from signs of UTI (e.g., no WBCs, culture less than 100,000 organisms/ml), complications of surgery.

Goal 5: Client will understand home care.

Plan/Implementation
- Refer to General Nursing Goal 3 page 242.
- Teach client how and why to avoid upper respiratory tract infection.
- Tell client to avoid heavy lifting for 4–8 weeks post-op.

Evaluation: Client lists home health measures.

☐ Cancer of the Bladder

1. General Information

a. Characteristics
1) more than 66% occur in men
2) most tumors start as benign papillomas or as leukoplakia
3) multiple tumors frequent
4) tumors often recur

b. Risk factors: probably a disease of multiple etiologies, not yet specifically identified; industrial carcinogens, smoking, aniline dyes, benzine, asbestos, and alcohol have been implicated

c. Medical treatment
   1) surgical intervention
      a) transurethral bladder resection if tumors are of the trigone or posterior bladder wall (85%)
      b) complete cystectomy when cure highly probable
      c) urinary diversion
         - *Ileal conduit*: a portion of the ileum becomes a conduit; the ureters are transplanted into one end and the other end becomes an external stoma
         - *cutaneous ureterostomy*: dissection of one or both ureters, bringing them to the skin, forming one or two stomas (for inoperable tumors)
   2) radiation therapy
      a) pre-op irradiation improves survival in clients with high-grade tumors
      b) external or internal radiation therapy for nonoperable tumors or clients who refuse surgery

2. Nursing Process

a. **Assessment/Analysis**
   1) painless hematuria
   2) abnormal cystogram
   3) abnormal blood and urine studies
   4) cystoscopy, biopsy results

b. **Plans, Implementation, and Evaluation**

Goal 1: Client will be prepared for surgery.

Plan/Implementation
- Refer to *Surgery* page 158.
- Give or arrange for sexual counseling regarding impotence (in men).
- Give bowel prep as ordered.
- Arrange for introduction to diversionary appliance.
- Ensure stoma site (RLQ) is marked.

Evaluation: Client discusses planned surgery and its implications; inspects diversionary appliance.

Goal 2: Client will remain free from post-op complications.

Plan/Implementation
- Refer to *Surgery*, page 159.
- Check ureteral splints for patency, output and color of urine qh.
- Monitor stoma for normal color (pink to red; dark purplish color indicates vascular compromise).
- Record I&O for at least 3 days; encourage up to 3,000 ml fluid intake/day.
- Offer psychologic support as needed.

Evaluation: Client maintains intake of 3,000 ml/day; shows no signs of shock or hemorrhage (e.g., tachycardia, hypotension, apprehension, cold clammy skin, decreased BP, increased pulse).

Goal 3: Client will learn care of urinary diversion appliance and will begin to adjust to alteration in body image.

Plan/Implementation
- Have enterostomal therapist orient client to appliance and its care.
- Reinforce all teaching regarding skin care, cleanliness, odor control.
- Allow client an opportunity to express feelings and concerns regarding changed body image.
- Encourage client to assume full care of appliance as soon as possible.

Evaluation: Client begins to adapt to body-image change (e.g., discusses change, cares for appliance); achieves self-care management of appliance with successful odor control.

☐ Acute Renal Failure

1. General Information

a. Definition: a sudden and potentially reversible loss of kidney function
b. Categories and causes of renal failure
   1) *prerenal* (outside kidney): poor perfusion, decrease in circulating volume
   2) *renal*: structural damage to kidney resulting from acute tubular necrosis
   3) *postrenal*: obstruction within urinary tract
c. Risk/predisposing factors
   1) prerenal
      a) reduction in blood volume (shock)
      b) trauma
      c) septic shock
      d) dehydration
      e) cardiac failure
   2) renal
      a) hypersensitivity (allergic disorders)
      b) obstruction of renal vessels (embolism, thrombosis)
      c) nephrotoxic agents (bacterial toxins, drugs)
      d) mismatched blood transfusion
      e) glomerulonephritis
   3) postrenal
      a) kidney stones or tumors

b) benign prostatic hypertrophy or obstruction

2. Nursing Process

a. Assessment/Analysis

1) oliguric phase (urine volume less than 400 ml/24 hours)
   a) decreased serum sodium and increased potassium; decreased calcium, bicarbonate
   b) increased BUN, creatinine maintaining a 10:1 ratio (normally 20:1 ratio)
   c) increased specific gravity
   d) hypervolemia, hypertension
   e) usually lasts 8 days–3 weeks
2) diuretic phase (urine volume greater than 3,000 ml/24 hours)
   a) serum sodium and potassium may return to normal, stay elevated, or decrease
   b) increased BUN and serum creatinine
   c) decreased specific gravity of urine
   d) hypovolemia
   e) weight loss
   f) usually lasts few days–1 week
3) recovery phase: gradual return of normal function over period of 3–12 months

b. Plans, Implementation, and Evaluation

Goal 1 (if prerenal failure): Client will experience increased renal blood flow through an increased circulating blood volume.

Plan/Implementation

- Monitor vital signs as ordered, especially BP and pulse.
- Maintain strict I&O; monitor urinary output hourly.
- Administer IV fluids as ordered.
- Treat shock if present.
- Administer prescribed medications to increase renal flow (e.g., dopamine 2–5 mcg/kg/minute).
- Administer prescribed diuretics to increase production of urine (e.g., mannitol, furosemide) if client still has output (see Table 3.37 on page 246).

Evaluation: Client has adequate circulation (normal BP, palpable pulse with regular rate and rhythm, skin warm, oriented in 3 spheres); urine output greater than 30 ml/hour.

Goal 2: Client will maintain fluid, electrolyte, and nitrogen balance.

Plan/Implementation (oliguric phase)

- Weigh client daily.
- Measure I&O carefully.
- Administer only enough fluid to replace losses.
- Include insensible losses in measurement of output
  - 500 ml/day if less than 5,000 ft above sea level
  - 1,000 ml/day if more than 5,000 ft above sea level
- Observe for edema and electrolyte imbalance.
- Monitor serum lab test results.
- Administer 50% dextrose with 5–10 units regular insulin as ordered, to drive potassium into cells.
- Administer ion-exchange resin Kayexalate enema as ordered, to lower high potassium levels.
- Reduce potassium, sodium, phosphorus in diet.
- Administer IV sodium bicarbonate for acidosis.
- Administer phosphate binders such as

Table 3.37 Diuretic Drugs

Name	Action	Side Effects	Nursing Implications
Osmotic Diuretics			
Mannitol (Osmitrol)	Draws water from the cells and extracellular spaces into the intravascular. Used to treat/prevent oliguric phase of acute renal failure. Reduces intra-ocular and cerebrospinal fluid.	Transient circulatory overload and edema, headache, confusion, blurred vision, thirst, nausea, vomiting, fluid/electrolyte imbalance, water intoxication, cellular dehydration	• Monitor I&O. • Check for electrolyte imbalance, water intoxication, cellular dehydration. • Be aware of renal and cardiovascular function. • Give frequent mouth care to relieve thirst.
Thiazide Diuretics see Table 3.16			
Potent Diuretics see Table 3.16			
Potassium-sparing Diuretics see Table 3.16			

aluminum hydroxide (Amphojel) or aluminum carbonate (Basaljel) for hyperphosphatemia.

- Reduce protein in diet and teach client rationale; provide high biologic value protein for diet (see Table 3.38 page 247).

Plan/Implementation (diuretic phase)

- Prevent dehydration; balance I&O.
- Increase dietary sodium and potassium to normal levels.
- Maintain positive nitrogen balance and sufficient calories to prevent body protein from being metabolized.
- Prevent infection.

Evaluation: Client maintains approximately equal intake and output and stable weight; remains free from signs of electrolyte imbalance, edema, and dehydration; lists foods on a low-potassium, low-protein diet.

Table 3.38 Low-protein Diet Sample Menu

	Serving	Gm of Protein
Breakfast		
Orange juice	½ glass	1
Farina	½ cup	1
Margarine	1 tbsp	Trace
Sugar	1 tbsp	—
Low-protein bread	1 slice	1
Jelly	1 tbsp	—
Milk	½ cup	3.5
Coffee		—
Lunch		
Fruit salad:		
Peaches (canned)	1	Trace
Pears (canned)	1	Trace
Apple (fresh)	1	Trace
Low-protein bread, toasted	1 slice	1
Margarine	1 tbsp	Trace
Jelly	1 tbsp	—
Sherbet	½ cup	1
Ginger ale with added sugar	1 glass	—
Tea		—
Dinner		
Omelette	2 eggs	13
Asparagus	½ cup	Trace
Carrots	⅔ cup	1
Baked potato	1	3
Margarine	1 tbsp	Trace
Ginger ale with added sugar	1 glass	—
Coffee	—	—
Cantaloupe	¼	½
	TOTAL	26 gm

Usual protein intake: 40–60 gm

Goal 3: Client will be free from infection and further damage to kidneys (refer to General Nursing Goal 1 page 241).

☐ Chronic Renal Failure

1. General Information

a. Definition: a progressive, irreversible deterioration of renal function that ends in fatal uremia unless kidney transplant or dialysis is performed

b. Risk/predisposing factors

1) urinary tract obstruction and infection
2) infectious diseases that cause hypertension and increased catabolism with retention of metabolites (glomerulonephritis)
3) metabolic disease (diabetes)
4) nephrotoxic agents (bacterial toxins, drugs)
5) acute renal failure

c. Pathophysiology

1) kidneys lose their ability to reabsorb electrolytes
2) urine output is decreased
3) anemia (thought to be caused by inadequate production of erythropoietin and depression of bone marrow as uremia increases)
4) end products of protein metabolism accumulate in blood (BUN, creatinine)
5) reduced resistance to infection
6) complications: acidosis, pericarditis, and renal osteodystrophy (abnormal calcium metabolism)

2. Nursing Process

a. Assessment/Analysis

1) urine output: oliguria, anuria
2) metabolic indicators
   a) elevated BUN, creatinine
   b) hyperphosphatemia
   c) hyperkalemia
   d) hypocalcemia
   e) metabolic acidosis
   f) elevated, normal, or decreased serum sodium depending on water retention
3) cardiovascular indicators
   a) hypertension
   b) congestive heart failure
   c) pericarditis
4) hematologic indicators
   a) anemia (decreased renal production of erythropoietin)
   b) alteration of platelet function leading to bleeding tendencies

c) susceptibility to infection (changes in leukocyte function)

5) respiratory indicators
   a) pulmonary edema
   b) uremic pneumonitis
   c) uremic pleurisy
6) gastrointestinal indicators
   a) mucosal irritation in GI tract
   b) ammonia on breath (uremic fetor)
   c) anorexia, nausea, vomiting, hiccoughs
7) central nervous system indicators
   a) early: mild deficit in mental functioning
   b) late: altered sensorium, slurred speech, generalized seizures, encephalopathy with toxic psychosis, coma
8) peripheral nervous system indicators
   a) peripheral neuropathy involving all extremities
   b) burning, painful paresthesias
9) musculoskeletal indicators
   a) renal osteodystrophy
   b) bone pain in feet and legs upon walking and standing, pathologic fractures
10) dermatologic indicators
   a) pruritus
   b) dry skin: caused by atrophy of sweat glands
   c) easy bruising, petechiae, and purpura
   d) pallor related to anemia
   e) sallow, yellow-tan color to skin
   f) brittle, dry hair
   g) dry and ridged nails
   h) uremic frost: crystalization of urea on skin (late sign)
11) endocrine indicators
   a) hypothyroidism
   b) decreased T_4 level
12) reproductive indicators
   a) infertility
   b) loss of libido
   c) amenorrhea in women
   d) decreased testosterone and sperm count in men

b. Plans, Implementation, and Evaluation

Goal 1: Client will maintain fluid and electrolyte balance (refer to "Acute Renal Failure" Goals 1 and 2 page 246).

Goal 2: Client will remain free from infection (refer to General Nursing Goal 1 page 241).

Goal 3: Client will maintain adequate caloric intake to prevent muscle wasting and prevent own body stores from being metabolized.

Plan/Implementation
- Initiate daily calorie count.
- Give medication to control nausea and vomiting before meals.
- Adjust level of protein in diet to client's serum levels of BUN and creatinine.
- Encourage protein of high biologic value (essential amino acids).
- Serve food attractively and at appropriate temperature.

Evaluation: Client's BUN and creatinine levels remain within normal limits or stable; calorie count is 35–40 calories/kg body weight.

Goal 4: Client will be protected from self-injury during period of altered sensorium.

Plan/Implementation
- Restrain if necessary.
- Institute seizure precautions.
- Perform neurologic checks frequently.
- Monitor BUN and creatinine closely.
- Teach significant others about cause of altered sensorium.

Evaluation: Client is free from injury during periods of confusion; significant others state awareness of relationship between disease process and altered sensorium.

Goal 5: Client will be relieved of itching and maintain skin integrity.

Plan/Implementation
- Avoid soap.
- Use soft cloth.
- Add oil to tepid bath water (baking soda in water may help).

Evaluation: Client's itching is relieved; skin remains intact.

Goal 6: Client and significant others will be supported emotionally (refer to General Nursing Goal 4 page 242 and Table 2.4 on page 24).

Goal 7: Client will adapt to altered sexual functioning.

Plan/Implementation
- Teach client and significant other about alterations in sexual functioning.
- Provide or arrange sexual counseling if necessary.

- Encourage client and significant other to discuss the problem.

Evaluation: Client and significant other discuss change and alteration in sexual expression.

☐ Dialysis

Dialysis is the passage of particles (ions) from an area of high concentration to an area of low concentration (diffusion) across a semipermeable membrane; simultaneously water moves (osmosis) toward the solution in which the solute concentration is greater. When dialysis is used as a substitute for kidney function, the semipermeable membrane used is either the peritoneum (peritoneal dialysis) or an artificial membrane (hemodialysis). The principle of exchange is the same with both methods. The pores in the membrane are large enough to allow the passage of urea, electrolytes, and creatinine, but are too small to allow the passage of blood cells and other protein molecules.

1. General Information: peritoneal dialysis

a. Definition: placement of catheter through abdominal wall into peritoneal space.

b. Procedure: body or room temperature dialysate is allowed to flow into the peritoneal cavity by gravity. The solution remains in the abdomen for exchange to occur and then is drained from the peritoneal cavity by gravity. It carries with it waste products and excess electrolytes. Can last from 12–24 hours.

c. Number of cycles: varies according to the client's problems, tolerance, response, and type of solution

d. Types

- **1)** intermittent manual
- **2)** intermittent automatic
- **3)** continuous ambulatory (CAPD)
  - **a)** dialysate remains in peritoneum 24 hr/day with several dialysate exchanges per day
  - **b)** advantages
    - lower BP (9 out of 10 clients can come off BP meds)
    - increased Hct and Hgb
    - less expensive
    - greater freedom for client
    - weight gain from glucose absorbed from dialysate (later can become a disadvantage)
  - **c)** disadvantages and risks
    - peritonitis
    - infection at catheter exit site
    - dialysate leakage
    - hypotension
    - hypoalbuminemia (caused by increased loss of protein from repeated peritonitis and large pores in peritoneum)

Figure 3.16 Schematic Representation of Dialysis

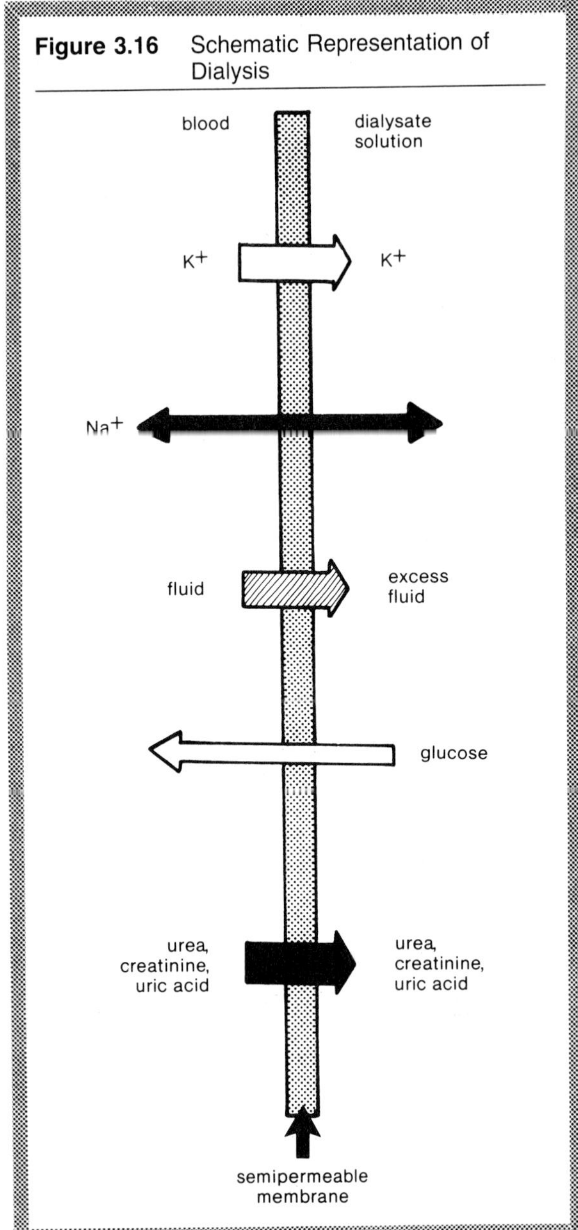

e. peritoneal access (e.g., Tenckhoff peritoneal catheter extends access to the peritoneal cavity for weeks to months)

2. Nursing Process

a. Assessment/Analysis

- **1)** temperature, pulse, respirations, and blood pressure

2) blood chemistries (electrolytes, BUN, creatinine, glucose)
3) daily I&O
4) daily weight (after fluid is drained from cavity)
5) catheter site for signs of infection or leakage (redness, tenderness, pain, or exudate)

b. **Plans, Implementation, and Evaluation**

Goal 1: Client will be protected from peritonitis.

Plan/Implementation
- Use scrupulous aseptic technique throughout dialysis.
- Check dialysate for cloudiness (sign of infection).
- Notify physician immediately if peritonitis is suspected (cloudy peritoneal fluid, fever, chills).
- Obtain peritoneal fluid sample for fluid analysis, culture and sensitivity.
- Initiate antibiotic therapy as ordered (cephalosporins or aminoglycosides either systemically or instilled into dialysate).
- Take temperature q4h.
- Change catheter site dressing at least qd; cleanse with iodine solution and apply topical antibiotic ointment.

Evaluation: Client's peritoneal fluid remains clear; temperature remains within normal limits.

Goal 2: Client will experience successful intermittent dialysis and maintain optimal concentrations of serum electrolytes.

Plan/Implementation
- Weigh client prior to dialysis and daily.
- Have client empty bladder and bowel prior to paracentesis.
- Place client in comfortable supine position.
- Warm dialysate in water or microwave to body temperature before instilling.
- Permit 2 liters dialysate to flow unrestricted into peritoneal cavity (inflow).
- Leave fluid in peritoneal cavity for 30–45 minutes so that solution can equilibrate (dwell time).
- Drain equilibrated fluid from peritoneal cavity.
- Record amount of fluid loss or gain; outflow should be approximately 100–200 ml more than inflow; have client turn on sides to localize fluid and promote drainage; if retention continues, notify physician.
- Repeat cycle as ordered.
- Perform blood chemistries as ordered.
- Maintain client comfort during dialysis.

Evaluation: Client's weight decreases after each dialysis session; has larger output than inflow.

Goal 3: Client will be free from hypertension.

Plan/Implementation
- Monitor BP standing and sitting.
- Monitor BP during dialysis (should decrease as fluid volume is reduced).
- Use a more hypertonic dialysate if hypertension persists.
- Restrict fluid and sodium intake.
- Give antihypertensive medications as ordered.
- Notify physician if symptoms of hypotension occur during procedure; treat by administering normal saline directly into the arterial or venous line and slowing the dialyzing procedures.

Evaluation: Client's BP remains within predetermined guidelines.

Goal 4: Client will be successful with CAPD at home if client's condition requires chronic dialysis.

Plan/Implementation
- Educate client and significant others in the principles, process, and techniques of CAPD
  - instill 2 liters room temperature dialysate
  - leave in peritoneal cavity 4–8 hours
  - go about daily activities
  - drain fluid and discard
  - replace with 2 liters fresh dialysate
  - repeat procedure 4 times/day
  - leave dialysate in peritoneal cavity overnight
- Educate about sterile technique and its importance in preventing peritonitis.
- Have client keep a written record of daily weight and BP.
- Provide diet instruction to replace lost protein; liberalize protein, potassium, salt, and water intake.
- Teach the importance of regular medical and nursing follow-up for lab work, catheter change, evaluation of dialysis technique, monitoring of weight and BP, and any other problems.

Evaluation: Client uses CAPD at home free from any problems; explains proper diet and the importance of follow-up.

Goal 5: Client will be assisted to cope psychologically with ongoing dialysis treatments (refer to ''Hemodialysis'' Goal 3 page 250).

3. General Information: hemodialysis

a. Definition: passage of heparinized blood from client through a tube consisting of a semipermeable membrane immersed in a dialysate bath composed of all important electrolytes in their ideal concentration. Diffusion and ultrafiltration occur between the client's blood and the dialysate. Protamine sulfate may be used to counteract the heparin effects.

b. Procedure: fresh dialysate is used continuously until the client's electrolyte and fluid balances are within safe levels.

c. Schedule varies with clinical condition and type of dialyzer

- **1)** up to 3 times/week
- **2)** 4–6 hours/day is possible for coil and hollow-fiber dialyzers; 10–12 hours/day is necessary for plate-type dialyzers

d. Access to client's circulation

- **1)** arteriovenous (AV) shunt
  - **a)** external device
    - ■ composed of two nonthrombogenic silastic rubber tubes or cannulas with Teflon tips, one sutured in artery, the other in vein
    - ■ between dialysis, the two tubes are joined by Teflon connector
    - ■ most commonly used vessels are the radial artery and cephalic vein of forearm
  - **b)** advantages
    - ■ can be used immediately after insertion
    - ■ use is relatively simple
  - **c)** disadvantages
    - ■ clotting
    - ■ infection
    - ■ accidental dislodgment with hemorrhage
    - ■ limited longevity
- **2)** arteriovenous (AV) fistula: access of choice for hemodialysis
  - **a)** internal access
    - ■ created by side-to-side or end-to-end anastomosis between adjacent vein and artery (often radial artery and cephalic vein)
    - ■ creates enlarged superficial vein with easy access for venipuncture
  - **b)** advantages
    - ■ longevity
    - ■ no danger of disconnection
  - **c)** disadvantages
    - ■ must be constructed 4–12 weeks in advance
    - ■ needs time to mature
    - ■ complications
      - – thrombosis
      - – venous hypertension distal to anatomosis
      - – ischemia of extremity
      - – infection (less frequent than AV shunts)
- **3)** graft
  - **a)** internal access (e.g., piece of bovine carotid artery or Gore-Tex material)
  - **b)** usually done when client's vessels are unsuitable to be used as a fistula
  - **c)** advantages
    - ■ not dependent on adequate client circulation for placement
    - ■ diameter is predetermined
  - **d)** disadvantages
    - ■ does not have healing properties (e.g., more chance of bleeding, infection, aneurysm formation)
    - ■ cannot be used for several weeks
    - ■ not used for clients awaiting transplants since bovine grafts can be rejected

4. Nursing Process

a. Assessment/Analysis

- **1)** arterial flow of AV shunt, AV fistula, or graft
  - **a)** palpate for thrill
  - **b)** listen for bruit
  - **c)** check skin temperature and pulses distal to access site
  - **d)** color of blood should be bright, cranberry red (shunt only)
- **2)** check client's temperature and BP
- **3)** check dialysate composition and temperature
- **4)** client's psychologic reaction to dialysis
  - **a)** reaction to physical condition
  - **b)** predialysis personality
  - **c)** family support system
  - **d)** financial status
  - **e)** signs of depression, fear, anxiety, denial, and regression
  - **f)** noncompliance with diet or fluid restrictions
  - **g)** verbalization of self-deprecation
  - **h)** relinquishment of decision making to family or staff

i) suicidal ideation
j) reaction to sexual dysfunction

b. **Plans, Implementation, and Evaluation**

Goal 1: Client will have access site protected from trauma.

Plan/Implementation

- Keep extremity elevated several hours after insertion.
- Instruct client to keep affected arm or leg as straight as possible at all times.
- Have clamps or tourniquet available at all times to control any severe bleeding from accidental dislodgment of shunt.
- Notify physician immediately of severe bleeding or clotting of cannula.
- Instruct client to avoid lifting heavy objects with affected arm.
- Do not use affected arm for BP or venipuncture.
- Instruct client to avoid constrictive clothing over shunt site.
- Instruct client to avoid exposing access site to extreme cold.

Evaluation: Client's blood flow to access site remains cranberry red with palpable thrill, audible bruit, and warm temperature.

Goal 2: Client will remain free from infection at access site.

Plan/Implementation

- Check site frequently for signs of infection (pain, redness, tenderness, or increase of temperature).
- Perform suture line care (10–14 days until sutures are removed)
  - remove old dressing
  - clean suture line with povidone-iodine solution
  - apply new sterile dressing
- Instruct client not to irritate scabs that form over needle insertion sites.
- Apply skin softening cream to scabs.
- Wash the affected limb with antibacterial soap (e.g., Dial, Safeguard) and water daily.

Evaluation: Client remains free from pain, redness, and tenderness, at site of shunt.

Goal 3: Client will be assisted to cope psychologically with ongoing dialysis treatments.

Plan/Implementation

- See Table 2.4 on page 24.
- Encourage client to express concerns, feelings and to ask questions re procedures and lifestyle adaptations.
- Educate client concerning treatments and rationale behind restrictions.
- Give consistent information to client and significant others.
- Encourage client to maintain as active and productive a life as possible, and to plan daily activities around treatments.
- Encourage client to be as independent and responsible for care as possible.
- Encourage significant others to express their feelings.
- Counsel significant others to avoid unrealistic expectations and overprotectiveness.
- Assist client to move from depression, despair, and defeat to acceptance of illness by exhibiting hope and planning for realistic goals.
- Refer for vocational rehabilitation, shelter workshops, or special services as needed (e.g., financial).
- Provide marital or sexual counseling.
- Conduct regular team conferences to discuss care of clients.

Evaluation: Client leads as active and productive a life as possible within the constraints of the illness; shows acceptance of disease by managing care and setting realistic goals.

☐ Kidney Transplantation

1. General Information

a. Definition: the surgical implanation of a donated, allogenic kidney to restore kidney function in a client with end-stage renal failure

b. Donor
  1) live
  2) cadaver

c. Rejection of the grafted kidney is a significant problem
  1) attempts to minimize: tissue typing prior to transplantation (must indicate high degree of histocompatibility)
  2) types of rejection
    a) *hyperacute*: occurs on the operating room table
    b) *acute*: 1st episode can occur 5–7 days posttransplant; subsequent episodes can occur within the 1st year
    c) *chronic*: rejection continues despite repeated attempts at immunosupression
    d) rejection rates
      - 20%–25% of cadaver grafts
      - 5%–10% of live donor grafts

- greatly increased by the presence of diabetes

d. Immunosupressive drugs are given to all transplant recipients; see Table 3.39 below.

2. Nursing Process

a. Assessment/Analysis

1) metabolic state
2) tissue histocompatibility
3) immunologic defense status
4) psychologic and emotional status
5) potential sources of post-op infection (carious teeth, infected donor kidneys) since client will be immunosuppressed
6) age; desires of the client regarding this risk-filled procedure

b. Plans, Implementation, and Evaluation

Goal 1: Client will be adequately prepared preoperatively to maximize the chances of a successful outcome.

Plan/Implementation

- Refer to *Surgery* page 157.
- Maintain accurate I&O; adhere to fluid restriction.
- Know that the client may need to undergo pre-op hemodialysis to achieve an optimal metabolic state.
- Protect client from possible sources of infection.

Evaluation: Client is able to describe the postoperative routine.

Goal 2: Client will be psychologically prepared for the surgery.

Plan/Implementation

- Refer to *Surgery* page 158.
- Allow client the opportunity to discuss feelings and concerns regarding the surgery and its chances of success.
- Answer client's questions as honestly and completely as possible.
- Allow client an opportunity to discuss any ambivalent feelings about the donor (may be a very close relative).
- Know that significant others also need support and information.

Evaluation: Client experiences only a moderate level of anxiety preoperatively; expresses realistic hope regarding outcome of transplant.

Goal 3: Client will be free from post-op complications.

Plan/Implementation

- Refer to *Surgery* page 159.
- Assess fluid and electrolyte balance carefully
  - measure urine output (may range from massive diuresis [live donor] to aneuresis [cadaver donor])
  - may require hemodialysis
- Protect client from infection
  - give Foley care
  - may be in reverse isolation
  - monitor temperature
- Observe for signs of acute rejection of transplant

Table 3.39 Immunosuppressive Drugs

Generic Name (Trade Name)	Action	Side Effects	Nursing Implications
Azathioprine (Imuran)	Inhibits RNA and DNA synthesis. Inhibits lymphoid tissue (where cells divide rapidly during the rejection process) thereby diminishing the rejection process.	Skin rash, alopecia, nausea, vomiting, leukopenia, thrombocytopenia	• Begin drug 1–5 days before surgery and continue afterwards. • Monitor hematologic status. • Institute reverse isolation if needed. • Monitor for fever, chills, unusual bleeding, bruising, and sore throat.
Cyclosporin (Sandimmune)	Strongly inhibits the antibody production that leads to graft rejection. Use should be accompanied by adjunct steroid administration.	Nephrotoxicity, hypertension, tremor, gum hyperplasia, hepatotoxicity, hirsutism	• Monitor kidney and liver function. • Dilute oral solution with milk or orange juice and give at room temperature. • Observe for anaphylaxis for at least 30 minutes after start of IV infusion of drug.

Steroids see Table 3.28.

- oliguria, anuria
- fever
- increased blood pressure
- swollen, tender kidney
- flu symptoms
- ■ Maintain integrity of venous access.

Evaluation: Client has vital signs within normal limits; output equivalent to fluid intake; remains free from infection.

Goal 4: Client will take medications correctly.

Plan/Implementation

- ■ Teach client that immunosuppressive drugs are the main defense against transplant rejection.
- ■ Teach side effects and complications of these drugs and that withdrawal (if it is ever appropriate) must be done gradually.
- ■ Tell client that he is more susceptible to infection while taking these drugs and to notify physician at the 1st sign of a cold or infection.
- ■ Teach client how to avoid or at least decrease exposure to sources of infection

Evaluation: Client lists side effects of all drugs; knows when to call physician regarding drug-related problems; states an awareness of administration schedule and importance of maintaining it.

☐ Benign Prostatic Hypertrophy (BPH)

1. General Information

a. Incidence: more than 50% of all men over 50

b. Predisposing factors: unknown

c. Medical treatment: surgical intervention

1) transurethral resection of prostate (TURP) is most common
2) suprapubic and retropubic approaches also used

2. Nursing Process

a. Assessment/Analysis

1) urinary dysfunction
2) symmetrical, smooth enlargement of prostate
3) signs and symptoms of hydronephrosis followed by renal failure (late)

b. Plans, Implementation, and Evaluation

Goal 1: Client will have adequate urinary flow preoperatively.

Plan/Implementation

- ■ Insert Foley catheter
  - on initial insertion: prevent bladder collapse by clamping draining tube after 1,000 ml urine is drained

Figure 3.17 Normal Male Anatomy

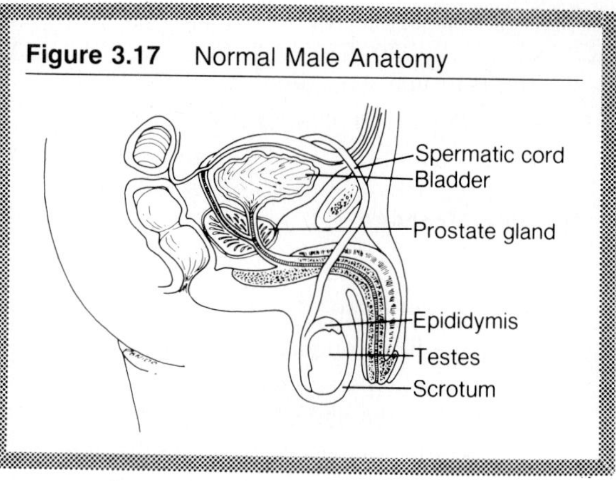

  - unclamp tube after 1 hour and repeat protocol
- ■ Measure I&O.
- ■ Know that a suprapubic catheter may be necessary.

Evaluation: Client's intake and output remains balanced.

Goal 2: Client will be able to describe surgical approach and post-op care (see Table 3.40 page 255).

Plan/Implementation

- ■ Teach client that vasectomy is usually done to reduce chance of epididymitis.
- ■ Know that most prostatectomies produce retrograde ejaculation and sterility.

Evaluation: Client describes a TURP; knows what to expect postoperatively (e.g., pain and discomfort, ambulation).

Goal 3: Client will have normal urinary drainage, clear to lightly pink-tinged in color; will be free from hemorrhage.

Plan/Implementation

- ■ Know that a 3-way Foley catheter with 30 ml balloon will be inserted post-op.
- ■ Ensure Foley is patent.
- ■ Apply traction on the Foley for 24 hours (puts pressure on prostatic bed).
- ■ Maintain constant bladder irrigation (CBI).
- ■ Increase speed of irrigation if increased blood seen; notify physician if this is not effective.
- ■ Measure I&O each shift.
- ■ Monitor urinary output after Foley is removed (2–3 days).
- ■ Care for dressing around suprapubic catheter if suprapubic prostatectomy done.

Evaluation: Client's urine remains clear and amber-colored.

Table 3.40 Prostatectomies

Type	Surgical Approach	Common Problems	Nursing Implications
Transurethral resection (TUR)	Client in lithotomy position Gland removed through resecting cystoscope Most common approach	Not all gland removed	Explain that benign prostatic hypertropy can recur.
		Constant bladder irrigation to decrease bleeding	Ensure catheter patency. Run irrigant at rate to keep urine light pink. Use only isotonic solution to prevent water intoxication.
		May damage internal sphincter leading to incontinence or bladder-neck strictures	Teach perineal exercises.
		May or may not cause sterility	Reassure client potency *not* affected.
Suprapubic	Abdominal approach Bladder is opened Allows abdominal exploration	Suprapubic catheter or drain with urinary drainage	Do frequent dressing changes. Prevent infection or irritation.
		Hemorrhage common; large-balloon Foley with traction is used to stop bleeding	Watch closely for bleeding. Check catheter patency. Irrigate with saline prn to prevent clots.
		Bladder spasms common	Reposition client. Give propantheline bromide (Pro-Banthine).
		Causes sterility	Reassure potency not affected.
Retropubic	Low abdominal incision; no bladder incision Allows complete, direct removal of gland with less bleeding	Can be done for cancer or BPH Causes sterility	Assure client potency *not* affected.
		Less chance of bleeding; sometimes constant bladder irrigation is ordered for 24 hours	Watch for bleeding.
		Few spasms	Medicate prn.
Perineal, radical (for cancer)	Incision in perineum between scrotum and rectum Client in lithotomy position	Causes impotence, sterility, and some incontinence	Allow expression of feelings. Teach perineal exercises.
		Large perineal wound with risk of infection and bleeding	Clean well. Check and change dressing prn.
		Straining or rectal trauma may increase bleeding	Avoid rectal temperature or tubes. Give stool softeners.
		May be done for castration for carcinoma	Talk to client. Explain changes.

Goal 4: Client will have minimal discomfort from bladder spasms.

Plan/Implementation

- Know that a large balloon on the Foley can stimulate spasms (more likely to be used with TURP).
- Administer narcotics plus anticholinergic drugs as ordered.

Evaluation: Client's post-op bladder spasms are controlled.

Goal 5: Client will remain free from undetected complications.

Plan/Implementation

- Observe for signs of osteitis pubis after a retropubic prostatectomy.

Figure 3.18 Types of Prostatectomies

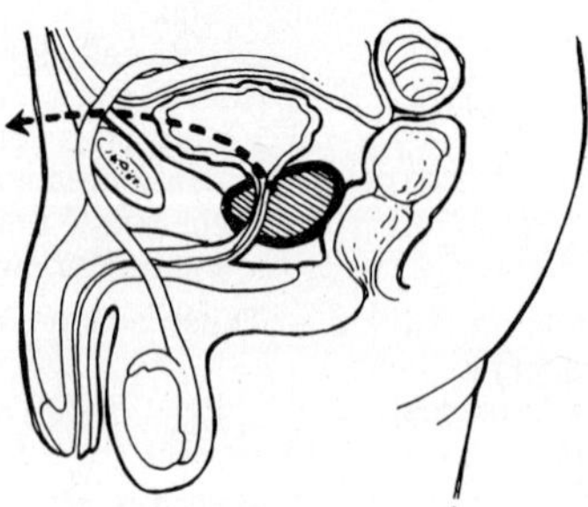

Suprapubic Prostatectomy

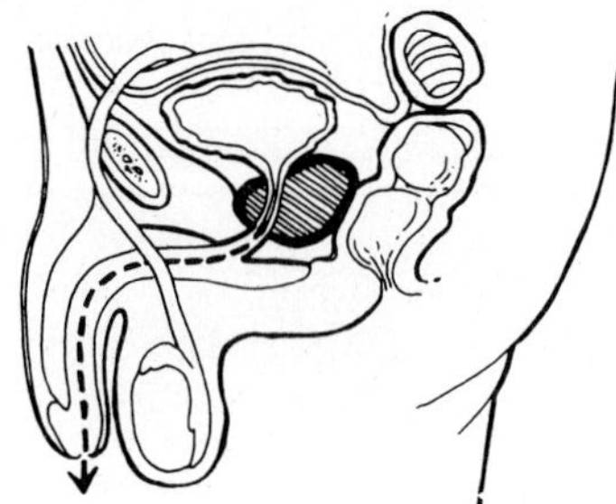

Transurethral Resection

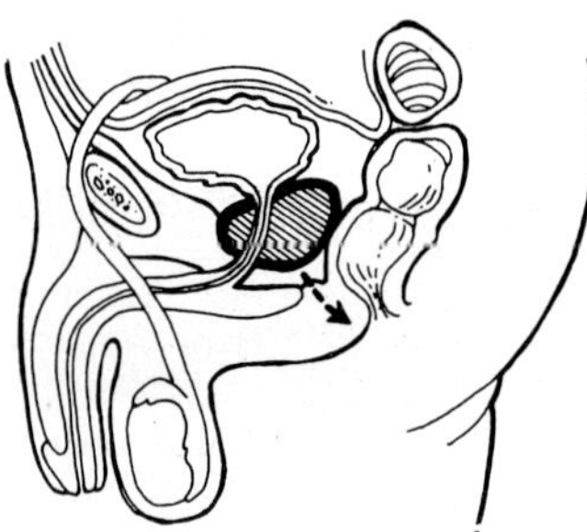

Perineal Prostatectomy

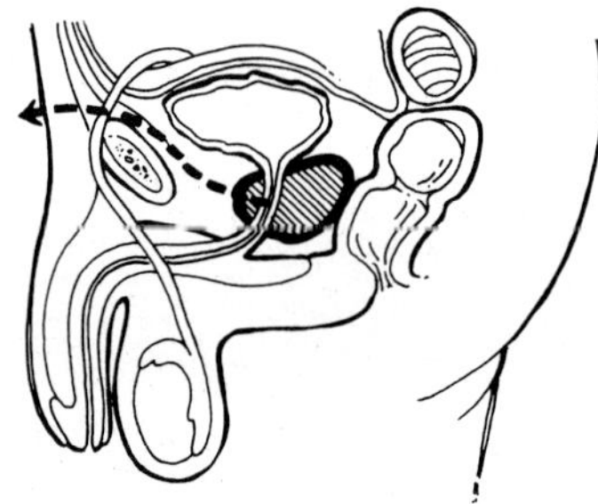

Retropubic Prostatectomy

- Institute strategies to prevent thrombophlebitis.
- Know that incisional infection is more frequent with suprapubic prostatectomy.
- Observe for signs of epididymitis (swelling, pain of scrotum, testes) if vasectomy was not done.
- For epididymitis place ice pack under testes and scrotum.

Evaluation: Client is free from post-op infections, signs of epididymitis.

Goal 6: Client will understand postdischarge activities allowed.

Plan/Implementation

- Tell client to refrain from sexual activity until approximately 6 weeks post-op.
- Have client avoid heavy lifting, straining, driving car for approximately 6 weeks.
- Monitor urine: should be continually clear.
- Teach client to increase fluid intake (i.e., 1 glass of fluid qh).
- Teach client to avoid alcohol for 6 weeks.
- Teach client that dribbling may occur after removal of catheter and that perineal exercise can help increase sphincter tone.

Evaluation: Client describes activity restrictions; states intent to monitor urine at home.

☐ Cancer of the Prostate

1. General Information

a. Incidence

1) increasing

2) 2nd most common cancer in men

3) most frequent in 50+ age group

b. Predisposing factors

1) family tendency

2) environmental risks and oncogenic virus suspected

c. Other information
   1) usually starts in posterior lobe
   2) most commonly adenocarcinoma
   3) usually palpable on rectal exam

d. Medical treatment: surgical intervention
   1) radical perineal prostatectomy
   2) radical retropubic prostatectomy
   3) TURP for palliation followed by hormonal manipulation (DES or bilateral orchiectomy)

2. Nursing Process

a. **Assessment/Analysis:** findings depend on size of tumor
   1) if large, tumor will cause obstruction and findings similar to those in BPH
   2) if small, no findings except hard nodule when prostate palpated rectally
   3) prostate-specific antigen (PSA) elevated
   4) positive biopsy
   5) acid phosphatase increased with spread beyond capsule; alkaline phosphatase increased with bony metastasis
   6) metastasis is usually to spine

b. **Plans, Implementation, and Evaluation**

Goal 1: Client will understand the planned surgery and what to expect postoperatively.

Plan/Implementation
- Refer to *Surgery* page 157.
- Counsel client regarding impotence and/or available penile prosthetic devices.
- Include significant others in pre-op discussion.

Evaluation: Client describes planned surgery in own words.

Goal 2: Client's incision will be kept clean and remain intact.

Plan/Implementation
- Do not take rectal temperatures or insert rectal tubes.
- Use T-binder if indicated.
- Give sitz baths after drains removed.
- Maintain patency of Foley.

Evaluation: Client's incision heals well.

Goal 3: Client will remain free from post-op complications.

Plan/Implementation
- Refer to *Surgery* page 159.
- Monitor for lymphedema if pelvic lymph nodes removed.

Evaluation: Client is afebrile, maintains clear lung sounds; is free from leg edema.

Goal 4: Client will regain perineal muscle tone and urinary continence.

Plan/Implementation
- Teach perineal and buttock-tightening exercises.
- Institute exercises 48 hours post-op; have client do them qh.
- Reassure client that some urinary control can be obtained.

Evaluation: Client demonstrates perineal exercises; expresses a positive attitude about regaining continence.

Goal 5: Client will be able to explain alternate ways of sexual expression.

Plan/Implementation
- Encourage client to discuss concerns/fears.
- Encourage client to discuss sexuality with significant other; have them explore different ways to satisfy each other sexually.

Evaluation: Client shows a willingness to discuss sexual concerns.

Goal 6: Client and significant other will understand the therapy for advanced disease.

Plan/Implementation
- Explain hormonal manipulation and side effects of female hormones.
- Prepare client for bilateral orchiectomy if indicated. Answer questions concerning prosthetic devices and the inguinal incision.
- Prepare client for TURP if cancer is causing obstruction but is not surgically treatable.

Evaluation: Client describes future care needs.

The Large Bowel

General Concepts

Overview/Physiology

1. The large intestine extends from the ileocecal valve to the anus (cecum, ascending colon, transverse colon, descending colon, sigmoid colon, rectum, and anal canal).
2. The major functions of the colon are the absorption of water and electrolytes in the proximal half of the large intestine and storage of feces in the distal half until defecation occurs.
3. Bacterial action in the large bowel not only provides gases to increase the bulk of and propel the feces but also facilitates synthesis of vitamin K, thiamine, riboflavin, vitamin B_{12}, folic acid, biotin, and nicotinic acid.

Application of the Nursing Process to the Client with Large Bowel Problems

1. **Assessment**
   a. Health history
      1) bowel habits: frequency and character of stool patterns
      2) changes in bowel habits: decrease or increase in frequency, change in consistency (more liquid → diarrhea; less liquid → constipation)
      3) presence of blood or change in color of stool
      4) use of laxatives or other methods that affect elimination
      5) effect of dietary habits on elimination
      6) presence of abdominal or rectal pain
      7) altered weight
   b. Physical examination
      1) inspection
         a) abdomen
            - scars, striae, wounds, fistulas, and/or ostomy
            - engorged veins
            - skin characteristics
            - visible peristalsis and pulsations
            - visible masses and altered contour
         b) anus
            - presence of dilated veins
            - constipation
            - breaks in skin, fissures
      2) auscultation
         a) bowel sounds
         b) bruit
         c) hum and friction rub
      3) percussion
         a) liver size
         b) presence of fluid
      4) palpation
         a) masses
         b) rigidity of abdominal muscles
         c) pain/tenderness
         d) fluid waves
   c. Diagnostic tests
      1) stool examinations
         a) odor, consistency, color
         b) presence or absence of mucus
         c) occult blood (by guaiac exam)
         d) ova and parasites
      2) barium enema
         a) definition: barium is instilled in the rectum through a rectal catheter
            - permits x-ray visualization of large intestine
            - used to detect polyps, tumors, diverticula, positional abonormalities (e.g., malrotation)
         b) nursing care pretest
            - explain procedure
            - administer cathartics as ordered the day prior to procedure
            - administer a suppository if ordered on the day of the procedure
            - may restrict diet to clear liquids for 24 hours prior to exam
            - keep NPO after midnight
         c) nursing care post-test
            - administer laxatives following procedure as ordered, to prevent impaction
            - instruct client that stool will remain light colored for 24–72 hours
      3) proctoscopy, sigmoidoscopy, colonoscopy
         a) definition: visualization of inside of entire colon (colonoscopy), sigmoid colon (sigmoidoscopy) or rectum (protoscopy) through a lighted scope
            - proctoscopy and sigmoidoscopy: rigid scope
            - colonoscopy: flexible scope
         b) nursing care pretest
            - explain procedure
            - give clear liquids 24–48 hours prior to exam
            - prepare bowel with laxatives, enemas, or suppositories as ordered
         c) nursing care post-test
            - observe for hemorrhage, abdominal distention, pain
            - check for return of normal bowel function postprocedure
      4) biopsy
         a) definition: removal of polyps or biopsy specimens through a specialized piece of equipment inserted during endoscopy
         b) nursing care
            - same as for proctoscopy
            - monitor carefully for hemorrhage
2. **Analysis**
   a. Safe, effective care environment
      1) potential for infection
      2) knowledge deficit
   b. Physiological integrity
      1) constipation, diarrhea, bowel incontinence
      2) altered nutrition: less than body requirements
   c. Psychological integrity
      1) anxiety
      2) body image disturbance
      3) altered pattern of sexuality

d. Health promotion/maintenance
   1) altered health maintenance
   2) knowledge deficit
   3) impaired adjustment

3. **General Nursing Plans, Implementation, and Evaluation**

Goal 1: Client's bowel elimination will follow a normal pattern.

Plan/Implementation
- Instruct client how to promote proper bowel function; adjust teaching if client has an ileostomy or colostomy.
- Teach client to respond to defecation reflex since holding feces can contribute to constipation.
- Instruct client on the use of foods high in bulk and roughage: skins and fibers of fruits and vegetables.
- Increase fluid intake if allowed.
- Encourage regular exercise to aid in elimination.
- Teach about the relationship of stress to altered bowel function.
- Prevent diarrhea through proper sanitation and hygiene.
- Restrict fruit juices and raw fruits and vegetables that contribute to diarrhea.
- Observe client with diarrhea for signs of fluid and electrolyte imbalance.
- Administer antidiarrheals (see Table 3.41 on page 260).
- Encourage intake of electrolyte-containing drinks (e.g., Gatorade).

Evaluation: Client establishes a normal pattern of bowel elimination; lists and consumes foods that promote bowel evacuation; establishes a pattern of regular exercise; passes stool of normal consistency.

Goal 2: Client's dietary intake will follow prescribed restrictions yet provide all needed nutrients.

Plan/Implementation
- Increase or decrease dietary nutrients as ordered.
- Teach client rationale for restrictions.
- Explore with client means of fostering compliance.
- Provide needed support and encouragement.

Evaluation: Client selects appropriate diet from sample menus; verbalizes rationale for restrictions; expresses a positive attitude toward diet alteration.

Goal 3: Client will be knowledgeable about disease process, medications, and the prevention of complications.

Plan/Implementation
- Explain disease process and its relationship to medications.
- Discuss rationale for ordered treatment regimen.
- Provide data concerning the administration and side effects of all medications.
- Assist client to identify potential stressors in life-style that might trigger complications of the disease; discuss appropriate client actions.

Evaluation: Client takes medications as ordered, returns for follow-up care; remains free from preventable complications.

Selected Health Problems Resulting in Alteration in Large Bowel Elimination

☐ Alteration in Normal Bowel Evacuation

1. **General Information**
   a. Definitions
      1) *constipation*: difficult or infrequent defecation with passage of unduly hard and dry fecal material
      2) *diarrhea*: frequent passage of abnormally watery bowel movements
      3) normal bowel evacuation: 2–3 movements/day to 2/week; varies in healthy individuals
   b. Precipitating factors
      1) constipation: worry, anxiety, fear, improper diet, intestinal obstruction, tumors, excessive use of laxatives, use of certain drugs, atony or spasticity of intestinal musculature
      2) diarrhea: diet, inflammation or irritation of intestinal mucosa, GI infections, use of certain drugs, psychogenic factors

2. **Nursing Process**
   a. **Assessment/Analysis**
      1) stool consistency, appearance
      2) acute or chronic pain, rebound tenderness
      3) weight loss, malnutrition
      4) dehydration
      5) nausea, vomiting; projectile vomiting
      6) electrolyte imbalance, especially sodium, potassium, chloride
      7) aggravation by certain foods and milk products

Table 3.41 Antidiarrheal and Laxative Drugs

Drug	Action	Use	Side Effects	Nursing Implications
Antidiarrheals				
Local acting: Kaopectate (Kaolin & Pectin) Pepto-Bismol (Bismuth subsalicylate)	Reduce liquidity of feces. Act within the bowel to soothe the intestinal tract and increase the absorption of water, electrolytes, and nutrients.	Treat acute and chronic diarrhea	Constipation Intestinal obstruction in chronic use Drug absorbs nutrients	• Advise patient to stop the medication and notify physician if drug is not effective in 48 hours. • Advise to maintain fluid intake during diarrhea. • Instruct to shake well before taking a liquid drug. • Check for presence of glaucoma; if present do not give meds containing atropine. • Hold drug and call physician if abdomen becomes distended, if bowel sounds diminish or are absent, if impaction is suspected.
Systemic acting: Lomotil (Diphenoxylate HCl with atropine sulfate) Imodium (Loperamide) Paragoric (also called camphorated tincture of opium)	Act systemically to inhibit the peristaltic reflex and reduce GI motility.	Same as above	CNS: drowsiness, headache, sedation, dizziness CV: tachycardia GU: urinary retention GI: dry mouth, nausea/vomiting, constipation	
Laxatives				
Bulk formers: Psyllium (Metamucil) Methylcellulose (Citrucel) Bran	Produce soft stool by retaining fluid. Working Time: 1–3 days	Prophylaxis and treatment of functional constipation	GI: abdominal cramps, diarrhea, nausea/vomiting; intestinal obstruction if taken dry or chewed	• Discontinue drug if abdominal pain occurs. • Advise to take 1 hour apart from other oral meds to prevent absorption of drugs by laxative.
Emollients: Colace (docusate sodium) Surfak (docusate calcium) Dialose (docusate potassium)	Docusate salts act as detergents in the intestine, reduce surface tension of interfacing liquids, thus, promoting incorporation of fat and additional liquid, softening the stool.	For clients who must avoid straining at stool	Increased absorption if used with mineral oil. Throat irritation if liquid used. Mild abdominal cramping	• Advise loss of effectiveness with long-term use. • Dilute liquid but not the syrup preparations to improve taste. • Discontinue if severe abdominal cramping.
Irritants: Cascara (Cas-Evac) Senna (Senokot) Castor oil (Alphamul) Bisacodyl (Ducolax)	Stimulates intestine, promotes peristalsis. Working time: 1–3 hours	Cleansing for pre-op, diagnostic studies; treat constipation unresponsive to other agents	Abdominal cramps, diarrhea. In excessive use: electrolyte imbalance. Constipation after carthARSis. Laxative dependence.	• Advise cascara may color urine reddish-pink or brown depending on urine pH. • Monitor for electrolyte imbalance or laxative dependence.

(continued)

Table 3.41 Continued

Drug	Action	Use	Side Effects	Nursing Implications
Lubricant: Mineral oil	Acts in the colon, lubricates the intestine, and retards colonic fluid absorption. Working time: 6–8 hours	Cleansing enema, preparation for bowel studies, constipation	Impaired absorption of fat-soluble vitamins, digitalis glycosides, sulfonamides, anticoagulants, oral contraceptives. Potential toxic absorption levels of mineral oil if taken with stool softeners. Nausea, vomiting.	• Prevent aspiration by not allowing the patient to lie flat during or after drug administration. • Monitor patients for impaired absorption of meds/vitamins. • Obtain detailed history if patient takes mineral oil as a regular laxative.
Saline/osmotics: Milk of Magnesia Magnesium sulfate Magnesium citrate (Epsom salt) Lactulose (Cephulac)	Produce watery stools that distend the bowel. This promotes peristalsis and bowel evacuation. Working time: 1–6 hours	Preprocedure cleansing, constipation	Abdominal cramps. Flatulence. Diarrhea with dehydration and loss of electrolytes.	• Monitor for fluid and electrolyte balance and dehydration.

For all laxatives: 1. Teach clients the importance of exercise, proper fluid intake and high fiber diet to prevent constipation. Avoid routine use of all laxatives except bulk formers.
2. Do not use any laxative if obstruction is suspected.

8) drug history
9) malabsorption of foods
10) mass in abdomen
11) low-grade fever
12) anemia
13) anorexia
14) presence of bowel sounds: increased or decreased
15) abdominal distention
16) decreased flatus

b. Plan, Implementation, and Evaluation (refer to General Nursing Goal 1 page 259)

☐ Inflammatory Bowel Disease (Regional Enteritis, Ulcerative Colitis)

1. General Information

a. Definition
  1) *regional enteritis* (Crohn's disease) is a segmental transmural inflammatory process that may involve any part of the alimentary tract; the ileum is the principal site
  2) *ulcerative colitis* is a continuous inflammatory process of the mucosa, primarily of the colon and rectum

b. Incidence: young people between 20 and 40 years of age

c. Etiology: unknown: possibly result of infection, stress, and/or autoimmunity; familial tendency

d. Pathophysiology
  1) regional enteritis presents with marked thickening of the submucosa with lymphedema, hyperplasia, granulomas, ulcerations, and fissures; the longitudinal ulcers and transverse fissure produce a cobblestone effect; in the later stages, full thickness penetration of the intestinal wall results in the formation of fistulas and abscesses
  2) ulcerative colitis presents with congestion, edema, multiple superficial ulcerations, and crypt abscesses in the rectum and distal colon and spreads upward; characterized by profuse watery diarrhea containing blood, mucus, and pus.

e. Diagnostic tests
  1) stool for blood, fat, and culture
  2) proctosigmoidoscopy with biopsy
  3) barium enema (cathartics are contraindicated as a prep)

2. Nursing Process

a. Assessment/Analysis
  1) rectal bleeding
  2) diarrhea: frequent liquid stools with

Table 3.42 Comparison of Crohn's Disease and Ulcerative Colitis

	Crohn's Disease	Ulcerative Colitis
General appearance	Usually normal	May feel and look ill
Age	Bimodal: 20–30 yr and 40–50 yr	Mostly young adults
Area affected	Mainly terminal ileum, cecum, and ascending colon (right side)	Colon only, primarily the descending colon (left side)
Extent of involvement	Segmental areas of involvement	Continuous, diffuse areas of involvement
Inflammation	Mostly submucosal	Mostly muscosal
Mucosal appearance	Cobblestone effect; granulomas	Ulcerations
Cancer potential	Normal incidence	Increased incidence
Character of stools	No blood; may have some fat; 3–4 semisoft/day	Blood present; no fat; frequent liquid stools
Reasons for surgery	Fistulas; intestinal obstruction	Poor response to medical therapy; hemorrhage; perforation
Complications	Fistulas; perianal disease; strictures; vitamin and iron deficiencies; fistulas to other organs	Pseudopolyps; hemorrhage; toxic megacolon; cachexia; perforation less often, causes peritonitis

Note: From *Mosby's Medical and Nursing Dictionary*, 1983, St. Louis: Mosby. Used with permission.

tenesmus; may contain blood, mucus, or pus

3) abdominal cramps before bowel movement; colicky cramping with urgency to defecate
4) pain, usually located in the left lower quadrant, with ulcerative colitis
5) anorexia, nausea, vomiting
6) dehydration
7) electrolyte imbalance (e.g., decreased potassium and sodium, metabolic acidosis)
8) weight loss
9) weakness, debilitation, malnutrition
10) anemia
11) fever
12) emotional concerns, immature and dependent personality
13) dietary habits

b. Plans, Implementation, and Evaluation

Goal 1: Client will be well nourished and hydrated.

Plan/Implementation
- Weigh client daily.
- Keep NPO in acute stage; give parenteral fluids with vitamins and minerals as ordered.
- Administer total parenteral nutrition (TPN) as ordered.
- Initiate high-protein, low-residue, high-calorie bland diet as tolerated (see Table 3.43 on page 263).
- Avoid gas-producing or irritating foods and milk products.
- Offer small feedings as necessary.
- Replace deficiency of fat-soluble vitamins (A, D, E, and K).
- Record caloric intake.
- Avoid too hot or too cold foods.
- Urge up to 3,000 ml fluid intake/day (if not contraindicated); keep I&O (include measurement of liquid stools).
- Involve client and significant others with dietitian for proper diet instructions.

Evaluation: Client maintains weight; states meal plan utilizing high-protein, low-residue, high-calorie, bland diet; maintains at least 2,500 ml fluid intake daily.

Goal 2: Client will be free from infection.

Plan/Implementation
- Prevent and treat secondary infection through use of sulfonamides (e.g., sulfasalazine [Azulfidine]) as ordered (see Table 3.36 on page 241).
- Assist and teach client to turn, cough, and deep breathe q2–4h (during acute stage).
- Check temperature q4h, avoid taking rectal temperature if anus is excoriated.
- Administer oral hygiene as necessary.
- Provide good skin care.

Evaluation: Client remains free from signs of infection (e.g., increased temperature, infiltrate in lungs, or secondary infection in mucous membranes of mouth, skin, or colon).

Goal 3: Client will experience reduced physical and psychologic stress.

Plan/Implementation
- Enforce bedrest to decrease intestinal motility in acute stage.

Table 3.43 Foods to be *Avoided* on Low Residue Diets

Types of Foods	Foods to be Avoided
Beverages	Milk in excess of 2 cups
Breads and cereals	Whole grain or bran
Desserts	Any containing fruits and nuts
Fruits	Any with seeds or skins, raw fruits except bananas
Meats, fish, poultry, cheese, eggs	Tough meats, pork, fried or highly seasoned meats, fish, cheese
Vegetables	Raw vegetables

- Maintain quiet, comfortable, nonstressful environment.
- Keep room odor free.
- Empty bedpan promptly and have within easy reach of client during acute episodes.
- Keep perianal area clean and dry, applying lubricant or ointments as necessary.
- Administer pain medications as ordered.
- Give sitz baths at least 3 times/day or as needed.

Evaluation: Client states relief of pain; rests comfortably.

Goal 4: Client will have fewer bowel movements than when admitted.

Plan/Implementation

- Administer antidiarrheal medications as ordered
  - opium alkaloids (paregoric)
  - diphenoxylate (Lomotil)
  - anticholinergic drugs (tincture of belladonna, Donnatol)
  - kaolin and pectin (Kaopectate)
  - see Table 3.41
- Reduce inflammation by administration of
  - azathioprine (Imuran) (immunosuppressive agent, see Table 3.39)
  - 6-mercaptopurine (see Table 5.22)
  - corticosteroids as ordered
- Check bowel sounds q2–4h; report increase or decrease to physician.
- Note frequency, color, and amount of stools.
- Report increase in abdominal distention to physician.
- Reduce emotional stress (direct influence on course of illness).

Evaluation: Client has a decrease in frequency and amount of stools; has no increase in abdominal distention.

Goal 5: Client will maintain a balance of adequate rest and exercise.

Plan/Implementation

- Encourage rest after meals.
- Do not confine to bed unless very weak.
- Provide calm, reassuring environment.
- Give sedation as necessary to provide adequate night's sleep.
- Initiate ambulation at short, frequent intervals.
- Allow for frequent rest periods.

Evaluation: Client verbalizes feeling rested; sleeps through the night; increases periods of ambulation as strength returns.

Goal 6: Client will accept alteration of life-style imposed by chronic illness.

Plan/Implementation

- Provide teaching regarding
  - how to live with chronic disease
  - factors in environment that aggravate colitis (emotional stress, dietary indiscretion, ingestion of irritants, overfatigue, infections, or pregnancy)
  - how to maintain nutrition
  - importance of medical management of the disease
  - need for biannual sigmoidoscopy and barium enema (increased incidence of carcinoma of large intestines)
- Provide emotional counseling and support as needed.
- Encourage verbalization of anxieties.
- Provide diversional activities.

Evaluation: Client verbalizes acceptance of disease; lists life-style modifications to be initiated.

☐ Total Colectomy with Ileostomy

1. General Information

a. Definition: surgical removal of the entire colon, rectum, and anus with the construction of permanent ileostomy to provide for passage of feces

b. Indications: when medical management fails and constant relapses with intractability occur; occurrence of complications (e.g., perforation, hemorrhage, obstruction, toxic megacolon, abscess and fistula); more effective as a treatment for ulcerative colitis

2. Nursing Process

a. Assessment/Analysis

1) physical status
2) emotional status
3) acceptance of ostomy
4) understanding of ostomy function
5) ability to verbalize feelings

b. Plans, Implementation, and Evaluation

Goal 1: Client will be physically and psychologically prepared for surgery.

Plan/Implementation

- Refer to *Surgery* page 158.
- Give TPN as ordered, to improve nutritional status pre-op.
- Prepare bowel for surgery: low-residue diet, clear liquids, oral antibiotics, cathartics, enema.
- Obtain help of an enterostomal therapist, if available, to plan site of stoma placement and to introduce client to appliance.
- Encourage client to express fears and concerns regarding change in body image.
- Introduce client to concept of ostomy support groups; obtain volunteer if desired.

Evaluation: Client views appliances; expresses positive reaction to outcomes of surgery.

Goal 2: Client will remain free from infection and complications postoperatively.

Plan/Implementation

- Refer to *Surgery* page 159.
- Observe stoma size, color.

Evaluation: Client remains free from any signs of post-op infection or complications (e.g., has normal temperature, clear lungs).

Goal 3: Client will maintain normal fluid and electrolyte balance.

Plan/Implementation

- Monitor I&O, weigh daily, NG tube drainage.
- Monitor state of hydration (skin turgor and condition of mucous membranes), urine output.
- Monitor serum electrolyte levels.
- Monitor ileal output; drainage begins immediately post-op.
- Administer IV fluids as ordered, until client can take oral nourishment.

Evaluation: Client's I&O, electrolytes remain within normal limits.

Goal 4: Client will understand dietary restrictions.

Plan/Implementation

- Teach client that food ingested will pass through the ileostomy within 4–6 hours.
- Teach client that each individual has different food tolerances.
- Provide diet information: most ostomy clients are discharged on a low-residue, high-protein, high-carbohydrate diet rich in high-potassium foods and low in gas-producing, highly seasoned, or fried foods.
- Know that vitamin supplements A, D, E, K, and B_{12} may be necessary.
- Prepare client for possible weight gain resulting from increased food tolerance post-op.
- Refer to dietitian as necessary.

Evaluation: Client states dietary changes; verbalizes intent to work out a diet plan within the limits of the individual variations.

Goal 5: Client will achieve self-care management.

Plan/Implementation

- Instruct client (step by step) and receive return demonstration on stoma care including
  - equipment: type, how to use, and where to purchase
  - skin care: ileostomy drainage is erosive and continuous
  - application of appliance
  - odor control
  - use services of enterostomal therapist if available
- Refer to visiting nurses (VNA) for home follow-up or continue following up by enterostomal therapist.

Evaluation: Client successfully manages self-care of ileostomy.

Goal 6: Client will successfully cope with altered body image.

Plan/Implementation

- Encourage verbalization of concerns.
- Assure client that major change in life-style is not necessary.
- Encourage involvement in ostomy club.
- Provide emotional support to the significant other in adjusting to ostomy.
- Obtain sexual counseling for client, if needed.

Evaluation: Client discusses altered body image; shows evidence of coping with change and resumption of normal activity.

☐ Mechanical Obstruction of the Colon

1. General Information

a. Pathophysiology

1) obstruction can be partial or complete
2) emergency situation if blood supply is compromised
3) if blood supply is not compromised, fluid and electrolyte deficiency becomes the major problem
4) absorption decreases and fluids and electrolytes accumulate in GI tract
5) fluid will either stay in GI tract or be lost through vomiting
6) subsequent decrease in extracellular fluid volume (dehydration)
7) metabolic acidosis results

b. Risk/causative factors
1) small intestine: adhesions, hernia, volvulus
2) large intestine: neoplasm, stricture, diverticulitis

c. Medical treatment
1) medical intervention
a) decompression with intestinal tubes
■ Cantor tube: permanent mercury weighted tip
■ Miller-Abbott tube: has port for injection of mercury
■ Length to be passed is determined by physician
b) fluid and electrolyte replacement
2) surgical intervention
a) colon resection with end-to-end anastomosis or temporary/permanent colostomy
b) abdominoperineal resection with permanent colostomy

2. Nursing Process

a. Assessment/Analysis

1) abdomen distended; altered bowel habits; most common with large intestine obstruction
2) projectile vomiting and severe pain, most common with small intestine obstruction
3) decreased or increased bowel sounds
4) decreased flatus

b. Plans, Implementation, and Evaluation

Goals 1 through 4 (refer to "Total Colectomy with Ileostomy" page 264).

Plan/Implementation
■ Attach NG tube to intermittant suction.
■ Care for intestinal tube if ordered
– after the tube is passed, tell client to lie 2 hours in each of the following positions in order: right side, back, left side, to facilitate passage of the tube into the intestine (usually passes at a rate of 2–3 inches/hour)
– do not allow tube to pass rapidly since twisting and knotting may result
– monitor for correct tube placement by testing for ph of aspiration contents (>7 = tube is in small intestine; <7 = tube is in stomach)
– DO NOT tape tube until it has passed into the small intestine
– if massive stomach content loss occurs, monitor for metabolic alkalosis (see Table 3.34); if massive intestinal loss, monitor for acidosis
– remove slowly when ordered to prevent twisting the intestine
■ Know that in addition, the client will undergo pre-op bowel preparation that will include
– clear liquids several days pre-op; then NPO
– bowel sterilization routine as ordered with neomycin and sulfonamides
– several enemas and cathartics
■ Monitor I&O, urine specific gravity, and gastric output.
■ Give narcotics sparingly (may mask symptoms); avoid morphine (decreases intestinal motility).

Evaluation: Client's bowel is clean and prepared for surgery.

Goal 5: Client will cope successfully with altered body image.

Plan/Implementation
■ See "Total Colectomy with Ileostomy" Goal 6 page 164.
■ Instruct client about irrigation and dietary management for regulation of colostomy.
■ If the colostomy is to be closed at a future date, encourage client to work for that day while at the same time reinforcing the importance of good daily care and adjustment to a temporarily changed body image.

Evaluation: Client discusses altered body image; expresses a willingness to adjust and to maintain colostomy until closure can be accomplished.

□ Cancer of the Colon

1. General Information

a. Definition: malignant neoplasm of the large bowel; 70% of cases occur in the rectosigmoid area
b. Incidence
1) 2nd most common malignancy in adults
2) equal in both sexes
3) occurs after 4th decade; peaks in the 7th decade

4) most are adenocarcinoma

c. Risk factors
   1) family history
   2) history of ulcerative colitis, polyps
   3) possibly related to increased fat in diet, food additives, low-fiber diet, or chronic constipation

d. Metastasis
   1) lymph nodes
   2) liver via the bloodstream

e. Diagnostic tests
   1) rectal exam (almost 50% of these tumors are palpable on digital exam)
   2) sigmoidoscopy, colonoscopy
   3) barium enema
   4) stool exam for occult blood
   5) alkaline phosphatase and SGOT: metastasis to liver
   6) carcinoembryonic antigen (CEA) level: elevated in advanced adenocarcinoma

f. Medical treatment
   1) surgical intervention: colon resection
      a) colectomy with anastomosis of the remaining colon or colostomy
      b) abdominal-perineal resection (removal of anus and rectum) with a permanent colostomy
   2) medical intervention
      a) radiation therapy
      b) chemotherapy

2. Nursing Process

a. Assessment/Analysis

1) change in bowel habits; blood in stool (more likely with left colon and rectal involvement)
2) vague, dull pain (more likely with ascending-colon involvement)
3) anorexia, weight loss, weakness, and anemia
4) signs of obstruction
5) hemorrhage
6) perforation with peritonitis, abscess and fistula formation

b. Plans, Implementation, and Evaluation

Refer to "Total Colectomy with Ileostomy" page 264 and "Mechanical Obstruction of the Colon" page 264. Refer to *Cellular Aberration* for information and goals pertinent to chemotherapy and radiation therapy.

☐ Hemorrhoids or Anal Fissure

1. General Information

a. Definitions
   1) *hemorrhoids*: dilated veins under the mucous membranes in the anal area; may be either internal or external
   2) *anal fissure*: linear ulceration on the margin of the anus

b. Predisposing factors
   1) straining at stool
   2) pregnancy
   3) portal hypertension
   4) congestive heart failure

c. Complications
   1) bleeding
   2) thrombosis
   3) strangulation
   4) infection

d. Medical treatment
   1) medical intervention
      a) high-roughage diet and 6–8 glasses of fluid/day
      b) stool softeners
      c) ointments or suppositories to shrink hemorrhoids
      d) warm sitz bath
      e) injection of a sclerosing substance into the tissues at the base of the vein
      f) rubber band ligation
   2) surgical intervention
      a) hemorrhoidectomy: excision of dilated veins
      b) fissurectomy: excision of fissure

2. Nursing Process

a. Assessment/Analysis

1) pain and pruritus around anus
2) character and amount of rectal drainage
3) usual bowel habits
4) abdominal distention
5) urinary retention
6) anemia caused by chronic bleeding

b. Plans, Implementation, and Evaluation

Goal 1: Client will remain free from post-op complications.

Plan/Implementation
- Refer to *Surgery* page 159.
- Avoid sitting for prolonged periods; while sitting, use flotation pad.
- Prevent infection
  - initiate procedures as ordered for thorough pre-op bowel cleansing
  - DO NOT take rectal temperature
  - administer perineal care with antiseptic solution after each stool

– administer sitz baths as necessary to clean incision

Evaluation: Client remains free from complications (e.g., infection).

Goal 2: Client will experience relief of pain.

Plan/Implementation

- Give analgesics as ordered.
- Avoid supine position; if supine position is unavoidable, use flotation pad under buttocks.
- Apply ice packs or warm, moist compresses if ordered.
- DO NOT use rubber rings.
- Administer topical anesthesia as ordered.

Evaluation: Client states pain is controlled; is comfortable in all positions.

Goal 3: Client's bowel function will return to normal.

Plan/Implementation

- Give low-residue, soft diet as tolerated for 1st week post-op; then advance diet to include roughage and fresh fruits.
- Force fluids to 2,500–3,000 ml/day unless contraindicated.
- Administer stool softener/lubricant or laxative as ordered (see Table 3.41).
- Provide support during initial BM, noting presence of blood in stool; be alert for vertigo; and administer analgesic as necessary.
- Teach client how to avoid constipation after discharge.
- Watch for and teach client symptoms of anal stricture (and report to physician)
  - – increased pain with BM
  - – difficulty passing stool

Evaluation: Client passes soft, brown, formed stool on 3rd post-op day with minimal discomfort; lists ways to prevent constipation; states signs of anal stricture.

References

Alterescu, K. (1985). The ostomy: What about special procedures? *American Journal of Nursing*, *85*, 1363–1367.

Alterescu, K. (1985). The ostomy: What do you teach the patient? *American Journal of Nursing*, *85*, 1250–1253.

Ash, S., Wimberly, A., & Mertz, S. (1983). Peritoneal dialysis for acute and chronic renal failure: An update. *Hospital Practice*, *18*(1), 179–210.

Bates, P. (1984). Three post-op perils of prostate surgery. *RN*, *47*(2), 10–43.

Becker, K. (1988). Performing in-depth abdominal assessment. *Nursing88*, *18*(6), 59–63.

Boarini, J. (1985). The ostomy: What can go wrong? *American Journal of Nursing*, *85*, 1358–1362.

Brogna, L., & Lakaszawski, M. (1986). The continent urostomy. *American Journal of Nursing*, *85*, 160–163.

Casadonte, L. (1984). The patient with a fistula, a colostomy, and an ileal conduit. *RN*, *47*(9), 42–46.

*Chambers, J. (1983). Bowel management in dialysis patients. *American Journal of Nursing*, *83*, 1051–1052.

Fleming, L., & Kane, J. (1984). Step-by-step guide to safe peritoneal dialysis. *RN*, *47*(2), 44–47.

Frank, A. & Murray, S. (1988). A no guess guide for urinary color assessment. *RN*, *51*(6), 46–51.

Ghiotto, S. (1988). A full range of care for nephrostomy patients. *RN*, *51*(4), 72–77.

Given, B., & Simmons, S. (1984). *Gastroenterology in clinical nursing* (4th ed.). St. Louis: Mosby.

Gloeckner, M. Perceptions of sexual attractiveness following ostomy surgery. *Research in Nursing and Health*, *7*, 87–92.

McConnell, E. (1987). Meeting the challenge of intestinal obstruction. *Nursing87*, *17*(7), 34–42.

McConnell, E., & Zimmerman, M. (1983). *Care of patients with urologic problems*. Philadelphia: Lippincott.

Murphy, L., & Cole, M. (1983). Renal disease: Nutritional implications. *Nursing Clinics of North America*, *18*, 57–70.

Neal, M., Cohen, P., & Reighley, J. (1983). *Nursing care planning guides, set 3* (2nd ed.). Baltimore: Williams & Wilkins.

Office of Medical Applications of Research. (1988). Prevention and treatment of kidney stones. *JAMA*, *260*, 977–981.

Pagana, K. (1987). Preventing complications in jejunostomy tube feedings. *Dimensions of Critical Care Nursing*, *6*(1), 28–38.

Pagana, K., & Pagana, T. (1986). *Diagnostic testing and nursing implications: A case study approach* (2nd ed.). St. Louis: Mosby.

Plantemoli, C. (1984). When the patient has a Foley. *RN*, *47*(3), 42–43.

Pritchard, V. (1988). Geriatric infections: the urinary tract. *RN*, *51*(5), 36–38.

Quinlan, M. (1984). UTI: Helping your patients control it once and for all. *RN 47*(3), 38–42.

Reilly, N., Torosian, L. (1988). The new wave in lithotripsy: Implications for nursing. *RN*, *51*(3), 44–50.

Ruge, C. (1987). Catheter-related UTIs: What's the best way to prevent them? *Nursing87*, *17*(12), 50–51.

Smith, D. (1985). The ostomy: How is it managed? *American Journal of Nursing*, *85*, 1246–1249.

Stark, J. (1988). A quick guide to urinary tract assessment. *Nursing88*, *18*(7), 56–58.

Watt, R. (1985). The ostomy: Why is it created? *American Journal of Nursing*, *85*, 1241–1245.

*See Reprint Section

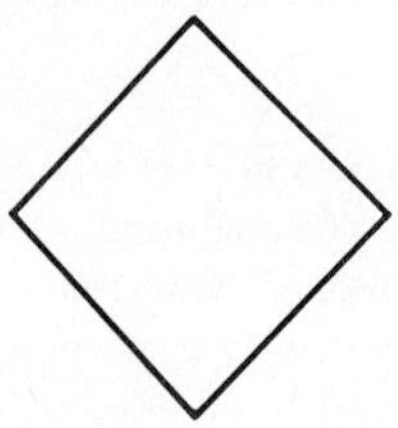

Safety and Security

(The nursing care presented in this unit concerns selected health problems related to disturbances in the nervous system, eye, ear, nose, and throat.)

General Concepts

Overview/Physiology

1. Nervous system: like an electrical conductance system; coordinates and controls all activities of the body
   a. Receives stimuli or information from internal and external environments over varied sensory pathways
   b. Communicates information between distant parts of body (periphery) and central nervous system
   c. Computes or processes information received at various reflex (spinal cord) and conscious (higher brain) levels to determine responses appropriate to existing situations
   d. Transmits information rapidly over varied motor pathways to effector organs for body-action control or modification
2. Central nervous system
   a. Brain
      1) cerebrum or cerebral cortex
         a) frontal lobe: functions
            ■ personality
            ■ higher intellectual functions (e.g., learning, problem solving)
            ■ ethical, social, and moral behavior
            ■ posterior edge of frontal lobe: center for initiation of motor function
         b) parietal lobe: responsible for interpretation of sensory input
         c) temporal lobe: center for hearing, taste, and smell
         d) occipital lobe: visual center
         e) structure
            ■ skull
            ■ meninges: connective tissue covering brain and spinal cord
            ■ layers of brain
               – dura mater
                  * extradura
                  * epidura
                  * inner dura (tentorium)
                  * subdura
               – arachnoid
               – pia mater
            ■ blood-brain barrier
            ■ brain tissue
      2) brainstem: contains midbrain, pons, and medulla oblongata
         a) relays impulses from spinal cord to cerebrum
         b) controls basic body functions (cardiac, respiratory, and vasomotor centers [medulla])
      3) cerebellum
         a) orientation of body in space (equilibrium)
         b) coordination and inhibition of movement
         c) control of antigravity muscles
         d) coordination of muscle tone
   b. Spinal cord
      1) 31 segments (do not correspond in name to the vertebral segments)
         a) 8 cervical: supply neck and upper extremities, diaphragm, and intercostals
         b) 12 thoracic: supply thoracic and abdominal areas
         c) 5 lumbar: supply lower extremities
         d) 5 sacral: supply lower extremities; urinary tract and bowel control
         e) 1 coccygeal
      2) anterior portion of cord carries motor information (descending tracts)
      3) posterior section of cord carries sensory information (ascending tracts)
      4) lateral columns contain preganglionic fibers for autonomic nervous system
3. Peripheral nervous system
   a. Cranial nerves (12): classified in order of their arising from the brain (number) and by describing their nature, function, and distribution (name) (see Table 3.44)

Table 3.44 Cranial Nerves

Number	Name	Type
I	Olfactory	Sensory
II	Optic	Sensory
III	Oculomotor	Motor, parasympathetic
IV	Trochlear	Motor
V	Trigeminal	Sensory, motor
VI	Abducent	Motor
VII	Facial	Sensory, motor, parasympathetic
VIII	Acoustic or auditory	Sensory
IX	Glossopharyngeal	Sensory, motor, parasympathetic
X	Vagus	Sensory, motor, parasympathetic
XI	Accessory	Motor
XII	Hypoglossal	Motor

b. Spinal nerves (31 pairs)

4. Autonomic nervous sytem: concerned with the control of involuntary bodily functions; divided into parasympathetic (craniosacral) and sympathetic (thoracolumbar) divisions (see Table 3.45)

a. Divisions

1) parasympathetic or craniosacral division controls normal body functioning

2) sympathetic or thoracolumbar division prepares body for fight or flight

b. Most effector organs receive innervation from both sympathetic and parasympathetic fibers

c. Vascular supply of skeletal muscle receives only sympathetic innervation

5. Vision

a. Major function of eyes is to produce vision: lightwaves → cornea → lens → retina → optic nerve (II) → occipital lobe of brain

b. Cranial nerves of the eye

1) optic (II): vision

2) oculomotor (III), trochlear (IV), abducent (VI): external muscles of the eye

3) oculomotor (III) also controls pupil size

c. Exterior of eye

1) tears secreted by lacrimal glands to lubricate lids and keep corneas moist; excess tears drain through lacrimal ducts into nasal cavity

2) six extrinsic eye muscles produce movements of eyeball

3) outer layer of eye

a) cornea: transparent covering of eye, called "window of the eye"

b) sclera: opaque, connective tissue covering all of eye except cornea

d. Interior of eye (see Figure 3.19)

1) iris: circular muscle that constricts or dilates pupil

2) lens: focuses image accurately on retina

3) aqueous humor and vitreous humor: liquids acting along with lens as refracting media

4) choroid: black, inner surface of eye that prevents scattering of light rays

5) retina: light-sensitive layer of eye; sensations of vision result from retina's focused response to image

6) optic disk: entrance of optic nerve into eyeball

7) optic pathway: transmits visual data to occipital lobe of the brain

Table 3.45 Parasympathetic and Sympathetic Effects of the Autonomic Nervous System

Site	Parasympathetic Effect	Sympathetic Effect
Eye	Pupils constricted Ciliary muscles excited	Pupils dilated
Nasal mucosa	Thin, copius muscus secreted	Vasoconstriction in nasal mucosa
Lungs	Bronchoconstriction	Bronchodilation
Heart	Cardiac rate slowed Contraction force decreased	Cardiac rate increased Contraction force increased Coronary arteries dilate
Liver		Hepatic glycongenolysis and lipolysis
Gallbladder	Biliary ducts stimulated	
Intestine	Peristalsis stimulated	Peristalsis inhibited
Urinary bladder	Detrusor muscle excited Trigone inhibited Urinary excretion promoted	Detrusor muscle inhibited Trigone excited Urinary retention promoted
Adrenal hormones	Secretion inhibited	Secretion increased

Figure 3.19 The Eye (Horizontal Section)

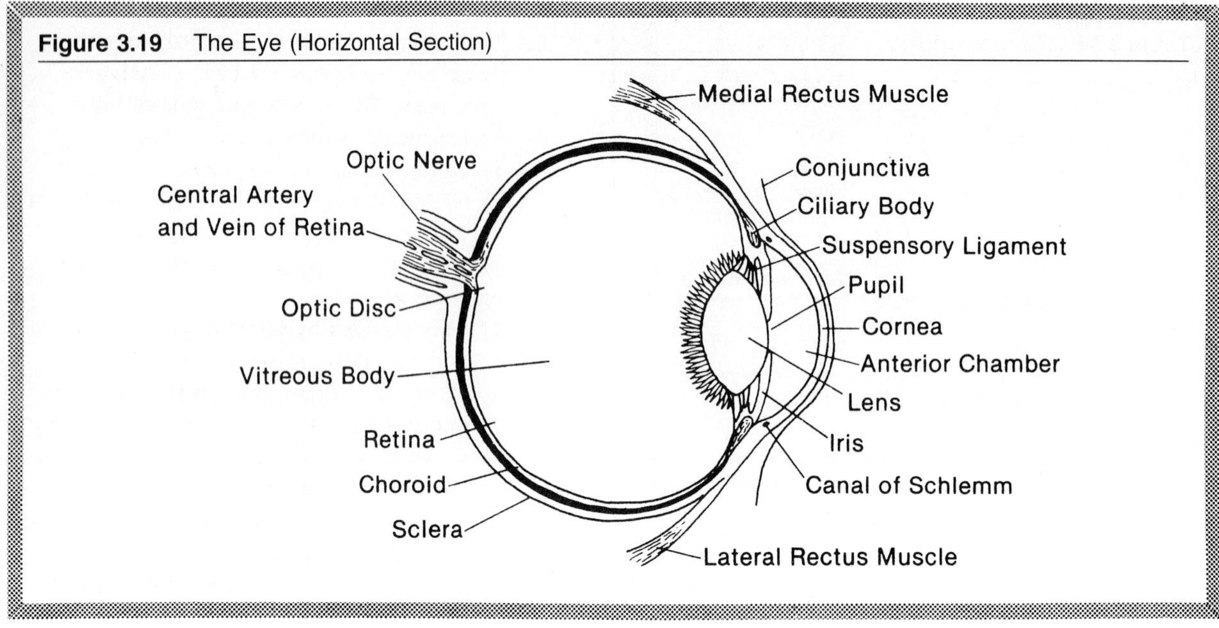

- **e.** Cerebrum/occipital lobe: interprets visual information

6. Hearing
- **a.** The major functions of the ears are balance and hearing; hearing pathway: sound waves → pinna → external ear canal → tympanic membrane → ossicles in middle ear → cochlea → auditory nerve (VIII) → auditory cortex in temporal lobe
- **b.** External ear
  - **1)** pinna: external flap of cartilage covered with skin that gathers and concentrates sound waves
  - **2)** external ear canal (auditory meatus): cavity in skull lined with skin; ceruminous glands produce cerumen (wax) to assist in protecting the canal from small foreign particles; conveys sound waves from pinna to tympanic membrane
  - **3)** tympanic membrane: flexible membrane that closes distal end of external auditory canal; membrane vibrates in response to sound, transmitting vibrations to middle ear
- **c.** Middle ear
  - **1)** ossicles: malleus, incus, and stapes
  - **2)** set into motion by sound waves from tympanic membrane
  - **3)** amplifies sound waves and transmits them to inner ear
  - **4)** connected with nasopharynx by eustachian tube
- **d.** Inner ear
  - **1)** cochlea: organ of sound perception
  - **2)** innervated by the auditory nerve VIII
    - **a)** cochlear branch: transmits auditory impulses from the cochlea to auditory cortex of brain
    - **b)** vestibular branch: controls balance
- **e.** Auditory portion of cerebral cortex interprets auditory information (temporal lobe)

7. Nose
- **a.** Air passageway
- **b.** Contains sensory receptors for smell
- **c.** Lined with mucosa, hair
  - **1)** secretes mucus
  - **2)** filters, warms, and humidifies inspired air
- **d.** Paranasal sinuses drain into nasal cavity

8. Throat
- **a.** Contains pharynx with tonsils and larynx with vocal cords
- **b.** Glottis closes over larynx during swallowing to prevent aspiration
- **c.** Chief function: passageway for air; filters and humidifies air

Application of the Nursing Process to the Client with Problems of Safety and Security

1. Assessment
- **a.** Health history
  - **1)** family history
  - **2)** history of problem: date of onset, precipitating factors, extent, duration or frequency, interventions that have been effective, location, any changes in description
  - **3)** headaches

4) seizures
5) medications: prescription and nonprescription
6) recent change in behavior or personality

b. Physical examination

1) neurologic examination
   a) cognitive function
      ■ general behavior, emotional status
      ■ level of consciousness (LOC): major index of client's neurologic status
        – *level 1*: consciousness (oriented to person, place, and time)
        – *level 2*: lethargy, somnolence, drowsiness, or obtundation
        – *level 3*: stupor (can be aroused by verbal stimuli but responds poorly or inappropriately)
        – *level 4*: light coma, semicoma (no response to verbal stimuli but responds to painful stimuli)
        – *level 5*: deep coma (no reaction to painful stimuli)
      ■ attention span
      ■ ability to follow commands
      ■ memory: short and long term
      ■ arithmetic ability
      ■ abstract thinking
      ■ language/speech
        – *motor aphasia* (expressive): inability to speak or write words
        – *sensory aphasia* (receptive): inability to comprehend written words (visual) or spoken words (auditory)
        – *dysarthria*: difficult speech caused by paralysis of muscles
   b) cerebellar function
      ■ balance
      ■ coordination
   c) motor function
      ■ muscle size, tone, and strength
      ■ involuntary movements (e.g., tremors)
      ■ coordination and accuracy of movement
      ■ motor integration
      ■ bowel and bladder function
   d) sensory function
      ■ superficial sensation: touch and pressure
      ■ superficial pain
      ■ sensitivity to temperature and vibration
      ■ deep pressure, pain
      ■ motion and position sense
      ■ vision
        – amount of sight with or without glasses or contact lenses
        – distortion
          * halos around lights
          * difficulty adjusting to dark room
          * diplopia
          * floaters
      ■ hearing
        – amount of hearing
          * use of hearing aid
          * tinnitus or other noises
        – conductive deafness (common causes: otosclerosis, otitis media)
          * impairment of outer- and middle-ear conduction of sound waves
          * causes problems of perception of volume, not discrimination of sounds
          * can benefit from hearing aid
          * benefits from increased decibels (dB) and high frequencies (cps)
        – sensorineural deafness (common causes: old age, noise, drug toxicity)
          * impairment of inner-ear nerve conduction
          * causes problems of loss of sensitivity to and discrimination of sounds
          * hearing aid not beneficial
          * benefits from decreased decibels and low frequencies
        – combined (conductive and sensorineural)
        – general speech pattern
        – indications of hearing loss
          * says "huh" frequently
          * asks you to repeat what you said
          * does not respond to questions or conversation
          * responds inappropriately to questions or comments
   e) reflexes: superficial and deep tendon
   f) cranial nerves (see Table 3.44)
2) neuro check
   a) LOC: *most reliable indicator of neurologic status* (see cognitive function above)
   b) vital signs
   c) pupils: size and reaction to light

d) motor function
- move all extremities
- muscle strength (grip)

e) sensory function: response to touch or painful stimuli

f) seizures

g) blood or fluid leakage from nose or ear(s)

h) posturing
- decorticate posture (corticospinal tract): rigid flexion of head, arms, wrists, and fingers, and extension with internal rotation of legs (see Figure 3.20)
- decerebrate posture (midbrain and pons): rigid extension of head, neck, back, arms, and legs, with hyperpronation of arms and plantar flexion of feet (see Figure 3.21)

c. Diagnostic tests

1) lumbar puncture (LP)

a) description
- collection of cerebrospinal fluid (CSF), measurement of pressure and characteristics of spinal fluid
- Queckenstedt's test can be done during LP: with manometer still in place, compress jugular veins for 10 seconds
  - normal response: increase in spinal fluid pressure of approximately 100 mm H_2O within 10 seconds and return to normal within 30 seconds after compression is removed
  - abnormal response: drop in spinal fluid pressure or no rise in pressure; indicates complete obstruction of flow of spinal fluid

b) nursing care
- explain procedure carefully to client prior to procedure
- position client on side with legs flexed onto abdomen and head bent down
- keep client flat in bed up to 24 hours after test to avoid a headache caused by fluid-tension change
- review CSF characteristics
- force fluids to replace loss and restore fluid balance
- observe for headache

2) radiologic exams

a) x-rays of skull and spine

b) computerized axial tomogram (CAT scan)
- description: 360° photographed view of brain in 1° angles; provides data on integrity of intracranial structures and precise location of abnormalities; used with or without contrast medium
- nursing care
  - explain procedure to client beforehand
  - client needs to lie still on table for 30–60 minutes

c) brain scan
- description: following administration of oral or IV radiopharmaceutical, the head is scanned and uptake of the material is recorded
- nursing care
  - explain procedure to client
  - reassure about radioactivity

d) magnetic resonance imaging (MRI)

e) cerebral arteriogram
- description: injection of a radiopaque dye through a catheter inserted into femoral, carotid, or vertebral artery; aortic arch; or brachial vessels to study cerebral circulation
- nursing care

Figure 3.20 Decorticate Posturing

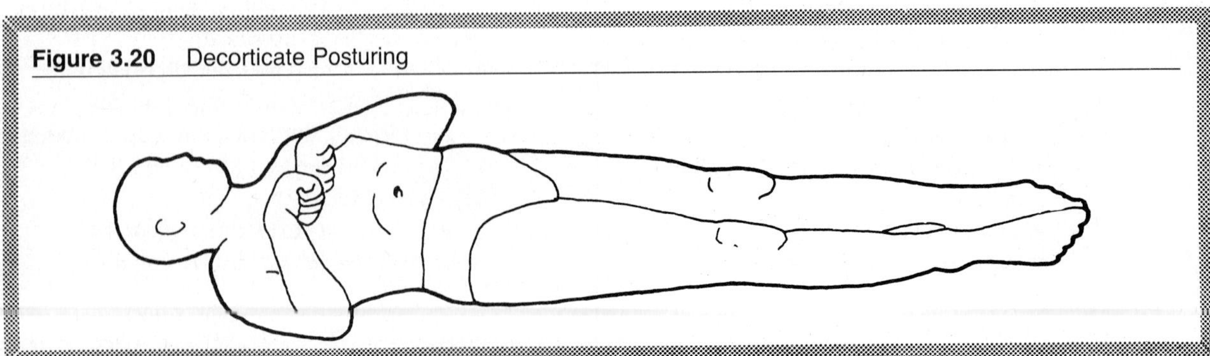

Figure 3.21 Decerebrate Posturing

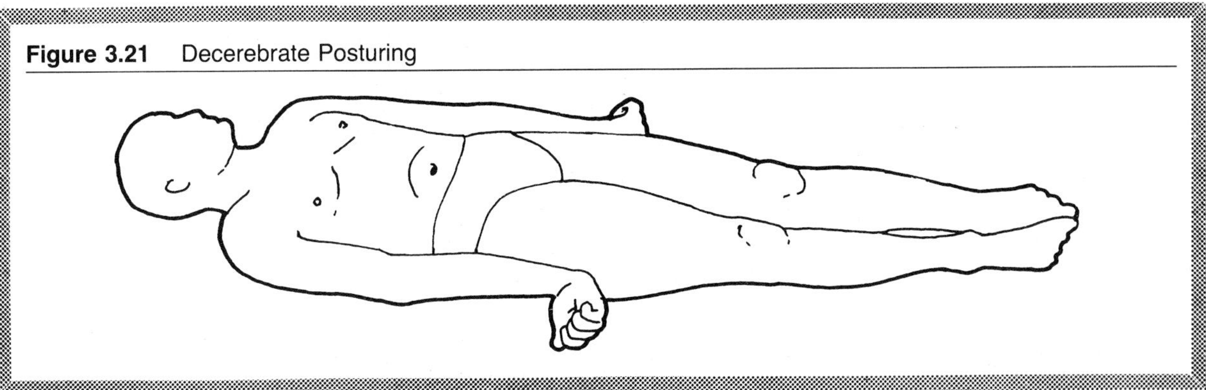

- explain procedure and post-test routine to client before test
- ensure pretest baseline neurologic status is documented
- check for allergies to iodine and report if present
- remove hairpins and dentures as ordered
- bedrest 8–24 hours after test with head of bed elevated 30°
- check incision for hemorrhage frequently
- maintain pressure dressing to incision site if femoral or brachial artery used; apply ice bag to reduce swelling
- watch for symptoms of sensitivity to dye (urticaria, pallor, respiratory difficulty) and report immediately
- watch for neurologic changes that indicate emboli in cerebrovascular system (limb weakness or paralysis; facial paralysis; speech difficulty; disorientation; change in level of consciousness) and report immediately
- observe and record vital signs and neurologic signs per protocol (usually q15min until stable than q1h for several hours, then q4h)

f) ventriculogram

g) pneumoencephalogram

3) electroencephalogram (EEG)

a) description: study of electrical activity of brain

b) nursing care

- ■ give information to client to allay fear of being electrocuted
- ■ clean client's hair before the test
- ■ continue anticonvulsants
- ■ have client remain on anticonvulsant
- ■ have client eat meal prior to test (fasting affects electrical pattern) but avoid stimulants (e.g., coffee, tea, Coke, cocoa)
- ■ tell client to remain calm and quiet during the test
- ■ remove EEG paste from hair after test

4) eye tests

a) Snellen test (eye chart) (see *Nursing Care of the Child* page 526)

b) ophthalmoscopic exam

c) intraocular pressure (normal: 12–20 mm Hg)

5) ear/hearing tests

a) otoscopic exam

b) whisper test for gross hearing: cover the ear not being tested and whisper words into the other ear or hold a ticking watch near the ear

c) audiogram

- ■ client wears earphones in soundproof room and signals when tone is heard, when tone disappears, and in which ear the tone is heard
- ■ hearing is measured in *intensity* (dB = decibels) and *frequency* (cps = cycles per second)

d) Weber and Rinne tests (see *Nursing Care of the Child* page 526)

6) nose/sense of smell tests: provide various scents for client to identify with eyes closed (e.g., alcohol, chocolate, tobacco)

7) mouth and throat/sense of taste tests: provide various things for client to taste with eyes closed (e.g., chocolate, peppermint)

2. Analysis

a. Safe, effective care environment

1) potential for injury

2) potential knowledge deficit
3) potential sensory-perceptual alteration (specify)

b. Physiological integrity
1) potential activity intolerance
2) potential for aspiration
3) pain
4) impaired physical mobility
5) ineffective breathing pattern
6) impaired verbal communication
7) hyperthermia

c. Psychological integrity
1) fear
2) altered thought processes
3) social isolation

d. Health promotion/maintenance
1) ineffective family coping: disabled
2) altered health maintenance
3) knowledge deficit
4) self care deficit

3. General Nursing Plans, Implementation, and Evaluation

Goal 1: Client will be free from increased intracranial pressure.

Plan/Implementation

- Monitor for early signs of increased intracranial pressure
  - changes in level of consciousness
  - vital signs changes
    * BP: widening of pulse pressure; systolic increases, diastolic remains the same
    * rise in temperature with failing thermoregulator
    * bradycardia
    * slow, deep irregular respirations
  - pupils: unequal, progressing to fixed and dilated
  - other clinical signs and symptoms (classic triad)
    * headache (generalized)
    * projectile vomiting
    * papilledema
- Assess at least q15min.
- Administer osmotic diuretics (e.g., mannitol) as ordered (see Table 3.36) and then monitor urine output qh.
- Keep client slightly dehydrated to reduce or prevent cerebral edema.
- Administer corticosteroid therapy, if ordered.
- Prevent transient increases in intracranial pressure
  - elevate head of bed 15°–30°
  - avoid neck flexion
  - maintain calm environment
  - avoid Valsalva maneuver (straining)
  - administer stool softeners and teach client not to strain with bowel evacuation
  - avoid bending over, coughing, sneezing, or vomiting
  - avoid isometric contraction of muscles (e.g., pushing up in bed on elbows, pressing feet against a footboard)

Evaluation: Client's intracranial pressure remains within normal limits (5–10 mm Hg); increase in intracranial pressure is immediately detected.

Goal 2: Client will remain free from complications of unconsciousness.

Plan/Implementation

- See General Nursing Goal 4, *Activity and Rest*, page 295.
- Prevent contractures and immobile joints (e.g., use range-of-motion exercises).
- Keep skin clean, dry, and intact.
- Keep mucous membranes clean, moist, and intact.
- Maintain adequate bowel and bladder function.
- Ensure normal respiratory function (e.g., turn client frequently).
- Provide safe environment (e.g., side rails).
- Administer feedings per NG tube as ordered
  - put client in high-Fowler's position if allowed
  - check to be sure tube is in stomach and not lungs (aspirate stomach contents; inject 5 ml of air while listening with a stethoscope over the gastric area for a swishing sound)
  - give feeding at slow rate
  - observe for regurgitation during and after feeding
  - observe for gastric retention
  - give feedings at room temperature
  - know that client will probably be given no more than 2 liters/day of a liquid feeding with a concentration of 0.5–1 kilocalorie/ml
- Administer total parenteral nutrition (TPN) as ordered (see reprint page 351).
- Check tissue hydration.
- Monitor fluid and electrolyte balance.
- Prevent corneal damage (e.g., use eye patches as needed).
- Maintain communication with client.

Evaluation: Client is free from contractures, immobile joints, pressure sores, fecal impactions, respiratory distress, injuries, malnutrition, and fluid and electrolyte imbalances.

Goal 3: Client with aphasia will maximize ability to use and understand written and spoken words.

Plan/Implementation

- Determine client's level of understanding.
- Determine client's use of speech or communication skills.
- Use gestures if client understands that best.
- Use aids to increase and improve communication: word cards, pictures, slate boards, and audiotapes.
- Talk slowly using natural tone (do not abbreviate, reducing sentences to a shorter, incomplete form; it does not help comprehension).
- Use simple words and phrases.
- Allow client time to respond; be patient.
- Listen and watch carefully when the client attempts to communicate.
- Keep distractions to a minimum.
- Maintain a calm, accepting manner.
- Sit level with client and maintain eye contact.
- Arrange for referral to speech therapist as needed.

Evaluation: Client attempts to communicate using written and spoken words.

Goal 4: Disabled client will function as independently as possible.

Plan/Implementation

- Determine client's strengths and deficits.
- Establish realistic, long-range goals with client and significant other.
- Devise measures with client to achieve goals
  - institute measures for gaining bowel and bladder control if necessary
  - arrange for physical therapy
  - arrange for occupational and recreational therapy
  - give client and significant others emotional support (e.g., adapting to altered body image, see *Loss, Death and Dying* page 30)
  - refer to appropriate community agency

Evaluation: Client performs ADL, to extent possible, without assistance.

Goal 5: Client will adapt to visual deficits.

Plan/Implementation

- Call client by name when approaching.
- Identify yourself when approaching client.
- Communicate in usual manner.
- Ambulate with client.
- Teach client
  - how to summon staff
  - where possessions are
  - physical layout of room
  - placement of food on tray
  - arrangement of food on plate
  - use of cane to aid in walking
- Provide meaningful sensory input
  - interaction with staff, significant others
  - radio, records, TV
  - physical exercise
- Provide safe environment (e.g., remove unnecessary equipment).
- Refer to appropriate community agencies.
- Encourage and reinforce client's independence.

Evaluation: Client functions in hospital environment without difficulty.

Goal 6: Client will adapt to hearing loss.

Plan/Implementation

- Face client when speaking.
- Keep light on your own face so client can watch your mouth.
- Speak with normal speech pattern.
- Allow more time than usual for commuunication.
- Assist client to get a hearing aid if appropriate.

Evaluation: Client understands conversation.

Selected Health Problems Resulting in an Interference with Sensation and Perception

☐ Acute Head Injury

1. General Information

a. Clients with acute head trauma need close scrutiny immediately following trauma; shock is rarely seen

b. Types

1) *concussion*: no structural alteration, but immediate and transitory impairment of neurologic function resulting from mechanical force and release of enzymes

2) *contusion*: structural alteration (bruised cortex) characterized by extravasation of blood

3) *Laceration*: a tear in brain or blood vessel

4) *hemorrhage*

a) extradural or epidural: arterial blood collects between skull and dura rapidly; usually results from a tear in an artery

- may lose consciousness and regain it temporarily
- within few hours, rapid deterioration: lethargy, coma, hemiplegia

b) subdural: venous bleeding (hematoma) below dura accompanied by manifestations of increased ICP
   - acute: develops within few days after injury; surgical intervention needed
   - subacute: develops between few days to three weeks; surgical intervention follows
   - chronic: develops weeks to months after injury

2. Nursing Process

a. **Assessment/Analysis** (refer to neurologic exam page 271)

b. **Plans, Implementation, and Evaluation**

Goal 1: Client will have an open airway at all times.

Plan/Implementation
- Establish and maintain airway.
- Position client for optimum ventilation.
- Maintain adequate O_2 level through use of respiratory aids as necessary.

Evaluation: Client's airway remains unobstructed; color is normal; blood gases are within normal limits.

Goal 2: Client will be protected from increasing intracranial pressure.

Plan/Implementation
- Refer to General Nursing Goal 1, page 274.

Evaluation: Client is free from papilledema; maintains normal vital signs, stable LOC.

Goal 3: Client will maintain optimal fluid and electrolyte status.

Plan/Implementation
- Monitor and record I&O.
- Administer IV fluids as ordered (fluids are usually restricted because of fear of increased intracranial pressure).
- Give osmotic diuretics (e.g., mannitol) as ordered (see Table 3.37).
- Monitor serum electrolyte levels.

Evaluation: Client's output remains greater than intake.

Goal 4: Client will have any fluid or blood from nose or ears detected.

Plan/Implementation
- Observe and record at least qh any leak of blood or clear fluid from nose or ears.
- Do not pack nose or ear; have fluid drain onto sterile towel or dressing.
- Report to physician immediately if any drainage is found.

Evaluation: Client remains free from fluid or blood leakage from nose and ears.

Goal 5: Client will be free from infection or injuries.

Plan/Implementation
- Protect from chilling.
- Take seizure precautions: padded side rails, nonmetal airway and suction apparatus at bedside.
- Employ aseptic technique during all invasive procedures.
- Do not permit visitors with colds.

Evaluation: Client remains afebrile; has skin and mucous membranes free from cuts, ecchymosis, and abrasions.

☐ Intracranial Surgery

1. General Information

a. Definitions: surgery performed inside the cranial cavity
   1) *craniotomy*: any operation on the cranium
      a) tentorium: fold of dura mater between cerebellum and occipital lobes
      b) supratentorial: above the cerebellum (e.g., cerebrum, anterior 2/3 of brain)
      c) infratentorial: posterior cranial fossa (e.g., cerebellum, brainstem, posterior 1/3 of brain)
   2) *cranioplasty*: repair of cranial defect by inserting a bone graft or a plate made of a synthetic substance; protects the brain from trauma

b. Reasons for surgery
   1) to debride or repair any trauma to the skull and underlying structures
   2) to control intracranial hemorrhage (e.g., aneurysms)
   3) to remove space-occupying lesions (e.g., scar tissue, abscess, tumor)
   4) intracrainial neoplasms
      a) all potentially fatal unless treated, because of lack of space within skull
      b) more than 50% are malignant
      c) types
         - gliomas (within brain substance)
         - meningiomas (external to brain substance)

2. Nursing Process

a. Assessment/Analysis

1) establish baseline data preoperability (refer to neurologic exam page 271)
2) client and significant others' knowledge of procedure and expected outcome

b. Plans, Implementations, and Evaluation

Goal 1: Client and significant others will be able to explain pre-op/post-op care, and OR-RR-ICU environment and care.

Plan/Implementation

- Prepare client for surgery (see "Perioperative Period" page 157).
- Prepare client for the likelihood of periocular edema and photophobia post-op.

Evaluation: Client and significant others describe planned procedure, post-op routine.

Goal 2: Client will be physically prepared for surgery.

Plan/Implementation

- Refer to "Perioperative Period" page 157.
- Know that narcotics are contraindicated pre-op.
- Prepare scalp
  - wash hair
  - cut hair (save according to agency policy); shave scalp
  - wash head and cover with clean towel
- Carry out any special order (e.g., insert indwelling Foley catheter, give enemas slowly to avoid straining and increased intracranial pressure).

Evaluation: Client's scalp is prepared for surgery without nicks or cuts.

Goal 3: Client will remain free from respiratory, circulatory, renal, neurologic, or psychologic complications or any infections postoperatively.

Plan/Implementation

- Refer to "Perioperative Period" page 157.
- Perform frequent neuro checks; compare with pre-op baseline (refer to neurologic exam page 271).
- Observe for seizures.
- Monitor breathing; NO COUGHING.
- Support head when turning client.
- Position properly and frequently
  - supratentorial craniotomy: do not position on operative site if large tumor was excised; elevate head 45°
  - infratentorial craniotomy: keep head of bed flat and client's head aligned with vertebral column at all times; position on either side for 1st 24 hours, not on back; avoid flexion of neck (danger is brain-stem compression)
- Do not suction via nose.
- Do not use central nervous system depressants (e.g., opiates, sedatives).
- Check ears, nose, and dressing for drainage (blood/CSF leakage).
- Change dressings only when ordered; reinforce as needed.
- Use strict aseptic technique for all dressings and other procedures.
- Assess periocular edema; relieve with ice packs.
- Administer steroids as ordered (e.g, dexamethasone sodium [Decadron]) to prevent/relieve cerebral edema.
- Do not take oral temps.
- Give passive ROM exercises q8h.

Evaluation: Client remains free from complications in the post-op period.

Goal 4: Client and significant others will accept lengthy rehabilitation period.

Plan/Implementation

- See General Nursing Goal 4 page 275.
- Inform client of residual effects that may be temporary (e.g, diplopia) or permanent (e.g., aphasia, paralysis).
- Inform client of cosmetic protection available when indicated (e.g., hairpiece, wig).
- Prevent client from striking or bumping head.

Evaluation: Client and significant others express willingness to participate in rehabilitation program; verbalize understanding of the need for patience and persistence.

☐ Cerebrovascular Accident (CVA)

1. General Information

a. Definition: severe, sudden decrease in cerebral circulation caused by either a thrombus or hemorrhage resulting in a cerebral infarct (also called a stroke)

b. Incidence
   1) third leading cause of death in the United States
   2) ages 60–69: most frequent cause is thrombosis
   3) ages 30–60: most frequent cause is a ruptured aneurysm with hemorrhage

c. Symptomology is dependent upon
   1) location of the infarct (see Figure 3.22)
   2) amount of collateral circulation to affected area of the brain

Figure 3.22 Areas of the Brain that Control Certain Motor and Sensory Functions

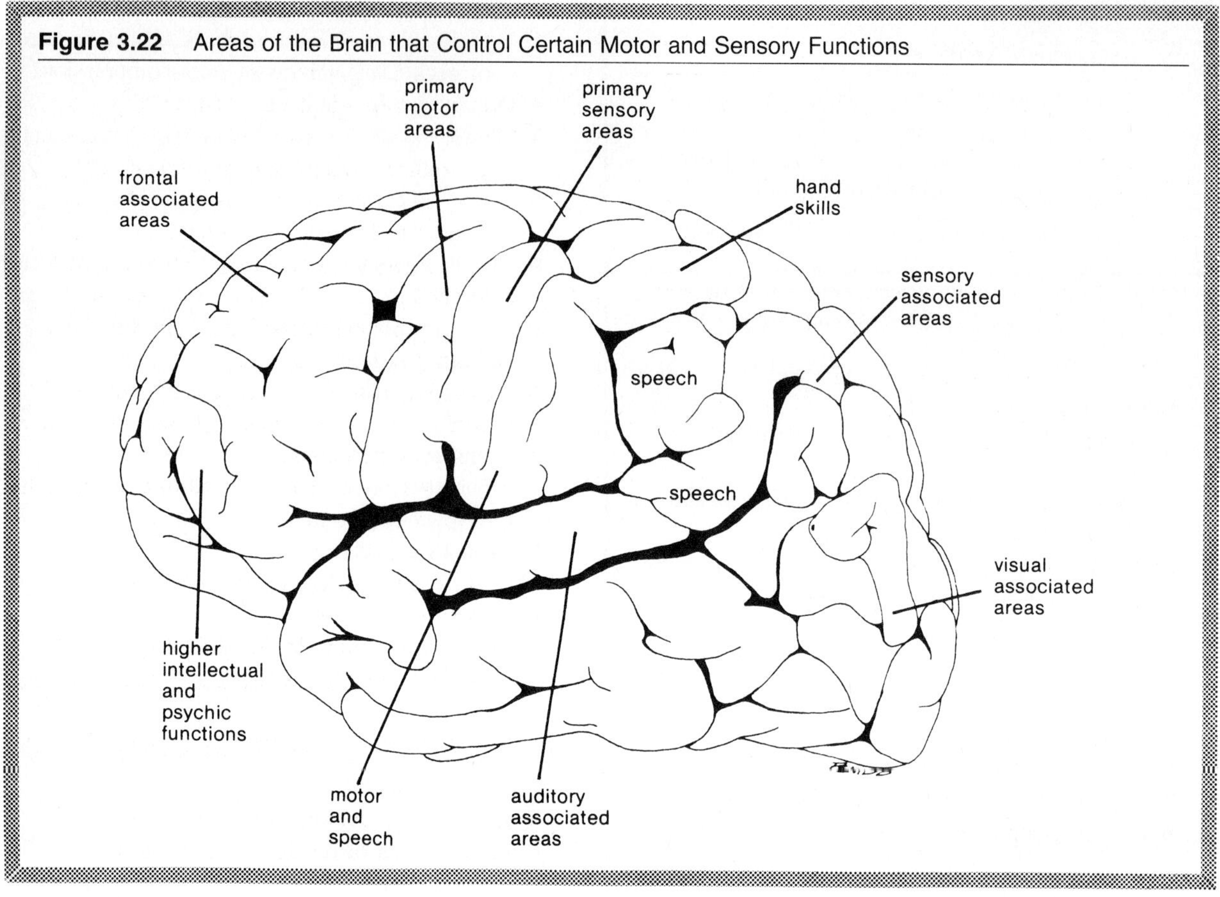

3) type of pathophysiology involved

d. Risk factors
   1) hypertension
   2) arteriosclerosis/atherosclerosis
   3) intracranial aneurysms
   4) diabetes mellitus
   5) peripheral vascular disease

e. Etiology
   1) rupture of the wall of a cerebral artery or an aneurysm
   2) trauma to a cerebral artery
   3) severe spasm of the cerebral artery
   4) embolus or thrombus blocking cerebral arterial system

2. Nursing Process

a. Assessment/Analysis

1) refer to neurologic exam page 271, and areas of the brain that control certain motor and sensory functions (Figure 3.22)
2) hemiplegia (paralysis) or hemiparesis (muscular weakness) of half of body
3) aphasia (most common with left cerebral infarct and right-handedness)
4) ataxia (staggering gait)
5) nuchal rigidity (with hemorrhage)
6) perceptual deficit
7) emotional lability
8) emotional needs of client/significant others
9) results of diagnostic studies
   a) CAT scan
   b) lumbar puncture

b. Plans, Implementation, and Evaluation

Goal 1: Client will be free from any additional cerebral damage.

Plan/Implementation

- Monitor neurologic status frequently until stable.
- Do not stimulate cough.
- Give passive ROM.
- If thrombus is cause of CVA: administer vasodilators and anticoagulants as ordered.
- If hemorrhage is cause of CVA
  - elevate head of bed 30°–45° (to improve venous drainage)
  - turn *gently*
  - decrease environmental stimuli (e.g., keep room semidark)

- maintain complete bedrest until bleeding has been controlled and client's condition is stable

Evaluation: Client remains stable, free from additional cerebral damage.

Goal 2: Client will ingest adequate fluids and food.

Plan/Implementation

- Help client feed self as needed.
- Provide adequate fluids to maintain skin turgor and sufficient output.
- Give small, frequent feedings as indicated (more easily tolerated than 3 large meals).
- Administer tube feedings if client is unable to take food and fluids orally (see General Nursing Goal 2 page 274).
- Monitor electrolyte levels.

Evaluation: Client's weight remains stable; skin turgor is firm; urinary output is greater than 30 ml/hour; urine is clear, straw colored, free from pus and blood.

Goal 3: If unconscious, client will remain free from complications (refer to General Nursing Goal 2 page 274).

Goal 4: Client will become as independent as possible (refer to General Nursing Goals 3 and 4 page 275).

Plan/Implementation

- Explain prognosis: lengthy rehabilitation, potential lifetime implications.
- Expect labile emotions (depression is common).
- Prevent deformities
- Make referral to speech therapist.
- Arrange for gait training; if fatigued from exercises, monitor for potential injury.

☐ Meningitis (refer to *Nursing Care of the Child* page 563)

☐ Spinal Cord Injuries (refer also to reprint page 361)

1. General Information

a. Definition: fracture or displacement of one or more vertebrae, causing damage to spinal cord and nerve roots with resulting neurologic deficit and altered sensory perception or paralysis or both. There will be total or partial absence of motor and/or sensory function below the level of the injury.

b. Types of injuries
  1) fracture of vertebral body (excessive vertical compression)
  2) compression of vertebral body (excessive flexion of vertebral column)
  3) spinal malalignment or vertebral body displacement (rotational injury)
  4) partial or complete dislocation of one vertebra onto another
  5) disruption of intervertebral disk and compressed interspinous ligament (hyperextension injury)

c. Incidence: estimated 10,000–20,000 people affected annually; usually younger age group

d. Predisposing factors
  1) trauma: car or motorcycle accidents, falls, or diving accidents
  2) tumors
  3) congenital defects; spina bifida
  4) infectious and degenerative diseases
  5) ruptured intervertebral disks

e. Immediately after an accident, care must be taken to prevent further damage to the spinal cord while patent airway and circulation are maintained

2. Nursing Process

a. Assessment/Analysis
  1) respiratory function
  2) cardiovascular function
  3) loss of sensation and motor function in body parts below injury level (see Table 3.46)
  4) loss of perspiration below injury level with resultant inability to cool body (autonomic responses become unpredictable)
  5) bowel and bladder control (assess for paralytic ileus and urine retention)
  6) pain
  7) edema
  8) nutritional status
  9) fever
  10) psychologic needs
  11) remaining sensory and motor function
  12) diagnostic tests
    a) neurologic exam
    b) x-ray of spine

b. Plans, Implementation, and Evaluation

Goal 1: Client will be free from further injury to spinal cord.

Plan/Implementation

- Immbolize the head and entire spine.
- Keep client's body and head in even alignment.

Table 3.46 Spinal Cord

Area of Spinal Cord	Gross Movements Controlled
Upper cervical	Neck and head movement; elevation of the shoulders.
Middle cervical	Movement of the upper arms and forearms; diaphragmatic breathing.
Lower cervical	Movements of fingers and hands.
Thoracic	Intercostal muscles involved in respiration; muscles involved in abdominal contractions.
Upper lumbar	Leg flexion at hip; adduction of thigh.
Lower lumbar	Remaining thigh movements; movements in lower legs.
Sacral	Foot and toe movements; sphincter and perineal muscle contraction.

- "Logroll" if moving client is necessary.
- Use specialized equipment for turning: Stryker frame, Foster frame, CircOlectric bed.
- Apply cervical traction for cervical lesion.
- Know that a laminectomy may be done to prevent further compression of spinal cord.
- Administer steroids (dexamethasone sodium [Decadron]) or osmotic diuretic (e.g., mannitol) IV as ordered, to reduce cerebral edema and edema of spinal cord.

Evaluation: Client shows no signs of progression of paralysis.

Goal 2: Client will maintain adequate respiratory function.

Plan/Implementation

- Observe respirations frequently (client may have spontaneous respirations after an accident but lose them later).
- Maintain respiratory function through use of a respirator if necessary.
- If respirations are spontaneous, have client deep breathe and cough qh.
- Care for and suction tracheostomy tube if in place.

Evaluation: Client's respiratory rate remains within normal limits.

Goal 3: Client will be free from undetected spinal shock.

Plan/Implementation

- Expect spinal shock to develop 30–60 minutes postinjury and to last 2–3 days to 3 months.
- Observe for
  - hypotension
  - dyspnea
  - flaccid paralysis
  - urinary retention
  - absence of sweating
- Administer colloid fluids and analgesics prn as ordered.

Evaluation: Client's spinal shock is detected promptly.

Goal 4: Client's fluid and electrolyte balance will remain within desired range.

Plan/Implementation

- Observe qh for signs of fluid and electrolyte balance until stable and then q4–8h.
- Replace fluids and electrolytes as needed.

Evaluation: Client's fluid and electrolytes are in desired balance; has had any imbalance detected and corrected immediately.

Goal 5: Client with cervical or high-thoracic injury will remain free from autonomic dysreflexia.

Plan/Implementation

- Observe for
  - rapidly increasing BP
  - bradycardia
  - severe headache
  - flushing
  - profuse sweating
  - goose pimples
- Take preventive measures
  - prevent bowel and bladder distention (chief causes of this phenomenon)
  - observe urinary drainage from catheter frequently
  - prevent pressure sores, pain in lower extremities, or pressure on penis or testes when client is in prone position
- Initiate treatment immediately (medical emergency)
  - remove the cause
  - check the bladder for distention
  - elevate head of bed to lower blood pressure

- look for sources other than bladder distention (e.g., cold air, drafts, sharp objects pressing on skin below level of injury)
- administer ganglionic-blocking agents as ordered

Evaluation: Client remains free from signs of autonomic dysreflexia; maintains bowel and bladder function.

Goal 6: Client will ingest adequate fluids and nutrition.

Plan/Implementation
- Give liquid diet until possiblity of paralytic ileus has passed, then diet as tolerated.
- Administer vitamin supplements as ordered.
- Encourage fluid intake.
- Monitor I&O.

Evaluation: Client's weight remains within desired range; skin turgor is firm.

Goal 7: Client will be free from urinary tract infection.

Plan/Implementation
- Insert Foley catheter or use intermittent catheterization as ordered, using sterile technique.
- Give aseptic care to Foley catheter.
- Observe client for signs of bladder infection (e.g., fever; abnormal UA, urine C&S).
- Encourage fluid intake to 3 liters/day.
- Observe odor, appearance, and amount of urine.
- Monitor I&O carefully.

Evaluation: Client drains normal urine; has no fever.

Goal 8: Client will be free from stress ulcer.

Plan/Implementation
- Monitor for complaints of ulcerlike pain.
- Observe for melena, hematemesis.
- Administer antacids frequently as ordered, to prevent gastric irritation.

Evaluation: Client offers no complaints of stomach pain; has stools negative for occult blood.

Goal 9: Client will be free from pain in paralyzed limbs.

Plan/Implementation
- Handle the affected limbs gently to avoid muscle spasms.
- Identify and eliminate stimuli that cause spasms.
- Medicate as ordered, to control spasms and pain.

Evaluation: Client experiences relief of pain.

Goal 10: Client will become as independent as possible. Refer to General Nursing Goal 4 page 275.

☐ Parkinson's Syndrome (Parkinsonism)

1. General Information

a. Definition: a progressive debilitating syndrome in which there is degeneration of nerve cells in the basal ganglia that impairs
   1) important centers of coordination, especially control of associated automatic movements
   2) control of muscle tone to produce finely coordinated movements
   3) control of initiation and inhibition of gross, intentional movements

b. Incidence: one of the major causes of neurologic disability; estimated to affect more than a half-million people in the United States

c. Onset: usually 50–60 years of age

d. Etiology
   1) unknown (i.e., idiopathic)
   2) it is hypothesized that these clients have a deficiency of dopamine, which is required for normal functioning of the basal ganglia; drug therapy aims at returning dopamine levels to normal to control symptoms of the syndrome

e. Precipitating factors
   1) drug-induced: phenothiazines and Rauwolfia alkaloids
   2) atherosclerosis
   3) trauma (e.g., midbrain compression)
   4) encephalitis
   5) toxic poisoning: carbon monoxide

2. Nursing Process

a. **Assessment/Analysis**
   1) muscle rigidity
      a) major disability
      b) bradykinesia and akinesia
   2) tremors at rest (nonintentional)
      a) especially of hands (pill rolling), arms, and head
      b) rhythmic: regular and rapid
   3) facial mask
   4) speech difficulty

5) loss of automatic movements (e.g., blinking of eyes)
6) propulsive gait, shuffling in nature
7) emotional changes (mood disturbances) depression and confusion
8) autonomic nervous system dysfunction
   a) decreased salivation
   b) perspiration
   c) lacrimation
   d) constipation
   e) incontinence
   f) decreased sexual activity

b. Plans, Implementation, and Evaluation

Goal 1: Client will have optimal function of muscles and joints.

Plan/Implementation
- Administer prescribed medications (see Table 3.47).
- Observe for side effects of medications.
- Assist client to remain as active as possible (see General Nursing Goal 4 page 275)
  - frequent ambulation
  - attention to grooming

Evaluation: Client maintains movement in muscles and joints; continues to ambulate and participate in ADL.

Goal 2: Client will be free from injury.

Plan/Implementation
- Use ambulatory aids such as hand rails in all rooms and near bathtub or shower.
- Instruct client to walk slowly and carefully.
- Balance activity and rest to avoid fatigue.

Evaluation: Client is free from cuts, abrasions, and falls; has balance of activity and rest.

Goal 3: Client will maintain gastrointestinal integrity.

Plan/Implementation
- Provide adequate fluid intake.
- Give high fiber diet.
- Observe for constipation.

Table 3.47 Drugs Used to Treat Parkinsonism

Name	Action	Side Effects	Nursing Implications
Levodopa (Larodopa)	Converts to dopamine in basal ganglia.	Gastrointestinal irritation (e.g., nausea, anorexia, vomiting); gastrointestinal hemorrhage; psychiatric symptoms; orthostatic hypotension	Begin with low dosage: gradually increase to therapeutic level. Give meds with meals. Use cautiously in clients with cardiovascular, respiratory, endocrine, hepatic peptic ulcer disease. Avoid vitamin B_6 (reverses effects of levodopa).
Carbidopa and levodopa (Sinemet)	Combined drugs provide same action as above at lower levels.	Same as levodopa	Same as levodopa.
Amantadine (Symmetrel)	Unknown	Restlessness, mental and emotional changes	Well tolerated (less effective than levodopa).
Trihexyphenidyl (Artane)	Anticholinergic: blocks muscarinic receptors at cholinergic synapses with CNS: relieves tremor, rigidity. Minimal effect on akinesia	Dry mouth; blurred vision; constipation; urinary retention; mental dullness, confusion. Sudden withdrawal precipitates sudden, incapacitating increase in symptoms	Begin using small doses; increase dosages gradually. Avoid sudden withdrawal of meds; withdrawal of drug reverses side effects. Monitor client with psychosis, wide-angle glaucoma, diabetes. Administer after meals to avoid GI irritation.
Procyclidine (Kemedrine)	Same as Artane	Same as Artane	Same as Artane.
Benztropine mesylate (Cogentin)	Same as Artane	Same as Artane	Same as Artane.

- Administer stool softeners or laxatives as ordered PRN.
- Give oral hygiene to relieve dryness of the mouth.
- Keep urinal and bedpan handy in case client is unable to reach bathroom in time.

Evaluation: Client is free from constipation and impactions; has adequate bowel function.

Goal 4: Client will maintain positive body image/self-concept.

Plan/Implementation

- Provide assistive devices to make ADL easier.
- Teach about/provide clothes that are simple and easy to put on.
- Allow sufficient time for meals.
- In general, do *not* hurry client.
- Supervise and assist in skin care and personal hygiene.
- Allow expression of depression and hopelessness (see "Depression" page 53).
- Reward attempts at activity that the client makes.
- Arrange for speech therapy for dysarthria.

Evaluation: Client's grooming projects positive self-concept; accepts responsibility for ADL to the extent possible.

Goal 5: Client and significant others will express fears and other feelings about present and future.

Plan/Implementation

- Assess level of anxiety.
- Give emotional support/relieve anxiety (see *Anxious Behavior* page 36).
- Explain disease and drug therapy.
- Clarify misconceptions and lack of information.
- Explain prognosis.

Evaluation: Client and significant others express feelings (e.g., fear, sadness, anger); state what to expect in the future.

☐ Multiple Sclerosis

1. General Information

a. Definition: chronic progressive nonvascular disease of the central nervous system characterized by unpredictable exacerbations and remissions; typically demyelinization of the white matter of the spinal cord and brain occurs in multiple areas

b. Incidence
  1) disease of young adults
  2) more common in women

c. Risk factors
  1) living in the temperate zone 40°–60° north or south of the equator
  2) higher incidence among higher socioeconomic classes

d. Etiology
  1) unknown
  2) may be a virus that is latent for months or years before some other factor initiates disease
  3) possibly an autoimmune disorder
  4) mineral deficiency, toxic substances

2. Nursing Process

a. Assessment/Analysis

1) at onset: vague symptoms
  a) diplopia
  b) awkwardness in handling articles and frequent dropping of articles
  c) stumbling or falling with no apparent cause

2) symptoms vary depending on location of myelin or nerve fiber destruction
  a) classic symptoms
  - nystagmus (rapid, involuntary movements of eyes)
  - intention tremors, absent at rest
  - scanning speech (slow enunciation with tendency to hesitate at beginning of a word or syllable, speech with pauses between syllables)

  b) sensory disorders
  - paresthesias (numbness, tingling, "dead" feeling, "pins and needles")
  - diminished vibration sense
  - impaired proprioception

  c) visual disorders
  - optic neuritis
  - diplopia
  - scotomata (blind spots)

  d) motor disorders: spastic weakness or paralysis of limbs
  e) cerebellar dysfunction: cerebellar ataxia
  f) bowel and bladder dysfunction
  - hesitancy, urgency, frequency
  - retention, incontinence
  - constipation

  g) emotional disorders: euphoria, mood swings

3) long-term effects of progressive disease
  a) spasticity
  b) paraplegia

c) speech defects
d) eating difficulties
e) extreme fatigue
f) vision difficulties
g) complete paralysis

b. Plans, Implementation, and Evaluation

Goal 1: Client will have optimal function of muscles and joints.

Plan/Implementation
- Arrange for physical therapy (muscle stretching and strengthening).
- Assist with gait retraining if ataxic.
- Encourage client to remain active and to do as many ADL as possible.

Evaluation: Client's joints and muscles function well; participates in ADL.

Goal 2: Client will maintain health-promoting habits in daily living.

Plan/Implementation
- Determine and encourage optimal activity level.
- Promote adequate rest periods to prevent exhaustion.
- Use safety devices such as hand rails and walkers to prevent falls.
- Maintain good nutrition and fluid intake.
- Supply self-help devices for eating, ambulation, reading.
- Provide pain medication and muscle relaxants (e.g., baclofen) as ordered.
- Attend to incontinence and pressure areas to maintain integrity of skin and mucous membranes.
- Make referral to community agencies (e.g., VNA, local branch of National Multiple Sclerosis Society) to help client/significant others in long-term management.
- Educate client/significant others about these aspects of care.

Evaluation: Client maintains good personal hygiene; eats a nutritious, well-balanced diet.

Goal 3: Client will maintain positive body image/ self-concept.

Plan/Implementation
- Provide assistive devices to make ADL easier.
- Promote as much independence in client as possible; teach significant others to do the same.
- Encourage hobbies and other pleasurable distractions.
- DO NOT hurry client.
- Supervise and assist in skin care and personal hygiene.
- Reward client's attempts at activity.
- Encourage and reinforce perseverance and hope.
- Help client identify realistic goals.

Evaluation: Client's grooming projects positive self-image; performs ADL within own limits.

Goal 4: Client and significant others will express fears about present and future.

Plan/Implementation
- Set aside time to talk to client and significant others, together and separately.
- Encourage expression of feelings.
- Convey that it is OK to express feelings.
- Clarify misconceptions and lack of information about present and prognosis.
- Allow expression of depression and hopelessness.
- Emphasize what the client can still do.

Evaluation: Client and significant others express fear about the disease; state what to expect in the future.

Goal 5: Client and significant others will learn to cope with illness-related problems and prevent complications.

Plan/Implementation
- Teach client/significant others information discussed in Goals 1 and 2.
- Evaluate knowledge and skills that client/ significant others have and go over areas where they have not retained information.
- Continue to teach and evaluate knowledge and skills related to Goals 1 and 2.

Evaluation: Client and significant others describe care needed because of disabilities; explain how to avoid complications related to disabilities.

☐ **Epilepsy** (see "Seizure Disorders" in *Nursing Care of the Child* page 560)

☐ Amyotrophic Lateral Sclerosis (ALS)

1. General Information

a. Definition: progressive, degenerative disorder of motor neurons in the brain, spinal cord, and motor cortex; remissions are uncommon; death occurs 2–15 years after onset.

b. Incidence
1) disease of middle age
2) more common in men
3) 3,000 new cases in US annually

c. Major complication: aspiration pneumonia

d. Etiology: unknown

e. Diagnosis
 1) electromyography (EMG)
 2) muscle biopsy to confirm diagnosis
 3) elevated serum creatinine phosphokinase (CPK)

2. Nursing Process

a. **Assessment/Analysis**
 1) at onset
  a) awkward fine hand movements
  b) weakness, wasting of hand muscles
  c) twitching, cramping
 2) atrophy of hand, forearms; hyperactive reflexes
 3) progresses to upper arms, neck, shoulders
 4) late stage: weakness involves lower extremeties
 5) remains alert and oriented
 6) bulbar palsy may be accompanied by erratic affective behavior (e.g., uncontrollable crying outbursts)
 7) impaired swallowing, palate, tongue, and pharynx

b. **Plans, Implementation, and Evaluation**
Refer to "Multiple Sclerosis" Goals 1–5 page 284.

☐ Myasthenia Gravis

1. General Information

a. Definition: a chronic, progressive neuromuscular disorder characterized by rapid exhaustion of voluntary muscles owing to a defect at the myoneural junction
b. Pathophysiology: transmission of impulse from nerve to muscle is impaired because of inadequate acetylcholine at the myoneural junction; contractions of voluntary muscles become progressively weaker and cease when the muscle is stimulated
c. Etiology
 1) unknown
 2) possibly an autoimmune disorder
 3) client may have a genetic predisposition

2. Nursing Process

a. **Assessment/Analysis**
 1) onset of symptoms insidious and gradual
 2) progressive voluntary-muscle weakness
 3) incapacitating fatigue
 4) ocular symptoms: ptosis, inability to open eyes, diplopia
 5) expressionless appearance with facial muscle involvement; characteristic "snarl" when client attempts to smile
 6) respiratory distress
 7) diagnostic test: positive Tensilon test (anticholinesterase): edrophonium chloride (Tensilon) injected IV produces increase in strength (see Table 3.48)

b. **Plans, Implementation, and Evaluation**

Goal 1: Client will have control of voluntary muscles.

Plan/Implementation
- Administer anticholinesterase medications to control symptoms (e.g., neostigmine methylsulfate [Prostigmin], pyridostigmine bromide [Mestinon]); see Table 3.48.
- Administer medications on individually adjusted schedule.

Evaluation: Client has control of voluntary muscles.

Goal 2: Client will remain free from respiratory impairment.

Plan/Implementation
- Observe respiratory status.
- Use postural drainage; turn frequently.
- Give prophylactic antibiotics to prevent respiratory infections.
- Instruct client to avoid exposure to people with URIs.
- Teach client diaphragmatic breathing exercises, to maintain strength with maximum ventilation and minimum energy expenditure.
- Balance physical activities with rest.
- Put client in a rocking bed.
- Know that client may require mechanical ventilation.

Evaluation: Client's lungs are clear; has no respiratory distress.

Goal 3: Client will remain well nourished.

Plan/Implementation
- Give anticholinesterase medications (e.g., pyridostigmine bromide [Mestinon]) 20–30 minutes before meals for full advantage.
- Provide small, frequent, semisolid, or fluid meals that are nutritious and high in potassium (adequate serum levels of potassium potentiate anticholinesterase effect).
- Provide IV or NG feedings if needed.
- Have suction equipment available.
- Allow client to eat meals without rushing.
- Observe for anorexia, nausea, diarrhea, abdominal cramping (common side effects of anticholinesterase drugs).

Evaluation: Client's weight remains stable.

Table 3.48 Drugs Used to Treat Myasthenia Gravis

Name	Action	Side Effects	Nursing Implications
Neostigmine bromide Neostigmine methylsulfate (Prostigmin)	Anticholinesterase: blocks breakdown of acetylcholine at myoneural junction	Nausea, vomiting, diarrhea, abdominal cramps, muscle twitching, weakness, hypotention *Toxic effect*: cholinergic crisis: increased myasthenia symptoms, vomiting, perspiration, salivation, bradycardia, muscle tightness, fasciculations May cause skin rash.	Give smallest dose that provides greatest strength; may give anticholinergics (e.g., atropine sulfate) to prevent side and toxic effects. Monitor vital signs; note CNS, irritability.
Pyridostigmine bromide (Mestinon)	As above	As above	As above Give 20–30 minutes ac.
Ambenonium chloride (Mytelase)	As above	As above	Less commonly used than above drugs; drug of choice if client is sensitive to bromides.
Endophonium chloride (Tensilon)	As above Short duration of action	As above	Useful in emergency treatment and as diagnostic agent. Differentiates disease from cholinergic crisis—watch for immediate relief of symptoms vs increased weakness due to medication overdose.

Goal 4: Client will receive psychologic and rehabilitative support.

Plan/Implementation

- Evaluate client and significant others' attitudes toward and knowledge of disease.
- Provide careful explanations of disorder.
- Offer opportunities for expressions of feelings.
- Promote a balance of rest and activities.
- Encourage healthy life-style.
- Refer to Myasthenia Gravis Foundation for information and support.

Evaluation: Client expresses positive outlook for future; has a plan for balancing activities with adequate rest periods.

Goal 5: Client remains free from an undetected ''cholinergic'' crisis.

Plan/Implementation

- Know that a ''cholinergic crisis'' (medical emergency) occurs when client cannot tolerate the dosage of anticholinesterase medications (see Table 3.48).
- Carefully monitor vital signs, including pupil checks, of client receiving increasing doses of anticholinesterases.
- Observe for dramatic increase in myasthenic symptoms accompanied by severe diarrhea, nausea and vomiting, hypersalivation, pallor, lacrimation, miosis, hypotension.
- Discontinue medications and give IV anticholinergic drug as ordered (e.g., atropine sulfate); see Table 3.49.

Evaluation: Client is free from symptoms of cholinergic crisis (no diarrhea, pallor).

☐ Cataracts

1. General Information

a. Definition: total or partial opacity of the normally transparent crystalline lens; the opacity of the lens interferes with light passage through the lens to the retina

b. Etiology: unknown

c. Risk factors

1) aging: onset usually after age 55
2) diabetes mellitus
3) intraocular surgery
4) previous injury to the eye

Table 3.49 Eye Medications

Name	Action	Side Effects	Nursing Implications
Cycloplegics			
Atropine sulfate	Parasympatholytic (anticholinergic) Dilation of pupil and paralysis of accommodation	Dryness of mouth, tachycardia, light sensitivity, inability to focus on near objects	Used to correct refractive errors, inflammations of the eye. Monitor for side effects, increased intraocular pressure (e.g., nausea, vomiting, pain). Inform of inability to accomodate for close-by objects, long duration of action, and photophobia. Contraindicated in glaucoma. Store in safe place out of reach of children.
Homatropine Hydrobromide	As above Slow onset; prlonged action	As above	As above plus use cautiously with older adults.
Miotics			
Pilocarpine hydrochloride	Cholinergic causes • contraction of sphincter muscle of the iris, resulting in pupil constriction (miosis) • spasms of ciliary muscle and deepening of the anterior chamber • vasodilation of vessels where intraocular fluids leave the eye	Headache	Drug of choice in treatment of glaucoma. Monitor for side effects, individual duration of action and tolerance and/or resistance. Inform of difficult adjustment to changes in illumination. Instruct regarding frequent instillation.
Carbachol (Carbacel, Isopto Carbachol, Miostat)	As above Produces intense and prolonged miosis.	Headache, conjunctival hyperemia	Used for glaucoma if pilocarpine is ineffective. As above
Physostigmine salicylate (Eserine)	Anticholinesterase Pupil constriction Spasm of accommodation Short duration of action	Conjunctivitis, allergic reactions	As above, plus give every 4–6 hr for wide-angle glaucoma.
Isoflurophate (Floropryl)	Anticholinesterase Pupil constriction Spasm of accommodation	Vomiting and diarrhea, tenesmus	Used for wide-angle glaucoma; plus above.
Neostigmine bromide (Prostigmin)	As above Short duration of action	Conjunctivitis	As above
Beta Blocking Agent			
Timolol maleate (Timoptic)	Beta adrenergic receptor blocking agent Reduces intraocular pressure by decreasing aqueous formation Acts in ½ hour	Headache, brochospasm, cardiac failure, hypotension, muscle weakness, dizziness	Generally well-tolerated. Contraindicated in clients with COPD; used cautiously in those with hyperthyroidism. Monitor for side effects.
Carbonic Anhydrase Inhibitors			
Acetazolamide (Diamox) Ethoxzalamide (Cardase) Methazolamide (Neptazane) Dichlorphenamide (Daranide)	Inhibit carbonic anhydrase, an enzyme necessary for formation of aqueous humor Result in reduced intraocular pressure	Lethargy, anorexia, numbness, tingling of face and extremities, acidosis, ureteral stones	Used for treatment of glaucoma. Monitor for side effects. Prohibit use in first trimester of pregnancy.

(continued)

Table 3.49 Continued

Name	Action	Side Effects	Nursing Implications
Osmotic Agents see Table 3.37			
Anti-infectives			
Bacitracin ophthalmic ointment* (Baciguent)	Bactericidal antibiotic; effective against gram-positive bacteria	No systemic effects	Preserve solutions with refrigeration; potency remains for 3 weeks. Ointment stable for 1 year at room temperature.
Neomycin sulfate (Myciguent)	Broad-spectrum bactericidal antibiotic	Minimal allergenic effects	Use cautiously with other systemically used antibiotics due to cross-sensitivity reactions. Effective for conjunctival and corneal infections.
Polymyxin B sulfate* (Aerosporin)	Bactericidal antibiotic; effective against gram-negative bacteria	Minimal	Often used in combination with above two to produce broader effects.
Tetracyclines (Achromycin) (Aureomycin) (Terramycin)	Bacteriostatic antibiotic for superficial infections	Rare	Monitor for effects.
Sulfacetamide sodium (Blefcon)	Bacteriostatic sulfonamide for surface infections	Local irritation	Monitor for ocular purulent drainage or exudate (interferes with sulfonamide's action).
Anti-inflammatories			
Cortisone acetate Fludrocortisone acetate	Decrease defense mechanisms and reduce resistance to pathogenic organisms Inhibit inflammatory response	Prolonged use increases susceptibility to glaucoma, cataracts, and fungus infection	Indicated for all allergenic reactions, nonpyogenic inflammation, and severe injury. Use for limited period. Monitor for increased intraocular pressure and secondary fungus function.

*See Table 3.20

5) prolonged treatment of glaucoma with topical preparations
6) radiation of the head for cancer
7) possibly steroid therapy

d. Medical treatment: surgical removal of lens
1) intracapsular extraction most common
2) extraction by cryosurgery
3) partial iridectomy done with lens extraction to prevent acute glaucoma
4) possible lens implantation

2. Nursing Process

a. Assessment/Analysis

1) distortion of vision
2) absence of red reflex (the red reflection seen with the retina is viewed through an ophthalmoscope)
3) gradual and painless loss of vision
4) knowledge of treatment modalities
5) knowledge of post-treatment course of recovery

b. Plans, Implementation, and Evaluation

Goal 1: Client and significant others will be able to explain pre-/post-op care, and the OR-RR environment.

Plan/Implementation

- Prepare client for surgery (see ''Perioperative Period'' page 157).
- Prepare client for pre-op instillation of eye medications (mydriatics and cyclopegics) as ordered (see Table 3.48).
- Teach about post-op procedures
  - bed position varies with type of surgery (usually head of bed up 30°)
  - no turning or turn only to unaffected side post-op
  - how to use call bell

- bed rails up at all times
- keep hands away from eyes to prevent infection
- ROM exercise routine

■ Review client knowledge.

■ Continue to explain areas client does not understand.

Evaluation: Client describes plan of treatment and post-op care; explains what will happen in OR-RR.

Goal 2: Client will be able, preoperatively, to explain how to prevent increasing intraocular pressure.

Plan/Implementation

■ Teach client before surgery
- no straining
- no coughing or sneezing
- no bending
- to prevent vomiting
- no squeezing shut of eyelids

■ Evaluate client knowledge after teaching.

■ Continue to explain areas client does not remember or understand.

Evaluation: Client explains how to prevent increased intraocular pressure.

Goal 3: Client will remain free from post-op complications.

Plan/Implementation

■ Refer to "Perioperative Period" page 157.

■ Provide adequate fluids.

■ Deep breathe qh, no coughing.

■ Elevate head of bed 30°–45°.

■ Turn only to *unaffected* side, if turning is permitted.

■ Check dressing frequently for bleeding (q15min for 2h, then qh for 8h).

■ Prevent increased intraocular pressure.

■ Give antiemetics prn.

■ Observe and report severe eye pain.

Evaluation: Client's vital signs are stable; has no complaints of pain; observes post-op activity restrictions.

Goal 4: Client will know the characteristics of the type of lenses or glasses to be worn for optimal vision.

Plan/Implementation

■ Teach according to client's situation
- cataract glasses (wear old glasses until curvature changes are complete: 12–14 weeks post-op)
  * magnify objects ⅓
  * clear vision only through center
- contact lenses (less vision distortion than glasses; more costly)
- intraocular lens
  * synthetic lens implanted into eye
  * designed for distance vision
  * for near vision, needs corrective glasses

■ Discuss with client a plan for obtaining new glasses or lenses.

Evaluation: Client describes type of protective eyewear prescribed.

Goal 5: Client will be discharged with a written rehabilitation plan and a physician's appointment for follow-up.

Plan/Implementation

■ Develop a plan for client to follow that explains
- progressively increased exercise
- return to sexual activity
- driving
- bending, stooping, and lifting restrictions
- dressing changes, eye meds as required

■ Instruct significant others in dressing change and medication administration.

■ Secure physician or clinic appointment for client.

Evaluation: Client states activity limitations upon discharge; significant others administer eye meds correctly.

□ Retinal Detachment

1. General Information

a. Definition: actual splitting of the retina between the rod and cone layers of the retina and the pigment epithelial layer. Partial separation becomes complete (if untreated) with subsequent total loss of vision.

b. Pathophysiology: vitreous humor seeps through opening and separates retina from pigment epithelium and choroid. Blindness results.

c. Types

  1) primary: from a break in the continuity of retina

  2) secondary: from intraocular disorders (e.g., post-cataract extraction, perforating injuries, severe myopia)

d. Early surgical repair imperative to avoid irreparable damage and irreversible blindness.

  1) cryosurgery: freezing stimulates inflammatory response leading to adhesions

2) photocoagulation: laser beam stimulates inflammatory response
3) electrodiathermy: creates inflammatory response
4) scleral buckling

2. Nursing Process

a. Assessment/Analysis

1) gradual or sudden onset
2) sudden flashes of light
3) blurred vision that becomes progressively worse
4) loss of portion of visual field
5) ophthalmologic examination: retina hangs like a grey cloud; one or more tears

b. Plans, Implementation, and Evaluation

Goal 1: Client will be able to explain pre-/post-op care, and the OR-RR environment.

Plan/Implementation

- Prepare client for surgery (see "Perioperative Period" page 157)
  - apply bilateral eye patches pre-op
  - protect client from injury
  - minimize stress on eye (e.g., avoid sneezing, coughing, sudden jarring)
  - instill pre-op meds as ordered (cycloplegics, mydriatics) (see Table 3.48)
- Teach client post-op positions, care.

Evaluation: Client explains surgical plan, pre-/post-op care, and the OR-RR environment.

Goal 2: Client will be able, preoperatively, to explain how to prevent increasing intraocular pressure (see "Cataracts" Goal 2 page 289).

Goal 3: Client will recover free from post-op complications.

Plan/Implementation

- Refer to "Perioperative Care" page 159.
- Avoid prone position.
- Speak before approaching client.
- Check eye patches frequently.
- Give antiemetics, analgesics prn.

Evaluation: Client is stable free from post-op complications.

Goal 4: Client will be discharged with a plan for rehabilitation.

Plan/Implementation

- Inform client of activities upon discharge
  - may watch television
  - avoid reading for 2–3 weeks
  - continue to avoid straining, injury to head
  - may shave, comb hair, bathe, and ambulate
- If pinhole glasses are prescribed, provide client with instructions for use.

Evaluation: Client describes activities and limitations upon discharge.

☐ Glaucoma

1. General Information

a. Definition: abnormal increase in intraocular pressure caused by any obstruction of the outflow channels of aqueous humor; uncontrolled glaucoma causes irreversible blindness as a result of atrophy of the optic nerve

b. Types
   1) *chronic* (wide angle): most common
      a) resistance to flow because of thickening of collecting channels, trabecular network, and canal of Schlemm
      b) insidious onset characterized by a decrease in peripheral vision
   2) *acute* (narrow angle)
      a) occurs when iris is abnormally structured in an anterior position
      b) exerts pressure on collecting channels and decreases size of anterior chamber
      c) sudden onset characterized by severe eye pain and rapid loss of vision

c. Risk factors
   1) heredity
   2) trauma
   3) tumor or inflammation of the eye
   4) vascular disorders
   5) diabetes
   6) prior eye surgery

d. Other information
   1) one of leading causes of blindness
   2) early detection is crucial (vision destroyed by optic nerve atrophy cannot be restored)
   3) regular eye exams that include tonometry (measure of intraocular pressure) are recommended for persons over age 35

2. Nursing Process

a. Assessment/Analysis

1) loss of peripheral vision; loss of central vision with progression
2) halos around lights
3) difficulty adjusting to dark rooms
4) difficulty focusing on close work
5) increased intraocular pressure (normal = 12–20 mm Hg)

6) client's support system
7) client's and significant others' coping mechanisms

b. Plans, Implementation, and Evaluation

Goal 1: Client's intraocular pressure will remain within normal limits.

Plan/Implementation
- Teach client
  - how to instill eyedrops correctly (e.g., Diamox)
  - how miotic eyedrops decrease intraocular pressure (e.g., pilocarpine); see Table 3.49
  - that emotional or stressful events can increase intraocular pressure
  - to avoid lifting, shoveling, wearing constrictive clothing around the neck

Evaluation: Client's intraocular pressure remains between 12–20 mm Hg.

Goal 2: Client will be free from further visual impairment.

Plan/Implementation
- Impress upon client that ocular damage that has already occurred is not reversible, but further visual impairment can be prevented by compliance with prescribed regimen.
- Emphasize importance of routine eye exams.

Evaluation: Client develops no further visual impairment.

☐ Nasal Problems Requiring Surgery

1. General Information

a. Definition: bone and soft tissue deformities requiring corrective surgery (usually under local anesthesia)

b. Precipitating factors
   1) fracture
   2) tumor
   3) foreign body
   4) deviated septum
   5) polyps
   6) cosmetic problems

c. Types of surgery
   1) submucous resection (rhinoplasty)
   2) reduction of a nasal fracture
   3) removal of polyps, tumors, foreign bodies

2. Nursing Process

a. Assessment/Analysis
   1) nasal obstruction
   2) pain (fractures)
   3) nasal congestion
   4) bleeding
   5) allergies
   6) self-concept/body image

b. Plans, Implementation, and Evaluation

Goal 1: Client and significant others will understand pre-/post-op care, and the OR-RR environment.

Plan/Implementation
- Prepare client for surgery (see "Perioperative Period" page 157).
- Teach about
  - mouth breathing post-op
  - no nose blowing
  - Fowler's position
  - post-op appearance (black eyes, dressing)
  - ice packs

Evaluation: Client and significant others describe the surgery and post-op course

Goal 2: Client will remain free from any post-op complications.

Plan/Implementation
- Refer to "Perioperative Care" page 159.
- Observe for frequent swallowing (hemorrhage).
- Check dressing frequently for bleeding.
- Change gauze pad under nose when saturated and note amount of bleeding.
- Apply ice continuously to the area for 1st 24 hours.
- Give frequent oral hygiene.
- Maintain Fowler's position to prevent aspiration.

Evaluation: Client has vital signs within normal limits; minimal periorbital edema and discoloration.

☐ Epistaxis

1. General Information

a. Definition: nose bleed

b. Risk factors
   1) trauma
   2) hypertension
   3) acute sinusitis
   4) deviated nasal septum
   5) nasal surgery

2. Nursing Process

a. Assessment/Analysis
   1) bleeding from nose
   2) frequent swallowing
   3) bright red vomitus

b. Plans, Implementation, and Evaluation

Goal 1: Client will experience control of epistaxis.

Plan/Implementation

- Utilize first-aid interventions: direct pressure, Fowler's position, ice pack.
- Know that cautery may be used.
- Monitor anterior and/or posterior nasal packing (removed in 48–96 hours to prevent infection).
- Give vasoconstrictors as ordered (e.g., topical phenylephrine HCl [Neo-Synephrine]).
- Observe frequently for bleeding.

Evaluation: Client has no further bleeding from nose.

Goal 2: Client will remain free from future attacks.

Plan/Implementation

- Teach client and significant others first-aid measures in event of future attack.
- Demonstrate proper nasal care.
- Help client identify precipitating factors.
- Monitor BP for hypertension.

Evaluation: Client states methods to prevent future attacks.

References

Agee, B., & Herman, C. (1984). Cervical logrolling on a standard hospital bed. *American Journal of Nursing, 84*, 314–318.

Callahan, M. (1984). Caring for a stroke patient like me. *Nursing84, 14*(5), 65–67.

Carver, J. (1987). Cataract care made plain. *American Journal of Nursing, 87*, 626–630.

†Coma (Continuing Education). (1986). *American Journal of Nursing, 86*, 541–556.

Fode, N. (1988). Subarachnoid hemorrhage from ruptured intracranial aneurysm. *American Journal of Nursing, 88*, 673–679.

Hanawalt, A., & Troutman, K. (1984). If your patient has a hearing aid. *American Journal of Nursing, 84*, 900–901.

Johnson, L. (1983). If your patient has intracranial pressure, your goal should be: No surprises. *Nursing83, 13*(6), 58–63.

Kess, R. (1984). Suddenly in crisis—Unpredictable myasthenia. *American Journal of Nursing, 84*, 994–998.

Meyd, C. (1978). Acute brain trauma. *American Journal of Nursing, 84*, 40–44.

Mizuki, J. (1984). There's no place like home. *American Journal of Nursing, 84*, 646–648.

Musolf, J. (1983). Chemonucleolysis. *American Journal of Nursing, 83*, 882–885.

*The person with a spinal cord injury (Continuing education). (1977). *American Journal of Nursing, 77*, 1319–1336.

Passarella, P., Gee, Z. (1987). Starting right after stroke. *American Journal of Nursing, 87*, 802–807.

Resler, M., & Tumulty, G. (1983). Glaucoma update. *American Journal of Nursing, 83*, 752–756.

Rubin, M. (1988). The physiology of bedrest. *American Journal of Nursing, 88*, 50–55.

Tilton, C., & Maloof, M. (1982). Diagnosing the problems in stroke. *American Journal of Nursing, 82*, 596–601.

Tooke, M., Elders, J., & Johnson, D. (1986). Corneal transplantation. *American Journal of Nursing, 86*, 685–687.

†Tumulty, G., & Resler, M. (1984). Eye trauma. *American Journal of Nursing, 84*, 740–744.

---

*see Reprint Section
†Highly recommended

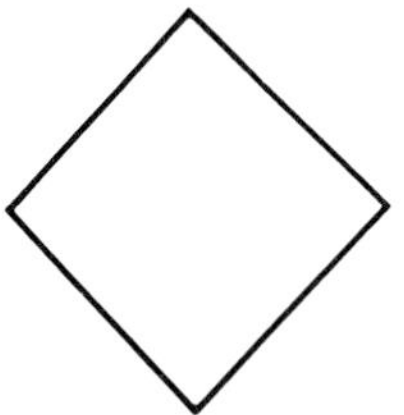

Activity and Rest

(The nursing care presented in this unit concerns selected health problems related to disturbances in the musculoskeletal system. The nurse plays an important role in maintaining musculoskeletal function by assessment, range-of-motion techniques, exercise, and early progressive ambulation.)

General Concepts

Overview/Physiology

1. Musculoskeletal system
   a. Muscles: contract and relax under the control of the nervous system to produce movement of the body as a whole or of its parts
      1) *fascia*: surrounds and divides muscles, main blood vessels, and nerves
      2) *tendons*: fibrous attachment between muscles and bones
      3) *ligaments*: fibrous connective tissue connecting bones, cartilage, and serving as support for or attachment of muscles and fascia
   b. Bones: for support and protection
      1) *joints*: junction between two bones
         a) synovium: lining of joints that secretes fluid to lubricate
         b) bursa: a closed cavity containing a gliding joint
      2) *cartilage*: dense connective tissue covering the ends of bones and at other sites where flexibility is needed
2. Terminology
   a. *Adduction*: movement toward the main axis of the body
   b. *Abduction*: movement away from the main axis of the body
   c. *Flexion*: act of bending
   d. *Extension*: stretching out into a straightened position
   e. *Strain*: trauma to the muscle caused by violent contraction or excessive forcible stretch
   f. *Sprain*: trauma to a joint with some degree of injury to the ligaments
3. Range-of-motion (ROM) exercises
   a. Uses
      1) prevent atrophy
      2) prevent weakness
      3) prevent contracture
      4) prevent degeneration of muscles and joints
   b. Types
      1) active
      2) passive
   c. Procedure
      1) stress importance of performing full ROM exercises
      2) perform ROM exercises at least twice daily, especially for clients on bedrest
      3) breathing should be as normal as possible (e.g., client should not hold breath)
      4) perform movements slowly and gently, especially with active ROM
      5) provide rest between each exercise
      6) perform each exercise same number of times on both sides of body; initially do each exercise three times, then work up to five times
      7) teach significant others to do ROM exercises for client
         a) demonstrate exercises
         b) allow return demonstration
         c) provide written instructions
4. Massage (centripetal: toward the heart)
   a. Uses
      1) increases circulation
      2) reduces edema
      3) relieves spasm
   b. May be used with heat
5. Isometric exercises
   a. Definition: alternately tightening and relaxing muscles without moving the joints
   b. Uses
      1) maintain muscle tone
      2) increase muscle strength

Application of the Nursing Process to the Client with Activity and Rest Problems

1. **Assessment**
   a. Health history

1) current health status
2) history of present complaint (e.g., weakness, stiffness, pain, swelling)
3) usual activities (e.g., work, social and recreational pursuits)
4) diet and sleep patterns

b. Physical examination
1) general inspection
   a) symmetry of the two sides of the body
   b) presence of spinal deformities, skin lesions, masses
   c) posture
2) gait and balance: watch for specific gait patterns associated with specific disorders
3) joints: active and passive ROM
4) muscle strength and bulk
5) vascular system of extremities
   a) pulses
   b) varicosities
   c) edema
6) deep tendon reflex testing (do not test in painful or arthritic joints)
   a) upper extremities
      - biceps
      - triceps
      - radial
   b) lower extremities
      - patellar
      - Achilles

c. Diagnostic tests
1) radiologic studies
   a) x-rays: detection of bone and soft tissue injury
   b) bone scan: detection of bone tumors
   c) myelogram
      - inspection of the spinal column
      - radiopaque medium injected into subarachnoid space of the spine
      - nursing care pretest:
        – check for iodine allergy
        – teach client regarding spinal tap and x-ray procedure
      - nursing care post-test:
        – keep flat in bed for 6–8 hours if client complains of a headache or if an oil-based medium was used
        – keep head of bed elevated at least 20° if a water-based medium was used
        – force fluids
   d) CAT scan
2) hematologic studies
   a) sedimentation rate: rheumatoid arthritis
   b) C-reactive protein in serum: rheumatoid arthritis
   c) serum uric acid: gouty arthritis
   d) CBC (increased WBC with gouty arthritis)
   e) serum globulin: protein
   f) antinuclear antibodies (ANA): positive with systemic lupus erythematosus (SLE)
3) electromyogram (EMG): a graphic record of the contraction of a muscle as a result of electrical stimulation

2. Analysis

a. Safe, effective care environment
1) potential for trauma
2) impaired physical mobility
3) knowledge deficit

b. Physiological integrity
1) pain
2) impaired physical mobility
3) potential for disuse syndrome

c. Psychological integrity
1) anxiety
2) ineffective individual coping
3) body image disturbance

d. Health promotion/maintenance
1) altered health maintenance
2) impaired adjustment
3) diversional activity deficit

3. General Nursing Plans, Implementation, and Evaluation

Goal 1: Client will achieve and maintain maximum physical mobility.

Plan/Implementation
- Teach client the proper use of assistive devices.
- Help client learn proper use of prosthetic devices.
- Provide needed support and encouragement.

Evaluation: Client expresses and demonstrates proper use of assistive devices; maintains maximum physical mobility.

Goal 2: Client will adapt to changes in body image.

Plan/Implementation
- Encourage client to verbalize concerns.
- Provide client with correct information about extent of body-image alteration.

Evaluation: Client expresses self-acceptance; engages in usual social activities.

Goal 3: Client will be knowledgeable about disease process, medications, and the prevention of complications.

Plan/Implementation
- Outine symptoms of disease.
- Outline progression of disease if applicable.
- Explain the rationale for ordered treatment regimen.
- Provide information regarding the administration and side effects of all medications.
- Discuss interventions that prevent the development of complications, including musculoskeletal damage and deficits.

Evaluation: Client takes medications as prescribed, returns for follow-up appointments; remains free from preventable complications.

Goal 4: Client will be free from complications of immobility.

Plan/Implementation
- See *Safety and Security*, General Nursing Goal 2 page 274.
- Prevent constipation
  - increase fluid intake, unless contraindicated
  - increase dietary roughage
- Assist with active ROM exercises as appropriate.
- Prevent urinary calculi with increased fluids.
- Prevent pressure sores
  - turn q2h
  - gently massage skin
  - keep skin clean and dry
- Prevent thrombophlebitis
  - apply antiembolic hose
  - encourage isometric exercises
  - avoid pillows behind the knees
- Prevent atelectasis by having client cough and deep breathe.

Evaluation: Client remains free from complications of immobility.

Selected Health Problems Resulting in an Interference with Activity and Rest

☐ Fractures

1. General Information

a. Types (can be assigned both classifications)
  1) classified according to severity
    a) *compound*: open
    b) *closed*: simple
    c) *complete*
    d) *comminuted*: fragmented
    e) *compression*: depressed
    f) *stress*: fatigue or sudden violent force
    g) *pathologic*: disease related, spontaneous
  2) classified according to direction of fracture line
    a) *linear, longitudinal (vertical)*: fracture runs parallel to long axis of the bone
    b) *transverse, horizontal*: fracture line runs straight across the bone
    c) *spiral*: twisted along shaft of the bone
    d) *oblique*: 45° angle

b. Risk factors
  1) old age
  2) active sports
  3) accidents
  4) osteoporosis from disease or steroid therapy

c. Medical treatment
  1) closed reduction (external fixation)
    a) manual manipulation of bone fragments into anatomic alignment
    b) immobilized in cast/traction
  2) open reduction (internal fixation)
    a) surgical procedure with direct visualization
    b) realignment of fracture fragments and immobilization with metallic device (e.g., plate, intramedullary rod)
    c) advantages: allows early weightbearing
    d) complications include post-op infections and delayed union
  3) ambulation with assistive devices
    a) crutches
      - non-weight bearing: 3-point gait
      - weight bearing
        - 2-point gait
        - 4-point gait
        - swing-to gait
    b) cane carried in hand opposite affected leg for support
    c) walker
    d) sling for arm
  4) traction (refer to *Nursing Care of the Child* page 606)

d. Emergency care of suspected fractures
  1) control of evident hemorrhage (most important problem); sterile bandage to open wound
  2) immobilize affected part (splint) before moving client
  3) do not attempt to reduce fracture
  4) apply ice pack to reduce swelling, hematoma, pain
  5) transport to medical facility as soon as possible

2. Nursing Process

a. Assessment/Analysis

1) age, developmental consideration
2) usual activity, recreational needs
3) circumstances of fracture occurrence (most result from accidents)
4) concurrent health problems (will affect healing)

b. Plans, Implementation, and Evaluation

Goal 1: If closed reduction is used, client's cast will dry properly.

Plan/Implementation

- Support cast on pillows along length of cast until dry (usually 24 hours).
- Know that drying creates heat, which causes cast to harden; heat should be uniform in nature, not felt as isolated hot spots.
- Use fan to stir air, but do not direct fan on the cast.
- *Never* use heat lamp or hair dryer on plaster cast.
- Do not completely cover the cast; when dry it is porous and will allow skin underneath to "breathe."
- Avoid weight-bearing on cast for 48 hours.
- Do not handle cast when wet, if possible; handle with palms, not fingertips.
- Do not place on hard surface while drying.
- Know that x-ray will be taken after cast application to ensure proper alignment.

Evaluation: Client's cast dries completely with fracture in proper alignment.

Goal 2: Client will maintain good circulation after cast is applied.

Plan/Implementation

- Observe circulatory status in exposed fingers or toes frequently during each shift
  - color: normal
  - temperature: warm and dry
  - swelling: minimal or none
  - circulation: good blanching; nail beds fill rapidly; adequate pulses
- Observe for neurologic impairment
  - presence of persistent, localized pain
  - ability to move digits
  - degree of sensation
- Avoid pressure areas on extremity
  - position client away from side on which he has a cast
  - support cast on pillow in a nondependent position
  - "petal" cast edges to eliminate rough, abrasive edges (see Figure 5.5.)

Evaluation: Client's toes (fingers) are warm, color good, blanch well.

Goal 3: Client's activity level will be safe and maintained to the extent allowed.

Plan/Implementation

- Know the instruction client has been given for crutch walking and reinforce teaching.
- Reinforce the principles of non-weight bearing or use of affected extremity.
- Instruct client in principles of safe movement (e.g., no hopping around).
- Instruct client in isometric, ROM exercises as appropriate.

Evaluation: Client uses crutches correctly and safely.

Goal 4: Client will experience relief of pain.

Plan/Implementation

- Administer pain medications as ordered.
- Know that pain should decrease after fracture is set (increasing pain may indicate that the cast is too tight or infection is beginning).
- Instruct client to notify nurse of any new pain or pain unrelieved by analgesics.
- Have client on crutches ambulate only with assistance after administration of pain medication.

Evaluation: Client is free from discomfort.

Goal 5: Client's rehabilitation course will remain free from complications.

Plan/Implementation

- Teach client signs and symptoms of complications (e.g., poor circulation, infection, nerve damage)
  - check for "hot spots" which indicate an area of inflammation beneath them
  - note odor under cast (necrotic tissue will produce malodor)
- Teach client principles of cast care
  - keep clean and dry
  - don't put objects (e.g., for scratching) down the cast
- Alert client to possible side effects of decreased mobility (e.g., weight gain, constipation)
  - increase fluids
  - readjust diet to include more protein and roughage, fewer carbohydrates

Evaluation: Client demonstrates methods of cast care; maintains weight; remains free from infection and constipation.

Goal 6: If open reduction with a cast or skeletal traction is utilized, client will be free from post-op complications.

Plan/Implementation

- Observe for post-op bleeding
  - draw circle around evidence of bleeding on cast; mark with date and time
  - check frequently
- Apply ice pack if ordered to reduce swelling and pain (protect cast from moisture).
- Administer analgesics as ordered.
- Maintain traction in proper alignment, with correct amount of weight.
- Prevent complications of immobilization
  - give frequent skin care over bony prominences to prevent decubitus ulcers; use sheepskin or egg-crate mattress
  - perform isometric and ROM exercises on unaffected extremities to prevent contractures, thrombophlebitis, foot drop
  - know that if the fracture occurred in the middle ⅓ of the femur, client may exercise ankle; if fracture is in the lower ⅓, no ankle exercise
  - increase fluids, roughage to prevent constipation, urinary calculi
- Observe carefully for post-op wound infection
  - provide pin care q8h if in skeletal traction
  - if client has a cast, observe for increased pain, swelling, or a malodor coming from cast
- Provide bedridden client with age-appropriate diversions/activities, as possible
  - arrange for school work for child/adolescent
  - arrange private time for adult clients and their visitors
- Be aware that prolonged bedrest may lead to sleep disturbances, sensory deprivation.

Evaluation: Client is free from complications during the recovery phase (maintains proper alignment, skin integrity); performs ROM exercises on unaffected extremities.

☐ Fractured Hip (Proximal End of Femur)

1. General Information

a. Definition: "broken hips" include fractures that are within the head of the femur, associated with osteoporosis and minor trauma; extracapsular fractures that occur below the capsule and are caused by severe trauma or a fall; and those of the greater or lesser trochanter

b. Incidence
   1) increases after age 60
   2) more common in women than men

c. Precipitating factors
   1) falls associated with osteoporotic and degenerative changes of the bone
   2) age-related physiologic changes in balance and perception

d. Medical treatment
   1) medical intervention: closed reduction achieved with traction (rare in older clients)
   2) surgical intervention: open reduction and internal fixation, or a prosthetic head-of-the femur

2. Nursing Process

a. Assessment/Analysis

1) affected leg
   a) shortened
   b) externally rotated
   c) abducted
   d) severe pain and tenderness
2) age of client and circumstances of injury
3) current health, mental status including degree of orientation
4) availability of family support mechanisms

b. Plans, Implementation, and Evaluation

Goal 1: Preoperatively, client will experience relief of symptoms and be protected from futher injury.

Plan/Implementation

- Administer analegesics as ordered.
- Use skin traction (Buck's) to relieve muscle spasms and reduce edema.
- Turn only 45° to affected side; may turn to unaffected side, with or without traction.
- Use fracture pan for elimination.
- Prevent external rotation of affected hip.
- Assess and monitor coexisting medical problems.

Evaluation: Client remains free from pain with affected leg in good alignment, preoperatively.

Goal 2: Postoperatively, client will maintain the proper position for functional healing of the hip.

Plan/Implementation

- Prepare client's bed (e.g., firm mattress, bed board, overhead trapeze, adjustable foot board, bed rails, and other decubitus ulcer-prevention aids).
- Know that rapid onset of sharp hip pain may indicate dislocation.

- Maintain abduction of affected leg at all times (e.g., use an abductor splint or pillows between legs).
- Prevent external rotation by placing a trochanter roll along affected side.
- Apply an antiembolic stocking from toes to groin on unaffected leg.
- Monitor Hemovac drainage; ensure that tubes remain patent.
- Prevent acute flexion of hip by keeping bed low (e.g., not higher than 35°–40°); elevate only for meals.

Evaluation: Client is afebrile postoperatively; has minimal pain; maintains affected leg in abduction.

Goal 3: Client will remain free from complications of immobility.

Plan/Implementation

- See General Nursing Goal 4 page 295.

Evaluation: Client's post-op course is free from complications (e.g., no fever, skin in good condition).

Goal 4: Client's activity level will increase progressively (depending on type of surgery and degree of bone healing).

Plan/Implementation

- Internal fixation with nails or pins
  - have client stand first
  - get client up in chair 1–2 days post-op
  - allow only partial weight bearing for 3 months
  - allow full weight bearing in 6 months
- Femoral-head prothesis
  - use measures to prevent dislocation at all times
  - have client stand at side of bed, starting 2–4 days post-op
  - allow partial weight bearing 4–10 days post-op
  - allow full weight bearing 2–6 months post-op
  - do not use wheelchair for 2 weeks to aid rising to a standing position and to prevent hyperflexion
  - prevent flexion greater than 90°
- Consult physician regarding muscle-setting exercises for gluteal and quadriceps muscles, movements of the affected leg, ambulation, and weight bearing on the nonaffected leg.
- Work with physical therapist to coordinate exercise and mobilization regimen.
- Perform full ROM exercises at least twice daily on unaffected limbs.
- Lead with unaffected leg when using transfer techniques.

Evaluation: Client ambulates with/without assistance and with/without partial weight bearing, depending on surgical intervention.

Goal 5: Client will remain free from psychosocial complications of hospitalization and immobility.

Plan/Implementation

- Refer to "Depression" page 53 and "Confused Behavior" page 48.

Evaluation: Client maintains contact with reality; is minimally confused, disoriented, dependent.

Goal 6: Client will regain use of joint to the maximum degree possible.

Plan/Implementation

- Get client out of bed as permitted, assisting with transfers.
- Keep leg abducted; avoid hip hyperflexion.
- Have client relax and contract gluteal and quadricep muscles 10 times/hour during the day.
- Teach client and family about precautions after discharge
  - avoid sleeping on operative side
  - use cane, walker, or crutches for support and partial weight bearing
  - do not cross or twist legs
  - do not lift heavy objects
  - observe carefully for signs of wound infection
- Reinforce need for continued exercise and maintenance of normal activities as possible.

Evaluation: Client uses rehabilitative measures to enhance recovery; pursues activities within range of ability, age, and level of interest.

Goal 7: Client will develop a workable plan for long-term convalescence.

Plan/Implementation

- Assist client and significant others regarding home care or decide where client will go upon discharge (e.g., home, extended-care facility).
- Teach client and significant others what they need to know about
  - length of convalescence and progress of weight-bearing ambulation
  - general health measures to be followed (e.g., medications, exercise, diet)
  - correct safety precautions for use of cane, walker, or wheelchair
  - persons and agencies who can be contacted for services

■ Help client and significant others develop a plan to eliminate unsafe environmental conditions that may have contributed to initial fracture.

Evaluation: Client makes adequate arrangements for long-term convalescence.

☐ Amputation

1. General Information

a. Definition: traumatic or surgical removal of an appendage or limb

b. Indications

1) certain tumors
2) severe traumatic injuries (usually affects upper extremities)
3) problems related to peripheral vascular disease (e.g., gangrene); usually affects lower extremities

2. Nursing Process

a. Assessment/Analysis

1) physical and psychologic strengths of client
2) support systems (e.g., family and friends)
3) health status, high-risk factors (i.e., smoking habits, cardiovascular disease, diabetes, cancer)
4) condition of affected appendage or limb
   a) color of skin
      ■ necrotic tissue may be blue or gray-blue
      ■ turns dark brown or black
   b) presence of infection
      ■ red streaks along lymphatic channels
      ■ systemic symptoms
5) availability of skilled rehabilitation team

b. Plans, Implementation, and Evaluation

Goal 1: Client will be physically and emotionally prepared for surgical outcome.

Plan/Implementation

■ Explain that surgery is performed above level of healthy tissue.
■ Explain that grieving is normal.
■ Allow client and significant others opportunities to express anger and fears.
■ Initiate exercises to develop strength in muscles that will be used in rehabilitation.
■ Prepare client for post-op stump care and prosthesis if appropriate.
■ Give prophylactic antibiotics as ordered.

Evaluation: Client expresses grief over anticipated loss.

Goal 2: Client's stump will remain free from contractures and will be reduced in size.

Plan/Implementation

■ Elevate stump for 24 hours (to hasten venous return and prevent edema).
■ Avoid elevation of stump after 1st 48 hours post-op to prevent hip contracture (most common post-op complication).
■ Keep stump in an extended position; have client with a leg amputation lie prone for short periods 2–3 times daily to prevent flexion contractures.
■ Use "shrinker sock" or elastic bandage if prosthetic fitting is delayed; apply in a figure-eight fashion to reduce size of stump in preparation for prosthesis; teach client how to apply properly (elastic bandages applied to above-the-knee amputations are also wrapped around the waist.
■ Know that an immediate prosthetic fit reduces the incidence of post-op complications, particularly incisional pain and phantom limbsensation.

Evaluation: Client applies shrinker sock properly; stump is clean, free from contractures; experiences minimal pain.

Goal 3: Client will recover from surgery free from complications.

Plan/Implementation

■ Refer to *Surgery* page 159.
■ Know that pain may be sharp and acute in the incisional area.
■ Assess for phantom limb sensation vs. phantom limb pain (limb sensation subsides with time).

Goal 4: Client will adapt to altered body image.

Plan/Implementation

■ Refer to General Nursing Goal 2 page 294.

Goal 5: Client will use prescribed prosthetic device.

Plan/Implementation

■ See General Nursing Goal 1 page 294.
■ Know that a good prosthetic fit takes time and adjustments.
■ Reinforce teaching done by the prosthetist.
■ Teach client to observe stump for signs of infection, irritation.
■ Teach client proper skin care: wash and dry daily, avoid use of skin creams.
■ Continue to offer encouragement and support to

client and significant others throughout the rehabilitation process.

- Reinforce client's efforts at maintaining balance and posture, and increasing auxiliary muscle strength.
- If prosthesis is not an option, assist client in safe use of wheelchair, transfer techniques.

Evaluation: Client adapts to prosthesis with few problems; transfers from bed to wheelchair safely.

Arthritis

1. General Information

a. Rheumatoid arthritis
  1) definition: a chronic, systemic, diffuse, collagen disease characterized by inflammatory changes in joints and related structures, resulting in crippling deformities
  2) incidence
    a) occurs 3 times more frequently in women
    b) peak incidence between 30 and 40 years of age
    c) primarily affects proximal joints and synovial membranes before involving larger weight-bearing joints
  3) predisposing factors
    a) possibly an autoimmune disorder
    b) stress, obesity, aggravation are implicated
  4) pathophysiologic sequence: synovitis → pannus formation → fibrous ankylosis → bony anklyosis (frozen joint)

b. Osteoarthritis
  1) definition: a chronic disease involving the weight-bearing joints; nonsystemic
  2) incidence
    a) occurs 5 times more frequently in women
    b) peak incidence between 50 and 70 years of age
  3) predisposing factors
    a) aging
    b) trauma
    c) excessive use of joint (e.g., worker who sews)
    d) obesity
  4) pathophysiologic sequence: degeneration of articular cartilage → new bone formation: Heberden's nodes (bony nodules or spurs on the dorsolateral aspects of distal joints of fingers)

c. Gouty arthritis
  1) definition: inflammation of a joint caused by gout (uric acid crystals deposited in joint)
  2) incidence
    a) 19 times more frequent in men
    b) peak incidence between 20 and 40 years of age
    c) often affects a terminal joint (e.g., great toe)
  3) predisposing factors
    a) hyperuricemia
    b) several metabolic disorders
  4) pathophysiology
    a) metabolic disorders of purine metabolism
    b) urate deposits in and around joints

d. Surgical interventions: for rheumatoid arthritis, osteoarthritis
  1) *tendon transplant*: from a normal muscle to another location to assume function of a damaged muscle
  2) *osteotomy*: cutting bone to correct bone or joint deformity
  3) *synovectomy*: removal of synovial membrane; helps prevent recurrent inflammation
  4) *arthroplasty*
    a) hemiarthroplasty: one part of a joint is replaced (e.g., head of femur)
    b) total hip replacement: head of the femur and the acetabulum are replaced
    c) total knee replacement: both articular surfaces of the knee are replaced
    d) interphalangeal joint replacement

2. Nursing Process: Rheumatoid Arthritis and Osteoarthritis

a. Assessment/Analysis
  1) rheumatoid arthritis
    a) stiffness, especially in morning
    b) proximal joint pain that decreases with use
    c) swollen joint
    d) limitation of muscle strength and atrophy; functional impairment caused by pain and muscle irritation
    e) acute and chronic episodes with remissions and exacerbations
    f) systemic symptoms (e.g., anemia, elevated body temperature)
    g) elevated sedimentation rate
    h) elevated C-reactive protein in serum
  2) osteoarthritis
    a) stiffness, especially in mornings
    b) joint pain that increases with use
    c) limitation of joint motion

d) aggravation of symptoms with temperature, humidity change, and weight bearing

b. Plans, Implementation, and Evaluation

Goal 1: Client will function as comfortably and as normally as possible.

Plan/Implementation

- Teach client to balance rest and activity
  - encourage to optimum level of functioning
  - exercise joint to point of pain—never beyond
  - perform PT and OT activities as prescribed
  - during acute phase maintain complete bedrest and wear splints on affected joints as prescribed
- Apply heat to provide analgesia and relax muscles.
- Teach client about medications and their side effects, see Table 3.50 below.
- Assist client to modify environment to accomplish activities easily.

Evaluation: Client maintains activity without undue stress; can state side effects of ordered medications.

Goal 2: Client will adjust to the chronicity of the condition.

Plan/Implementation

- Allow client to express fear and concerns.
- Encourage as much activity as possible.
- Teach client that continuous immobilization may cause increased pain.
- Teach client to avoid sudden jarring movements of joints.
- Warn client about "quacks" who promise miracle cures.
- Encourage continued follow-up to reevaluate progression of disease and efficacy of drug therapy.
- Counsel client and family regarding the need for a well-balanced diet and, if obesity is a problem, weight reduction.

Evaluation: Client states a willingness to continue with therapeutic regimen as prescribed; expresses concerns about chronicity of the disease; maintains maximum activity level.

Goal 3: Client will be prepared for surgery.

Plan/Implementation

- Refer to *Surgery* page 157.
- Usually joint surgeries require multiple preps, then covering with a sterile towel.

Evaluation: Client describes what to expect in immediate post-op period.

Table 3.50 Anti-inflammatory Drugs

Type	Side Effects	Nursing Implications
Acetylsalicylic acid (Aspirin)	Tinnitus, GI distress, nausea, vomiting, prolonged bleeding time	Give with food, milk, or antacids. Avoid use with oral or parenteral anticoagulants.
Phenylbutazone (Butazolidin)	Nausea, vomiting, diarrhea, bone-marrow depression, cardiac decompensation, salt and water retention, liver damage	Give with food, milk, or antacids. Monitor client for fever, sore throat, mouth ulcers, bleeding and weight gain. Monitor CBC. Record client's weight, I&O daily.
Ibuprofen (Motrin)	Epigastric distress, nausea, vomiting, occult blood loss	Give with food, milk, or antacids. Monitor for GI distress, weight gain. Check renal and hepatic function in long-term therapy.
Indomethacin (Indocin)	Headaches, dizziness, blurred vision, nausea, vomiting, severe GI bleeding, hemolytic anemia, bone-marrow depression	Give with food, milk, or antacids. Contraindicated in aspirin allergy and GI disorders. In long-term drug therapy, monitor CBC and renal function, and encourage eye examinations.
Naproxen (Naprosyn)	Epigastric distress, nausea, occult blood loss	Monitor for GI distress.
Sulindac (Clinoril)	Epigastric distress, nausea, occult blood loss, aplastic anemia	Give with food, milk, or antacids. Monitor for bleeding. Watch for edema and periodically check blood pressure.
Piroxicam (Feldene)	Same as Indocin	Same as Indocin.

Goal 4: If surgery is performed on the affected hip, client will remain free from post-op complications.

Plan/Implementation
- Refer to *Surgery* page 159.
- See Goal 2, "Fractured Hip" page 297.

Goal 5: Client will regain use of joint to the maximum degree possible.

Plan/Implementation
- Refer to Goal 6, "Fractured Hip," page 298.

3. Nursing Process: gouty arthritis

a. **Assessment/Analysis**
   1) pain, swelling, and inflammation of affected joint (usually great toe)
   2) increased serum uric acid, sedimentation rate, WBC count

b. **Plans, Implementation, and Evaluation**

Goals 1 and 2 refer to "Rheumatoid Arthritis" page 301.

Goal 3: Client will adjust diet and life-style to prevent future attacks.

Plan/Implementation
- Teach client about use of medications and their side effects.
- Obtain dietary counseling for client; instruct in a low purine diet (i.e., restrict meats, especially organ meats, and legumes).
- Encourage daily high intake of fluids to prevent precipitation of uric acid crystals in the kidney.
- Advise regarding weight control as needed.

Evaluation: Client lists foods to be avoided; has a plan for weight reduction, if indicated.

☐ Collagen Disease

1. General Information

a. Definition: a group of diseases characterized by widespread pathologic changes in connective tissue; these are difficult to diagnose, have no cure, and cannot be prevented
b. Systemic lupus erythematosus (SLE): generalized connective tissue disorder
   1) incidence
      a) affects women 4 times more frequently than men
      b) more likely to occur in young adults and adolescents
   2) etiology and risk factors are unknown; an autoimmune disease
c. Medical treatment: aim is temporary remission or slowing of collagen destruction
   1) high doses of steroids for exacerbation
   2) aspirin for pain
   3) nonsteroidal anti-inflammatory drugs
   4) plasmopheresis (plasma exchange)

2. Nursing Process

a. **Assessment/Analysis**
   1) arthritic-like symptoms
   2) sensitivity to sun
   3) presence of erythematous "butterfly" rash across bridge of nose
   4) alopecia
   5) involvement of other organ systems
      a) renal (leading cause of death)
      b) cardiovascular
      c) peripheral vascular
      d) nervous
      e) respiratory
   6) polymyositis (inflammation of skeletal muscle)
   7) Raynaud's Phenomenon
   8) diagnostic test results
      a) positive lupus erythematosus (LE) prep
      b) anemia
      c) proteinuria

b. **Plans, Implementation, and Evaluation**

Goal 1: Client will follow correct medication regimen.

Plan/Implementation
- Outline plan for steroid therapy.
- Minimize side effects through diet modification, time of administration, etc.
- Teach client safety precautions for steroid therapy (see Table 3.28 on page 226).

Evaluation: Client describes medications, expected side effects and ways to minimize them.

Goal 2: Client will understand disease and its complications.

Plan/Implementation
- See General Nursing Goal 3 page 294.

☐ Lumbar Herniated Nucleus Pulposus

1. General Information

a. Definition: a protrusion of the gelatinous cushion between vertebrae (intervertebral disk)

Table 3.51 Antigout Medications

Types	Uses	Action	Side Effects	Nursing Implications
Colchicine	Gout	Inhibits renal tubular reabsorption of urate	Nausea, vomiting, abdominal pain, diarrhea, aplastic anemia and agranulocytosis with prolonged use	Monitor for GI distress. Monitor fluid I&O. Keep daily output at 2,000 ml; force fluids to 6–8 glasses/day.
Allopurinol (Zyloprim)	Gout	Reduces the production of uric acid	GI distress, drowsiness, headache, dizziness, agranulocytosis, aplastic anemia, skin rash	Monitor for rash (may be first sign of severe hypersensitivity reaction). Give with or immediately after meals. Monitor I&O. Keep daily output at 2,000 ml; force fluids to 6–8 glasses/day. Periodically check CBC, hepatic and renal function.
Phenylbutazone (Butazolidin)	Acute gout	Anti-inflammatory, antipyretic analgesic	See Table 3.50 on page 301.	See Table 3.50 on page 301.

through surrounding cartilage causing pressure on nerve roots with resultant pain

b. Incidence
  1) more frequent in men
  2) commonly occurs in the space between the 4th and 5th lumbar vertebrae

c. Predisposing/risk factors
  1) sedentary occupations
  2) long-term driving (e.g., truck driver)
  3) infrequent physical exercise, certain sports (e.g., bowling, baseball)

d. Medical treatment
  1) medical intervention
    a) bedrest on a firm mattress with bed board
    b) pelvic traction
    c) proper body alignment (e.g., no prone position)
    d) medications
      - muscle relaxants
      - analgesics
      - non-steroidal anti-inflammatory agents
      - steroids
    e) physical therapy
      - diathermy
      - back exercises
      - braces
    f) weight reduction as needed
  2) surgical intervention
    a) indications
      - prevention of further nerve damage and deficits
      - severe back and leg pain that does not respond to conservative therapy
      - a totally extruded disk that causes sensory and motor deficits in the lower extremities, bowel, and bladder (an emergency)
    b) procedures
      - *laminectomy*: removal of the posterior arch of the vertebra to relieve pressure on the nerve root
      - *spinal fusion* (for additional stability): bone graft from iliac crest used to fuse two or more vertebrae together
      - chemonucleolysis: relieves pressure if pain persists (check for allergies to meat tenderizer or papaya)
    c) success rate ranges from 50%–90%

2. Nursing Process

a. Assessment/Analysis
  1) low back pain radiating down posterior thigh (sciatic nerve involvement)
  2) paresthesia of affected nerve roots
  3) muscle weakness, muscle spasm in lumbar region
  4) numbness, weakness, paralysis, or decreased reflexes along affected nerve pathway of leg, ankle, and foot
  5) character of pain
    a) intermittent; more frequent and severe depending on degree of herniation

b) may be related to a single traumatic event
c) get progressively worse
d) worsened by anterior and lateral flexion of the spine; rotational movements, laughing, sneezing, coughing, straining; straight leg raising to 80° or 90° while supine

6) diagnostic tests: CAT scan or MRI
7) client's occupation, exercise routine, physical status

b. Plans, Implementation, and Evaluation

Goal 1: Client will be relieved of pain.

Plan/Implementation

- Place on bedrest on a firm mattress with bed board, traction as ordered.
- Administer analgesics, msucle relaxants as ordered, noting client's response.
- Prevent twisting and straining.
- Use noninvasive methods to relieve pain (e.g, frequent back rubs, diversion).

Evaluation: Client experiences decreased pain; requires infrequent analgesia; maintains bedrest.

Goal 2: Client will learn how to care for back to prevent future episodes.

Plan/Implementation

- Observe and reinforce physical therapy regimens.
- Give warm bath and muscle relaxants prn prior to exercise sessions.
- Assist client to apply and wear back supports correctly, observing for any signs of skin irritation.
- Teach client to use appropriate body mechanics
  - use broad base of support
  - use large body muscles
  - maintain good posture
  - bring object close to the body before moving
  - pull rather than push an object
  - do not lift items
  - squat, do not bend over
- Walk rather than stand, but stand rather than sit.

Evaluation: Client demonstrates back exercises correctly and states a willingness to do them regularly; demonstrates use of appropriate body mechanics.

Goal 3: If surgery is required, client will be physically and psychologically prepared for surgery.

Plan/Implementation

- Refer to *Surgery* page 158.
- Explain importance and demonstrate post-op positioning, logroll turning, and body alignment.
- Explain that if spinal fusion is to be done, a turning frame may be used.
- Tell client about incision needed for bone graft and HemoVac that may be in place.
- Obtain pre-op neurologic assessment for post-op comparison.

Evaluation: Client verbalizes a positive attitude toward the surgical outcome; demonstrates understanding of planned procedure and immediate post-op care.

Goal 4: Client will remain free from post-op complications.

Plan/Implementation

- Refer to *Surgery* page 159.
- Keep client flat in bed for 1st 12 hours; then may raise head of bed to 30°.
- Know that client will usually get out of bed on 1st or 2nd post-op day (unless spinal fusion done).
- Use turning sheet and turn client by "logrolling."
- Tell client to report numbness or tingling in feet or legs.
- Give medications for pain and frequent muscle spasms as ordered.
- Provide laxative to avoid straining.
- When allowed to be up, have client stand and not sit.
- Apply antiembolic stockings and have client do leg exercises to prevent thrombophlebitis.
- When ambulating, have client wear shoes, not slippers, for better support.
- Prepare client for 3–6 month use of body cast or brace post-op if fusion was done.

Evaluation: Client has uneventful post-op course; maintains dry and intact dressing; has adequate sensation in toes; ambulates frequently with minimal discomfort.

Goal 5: Client and significant others will be adequately prepared for discharge.

Plan/Implementation

- Refer to General Nursing Goal 3 page 274.
- Provide client and significant others with written instructions regarding care of operative site, back-care regimen, and back exercises.
- Ensure that client knows proper application of back brace, if ordered.

- Provide client with a list of instructions or a timetable to resume activities such as driving, sexual intercourse, sports, housework, or job responsibilities.
- Ensure that client knows to report signs of illness, fever, increasing back pain, or muscle spasms to physician.

Evaluation: Client states schedule for exercising; applies back brace correctly; knows when to resume additional activities.

References

Adult arthritis. (1983). *American Journal of Nursing*, *83*, 253–278.

Evers, J., & Werpachowski, D. (1984). Dealing with fractures. *RN*, *47*(11), 53–57.

Faehnrich, J. (1983). When pathologic fractures threaten. *RN*, *46*(11), 34–37.

Farrell, J. (1984). Orthopedic pain—What does it mean. *American Journal of Nursing*, *84*, 466–469.

Gandy, E., & Veigh, G. (1984). Help the amputee stand on his own again. *Nursing84*, *14*(7), 46–49.

Harris, C. (1985). Rheumatoid arthritis and the pregnant woman. *American Journal of Nursing*, *85*, 414–417.

Hawley, D. (Ed.). (1984). Symposium on arthritis and related rheumatic diseases. *Nursing Clinics of North America*, *19*, whole issue.

Henning, L., & Burrows, S. (1986). Keeping up on arthritis meds. *RN*, *49*(2), 32–38.

Kutcher, J., & Bourne, D. (1985). Postop needs of the amputee. *RN*, *48*(2), 46–47.

Miller, R. & Evans, W. (1987). Immediate post-op prosthesis. *American Journal of Nursing*, *87*, 310–311.

Musolf, J. (1983). Chemonucleolysis: A new approach for patients with herniated intervertebral disks. *American Journal of Nursing*, *83*, 882–885.

Robinson, J., & Mary, L. (1985). A nail-safe method. *American Journal of Nursing*, *85*, 158–161.

Rubin, M. The physiology of bed rest. *American Journal of Nursing*, *88*, 50–56.

Searle, L., et al. (1985). Honoring the personal side of chronic illness. *Nursing85*, *15*(8), 53–57.

Walters, J. (1981). Coping with a leg amputation. *American Journal of Nursing*, *81*, 1349–1352.

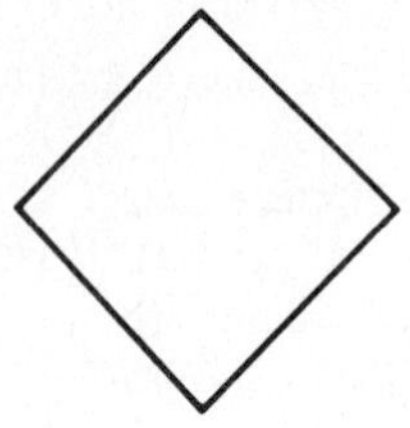

Cellular Aberration

(The nursing care presented in this unit contains selected health problems related to neoplastic disease.)

General Concepts

Overview/Physiology

1. Terms pertaining to neoplasia
   a. *Cancer*: a group of diseases characterized by uncontrolled growth and spread of abnormal cells
   b. *Neoplasm*: neo = new; plasm = formation
   c. *Carcinoma*: a malignant tumor arising from epithelial tissue
   d. *Sarcoma*: a malignant tumor arising from nonepithelial tissue
   e. *Differentiation*: degree to which neoplastic tissue resembles the parent tissue
   f. *Metastasis*: spread of cancer from its original site to other parts of the body
   g. *Adjuvant therapy*: therapy designed to be adjunctive or supplemental to primary therapy
   h. *Palliation*: relief or alleviation of symptoms without cure
2. Tumors are characterized by tissue of origin
   a. Adeno: glandular tissue
   b. Angio: blood vessels
   c. Basal cell: epithelium, mainly sun-exposed areas
   d. Embryonal: gonads
   e. Fibro: fibrous tissue
   f. Lympho: lymphoid tissue
   g. Melano: pigmented cells of epithelium
   h. Myo: muscle tissue
   i. Osteo: bone
   j. Squamous cell: epithelium
3. Incidence
   a. 2nd leading cause of death in the US
   b. One of every four Americans can expect to develop cancer
   c. Occurs in all age groups; incidence increases with age
4. Eitology: no *single* cause
5. Risk factors (American Cancer Society)
   a. Tobacco: smoking or chewing
   b. Alcohol: excessive intake
   c. Hormones (e.g., estrogen)
   d. Genetic predisposition
   e. Immune deficiency
   f. Age
   g. Occupational: exposure to carcinogens (e.g., asbestos, vinyl chloride)
   h. X-rays: overexposure
   i. Sunlight: long exposure
   j. Diet: high fat and/or high total calories
6. Physiology/pathophysiology (not a single disease)
   a. Cell cycle: five phases
      1) G_0 (G means gap): resting phase; minimal biologic activity
      2) G_1 (1st growth period): enzymes, RNA, structural protein are synthesized
      3) S: synthesis of DNA
      4) G_2 (2nd growth period): RNA and protein synthesis
      5) M (mitosis): cell division
   b. Characteristics of malignant cells
      1) anaplastic (loss of differentiation)
      2) disorderly division
      3) uncontrolled growth pattern
      4) loss of normal growth-limiting mechanisms
      5) nonencapsulated
      6) tend to metastasize
      7) may be necrotic from poor vascular supply
      8) often recur after treatment
7. Metastasis
   a. Modes
      1) lymphatic
      2) vascular
      3) direct extension
      4) seeding
   b. Site(s)
      1) usually determined by the lymph and blood drainage patterns of the original cancer site (e.g., primary tumors entering systemic venous circulation are apt to lodge in the lung)
      2) most common: lung, liver, bone, and brain
8. Classification

a. Histologic classification (grading of tumor appearance and degree of differentiation)
   1) grade 1: most differentiated (resembles parent tissue most closely), best prognosis
   2) grade 2: intermediate differentiation
   3) grade 3: essentially undifferentiated
   4) grade 4: highly undifferentiated (most unlike parent tissue), anaplastic, poorest prognosis
b. TNM classification: *t*umor, *n*odes, *m*etastasis
   1) tumor
      a) T_0: no evidence of primary tumor
      b) TIS: carcinoma in situ
      c) T_{1-4}: progressive increase in tumor size and involvement
      d) TX: tumor cannot be assessed
   2) nodes
      a) N_0: regional lymph nodes not demonstrably abnormal
      b) N_{1-3}: increasing degrees of demonstrable abnormality of regional lymph nodes
      c) NX: regional lymph nodes cannot be assessed clinically
   3) metastasis
      a) M_0: no evidence of distant metastasis
      b) M_{1-3}: ascending degrees of distant metastasis, including metastasis to distant lymph nodes

9. Prognosis
   a. Factors
      1) tumor size
      2) nodal involvement
      3) metastasis
   b. 5 year survival: approximately 1 out of 3 persons

Application of the Nursing Process to the Client with Cancer

1. **Assessment**
   a. Health history
      1) seven warning signs (CAUTION)
         a) *C*hange in usual bowel and bladder function
         b) *A* sore that does not heal.
         c) *U*nusual bleeding or discharge: hematuria, tarry stools, ecchymosis, bleeding mole
         d) *T*hickening or a lump in the breast or elsewhere
         e) *I*ndigestion or dysphagia
         f) *O*bvious change in a wart or mole
         g) *N*agging cough or hoarseness
      2) family history
      3) presenting symptoms
         a) appetite
         b) weight loss
         c) energy level
         d) pain (severe pain is *not* a common early problem)
   b. Physical exam
      1) general appearance
      2) percussion
         a) fluid waves (ascites)
         b) chest percussion
      3) palpation
         a) masses
         b) lymph nodes
   c. Diagnostic tests
      1) lab tests
         a) CBC, platelet count
         b) blood chemistries
         c) CEA (carcinoembryonic antigen)
         d) specific tests depending on suspected site of cancer
      2) cytologic studies (microscopic exam of body secretions for cancer cells) (e.g., Pap smear)
      3) biopsy of mass
      4) radiologic studies
         a) x-rays (e.g., mammogram)
         b) CAT scans
         c) radioisotope scanning
         d) ultrasound
         e) thermography
      5) endoscopic examinations (e.g., bronchoscopy, gastroscopy)
   d. Medical treatment
      1) surgery
         a) principles
            - excision/radical excision: tumor plus margin of healthy tissue must be excised
            - often results in some significant defect or loss of function
         b) uses
            - diagnosis
            - cure
            - palliation
              - remove obstruction
              - debulk large unresectable tumors
              - control pain (e.g., cordotomies, nerve blocks)
            - ablative: removal of hormone-producing organs to effect a response in hormone-dependent tumor
      2) radiation
         a) definition: the use of ionizing radiation

to cause damage and destruction to cancerous growths

b) effect: radiation causes damage at the cellular level
- indirectly: water molecules within the cell are ionized
- directly: causes strand breakage in the double helix of DNA
- not every cell is damaged beyond repair

c) uses
- cure
- palliation
- combined with surgery
  - pre-op: to reduce size of the tumor
  - post-op: to retard/control metastasis of tumor cells
- combined with chemotherapy

d) administration
- external (e.g., cobalt)
- internal (e.g., implants)

e) side effects
- radiation syndrome: effects not related to site treated (experienced to one degree or another by most clients receiving radiation therapy)
  - fatigue, malaise
  - headache
  - anorexia, nausea, vomiting
- specific side effects: related to site treated
  - cranium: transitory or permanent hair loss (i.e., alopecia)
  - mouth, rectum: mucositis, stomatitis
  - mouth, head and neck: taste alteration, reduced saliva production, dental caries
  - throat, esophagus: dysphagia
  - GI tract: nausea, vomiting, diarrhea
  - abdomen: malnutrition, anorexia
  - pelvis, long bones, sternum: bone-marrow suppression
    - * thrombocytopenia (platelets) → bleeding
    - * leukopenia (WBCs) → infection
    - * erythropenia (RBCs) → anemia
  - bladder, pelvis: cystitis
  - testicles, ovaries: sterility
  - rectum: proctitis
  - lungs, chest wall: pneumonitis

3) chemotherapy

a) definition: the use of drugs to retard the growth of or destroy cancerous cells

b) classification/effect (see Table 5.22 on page 614).
- antineoplastics
  - cell-cycle specific: attack cells at a specific point in the process of cell division
  - cell-cycle nonspecific: act at one time during cell division
- hormones
  - alter the hormone balance
  - modify the growth of some hormone-dependent tumors

c) combination chemotherapy
- two or more drugs used simultaneously
- each drug has different effect
- increases the effectiveness of the destruction/retardation of cancerous cells

d) uses
- cure
- palliation
- combined with surgery
- combined with radiation

e) administration
- intravenous infusion
  - most common route
  - diffuses drug throughout the entire body
- arterial infusion
  - drug is introduced through a catheter directly into the tumor via the main artery that supplies it
  - advantage: high proportion of drug is absorbed by tumor before it reaches systemic circulation
- regional perfusion
  - one extremity is isolated from the general circulation
  - advantage: systemic circulation of drug is diminished, thus systemic toxic effects are reduced
- oral, IM (less common)

f) side effects drug specific (see Table 5.22)
- nausea and vomiting
- bone-marrow depression
- alopecia
- fatigue, anorexia
- stomatitis
- menstrual irregularities, aspermatogenesis

4) supportive (e.g., nutrition, comfort, measures)

2. **Analysis**
   a. Safe, effective care environment
      1) potential for infection
      2) potential for injury
      3) sensory-perceptual alterations: visual, auditory, kinesthetic gustatory, tactile, olfactory
   b. Physiological integrity
      1) pain
      2) fatigue
      3) altered nutrition: less than body requirements
   c. Psychological integrity
      1) anxiety
      2) body image disturbance
      3) ineffective individual coping
   d. Health promotion/maintenance
      1) knowledge deficit
      2) ineffective family coping: compromised
      3) diversional activity deficit
3. **General Nursing Plans, Implementation, and Evaluation**

Goal 1: Client will know guidelines for early detection of cancer.

Plan/Implementation

- Use detection/screening services.
- Explain importance of American Cancer Society guidelines for early detection in asymptomatic individuals
  - cancer-related checkup
    * every 3 years ages 20–40
    * every year after 40
  - breast exam
    * by self (SBE, see page 389): every month after age 20
    * by physician: every 3 years ages 20–40; every year after 40
    * by mammogram: single baseline x-ray between ages 35–40; every 1–2 years between ages 40–50; every year after age 50
  - uterus
    * pelvic exam: every 3 years ages 20–40; every year after age 40
    * Pap smear: every 3 years after 2 initial negative tests one year apart, from onset of sexual activity throughout life
  - colon and rectum (men and women)
    * digital rectal exam: annually, beginning at age 40
    * guaiac test: every year after age 50
    * sigmoidoscopy: every 3–5 years after 2 initial negative exams one year apart, after age 50
- Refer client to American Cancer Society for information.

Evaluation: Client lists guidelines for early detection of cancer.

Goal 2: Client undergoing cancer surgery will be physically and psychologically prepared.

Plan/Implementation

- Refer to *Surgery* page 158.
- Assist client to deal with body-image changes.
- Arrange referral to appropriate agency (e.g., Lost Chord, Reach-to-Recovery).

Evaluation: Client describes surgery in own terms; expresses fears and concerns.

Goal 3: Client and staff will be knowledgeable about planned radiation treatment and how to minimize side effects.

Plan/Implementation

- Discuss reasons for radiation therapy and type to be used (e.g., external or internal).
- External radiation
  - tell client that although alone during the treatment someone will be watching closely
  - explain that skin markings must not be washed off for duration of therapy
  - teach proper skin care
    * avoid soaps and bathing the area unless approved by physician
    * avoid exposing area to sun and temperature extremes
    * expose area to air
    * wear nonconstrictive clothing
    * do not apply cosmetics, lotions, or powder to area unless directed to do so
  - maintain or improve client's nutritional status
    * administer antiemetics as needed before vomiting occurs; see Table 3.52 on page 310.
    * obtain nutritional counseling
    * observe for signs of mucositis
    * teach good oral hygiene
    * teach use of prescribed medications (e.g., viscious lidocaine [Xylocaine], oral antibiotics [nystatin (Mycostatin)] suspension)
    * advise small, low residue meals if diarrhea develops
    * encourage fluid intake
    * advise sweet foods if taste is altered
  - protect client from bleeding and/or infection
  - help client balance activity with rest

Table 3.52 Antiemetics

Generic Name (Trade Name)	Action	Side Effects	Nursing Implications
Phenothiazines			
Prochlorperazine (Compazine)	Acts on chemoreceptor trigger zone to inhibit nausea and vomiting	Drowsiness, dizziness, extrapyramidal symptoms, orthostatic hypotension, blurred vision, dry mouth	Dilute oral solution with juice, etc. Give deep IM only. Obtain baseline BP before administration. Monitor BP carefully.
Perphenazine (Trilafon)	Same as above	Same as above	Same as above.
Thiethylperazine (Torecan)	Same as above	Same as above	Same as above.
Nonphenothiazines			
Dimenhydrinate (Dramamine)	Inhibits nausea and vomiting via unknown mechanism	Drowsiness	Warn patient of decreased alertness. Dilute (very irritating to veins).
Benzquinamide (Emete-Con)	Acts on chemoreceptor trigger zone to inhibit nausea and vomiting	Drowsiness	Do not give IV in cardiovascular patients or with preanesthetic drugs. Do not reconstitute with 0.9% saline. Use large muscle for IM injection.
Trimethobenzamide (Tigan)	Same as above	Drowsiness	Do not give to children with viral illness (may contribute to Reye's syndrome). Warn patient of drowsiness. Give deep IM.
Diphenidol (Vontrol)	Inhibits vestibular cerebellar pathways and possibly chemoreceptor trigger zone to inhibit nausea and vomiting	Drowsiness, dry mouth, confusion	Monitor BP carefully. Use only on hospitalized patient. Observe for visual and auditory hallucinations.
Metoclopramide (Reglan)	Stimulates motility of upper GI tract; blocks dopamine receptors at chemoreceptor trigger zone to inhibit nausea and vomiting	Restlessness, anxiety, drowsiness, extrapyramidal symptoms	Give IV slowly over 15 minutes. Warn patient of decreased alertness.

- Internal radiation
  - tell client that once the radiation source is removed, the radioactivity is gone
  - protect staff and significant others from exposure to radiation source
    - * explain that three factors critical to safe care are *time, distance*, and *shielding*
    - * place client in private room
    - * mark room with signs regarding radiation therapy
    - * restrict visitors to one 15-minute visit/day
    - * allow only nonpregnant visitors
    - * use long forceps to handle a dislodged implant and place them in a lead-lined container
    - * handle client's body fluids and eating utensils as radioactive, if client has received oral or IV radioactive substances
  - prevent dislodgment of cervical implant
    - * maintain strict bedrest
    - * reduce residue in diet
    - * prevent bladder distention with Foley catheter

Evaluation: Client states reason for and undergoes radiation therapy with minimal side effects.

Goal 4: Client will understand the goals of chemotherapy, names of drugs, anticipated side effects, and treatment of side effects.

Plan/Implementation

- Discuss treatment plans with client.
- Tell client names of drugs prescribed and probable side effects.
- Maintain integrity of veins
  - use arm veins
  - discontinue infusion at first sign of infiltration, check patency by aspirating every 2–3 cc during I.V. push drugs
  - know drugs that are vesicants (e.g., nitrogen mustard, doxorubicin)
- Avoid prolonged, severe nausea and vomiting
  - use antiemetics preventatively
  - advise light food intake before treatments
  - avoid dairy products and red meats
  - encourage dry, bulky foods, sweet foods, clear fluids, and noncarbonated cola
- Prevent infection or bleeding
  - monitor client's bone-marrow function
  - obtain CBC and platelet count before treatments (WBC of at least 3,000 is needed before therapy is started)
- Prepare client for possible hair loss
  - explain that all body hair is susceptible to effects of chemotherapy but that the fastest growing hair is most affected
  - advise client to purchase a wig, hats, or scarves before losing hair
  - tell client that hair will grow back after chemotherapy is discontinued, but color and texture may be different
- Maintain good oral hygiene
  - teach client good oral hygiene
  - teach client signs and symptoms of stomatitis
  - teach client what to do if stomatitis develops

Evaluation: Client states the goals of chemotherapy and lists the drugs and measures to minimize side effects.

Selected Health Problems

☐ **Cancer of the Lung** see page 195

☐ **Cancer of the Bladder** see page 244

☐ **Cancer of the Prostate** see page 256

☐ **Cancer of the Colon** see page 265

☐ **Cancer of the Larynx** see page 196

☐ Hodgkin's Disease

1. General Information

a. Definition: malignancy of the lymphoid system characterized by a generalized painless lymphadenopathy; unkown etiology

b. Incidence
- **1)** peak incidence between 15–30 years of age
- **2)** more common in males
- **3)** non-Hodgkin's lymphomas (lymphosarcoma, reticulum cell sarcoma) are more common in children under age 15
- **4)** 5-year survival rate is 90%; late recurrences (after 5–10 years) are not uncommon

c. Medical treatment
- **1)** diagnostic tests
  - **a)** lymphangiography
  - **b)** inferior venacavogram
    - erythrocyte sedimentation rate (ESR): elevated
    - serum copper: elevated
- **2)** clinical staging: surgical laparotomy to determine stage of the disease and best course of treatment; staging determines prognosis (see Table 3.53)
  - **a)** lymph node biopsy for characteristic cell (Reed-Sternberg)
  - **b)** surgical clips are used to outline area for irradiation
  - **c)** splenectomy
- **3)** chemotherapy: combination drug MOPP (mechlorethamine [Mustargen], vincristine [Oncovin], prednisone, procarbazine) for 6–18 months
- **4)** radiation therapy

2. Nursing Process

a. Assessment/Analysis
- **1)** enlarged lymph nodes (most common sites: cervical, inguinal, mediastinal, axillary, retroperitoneal regions)
- **2)** anemia
- **3)** fever, infection (increased susceptibility to infection)
- **4)** anorexia, weight loss
- **5)** malaise
- **6)** night sweats

b. Plans, Implementation, and Evaluation

Goal 1: Client will be prepared for lymphangiography; will be free from complications.

Plan/Implementation

Pretest

- Explain the procedure in terms of what the client/family can expect
  - food/drink are usually not restricted

Table 3.53 Staging of Hodgkin's Disease

Stage 1	Involvement of a single lymph node area or one additional extralymphatic organ (liver, kidney, lung, or intestine)
Stage II	Involvement of two or more lymph node areas on the *same side* of the diaphragm or one additional extralymphatic organ on the same side of the diaphragm
Stage III	Involvement of lymph node areas on *both sides* of the diaphragm; may be accompanied by involvement of one extralymphatic organ, the spleen, or both
Stage IV	Diffuse involvement of one or more extralymphatic organs, with or without lymph node involvement
Each stage is also further categorized as subtype A or B:	
Subtype A	Absence of generalized symptoms
Subtype B	Presence of generalized symptoms, such as fever, weight loss, night sweats

- procedure last approximately 4 hours, may last longer
- feet are anesthetized and immobilized for lymphatic vessel catheterization
- client must lie still during procedure, sedation usually given
- the dye may cause the following normal reactions
  * unusual taste sensations
  * fever
  * headache
  * insomnia
  * retrosternal burning sensation
  * bluish-green discoloration of urine/stool for several days
  * bluish discoloration of skin, especially hands and feet, which may persist for weeks or longer

■ Check for allergies to iodine, seafood.
■ Ensure consent is on chart.
■ Have client void before test.

Post-test

■ Monitor for signs of complications
- bleeding or infection from cutdown site
- oil embolism (from oil-based dye)
  * fever, chills
  * dyspnea
  * cough
  * chest pain, soreness
  * hypotension

■ Maintain bedrest for 24 hours or as ordered.
■ Monitor vital signs frequently until stable, then every 4 hours for 48 hours.
■ Assess incision site for infection; dressing is usually not changed for 48 hours.
■ Do not get original dressing wet.
■ Check for leg edema; elevate lower extremities as necessary.

Evaluation: Client is prepared for procedure and develops no complications.

Goal 2: Client/family are prepared for staging and splenectomy.

Plan/Implementation

■ Refer to "Surgery" page 157.
■ Inform client of effects of splenectomy: increased susceptibility to infection.

Evaluation: Client/family states effects of splenectomy and implications for life-style (minimizing exposure to infection).

□ Cancer of the Cervix

1. General Information

a. Incidence
  1) second most common cancer location in women
  2) 100% cure if detected early (stage 0)
  3) squamous cell most common cell type

b. Classification: clinical stages
  1) stage 0: carcinoma in situ
  2) stage I: confined to cervix
  3) stage II: spread from cervix to vagina
  4) stage III: involves lower one-third of vagina and has invaded paracervical tissue to pelvic wall on one or both sides and is associated with palpable lymph nodes in pelvic wall
  5) stage IV: involves bladder and rectum and extends outside true pelvis

c. Predisposing factors
  1) early, frequent coital exposure to multiple partners
  2) pregnancy at young age
  3) history of sexually transmitted disease/herpes/venereal warts

d. Medical treatment
   1) stage 0: conization of the cervix
   2) stage I: hysterectomy or possible conization
   3) stage II or III: intracavitary and external beam irradiation; possible radical hysterectomy
   4) stage IV: radiation therapy followed by pelvic exenteration when there is persistent disease

2. Nursing Process

a. Assessment/Analysis
   1) menstrual history
   2) pain in back, flank, and legs
   3) vaginal discharge
   4) diagnostic tests: positive cytology (Pap smear); Schiller's test and punch biopsy

b. Plans, Implementation, and Evaluation

Goals: Refer to "Uterine Fibroid" page 452.

☐ Cancer of the Endometrium of the Uterus

1. General Information

a. Incidence
   1) ratio of cervical to endometrial cancer is 3:1
   2) About 50% of clients with postmenopausal bleeding have endometrial carcinoma
   3) diagnosis is made only after development of overt symptoms

b. Predisposing factors
   1) history of infertility
   2) dysfunctional uterine bleeding
   3) long-term estrogen therapy

c. Medical treatment: hysterectomy

2. Nursing Process

a. Assessment/Analysis
   1) menstrual history
   2) irregular uterine bleeding
   3) diagnostic tests: endometrial biopsy

b. Plans, Implementation, and Evaluation

Goals: Refer to "Hysterectomy" page 451.

☐ Cancer of the Breast

1. General Information

a. Incidence
   1) most common cancer in women
   2) can be bilateral
   3) highest incidence 40–49 and 65+
   4) incidence increasing, especially in women under age 40

b. Predisposing factors
   1) family history
   2) chronic irritation; fibrocystic disease
   3) menarche before age 11; menopause after age 50
   4) no children or 1st child after age 30
   5) previous breast cancer
   6) uterine cancer

c. Surgical/medical treatment
   1) surgical intervention
      a) modified radical mastectomy: breast, axillary contents
         - most commonly performed surgery
         - suitable for palpable, nonfixed tumors
      b) wedge (quadrant) resection of breast
         - a wide local excision
         - suitable for small (less than 1 cm) or nonpalpable tumors
         - usually followed by radiation and chemotherapy, hormonal manipulation
         - often done in combination with axillary lymph node dissection or sampling
         - remains somewhat controversial
      c) Halstead radical mastectomy; breast, axillary contents, pectoralis muscle
         - for advanced, fixed tumores
         - infrequently used
   2) adjuvant therapy
      a) chemotherapy: specifics of therapy vary from institution to institution
      b) hormonal manipulation done if tumor is known to be estrogen receptor positive
         - premenopausal women: anti-estrogen therapy
         - postmenopausal women: estrogen therapy

d. Sequence of surgery
   1) one-step: biopsy, frozen section, and mastectomy if positive; one anesthetic
   2) two-step: biopsy under local or general anesthetic; client is awakened and when pathology results are available (2–3 days), treatment options are discussed; mastectomy or definitive surgery under a second anesthetic

2. Nursing Process

a. Assessment/Analysis

1) dimpling of skin
2) retraction of nipple
3) hard lump; not freely movable
4) change in skin color
5) change in skin texture (peau d'orange)
6) alterations of contour of breast
7) discharge from nipple
8) pain (late sign)
9) ulcerations (late sign)
10) diagnostic tests: positive mammography, biopsy, and frozen section
11) symptoms of bone, lung, and brain involvement (common areas of metastasis)

b. Plans, Implementation, and Evaluation

Goal 1: Client will be able to explain proposed surgery, effects of surgery, and pre- and post-op care.

Plan/Implementation
- Refer to *Surgery* page 157.
- Explore client's expectations of what surgical site will look like.
- Discuss skin graft if one is a possibility.

Evaluation: Client describes treatment options and expresses satisfaction with treatment decision.

Goal 2: Client will remain free from post-op complications.

Plan/Implementation
- Refer to *Surgery* page 159 for common complications.
- Check under dressing, HemoVac and under client's back for bleeding.

Evaluation: Client is free from post-op complications, evidence of bleeding.

Goal 3: Client will regain use of arm, joint movement on side of surgery.

Plan/Implementation
- Position arm on operative side on a pillow.
- Encourage hand activity (e.g., squeeze small ball).
- Have client use arm and hand for daily activities (e.g., brush hair).
- Consult with physician regarding additional exercises.
- Instruct client in post-op exercises (e.g., wall climbing).

Evaluation: Client demonstrates appropriate post-op exercises; knows schedule for exercising.

Goal 4: Client will be able to explain incision care, prosthetic devices available.

Plan/Implementation
- Encourage client to look at incision.
- On discharge, have client wear own bra with cotton padding or Reach-to-Recovery prosthesis.
- Discuss with client plans for obtaining a permanent prosthesis.
- Teach client to wash incision with soft cloth using soap and water.

Evaluation: Client has viewed incision; explains wound care.

Goal 5: Client will describe lymphedema and list ways to prevent it.

Plan/Implementation
- Teach client reasons for lymphedema.
- Have client sleep with arm elevated on pillows.
- Elevate arm throughout day.
- Avoid any constriction around arm.
- Apply elastic bandage, arm stocking as needed.
- Decrease sodium and fluid intake.
- Obtain an order for a JOBST pressure machine if above methods are ineffective.

Evaluation: Client describes measures to prevent lymphedema, keeps arm elevated at rest.

Goal 6: Client will describe precautions necessary to prevent infections in arm on side of surgery.

Plan/Implementation
- Avoid BP measurements, injections, blood drawing in affected arm.
- Wear gloves when gardening, etc.
- Attend to any small cut or scrape immediately.
- Avoid biting, chewing nails.
- Prevent sunburn and any kind of regular burn.
- Do not shave axilla on affected side.

Evaluation: Client lists measures to avoid arm infection.

Goal 7: Client will demonstrate positive self-concept.

Plan/Implementation
- Encourage return to normal activities.
- Help plan for prosthesis fitting and discuss types of clothes she can wear.
- Discuss reconstruction possibilities.
- Encourage client to discuss operation and diagnosis with significant others.
- Spend time with significant others to allow discussion of concerns and fears, so they can provide support for client's needs.

■ Arrange Reach-to-Recovery visit.

Evaluation: Client has Reach-to-Recovery visit; discusses self in positive terms; has plans to obtain prosthesis.

Goal 8: Client will experience normal grieving.

Plan/Implementation

- Allow client to cry, withdraw, etc.
- Explain that these feelings are usual and expected, that other women in a similar situation feel the same way.
- Help client focus on future, but discuss loss.
- Let client know that sometimes grief is delayed 2 or 3 months, and that it is a normal experience nonetheless.

Evaluation: Client expresses grief over loss of breast, diagnosis.

Goal 9: Client and significant other can describe additional treatment when appropriate.

Plan/Implementation

- Refer to General Nursing Goals 3 and 4, page 309.

Evaluation: Client lists anticipated side effects of planned adjuvant therapy.

☐ Acquired Immune Deficiency Syndrome (AIDS)

1. General Information

a. Definition: A syndrome characterized by a defect in cell-mediated immunity: may have a long incubation period (from 6 months to 5 years). As the cell-mediated immunity becomes more impaired, the client becomes more likely to develop any of the opportunistic infections characteristically seen with the syndrome. To date there is no known cure and the syndrome is predominantly fatal.

b. Incidence: approximately 73% of adult AIDS clients are homosexual or bisexual males, 17% are men or women who have abused IV drugs; the remaining 10% is made up of persons with hemophilia who have received clotting factor products, newborns of high-risk or infected mothers, and sex partners of infected persons.

c. Causative agent: human immunodeficiency virus (HIV)

d. Mode of Transmission

1) sexual contact
2) exposure to HIV-infected blood or blood products
3) perinatally from mother to child
4) HIV found in blood, semen, vaginal secretions, saliva, tears, breast milk, cerebrospinal fluid, amniotic fluid, and urine; but studies to date have implicated only blood, semen, vaginal secretions, and possibly breast milk in transmission.

e. Diagnosis: Requires presence of

1) cellular immunodeficiency (confirmed by CBC, immune profile)
2) opportunistic infection or cancer
3) positive test result for antibody to HIV (confirmed by ELISA test or Western blot assay)

f. Complications

1) Kaposi's sarcoma (seen in 78% of clients)
2) pneumocystis carinii pneumonia (seen in 78% of clients)
3) cytomegalovirus, retinitis, encephalitis, colitis, or pneumonia
4) HIV encephalopathy
5) CNS toxoplasmosis

g. Medical treatment

1) none for HIV virus
2) treatment for opportunistic infections and cancer
3) zidovudine (Retrovir) has been approved by FDA for use in certain AIDS clients
4) supportive
5) other drugs are being researched

2. Nursing Process

a. Assessment/Analysis

1) fever
2) weight loss
3) fatigue
4) lymphadenopathy
5) diarrhea
6) night sweats
7) signs and symptoms of opportunistic infections or cancer

b. Plans, Implementation, and Evaluation

Goal 1: Significant others and staff will be protected from client's infection.

Plan/Implementation

- Implement Universal Precautions for body or body substance isolation secretions.
- Exercise care when handling sharp instruments during procedures, cleaning.
- Place needle disposal containers in client's room and do not recap needles.
- Dispose of used needles and syringes in puncture-resistant containers and incinerate.
- Use protective barriers when exposure to blood or body fluids is likely (e.g., gloves, masks, eyewear, face shields, gowns).

- Use gloves when inserting or discontinuing an IV or NG tube or when drawing blood.

Evaluation: Significant others and staff remain free from the client's infection.

Goal 2: Client will be free from respiratory infection and subsequent respiratory distress.

Plan/Implementation

- Provide oxygen as needed.
- Place in position of comfort and best respiratory effort.
- Pace activities so as not to cause or increase fatigue.
- Assess for signs and symptoms of respiratory infection, distress, and failure.
- Teach client/family signs and symptoms of respiratory complications.

Evaluation: Client breathes easily, remains afebrile; paces daily activities; reports early signs of respiratory complications.

Goal 3: Client will have adequate nutrition and hydration.

Plan/Implementation

- Monitor I&O, nutritional status, and electrolyte balance closely.
- Provide appropriate calorie intake if oral nutrition is tolerated.
- Provide antidiarreal drugs PRN.
- Administer TPN as ordered.
- Provide meticulous mouth care.
- Provide pain relief from mouth lesions if present, prior to attempts at oral feedings.

Evaluation: Client eats prescribed diet, has adequate calorie intake; maintains good urine output, moist mucous membranes; maintains desired weight.

Goal 4: Client will understand goals of therapy, anticipated side effects of drugs, and methods to prevent HIV transmission to others.

Plan/Implementation

- Assess client's knowledge of syndrome.
- Encourage client to discuss feelings, concerns about plan of therapy, changes in work, home, and life-style environment.
- Use a nonjudgmental approach during care.
- Tell client names of drugs prescribed and possible side effects.
- Teach signs and symptoms of infection and what steps to take if these symptoms occur.
- Teach how to avoid transmission of the illness.
- Warn not to share toilet articles or donate blood or organs.
- Advise client to inform physicians, dentists, and sexual partners of diagnosis and required precautions.

Evaluation: Client discusses goals of therapy, lists side effects of prescribed rugs; employs methods to prevent spread of virus.

Goal 5: Client will accept psychosocial support throughout illness.

Plan/Implementation

- Allow client to express fear and grief regarding the fact that illness is incurable.
- Assess client's adjustment to altered body image and self-concept.
- Spend time listening to concerns and feelings.
- Refer client to appropriate community agency for financial support as necessary.
- Encourage acceptance of support from significant others during illness.
- Teach significant others what they can do to help and support client, and to protect themselves from the virus.

Evaluation: Client expresses feelings, acknowledges efforts to support him/her through diagnosis and treatment.

References

AIDS precautions, changing practice. (1988). *American Journal of Nursing*, *88*, 372–390.

American Pain Society. (1988). Relieving pain: an analgesic guide. *American Journal of Nursing*, *88*, 815–826.

Bersani, G., Carl, W. (1983). Oral care for cancer patients. *American Journal of Nursing*, *83*, 533–536.

Birdsall, C. (1986). What are the do's and don'ts for the Hickman/Broviac catheters? *American Journal of Nursing*, *86*, 385.

Dugan, K. (1985). The bleak outlook on ovarian cancer. *American Journal of Nursing*, *85*, 144–147.

Frawley, L. (1986). Multi-lumen line—the Broviac and Hickman. *Infection Control*, *7*, 34–35.

Hassey, K. (1985). Demystifying care of patients with radioactive implants. *American Journal of Nursing*, *85*, 789–792.

Hughs, C. (1986). Giving cancer drugs IV. *American Journal of Nursing*, *86*, 34–38.

Irwin, M. (1987). Diet and cancer—what are the links. *American Journal of Nursing*, *87*, 1086–1088.

Mamaril, A. (1984). Preventing complications after radical mastectomy. *American Journal of Nursing*, *84*, 2000–2056.

Petton, S. (1985). Your role in radiation therapy. *RN*, *48*(2), 32–37.

Shapiro, T. (1987). How to help patients get through chemotherapy. *RN*, *50*(3), 58–60.

Wilkes, G., Vannicolo, P., Starck, P. (1985). Long term venous access. *American Journal of Nursing*, *85*, 793–796.

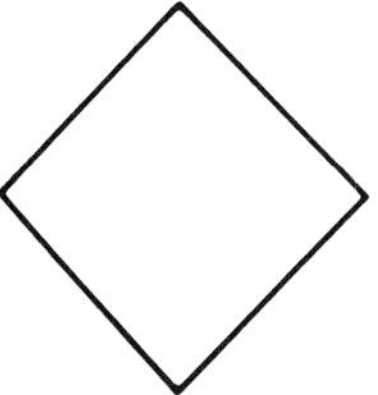

Reprints
Nursing Care of the Adult

CE Pain 320
Cohen, S. "How to Work with Chest Tubes" 331
Caine, R. & Bufalino, P. "The Patient Receiving Total Parenteral Nutrition" 351
Gavin, J. "Diabetes and Exercise" 356
Chambers, J. "Bowel Management in Dialysis Patients" 359
Larrabee, J., & Pepper, G. "The Person with a Spinal Cord Injury" 361

AMERICAN JOURNAL OF NURSING

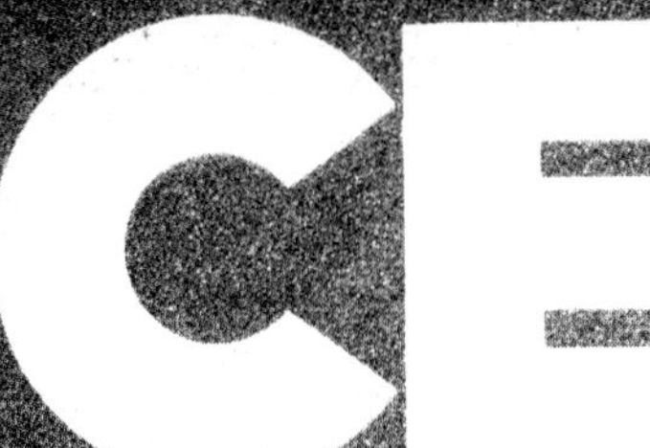

To earn continuing education credit for home study of this feature, send for the test. See page 826 for coupon and fee

RELIEVING PAIN

AN ANALGESIC GUIDE

PRINCIPLES OF ANALGESIC USE IN THE TREATMENT OF ACUTE PAIN AND CHRONIC CANCER PAIN

BY THE AMERICAN PAIN SOCIETY

After you study the material presented here, you will be able to:

1. Identify the key differences between acute pain and chronic pain.
2. Describe at least four effects of nonnarcotic analgesics.
3. List at least one advantage/disadvantage of each of five routes of administration of narcotic analgesics.
4. Name six of the basic principles of narcotic analgesic therapy.
5. Identify physical dependence, psychological dependence, and tolerance.
6. Recognize at least five categories of adjuvant analgesics.
7. Discuss at least two ways pain management varies with the age of the patient.
8. Describe the American Pain Society's stepwise approach to pain management.

Susan C. Schafer, RNC, MS, clinical research nurse at the Pain Research Clinic, National Institutes of Health, Bethesda, MD, served as consultant for this continuing education feature.

Officially Approved For

6

CE Contact Hours by the ANA Mechanism for Continuing Education.

CE PAIN

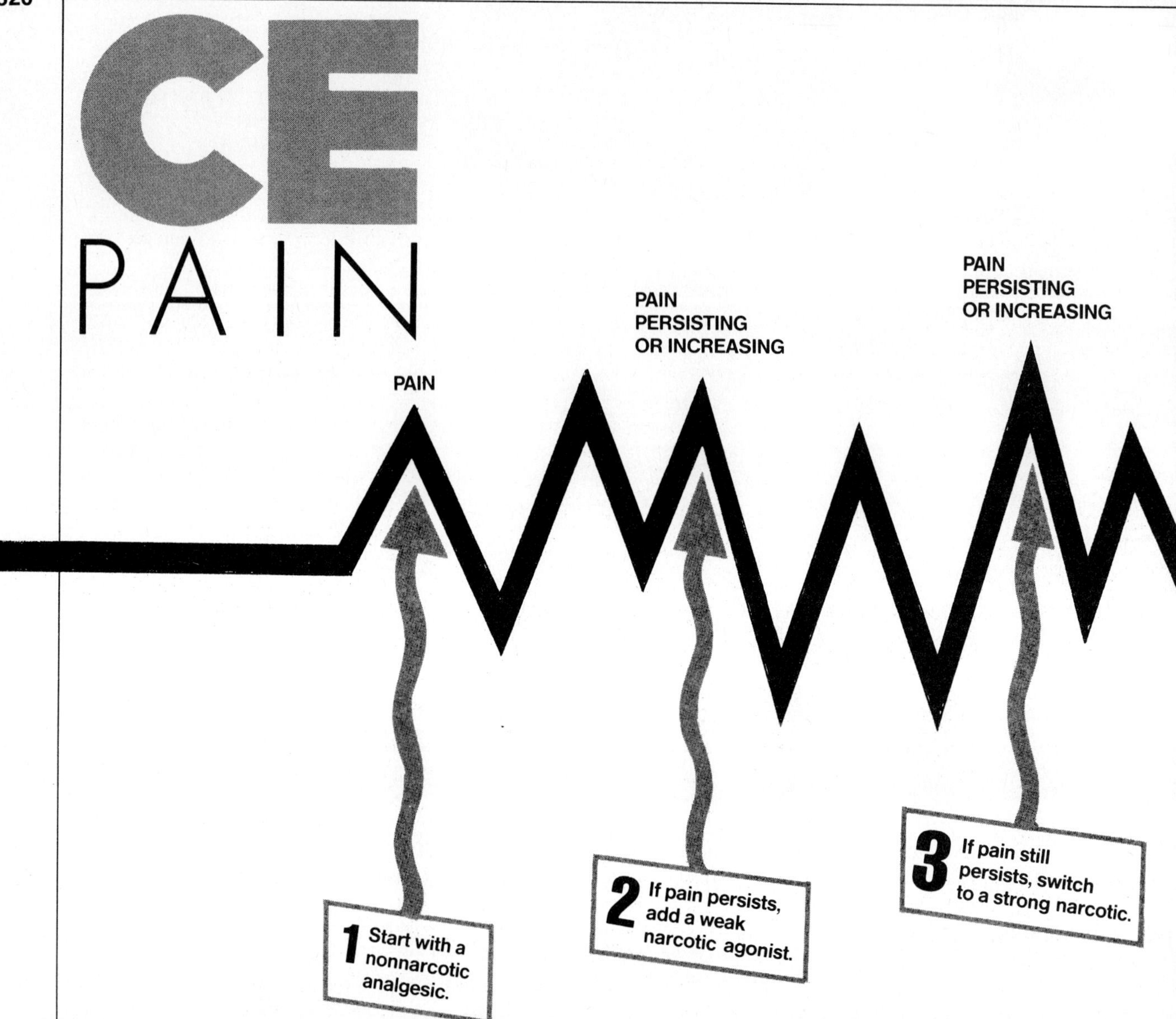
PAIN
PAIN PERSISTING OR INCREASING
PAIN PERSISTING OR INCREASING
1 Start with a nonnarcotic analgesic.
2 If pain persists, add a weak narcotic agonist.
3 If pain still persists, switch to a strong narcotic.

APS's stepwise approach to managing cancer pain provides a framework within which analgesia regimens can be tailored specifically for each patient.

ROBERT HARFORD

Pain may be defined as "an unpleasant sensory and emotional experience associated with actual or potential tissue damage, or described in terms of such damage"(1). Pain is always subjective. Objective signs such as grimacing, limping, and tachycardia may help in assessment, but such signs may not be seen in patients who have chronic pain caused by structural lesions. No neurophysiological or chemical test can measure pain. The question "Does the patient have real pain?" cannot be answered. The clinician must accept the patient's report of pain.

Acute pain follows injury to the body and generally disappears when the injury heals. It begins at a specific time, usually along with objective physical signs of autonomic nervous system activity—tachycardia, hypertension, diaphoresis, mydriasis, and pallor. These autonomic signs are similar to those of anxiety. Acute pain is best treated by recognizing and treating its cause—and relieving it temporarily with narcotic and nonnarcotic analgesics.

A patient whose pain lasts longer than several months often presents a different clinical picture. **Cancer pain** typically has a specific cause and is perhaps best considered acute recurrent pain. **Chronic pain** persists beyond the expected healing time and often cannot be ascribed to a specific injury. Chronic pain may or may not have a well-defined onset and by definition does not respond to treatments directed at its cause.

The cause of chronic pain due to nonmalignant disease may be difficult to identify, and in contrast to acute pain, chronic pain rarely triggers autonomic nervous system activity (sweating, tachycardia, dilated pupils). With few objective signs of pain, the inexperienced clinician may say the patient does not look as if he is in pain.

Further, chronic pain may effect some changes in personality, lifestyle, and ability to function, and may be associated with signs and symptoms of depression—hopelessness, helplessness, loss of libido and weight, and disturbed sleep.

Treating chronic pain involves identifying any potential tissue damage that might be causing the pain, recognizing associated affective and environmental factors, and doing whatever might help the patient continue personally meaningful activities without risking harm.

Children may have acute or chronic pain, but inadequate verbal skills or their misconceptions about the cause or consequences of pain may hamper assessment. For example, children may not report pain because they fear painful diagnostic evaluations. Abnormal gait, failure to move an extremity, or persistent crying may be the only clues that the child feels pain. Clinically, altered heart rate and blood pressure in acute pain, or changes in activity levels in both acute and chronic pain, provide the best means of assessing pain in children.

The mainstay of management of acute pain and chronic cancer pain is, of course, drug therapy. Using narcotic analgesics to control chronic pain not due to cancer is controversial (especially in the absence of structural lesions) and is generally not recommended(2).

Analgesic drugs fall into three classes: nonnarcotic analgesics, narcotic analgesics, and adjuvant analgesics.

NONNARCOTIC ANALGESICS

Nonsteroidal anti-inflammatory drugs (NSAIDs) and aspirin are "general purpose" analgesics used to treat acute and chronic pain due to surgery or trauma, as well as systemic diseases such as arthritis and cancer(3-6). They act on peripheral nerve endings at the injury site and produce analgesia by interfering with the prostaglandin system. Examples of nonnarcotic analgesics are aspirin, fenoprofen (Nalfon), ibuprofen (Motrin, Advil), diflunisal (Dolobid), and naproxen (Naprosyn).

Nonnarcotic analgesics have a ceiling effect—that is, raising the aspirin dose above 1,300 mg will not intensify peak effect but may prolong the duration of analgesia. Nonnarcotic analgesics have four major pharmacological actions: analgesic, antipyretic, antiplatelet, and anti-inflammatory.

These agents differ from narcotic analgesics in that they have a ceiling effect, they do not produce tolerance or physical or psychological dependence, and most of them presumably act by inhibiting the enzyme cyclooxygenase, thus preventing the formation of prostaglandin E_2 (PGE_2). PGE_2 sensitizes nociceptors on peripheral nerves to the pain-producing effects of substances such as bradykinin. Thus NSAIDs, by interfering with the formation of PGE_2, can influence pain at the level of the peripheral nervous system and may act synergistically with narcotic analgesics, which modulate pain in the central nervous system (CNS).

NSAIDs are used for mild-to-moderate pain, and all have been shown to be equal to or more effective than aspirin in clinical trials. They differ from each other pharmacokinetically and in duration of analgesia. Ibuprofen and fenoprofen have short half-lives and the same duration of action as aspirin; diflunisal and naproxen have longer half-lives and act longer than aspirin. NSAIDs may prolong bleeding times since they inhibit platelet cyclooxygenase and reduce formation of thromboxane A_2. Gastric irritation is a common side effect.

NSAIDs are especially effective for bone pain due to tumor metastasis and for joint inflammation—for example, from rheumatoid arthritis. The usefulness of NSAIDs in oncology is limited because their antipyretic effects may mask infection (especially in children) and because their effects on platelet function may promote hemorrhage in patients who already have thrombocytopenia and coagulation defects.

Acetaminophen (Tylenol, Panadol, Datril, Anacin-3) belongs in the nonnarcotic analgesic class as well. Roughly equipotent to aspirin in its analgesic and antipyretic potency, acetaminophen has no anti-inflammatory or antiplatelet effects. Side effects include hepatotoxicity at doses higher than 4 g per day.

Choline magnesium trisalicylate (Trilisate), 500 to 3,000 mg per day, is also an effective analgesic, has no antiplatelet effects, and has fewer gastrointestinal side effects than does aspirin(7).

NARCOTIC ANALGESICS

Narcotic analgesics are used to manage severe acute pain and chronic cancer-related pain. They act by binding to opiate receptors and activating endogenous pain-suppression systems in the central nervous system (CNS). The following principles emphasize tailoring narcotic analgesic therapy to each patient's needs(4,8-11).

Individualize the dosage. Choose

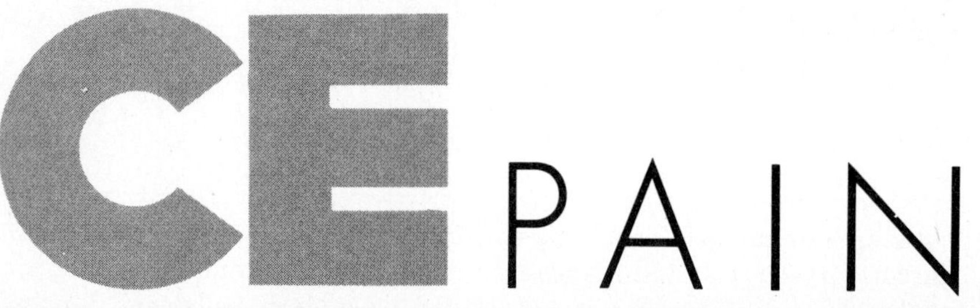

PAIN

ANALGESICS COMMONLY USED FOR MILD TO MODERATE PAIN

DRUG	APPROXIMATE EQUIANALGESIC PO DOSES (MG) TO 650 MG PO ASPIRIN[1]	STARTING ORAL DOSE RANGE (MG)	COMMENTS	PRECAUTIONS AND CONTRAINDICATIONS
NONNARCOTICS				
aspirin	650	650	often used in combination with narcotic analgesics	chronic excessive use may cause papillary necrosis and interstitial nephritis; avoid during pregnancy, in hemostatic disorders, and in combination with steroids
acetaminophen	650	650	like aspirin but no anti-inflammatory effects; does not affect platelet function	may damage liver in patients with preexisting liver disease
ibuprofen (Motrin)	ND[2]	200–400	probably more effective than aspirin	like aspirin
fenoprofen (Nalfon)	ND	200–400	like ibuprofen	like aspirin
diflunisal (Dolobid)	ND	500–1,000	like ibuprofen, but with longer duration of action	like aspirin
naproxen (Naprosyn)	ND	250–500	like diflunisal	like aspirin
choline magnesium trisalicylate (Trilisate)	ND	1,500	does not affect platelet function	
MORPHINELIKE AGONISTS				
codeine	30–60	30–60	often used in combination with nonnarcotic analgesics; biotransformed, in part, to morphine	use with caution in patients with impaired ventilation, bronchial asthma, increased intracranial pressure
oxycodone	5	5–10	shorter-acting; also used in combination with nonnarcotic analgesics (as in Percodan, Percocet), which limits dose escalation; oxycodone in 3 Percocet (15 mg) = 5 mg morphine IM	like codeine
meperidine (Demerol)	50	50–100	shorter-acting; biotransformed to normeperidine, a toxic metabolite	normeperidine accumulates with repetitive dosing causing CNS excitation; not for patients with impaired renal function or those receiving monoamine oxidase inhibitors
propoxyphene HCl (Darvon) propoxyphene napsylate (Darvon-N)	65–130	65–130	low analgesic efficacy; often used in combination with nonnarcotic analgesics; biotransformed to potentially toxic metabolite (norpropoxyphene)	propoxyphene and metabolite accumulate with repetitive dosing; overdose complicated by convulsions
MIXED AGONIST-ANTAGONIST				
pentazocine (Talwin)	50	50–100	oral form may be prepared in combination with naloxone to discourage parenteral abuse	may cause psychotomimetic effects; may precipitate withdrawal in narcotic-dependent patients

For these equianalgesic doses the time to peak analgesia ranges from 1.5 to 2 hours and the duration from 4 to 6 hours. Oxycodone and meperidine are shorter-acting (3 to 5 hours) and diflunisal, naproxen, and choline magnesium trisalicylate are longer-acting (8 to 12 hours).

[1]These doses are recommended starting doses from which the optimal dose for each patient is determined by titration.

[2]ND = not determined

NARCOTIC ANALGESICS COMMONLY USED FOR SEVERE PAIN

DRUG	APPROXIMATE EQUIANALGESIC IM DOSES (MG) TO 10 MG IM OR SC MORPHINE[1]	IM:PO POTENCY RATIO[2]	STARTING ORAL DOSE RANGE (MG)	COMMENTS	PRECAUTIONS AND CONTRAINDICATIONS
MORPHINELIKE AGONISTS					
morphine	10	3	30–60	standard of comparison for narcotic analgesics	use with caution in patients with impaired ventilation, bronchial asthma, increased intracranial pressure, liver failure
hydromorphone (Dilaudid)	1.5	5	4–8	slightly shorter duration than morphine	like morphine
methadone (Dolophine)	10	2	5–20	good oral potency; long plasma half-life (24–36 hours)	like morphine; may accumulate with repetitive dosing, causing excessive sedation (on days 2-5)
levorphanol (Levo-Dromoran)	2	2	2–4	long plasma half-life (12–16 hours)	like methadone; may accumulate on days 2–3
oxymorphone (Numorphan)	see comment	—	not available orally	5 mg rectal suppository = 10 mg morphine IM	like IM morphine
heroin	5	(6–10)	not recommended	slightly shorter-acting than morphine; not available in the United States	like morphine
meperidine (Demerol)	75	4	not recommended	slightly shorter-acting than morphine	normeperidine (toxic metabolite) accumulates with repetitive dosing causing CNS excitation; avoid in patients with impaired renal function or receiving monoamine oxidase inhibitors[3]
MIXED AGONIST-ANTAGONISTS					
pentazocine (Talwin)	60	3	50–100	used orally for less severe pain; less abuse liability than morphine; included in Schedule IV of Controlled Substances Act	may cause psychotomimetic effects; may precipitate withdrawal in narcotic-dependent patients; contraindicated in myocardial infarction[3]
nalbuphine (Nubain)	10	—	not available orally	like IM pentazocine but not scheduled	incidence of psychotomimetic effects lower than with pentazocine
butorphanol (Stadol)	2	—	not available orally	like IM nalbuphine	like IM pentazocine
PARTIAL AGONISTS					
buprenorphine (Buprenex)	0.4	—	not available orally	sublingual preparation not yet available in the United States; less abuse liability than morphine; does not produce psychotomimetic effects	may precipitate withdrawal in narcotic-dependent patients

For IM doses, time to peak analgesia ranges from one-half to one hour and duration, four to six hours. Peak analgesic effect is delayed and duration prolonged after oral administration.

[1]These doses are recommended starting IM doses from which the optimal dose for each patient is determined by titration and the maximal dose limited by adverse effects. Equianalgesic doses are based on single-dose studies in which an intramuscular dose of each drug listed was compared with morphine to establish relative potency.

[2]For example, 1.5 mg IM Dilaudid equals $1.5 \times 5 = 7.5$ mg PO Dilaudid

[3]Irritating to tissues with repeated IM injection

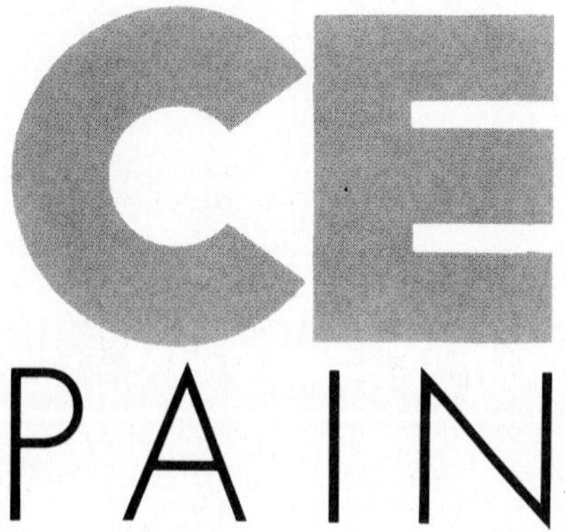

PAIN

the route that best suits the patient.

Oral (PO). This route is preferred because it is convenient and produces relatively steady blood levels. Drug effect peaks after 1½ to 2 hours for most analgesics.

Intramuscular (IM). Most commonly used for postoperative patients, this route has the disadvantages of wide fluctuations in absorption from muscle (a 30- to 60-minute lag to peak effect) and rapid falloff of action compared to the PO route.

Intravenous (IV) bolus. This route provides the most rapid onset of effect. Time to peak effect varies with drug lipid solubility, ranging from 1 to 5 minutes for fentanyl to 15 to 30 minutes for morphine. To start, use one-half the IM doses suggested in the table on the previous page.

Continuous IV infusion. This method provides steady blood levels and the ability to rapidly titrate relief for patients who have acute pain or acute exacerbations of chronic pain(12). In most cases, a drug with a short half-life (morphine, hydromorphone [Dilaudid]) is more easily titrated than one with a long half-life (methadone [Dolophine], levorphanol [Levo-Dromoran]). For stable chronic pain, the oral route is just as effective unless the patient cannot absorb PO medicines (for example, if he is vomiting or has dysphagia or bowel disease). Chronic subcutaneous (SC) infusion is an alternative to IV infusion for such patients.

Rectal. This is an alternative to the IV route for patients who cannot take PO medicine.

Epidural and intrathecal. Spinal analgesia is under clinical investigation for postop and chronic cancer-related pain. As yet we have no consensus on the choice of drug and indications for choosing that route over others.

The optimal dose of opiate analgesics varies widely among patients. A typical range of systemic morphine doses used for postoperative pain is 0.08 to 0.2 mg/kg IM q3 to 4h (5 to 15 mg for a 70-kg patient). Give each analgesic an adequate trial by titrating the dose—that is, raising the dose until limiting side effects appear—before switching to another drug.

Administer analgesic regularly (not PRN). Continuous pain requires continuous analgesia. First, though, establish the optimal dose by titration, especially when using a drug with a long half-life (levorphanol, methadone). Once you have identified dose requirements for a 24-hour period, you can give the analgesic around-the-clock (ATC) with fewer side effects. A PRN prescription for a supplementary opiate dose between regular doses is a useful backup. If *only* PRN meds are used, it may take several hours and higher doses of opiates to relieve the pain, leading to a cycle of undermedication and pain alternating with overmedication and drug toxicity.

Become familiar with the dose and time course of several strong narcotics. Although morphine is the standard strong narcotic, all morphinelike agonists provide a similar quality of analgesia and provoke similar side effects. In practice, though, people respond differently to specific narcotics. Choose a narcotic analgesic other than morphine if the patient has had a favorable experience with the drug or if you prefer a longer duration of action.

For example, methadone and levorphanol have much longer elimination half-lives (24 to 36 hours for methadone; 12 to 16 hours for levorphanol) than morphine (2 to 3 hours) and prolong analgesia, especially in the patient who is unused to opioids. Even so, constant pain relief requires giving methadone and/or levorphanol every 4 to 6 hours, since the analgesic duration of action is shorter than the plasma half-life.

You may also choose another analgesic to avoid an adverse effect of morphine. For example, although any narcotic may cause nausea, some patients are particularly sensitive to the emetic effects of morphine. Or you may take advantage of incomplete cross-tolerance among the morphinelike drugs by switching to an equianalgesic dose of another drug.

Choosing an alternative to morphine also widens the choice of dosage forms. Dilaudid-HP (10 mg/ml) is particularly useful for subcutaneous administration to an emaciated patient who needs a potent analgesic delivered in a limited volume. Hydromorphone (4 mg) and oxymorphone (Numorphan) (5 mg) come in rectal suppositories, as does morphine (5, 10, and 20 mg). Sustained-release morphine preparations, such as MS Contin and Roxanol SR are available as 30-mg tablets, with a duration of action of 8 to 12 hours.

To start a patient on a sustained-release morphine preparation, calculate the 24-hour dose of an immediate-release opioid preparation (in morphine-equivalents using the relative potency estimates given in the tables), then give one-third of that dose q8h or one-half q12h. If the patient has breakthrough pain and needs "rescue doses" of narcotics before the scheduled dose is due, give rescue doses of a standard morphine preparation.

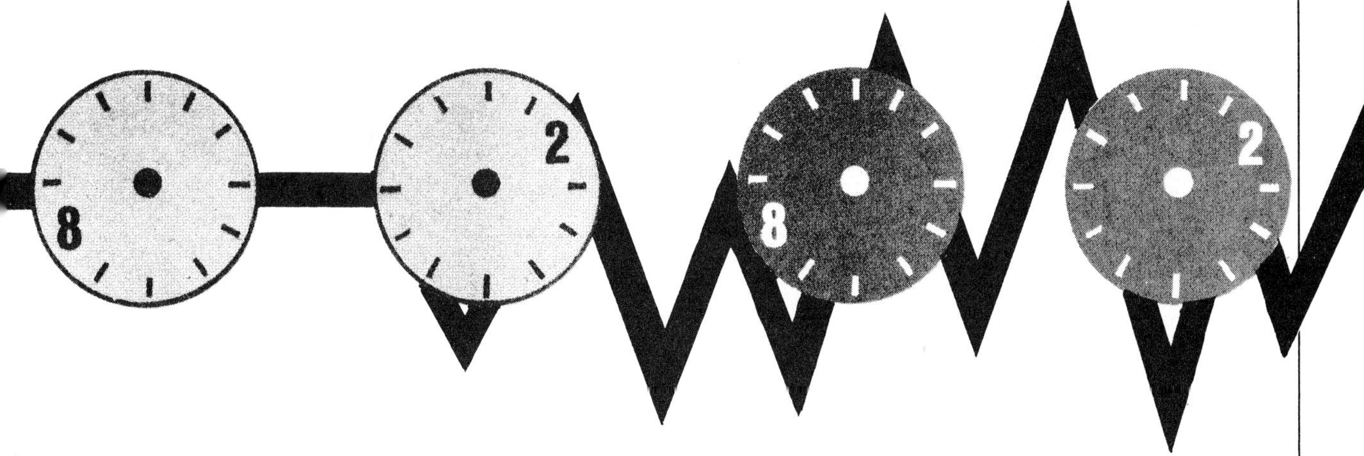

Continuous pain requires continuous analgesia. Giving only PRN doses alternates undermedication and pain with overmedication and toxicity. Around-the-clock dosing, on the other hand, keeps the patient on an even keel of relief.

A final reason for choosing an alternative opiate to morphine is to produce a more rapid onset of action. Lipophilic drugs such as methadone, meperidine, and fentanyl are good choices for premedicating a patient for a diagnostic or surgical procedure.

Be aware of the potential hazards of pentazocine and meperidine. Pentazocine (Talwin) is the only mixed agonist-antagonist narcotic analgesic available in oral form. The mixed agonist-antagonist drugs bind to opioid receptors to produce analgesia (and are therefore opioid agonists), but also have antagonist properties—they reverse opioid analgesia and can precipitate withdrawal in patients who are taking morphinelike agonists. Pentazocine may cause confusion and hallucinations and does not control severe pain. For these reasons, we cannot recommend the routine use of pentazocine.

Meperidine (Demerol) is a synthetic, short-acting narcotic with poor oral potency. In single-dose analgesic studies, 300 mg PO is roughly equivalent to 10 mg IM morphine.

Normeperidine, a metabolite of meperidine, is a CNS stimulant that produces anxiety, tremors, myoclonus, and generalized seizures if it accumulates during repetitive dosing(13). Patients with compromised renal function are at particular risk. The hyperexcitability is not reversed with naloxone (Narcan) and, in fact, giving naloxone to patients chronically on meperidine may exacerbate toxicity. For these reasons we recommend that meperidine not be used chronically.

Recognize and treat side effects appropriately. Sedation, constipation, nausea, vomiting, and respiratory depression are the most common effects. Treat sedation by reducing the dose and giving the drug more often. Dextroamphetamine (Dexedrine) 2.5 to 7.5 mg BID may improve alertness if the previous strategy does not. All patients taking narcotic analgesics are at risk for constipation; be sure to give stool softeners and laxatives.

A useful laxative regimen is docusate sodium (Colace) 100 to 300 mg per day and senna (Senokot) tablets or suppositories. Treat nausea and vomiting with hydroxyzine (Atarax, Vistaril) or a phenothiazine antiemetic (Compazine, Phenergan).

Use drug combinations that enhance analgesia.

Do not use placebos to assess the nature of pain.

Watch for tolerance and treat it appropriately.

Be aware of the development of physical dependence and prevent withdrawal.

Tolerance means that the patient needs a larger dose of narcotic analgesic to maintain the original effect. Tolerance may develop in any patient who takes narcotics chronically. Tolerance is usually associated with physical dependence, but does not imply psychological dependence.

The first sign of tolerance is a shortening of the duration of effective analgesia. In patients who have cancer, the need for more analgesics usually means progression of disease. To delay tolerance and to provide effective analgesia in the tolerant patient, combine narcotics with nonnarcotics.

Or, switch to an alternate narcotic and select one-half of the predicted equianalgesic dose as the starting dose, since cross-tolerance among narcotics is not complete.

A third alternative is to choose PO rather than IV dosing, as IV infusion of narcotics may produce rapid tolerance (since tolerance is a function of the dose and frequency of dosing).

Physical dependence is revealed in patients taking chronic opioids when abruptly stopping a narcotic (or when giving a narcotic antagonist) produces an abstinence syndrome. This syndrome is characterized by anxiety, irritability,

CE PAIN

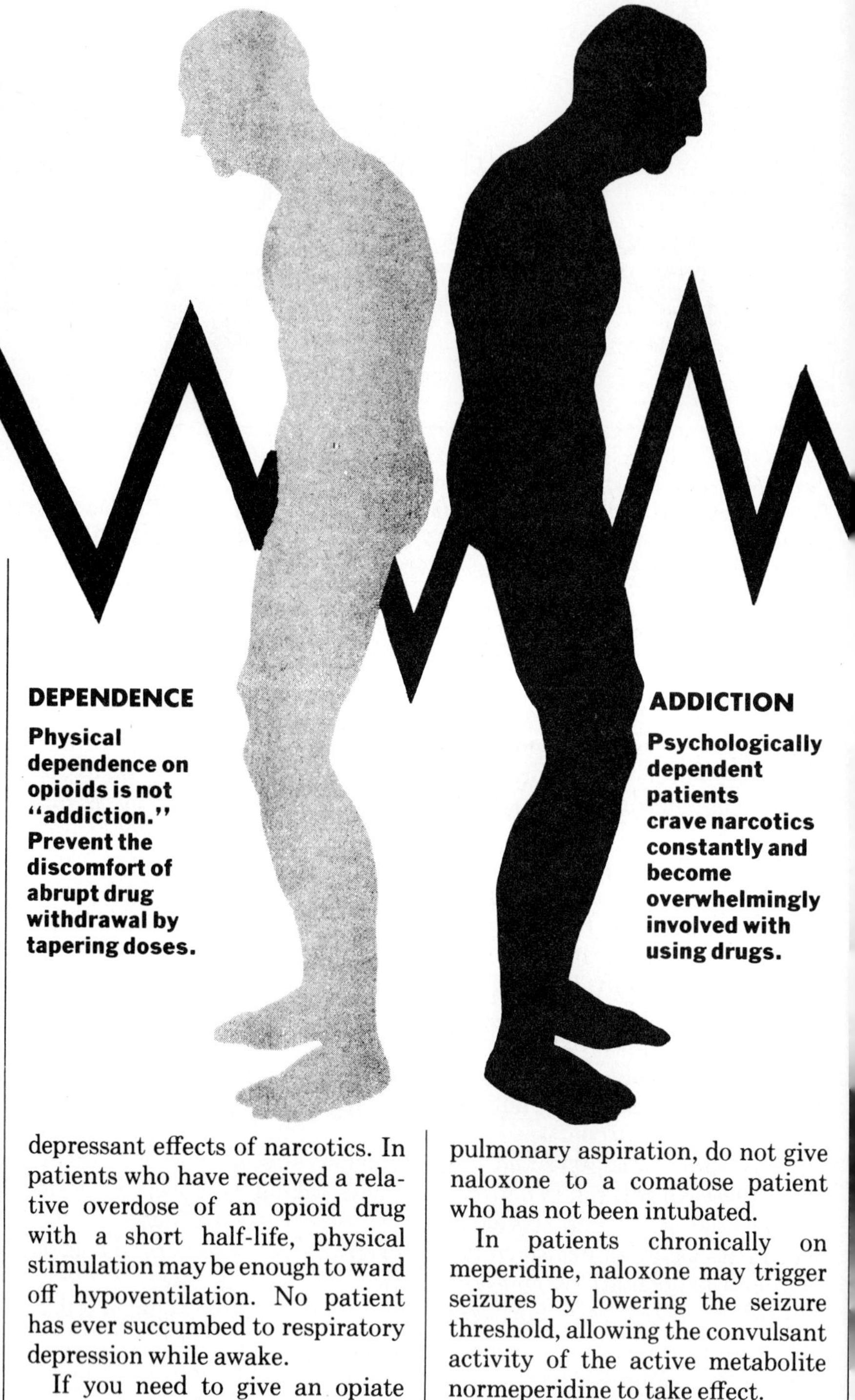

DEPENDENCE

Physical dependence on opioids is not "addiction." Prevent the discomfort of abrupt drug withdrawal by tapering doses.

ADDICTION

Psychologically dependent patients crave narcotics constantly and become overwhelmingly involved with using drugs.

chills alternating with hot flashes, salivation, lacrimation, rhinorrhea, diaphoresis, piloerection, nausea, vomiting, abdominal cramps, insomnia, and (rarely) multifocal myoclonus. The time course of the abstinence syndrome relates to the half-life of the narcotic. With drugs that have short half-lives (morphine, hydromorphone), the symptoms may appear in 6 to 12 hours and peak at 24 to 72 hours; with long-half-life drugs (methadone, levorphanol), the symptoms may be delayed several days and are usually less florid.

Avoid the abstinence syndrome by slowly withdrawing chronically used narcotics. About 25 percent of the previous daily dose is required to prevent withdrawal. Detoxify the patient as follows: give one-fourth of the previous daily dose in divided doses for the first two days and reduce it by 75 percent every two days. Continue this schedule until a total daily dose of 10 to 15 mg per day of IV morphine (or its equivalent) is reached. After two days at this minimum dose, stop the analgesic.

For an alternate method, switch to PO methadone (using the dose ratios provided in the table), giving one-fourth the equianalgesic dose as the initial "detoxification" dose and proceeding as above.

Patients on chronic opioids are often tolerant to the respiratory depressant effects of narcotics. In patients who have received a relative overdose of an opioid drug with a short half-life, physical stimulation may be enough to ward off hypoventilation. No patient has ever succumbed to respiratory depression while awake.

If you need to give an opiate antagonist to reverse respiratory depression or coma in a patient chronically on narcotics, be aware of the patient's exquisite sensitivity to antagonists. Use a dilute solution of naloxone (Narcan)—0.4 mg in 10 ml normal saline solution. Give 0.5 ml IV push every two minutes. Titrate the dose to avoid precipitating profound withdrawal, seizures, and severe pain. To avoid pulmonary aspiration, do not give naloxone to a comatose patient who has not been intubated.

In patients chronically on meperidine, naloxone may trigger seizures by lowering the seizure threshold, allowing the convulsant activity of the active metabolite normeperidine to take effect.

Psychological dependence ("addiction") is a pattern of compulsive drug use characterized by a continued craving for a narcotic and the need to use the narcotic for effects other than pain relief. The patient exhibits drug-seeking behavior and becomes overwhelmingly involved with using and procuring the drug. Physical dependence and tolerance are not equivalent to addiction. Although most psychologically dependent patients are also physically dependent, the reverse is rarely the case. The available data suggest that the risk of medically caused addiction is very small and the fear of narcotic addiction should not be a primary concern in treating acute pain and cancer pain(14). Drug use alone does not cause psychological dependence; medical, social, and economic factors contribute(15).

ADJUVANT ANALGESICS

Several other classes of drugs may enhance the effects of narcotics or aspirinlike drugs or have independent analgesic activity in some situations(16).

Tricyclic antidepressants include amitriptyline (Elavil), imipramine (Tofranil), desipramine (Norpramin), doxepin (Sinequan). These agents provide direct analgesic effects and may potentiate opiate analgesia, possibly by blocking the reuptake of serotonin and norepinephrine at CNS synapses. Amitriptyline has the best-documented analgesic action, but is also the least tolerated because of its potent anticholinergic effects—dry mouth, urinary retention, delirium(17-19). Sedation and orthostatic hypotension may also result with tricyclic compounds.

The analgesic effects are seen at lower doses (typically 25 to 150 mg per day for amitriptyline) than are the antidepressant effects. These drugs may ameliorate insomnia and may be given at bedtime. They are recommended for a wide variety of pain syndromes such as migraine headache, pain due to nerve injury (diabetic neuropathy, postherpetic neuralgia), and for prevention of migraine.

Antihistamines. The antihistamine hydroxyzine (Vistaril, Atarax) also has analgesic, antiemetic, and mild sedative effects. The usual dose is 25 to 50 mg PO or IM q4 to q6h PRN. Because hydroxyzine may produce analgesia when combined with narcotics, it is a useful adjuvant for the anxious or nauseated patient.

Caffeine. Doses of at least 65 mg of caffeine have been shown to enhance analgesia when given with aspirinlike or opiate drugs in patients with uterine cramping, episiotomy pain, dental pain, headaches, and other pain syndromes. The optimal daily dose of caffeine has not been established, but 100 to 200 mg per day seems well tolerated by most patients(20).

Dextroamphetamine (Dexedrine) may enhance postop analgesia when combined with narcotics(21). It also reduces the sedative effects of narcotics in cancer patients who have chronic pain.

Steroids have specific and nonspecific effects on acute and chronic cancer pain. They may directly lyse some tumors (such as lymphoma) and relieve painful nerve or spinal cord compression by reducing edema in tumor and nerve tissue. Their use is standard emergency treatment for suspected malignant spinal cord compression (dexamethasone, 16 to 96 mg per day or its equivalent). One to two weeks of dexamethasone, 24 mg per day or its equivalent, may relieve pain caused by malignant lesions of the brachial or lumbosacral plexus in patients who do not respond to large doses of opioids. In the moribund patient, steroids may provide euphoria, stimulate appetite, and relieve tumor-related pain. Chronic side effects are not an issue in this situation.

Steroids are also useful for managing acute exacerbations of vascular headache syndromes (migraine and temporal arteritis). Chronic use causes weight gain, Cushing's syndrome, proximal myopathy, psychosis (rarely), and possibly GI bleeding (especially when used with NSAIDs). Rapid withdrawal of steroids may exacerbate pain.

Phenothiazines include methotrimeprazine (Levoprome), chlorpromazine (Thorazine), fluphenazine (Prolixin), prochlorperazine (Compazine). Only methotrimeprazine (20 mg/ml, available in parenteral form only) is an analgesic; it doesn't cause constipation or respiratory depression, but sedation and orthostatic hypotension can result. These drugs are useful as antiemetics when used with narcotics. Use only if the patient is nauseated; only methotrimeprazine produces analgesia. All may exacerbate the sedative effects of narcotics.

Anticonvulsants include phenytoin (Dilantin), carbamazepine (Tegretol), valproic acid (Depakene), clonazepam (Klonopin). These drugs are especially useful for managing the brief lancinating pain of chronic neuralgias (such as trigeminal neuralgia, postherpetic neuralgia, glossopharyngeal neuralgia, posttraumatic neuralgias)(22). Carbamazepine, 400 to 800 mg per day or more, is the drug of choice for the pain of trigeminal neuralgia.

AGENTS TO AVOID

Benzodiazepines work well in acute anxiety attacks and muscle spasm, but do not have analgesic or coanalgesic properties. Their routine use is not recommended for chronic pain. Although acute pain is often associated with signs of anxiety, treatment is best focused on the cause of pain and controlling it with nonnarcotic and narcotic analgesics.

Sedative-hypnotic drugs (barbiturates) do not have intrinsic analgesic properties and are avoided in pain management. Many commonly used analgesics are combined with barbiturates (in

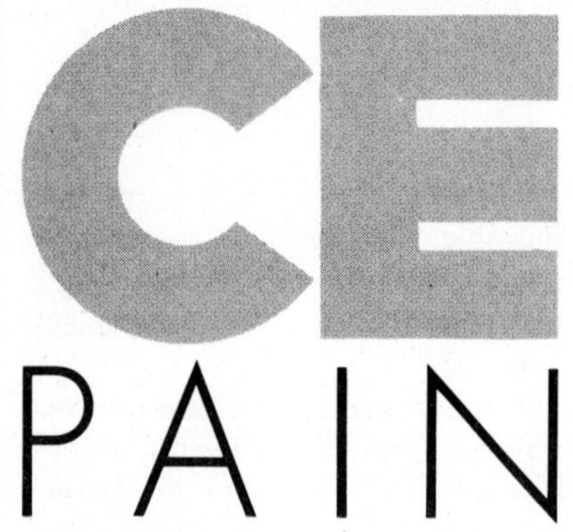

PAIN

preparations such as Belladenal, Fiorinal, Axotal) and must be given with caution.

Cannabinoids. Although tetrahydrocannabinol (THC), which is the active principle of marijuana, has been shown to have analgesic properties in controlled clinical studies, its side effects of dysphoria, drowsiness, hypotension, and bradycardia preclude routine use.

Cocaine has local anesthetic properties, but controlled trials have failed to demonstrate any analgesic or coanalgesic effects in combination with narcotics.

RELATED ISSUES

A positive analgesic effect from IM normal saline does not provide any useful information about the cause or severity of the patient's pain. In fact, many patients who have a documented organic basis for their pain do feel temporary relief from **placebo**. The deceptive use of placebos and the misinterpretation of the placebo response as evidence of "psychogenic" pain is inappropriate in any situation.

Pain and psychiatric disorders. Pain is the chief complaint of many patients who have psychiatric disorders. Without physical findings and a clear cause of pain, these patients need psychotherapy and pharmacotherapy for their psychiatric disorder(23). Meanwhile, continue to look for signs of organic lesions. If the patient with psychopathology has organic disease, treat him with analgesic regimens similar to those of other patients with the disease, even though his behavior and description of pain may be atypical.

Pain in children. Preverbal children feel pain. Give them narcotic analgesics when they undergo surgical procedures. Preadolescent and adolescent children given narcotics for pain are at no higher risk for addiction than the general population. Like adults, they develop tolerance during chronic narcotic treatment and may need larger doses to control their pain. This is especially true for children who have advanced cancer.

Young children may refuse PO medicine and intermittent injections. Thus, the IV route is often best. Narcotic infusions are indicated when pain control is unsatisfactory with intermittent dosing; continuous IV or SC infusion (using a portable syringe pump) has relieved pain in most of these patients.

In choosing the starting dose of narcotic analgesics for children who have postop or cancer pain, consider the age, weight, and prior narcotic experience of the child. Give children 12 years of age and older full adult doses. Children 7 to 12 years old usually need one-half the adult starting dose; children 2 to 6 years old need 20 to 25 percent of the adult starting dose. For infants under 2 years of age, the starting dose of morphine is generally 0.1 mg/kg. Remember, these are *starting* doses and, as for the adult patient, doses must be titrated up or down to obtain analgesia with minimal side effects.

Heroin for cancer pain. Heroin does not offer any unique or special advantages over morphine or other available narcotics for managing cancer pain. The effects of heroin

ABOUT THIS GUIDE

The American Pain Society (APS) prepared this analgesic guide to respond to the gap between basic knowledge of pharmacology and its application in clinical practice.

The committee preparing the syllabus consisted of: Richard Payne, MD, chair (Dept. of Neurology, Memorial Sloan-Kettering Cancer Center); Mitchell Max, MD (Neurobiology and Anesthesiology Branch, National Institute of Dental Research); Charles Inturrisi, PhD (Dept. of Pharmacology, Cornell University Medical College); Ada Rogers, RN (Pain Research Group, Dept. of Neurology, Memorial Sloan-Kettering Cancer Center); Angela Miser, MD (Pediatric Branch, National Cancer Institute); Samuel Perry, MD (Dept. of Psychiatry, Cornell University Medical College); and Ronald Kanner, MD (Dept. of Neurology, Albert Einstein School of Medicine). The committee's work was reviewed by outside consultants and has been approved by the Board of Directors of the American Pain Society.

The APS, a national chapter of the International Association for the Study of Pain, was incorporated on August 8, 1978, in Washington, DC, as a not-for-profit educational and scientific organization. APS membership represents many specialties in the fields of medicine, dentistry, psychology, nursing, other health professions, and the basic sciences. Members include both investigators and clinicians in the field of pain and its treatment. One of the major goals of the Society is to promote education and training in the field of pain. The development of this document is consistent with this goal. *AJN* reprints the analgesic guide, with minor modifications, with APS permission. For further information about APS, write American Pain Society, 1615 L St. NW, Suite 925, Washington, DC 20036, or call 202-296-9200.

The original publication of the analgesic guide was supported by a grant from the International Pain Foundation (IPF), incorporated in Washington, DC, on August 15, 1986, as a nonprofit, charitable, and educational organization. Close formal ties are maintained between the IPF and its parent organization, the International Association for the Study of Pain. The primary goal of the IPF is to support public and professional education about pain disorders and their treatment. For further information, please write or call International Pain Foundation, 909 NE 43d St., Rm. 306, Seattle, Washington 98105-6020, tel. 206-547-2157.

Copies of the original guide can be obtained at cost from the American Pain Society at the address above.

are due to its in-vivo biotransformation to morphine and 6-acetylmorphine(24-26).

Using analgesics for the elderly. Geriatric patients can take analgesics safely, but doses usually need adjustment(27). For example, in older patients, plasma levels of tricyclic compounds are usually higher for a given dose than they are in younger patients(27). IM morphine produces a longer duration of analgesia in older patients, in part related to prolonged elimination from the blood(28). Further, any patient with a CNS disorder may be more sensitive to opioids, making the titration of analgesic doses even more crucial.

A STEPWISE APPROACH

To treat patients who have acute pain or chronic cancer-related pain:

☐ Step One. Start with a nonnarcotic analgesic (for example, aspirin 650 mg or its equivalent q4h to q6h). Although nonnarcotic analgesics compare favorably with narcotics for wound pain, they are usually not used for postop pain management because they are not available in the United States in parenteral form. Aspirin, acetaminophen, and indomethacin (Indocin) are available in suppository form, however, and could be used to enhance the effects of narcotic analgesics.

☐ Step Two. If the patient needs more analgesia, add a weak narcotic agonist such as oxycodone or codeine. These drugs have no ceiling effect, but side effects such as nausea and mental clouding may preclude dose escalation.

☐ Step Three. If the patient still needs more analgesia, use a stronger narcotic—methadone, levorphanol, morphine, or hydromorphone. Morphine and hydromorphone are rapidly eliminated (half-life, two to three hours). Levorphanol and methadone are eliminated slowly and accumulate with repetitive dosing, reaching steady state after five to six half-lives (two to three days for levorphanol; five to six days for methadone).

☐ Be aware that in switching a patient from a short-half-life drug to a long-half-life drug you may need to reduce the dose after 24 hours since the long-half-life drug accumulates progressively over the first three to five days of therapy. Conversely, when you switch from a long- to a short-half-life drug, you may need to raise the dose as early as 12 hours after the change, as the former drug leaves the body.

☐ Respect differences among patients and expect to titrate the dose of analgesics to maximum effect. Ask the patient often if pain relief is adequate; many patients silently tolerate suboptimal doses of analgesics(29,30).

REFERENCES

1. Merskey, H., and others. Pain terms: a list with definitions and notes on usage. *Pain* 6:249-252, 1979.
2. Portenoy, R. K., and Foley, K. M. Chronic use of opioid analgesics in nonmalignant pain: report on 38 cases. *Pain* 25:171-186, May 1986.
3. Kantor, T. G. The control of pain by nonsteroidal anti-inflammatory drugs. *Med.Clin.North Am.* 66:1053-1059, Sept. 1982.
4. Foley, K. M. The treatment of cancer pain. *N.Engl.J.Med.* 313:84-95, July 11, 1985.
5. Flower, R. J., and others. Analgesic antipyretics and anti-inflammatory agents: drugs employed in the treatment of gout. In *Goodman*

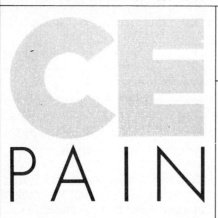

PAIN

Therapeutics, 7th ed., edited by A. G. Gilman and others. New York, Macmillan, 1985, pp. 674-715.

6. Moertel, C. G., and others. A comparative evaluation of marketed analgesic drugs. *N.Engl.J.Med.* 286:813-815, Apr. 13, 1972.
7. Ehrlich, G. E., ed. *The Resurgence of Salicylates in Arthritis Therapy.* Norwalk, CT, Scientific Media Communications, 1983, pp. 75-90.
8. Foley, K. M. The practical use of narcotic analgesics. *Med.Clin.North Am.* 66:1091-1104, Sept. 1982.
9. Houde, R. W. The use and misuse of narcotics in the treatment of chronic pain. *Adv.Neurol.* 4:527-536, 1984.
10. Payne, R., and Foley, K. M. Advances in the management of cancer pain. *Cancer Treat.Rep.* 68:173-183, Jan. 1984.
11. Twycross, R. G., and Lack, S. A. *Therapeutics in Terminal Cancer.* London, Pitman Publishers, Ltd., 1984.
12. Portenoy, R. K., and others. IV infusion of opioids for cancer pain: clinical review and guidelines for use. *Cancer Treat.Rep.* 70:575-581, May 1986.
13. Kaiko, R. F., and others. Central nervous system excitatory effects of meperidine in cancer patients. *Ann.Neurol.* 13:180-185, Feb. 1983.
14. Kanner, R. M., and Foley, K. M. Patterns of narcotic drug use in a cancer pain clinic. *Ann.N.Y.Acad.Sci.* 362:161-172, 1981.
15. Newman, R. G. The need to redefine "addiction." *N.Engl.J.Med.* 308:1096-1098, May 5, 1983.
16. Foley, K. M. Adjuvant analgesic drugs in cancer pain management. In *Evaluation and Treatment of Chronic Pain,* edited by G. M. Aronoff. Baltimore, MD, Urban and Schwartzenberg, 1985, pp. 425-434.
17. Max, M. B., and others. Amitriptyline relieves diabetic neuropathy pain in patients with normal or depressed mood. *Neurology* 37:589-596, Apr. 1987.
18. Watson, C. P., and others. Amitriptyline versus placebo in post-therapeutic neuralgia. *Neurology* 32:671-673, June 1982.
19. Couch, J. R., and others. Amitriptyline in the prophylaxis of migraine. Effectiveness and relationship of antimigraine and antidepressant effects. *Neurology* 26:121-127, Feb. 1976.
20. Laska, E. M., and others. Caffeine as an analgesic adjuvant. *JAMA* 251:1711-1718, Apr. 6, 1984.
21. Forrest, W. H., Jr., and others. Dextroamphetamine with morphine for treatment of postoperative pain. *N.Engl.J.Med.* 296:-712-715, Mar. 31, 1977.
22. Swerdlow, M. Anticonvulsant drugs and chronic pain. *Clin.Neuropharmacol.* 7(1):51-82, 1984.
23. Fordyce, W. E. *Behavioral Methods for Chronic Pain and Illness.* St. Louis, C. V. Mosby Co., 1976.
24. Inturrisi, C. E., and others. The pharmacokinetics of heroin in patients with chronic pain. *N.Engl.J.Med.* 310:1213-1217, May 10, 1984.
25. Inturrisi, C. E., and Foley, K. M. Narcotic analgesics in the management of pain. In *Analgesics: Neurochemical, Behavioral and Clinical Perspectives,* edited by M. J. Kuhar, and G. W. Pasternak. New York, Raven Press, 1984, pp. 257-288.
26. Kaiko, R. F., and others. Analgesic and mood effects of heroin and morphine in cancer patients with postoperative pain. *N.Engl.J.Med.* 304:1501-1505, June 18, 1981.
27. Nies, A., and others. Relationship between age and tricyclic antidepressant plasma levels. *Am.J.Psychiatry* 134:790-793, July 1977.
28. Kaiko, R. F., and others. Narcotics in the elderly. *Med.Clin.North Am.* 66:1079-1089, Sept. 1982.
29. Marks, R. M., and Sachar, E. J. Undertreatment of medical inpatients with narcotic analgesics. *Ann.Intern.Med.* 78:173-181, Feb. 1973.
30. Angell, M. The quality of mercy. (editorial) *N.Engl.J.Med.* 306:98-99, Jan. 14, 1982.

PROGRAMMED INSTRUCTION

How to Work With Chest Tubes

This programmed unit was prepared by Stephen Cohen, Stepdesign, Inc., New York, N.Y. Clinical consultant for this program was Madonna Stack, R.N., M.A., associate director of nursing, Brookdale Hospital Medical Center, Brooklyn, N.Y.

INTRODUCTION

In this course you will learn how to identify and repair malfunctions that can develop in a chest tube system. You will also learn about the effects of such malfunctions on the patient.

STUDY INSTRUCTIONS

The discussion takes two forms: essays and programmed instruction sequences. The programmed sequences consist of a series of teaching steps called frames. Each frame presents some information and calls for a written response on your part. In the format for this course, the correct responses will be found in a column on the right-hand side of each page opposite the frame.

Essays can be recognized by the absence of a correct response column. Such essays call for no active responses, though they should be read carefully.

From time to time, the information in a frame is supplemented by information in a panel. Each panel appears before the first frame to refer to it. When you come to a panel, read through the following frame first. Then refer to the panel as the frame instructs you.

SECTION 1—THE DESIGN OF CHEST TUBE SYSTEMS

Customarily, a chest tube system is used to evacuate air, or a combination of air and serosanguineous fluid, from a patient's intrapleural space. It is also sometimes used to evacuate serosanguineous fluid from his mediastinal space, but this situation will not be discussed in our course.

During inspiration, air enters the lungs because of the lower alveolar pressure. Air exits from the lungs when the alveolar pressure becomes positive.

The lungs are separated from the chest wall by two layers of pleura, visceral and parietal. The space between the pleurae is normally filled with a thin layer of serous fluid and contains no air. At the same time, the lungs, being elastic, tend to pull the visceral and parietal pleurae apart. This creates a suction force between the pleurae, which may be expressed as negative pressure.

The negative pressure between the pleurae maintains the lungs in full expansion. If there were no negative pressure in the intrapleural space, the lungs, being elastic, would recoil and collapse. The degree of negative pressure in the intrapleural space varies during the respiratory cycle. During inspiration, as the chest cavity expands, the negative pressure becomes greater; during expiration, less. Intrapleural pressure is thus continuously negative throughout the respiratory cycle (though varying in degree), while alveolar pressure goes from negative during inspiration to positive during expiration. The illustration at the top of the next page shows the wrong positions during respiration.

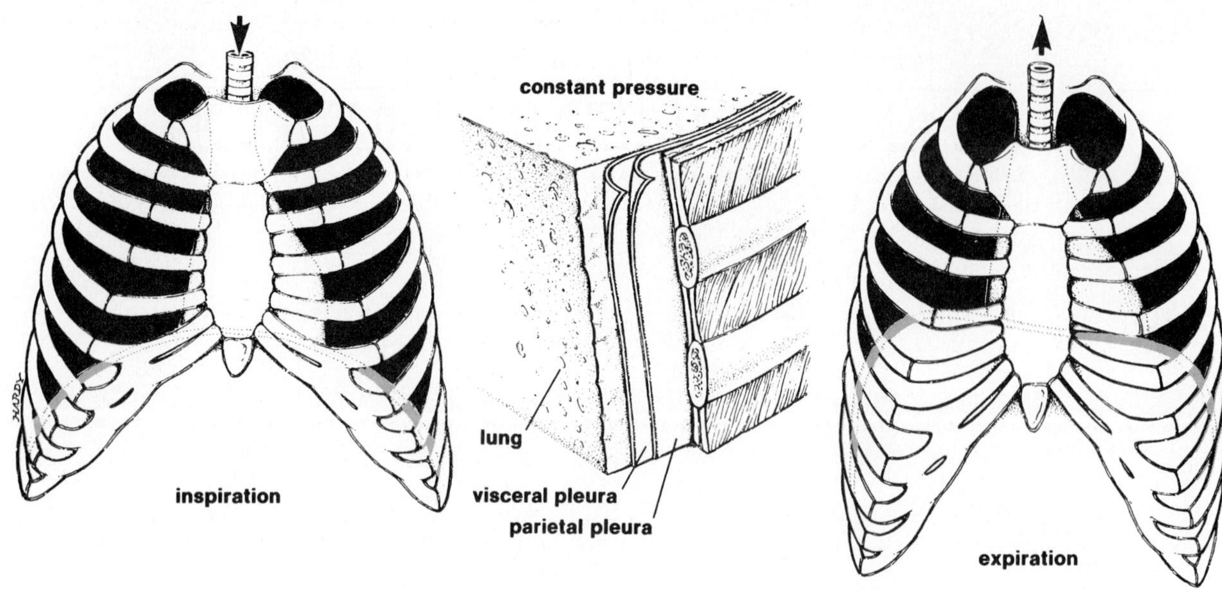

There are basically two abnormal conditions that concern us:

1. Some pathology causes an internal rupture in the surface of a lung or in the tracheobronchial tree, which permits the entry of air and varying amounts of serosanguineous fluid into the intrapleural space. The chest wall remains closed.

2. Accidental or surgical trauma causes an external rupture in the chest wall, again permitting the entry of air and varying amounts of serosanguineous fluid (from ruptured tissues) into the intrapleural space. Since the trauma is also likely to rupture the lung surface, it permits the entry of air, not only through the chest wall but internally through the surface of the lung. The internal rupture may persist for some time after the chest wall is closed. This situation thus comes to resemble the first one described above.

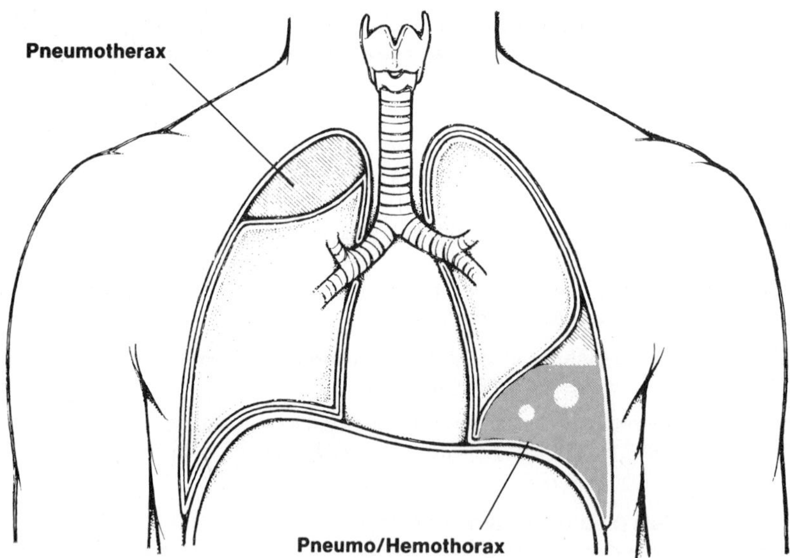

In either of these situations, the entry of air (with or without fluid) into the intrapleural space separates the visceral and parietal pleurae, and the intrapleural space becomes a compartment in the chest like the lungs themselves. The pressure in the intrapleural space then varies during the respiratory cycle in the same way pressure varies in the lungs; namely, during inspiration, when the chest wall expands, intrapleural pressure becomes negative, and during expiration, when the chest wall contracts, intrapleural pressure becomes positive. Where, under normal conditions, the intrapleural pressure was continuously negative throughout the respiratory cycle, it now goes from negative during inspiration to positive during expiration.

At the same time, since intrapleural pressure is no longer continuously negative, the lung on the affected side recoils and collapses. If such collapse results from the entry of air into the intrapleural space with little or no serosanguineous fluid, the condition is called pneumothorax. If it results from entry of a large amount of serosanguineous fluid with a smaller or equally large amount of air, the condition is called hemopneumothorax.

Following a pneumothorax or hemopneumothorax, there may be a further development. Assuming that a rupture persists in the affected lung or in the tracheobronchial tree, the intrapleural space continues sucking air in through the internal opening during inspiration (when intrapleural pressure is negative). It would also expel air back through this opening during expiration (when intrapleural pressure is positive) except that such an opening permits air more easily to enter than exit.

If at the same time the chest wall is closed (either initially or through repair), air that enters the intrapleural space has nowhere to exit and accumulates in the space. Ultimately, almost the entire pleural cavity on the affected side is filled with air (and fluid, if any), resulting in massive lung collapse and shift of the mediastinum. This is the condition known as tension pneumothorax.

Basic Functions of a Chest Tube System

With the setup of a chest tube system, one or more tubes are inserted through the chest wall to remove air from the intrapleural space, as well as to permit the drainage of any fluid. Such an insertion serves both to prevent a tension pneumothorax and to permit the affected lung to reexpand. As air and fluid are evacuated from the intrapleural space, the visceral and parietal pleurae are brought back into apposition, and the pressure in the intrapleural space once more becomes continuously negative throughout the respiratory cycle. Normal conditions are thus reconstituted.

At the same time, the insertion of a chest tube is itself a pathologic (that is, iatrogenic) event of some consequence. Though it has a therapeutic purpose, it creates a new external rupture in the chest wall. Thus, while air is expelled through the tube during expiration, it might also reenter through the tube during inspiration.

To prevent the reentry of air into the chest, the distal end of the chest tube (or of some tube in turn connected to it) is submersed under water. This water permits the patient's air to exit but not reenter, and it is thus called an underwater seal, or more simply, a water seal. The chest tube and the water seal together constitute the most basic components of any chest tube system.

Substances Being Evacuated

As noted previously, a pneumothorax involves an amount of air with little or no fluid, while a hemopneumothorax involves a large amount of fluid with a smaller or equally large amount of air. A chest tube system may thus be used to evacuate

— an amount of air initially large, with no fluid;

— mostly fluid, with an amount of air initially small;

— fluid and air in equally large amounts.

We will focus on the first two conditions in which either air alone or mostly fluid is being evacuated.

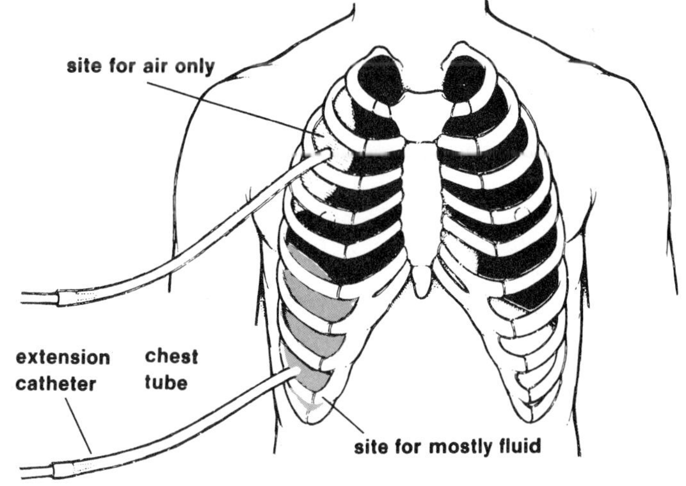

Evacuation Forces: Gravity Systems vs. Systems on Suction

As noted earlier, positive pressure develops in the intrapleural space during expiration when the space contains some air. Though such positive expiratory pressure is an abnormal condition, it actually serves a therapeutic purpose: it helps to expel the air, and to a lesser extent any fluid, that the space contains. Until such time as all the air is expelled and intrapleural expiratory pressure returns to normal (that is, becomes negative), the positive expiratory pressure serves as one of the evacuation forces upon which all chest tube systems depend.

A second evacuation force upon which all chest tube systems depend is gravity, which is exploited by arranging the chest tube so that it descends continuously from its insertion site. Unlike positive expiratory pressure, gravity serves primarily to evacuate fluid and, to a lesser extent, air.

A third evacuation force is suction, used in some systems, which evacuates fluid and air equally.

Based on the above, one may distinguish between the following chest tube systems:

— those that employ only positive expiratory pressure and gravity;

— those that employ positive expiratory pressure, gravity, and suction.

For convenience, we will refer to the first group of systems (employing two forces) as gravity systems, and to the second group (employing three forces) as systems on suction.

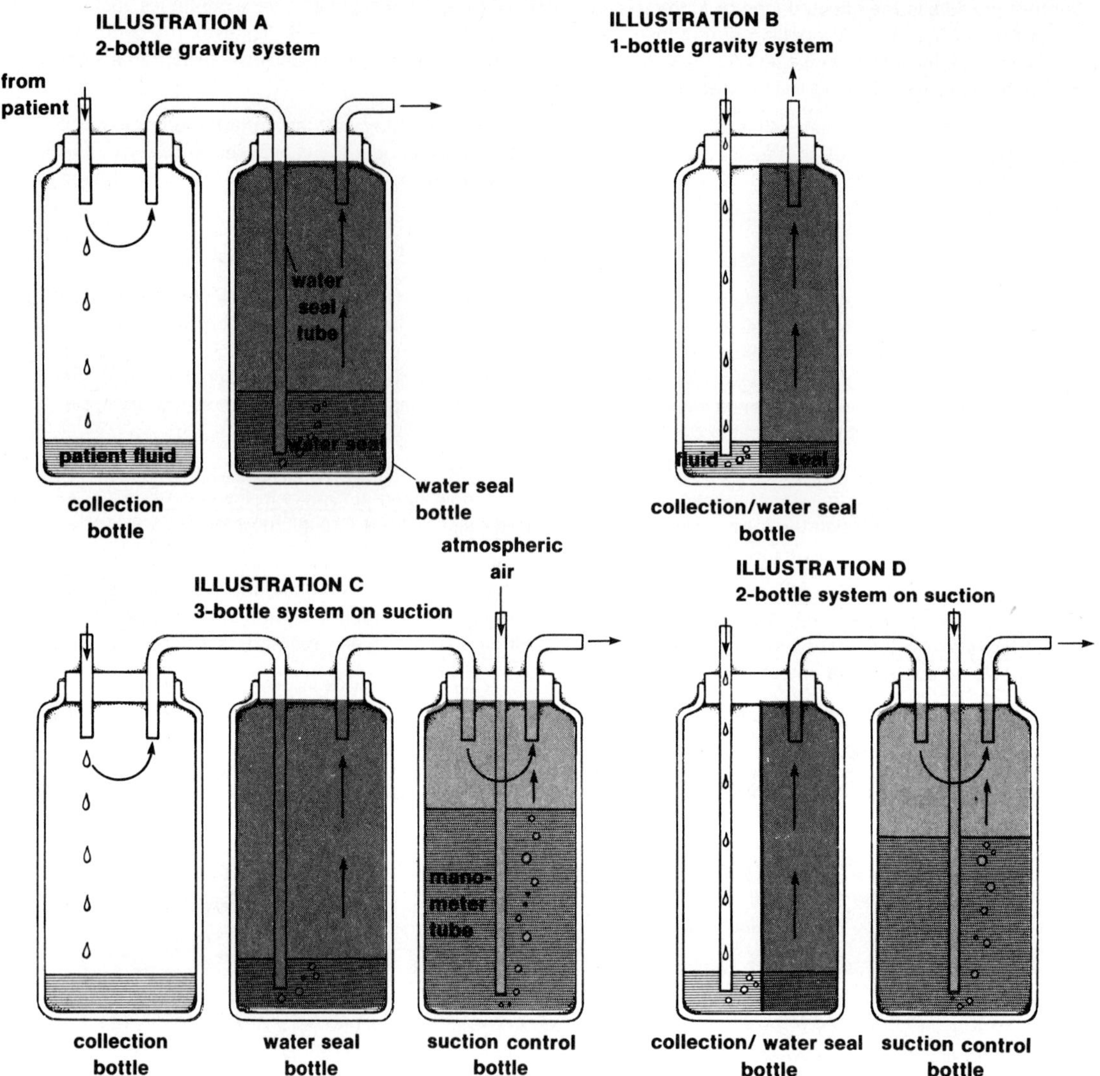

External Compartments

Moved by two or three forces, air (and fluid, if any) is conveyed from the patient's intrapleural space through the chest tube to one or more external compartments, either in bottles or chambers in a multichamber plastic unit, which is disposable.

Bottle systems

Illustration A shows a 2-bottle gravity system. In this system, the patient's air, or combination of air and fluid, is received initially by the collection bottle (sometimes called the drainage bottle), which traps the fluid and passes the air onward. The air (and fluid, if any) enters through the collection inlet, and the air exits through the collection outlet.

The patient's air then passes to the water seal bottle. The air is conveyed through the water seal in the bottom of this bottle by the water seal tube. The air enters the water seal bottle through the water seal inlet and exits through the water seal outlet.

The forces that move the patient's fluid (if any) into the collection bottle, and his air through both the collection and water seal bottles, consist of gravity and positive expiratory pressure.

Illustration B shows a 1-bottle gravity system. It is identical to a 2-bottle gravity system, except that the collection and water seal bottles are combined in a single bottle. As in a 2-bottle gravity system, air is also conveyed through the water seal by the water seal tube. But this tube now serves also to convey any fluid, which augments the water comprising the water seal.

Illustration C shows a 3-bottle system on suction. The first two bottles are identical to the two bottles making up a 2-bottle gravity system. Instead of passing from the water seal bottle into the atmosphere, however, air from the patient now passes into a third bottle, the suction control bottle.

Like the water seal bottle, the suction control bottle contains some water. It also has an opening for the entry

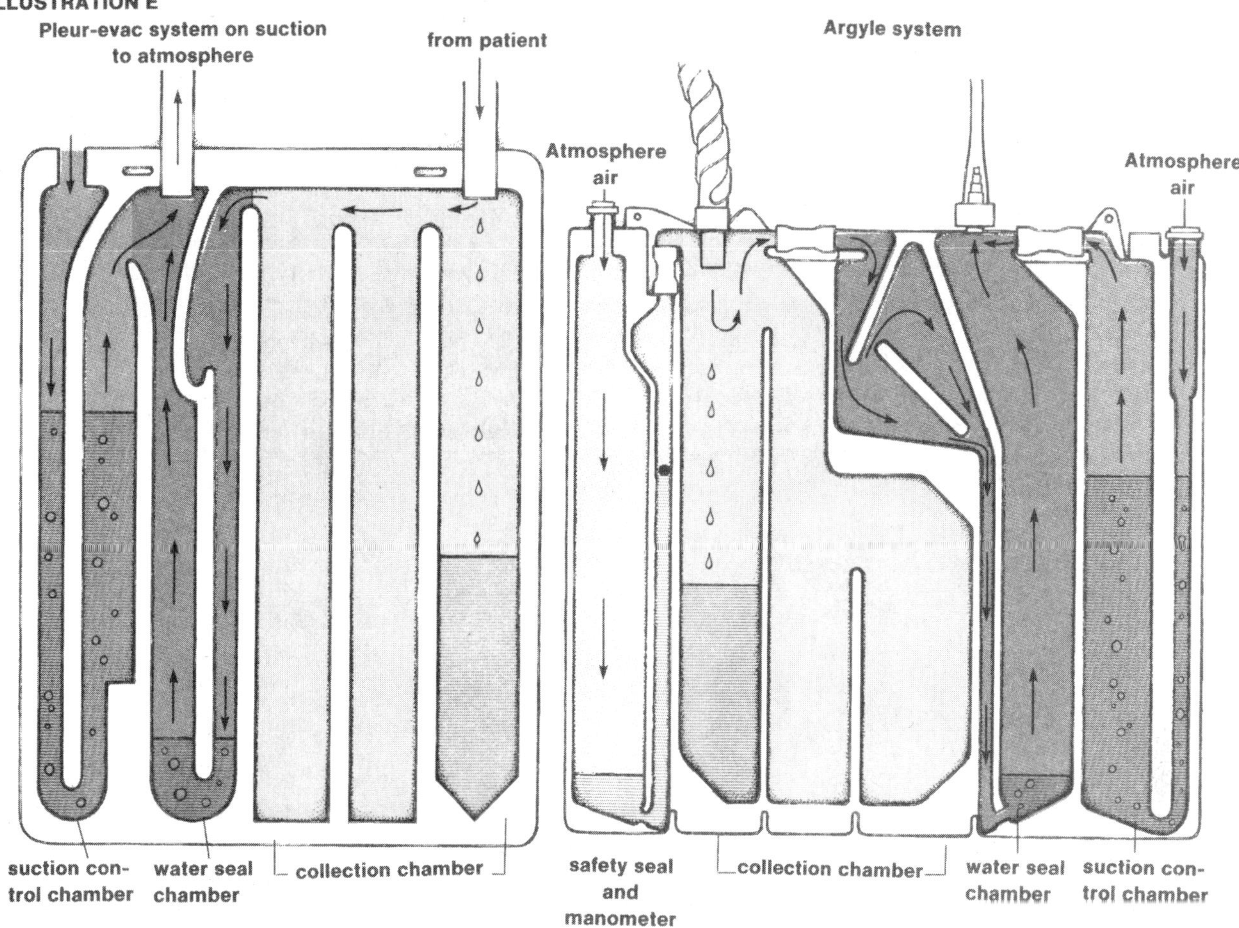

of air from the atmosphere. Air from the patient passes over the suction control water, while air from the atmosphere passes through it. Atmospheric air is conveyed through the suction control water by means of a tube, which is called a manometer tube. It is the depth to which this tube is submerged that determines the amount of suction pressure applied to the patient's intrapleural contents.

The suction control bottle has two inlets, one for the patient's air and the other for atmospheric air. It has a single suction control outlet for both. Because this system makes use of suction, three forces—gravity, positive expiratory pressure, and suction—move the patient's fluid (if any) into the collection bottle and his air through all three bottles into the suction source.

Illustration D shows a 2-bottle system on suction. It is identical to a 3-bottle system on suction, except that the collection and water seal bottles are combined in a single bottle.

Disposable unit systems

Illustration E shows a Pleur-evac system on suction. A Pleur-evac unit consists of three chambers arranged from right to left. The first chamber (right) is the collection chamber, which is equivalent to a collection bottle. The collection chamber is divided into three subchambers.

The patient's fluid (if any) is trapped in the collection chamber, while his air passes on to the water seal chamber. This chamber is U-shaped and is equivalent to the water seal tube in a bottle system. The patient's air enters the inlet side of the U, passes through the water seal, and then exits the outlet side of the U. The air then passes into the suction source.

The third chamber is the suction control chamber, which is also U-shaped and it is equivalent to the manometer tube in a bottle system. The height of the water in the chamber determines the amount of pressure applied to the patient. Atmospheric air enters the inlet side of the U (far left), passes through the suction control water, and exits the outlet side where it joins air from the patient, both passing into the suction source.

Illustration F shows an Argyle "Double Seal" system on suction, which consists of four chambers, whose sequence is also different. Reading from left to right, note the second chamber, the collection chamber, which is also divided into three subchambers. The next chamber to the right is the water seal chamber, whose shape is essentially that of a "U," except that the pathway through the chamber is more tortuous than in a Pleur-evac unit. The last chamber is the suction control chamber, which again is U-shaped.

The extra chamber in an Argyle unit is on the left. This chamber is also a water seal chamber, as is the third chamber. Customarily, the patient's air passes through the third chamber into the suction source. If, however, the passage into the suction source is accidentally obstructed, the patient's air can pass instead through the first chamber into the atmosphere. The first chamber thus provides a "safety" vent for the patient's air.

Suction Source

The suction source may be a wall or portable pump.

The air (atmospheric and patient's) exiting the suction control outlet is conveyed to the suction source by a suction tube. If the suction source is a portable pump, the suction tube is connected directly to the suction source inlet. If it is a wall pump, the suction tube is connected to a suction gauge, which in turn is connected to the suction source inlet.

Direction of Air Flow: The Terms "Proximal" and "Distal"

As you have seen, the patient's air enters through one end of a chest tube system (the open end of the catheter inside his chest) and eventually exits through the other (into either the atmosphere or a suction source).

Based on this direction of air flow, one may speak of proximal and distal ends of the chest tube system, the proximal end being the point at which the patient's air enters and the distal end being the point at which it exits.

One may similarly describe the relative positions of various sites in the system. For example, the catheter may be described as "proximal" to the extension, the extension as "distal" to the catheter or "proximal" to the collection inlet, the collection compartment as "distal" to the extension or "proximal" to the water seal compartment, and so forth.

SECTION 2—PROBLEMS THAT CAN DEVELOP IN A CHEST TUBE SYSTEM

PANEL 1

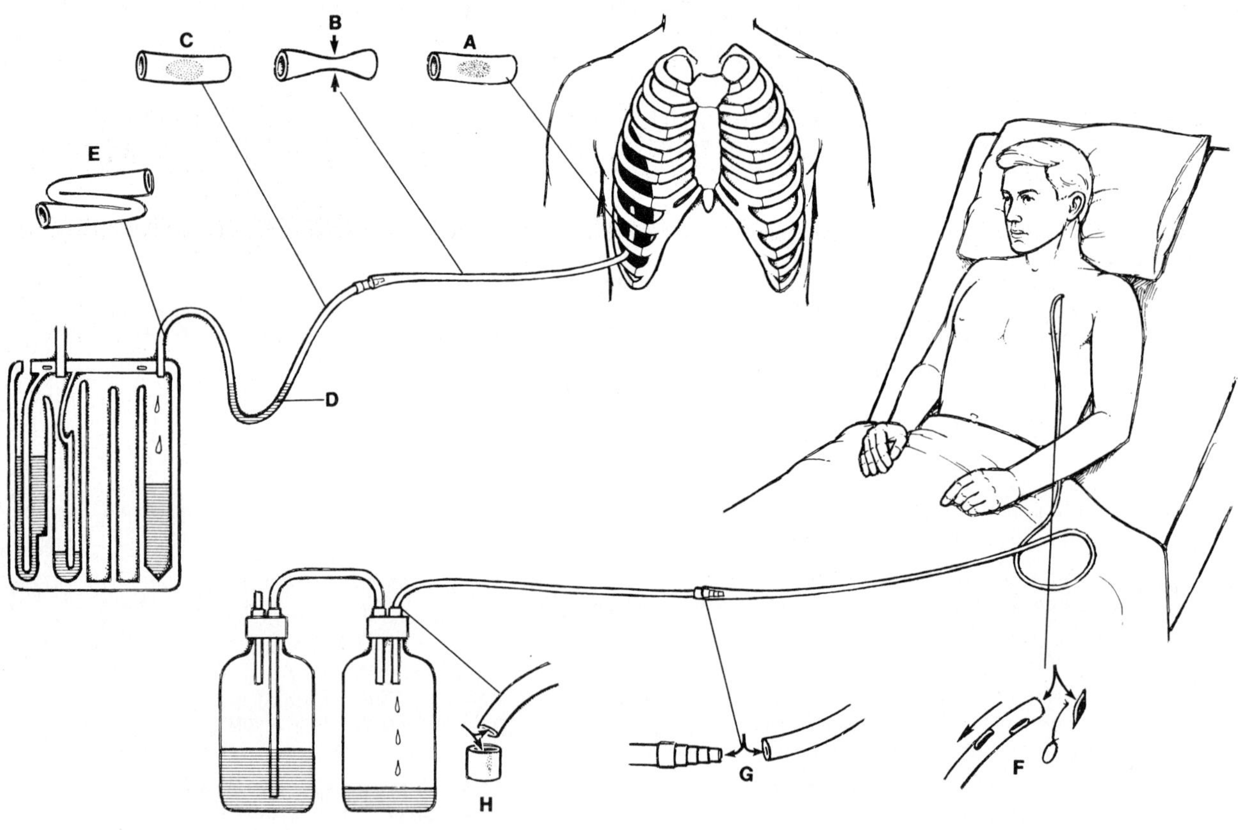

1.

Panel 1 illustrates some conditions that can develop after the setup of a chest tube system. The illustration of each condition is signified by a letter, and the various conditions are described below verbally. Write the letter that indicates the illustration of each condition:

clot in external portion of chest tube	________	C
clot in internal portion of chest tube	________	A
dependent loop in chest tube	________	D
disconnection of catheter from extension	________	G
disconnection of extension from collection inlet	________	H
dislodgement of catheter from inside patient's chest	________	F
kink in chest tube	________	E
pressure on chest tube	________	B

2.

Some of the conditions listed in the preceding frame can be grouped together under general headings. For example, each of the following conditions,

- disconnection of catheter from extension
- disconnection of extension from collection inlet
- dislodgement of catheter from inside patient's chest,

has the effect of opening the patient's intrapleural space completely to the atmosphere. These conditions may thus be classified generally as chest tube disconnections.

Similarly, each of the following conditions,

- clot in external portion of chest tube
- clot in internal portion of chest tube
- kink in chest tube
- pressure on chest tube.

has the effect of occluding the lumen of the tube. These conditions may thus be classified generally as chest tube obstructions.

By itself, a dependent loop is not an obstruction. Its effect is to convert gravity from a force that helps, into one that opposes, the evacuation of substances from the patient's intrapleural space. An obstruction may or may not ensue.

Referring again to Panel 1, write the letter of each illustration that shows a

chest tube disconnection _________ chest tube obstruction_________

FOOTNOTE

Any chest tube can develop a kink or be subjected to pressure. But only a chest tube that is draining fluid can develop clot. The specific obstructions that can develop in a chest tube thus vary with its contents.

PANEL 2

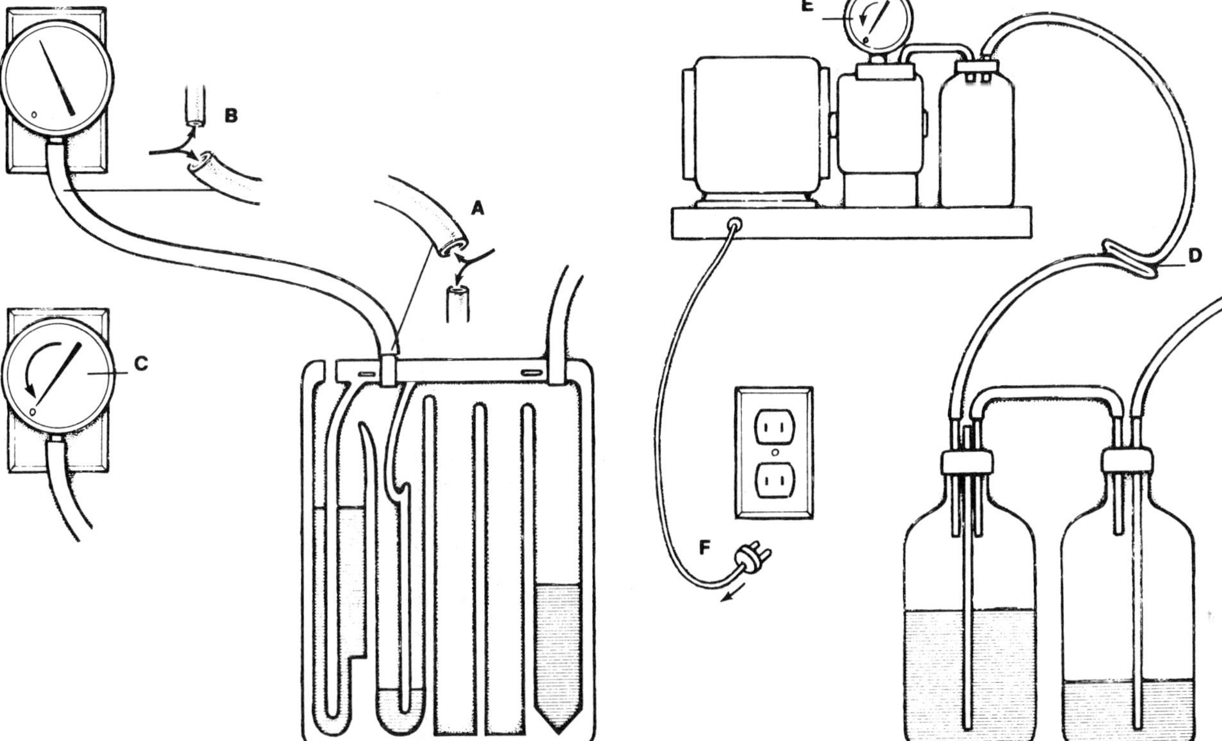

3.

Panel 2 shows some additional conditions that can develop after the setup of a chest tube system. Once again, the illustration of each condition is indicated by a letter. Write the letter of the illustration that shows each of the following:

defect in portable suction pump _________
defect in wall suction pump _________
disconnection from electrical outlet of cord from portable suction pump _________
disconnection of suction tube from suction control outlet _________
disconnection of suction tube from suction source inlet _________
kink in suction tube _________

E
C
F
A
B
D

4.

338 Each of the following conditions,

- defect in portable suction pump
- defect in wall suction pump
- disconnection from electrical outlet of cord from portable suction pump,

has the effect of terminating suction pressure at its source. These conditions may thus be classified generally as suction source breakdowns.

A kink in the suction tube does not terminate suction pressure at its source, though it does block the transmission of suction pressure to the suction control compartment.

Suction pressure also continues when there is a

- disconnection of suction tube from suction control outlet
- disconnection of suction tube from suction source inlet.

The effect of these conditions is to open the suction source completely to the atmosphere. These conditions may thus be classified generally as suction tube disconnections.

Referring again to Panel 2, write the letter of each illustration that shows a

breakdown in the suction source ________ C, E, F
disconnection in the section tube ________ A, B

PANEL 3

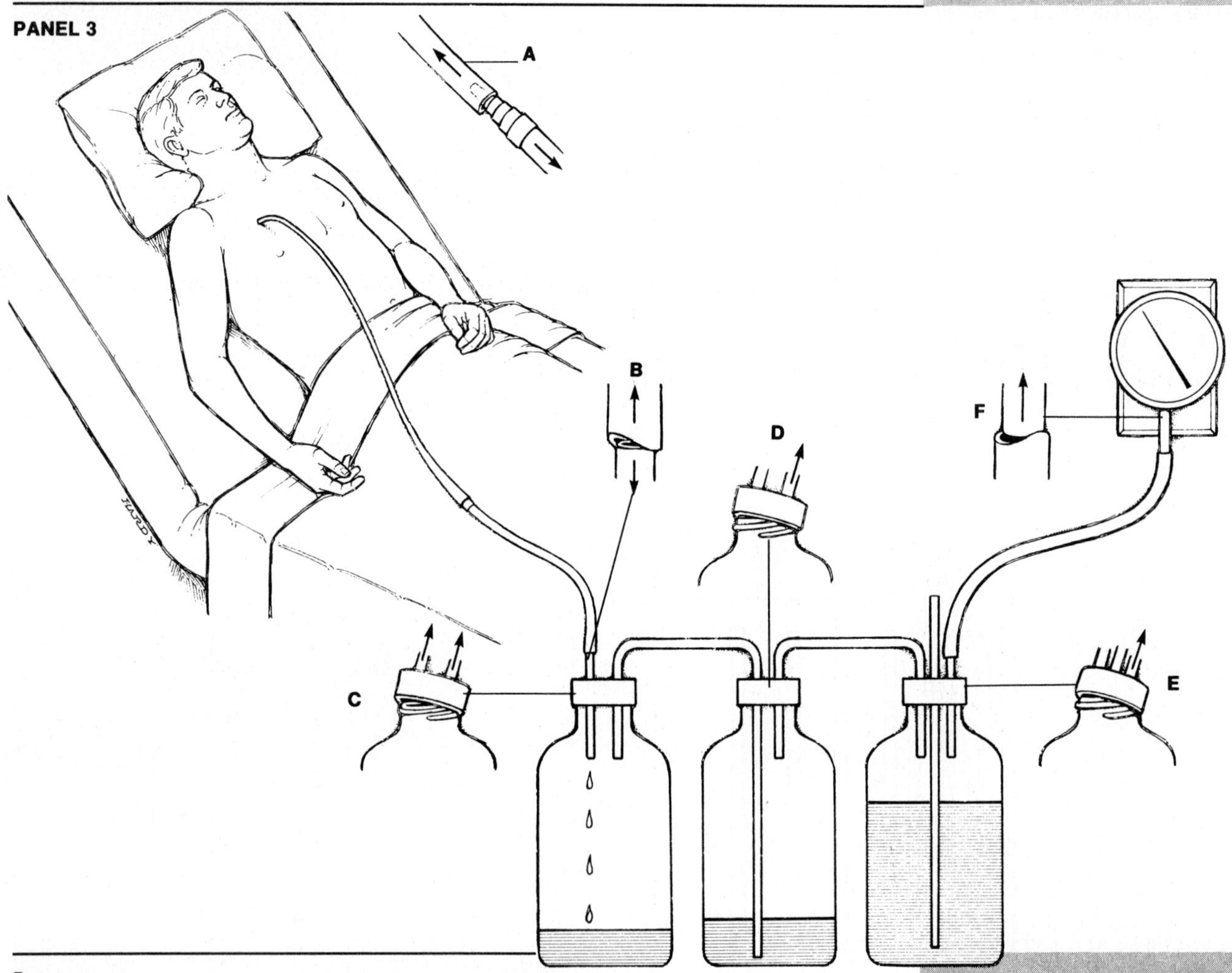

5.

Panel 3 shows some more conditions that can develop after the setup of a chest tube system. Write the letter of the illustration that shows a

loose cap on collection bottle ________ **C**
loose cap on suction control bottle ________ **E**
loose cap on water seal bottle ________ **D**
loose junction (but not complete disconnection) between catheter and extension ________ **A**
loose junction (but not complete disconnection) between extension and collection inlet ________ **B**
loose junction between suction gauge and inlet of pump ________ **F**

6.
In contrast to the complete disconnections in a chest tube or suction tube shown earlier, the conditions shown in Panel 3 open a chest tube system only partially to the atmosphere. Consequently, they should be called leaks rather than disconnections.

Look again at illustration A which shows a loose junction between the catheter and the extension. As the arrows show, some of the leaking air can pass up the chest tube toward the patient.

The same applies to air leaking through a loose junction between the extension and collection inlet (illustration B) and under a loose top on the collection bottle (illustration C).

Check each illustration, if any, that shows a leak that permits the reentry of atmospheric air into the patient's intrapleural space:

☐ A ☐ B ☐ C ☐ none of these

A, B, C

7.
Now look again at illustration F which shows a loose junction between the suction control tube and suction source inlet. As the arrow shows, the leaking air passes into the suction source. Even if some of the air were to pass back into the suction control and water seal bottles, it would be barred by the water seal from going any farther.

The same applies to air leaking under a loose cap on either the suction control bottle (illustration E) or on the water seal bottle (illustration D). In the latter instance, air leaks into the water seal bottle but it cannot gain access to the water seal, which is still submersed under water.

Check each illustration, if any, that shows a leak that permits the reentry of atmospheric air into the patient's intrapleural space:

☐ D ☐ E ☐ F ☐ none of these

none of these

8.
If atmospheric air that leaks into a chest tube system is barred by the water seal from reentering the intrapleural space, the leak may be considered distal to the water seal.

If atmospheric air that leaks into a chest tube system is not barred by the water seal from reentering the intrapleural space, the leak may be considered proximal to the water seal.

Referring again to Panel 3, write the letter of each illustration that shows a

leak distal to the water seal ________

leak proximal to the water seal ________

D, E, F

A, B, C

9.
If a leak is distal to the water seal, the leaking atmospheric air is:

☐ barred by the water seal from reentering the intrapleural space

☐ not barred by the water seal for reentering the intrapleural space

barred by the water seal from reentering the intrapleural space

If a leak is proximal to a water seal, the leaking atmospheric air is:

☐ barred by the water seal from reentering the intrapleural space

☐ not barred by the water seal from reentering the intrapleural space

not barred by the water seal from reentering the intrapleural space

FOOTNOTE

Among the leaks that can develop proximal or distal to a water seal, the following,

- loose cap on collection bottle
- loose cap on water seal bottle
- loose cap on suction control bottle,

can obviously develop only in a bottle system. The remaining leaks,

- loose junction between catheter and extension
- loose junction between extension and collection inlet
- loose junction between suction gauge and wall inlet,

can develop in either a bottle or a disposable system.

10.

First, consider the effect on the patient of a disconnection in the chest tube or a leak proximal to the water seal.

As noted earlier, each condition opens the patient's intrapleural space to the atmosphere—completely with a disconnection, partially with a leak. With either condition, atmospheric air is thus sucked into the intrapleural space during inspiration (when intrapleural pressure is negative).

Suppose the chest tube is disconnected. The patient's pneumothorax will be:

☐ rapidly replenished ☐ slowly replenished ☐ depleted

rapidly replenished

Suppose a leak develops proximal to the water seal. The patient's pneumothorax will be:

☐ rapidly replenished ☐ slowly replenished ☐ depleted

slowly replenished

11.

Now consider the effect on the patient of an obstruction or dependent loop in the chest tube.

As noted earlier, an obstruction is, by definition, any condition that occludes the lumen of the tube. By itself, a dependent loop does not occlude the lumen; its effect is to convert gravity from a force that helps into one that opposes the evacuation of substances from the patient's intrapleural space.

The eventual outcome of a dependent loop varies with the weight of the substances being evacuated. Air is light, and if only air is being evacuated, gravity opposes, but does not overcome, the evacuation forces of positive expiratory pressure and suction (if it is being used).

On the other hand, fluid is heavy, and if mostly fluid is being evacuated, gravity does overcome the other evaluating forces. The result is a pooling of fluid in the loop, which will eventually obstruct the further evacuation of both fluid and air.

Suppose an obstruction develops in a chest tube. The evacuation of any fluid will be:

☐ terminated ☐ retarded, but not terminated ☐ unaffected

terminated

and the evacuation of air will be:

☐ terminated ☐ retarded, but not terminated ☐ unaffected

terminated

Suppose a dependent loop develops in a chest tube evacuating mostly fluid. The evacuation of the fluid will be:

☐ terminated ☐ retarded, but not terminated ☐ unaffected

terminated

and the evacuation of air will be:

☐ terminated ☐ retarded, but not terminated ☐ unaffected

terminated

Suppose a dependent loop develops in a chest tube evacuating only air. The evacuation of the air will be:

☐ terminated ☐ retarded, but not terminated ☐ unaffected

retarded, but not terminated

FOOTNOTE

If the evacuation of air is accidentally terminated, a serious complication may ensue in the patient. Assuming there is still an opening in the surface of his affected lung or in his tracheobronchial tree, air will leak through the opening, accumulate in the intrapleural space, and eventually cause a tension pneumothorax.

12.

Next consider the effect on the patient of a breakdown in the suction source or a kink in the suction tube.

As noted earlier, a breakdown terminates suction at its source, while a kink blocks the transmission of suction pressure to the suction control compartment.

The effect is thus to remove suction as a force helping to evacuate substances from the patient's intrapleural space. Other forces continue to act, however. Thus, gravity (and to a lesser degree, positive expiratory pressure) continues the evacuation of fluid, and positive expiratory pressure (and to a lesser degree, gravity) continues the evacuation of air.

At the same time, the distal end of the chest tube system remains closed. Thus, air from the patient that continues to pass through the water seal accumulates over the water in the water seal and suction control compartments.

As the air accumulates, air pressure over the water increases. While this "back pressure" never equals the forces continuing the evacuation of fluids (which is heavy), it will eventually equal the forces continuing the evacuation of air.

The effect of a breakdown in the suction source or a kink in the suction tube thus varies over time.

Suppose the suction source breaks down or a kink develops in the suction tube. Assuming that the breakdown or kink is recent, the evacuation of any fluid will be:

☐ terminated ☐ retarded, but not terminated ☐ unaffected — retarded, but not terminated

and the evacuation of air will be:

☐ terminated ☐ retarded, but not terminated ☐ unaffected — retarded, but not terminated

Now, assuming that the breakdown or kink is long-standing, the evacuation of any fluid will be: ☐ terminated ☐ retarded, but not terminated ☐ unaffected — retarded, but not terminated

and the evacuation of air will be:

☐ terminated ☐ retarded, but not terminated ☐ unaffected — terminated

---

13.
Finally, consider the effect on the patient of a disconnection in the suction tube or a leak distal to the water seal.

As noted earlier, each condition opens the suction source to the atmosphere—completely with a disconnection, partially with a leak. With either condition, the suction can draw air directly from the atmosphere more freely than it can draw atmospheric air through the suction control water or air from the patient.

Once again, the effect is to remove suction as an evacuation force, while other forces continue to act. The situation thus resembles one involving a breakdown in the suction source or kink in the suction tube.

But the situation differs in that a disconnection or leak opens the distal end of the chest tube system. Thus, air from the patient that continues to pass through the water seal can exit the system. No air accumulates over the water in the water seal and suction control compartments, and no back pressure builds up.

Suppose the suction tube is disconnected, or a leak develops distal to the water seal. Assuming the disconnection or leak is recent, the evacuation of any fluid will be:

☐ terminated ☐ retarded, but not terminated ☐ unaffected — retarded, but not terminated

and the evacuation of air will be:

☐ terminated ☐ retarded, but not terminated ☐ unaffected — retarded, but not terminated

Now, assuming the disconnection or leak is long-standing, the evacuation of any fluid will be:
☐ terminated ☐ retarded, but not terminated ☐ unaffected — retarded, but not terminated

and the evacuation of air will be:

☐ terminated ☐ retarded, but not terminated ☐ unaffected — retarded, but not terminated

---

14.
Each condition below removes suction as an evacuation force. Check each condition, if any, whose effect on the evacuation of air varies over time:

☐ breakdown in suction source ☐ leak distal to water seal
☐ disconnection in chest tube ☐ none of these
☐ kink in suction tube

Answer: breakdown in suction source; kink in suction tube

Now check each condition, if any, whose effect on the evacuation of fluid varies over time:

☐ breakdown in suction source ☐ leak distal to water seal
☐ disconnection in chest tube ☐ none of these
☐ kink in suction tube

Answer: none of these

FOOTNOTE

Each condition listed in the preceding frame removes suction accidentally. In some situations, suction is removed by choice. In these situations, the distal end of the chest tube system should simultaneously be opened to the atmosphere, to prevent the buildup of back pressure. This can be accomplished simply by disconnecting the suction tube.

Note that, in a bottle system, the manometer tube submersed in the water of the suction control bottle does <u>not</u> vent the patient's air into the atmosphere. Its purpose is to permit the entry of atmospheric air when suction is on. The patient's air, which passes over the suction control water, has no access to the manometer tube; the manometer tube may not be viewed as a safety vent when suction is, for any reason, discontinued.

15.
Using the following code,

1 — replenishes patient's pneumothorax (rapidly or slowly)
2 — retards, but does not terminate, evacuation of any fluid
3 — retards, but does not terminate, evacuation of air
4 — terminates evacuation of any fluid
5 — terminates evacuation of air,

indicate the effect or effects on the patient of each condition described below:

Condition		Answer
breakdown in suction source (recent)	________	2, 3
breakdown in suction source (long-standing)	________	2, 5
dependent loop in chest tube evacuating mostly fluid	________	4, 5
dependent loop in chest tube evacuating only air	________	3
disconnection in chest tube	________	1
disconnection in suction tube	________	2, 3
kink in suction tube (recent)	________	2, 3
kink in suction tube (long-standing)	________	2, 5
leak distal to water seal	________	2, 3
leak proximal to water seal	________	1
obstruction of chest tube	________	4, 5

FOOTNOTE

As noted, there are several conditions that retard without terminating the evacuation of fluid. If the fluid includes a large amount of blood, the slow up in its evacuation promotes coagulation. Thus, a slow up in the evacuation of fluid can ultimately lead to an obstruction.

SECTION 4—REPAIRING MALFUNCTIONS IN THE CHEST TUBE SYSTEM

PANEL 4

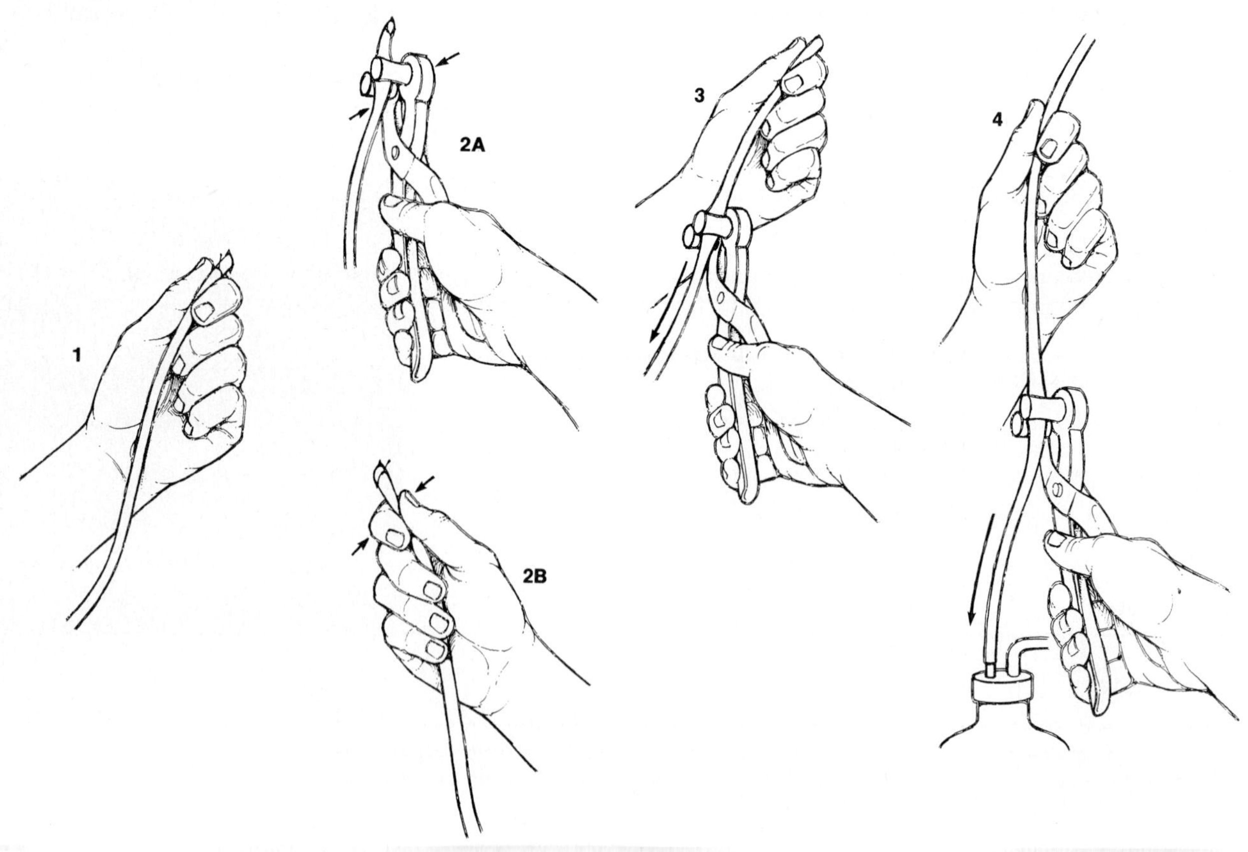

16.
The first malfunction whose repair we will discuss is a clot in the external portion of the chest tube.

The procedure for expressing such a clot from the tube is illustrated in Panel 4. This procedure is called milking, and it can be understood best by beginning at the end. So look first at Steps 3 and 4.

Note that the chest tube is milked away from the patient, beginning at:

☐ a point distal to the insertion site by a few inches
☐ the insertion site

and ending at:

☐ a point proximal to the collection inlet by a few inches
☐ the collection inlet

the insertion site

the collection inlet

17.
Only by starting the milking process at the insertion site can a nurse be certain of removing all occlusive matter from the tube, including not only the clot but any matter proximal to it.

Only by ending the process at the collection site can she be certain of expressing all such matter, including the clot, from the tube.

Milking the entire length of the tube, from its insertion site down to the collection inlet, is thus:

☐ essential ☐ not essential

essential

18.
Now look at Steps 2A and 2B in Panel 4. These illustrations show how pressure can be applied to the chest tube during the milking process. As you can see, a nurse can squeeze the tube using:

☐ a special implement ☐ her fingers

Both choices should be checked.

19.
The special implement shown in Panel 4 has a variety of names; we will call it simply a milker.

A milker is designed especially for the milking process. But your fingers can serve as well, providing you use them to apply pressure that is firm and steady throughout the milking.

The use of a milker is thus: ☐ essential ☐ not essential

At what site should pressure be initially applied to the chest tube? ________________

not essential

the insertion site

20.
A nurse uses one hand to squeeze the chest tube with a milker or her fingers.

Look at Step 1 in Panel 4, which shows the use of her other hand. As you can see, the other hand is:

☐ idle
☐ used to immobilize the chest tube at its insertion site
☐ used to immobilize the chest tube at some point distal to the insertion site.

used to immobilize the chest tube at its insertion site

21.
Customarily, a catheter is secured inside a patient's chest only by a single suture at the insertion site. The catheter can thus be easily extracted from the patient's chest during a milking procedure, which exerts a pulling force away from the patient.

Immobilizing the chest tube at its insertion site before milking the tube is thus:

☐ essential ☐ not essential

essential

FOOTNOTE

Immobilization and milking of the chest tube occur in stages. Initially, the nurse places one hand on the chest tube, near the insertion site, to stabilize it while the other hand milks the tube. When the nurse finishes milking one section, she moves the stabilizing hand to the end of that section and then milks the next section. This procedure is followed until the entire length of tube has been milked. The illustrations in Panel 4 thus show the initial steps only.

22.
Listed below, in alphabetical order, are the initial steps involved in milking a chest tube to express a clot:

A — milk chest tube from its insertion site down to collection inlet
B — use one hand to immobilize chest tube at its insertion site
C — use one hand to squeeze chest tube at its insertion site, using milker or fingers

Using the letters, write the steps in the order of performance: ________________

B, C, A

FOOTNOTE

A chest tube can be milked, not only to express an external clot, but to prevent one from developing. As a preventive measure, milking is performed routinely at a frequency that varies with the rate and composition of the patient's drainage. Thus, during an early phase of drainage, when its rate is likely to be high and blood its largest component, milking should be performed every one to two hours. During a later phase, when the rate of drainage is likely to be low and serum its largest component, milking should be performed every four to eight hours.

PANEL 5

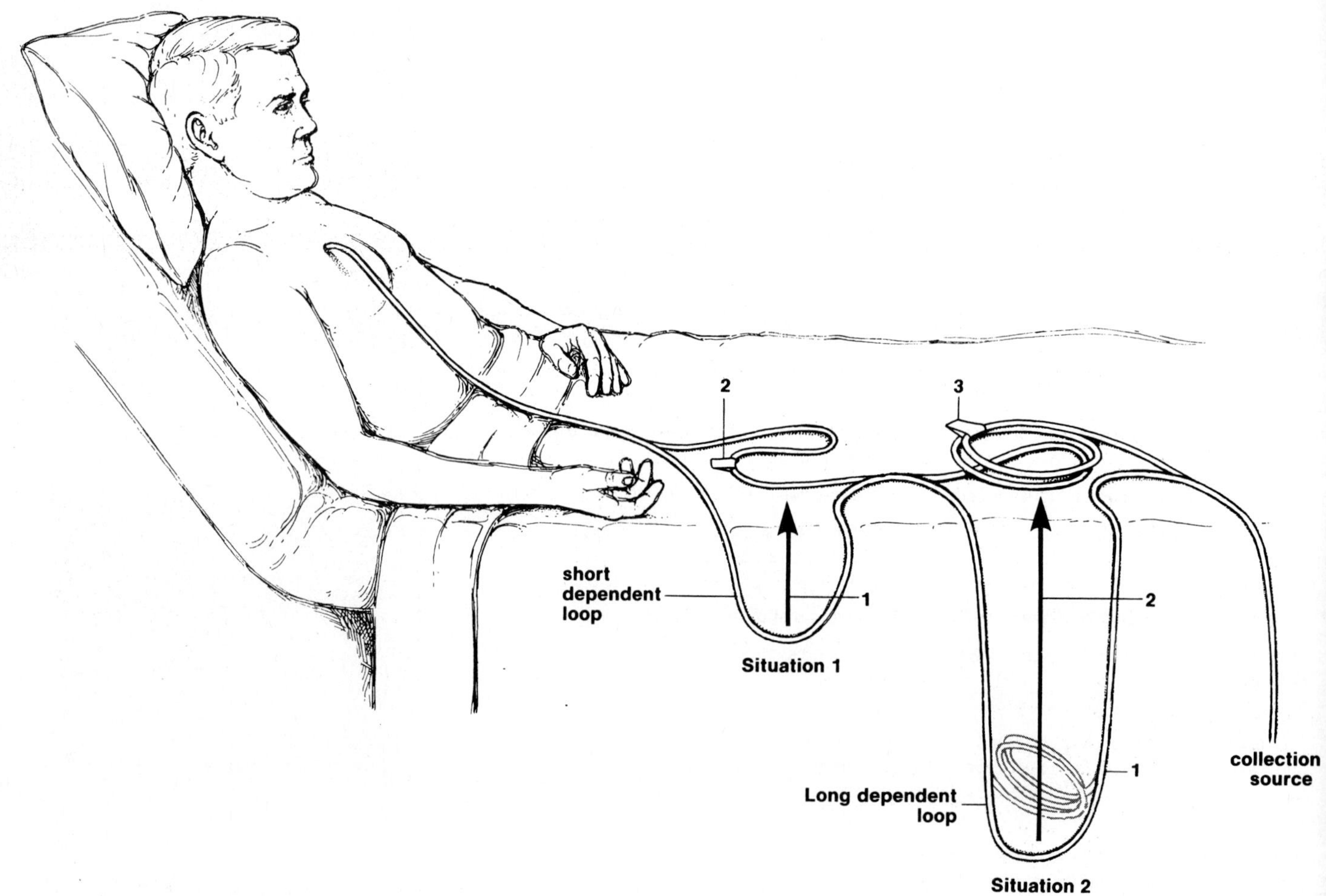

23.
The next malfunction whose repair we will discuss is a dependent loop.

Panel 5 shows how a dependent loop is repaired. Note that the procedure varies with the length of the loop.

Look at Situation 1 involved in repairing a loop that is short and at Situation 2 involved in repairing a loop that is long.

ıs you can see, these steps each consist of:

☐ lowering the dependent section
☐ raising the dependent section

raising the dependent section

o a level that is:

☐ above the insertion site of the tube
☐ below the insertion site of the tube

below the insertion site of the tube

☐ above the collection inlet
☐ below the collection inlet

above the collection inlet

4.
ıs noted in Section 1, gravity is used for evacuation by arranging a chest tube so that it escends continuously from its insertion site.

ı the repair of a dependent loop, raising and looping the dependent section to a level above ne collection inlet but below the insertion site is thus: ☐ essential ☐ not essential

essential

5.
.ook again at Panel 5. Which procedure, if either, involves a first step that consists of making ircular loops from the dependent section?

☐ repairing a long dependent loop
☐ repairing a short dependent loop
☐ neither of the above

repairing a long dependent loop

6.
;hest tubes are usually quite long to permit the patient some freedom of movement. Unless ıny excess length is converted into circular loops, there is virtually no way to arrange the tube o that it descends continuously from its insertion site.

ı the repair of a long dependent loop, making circular loops from the dependent section efore raising it is thus:

☐ essential ☐ not essential

essential

7.
low, look at the last step involved in repairing either a short or a long dependent loop. As you an see, after the dependent section has been raised to a new level, it is:

☐ affixed in place ☐ left simply resting in place

affixed in place

8.
hat a dependent loop developed indicates that the chest tube was not sufficiently secured vhen first arranged. Affixing the dependent section at its new level is thus:

☐ essential ☐ not essential

essential

FOOTNOTE

The illustration in Panel 5 shows the repair of a dependent loop while the patient is lying in bed. A dependent loop can, of course, also develop while the patient is sitting up in a chair. In that event, the dependent section can be affixed only to the chair arm. Otherwise, the procedure with a chair is the same as the one with a bed.

9.
.isted below are steps involved in repairing a dependent loop of one or another length:

A — affix dependent section
B — make circular loops out of dependent section
C — raise dependent section to level above collection inlet but below insertion site

Vrite the steps involved in repairing each dependent loop described below. Write the steps in heir order of performance:

long dependent loop ________ B, C, A
short dependent loop ________ C, A

30.

The next malfunction whose repair we will discuss is a disconnection of the catheter from its extension or of the extension from the collection inlet.

As noted earlier, a disconnection permits the reentry of atmospheric air into the patient's intrapleural space. At the same time, it exposes the lumen of the chest tube to ambient bacteria along its entire length. This is true whether the disconnection occurs between the catheter and extension or between the extension and collection inlet.

Check each disconnection, if either, that results in contamination of the catheter:

☐ disconnection of catheter from extension
☐ disconnection of extension from collection inlet
☐ neither of the above

disconnection of catheter from extension
disconnection of extension from collection inlet

Now check each disconnection, if either, that results in contamination of the extension:

☐ disconnection of catheter from extension
☐ disconnection of extension from collection inlet
☐ neither of the above

disconnection of catheter from extension
disconnection of extension from collection inlet

31.

When the lumen of a chest tube is contaminated, there is a risk of infection to the patient.

This risk can be reduced by replacing the extension, which is a simple procedure.

The risk of infection could also be reduced by replacing the catheter. But this is not a simple procedure. It would require a new insertion site (the old one cannot be used), and the surgery, like the disconnection that prompted it, would open the patient's intrapleural space to atmospheric air (not to mention introducing a risk of infection of its own).

Check each component of a chest tube, if either, that should be replaced when the catheter is disconnected from the extension:

☐ catheter ☐ extension ☐ neither

extension

Now check each component, if either, that should be replaced when the extension is disconnected from the collection inlet:

☐ catheter ☐ extension ☐ neither

extension

32.

With a disconnection of the catheter from the extension, the latter remains connected to the collection inlet; with a disconnection of the extension from the collection inlet, the extension remains connected to the catheter.

Check each step below that should be part of repairing a disconnection:

☐ disconnect old extension from end still connected
☐ connect new extension at both ends
☐ reconnect old extension at disconnected end

disconnect old extension from end still connected
connect extension at both ends

33.

While the extension is being replaced, atmospheric air can continue to reenter the patient's intrapleural space during inspiration unless the catheter is clamped. Clamping the catheter can thus minimize the degree to which the patient's pneumothorax is replenished.

At the same time, clamping the catheter will prevent the exit of air from the intrapleural space during expiration, and prolonged clamping (like any chest tube obstruction) can lead to a tension pneumothorax.

Taking into account the risk on one hand of fully replenishing the patient's pneumothorax and the risk on the other of producing a tension pneumothorax, check the procedure below that seems best to you:

☐ clamp catheter before replacing extension and leave clamp in place for some time afterward
☐ clamp catheter before replacing extension and unclamp it immediately afterward
☐ do not clamp catheter at all

We think the following is the best procedure:
clamp catheter before replacing extension and unclamp it immediately afterward

34.

When a clamp is applied to a catheter, its weight tends to extract the catheter from the patient's chest, the more so if the clamp is swinging freely, as it would if applied far from the insertion site of the catheter.

The clamp should thus be applied:

☐ far from the catheter's insertion site
☐ near the catheter's insertion site

near the catheter's insertion site

35.
It may be necessary to repair a disconnected chest tube in either a gravity system or a system on suction.

The steps discussed so far are sufficient for repairing the tube in a gravity system, and they are listed below in alphabetical order:

A — clamp catheter near its insertion site
B — connect new extension at both ends
C — disconnect old extension from end still connected
D — unclamp catheter immediately

Using the letters, write the steps in the order of performance: ________________

A, C, B, D

36.
When suction is being used, there are a few additional steps.

If the suction source is on when the catheter is unclamped (following the repair), then the patient's intrapleural space will go abruptly from zero to full suction, which can damage pulmonary tissue that is fragile or dislodge clots in the lung surface that are recent.

Consequently, the suction should be:

☐ maintained at its initial level throughout the procedure
☐ turned down before the catheter is unclamped and gradually turned back up afterward
☐ turned down before the catheter is unclamped and quickly turned back up afterward

turned down before the catheter is unclamped and gradually turned back up afterward

37.
Suction makes a distracting noise when a chest tube system is open to the atmosphere. So it is advisable to turn the suction down early in the procedure. But closing the patient's intrapleural space to the atmosphere has first priority.

Listed below, in the order of performance, are steps involved in repairing a disconnected chest tube in a system on suction. Using the margin on the left, insert an arrow to indicate the point at which you would turn down the suction:

clamp catheter near insertion site
disconnect extension from end still connected
connect new extension at both ends
unclamp catheter immediately
gradually turn suction back up

clamp catheter near insertion site
→
disconnect extension from end still connected

38.
Listed below, in alphabetical order, are the steps involved in repairing a disconnected chest tube in a system on suction:

A — clamp catheter near insertion site
B — connect new extension at both ends
C — disconnect old extension from end still connected
D — gradually turn suction back up
E — turn suction down
F — unclamp catheter immediately

Using the letters, write the steps in the order of performance: ________________

A, E, C, B, F, D

FOOTNOTE

Before turning the suction down, note the setting on the suction gauge, and turn the suction back up to this setting afterward. You can verify that your setting is proper by looking at the water in the suction control compartment; when the suction is functioning properly, there will be vigorous, though not excessive bubbling, in this compartment.

Incidentally, after a disconnected chest tube had been repaired, it may be useful to secure its junctions against disconnections in the future. This can be done by twisting a wire-tie around each junction, or wrapping each junction in clear tape. Opaque tape should not be used because a subsequent disconnection occurring beneath it may go undetected.

39.
The next malfunction whose repair we will discuss is a dislodgement of the catheter from inside the patient's chest.

In this situation, the catheter must be replaced, and a new insertion site must be created in the chest wall. The old site cannot be used.

This repair thus requires the intervention of:

☐ a nurse only ☐ both a nurse and a physician

both a nurse and a physician

40.
The old site is an opening in the chest through which atmospheric air can enter the patient's intrapleural space.

The old site should thus be:

☐ left open ☐ sealed

sealed

41.
Air can pass through a piece of plain gauze, but it cannot pass through a piece of petrolatum gauze.

Which material, if either, is sufficient to seal an old insertion site prior to its closure?

☐ petrolatum gauze ☐ plain gauze ☐ neither

petrolatum gauze

42.
Listed below are steps involved in repairing a catheter that has been dislodged from inside the patient's chest:

A — notify patient's physician
B — seal old insertion site with petrolatum gauze

The longer the delay in sealing the old insertion site, the more air will enter the patient's intrapleural space. Which step above has the higher priority? Letter ________

B

REPAIRING OTHER MALFUNCTIONS

Malfunction	Nursing Action
clot in internal portion of chest tube	Notify the patient's physician immediately.
defect in portable suction pump	Simply replace the pump.
defect in wall suction pump	Notify the engineering department. Use a portable pump (if available) in the meantime.
disconnection from electrical outlet of cord from portable pump	Plug it back in.
disconnection of suction tube from suction control outlet or from suction source inlet	If the tube has touched the floor, it should be replaced before it is reconnected. Otherwise, simply reconnect it.
kink in chest tube or in suction tube	Simply remove the kink.
loose cap on collection, water seal, or suction control bottle	Simply tighten the cap.
loose junction (though not complete disconnection) between catheter and extension or between extension and collection inlet	Simply tighten the junction. Again, it may be useful to secure the junction against future loosening by using a wire-tie or piece of clear tape.
loose junction between suction gauge and inlet of wall pump	Simply tighten the junction.
pressure on chest tube	Simply relieve the pressure. Take steps during future changes in the patient's body position to prevent new pressure from being exerted on the tube.

SECTION 5—RECOGNIZING MALFUNCTIONS IN A CHEST TUBE SYSTEM

Some malfunctions, such as a disconnection or dependent loop in the chest tube, may be self-evident. But these as well as others may first be signified by activities elsewhere in the system or in the patient.

Conditions to Be Considered

You have already been introduced to the various malfunctions. Some of these malfunctions pertain to both gravity systems and systems on suction, whereas others pertain only to systems on suction:

Gravity Systems or Systems on Suction	Systems on Suction Only
dependent loop in chest tube	breakdown in suction source
disconnection in chest tube	disconnection in suction tube
leak proximal to waste seal	kink in suction tube
obstruction of chest tube	leak distal to water seal

Of the malfunctions that pertain only to systems on suction, there are two—a breakdown in the suction source and a kink in the suction tube—whose signs vary with the duration of the malfunction. Of the malfunctions that pertain to all systems, there is one—a dependent loop—whose signs vary with duration, and another—a leak proximal to the water seal—whose signs vary with size. Our discussion will thus cover the following variations:

Gravity Systems or Systems on Suction	Systems on Suction Only
dependent loop (recent) in chest tube	breakdown (recent) in suction source
dependent loop (long-standing) in chest tube	breakdown (long-standing) in suction source
leak (large) proximal to water seal	kink (recent) in suction tube
leak (small) proximal to water seal	kink (long-standing) in suction tube

Finally, some malfunctions give rise to signs that resemble those of a normally operating system that has evacuated all air from the patient's intrapleural space. Our discussion will thus cover the following normal conditions in addition to malfunctions:

normal status, with some air left in intrapleural space
normal status, with no air left in intrapleural space

Basic Situations

The difference between gravity systems and systems on suction affects not only the kinds of malfunctions that can develop but the signs that each malfunction can produce.
The signs also vary with the substances initially contained in the patient's intrapleural space; that is, a large amount of air with no fluid, or mostly fluid with a small amount of air.

There are thus four basic situations, as follows:

- gravity system evacuating an amount of air initially large, with no fluid;
- gravity system evacuating mostly fluid, with an amount of air initially small;
- system on suction evacuating an amount of air initially large, with no fluid;
- system on suction evacuating mostly fluid, with an amount of air initially small.

Whether a system is based on a disposable, multichambered unit or bottles is less important. This difference does not affect the signs so much as the kinds of malfunctions that can develop. For example, a loose cap can develop only in a bottle system.

The Signs

Two or more of the following observations should be made during a routine assessment of a patient who is on a chest tube system. The exact number of observations, and sometimes their order, depends on the basic situation (see above) and on the results as they accumulate. As a general rule, the observations should proceed in the following sequence:

1. Observe patient for respiratory distress.

At the time an evacuation is started, severe respiratory distress will be evident in the patient, as the result of his pneumothorax or hemopneumothorax. With insertion of a chest tube, the distress will at first rapidly diminish. Thereafter, continued progress will depend on the function of the chest tube system (among other factors, such as pulmonary congestion, acid-base balance, and so forth).

Since the patient's respiratory progress provides some evidence of how the chest tube system is functioning, every routine assessment should begin with an observation of his respiratory distress. Comparing the current with former assessments, the patient will then be found in either of the following:

- diminishing respiratory distress;
- increasing respiratory distress.

While diminishing distress is a "good" sign, it is nevertheless compatible with some malfunctions in a chest tube system, especially those that retard without terminating the evacuation. Diminishing distress thus does not exclude a condition that requires repair.

On the other hand, increasing distress may signify some condition other than a malfunction in the chest tube system. There are many conditions that can compromise a patient's respirations, including pulmonary congestion or embolism, incisional pain, cardiac tamponade, and so on. For the sake of discussion, we are going to assume that a patient's respiratory status depends solely on the function of his chest tube system. But you should bear in mind that other factors can also play a significant role.

2. Inspect chest tube for disconnection or dependent loop.

These malfunctions are the ones mostly likely to be self-evident upon simple inspection. As the result of the inspection, the following results are possible:

- disconnection seen, or no disconnection seen:
- dependent loop seen, or no dependent loop seen.

3. Observe water seal for bubbling.

The function of the chest tube system affects activity in the water seal compartment, and in particular, the bubbling of air through the water seal. As the result of your observation, one of the following results may be obtained:

- continuous, noisy, turbulent bubbling;
- continuous, silent, turbulent bubbling;
- intermittent, silent, turbulent bubbling;
- intermittent, silent, placid bubbling;
- no bubbling.

Note that the bubbling (if any) must be evaluated in three respects: continuous vs. intermittent; noisy vs. silent; and turbulent vs. placid. Each variation is significant.

4. Observe fluid in chest tube, or water in water seal tube, for fluctuations.

The function of the chest tube system also affects the movement of fluid in a chest tube or of water inside a water seal tube. Depending on the status of the system, one may observe the fluid or water to rise and fall repetitively. We will refer to such movements as fluctuations. (For the rise and fall of water in a water seal tube, the term tidalling is sometimes also used.)

Whether in fluid in a chest tube or water inside a water seal tube, fluctuations have the same significance. But it is preferable to observe the fluid in a chest tube because fluctuations of water in a water seal tube can be obscured by the bubbling of air through the water seal. Also, some water seal tubes are opaque.

By the same token, fluid can be observed in a chest tube only if fluid is being evacuated by the system. If the system is evacuating only air, fluctuations can be sought only in the water in the water seal tube.

Fluctuations may be observed in either a gravity system or a system on suction. But they are more important in tracing a malfunction in the latter.

Based on all the above, the following observations are called for:

system on suction evacuating mostly fluid, with an amount of air initially small	observe fluid in chest tube for fluctuations
system on suction evacuating an amount of air initially large, with no fluid	observe water in water seal tube for fluctuations

In referring to a "water seal tube," we are obviously speaking of a bottle system; there is no water seal tube in a disposable system. But a disposable unit does have a U-shaped water seal chamber with inlet and outlet sides. Just as water may fluctuate inside a water seal tube, so it may fluctuate on the inlet side of a disposable water seal chamber (with opposite fluctuations on the outlet side of the chamber). We will continue referring only to a "water seal tube," but our comments apply equally to the inlet side of a disposable water seal chamber.

In summary, the observation of fluid in a chest tube, or of water in a water seal tube, may result in either of the following:

- fluctuations;
- no fluctuations.

5. Observe suction control water for bubbling.

This last sign also pertains only to systems on suction, and as with other signs, it can vary with the function of the system. As a result of the observation, either of the following results may be obtained:

- continuous bubbling;
- no bubbling.

The Patient Receiving Total Parenteral Nutrition

Definition/Discussion

Total parenteral nutrition (TPN), sometimes called hyperalimentation, is the infusion of hypertonic solutions of dextrose, nitrogen, and additives (vitamins, minerals, electrolytes, essential trace elements) directly into the blood stream through an indwelling venous catheter in order to restore/maintain normal body composition and nutrition in individuals who are unable to meet their needs via the gastrointestinal (GI) tract. TPN is usually administered via an established central venous line or a right atrial catheter. Hypertonic solutions need to be infused directly into a central vein with high blood flow. Less concentrated solutions may be given via a peripheral vein.

Nursing Assessment

☐ PERTINENT HISTORY

Health problem that interferes with normal nutrition (e.g., Crohn's disease, chemotherapy, surgical manipulation of GI tract); anticipated duration of treatment (short-term during acute illness or lifelong); previous parenteral nutrition experiences; other chronic illnesses that may affect treatment (e.g., diabetes mellitus, renal disease requiring protein and calcium restrictions, cardiac disease requiring sodium restriction)

☐ PHYSICAL FINDINGS

Height and weight; muscle mass; serum proteins, electrolytes, minerals; fluid status (skin turgor, edema, diaphoresis); ability to ingest oral foods; method of elimination (usual urinary and GI patterns, ostomies, abnormal losses via vomiting); presence of wounds or fistulas that increase nutritional requirements for tissue repair and growth; anticipated caloric and nitrogen needs; established venous access

☐ PSYCHOSOCIAL CONCERNS/ DEVELOPMENTAL FACTORS

Age; sex; usual coping mechanisms; stage of grief response to loss of normal body functioning; changes in role, family dynamics, daily activities, and employment; mental stability, personal resources to perform home parenteral nutrition

☐ PATIENT AND FAMILY KNOWLEDGE

Level of knowledge; patient acceptance of health problem necessitating parenteral nutrition; understanding of purpose and mechanics of parenteral nutrition, patient role, and problems to report; readiness and willingness to learn

Nursing Care

☐ LONG-TERM GOAL

The patient will receive total parenteral nutrition infusion free from preventable complications.

NURSING DIAGNOSIS #1

Alteration in nutrition: less than body requirements related to inability to absorb nutrients via GI tract, inability to ingest sufficient nutrients

Rationale: *Pathophysiology making GI absorption of nutrients a problem for the patient will vary depending on specific health problem. Regardless of the specific situation, a person needs enough protein for tissue repair and growth, enough calories for energy (both carbohydrate and fat sources), and enough electrolyte, vitamins, minerals, and trace elements* *for normal body functioning. The specific health problem determines exact amount of nutrients needed. General guidelines for daily parenteral nutrition (for adults) are: amino acids—1-1.5 gm/kg; glucose and lipids—25 cal/kg + 10%-30%; sodium—50-120 mmol; potassium—80-120 mEq.*

☐ GOAL

The patient will receive adequate nutrition to restore/maintain health.

☐ IMPLEMENTATION

- Assist with assessment of nutrition needs by
  - measuring height and daily weight
  - accurately recording foods eaten
  - collecting ordered laboratory studies
  - observing fluid status via intake and output (include unusual losses such as vomiting, diarrhea, ostomies, and wounds)
  - performing a daily physical assessment
- Administer using an electronic infusion pump to accurately control rate.
- If solution infuses too slowly do not increase rate to catch up; if solution infuses ahead of schedule, infuse 20% dextrose in water to keep system open until time to resume TPN.
- Monitor blood sugar according to method ordered (e.g., Accucheck, serum glucose) closely during this interim and when TPN is resumed (there may be decreased blood sugar when TPN is not infusing because 20% dextrose is usually a less concentrated glucose solution and it will be infusing at a slower rate).
- Administer intralipids as ordered using an electronic infusion pump (intralipids may be given via a peripheral vein because these solutions are isotonic; they are occasionally piggybacked into TPN solution, sometimes given simultaneously via a second intravenous access site, and sometimes given while TPN is turned off).
  - do not use an IV filter because particles are too large to pass through filter
  - take baseline vital signs and repeat every 10 minutes during first 30 minutes of infusion to monitor for side effects (chills, fever, flushing, diaphoresis, allergic reactions, chest and back pain, nausea and vomiting, headache, vertigo, pressure over the eyes)
  - discontinue infusion if side effects occur
- Monitor patient for hyper/hypoglycemia refer to Nursing Diagnoses #2.

☐ EVALUATION CRITERIA/DESIRED OUTCOMES

The Patient

- Receives infusions on time, free from side effects
- Maintains ideal body weight
- Heals existing wounds
- Is free from electrolyte imbalance or excess/deficit of vitamins and minerals

NURSING DIAGNOSIS #2

a. **Potential for injury** (air embolism, glucose imbalance, impaired catheter integrity) related to infusion of TPN via a central line

b. **Potential for infection** related to central line, TPN

Rationale: *Patients receiving TPN are frequently malnourished and at risk for infection. Hypertonic glucose solution is an excellent culture medium for bacteria and yeast. Poor aseptic technique may result in contamination of catheter or solution. In addition, TPN bypasses the normal defenses of the GI tract. Disconnection of IV tubing attached to a central line without proper clamping may result in air embolism. Inconsistent rate of infusion and inadequate or overdosage of insulin to cover glucose load may lead to hyper/hypoglycemia. Improper clamping or inadequate heparinization of catheter may result in breaks in catheter integrity. Any of these problems may result in breaks and interruption of needed nutrition and can cause serious, even life-threatening problems for the patient.*

☐ GOAL

The patient will be free from complications associated with parenteral nutrition.

☐ IMPLEMENTATION

- Use strict aseptic technique when handling catheter; follow established hospital protocol; refer to *The Patient with a Right Atrial Catheter*, page 576.

- Check temperature every 4-6 hours and report elevations above 100°F (37.8°C).
- Culture any purulent drainage from any part of body; perform routine blood and urine cultures as ordered.
- Refrigerate TPN solution (which has been prepared by pharmacist under laminar flow hood) until 1 hour before administration to retard the growth of yeast that grows easily in high dextrose solution; inspect solution for turbidity, precipitates, or cracks in the bottle before administration.
- Administer solution via IV tubing with 0.22 micron in-line filter to remove impurities; do not allow solution to hang for more than 12 hours.
- Tape all catheter connections securely to avoid inadvertent disconnections; instruct patient to bear down and/or hold breath when changing IV tubing to avoid air embolism; if patient becomes short of breath with chest pain, coughing, or cyanosis, clamp catheter and position on left side to keep air from going into pulmonary circulation, left heart, and into arterial circulation; report immediately.
- Check fingerstick blood sugar or urine sugar/acetone every 4 hours during therapy; administer insulin coverage as ordered; observe for manifestations of hypoglycemia (sweating, pallor, palpitations, nausea, headache, hunger, shakiness, blurred vision) or hyperglycemia (nausea, weakness, thirst, headache, polyuria).
- Flush catheter with heparin solution between infusions if treatment is intermittent rather than continuous; clamp catheter with specially designed toothless nontraumatic clamp between infusions; clamp tubing at a different place each time to prevent clot formation within catheter and breaks in catheter.

☐ EVALUATION CRITERIA/DESIRED OUTCOMES

The Patient

- Is afebrile
- Has no redness, swelling, or discharge at catheter insertion site
- Maintains negative urine and blood cultures
- Is free from shortness of breath, chest pain
- Maintains serum glucose between 80-120 mg%; urine sugar less than 3+

NURSING DIAGNOSIS #3

a. **Alteration in health maintenance** (need for parenteral nutrition) related to digestive dysfunction
b. **Social isolation** related to fear of being different
c. **Grieving** related to lost body function and inability to eat normally
d. **Ineffective individual coping** related to altered health status

Rationale: *Eating is both a time to meet the body's need for nutrition and a time for social interaction. The person who is unable to eat normally due to dysfunction of the digestive system may experience a grief process over the loss. This may progress normally with development of alternative behaviors to deal with the loss or may develop into ineffective coping behaviors. The patient may feel so abnormal that s/he avoids social contact with others. Whatever the response, the patient will need to adjust to a new method of health maintenance regarding diet.*

☐ GOAL

The patient will develop effective coping behaviors to deal with a new method of nutritional support.

☐ IMPLEMENTATION

- Be an empathic and supportive listener during the patient's stages of grief (patient may be in shock; may be mistrustful of an artificial method of nutritional support); use open-ended, leading statements to facilitate expressions of feelings.
- Assess for fluid and electrolyte balance, sepsis, protein imbalance if patient demonstrates delirium; if no metabolic cause or evidence of substance abuse, consult psychologic professionals; refer patient as necessary.
- Assess for signs of depression and hopelessness; provide support and clarify facts as needed.
- Educate patient regarding the treatments and long-term needs; assist in the resumption of normal social contacts.
- If family is overprotective, work with members to encourage patient progress toward an independent life-style.

- Encourage patient to participate in meals; patients can often tolerate small amounts of clear liquids and can schedule this during usual mealtimes.
- Encourage resumption of normal work and leisure activities
  - most patients infuse their solutions at night and are able to conceal catheter beneath clothing during the day
  - contact sports are not allowed due to possibility of damage to the catheter
  - if swimming, cover dressing with plastic wrap and change dressing right after swimming
  - travel is possible with planning
  - sexual activity is also possible with good communication and planning in terms of how to avoid catheter displacement
- Ensure patient has address of a national organization such as Lifeline Foundation, Inc. (2 Osprey Rd., Sharon, Maine 02067) in order to obtain support and ideas for adaptation to condition (local health care centers may also have support groups available).

☐ EVALUATION CRITERIA/DESIRED OUTCOMES

The Patient

- Progresses normally through grief response
- Utilizes effective coping behaviors to deal with alteration in diet
- Participates in family meals and social situations that include food
- Resumes preillness work and leisure activities, making changes as needed to protect catheter
- Expresses feelings to staff and family

NURSING DIAGNOSIS #4

Knowledge deficit regarding new method of nutritional support

Rationale: *The patient/family who understands health problems and treatment will be better able to participate in therapy. They will be willing to ask questions, avoid many problems (e.g., sleep pattern disturbances, sexual dysfunction, noncompliance with treatment), and know how to recognize and deal with complications.*

☐ GOAL

The patient will verbalize need for parenteral nutrition; will cooperate with treatment.

☐ IMPLEMENTATION

- During the acute phase of illness, explain treatments as patient is interested; keep explanations brief; including
  - need to keep head turned away from insertion site during dressing changes to maintain asepsis
  - that TPN is a method of supplying complete nutritional need
  - importance of not turning suddenly or pulling at dressings to avoid dislodging the catheter
- Teach technique of TPN administration to patients who will receive it at home; include
  - reason for TPN
  - dressing change technique and symptoms to report to physician
  - how to irrigate the catheter with heparinized saline between infusions and how to change catheter cap
  - how to set up infusion and deliver it via an infusion pump
  - how to identify complications and what to do about them
- Teach patient how to monitor blood/urine glucose at home and administer insulin as needed.
- Teach to weigh every other day to detect fluid retention and assess nutritional status.
- Teach to infuse solution at night while sleeping; reassure patient that infusion pump has an alarm if problems with flow occur; ensure patient knows how to set alarm.
- Teach in several, short teaching sessions; demonstrate techniques and have patient give a return demonstration.
- Assess patient's usual routine and help incorporate TPN into usual work and social schedule.
- Include family members in the instruction.
- Refer patient/family to support groups appropriate to their needs, as necessary.
- Ensure patient has an appointment for return visit to physician.

☐ EVALUATION CRITERIA/DESIRED OUTCOMES

The Patient

- Explains reasons for TPN and how to perform procedure at home

- Demonstrates procedures before discharge including
  - dressing change and observations of site
  - heparinization of catheter
  - changing catheter cap
  - setting up infusion, including adding vitamins, minerals, and elements to solution
  - blood/urine glucose testing and insulin administration
- Lists complications that may occur and how to deal with them
- States when and how to notify physician of progress or problems; lists health agencies and support groups (at least one of each) available for assistance
- Asks questions and discusses concerns freely
- Shows evidence of maintained or improved nutritional status during follow-up care

DIABETES AND EXERCISE

BY JAMES R. GAVIN III

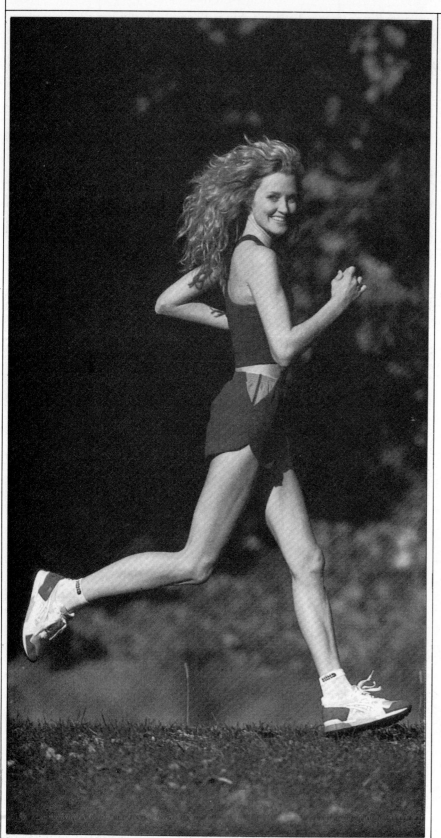

RODALE PRESS, INC.

Regularly performed aerobic exercise—exercise that involves the use of large numbers of muscles and that elevates the pulse to 70 to 80 percent of its maximum attainable rate—can be as complex to prescribe as it is crucial in both insulin-dependent (IDDM) and non-insulin-dependent (NIDDM) diabetes mellitus.

One must draw a fundamental distinction between the effects of random physical activity—for example, running to catch the bus or walking up one flight of stairs because the elevator just left—versus regular exercise or exercise training. The former produces acute, short-lived responses by muscles and other organ systems, but confers little in the way of lasting benefits.

Endurance training, on the other hand, lowers triglycerides and blood glucose, heightens sensitivity to insulin, and lowers blood pressure. Many of these changes are exactly the types of modifications that would be expected to reduce the risk of atherosclerosis, a desirable goal in diabetes mellitus.

WHETS THE APPETITE

When a person begins to exercise, muscle glycogen is the primary fuel. After 5 to 10 minutes, glucose uptake from blood is 7 to 20 times the resting rate, depending on how strenuous the exercise is. By 40 minutes or so of continuous exercise, blood glucose provides 75 to 90 percent of the total carbohydrate consumed by muscle, since muscle glycogen is depleted.

Patients with diabetes can benefit from this uptake of glucose from the blood during exercise—but

James R. Gavin III, MD, PhD, is presently professor of medicine and chief, diabetes section, Division of Endocrinology, Metabolism and Hypertension of Oklahoma University Health Sciences Center, Oklahoma City, OK.

Without enough insulin, exercise can make a diabetic ketotic and hyperglycemic.

only if they have adequate insulin available. Without adequate circulating insulin levels, insulin-dependent diabetics actually become *more* ketotic and *more* hyperglycemic with vigorous exercise.

How is it that blood sugar can actually rise, instead of fall, in the insulin-deficient person? During the early phases of exercise, the liver steps up its rate of glycogen breakdown to keep pace with muscle uptake of glucose. With prolonged exercise, gluconeogenesis from circulating substrates including alanine, lactate, pyruvate, and glycerol provides more of the glucose produced.

Insulin promotes uptake of glucose by muscles and prevents excessive glycogen breakdown and gluconeogenesis in the liver. If a person is insulin deficient, exercise can paradoxically create an overload of glucose in the blood. Without sufficient insulin, the muscles are not able to use as much glucose and the liver has no check on its glucose production.

EXERCISE AND IDDM

The absolute requirement for exogenous insulin means that IDDM patients must carefully coordinate the dose and the timing of insulin injections with the exercise program. Exercise works almost like insulin. Taken to the extreme, diabetics participating in marathons or triathlons need only two to five units of insulin *per day* during competition to maintain normal blood sugar levels. The key is to ensure adequate insulin levels so the exercise can be beneficial.

Unfortunately, one cannot look to blanket guidelines for determining how to adjust the insulin.

Since vigorous exercise of the injection site can speed the rate of insulin absorption, the patient is taught to avoid injections into the arms or legs before vigorous physical activity. Absorption also can be faster when blood flow to and from the injection site increases, such as when exercising in warm outdoor temperatures or in vinyl clothing. The problem with rapid absorption of insulin is the high probability of transient hypoglycemia.

IDDM diabetics must check their blood glucose within 30 minutes before exercise and an hour after exercise.

Before exercise, if the blood sugar exceeds 225 mg/dl and the person has not taken a short-acting insulin in the last two hours or an intermediate-acting drug in the last five to six hours, he should take Regular insulin to reduce blood sugar below 200 mg/dl before exercising. However, if Regular insulin has been taken within the last 1½ hours, or intermediate-acting insulin within the past five hours, the person should just delay exercise until the blood sugar responds to the insulin.

Of course, some patients become so adept at recognizing their own response patterns that they can exercise safely even when their blood sugars fall outside these guidelines.

At the other extreme is the blood sugar below, for example, 100 mg/dl. In this case, extra carbohydrate should be consumed or carried to prevent exercise-induced hypoglycemia. Since hypoglycemia may occur or persist several hours after exercise, the diabetic needs to ingest enough carbohydrates to replenish expended stores within the first few hours after exercise.

Patients with proliferative retinopathy should avoid exercises that jar the body (jumping rope, jogging, aerobic dancing) or that require a head-down position or the Valsalva maneuver (bench-pressing, floor exercises for abdominal muscle strengthening). These exercises may result in retinal detachment or increased intraretinal vascular pressure with subsequent hemorrhage.

Patients with significant nephropathy may spill more protein into their urine with vigorous, high-impact physical activities. Diabetics with peripheral neuropathy should exercise with caution because their impaired sensations can mask lower-extremity injuries. Patients with autonomic neuropathies should avoid vigorous exercise that elevates heart rate or increases sweat response—functions that may be impaired in such patients. In these patients, the benefits of vigorous aerobic exercise are likely to be outweighed by the risks involved.

EXERCISE FOR NIDDM

Because insulin resistance is a problem, any therapeutic exercise for NIDDM patients must overcome this resistance. For many with NIDDM, regular physical exercise eliminates the need for an intense campaign of food restriction for weight loss—not to mention the way exercise improves blood lipid levels, hypertension, and overall well-being.

All diabetics need a physical examination before starting an exercise program. For NIDDM patients, who are older, more obese, sedentary, and in a high-risk group for cardiac disease, this is especially important. They need to be checked for ischemia, angina pectoris, and arrhythmias.

Patients—especially those who have heart-disease symptoms, elevated blood lipids, or strong family histories of heart disease—should be assessed for exercise tolerance as they do graded exercise tests.

Patients who have not been exercising must build up their exercise intensity gradually, monitoring their heart rates to measure progress. The patient is taught to stop for 15 seconds at the peak of exercise, counting the pulse for 10 seconds, and multiply by six. Comparing the pulse at peak with the target pulse rate (usually 65 to 80 percent of maximum) set with the clinician determines whether or not the intensity of the patient's exercise is appropriate.

Studies have shown that the target pulse must be maintained for 15 to 30 minutes three to four times per week for exercise to be beneficial. Also, the effects of exercise on sensitivity to insulin are lost if exercise is stopped for 72 hours. Those effects are quickly regained when exercise is resumed.

Our studies of sedentary NIDDM patients showed that they needed 10 to 12 weeks of slowly progressing exercise before they could exercise at recommended intensity and duration. Attempts to shorten the time resulted in sore joints and muscles, fatigue, and failure to continue the program.

NIDDM patients on insulin or oral hypoglycemic drugs are taught to monitor their pre- and postexercise blood sugars and adjust drug timing and dose accordingly. NIDDM patients on small doses of insulin or oral drugs can often stop the drugs entirely once regular exercise is established.

PRESCRIBING EXERCISE

A 26-year-old IDDM woman with no known complications decides to exercise. She takes 15 units NPH and 8 units Regular insulin every morning, plus 10 units NPH and 5 units Regular insulin every evening.

She prefers running, so a jogging program is prescribed. She is told to begin with a walk/run routine for 15 minutes and gradually increase duration and intensity over four to six weeks.

She is instructed to check her blood sugar just before exercise. If it is 220 mg/dl or higher, she takes three to four units Regular insulin in an abdominal injection site. If her pre-exercise glucose is 100 mg/dl or less, she is to take some concentrated carbohydrate, such as a fast-dissolving mint, along during the run. If blood glucose is 80 mg/dl or less, she ingests 20 to 30 g of carbohydrate before the run.

After jogging, she is advised to check her BS within an hour. Deciding whether she needs extra calories or extra insulin is done on the basis of her blood glucose pre- and postexercise. Since she will exercise prior to the evening meal, her insulin requirements at this time will be expected to decrease as the intensity and duration of her exercise sessions increase.

> **Be precise in the exercise prescription: type, mode, intensity, duration, and frequency.**

The symptoms of hypoglycemia are carefully reviewed with her and she is advised that if such symptoms occur during or after exercise, she must stop immediately and ingest some carbohydrate (or the most immediately available fuel). She is reminded that such symptoms may occur for several hours postexercise. She learns to keep a diary of her exercise activity, her blood glucose readings, and any symptoms of hypoglycemia.

Contrast this to NIDDM. For example, a 49-year-old man with NIDDM elects to increase his exercise and reduce his calories to lower his blood sugar and body weight. He is in good general health except for diabetes, obesity, and his sedentary life-style.

After a discussion of the various options for aerobic exercise, he chooses an exercise bicycle. The staff teach him to take his pulse and give him a booklet that describes warm-up routines. For the first week he is advised to do stretch/flex exercises for 10 to 15 minutes and to begin low-intensity cycling for 10-minute periods at a workload of 60 to 65 percent of his maximum heart rate (MHR). His MHR is calculated by subtracting his age from 220: 220 − 49 = 171. Multiplying his MHR by 0.65, his pulse rate at peak exercise ought to be about 110.

He is provided a three-times-a-week schedule in which his exercise periods are increased by three to five minutes per session with a workload of 70 to 75 percent of maximum heart rate by the end of week three. By the end of week six, he is advised to have reached a duration of 30 to 45 minutes of cycling activity with a peak pulse rate of 80 to 85 percent of MHR.

He maintains a diary containing results of SMBG, weights, and any reports of incidents that may be of interest or concern to the patient. Data from the diary is reviewed with the clinician by telephone biweekly and during visits.

When you teach a patient to exercise, give him a regimen no less detailed than one for a drug. Specify the type, mode, intensity, frequency, and duration, and discuss the benefits and risks. With reasonable goals, the patient can soon learn that exercise is one of the very few forms of therapy that is certain to work and that can also be fun.

BIBLIOGRAPHY

Felig, P., and Wahren, J. Fuel homeostasis in exercise. *N.Engl.J.Med.* 293:1078-1084, Nov. 20, 1975.

Vranic, M., and Berger, M. Exercise and diabetes mellitus. *Diabetes* 28:147-163, Feb. 1979.

Zinman, B., and others. Comparison of the acute and long-term effects of exercise on glucose control in Type I diabetes. *Diabetes Care* 7:515-519, Nov.-Dec. 1984.

Zinman, B., and others. The role of insulin in the metabolic response to exercise in diabetic man. *Diabetes* 28(Suppl. 1):76-81, Jan. 1979.

Bowel Management In Dialysis Patients

Reprinted from American Journal of Nursing, July 1983.

By Jeanette K. Chambers

Yes, dialysis sustains life by removing metabolic wastes and restoring fluid and electrolyte balance. But most people who have end-stage renal failure also learn to live with a number of other treatment measures. These measures include using phosphate-binding agents to counteract hyperphosphatemia, controlling fluid intake, and restricting the diet. All of these measures lead to constipation, a common problem experienced by most patients requiring dialysis. At the same time, the usual guidelines for teaching normal bowel management do not apply to these patients.

For instance, health teaching for regular bowel elimination in most people typically includes such suggestions as getting plenty of rest and exercise, drinking large amounts of fluid, and eating a diet high in fiber. And if constipation occurs at times, laxatives or enemas can be used. But these measures may all be specifically harmful for the chronic renal failure patient.

Since end-stage renal disease patients develop hyperphosphatemia, elevated serum levels of phosphorus are treated by phosphate-binding agents, which are aluminum hydroxide compounds, such as ALternaGEL, Amphojel, or Alu-Caps. These agents must be taken regularly to achieve a normal phosphorus level, but the primary side effect is constipation. Phosphorus is a chemical element distributed so widely in food that restriction of these foods is impractical.

JEANETTE K. CHAMBERS, MDN, RN, CS, is a renal clinical nurse specialist, Riverside Methodist Hospital, Columbus, Ohio.

If untreated, hyperphosphatemia has serious consequences. Normally calcium and phosphorus exist in a 2:1 ratio; that is, the calcium level is twice that of the phosphorus level. If this 2:1 balance is disturbed, the body will attempt to restore the normal balance.

When the phosphorus level becomes elevated, calcium binds with the phosphorus to form calcium phosphate. Calcium phosphate precipitates and may produce renal calculi and soft tissue calcifications. But in such binding, only the serum calcium level is lowered; the phosphorus level is too high to be reduced significantly. The parathyroid glands monitor the serum calcium level and are sensitive to lowered levels of calcium. Thus, when the serum becomes hypocalcemic, the parathyroid glands produce parathormone in an attempt to raise the low calcium level. Parathormone mobilizes calcium from bone cells. However, the all-too-available phosphorus also overwhelms this newer mobilized supply of calcium.

Failure to control hyperphosphatemia and the resultant hypocalcemia can lead to long-term problems for the chronic dialysis patient. Constant stimulation of the parathyroid glands results in secondary hyperparathyroidism. Calcium depletion leads to bony deformities and pathological fractures in a condition known as renal osteodystrophy.°

Calcium phosphate is also deposited in the arteriolar smooth muscle and in the conduction system of the heart. The resultant arteriolar rigidity heightens vascular resistance, thus making blood pressure even more difficult to control. Deposits in the cardiac conduction system cause arrhythmias. Soft tissue deposits in the hips, thighs, and conjunctiva produce painful irritated areas that can become potential sites for infection. Therefore, management of the initial problem, high serum phosphorus, is important in preventing this sequence of pathology, but the remedy—the phosphate binders—also causes constipation.

°Binkley, Lowanna F., ed., Renal Osteodystrophy, *J.Nephr.Nurs*, Sept./Oct. 1979, p. 45.

Modifying the Rules

Getting plenty of fluids, particularly water, is probably the most common advice given for managing constipation. Fluids, however, are restricted for those dialysis patients who are oliguric or anuric—and most are. By definition, oliguria refers to the production of less than 400cc urine in 24 hours and anuria refers to the production of less than 100cc in 24 hours. In general, end stage renal failure patients are restricted to a 24-hour fluid intake equal to the amount of their urine output for 24 hours plus 600cc. The goal is to control the patient's water weight gain to 0.45 to 0.68 kg (1 to 1½ lb.) per day between dialyses. Fluid overload will all too quickly result in peripheral edema, hypertension, heart failure, and pulmonary edema. Frequent volume overload will make dialysis treatment uncomfortable because of muscle cramping associated with shifts in fluids and electrolytes. Consequently, dialysis patients do not have the option of increasing fluid intake to combat constipation.

The second most common advice is to eat foods high in fiber. Sources of fiber are generally fresh fruits and vegetables and bran products. But these foods are also high in potassium and phosphorus. Because it is not excreted by the kidneys, serum potassium increases between dialysis treatments. The rate of increase is directly related to the patient's dietary intake. Foods high in potassium must be limited. Depending on the patient, however, bran may be used as a cereal additive or mixed in applesauce, if necessary. Although patients with chronic renal failure tolerate slightly higher serum potassium levels—6.0mEq/L or perhaps even 6.5mEq/L—than the normal 3.5-5.0 mEq/L, they run the risk of arrhythmias when the serum potassium approaches 7mEq/L or higher, and cardiac arrest may result. In addition, such higher levels allow little safety margin and do not represent ideal management.

Finally, the third recommendation is to get plenty of exercise, balanced by rest. End-stage renal disease results in chronic anemia that is both normocytic and normochronic. The anemia is mainly caused by the lack of erythropoietin production that is needed in turn to stimulate the bone marrow to produce red blood cells. Some blood is also lost through hemodialysis and frequent lab work. Obviously, then, fatigue is one of the most noticeable symptoms in patients requiring dialysis. Although the fatigue may be influenced by the patient's psychological adjustment to his illness and by the quality of his support system, it is real and must be addressed in counseling the patient. Therefore, advising exercise as a method of managing constipation is not likely to be realistic. Encouraging the patient to make some effort in physical activity should be offered, however, since the adage "If I think I can, I can" is often true.

Management is most effective when a plan of aggressive prevention is used. Contrary to usual bowel management that suggests minimal reliance on stool softeners, people on dialysis often require such softeners. However, careful consideration must be given to the types of available agents, their mode of action and their potential side effects. Random selection of over-the-counter products and reliance upon recommendations of family and friends will probably yield less satisfactory results and may cause electrolyte imbalance.

Stool softeners are classified as emollients; they alter the surface tension of the feces and promote entry of water and fats into the fecal contents. Since these agents require 24 to 48 hours to act, their use is to prevent constipation, not to treat hardened stool.

Two common examples of emollient/stool softeners are docusate calcium (Surfak) and docusate sodium (Colace). The sodium and calcium in these products are not sufficient to warrant concern.

The usual advice for constipation—fluids, exercise, high fiber foods—may create new problems for the dialysis patient.

Bulk laxatives, such as psyllium hydrophilic mucilloid (Metamucil) may also be used regularly for management of chronic constipation. Such laxatives act by increasing the water content and, thus, the bulk of the stool. In turn, peristalsis is stimulated by mechanical distension of the bowel. Bulk laxatives are mild in the gastrointestinal tract; however, their effectiveness depends on fluid intake. Generally, the person is advised to take the laxative with a full glass of water. For renal patients who are restricted to 1000-1200cc of fluids per day, the glass of water, 240cc, would have to be included in their fluid allotment. Although bulk laxatives contain sodium, the amounts are minimal.

Stimulant laxatives should generally be reserved for acute constipation. If emollients and bulk agents become temporarily ineffective, a stimulant laxative may be indicated. Examples include castor oil, senna preparations (Senokot), danthron (Doxidan, Modane), and bisacodyl (Dulcolax). They act by stimulating sensory nerves, which in turn stimulate parasympathetic reflexes via Auerbach's plexus, which controls peristaltic activity in the large colon. Stimulant laxatives are site specific and do not alter motility in the stomach or small intestine.

Lubricant laxatives such as mineral oil alter the consistency of the feces, but do not influence peristalsis. The coating on the stool prevents the absorption of water by the intestinal mucosa; thus, feces do not become dry and hardened. Mineral oil is best used occasionally, since long term use is believed to interfere with absorption of the fat soluble vitamins. For this reason, mineral oil should be taken at bedtime, not immediately before or after meals. Some patients might also run the risk of aspirating the oil, which could cause pulmonary problems.

Laxatives and/or cathartics should be carefully selected. Compounds containing magnesium (milk of magnesia, Maalox) or phosphorus (Fleet's Phospho-Soda) can cause electrolyte toxicities. Serum magnesium levels can become elevated with repeated use of magnesium compounds. Attaining normal phosphorus levels will be further compromised by the ingestion of phosphorus compounds. Occasional use of these products may be necessary because of their stonger laxative properties. In such case, electrolyte levels must be monitored. Chronic use should be discouraged.

Caution is also needed regarding enemas. The usual rule of avoiding regular use also applies to the patient with renal failure. Generally small volume, gentle stimulant enemas, such as a Fleet or oil retention enema, are acceptable if used sparingly. They provide minimal fluid and interfer least with the electrolyte balance. Large volume saline or water enemas must be avoided; the fluid and saline may be absorbed through the intestines causing volume overload and sodium imbalance.

Patients and their families can learn effective bowel management and ways to alleviate constipation problems. The key is recognizing that the usual guidelines must be modified when the patient has renal disease.

The Person with a Spinal Cord Injury

Physical Care During Early Recovery

Reprinted from American Journal of Nursing, August 1977.

Whether the nurse works in an emergency room, intensive care unit, or on a general unit, she helps the patient to survive initially and to be ready eventually for the extensive rehabilitation that follows the intermediate stage of spinal cord injury. The complications that can delay rehabilitation are time-consuming and costly, and may be fatal. Good nursing in the general hospital can prevent or relieve most of them.

JUNE HANSEN LARRABEE

John's mind was on the party as he drove away from the fraternity house that May night. The road was a bit hazy to the 20-year-old, due to all the beer he'd drunk. He did not notice the embankment looming ahead until it was too late. When he regained consciousness, he had severe pain in his neck and some tingling in his arms. Rescue workers carefully secured him on a rigid stretcher and rushed him by ambulance to the nearest emergency room. The neurosurgeon who examined John in the ER thought he might have a spinal column fracture even though he had the full use of his fingers and toes.

John was taken to the x-ray department and transferred from the rigid stretcher to an x-ray table. After several exposures were taken, he was put back on the stretcher, returned to the ER, and transferred to a bed in the holding area. When room was available in the intensive care unit, he was transferred to a regular hospital bed and taken to the ICU.

The neurosurgeon reexamined John on arrival in the ICU and found that he had lost all sensation and movement in his arms, trunk, and legs. What had gone wrong? Why did he now have a neurological deficit when he had not on reaching the ER? Did everyone handling John know how to prevent neurological damage in a person with a suspected spinal fracture?

Knowledge about spinal cord injury (SCI) and its management, especially during the acute phase, is a growing need. Before the advent of antibiotics, most people who sustained an SCI died from urinary tract or respiratory infections, or from septicemia generated by decubitus ulcers. Over the past 30 years, specific antibiotic therapy and rapid advances in rehabilitation medicine have greatly increased the long-term survival rate of people with SCI(1).

The impact of SCI on the individual is immeasurable. It can only be worsened by an increase in neurological deficit or by urinary, respiratory, or skin infections. To enhance the patient's well-being, both physical and psychological, and to prevent unnecessary complications, the nurse must intervene knowledgeably.

The goal of care during the acute and intermediate phases following SCI is twofold: first, to resolve any life-threatening situation caused by or occurring with the injury; second, to provide care that prevents complications and moves the patient toward readiness for rehabilitation.

Transfer After Injury

When a patient is brought to an ER with a suspected SCI, the neurological deficit may or may not be the primary concern. Massive hemorrhage from other wounds; head injury, often associated with spinal cord trauma; and other problems may demand immediate attention if the patient is to survive.

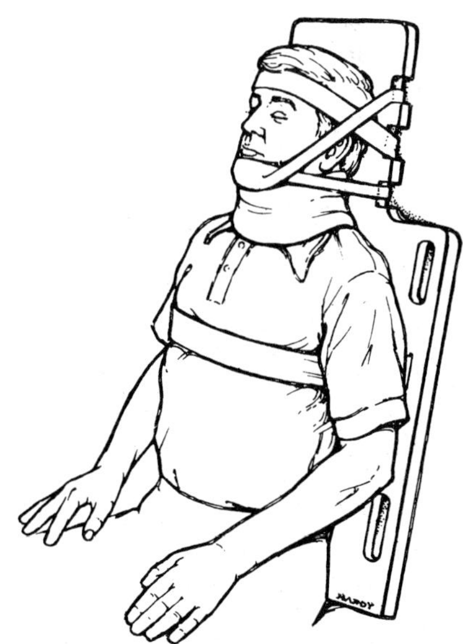

Before removing person with suspected back injury from car, (1) stabilize cervical spine with improvised collar (heavy towel, scarf); (2) slide rigid support (door, board, table leaf) behind him; (3) secure him to board with broad straps (wide belts, ties).

JUNE LARRABEE, R.N., M.S.N., was a surgical clinical nurse specialist at St. Vincent's Medical Center, Jacksonville, Fla., when she wrote this article. Now she is medical-surgical clinical nurse specialist at Kennestone Hospital in Marietta, Georgia.

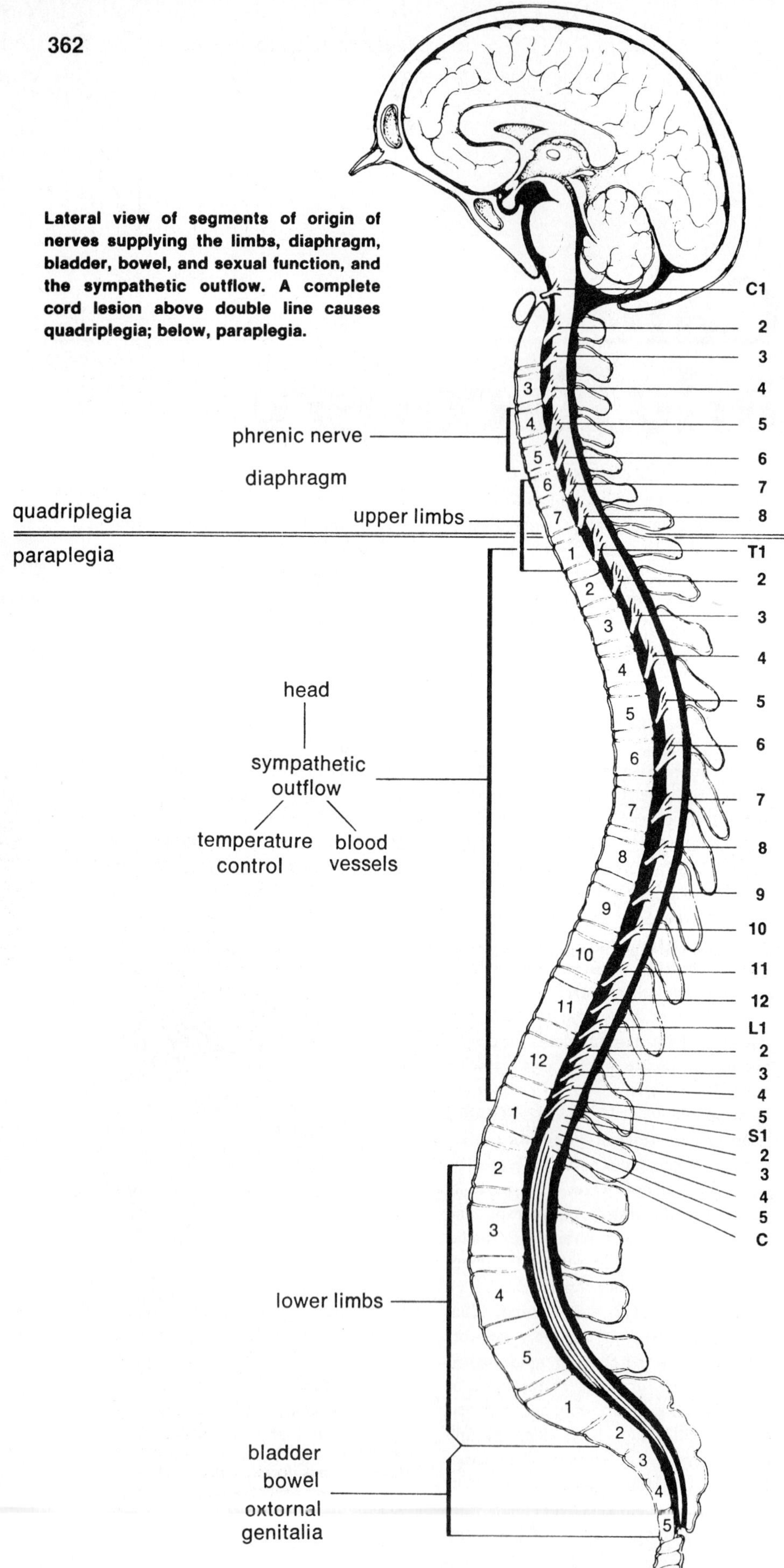

Lateral view of segments of origin of nerves supplying the limbs, diaphragm, bladder, bowel, and sexual function, and the sympathetic outflow. A complete cord lesion above double line causes quadriplegia; below, paraplegia.

However, efforts to prevent further neurological damage must be started along with the management of life-threatening injuries.

From the time of injury until the patient's spine has been immobilized, all transfers must avoid any movement, particularly flexion, of the spinal column.

Any person with a possible spinal injury, including all patients with head injuries, should be placed immediately on a rigid surface—a board, door, or table leaf. Transfer to this surface must be accomplished without flexing the spine. The patient should remain on the board until he arrives at the hospital unit where he will be cared for.

The only truly effective way to ensure that the patient's cervical spine is kept immobile is for a nurse or other responsible person to accompany him during all transfers, supporting his head to prevent flexion or extension, which might further traumatize the cord. Because the patient may have difficulty managing secretions in this position, suction equipment must be at hand to clear his airway and to prevent aspiration if he vomits.

If the person has sustained a cervical cord injury, a primary concern is the possible interruption of automatic respiration, secondary to lost or depressed innervation of the intercostal muscles, the diaphragm, or both. Weak or labored respirations or diaphragmatic breathing usually indicate the need for a tracheostomy. Endotracheal intubation is contraindicated as the need to hyperextend the neck while placing the tube could damage the cord further.

Because most spinal cord injuries are caused by accidents, the presence of severe wounds elsewhere in the body is a distinct possibility and should be investigated. Any hemorrhaging must be controlled immediately. If a frank bleed is not obvious and the patient does not have hemothorax, an abdominal tap usually is done to rule out that site. Intracranial hemorrhage is not sufficient to cause hypovolemic shock.

The management of fluid replacement is a difficult medical problem because the patient's shock with low blood pressure may be due to a frank bleed ((hypovolemic shock), to massive vasodilation secondary to the loss of

SCI - Physical Care

sympathetic tone caused by the cord injury (vasomotor shock), or to both bleeding and vasodilation(2).

Because the hypotension due to vasodilation usually is not severe enough to require support and because it is self-correcting over time, many physicians treat with fluid replacement, supplementing with steroid therapy.

Fluids extravasate from the microvasculature of the spinal cord within 30 minutes after it is injured. This edema, if allowed to run its full course, will cause local damage to the cord, called traumatic necrosis. Overhydration tends to exacerbate this condition. To prevent the edema responsible for traumatic necrosis, large doses of steroids may be administered.

A still-experimental method for reducing traumatic necrosis is to perfuse cold normal saline into the subarachnoid or epidural space. This produces local hypothermia of the cord(3,4).

Stabilization of Injury

After any life-threatening disorders have been controlled, the specific vertebral and cord injury is attended to. X-rays will help in determining the type of fracture. Basically, there are four types of spinal column injuries:

- *wedge or compression fracture*—the anterior portion of the vertebral body is compressed between the upper and lower vertebral bodies; posterior portion is intact and stable
- *burst fracture*—one or more intervertebral discs are forced through the end plate of the vertebrae by a vertical force on the whole spine
- *dislocation and rotational fracture dislocation*—one or more vertebrae are displaced or displaced and fractured by flexion and rotation of the spine or by a severe, direct, shearing force.

Dislocation and fracture dislocation are grossly unstable injuries because the ligament complex, which gives stability to the spine, is severed. They are the injuries that most often damage the

Flexion Injuries

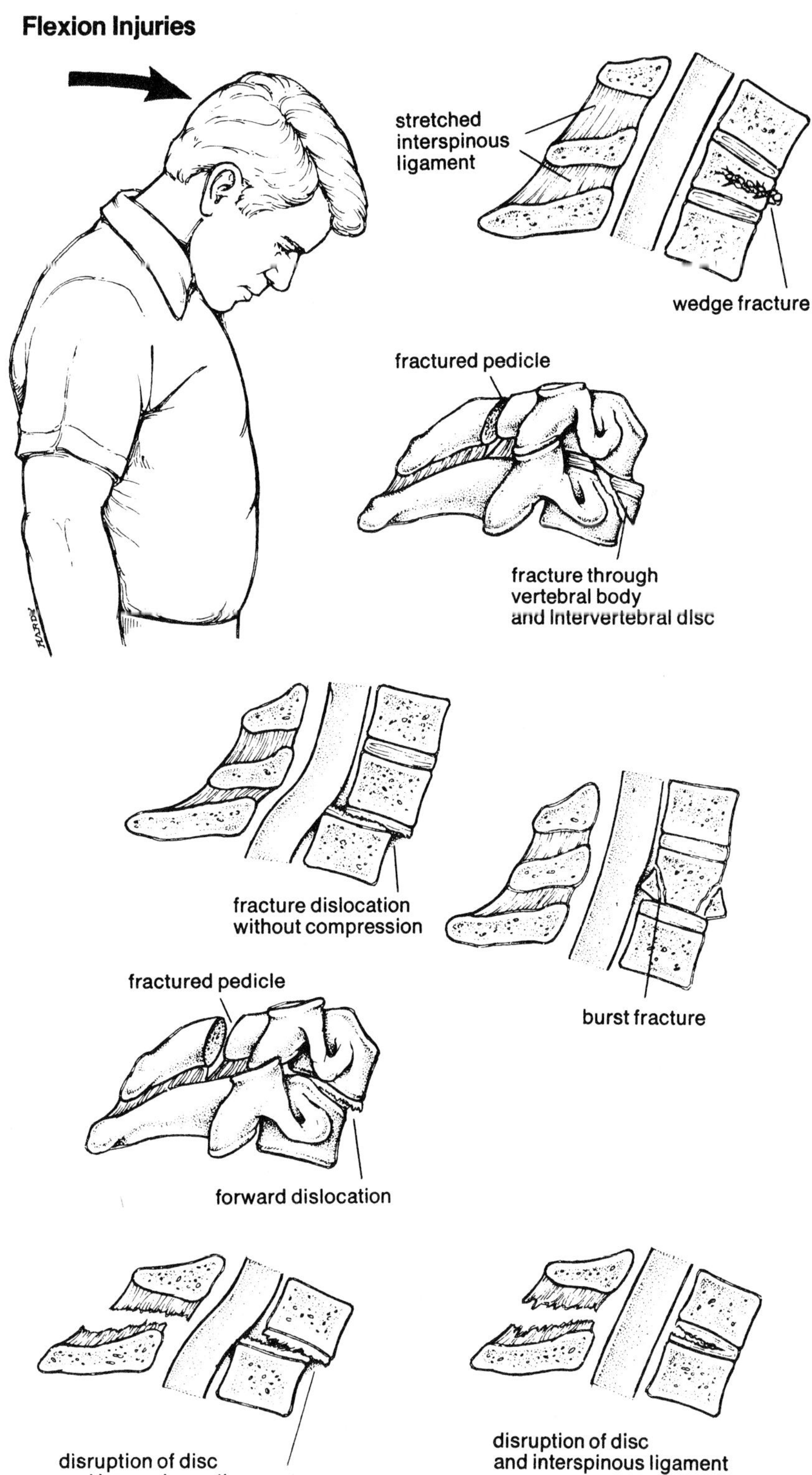

Rotation with Flexion Injury

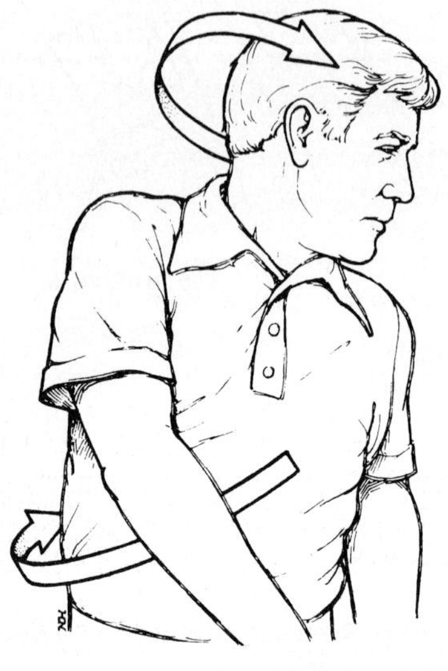

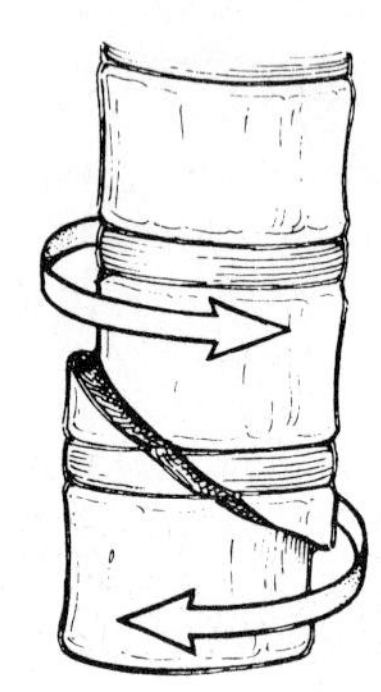

displacement of vertebrae with fracture of 2 vertebral bodies and 1 disc

Lateral Flexion Injury

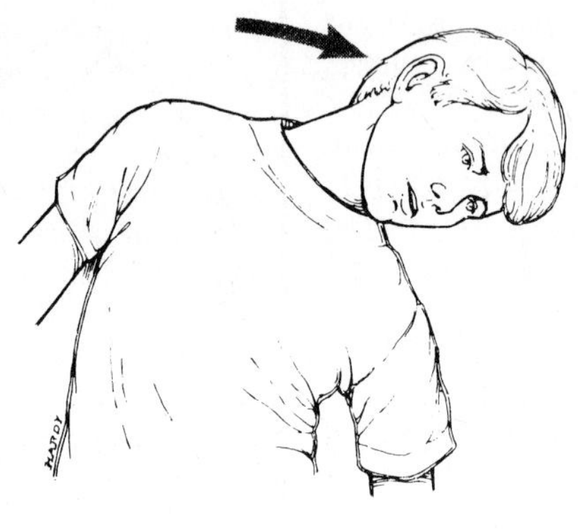

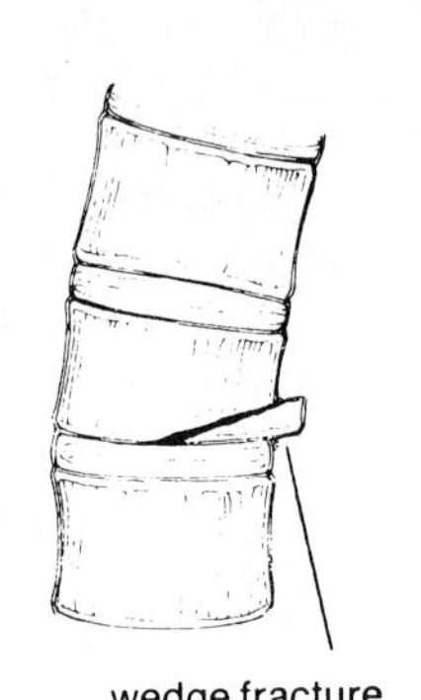

wedge fracture of vertebral body

Vertical Compression Injury

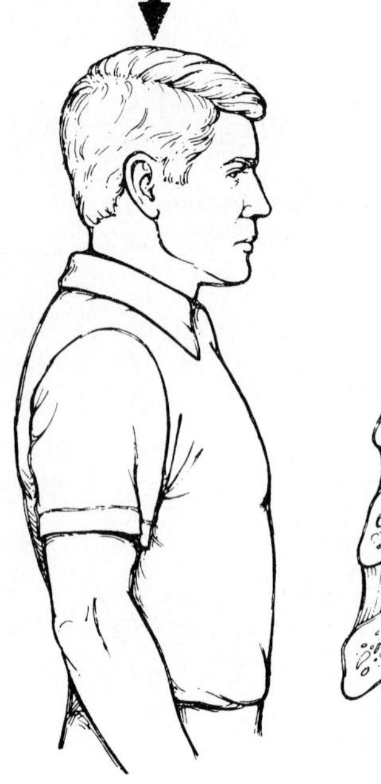

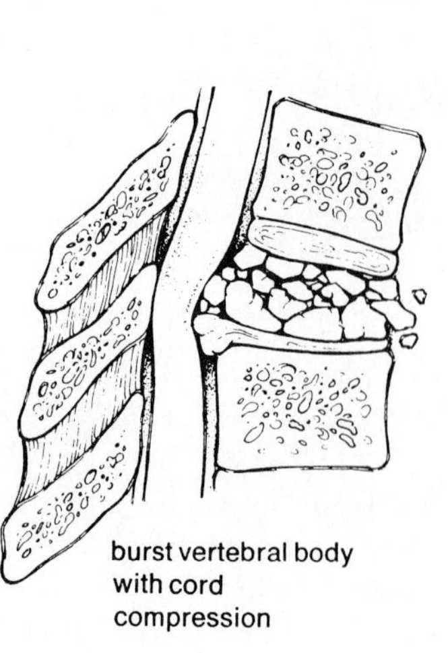

burst vertebral body with cord compression

Hyperextension Injury

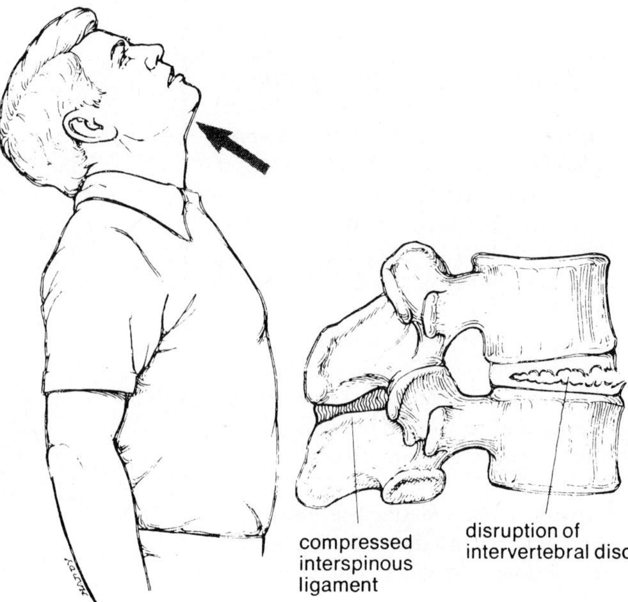

SCI - Physical Care

spinal cord and nerve roots, with resulting neurological deficit. Injudicious movement of the patient can increase the pressure of the vertebral body or bony fragments on the spinal cord and change an incomplete lesion, which damages part of the cord, into a complete lesion, which damages most or all of the cord.

Whether the physician uses medical or surgical treatment depends on the stability or instability of the spinal column injury and on the possibility that bone fragments are compressing the cord. If cord compression is a possibility, a decompression laminectomy may be necessary, particularly if the neurological deficit becomes progressively worse. Decompression laminectomy also would be indicated if an increase in neurological loss was accompanied by evidence of blockage of the cerebrospinal fluid, such as a positive Queckenstedt sign.

To test for this sign, a lumbar puncture may be done and the CSF pressure determined. The patient's internal jugular veins are then compressed manually and changes in CSF pressure observed. Normally, pressure rises with jugular compression and returns to normal when it is released. Absence of this response indicates a block in the circulation of CSF.

The Queckenstedt test would be omitted if the patient had a concomitant head injury and a possibly elevated CSF pressure, because of the risk that brain tissue might herniate into the foramen magnum.

If the fracture is stable, the patient can be treated medically by stabilization of the spine with Crutchfield tongs or a halo body cast. The patient with Crutchfield tongs has to remain in bed for six to eight weeks, or until a stabilizing callus forms at the fracture site. A person wearing a halo body cast can be out of bed much sooner.

For an unstable fracture, surgical stabilization is required, by the placement of Harrington rods, by laminectomy and fusion, or by anterior fusion, in which the lamina are not encountered. The bone to be grafted is taken from the iliac crest, tibia, fibula, or ribs. About a week after such a procedure, the patient can be out of bed in a brace, which he will wear for three to four months(5-7).

ACUTE CARE

Once the nature of the spinal injury has been determined and the appropriate management begun, the patient can be placed on a hospital bed and transferred to the ICU. The bed must provide firm support and, if possible, some means of turning the patient. A CircOlectric, Stryker, Foster frame, Roto-rest, or regular hospital bed with bed boards may be used. An alternating pressure or a flotation mattress and pad should be put on the bed before the patient is placed on it.

The most obvious disability following SCI is paralysis of the extremities,

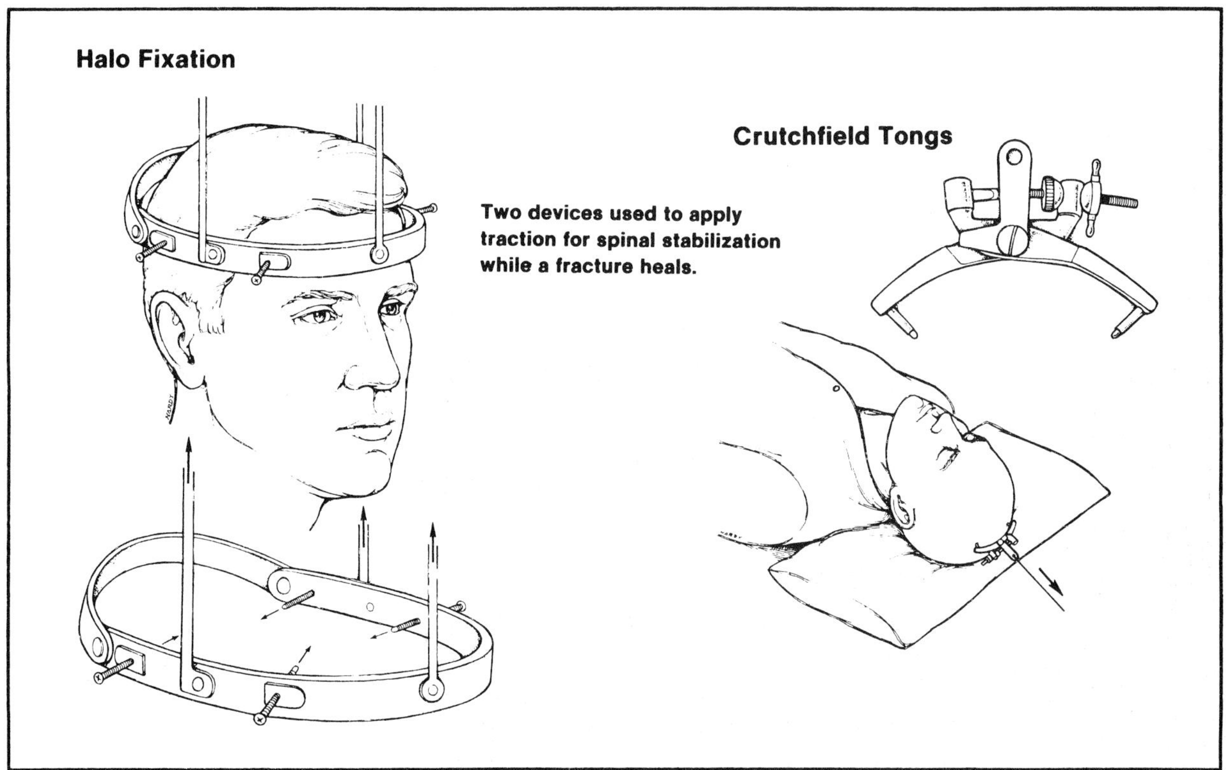

Two devices used to apply traction for spinal stabilization while a fracture heals.

but this is only one manifestation of the injury and not necessarily the chief threat to survival. Other disorders occur as direct or indirect results of neurological trauma. Some of these problems reflect disturbances of nervous system function; others are secondary to the trauma and are manifested by symptoms related to other body systems. Each disorder must be managed if the person is to survive.

Many problems during the acute phase are due to spinal shock and to edema surrounding the site of injury. Although they may be serious and even life-threatening at this time, the deficits caused by spinal shock are transient. Edema can cause permanent damage.

Spinal shock involves the complete or nearly complete suppression of all reflexes at all spinal segments below the level of injury. The suppression is caused by "jamming" of neurological mechanisms. It results in the loss of temperature control, vasomotor tone, and sweating, as well as in the retention of feces and urine. Jamming is caused by the sudden cessation of efferent impulses and by inadequate microcirculation to the cord.

Spinal shock and edema develop within 30 to 60 minutes postinjury. Therefore, a person who *gradually* loses neurological function after an accident has some chance of recovering at least partial function when spinal shock dissipates. Return of function is not due to regeneration. Any patient who eventually demonstrates an improvement in level of function had an incomplete or partial lesion that appeared to be complete because of spinal shock.

Spinal shock wears off any time from two weeks to two years after an accident; three months is average. Edema resolves more quickly if steroids and proper alignment are used. Because some patients do have a chance of regaining some neurological function, the nurse must ensure maintenance of straight spinal alignment until this occurs.

The antacid Maalox (magnesium and aluminum hydroxide) may be given by nasogastric tube or orally to prevent the development of stress ulcers secondary to high-dose steroid therapy and to the emotional impact of the injury.

Maintaining Respiratory Function The nature and extent of respiratory involvement depend on the level of the spinal cord lesion. The diaphragm and the intercostals are the major muscles of respiration. Impulses are delivered to the intercostals by spinal nerves in the thoracic segments of the cord. The diaphragm receives its motor impulses via the phrenic nerve, which arises from the cervical plexus (C1-C4). If a person has a cervical injury, intercostal muscle function is lost, along with the ability to cough and take a deep breath.

If the injury is at the level of the cord involving the phrenic nerve, or if posttraumatic edema extends involvement to that level, the person loses involuntary control of respiration. To maintain life, artificial respiration must be provided. Some patients require respirator assistance for the rest of their lives; others recover involuntary respiratory control, particularly if their loss of respiration was gradual and caused by cord edema.

Another consequence of SCI is a susceptibility to pneumonia. Some patients arrive on a nursing unit without a reliable history about possible aspiration after the SCI. The breath sounds of such patients should be auscultated at least every eight hours, more frequently if the nurse detects changes. The tendency to develop pneumonia continues and is related to the impairment of intercostal muscle function and to the patient's supine position while at bed rest. Paraplegics may develop pneumonia, but quadriplegics and patients with higher thoracic injuries are more prone to do so.

Pneumonia develops by the following mechanisms. When a person is in the upright position, the bronchioles are held open by the outward traction of negative intrapleural pressure. The supine position, on the other hand, causes the diaphragm to rise because of greater pressure from abdominal contents. The great vessels of the chest fill with blood and the negative pressure falls. This reduces the diameter of the bronchioles, increasing their tendency to be obstructed by mucus.

When the person is upright, mucus coats the walls of the bronchioles evenly; when the person is supine, gravity pulls the mucus to the dependent side of the bronchioles. The upper surface of the bronchiole dries out and may crack, providing a site for infection. The lower surface is covered with a pool of mucus, increasing the chances of a mucous obstruction.

Coupled with the narrowing of the bronchioles and the pooling of mucous secretions is the patient's inability to cough effectively, due to neurological deficit. These events predispose him to develop hypostatic pneumonia.

For these reasons, it is essential to prevent excessive drying or pooling of secretions. If the patient must be maintained on bed rest, it is crucial to turn him every two hours around the clock. He also should receive chest physiotherapy as soon as possible and be mobilized as soon as spinal stabilization has been accomplished.

Maintaining Hydration and Nutrition Adequate hydration and nutrition must be provided parenterally until the patient can eat and drink. Overhydration is avoided because it promotes traumatic necrosis of the cord in the early postinjury period. Not uncommonly, cord-injured patients have paralytic ileus, so they should be tolerating clear liquids before progressing to a regular diet.

Maintaining Elimination A major risk immediately after injury is the possibility of overdistention and rupture of the bladder. Spinal shock prevents the involuntary reflex emptying of the bladder in a person who has lost voluntary control. Catheterization to prevent overdistention must be done in the emergency room, then repeated until reflex functioning has returned and

SCI - Physical Care

bladder retraining has been accomplished. An indwelling catheter or intermittent catheterization are used to prevent overdistention.

INTERMEDIATE CARE

After the acute phase of SCI has passed and life-threatening disorders are controlled, attention is turned to preparing the patient for rehabilitation while preventing complications that might result from the neurological deficits and from prolonged bed rest.

Neurogenic Bowel and Bladder Despite specific antibiotic therapy, recurrent bladder infections and their sequelae are still the leading threat to the long-term survival of spinal-cord-injured persons. Intermittent (every eight hour) straight catheterization with aseptic technique is recommended. Research has shown that this method is far superior to indwelling catheter drainage in lowering the incidence of urinary tract infections(8-10).

Intermittent catheterization prevents the hazards of reflux of the urine accumulated in a drainage bag or tube, and the inevitable trauma at the meatus produced by indwelling catheters. Then, too, because an indwelling catheter keeps the bladder constantly empty rather than alternately stretched and contracted as in normal function, prolonged use of an indwelling catheter can lead to a contracted, atonic bladder that is not easily retrained. If the patient must wear an indwelling catheter, bladder atony can be prevented by instituting a regular clamping-unclamping routine.

Measures are taken to discourage bladder infection in persons with indwelling catheters. For example, the catheter and collection system should be changed every two weeks, and a closed system of drainage used, with no break, ever, in its connections.

Urine specimens are obtained through sampling ports or by needle-and-syringe aspiration if special ports are not available. Collection systems with a drip chamber are preferable, as these prevent backflow of urine from the bag into the tubing and, possibly, the bladder. The tubing is positioned to allow drainage by gravity and taped securely to prevent the trauma of traction on the urethra and bladder. The urinary meatus is cleaned at least twice daily with a povidone-iodine (Betadine) solution, and Betadine ointment is applied lightly.

To help prevent bladder infection and renal calculi, the patient is encouraged to drink at least 3,000 ml. of fluids daily. Drinking cranberry juice several times a day helps keep the urine acidic, which discourages bacterial growth and bladder stone formation. The consumption of such alkaline ash foods as orange juice and grapefruit juice should be avoided or at least limited.

During the period of spinal shock, bowel function is affected in much the same way as bladder function. There is no voluntary or involuntary elimination, so impactions can occur. Soap suds enemas or saline enemas must be given about every three days during this period, simply to wash out the bowel. As spinal shock dissipates, the patient begins to have reflex emptying of the bowel following a stimulus, such as a meal, abdominal effleurage, or light tugging on the pubic hair.

After spinal shock has dissipated, bowel function is stimulated by using stool softeners, abdominal massage, and glycerin or bisacodyl (Dulcolax) suppositories. If evacuation does not occur with this regimen, a small enema—sodium biphosphate and sodium phosphate (Fleet, Phospho-Soda)—may be required. Some SCI centers prefer that staff remove the fecal mass digitally. At this stage, soap suds enemas should be given only as a last resort, not routinely(11).

A record is kept to document evacuations and the aids used to accomplish them. At this time a bowel retraining program can be started, taking into consideration the person's preinjury bowel habits(11-13).

Bladder and bowel as well as sexual function are innervated through S 2-4 (the sacral micturition center). During the period of spinal shock, there is no voluntary or reflex activity because both the upper and lower motor neurons are affected.

The upper motor neuron consists of the motor cell body in the cerebral cortex and its axon in the descending motor pathway (the pyramidal tract or corticospinal tract) to its synapse with the anterior horn cell in the spinal cord. Interruption of this neuron disrupts regulation by higher nervous system centers and leads to reflex activity.

The lower motor neuron consists of the anterior horn cell in the spinal cord and its efferent motor axon to its synapse with peripheral cells. Interruption of the lower motor neuron disrupts reflex activity *at the level of the lesion.* If the spinal cord lesion is above the sacral micturition center (S 2-4), reflex activity of bowel, bladder, and sex organs may occur after spinal shock resolves. For example, if the lesion is cervical, thoracic, or high lumbar, a man may have reflex penile erection after spinal shock has passed. Some may even attain reflex ejaculation.

A lesion above the sacral micturition center results in reflex urination, and the bladder is called an "upper motor neuron" or "automatic" bladder. If the lesion is at the level of the sacral micturition center, the reflex arc is disrupted, no reflex activity can occur, and the results are a "lower motor neuron" or "autonomous" bladder and bowel. Any functioning is merely the organ's response to filling, and consists of weak, asynchronous, incomplete contraction.

The lower motor neuron, or asynchronous, bladder or bowel cannot be retrained. A person with automatic bowel, bladder, and sexual function, on the other hand, is more likely to experience some success with retraining.

Skin and Musculoskeletal Complications Septicemia secondary to decubitus ulcers is another threat to the patient's long-term survival. These ulcers can be prevented through conscien-

Posturing the Patient to Prevent Decubitus Ulcers

SUPINE **Distribute body weight evenly, align correctly, and prevent pressure on bony prominences and genitalia (males) by placing patient on firm pillows or foam cushions (2″-4″ thick depending on body weight). Support feet in dorsiflexion with padded footboard, bolster, or sandbags, with heels off mattress.**

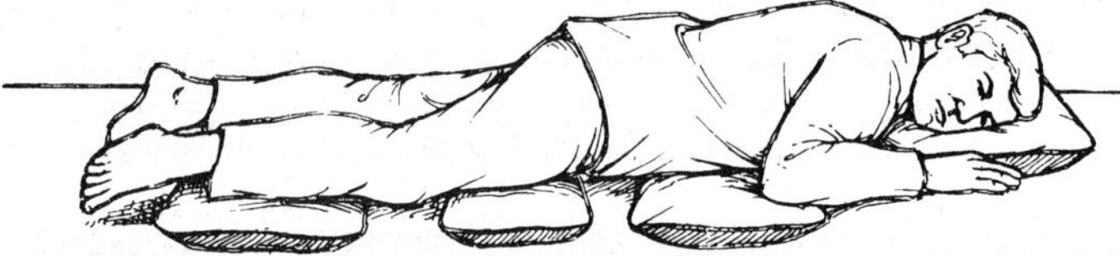

PRONE **Arrange cushions to prevent or decrease pressure on insteps, toes, knees, genitalia, iliac crests, ribs, and the female breasts. Encourage face lying as patient's condition permits.**

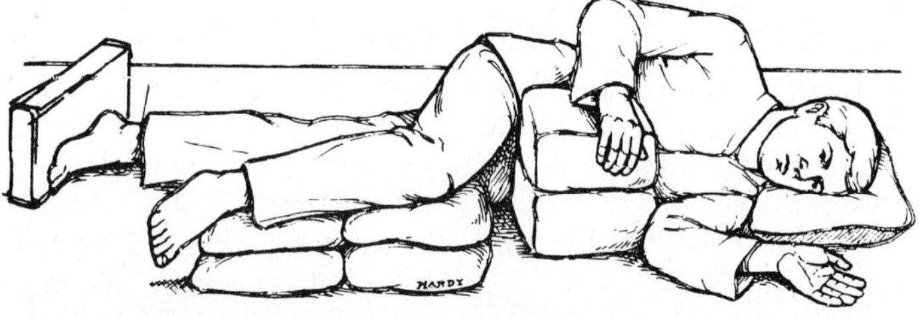

SIDE LYING **Support upper extremities on firm, double pillows to prevent overstretching shoulder and hip muscles. Place lower leg in slight hyperextension, flat on bed, with foot supported at right angle to leg, and malleolus protected. Usually, no back support is needed if the patient has been correctly postured.**

Suggested by Nicholas F. Saverine, L.P.N., New Jersey

tious nursing care. The greatest contributor to decubitus ulcers in any patient is prolonged pressure, especially over bony prominences.

For the spinal-cord-injured patient, who cannot move in bed, pressure is a special problem. His paresthesias or sensory losses prevent him from feeling the discomfort that prolonged pressure causes, so he does not recognize the need to be turned. Also, circulation to all areas below the level of the spinal lesion, including the skin, is decreased by the depressed autonomic nervous system function and decreased muscle tone.

Bedfast patients are in a metabolic state of catabolism, in which body cells break down faster than they cán be built. This means that the nitrogen balance is negative rather than positive. Consequently, if the SCI patient develops a decubitus ulcer, it is difficult to heal. Prevention is imperative.

The best way to prevent prolonged pressure is to turn the patient frequently and mobilize him as soon as possible. The *maximum* time any paralyzed person should stay in the same position is two hours. Beyond that time, irreversible changes may take place in the integrity of the dependent tissues. If the patient in Crutchfield tongs and traction is on a turning bed or frame, the nurse's task is simplified. If the patient is on a regular hospital bed with bed boards and an alternating pressure mattress, turning him is more difficult but no less important.

Before changing the patient's position for the *first* time, the nurse must verify with the physician the amount and extent of turning that are safe. These limits are communicated to all personnel involved in changing the patient's position. If he cannot be turned at all, even more diligence is required to prevent skin breakdown. Skin care can be given by depressing the mattress with one hand and applying massage with the other. Particular care is taken to keep the back relatively dry, because excessive moisture will macerate the skin.

Turning also helps maintain adequate respiration, facilitates drainage of urine from the kidneys into the ureters, and provides an opportunity to carry the patient's limbs through their range of motion. When positioning the patient, the nurse aligns the extremities carefully.

A footboard is used to prevent footdrop; splints to prevent wristdrop, and the feet positioned so that the heels do not rest on the mattress. While the patient is on his side, his upper arm and leg are supported on pillows to prevent overstretching of muscles. If the patient receives adequate attention to joint mobility during the intermediate phase of care, he can progress more rapidly into the rehabilitation phase.

Muscle spasms that may be strong enough to cause violent contracture of the limbs and trunk often develop after

SCI - Physical Care

spinal shock dissipates. Spasticity occurs only when lower motor neurons are intact. The higher the cord injury, the more lower motor neurons remain intact and the greater the body area involved in spasms. In one study, all patients with cervical-cord injury had spasms; 75-80 percent with thoracic cord lesions had spasms, and 44 percent with lumbar lesions had spasms(15).

Spasm occurs spontaneously or in response to such external or internal stimuli as pressure of bed clothing, a decubitus ulcer, tight shoes or clothing, ill-fitting braces, renal calculi, and range of motion exercises. Whatever the stimulus, it causes the lower motor neuron to fire impulses that result in contraction of skeletal muscles. The normal dampening control from the cerebellum and brainstem structures has no influence over these lower motor neurons below the level of the spinal cord lesion, so impulses for muscle contraction continue to be fired for a prolonged period, often until the stimulus is identified and removed.

Mild spasticity can benefit the patient. It helps prevent disuse atrophy of muscles and osteoporosis, and may aid in maintaining trunk posture. Extensor spasticity of the legs allows for weight bearing. If the spasticity is severe, however, its detrimental effects far exceed its benefits. Severe spasticity can make it difficult to stay in a wheelchair or even in bed. Reflex resistance to passive ROM exercises causes stiffness of the extremities and trunk, and interferes with proper positioning and, later, with vocational rehabilitation.

Although strong spasms often subside when the offending stimulus is removed, in many patients spasticity increases, and may prevent participation in their rehabilitation programs. No antispasmodic drug controls spasticity without impairing mental functions, so other medical or surgical means must be employed. These include rhizotomy, cordectomy, and subarachnoid alcohol or phenol blocks.

Such procedures obliterate or sharply decrease lower motor neuron function. Therefore they are used only after the patient has considered the alternatives. If he decides to keep the spasticity, his activities will be hindered greatly. If he eliminates spasticity, he will sacrifice those activities that the intact lower motor neurons allowed him to have. Among those activities are reflex bowel, bladder, and sexual function(16).

Metabolic Disturbances Research has demonstrated that the stress of trauma and surgical procedures stimulates an overproduction of adrenocortical hormones(14). One result is the conservation of fat and glucose while protein stores are used for energy. The breakdown of large amounts of amino acids for energy produces a negative nitrogen balance. This leads to anemia, loss of muscle mass, decreased healing power, and lowered resistance to infection. Routine analysis of blood-nitrogen and urine-nitrogen levels will indicate whether nitrogen intake and depletion are balanced. If nitrogen balance becomes negative, the patient should be placed on a high protein diet with protein supplements.

Experts disagree on the desirability of encouraging milk as a protein supplement. Some believe milk should be urged during the intermediate phase of recovery, to combat nitrogen depletion. Others restrict or prohibit milk and milk products, because their high calcium content may contribute to renal calculus formation. After the SCI patient is eating a regular diet and has progressed to a specialized rehabilitation program (beyond the acute and intermediate phases of recovery), milk consumption usually is sharply restricted(17).

Another major metabolic change related to immobility is the absorption of calcium from the bones into the circulatory system, which occurs in the absence of weight bearing. Decalcification causes two complications: (a) pathological fracture or increased susceptibility to fracture under minimal trauma, and (b) the formation of renal calculi(18). As soon as the patient's spine is stabilized, physical therapy should be started with tilt-table exercises to provide for some weight bearing.

Managing Autonomic Nervous System Disturbances These are most common in patients with injuries in the cervical or thoracic cord. Such disturbances may be manifested by flushing, occasional mild headaches, and goose pimples. All are caused by marked sympathetic stimulation. Sweating may constitute a major problem, by its presence or its absence.

Excessive sweating, besides being uncomfortable, can endanger the patient's health, especially if he is exposed to drafts. Sweating usually can be controlled by various drugs of the atropine group, but extreme sweating may require sympathectomy. Excessive sweating may diminish over a period of years.

Absence of sweating disturbs the patient's thermoregulatory mechanism, particularly in extremely hot weather. Because patients who cannot sweat cannot release excess body heat, they need closely regulated environmental temperatures(19).

The most serious manifestation of autonomic dysfunction is the alternations in blood pressure that may occur. *Postural hypotension*—a fall in blood pressure when the patient moves from a horizontal to a vertical position—results from depressed sympathetic control over blood-vessel contractility.

When light-headedness or syncope occurs, the patient must be returned to the horizontal position immediately. Vasopressor drugs may be required to support the blood pressure following such an episode. Postural hypotension and syncope can be prevented by using support hose and by raising the patient very gradually on a tilt table to a vertical position.

Autonomic dysreflexia (hyperreflexia or pressor reflex) is a rise in blood pressure to uncomfortable, sometimes fatal, levels. It is a medical emergency. Hyperreflexia is a reflex response to stimulation of the sympathetic nervous system. If the stimulus is not removed, the blood pressure continues to rise. The normal dampening control over such reflex activity is located in higher centers of the central nervous system, which cannot influence areas below the level of the spinal cord lesion.

Most often, the stimulus responsible for autonomic dysreflexia is a distended bladder or rectum, but it can be spasticity, decubitus ulcers, infection of the bladder, chilling, or even pressure on the skin. Symptoms include extremely severe headache, paroxysmal hypertension, bradycardia, profuse sweating, flushing, pilo-erection, and nasal congestion. Immediate intervention is necessary to avert a cerebrovascular accident(19).

The cycle of stimulus-response must be broken by removing the stimulus, administering a ganglionic-blocking agent, or both. The nurse's first intervention is to check the patient's bladder for distention; second, to catheterize the bladder if it is distended or to irrigate the indwelling catheter, if present, to clear it and allow the bladder to empty(20). If symptoms are not alleviated promptly by such measures, the intravenous administration of a ganglionic-blocking agent like hexamethonium. chloride may be necessary. Once the stimulus has been identified, efforts are made to prevent future episodes. If the stimuli are too numerous to eliminate, the patient may require daily maintenance with hexamethonium chloride, or surgical intervention as described for the elimination of spasms.

Autonomic hyperreflexia rarely occurs until after spinal shock has subsided and usually is first seen when the patient enters an active rehabilitation program. Unlike postural hypotension, autonomic hyperreflexia does not tend to correct itself over time. It is such a constant problem for some patients that the reflex arc must be interrupted surgically.

Emotional Support The nursing care to aid the patient's emotional adjustment is discussed in detail in the following article. Briefly, the emotional adjustment faced by a spinal-cord-injured person parallels the grief experience of those who have lost a loved one.

The injured person needs to recognize and come to accept the loss or "death" of portions of his previous self-image before he can begin to establish a new self-image. Lindemann has described the grieving process as consisting of stages, including initial realization, denial, realization, anger and dismay, and acceptance(21). The literature indicates that denial is the stage of grief at which many SCI patients become fixed during the acute and intermediate care periods(22). A healthy emotional adjustment cannot occur unless the person goes through all stages of the grieving process. The nurse supports the patient as he adjusts—a process that may take months to years—and is careful not to "push" him faster than he can progress.

Immediately following injury, the patient is overwhelmed by the personal and social implications of the lost body functions. Often, the patient copes by denying that the injury happened or that it is permanent.

Denial, the second step the paralyzed person must go through in the grieving process, is a normal reaction. Most patients believe that they eventually will recover completely. They tend to think that their early rehabilitation efforts are not very important —that time will work miracles. Because denial is a defense mechanism, health personnel must be careful not to strip the patient of this means of coping until he is able to deal with reality.

When the patient moves from denial in the grieving process, he faces, once again, all the implications of his loss. The normal emotional reaction is anger, then despair. The person may send out "SOS" signals to relatives, friends, or hospital personnel. It is essential, during this time, that the staff and family help the patient recognize that they consider him worthwhile and "good" despite his loss. Over time, these efforts can help the patient reassess his values, changing some, adding or dropping others, as he develops a self-image that reflects and emphasizes his essential worth rather than his status as a disabled person.

References

1. ABRAMSON, A. S. Modern concepts of management of the patient with spinal cord injury. *Arch.Phys.Med.Rehabil.* 48:113-121, Mar. 1967.
2. MCKIBBEN, B., AND BROTHERTON, B. J. The early management of cervical spine injuries. *Resuscitation* 2:245, Dec. 1973.
3. OSTERHOLM, J. L. The pathophysiological response to spinal cord injury. *J.Neurosurg.* 40:7-9,23-25, Jan 1974.
4. NEGRIN, JUAN, JR. Spinal cord hypothermia in the acute and chronic post-traumatic paraplegic patient. *Paraplegia* 10:336-343, Feb. 1973.
5. BEDBROOK, G. M. Pathological principles in the management of spinal cord trauma. *Paraplegia* 4:43-56, May 1966 .
6. LUSSKIN, RALPH, AND PENA, ARTURO. Orthopedic management of transverse myelopathies. *NY J.Med.* 68:2046-2049, Aug. 1, 1968.
7. ALPERS, B. J. *Clinical Neurology.* 5th ed. Philadelphia, F. A. Davis Co., 1963, p. 359.
8. GUTTMANN, L. Statistical survey of one thousand paraplegics. *Proc.R.Soc.Med.* 47:1,101, June 19, 1954.
9. BORS, E. Intermittent catheterization in paraplegic patients. *Urologia Internationalis* 22:236-249, 1967.
10. TALBOT, H. S. Pathogenesis of renal infection in spinal cord injury. *Paraplegia* 7:101-110, Aug. 1969.
11. ROSSIER, A. B. Rehabilitation of the spinal cord injury patient. *Documenta Geigy:Acta Clinica.* No. 3, North American Series, 1963.
12. CORNELL, S. A., AND OTHERS. Comparison of three bowel management programs. *Nurs.Res.* 22:321-328, July-Aug. 1973.
13. TALBOT, H. S. Adjunctive care of the spinal cord injury. *Surg.Clin.North Am.* 48:754-755, Aug. 1968.
14. GUYTON, A. C. *Textbook of Medical Physiology.* 3d ed., Phila., Pa., W.B. Saunders, 1967, pp. 1055-1056.
15. RUGE, DANIEL. *Spinal Cord Injuries.* Springfield, Ill., Charles C Thomas, Publisher, 1969, pp. 148-152.
16. HIRSCHBERG, G. G., AND OTHERS. *Rehabilitation.* 2nd ed., Phila., Pa., J. B. Lippincott Co., 1976, pp. 286-288.
17. KRAUSE, M. V., AND HUNSCHER, M. A. *Food, Nutrition and Diet Therapy.* 5th ed., Phila., Pa., W.B. Saunders, 1972, pp. 324-325.
18. BROWSE, N. L. *The Physiology and Pathology of Bedrest.* Springfield- Ill., Charles C Thomas, Publisher, 1965, pp. 95-96.
19. RUGE, DANIEL. *op.cit.* pp. 110-113, 133.
20. FEUSTEL, DELYCIA. Autonomic hyperreflexia. *Am.J.Nurs.* 76:228, Feb. 1976.
21. LINDEMANN, ERICH. Symptomatology and management of acute grief. *Am.J. Psychiatry* 101:143, Sept. 1944.
22. NAGLER, BENEDICT. Psychiatric aspects of cord injury. *Am.J.Psychiatry* 107: 49-56, July 1950.

The Person with a Spinal Cord Injury

Psychological Care

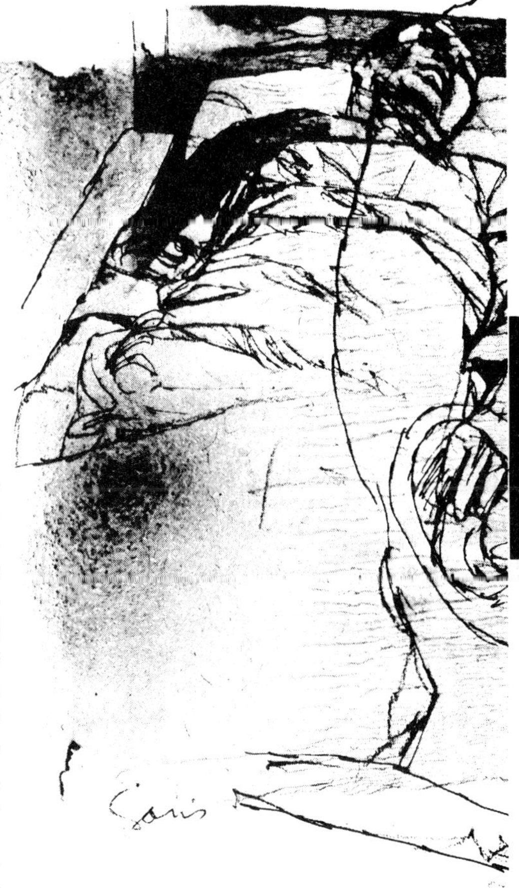

Correlating the emotional adjustments of the severely injured person with the developmental tasks of the infant, child, and adolescent may help nurses understand the disabled person's often perplexing behavior.

GINETTE A. PEPPER

Persons who become physically disabled from a sudden catastrophe, such as paralysis or loss of a limb after an accident, experience intense psychological reactions. The abrupt, overwhelming onset of the disability prevents the gradual development of awareness and acceptance that disorders with a slower onset may allow.

The variety and intensity of the patient's emotional reactions, coupled with the nurse's personal and culturally determined attitudes toward the deformed and disabled, may challenge the nurse's perceptions of her professional competence, and lead to frustration, anger, or avoidance.

"I feel terrible after I take care of him," a nurse said of a quadriplegic patient. "I can't even begin to meet his needs."

Nurses in rehabilitation centers can rely on an established approach to care that emphasizes patient independence, an approach that usually succeeds. However, in acute care hospitals as well as in rehabilitation centers, several important questions arise: What are the ranges of normal behavior following sudden catastrophic injury? Is the emphasis on independence appropriate at all times during the postinjury course? If not, how does the nurse determine when to alter her approach?

The theoretical model presented here proposes that a similarity exists between the psychosocial developmental stages postulated by Erikson and the adjustment phases experienced by patients who suddenly become paralyzed or severely disfigured. The model is based on the assumption that there is a natural regression and an obligatory reworking of some previously surmounted developmental tasks, namely, the first three stages described by Erikson.

Although the assumption that regression is normal or even requisite is far from universally accepted, much evidence supports the assumption. The dependent position into which the necessarily intense medical and nursing care places a severely injured person, as well as the devastating impact of the injury, demand a realignment of self-concept and body image.

Regression may allow the person time to reintegrate his ego in light of his new body image and curtailed abilities, then to align with a new social identity as a member of the disabled minority, and, finally, to form new expectations for himself.

Correlating this process with the psychosocial development process described by Erikson and others(1,2) accounts for many of the behaviors nurses see as they care for disabled patients, and begins to answer many questions about dependence and independence. Also, a valid theoretical model may aid in reducing the nurse's uncertainty about her ability to help a patient who is adjusting to severe disability, thereby reinforcing rather than threatening her feelings of competence.

Erikson's psychosocial stages are based on the psychosexual phases identified by Freud. The stages follow the epigenetic principle which maintains that psychosocial progress re-

GINETTE PEPPER, R.N., M.S., a senior instructor at the University of Colorado School of Nursing, Denver, has practiced as staff and head nurse in several orthopedic/neurologic units. She coauthored "Geriatric Nurse Practitioner in Nursing Homes," *AJN*, Jan., 1976.

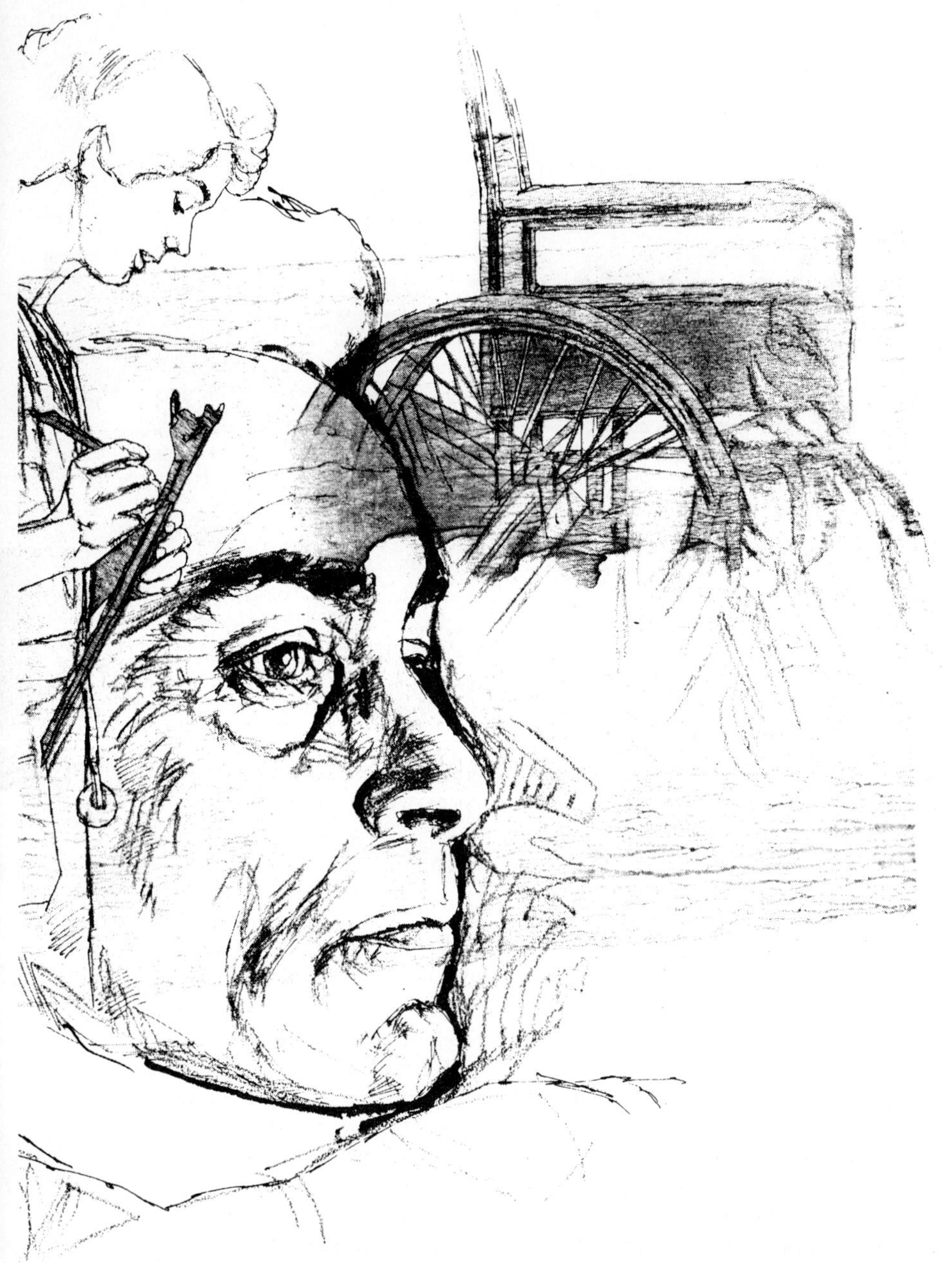

quires a person to surmount the critical task of each developmental phase at the proper time and in the proper sequence.

For each of eight phases, Erikson postulated a psychosocial task, expressed as a dichotomy (for example, a sense of basic trust or a sense of mistrust in the oral stage). The overall personality is determined by a favorable ratio of one to the other; but in each person the negative sense continues to exist as a dynamic counterpart of the positive sense.

Erikson related each "crisis," or dichotomy, to an ego strength, an organ mode, and a psychopathology (see table). The "eight ages of man," from birth to old age, are basic trust versus mistrust; autonomy vs. shame and doubt; initiative vs. guilt; industry vs. inferiority; identity vs. role confusion; intimacy vs. isolation; generativity vs. stagnation; and ego integrity vs. despair.

This discussion is limited to the first three crises, for several reasons. First, the person who sustains a catastrophic injury usually is an adolescent or young adult. Consequently, he may not have surmounted more than the third or fourth task at the onset of the disability. Second, more is known about early adjustment to such injuries, as indicated by the relative emphasis on this period in the literature. Finally, except for occasional encounters with community-based nurses, these people seldom interact with nurses after mastering the first three developmental stages following injury. As a result, there is little case material to draw on in explaining these persons' progress through later stages.

Trust: The First Task. The infant's need and ability to take in by mouth become the focus of the first approach to life, the *incorporative* approach. Initially, the pattern is receptive incorporation, not only of food but of other stimuli, through the senses. Later, the child becomes more assertive in seeking stimuli. To gain a sense of trust, the infant must have his needs met fairly readily and consistently, and must have an expectation that they will continue to be met. When this occurs, he gains a sense of outer predictability and a recognition that there is a corresponding inner certainty of remembered and anticipated sensations and images. These result in a basic sense of his own trustworthiness.

If an infant's needs are sporadically met, he may never experience the necessary consistency and constancy, and therefore may grow to mistrust others and himself. Temporal organization and willingness to let the mother out of his sight are important achievements of this stage.

Mahler postulates a period of *normal autism* in the newborn infant, when the primary task is maintaining inner homeostasis and he is shielded naturally against the bombardment of external stimuli. During the next period, which Mahler calls *normal symbiosis,* the child becomes aware that nurture comes from outside himself, and regards himself and his mother as one. It is the mother who screens the external stimuli at this stage.

SCI - Psychological Care

Immediately following the sudden onset of disability, the patient is acutely ill and in a situation analogous to the infant's. He receives all therapy from others, including medication, intravenous infusion, oxygen, respiratory assistance, and frequent position changes. His relationship to his environment becomes literally incorporative. The physical limitations, the restrictions imposed by therapy, and the overwhelming psychological assault combine to enforce dependence. Camille Cayler, a psychiatrist who became paraplegic following an accident, stated:

The first phase is dominated by severe bodily discomfort, shock, confusion, excitement. The patient suddenly becomes the center of worried attention of doctors, family and friends. This may provide him with some narcissistic gratification and draw his attention away from the outside world, the tragic consequences of his disability, and the difficult future. . . . Because of psychological traumata, and dependency on others . . . the patient's ego has, as a rule, been weakened. Because he cannot take care of himself physically he regresses to the position of a child not only physically but also psychologically. His dependency on the hospital, where he literally has to repeat the training procedures of his childhood, fosters much emotional regression. (3)

During this initial shock period, the patient is protected from external stimuli much as an infant is protected. Each has the major task of establishing or reestablishing homeostasis. Several researchers have documented a dissociation from self and the development of infantile thought patterns. Studies of persons with spinal cord injury and poliomyelitis have revealed that patients have a tendency toward immature emotional behavior, including impulsive, egocentric explosiveness; ambivalence; and a tendency to think autistically about future problems(4,5).

A patient implied this in describing her reactions during the acute phase: "I had a peculiar inability to identify myself with my name; we didn't come together, my name and I." Noreen Linduska wrote of her experience in the acute stage of polio, "Something happened and I became a stranger. I was a greater stranger to myself than to anyone"(6). This absence of ego boundaries, comparable to the situation of the infant who has not yet defined his, may allow the patient to form a symbiotic relationship with the nurse until he is again able to cope.

After the initial shock, the patient becomes more aware of his environment. This contributes multiple stimuli that are meaningless to anyone unfamiliar with hospital equipment and routines, and the patient must begin to organize them. In an intensive care unit, where there often are no windows and the activity level is always high, it is difficult for the patient to gain temporal organization(7). The incorporative relationship becomes less receptive and the patient begins to indicate his needs more aggressively as he becomes less acutely ill.

Nursing Implications

Independence is *not* a realistic goal during this stage, but neither should the goal of nursing care be to maintain dependence. Rather, the primary goal is to establish the *dependability* and *consistency* of nursing care. Dependence is caused and maintained by the physical and psychological assault. Purposefully consistent nursing care helps the patient acquire a sense of trust in the nurse and in himself—the foundation for successful rehabilitation.

In responding to the patient's serious and often labile condition, the nurse constantly and regularly meets his physical needs through observation, hygiene and nutrition measures, and the alleviation of discomfort. These very actions also help to satisfy his psychological needs.

During this early period, the patient rarely initiates futuristic discussion of sexual and vocational adjustment, and it is rarely appropriate for the nurse to begin such a discussion or to feel that she is not providing an accepting atmosphere if the patient does not do so. Similarly, the patient should not be forced to perform all the self-care which he appears to be physically able to perform. As the patient gains a sense of trust, he will assume these responsibilities. The nurse offers him opportunities to perform these tasks as he is ready.

Mathews demonstrated the importance of consistency in care of the quadriplegic(8). Designating one nurse to provide care helps ensure a constant approach. However, the approach must be consistent among shifts and when the designated nurse has a day off. This underlines the need for written care plans and intra- and intershift conferences.

The professional nurse is best qualified to deal with the complex needs of these patients and to plan care based on accurate assessment of their psychological adjustment, but this may not always be feasible outside the ICU. Regardless of the setting, it remains the nurse's responsibility to understand thoroughly the patient's physical and emotional status, to ascertain if care is effective, and to reinforce and support those who provide the care. Although it is best that the nurse give the actual care, especially during the early period, one indication of the patient's developing sense of trust is the ease with which he accepts less attention from the nurse and more attention from other members of the staff.

As the shock wears off and the patient becomes aware of the environment, screening and interpreting the many stimuli which bombard him become important nursing functions. Clocks, calendars, and familiar personal items encourage temporal perspective and reality orientation. Family members, too, need to be included in the care, and their part in each phase of adjustment must be explained. The experience of C.M. demonstrates the importance of the development of trust and temporal organization.

C.M., a 17-year-old female, sustained a head injury in a motorcycle accident. Ultimately this resulted in left hemiparesis with severe spasticity and motor aphasia. Tests revealed that her intelligence level was essentially unchanged despite a long period of unconsciousness during her stay in a neurological ICU. On transfer to the rehabilitation unit shortly after she regained consciousness, C.M. showed extreme regression. A nurse began to work with C.M. and her family.

Initially, C.M. covered her head with a blanket when anyone approached. She confused day and night, and responded to questions or discomfort with a piercing wail. The nurse began by telling C.M. how long the visit would last, and sat quietly beside the bed. On leaving, she said when she would return. Family members did the same.

After several days, C.M. came out from under the blanket and grasped the nurse's hand. The staff then began to interpret and explain daily routines and expectations to her. Her eating and sleeping patterns became normal after two weeks, but she continued to be easily frustrated and lacked restraint in expression. At first she ignored her disability, but did permit therapy. After C.M. noted her deformed hand, she tried to persuade everyone to exercise it, often refusing therapy to her other extremities. Ultimate rehabilitation was considered very successful because C.M. was employed one year later.

When the patient begins to express his needs more assertively, staff may be annoyed that this person, in whom they have invested so much care, has become difficult to satisfy. The staff's response is often negativism and avoidance or a demand that the patient assume more independence in self-care.

Unfortunately, just at this time, when aggressiveness corresponds with improved physical condition, the patient often is transferred to a different unit. Here, he meets a new staff whom he is uncertain about, and the staff meets a demanding and testing patient whom they do not understand and tend to avoid.

This avoidance further threatens the patient. Nursing care should continue to emphasize consistency, which not only reaffirms the patient's sense of trust in others and himself but also sets limits that provide predictability in the new environment. Until trust and predictability have been established, emphasis on independence is still premature.

The patient whose needs are met consistently develops a hope for successful rehabilitation. If he finds that he must often wait for care, he develops behaviors indicating a lack of trust and he may be unable to move on from dependence. He may despair or express unrealistic hope, such as the expectation of complete recovery. L.H. was a patient who maintained extreme overdependence, based on a lack of trust.

A leader in family, church, and community, L.H., aged 46 and father of five, sustained a spinal cord injury at work. On admission, he had no motion or sensation below C-6 (quadriplegia). Because the census was low in the ICU, he received much attention from staff.

On transfer to a busy orthopedic ward, L.H. became demanding, required many hours to be bathed or fed, and was uncomfortable if not turned at least every hour—a difficult task due to his large size.

No staff member could care for anyone in the room without constant interruption, and most staff began to avoid L.H. Finally, he demanded the total attention of a nurse, refusing care from

ERIKSON'S PSYCHOSOCIAL STAGES*

Psychosexual Stage	*Organ Mode*	*Psychosocial Stage*	*Rudimentary Ego Strength*	*Relation to Psychopathology*
oral sensory cutaneous	incorporative	basic trust vs. basic mistrust	hope	addictive psychotic
muscular anal urethral	retentive-eliminative	autonomy vs. shame and doubt	will	compulsive impulsive
phallic-locomotor	intrusive	initiative vs. guilt	purpose	hysterical phobic

*Adapted from Erikson, E. Insight and Responsibility, W. W. Norton, 1964, p. 186.

The phases of a patient's emotional adjustment following sudden catastrophic injury resemble the psychosocial developmental stages described by Erikson.

SCI - Psychological Care

aides and orderlies. Because of his generally apprehensive behavior, episodes of dyspnea were discounted until he became so ill that he was transferred back to the ICU. There, multiple pulmonary emboli were diagnosed.

When L.H. returned to the orthopedic ward, the staff was defensive and rejecting. L.H. expressed his mistrust of staff and continued to demand and manipulate. His commitment to physical therapy was minimal as he waited passively for return of function. Although much function actually did return, he left the hospital almost completely dependent on others for care.

Autonomy: The Second Task. Erikson says that muscular maturation establishes holding on (*retentive*) and letting go (*eliminative*) as the social modalities of the second psychosocial stage (Freud's anal stage). In this stage the child discovers conflict between his desires and his mother's. The dichotomy of this stage is autonomy—the lasting sense of pride, goodwill, and self-control without loss of self-esteem— versus the shame and doubt that result from a loss of self-control and from foreign overcontrol. For the child, the focus of conflict and control often is bowel and bladder training. Mahler describes this phase as *separation-individuation,* a time of moving away but constantly checking to gain reassurance from the mother's presence. It is a time of negativism.

Following transfer to a general unit or rehabilitation center, the disabled person usually is placed on a fairly rigid therapy schedule, and bowel and bladder retraining is begun. Therefore, progress in bowel and bladder training and in physical mobility represents progress in self-control and influences the patient's self-esteem and ego reformation.

Cayley stressed the significance of this phase: " . . . specific areas of the body and bodily functions assume tremendous psychological importance. These are the excretions. . . . Some patients overcome gradually the exaggerated value of their excretory functions, while the lives of others continue to revolve around their urination and defecation"(9).

Another important factor during this stage of recovery is control by hospital staff as opposed to self-control. "Most patients want to be 'good patients'," Cayley said, "to accept the routine of the hospital blindly, in order to please the paternalistic hospital authorities. They do it at the expense of their spontaneity" (9). Too strong control by the staff may become internalized, creating a compulsive patient who is unable to adapt to change.

While many patients exhibit a certain compulsiveness which may actually benefit rehabilitation at this point, too much compulsiveness may halt progress by limiting the desire to take the gambles necessary to improve.

Patients may react to a strongly controlling staff by becoming negative and rejecting therapy or by demonstrating overt anger or prolonged depression. On the other hand, too little guidance and control, infrequent though this may be in the average institution, forces the patient to flounder in a sea of uncertainty.

If there is adequate—not excessive—control, the patient gains a sense of pride in his ability to cope and in his self-control, and a goodwill toward others. When control is rigid, he becomes compulsive, angry, and anxious from a sense of doubt in his ability to cope and in others' ability to help him. R. S. typifies this stage:

A 30-year-old man with two children, R. S. became paraplegic following a car accident. His relationship with the nursing staff was warm and trusting. Because he was in a private room and unable to compare himself with other patients, he questioned staff on all shifts to learn whether he was a "good patient." He established strict routines for eating, bathing, and transfer to a wheelchair; he seemed lost if this routine was broken. One night he was unable to sleep because a small sore on his foot, which previously had been open to air at night, had been rebandaged by a new nurse.

When the indwelling catheter was removed, R. S. achieved bladder control readily, an accomplishment he had been worried about. Now his pride was evident and for two weeks he quoted his intake-output total to anyone who would listen. Within a month, however, he began to adjust and the topic of excretion no longer occupied his attention.

Nursing Implications

To gain a sense of mastery, the patient must experience success. Hence, the nurse helps him establish reasonable early goals so that he does not learn failure. She does not expect him to assume too many or too complex tasks rapidly. At this point, the patient begins to be a full member of the health care team.

He makes decisions, an important component of independent functioning that is often overlooked. While the decisions should be small in scope initially, they should not be confined for too long to inconsequential matters. After the patient has resolved dependency needs, the nurse does not foster dependence in order to meet her needs. As he becomes increasingly autonomous, she remains available, reassuring him and coordinating his widening experiences.

The importance of bowel and bladder control to the patient's growing sense of autonomy dictates that nursing staff never show revulsion or foster shame by word or action. Responsibility for helping him regain bowel and bladder control rests primarily with the nurse. Control of elimination is a strong determinant of rehabilitation outcomes, so the nurse continually updates her knowledge about techniques of training, to afford patients the maximum opportunity for success. When the patient soils himself, this may threaten his developing sense of control; inappropriate emphasis by nursing staff on control of elimination can foster a life that revolves around elimination.

Extreme, persistent, obsessive-compulsive behavior is abnormal. But in relation to physical therapy, the transient compulsiveness of many patients may be beneficial. If a patient is learning one method of transfer in the physical therapy department, nursing staff should use the same method on the unit because learning a second method is confusing and potentially dangerous.

Reinforcement and practice of activities learned in the various therapy departments are included in the patient's nursing care. This requires open communication among all disciplines. The nurse does not challenge the patient's compulsions. Necessary changes in therapy or routine are explained thoroughly before they are implemented. Again, a limited number of staff who know the patient well should provide his nursing care.

Many disabled persons say that at one time they felt overwhelmingly ashamed, as though they had committed a terrible crime against society. Rigid expectations, rules, and a prison-like atmosphere foster this feeling. Nurses must evaluate the rules governing patients' lives, then work to eliminate all but those that are essential for people who must live for months in an environment where eating, sleeping, and even social contact are controlled.

Part of the patient's adjustment entails a change in value system. Therefore, nurses provide a value system that serves as a reference point; other patients may serve as models (see "Eddie—A Successful Quad"). Wright suggests that the disabled must subordinate physique, enlarge the scope of values to include those still available, and contain the disability effects(10). A sense of autonomy and containment of disability effects—that is, belief that the whole self is not worthless because a part does not function—developed simultaneously in M. D., a 19-year-old soldier wounded in Vietnam.

On return to a stateside hospital, M. D. had an above-knee amputation. On the stump sock he drew the cartoon figure Snoopy. Soon everyone called him Snoopy, and he introduced himself that way.

On this orthopedic unit, the patients, mostly veterans, were given weekend passes. Those who lived far from home went out in groups—usually with patients who had been around longer—to parties, discotheques, and the beach.

"Snoopy" had gone with the group on several weekends before the time he became separated and walked several miles back to the hospital on a temporary prosthesis. Shortly thereafter, he asked that he not be called Snoopy, but by his legal name. This request suggested that he no longer considered himself and the disability as synonymous.

Initiative: the Third Task. Mahler and Erikson believe that the child becomes a more distinct individual during the next period. The organ mode for this stage is *intrusive*: the male "making" and the female "on the make." Freudian theory calls this the oedipal stage, in which the child loves the opposite-sexed parent but, fearing retaliation by castration, represses the love for the opposite-sexed parent and identifies with the same-sexed parent.

The oedipal stage has been called the "self-centered sexual stage," because many advantages of loving augment personal worth rather than the desire to give. Erikson identified the danger of this stage as guilt—guilt over the goals contemplated or the inability to achieve them. The child gains a basic sense of initiative through awareness of moral responsibility, roles, and institutions. He finds accomplishment in manipulating tools and weapons.

By the time the disabled person has resolved dependence and gained some measure of self-control, he has begun to question the effect of the disability on his sexual functioning and desirability. Confusion and conflict in this area may complicate the interpersonal situation. To prove or test their sexual desirability, patients often express romantic or sexual desire for a staff member.

The loss of sexual function or fear of its loss may reawaken the guilt of the oedipal phase; the patient may believe that his injury is punishment for wrongdoing. This can impede rehabilitation, for it limits initiative. Cayley says that patients who lose sexual function "are then inclined to consider themselves as failures, and feel inadequate not only sexually, but in every respect"(11).

Some patients become obsessed with sexuality while others sublimate it completely. Comarr and Gunderson described a paraplegic who invested his total energy in job, church, and school, a behavior that caused severe marital stress(12). Other patients identify with a staff member of the same sex, and the desire to become a nurse or therapist often is voiced.

C. M., for instance, had a crush on an intern for some time and carried his picture with her. Shortly after the crush terminated, she spoke of becoming a nurse. Eventually she was employed in the hospital in a clerical position.

The re-alignment of the value system continues. The patient begins to sever ties with the staff, for soon he will leave the hospital. This may cause some ambivalence. He may revert temporarily to dependence, but will recover his initiative after a period of reassurance. This is the time he will begin to consider his societal role and to prepare for a job.

Nursing Implications

If the patient is ambivalent and retreats to dependence, the nurse offers the support he needs, recognizing that this is not an unusual reaction. If a sexual counselor and vocational counselor are available, the nurse may only need to coordinate and augment their contributions. If such counselors are not available, she will need to work closely with other health care professionals and may need to assume these functions herself to ensure that total rehabilitation is achieved.

Role definition by patients is more than merely vocational; it requires a

SCI - Psychological Care

total interaction with family and community, and always entails anticipatory guidance. Some institutions use role playing successfully to help patients and families identify future problems.

Because sexuality is an emotion-laden topic for patient and nurse, sex counseling is difficult, but it should not be avoided. Ideally, counseling is based on a physiological and humanistic approach. Rather than leave sex counseling to physicians by default, Smith and Bullough recommend a system that uses a primary sex counselor, who can be a specially prepared nurse, with secondary support by other team members(13). These authors state that a generally hopeful attitude characterized by interest and concern is the best approach to the topic of sexuality, and they stress the need to include the patient's partner, if possible.

When a patient attempts to form a romantic relationship with the nurse, she recognizes the need this demonstrates and maintains her acceptance while assisting him to channel these energies elsewhere. A patient's identification with the nursing role can be used as a positive force in rehabilitation if the goal is not unrealistic. Referral to a psychiatrist is appropriate for any patient with severe, prolonged guilt feelings.

The astute nurse can use the theoretical framework presented here to identify the patient's progress and needs, and to determine what approaches best foster his ultimate independence. The limitations of using any model include the tendency to fit patient to model by ignoring important individual variations. This particular developmental model could introduce the risk of treating patients like children rather than adults with established personalities who have suffered overwhelming physical and psychological assault.

The nurse's day-by-day sensitivity to the patient's feelings and unique pace in adjusting are the best assurance that the patient gradually will again become a "whole" human being, no matter how devastating the injury.

References

1. ERIKSON, E. H. *Identity: Youth and Crisis.* New York, W. W. Norton, 1968.
2. MAHLER, M. S., AND FURER, MANUEL. *On Human Symbiosis and the Vicissitudes of Individuation.* New York, International Universities Press, 1968.
3. CAYLEY, C. K. Psychiatric aspects of rehabilitation of the physically handicapped. *Am.J.Psychotherapy* 8:518-529, July 1954.
4. MUELLER, A. D. Personality problems of the spinal cord injured. *J.Consult. Psychiatry* 14:189-192, 1950.
5. ARNOLD, N. Adjustment of adolescents to poliomyelitis; A study of six patients. *J.Pediatr.* 45:347-361, Sept. 1954.
6. LINDUSKA, NOREEN. *My Polio Past.* New York, Pellegrini and Cudahy Co., 1947.
7. SORENSEN, K. M., AND AMIS, D. B. Understanding the world of the chronically ill. *Am.J.Nurs.* 67:811-817, Apr. 1967.
8. MATHEWS, N.C. Helping a quadriplegic veteran decide to live. *Am.J.Nurs.* 76:441-443, Mar. 1976.
9. CAYLEY, *op.cit.*, p. 519.
10. WRIGHT, B. A. *Physical Disability, a Psychological Approach.* New York, Harper & Row, 1960.
11. CAYLEY, *op.cit.*, p. 520.
12. COMARR, A. E., AND GUNDERSON, B. B. Sexual function in traumatic paraplegia and quadriplegia. *Am.J.Nurs.* 75:250-253, Feb. 1975.
13. SMITH, JIM, AND BULLOUGH, BONNIE. Sexuality and the severely disabled person. *Am.J.Nurs.* 75:2194-2197, Dec. 1975.

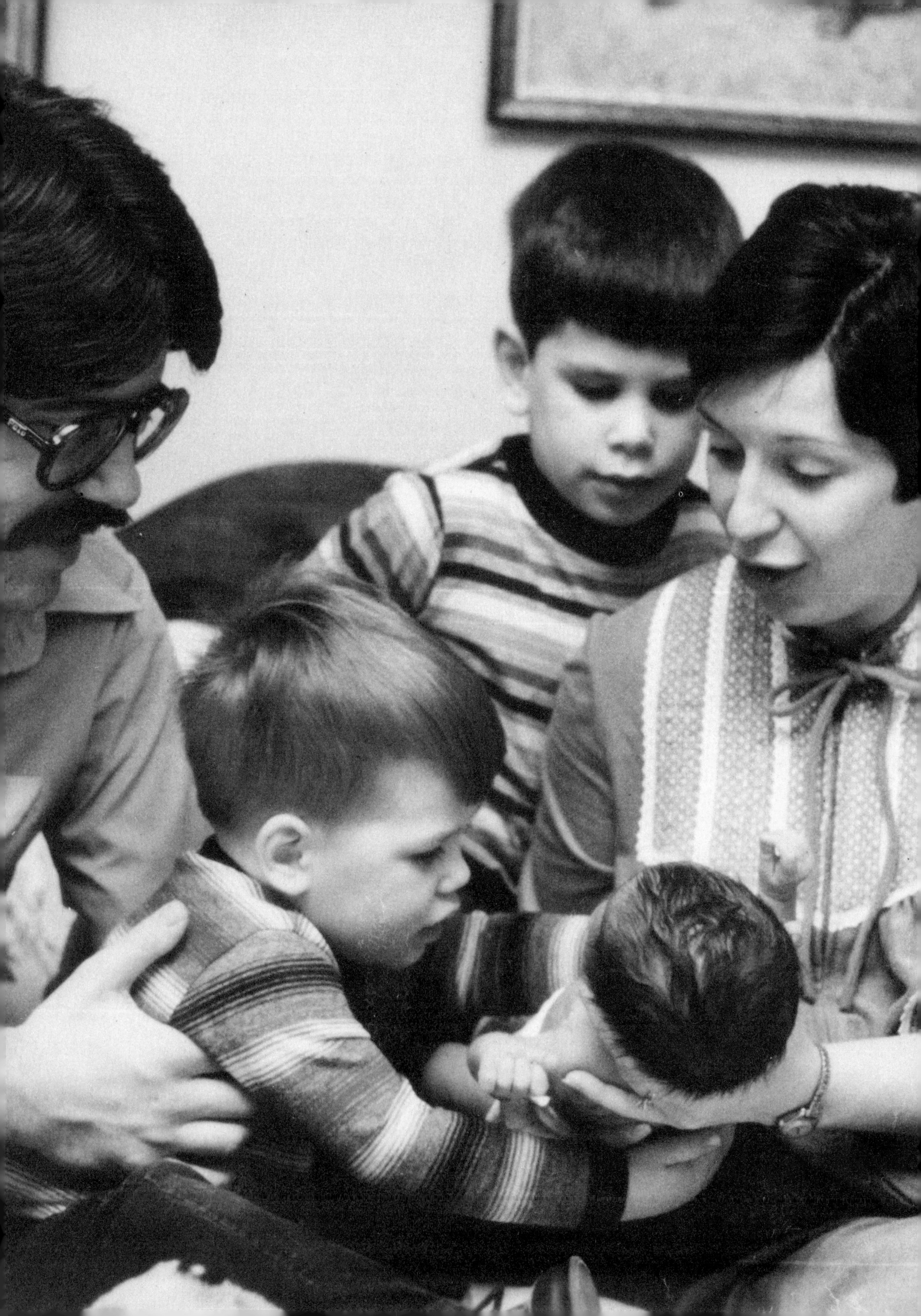

4 Nursing Care of the Childbearing Family

Coordinator

Marybeth Young, MSN, RNC

Contributors

Quilla D. Bell-Turner, PhD, RN
Gita Dhillon, EdD, RNC
Roberta Kordish, MSN, RN
B. Patricia Nix, MSN, RN
Karen Stefaniak, MSN, RN
Deborah L. Ulrich, PhD, RN

Section 4: Nursing Care of the Childbearing Family

FEMALE REPRODUCTIVE ANATOMY AND PHYSIOLOGY 383

General Concepts 383

Overview/Physiology 383

Application of the Nursing Process to Reproductive Health Maintenance/Health Promotion of Adult Women 385

ANTEPARTAL CARE 390

General Concepts 390

Normal Childbearing 390

Overview of Management 395

Application of the Nursing Process to Normal Childbearing, Antepartal Care 395

High-risk Childbearing 399

Application of the Nursing Process to the High-Risk Pregnant Client 403

Selected Health Problems in the Antepartal Period 404

Abortion 404

Incompetent Cervical Os 404

Ectopic Pregnancy 405

Hydatidiform Mole 405

Placenta Previa 406

Abruptio Placentae 407

Pregnancy-Induced Hypertension 408

Diabetes 410

Cardiac Disorders 412

Anemia 413

Hyperemesis Gravidarum 414

Infections 414

Multiple Gestation 416

Adolescent Pregnancy 416

INTRAPARTAL CARE 419

General Concepts 419

Normal Childbearing 419

Ongoing Management and Nursing Care 422

Application of the Nursing Process to Normal Childbearing, Intrapartal Care 426

Application of the Nursing Process to the High-risk Intrapartal Client 431

Selected Health Problems in the Intrapartal Period 432

Dystocia 432

Premature Labor 434

Emergency Birth 435

Episiotomy 436

Forceps 436

Vacuum Extraction 437

Cesarean Birth 438

Vaginal Birth After Cesarean Delivery 439

Rupture of the Uterus 439

Amniotic Fluid Embolism 440

POSTPARTAL CARE 441

General Concepts 441

Normal Childbearing 441

Application of the Nursing Process to Normal Childbearing, Postpartal Care 443

Application of the Nursing Process to the High-risk Postpartal Client 442

Selected Health Problems in the Postpartal Period 447

Postpartum Hemorrhage 447

Hematoma 448

Pulmonary Embolus 448

Puerperal Infection 448

Mastitis 449

Postpartum Cystitis 450

Psychological Maladaptations 450

Selected Long-term Problems Associated with Childbearing 451

Uterine Prolapse with or without Cystocele or Rectocele 451

Uterine Fibroids 452

NEWBORN CARE 454

The Normal Newborn 454

General Characteristics 454

Specific Body Parts 455

Systems Adaptations 458

Gestational Age Variations 460

Application of the Nursing Process to the Normal Newborn 463

Application of the Nursing Process to the Newborn at Risk 466

Selected Health Problems in the Newborn 466

Hypothermia 466

Neonatal Jaundice 467

Respiratory Distress 469

Neonatal Necrotizing Enterocolitis 470

Hypoglycemia 471

Newborn Infection 472

Neonatal Drug and Alcohol Addiction 472

Acquired Immune Deficiency Syndrome 473

Birth Injuries/Congenital Anomalies 474

Parental Reaction to a Sick, Disabled, or Malformed Newborn 475

REPRINTS 477

Section 4 Tables

4.1 Assessment of Fertility/Infertility 386
4.2 Family Planning 387
4.3 Interpretation of Pap Test Results 389
4.4 Health Teaching to Reduce Risk of Osteoporosis 389
4.5 Signs and Symptoms of Pregnancy 393
4.6 Naegele's Rule 395
4.7 McDonald's Rule 396
4.8 Recommended Dietary Allowances for Females Aged 11–50 398
4.9 Selected Nutrients Essential for Health in Pregnancy and Lactation 399
4.10 Pregnant Woman's Daily Food Intake 399
4.11 Childbirth Preparation 400
4.12 Laboratory Studies of Fetal Well-Being 403
4.13 Classification of Pregnancy-Induced Hypertension 409
4.14 Anticonvulsive Agents 410
4.15 Baseline Fetal Heart Rate 422
4.16 Decelerations in Fetal Heart Rate 424
4.17 Stages and Phases of Labor 425
4.18 Uterine Smooth Muscle Stimulants 431
4.19 Uterine Dysfunction in Labor 432
4.20 Oxytocin 433
4.21 Tocolytic Agent 436
4.22 Lochia Changes 442
4.23 Maternal Psychological Adaptation (Rubin) 443
4.24 Rh O (D) Human Immune Globulin 444
4.25 Lactation Suppressant Drugs 445
4.26 Postpartum Depression 451
4.27 Nutritional Comparison of Human and Cow's Milk 460
4.28 High-Risk Conditions for Newborns by Gestational Age and Growth Classifications 462
4.29 Apgar Scoring Chart 464

Section 4 Figures

4.1 Female Pelvis 384
4.2 Female Internal Reproductive Organs (Side View) 384
4.3 Basal Body Temperature (30 Day Cycle) 386
4.4 Common Site of Ectopic Pregnancy 405
4.5 Hydatidiform Mole 405
4.6 Placenta Previa 406
4.7 Abruptio Placentae 407
4.8 Selected Categories of Presentation 420
4.9 Tracing of Normal Fetal Heart Rate 421
4.10 Acceleration of Fetal Heart Rate in Response to Uterine Activity 422
4.11 Types of Deceleration in Fetal Heart Rate 423
4.12 Assessment of Uterine Contractions 426
4.13 Leopold's Maneuvers 427
4.14 Site of Auscultation of FHR with Fetus in ROA Position 429

4.15 Friedman Curve 434
4.16 Types of Episiotomies 437
4.17 Types of Cesarean Incisions 438
4.18 Bones, Fontanels, and Sutures of Newborn's Skull 456
4.19 Fetal Circulation 459
4.20 Newborn Maturity Rating and Classification 461
4.21 Rh Sensitization 467
4.22 Silverman-Andersen Scale 470

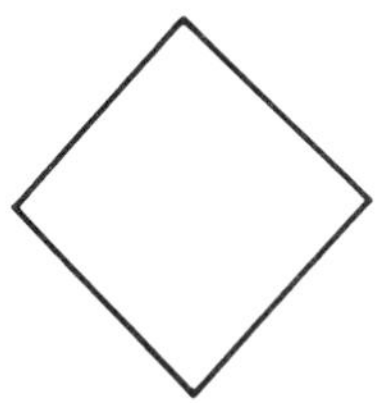

Female Reproductive Anatomy and Physiology

General Concepts

(*NOTE*: The concept development in the sections on the Adult, Child, and the Client with Psychosocial Problems also applies to the mother and her newborn. However, this section has been organized according to the normal childbearing cycle, from conception to postpartum.)

Overview/Physiology

1. Structure of the female pelvis
- **a.** Pelvic structure (four united bones): two hip bones (right and left innominate), the sacrum, and the coccyx
- **b.** Pelvic divisions: two parts divided by the inlet or brim
  - **1)** false pelvis: upper portion above brim; supports uterus during late pregnancy
  - **2)** true pelvis: located below brim; composed of three parts: the pelvic inlet, the mid-cavity, and the pelvic outlet; forms birth canal through which fetus passes during parturition
- **c.** Pelvic variations: pelvic structures differ in shape and size
  - **1)** android: normal male type; heart-shaped inlet, narrow pubic arch; influence on labor/delivery is not favorable
  - **2)** gynecoid: true female type; slightly ovoid or rounded inlet; influence on labor/delivery *most favorable*
  - **3)** platypelloid: flattened anteroposteriorly, oval-shaped inlet; influence on labor/delivery not favorable
  - **4)** anthropoid: apelike type; inlet oval shaped; influence on labor/delivery favorable
- **d.** Pelvic measurements
  - **1)** diagonal conjugate (DC): distance between sacral promontory and lower margin (inferior border) of symphysis pubis; adequate size for childbirth is 12.5 cm or more, depending on fetal size, position; *estimated on pelvic exam*
  - **2)** true conjugate or conjugate vera (CV): distance between upper margin, superior border of symphysis pubis to sacral promontory; adequate size for childbirth 11 cm or more (1.5–2 cm less than diagonal conjugate); *measured accurately by x-ray*
  - **3)** obstetric conjugate: the shortest distance between the inner surface of the symphysis and the sacral promontory; *measured by x-ray*
  - **4)** tuber-ischial diameter: transverse diameter of the outlet, the distance between the ischial tuberosities; adequate size for childbirth 9–11 cm or more; *estimated on pelvic exam*
  - **5)** assessment of size
    - **a)** estimate of pelvic dimensions: diagonal conjugate and tuber-ischial diameter on pelvic exam
    - **b)** x-ray or internal pelvimetry: use is limited to suspected pelvic bony contractions and suspected cephalopelvic disproportion (most accurate measurement of pelvic size)
    - **c)** ultrasonography: employs use of high-frequency sound waves for determination of gestational age

2. Female external organs
- **a.** Mons veneris or pubis: rounded, soft, fatty pad over symphysis pubis, covered by coarse hair in adult
- **b.** Labia majora: two folds of skin containing fat and covered with hair; located on either side of the vaginal opening
- **c.** Labia minora: two thin folds of delicate tissue without hair; located within labia majora
- **d.** Glans clitoris: a small body of erectile tissue partially hidden between the anterior ends of the labia minora; highly sensitive to touch, temperature, and pressure
- **e.** Hymen: thin mucous membrane; located at the opening of the vagina, can be stretched or torn during intercourse, physical activity, tampon insertion, or vaginal examination

Figure 4.1 Female Pelvis

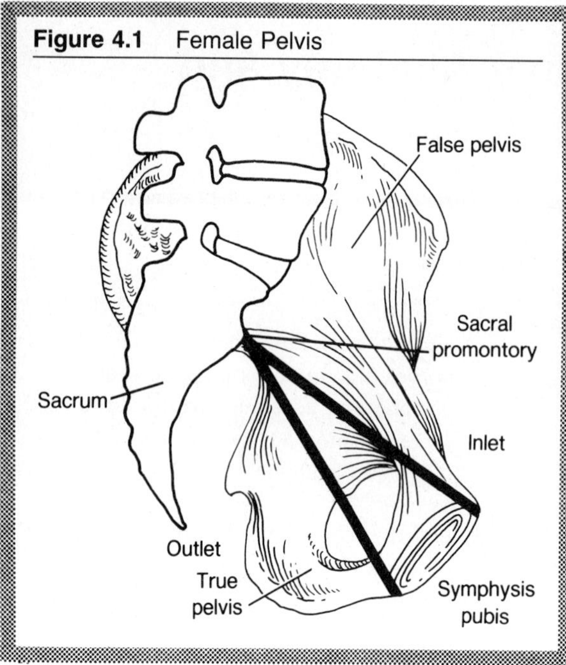

f. Urinary meatus: external opening of the urethra
g. Openings of vulvovaginal or Bartholin's glands: two small glands situated between the vestibula on either side of the vaginal orifice; secrete alkaline mucus during coitus
h. Openings of Skene's ducts: two paraurethral glands open onto posterior urethral wall
i. Perineum: area between vagina and rectum consisting of fibromuscular tissue

3. Female internal organs
   a. Ovaries: two oval-shaped organs located on either side of the uterus in the upper pelvic cavity; responsible for producing the ovum and the female hormones, estrogen and progesterone
   b. Fallopian or uterine tubes: two thin muscular canals extending from the cornua of the uterus to the ovaries; responsible for transport of the ovum from the ovaries to the uterus; fertilization occurs in middle 3rd (ampulla) of either fallopian tube
   c. Uterus: a hollow muscular organ that is the site of implantation, retainment, and nourishment of the products of conception. It is also the organ of menstruation in the nonpregnant female. The larger, upper portion of the uterus is known as the *body* and the smaller, lower segment is called the *cervix*. The convex, upper part between the insertion of fallopian tubes is the *fundus*. In the nonpregnant female, the uterus is located in the pelvic cavity between the bladder and rectum and weighs approximately 60 gm. The uterus is composed of smooth muscle (myometrium) and an inner mucoid lining (the endometrium), which responds to estrogen and progesterone during the menstrual cycle.

Figure 4.2 Female Internal Reproductive Organs (Side View)

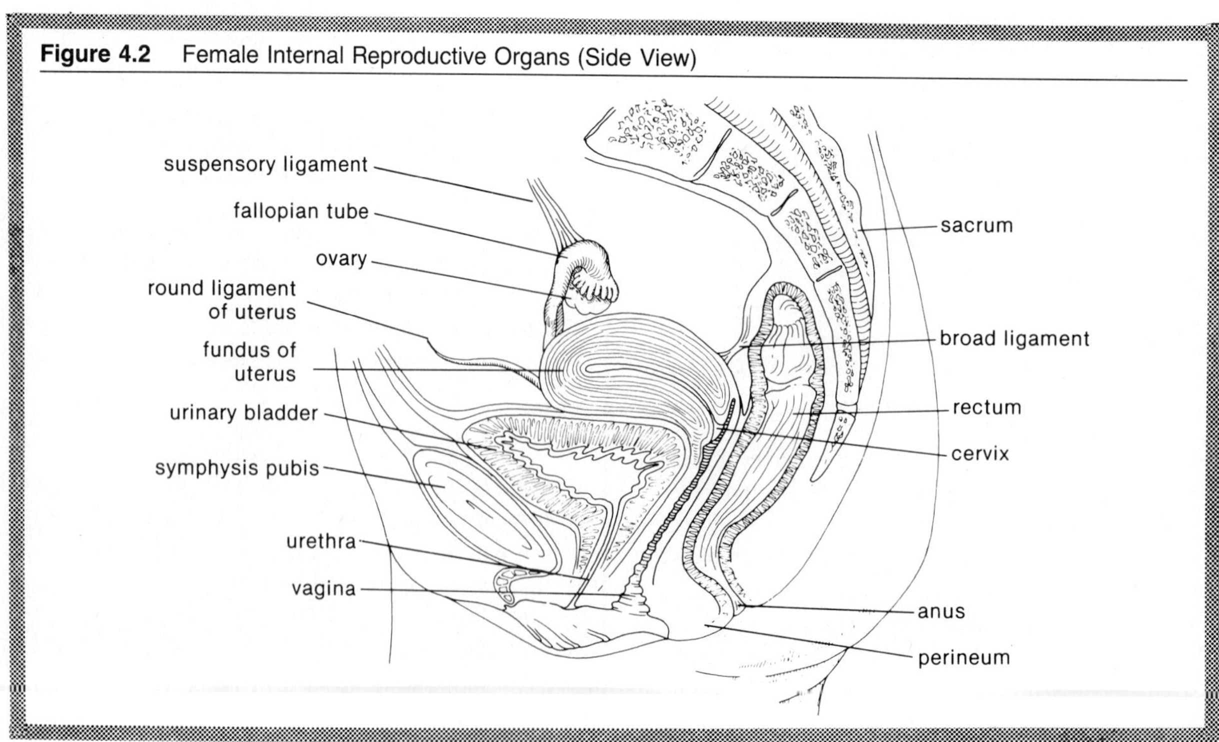

d. Vagina: a thin-walled dilatable canal located between the bladder and rectum that serves as the passageway for menstrual discharge, copulation, and the fetus
e. Accesory structures (breasts): two mammary glands composed of glandular tissue and fat, which are capable of producing and secreting milk for nourishment of the infant

4. Menstrual cycle
   a. Reproductive hormones (all are affected by thyroid function)
      1) follicle-stimulating hormone (FSH): secreted by anterior pituitary gland during the first half of the menstrual cycle; stimulates development of graafian follicles and thins the endometrium
      2) interstitial-cell stimulating hormone (ICSH) or luteinizing hormone (LH): secreted by the pituitary; stimulates ovulation and development of the corpus luteum; causes the endometrium to thicken
      3) estrogen: secreted primarily by the ovaries and by the adrenal cortex (in small amounts), and by the placenta in pregnancy; assists in maturation of ovarian follicles, stimulates thickening of the endometrium, causes suppression of FSH secretion, and is responsible for development of secondary sex characteristics; in pregnancy, it maintains the endometrium, causes fatigue, and stimulates contraction of smooth muscle
      4) progesterone: secreted by corpus luteum and by the placenta during pregnancy; supplements estrogen effect on endometrium by facilitating secretory changes; relaxes smooth muscle; decreases uterine motility; has thermogenic effect (i.e., increases temperature); causes cervical secretion of thick viscous mucus; allows pregnancy to be maintained
      5) prostaglandins: fatty acids categorized as hormones, produced by many organs of the body, including the endometrium; affect the menstrual cycle and may influence the onset and maintenance of labor
   b. Ovulation: growth and release of a nonfertilized ovum from the ovary after puberty; generally occurs 13–15 days prior to next menses in regular cycle; presence of stretchable cervical mucus (Spinnbarkheit) observed at ovulation; purpose to enhance sperm motility and permit fertilization
   c. Menstruation: cyclic vaginal discharge of blood and superficial fragments of endometrium and other secretions in response to falling levels of estrogen and progesterone after puberty
   d. Menopause: cessation of menses at the end of fertility cycle
5. Fertilization: impregnation of an ovum by a spermatozoon, occurring in the ampulla of the fallopian tube; egg life span is 24–36 hours after ovulation; sperm life span is 48–72 hours or more after ejaculation; usual sperm count: 250–400 million
6. Implantation: the imbedding of the fertilized ovum into the uterine mucosa (usually in the upper segment); occurs approximately 7–10 days after ovulation (also known as nidation)
7. Menopause: cessation of menses at end of fertility cycle
   a. Occurrence: normal developmental process that occurs naturally between the ages of 35 and 60 (average age: 53)
   b. Alterations: early menopause may be stimulated by
      1) multiple, frequent pregnancies or abortions
      2) hypothyroidism with obesity
      3) surgical removal of ovaries
      4) hard physical work or very active exercise
      5) overexposure to radiation
   c. Medical treatment: for symptom relief
      1) estrogen replacement therapy: often controversial
      2) vitamins: increased doses of B complex and vitamin E for symptoms such as hot flashes
      3) hormonal vaginal creams and water-soluble lubricants for painful intercourse (dyspareunia)
      4) emotional support during this developmental change/crisis

Application of the Nursing Process to Reproductive Health Maintenance/Health Promotion of Adult Women

1. **Assessment/Analysis**
   a. Health History: Onset of menarche, duration of menstrual periods, menstrual problems (e.g., amenorrhea: absence of menses as a result of hormonal problems or surgery; dysmenorrhea: painful menses), premenstrual tension, osteoporosis (decrease in skeletal bone mass), use of family planning, past and current pregnancies, infertility problems (see Table 4.1), symptoms such as hot flashes, dizzy spells, palpitations; identification of risk factors

Figure 4.3 Basal Body Temperatue (30 Day Cycle)

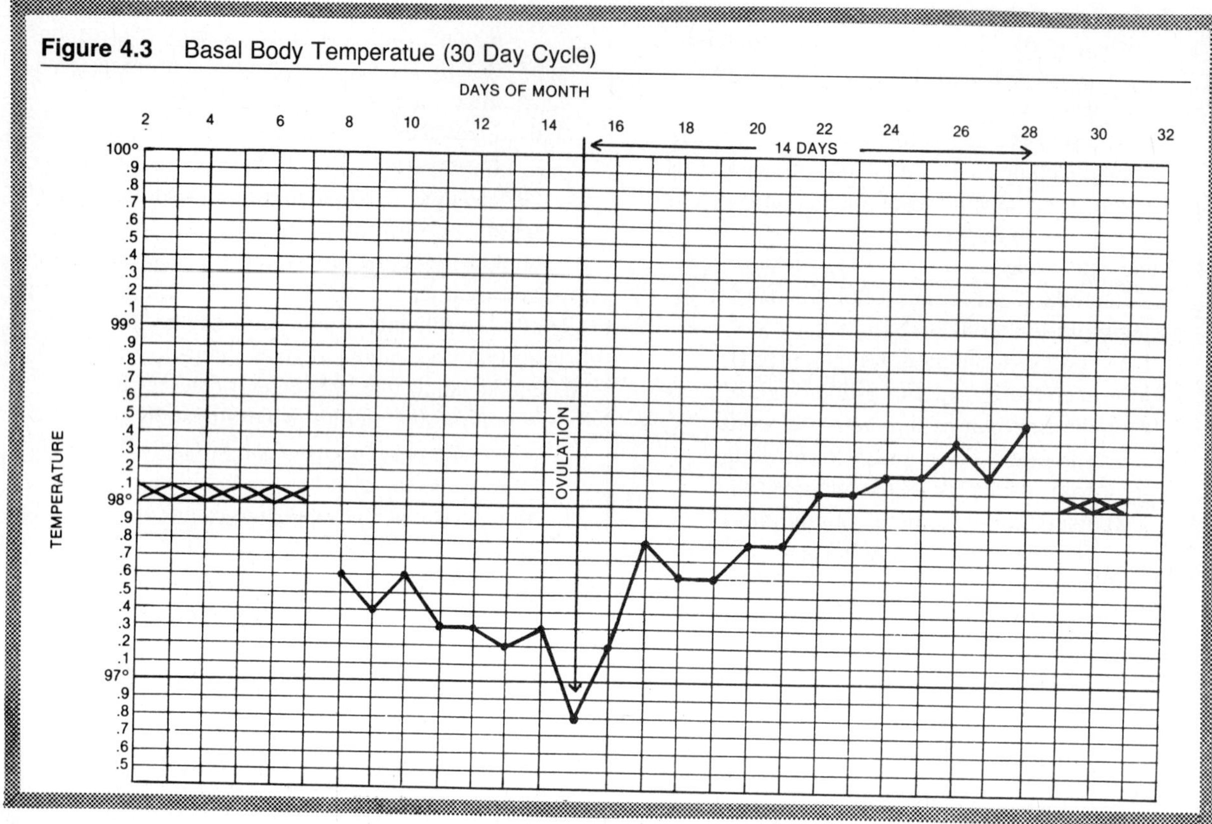

Table 4.1 Assessment of Fertility/Infertility

Test	Purpose	Nursing Implications
Male		
Semen analysis	To determine sperm count, motility	Take careful history of both partners • chronic health problems • medications • drug use • exposure to chemicals, radiation
Female (simplest to more complex)		
Basal body temperature	To determine time of ovulation	
Cervical-mucus examination (self-done, basis for natural family planning)	To determine elasticity for sperm motility	Provide detailed explanation of all tests to couple.
Pelvic examination (bimanual)	To identify obvious reproductive problems	Know that process of assessment of fertility and subsequent interventions may be lengthy and, for the couple, frustrating.
Blood hormone levels and thyroid function tests	To measure levels of estrogen and progesterone, and influence of the thyroid	
Sims-Huhner test (postcoital cervical mucus test)	To determine pH of cervical mucus, effects of hormones	
Tubal patency tests • hysterosalpingogram (x-ray) • laporoscopic exam (direct visualization)	To determine condition, patency of Fallopian tubes	
Endometrial biopsy	To determine condition of endometrium	
Culdoscopy (examination through cul-de-sac with dye injection)	To determine function of Fallopian tubes	

b. Physical assessment of external reproductive organs (by physician or nurse); breast palpation for masses; bimanual internal examination; and observation of cervical-vaginal discharge

2. General Nursing Plans, Implementation, and Evaluation

Goal 1: Client will understand her reproductive system; will report gynecologic problems to the physician.

Plan/Implementation

- Discuss anatomy and physiology of female reproductive system.
- Review menstrual cycle, ovulation, and fertilization.
- Teach client reportable problems.

Evaluation: Client gives a basic explanation of reproductive anatomy and physiology; explains relationship of menstrual cycle, ovulation, and fertilization.

Goal 2: Client will be knowledgeable about various methods of family planning.

Table 4.2 Family Planning

Method and Mode of Action	Characteristics	Nursing Implications
Temporary Methods		
Oral contraceptives (birth control pills): May be single hormone or combination of estrogen and progesterone • prevent ovulation by inhibiting FSH • change cervical mucus	*Effectiveness:* 99% if used as directed *Advantages:* Convenient, effective *Disadvantages:* Increased risk over age 35; smokers; women with risk/history of vascular disease, hypertension, respiratory problems, breast cancer in family	Teach proper and regular use • action to take if one or more pills are missed • side effects; reportable signs (e.g., headaches, chest or calf pain, heavy bleeding). Recommend regular Pap smears. Caution against use of antibiotics unless physician is aware client uses oral contraceptives. Increase folic acid, vitamins B and C. Advise client to notify physician and discontinue oral contraceptives if pregnancy is suspected.
Intrauterine device (IUD) • causes local inflammatory response inhibiting implantation • several IUD products have been withdrawn by manufacturer	*Effectiveness:* 90%–99% *Advantages:* Convenient, long term, effective *Disadvantages:* Increased risk for pelvic infection, ectopic pregnancy; subsequent infertility	Teach • compliance with regular health care visits • reportable signs (e.g., abdominal pain, foul discharge) • to check for presence of string before coitus. Must be removed by health care provider.
Diaphragm • barrier to seminal fluid, sperm when used with spermicidal cream	*Effectiveness:* 83%–95% if correctly fit and properly used *Advantages:* Side effects are rare *Disadvantages:* Requires motivation and planning; may interfere with spontaneity; must remain in place several hours after coitus	Teach proper use with spermicide (not KY jelly). Suggest that client be refitted after pregnancy, weight changes. Report problems with fit, removal, vaginal discharge.
Vaginal contraceptive sponge	*Effectiveness:* 84%–97% *Advantages:* Convenient; no additional creams needed; may leave in place up to 24 hours; barrier to seminal fluid, sperm; economical *Disadvantages:* Increased risk of allergies, toxic shock; removal may be difficult	Teach proper use and insertion. Avoid use for over 30 hours. Avoid use during menses. Urge immediate reporting of problems/symptoms.
Cervical cap • barrier to seminal fluid and sperm • FDA approval for research • used with spermicidal cream	*Advantages:* Side effects are rare; unlikely to dislodge during coitus *Disadvantages:* Increased risk of cervical erosion, inflammation; may be difficult to remove	Teach proper use. Report signs of vaginal infection or other problems. Seek regular health care

(continued)

Table 4.2 Continued

Method and Mode of Action	Characteristics	Nursing Implications
Temporary Methods (continued)		
Condom • barrier to passage of sperm when slipped over erect penis	*Effectiveness:* 64%–98% when used with spermicides *Advantages:* Involves male in family planning; protects against some sexually transmitted diseases; easily available *Disadvantages:* Requires motivation and planning; may tear during use; rare allergic reactions	Teach proper use. Discuss role in prevention of transmission of sexually transmitted diseases, AIDS.
Spermicides • immobolizes or destroys sperm	*Effectiveness:* 70%–98% depending on use; more effective with other methods (e.g., condom, diaphragm) *Advantages:* Easily available; few side effects *Disadvantages:* Inconvenient; may cause allergic reaction; there is concern (unproven) about potential risk of birth defects in some users	Teach proper use after reading specific product directions. Avoid douching after coitus. Report problems (e.g., itching, burning).
Natural family planning • abstinence from coitus during the fertile (ovulation) phase of the menstrual cycle (the couple trying to conceive may also plan optimal time for coitus to achieve pregnancy) • assessment of ovulation is based on – daily basal body temperature (BBT) to monitor changes before and at ovulation (slight drop, then rise after ovulation) – cervical mucus characteristics: clear, slippery, elastic at ovulation (Billings method) – calendar recording based on usual menstrual pattern – symptothermal method: a combination of calendar tracking of monthly fertility cycle, BBT, and cervical mucus self-exam • research has led to development of several OTC products for self-assessment of ovulation	*Effectiveness:* 75%–98% depending on accuracy of observations, motivation of both partners *Advantages:* Inexpensive; involves both partners; no chemical or mechanical barrier to sperm movement; no health risk *Disadvantages:* Requires motivation of both partners; may be less effective in presence of infection or during menopause	Teach and reinforce information to both partners.
Permanent Methods		
Tubal ligation/vasectomy • ligation/severance of fallopian tube or vas deferens for permanent sterilization	*Effectiveness:* Greater than 99.5% (reversing the procedure is difficult, outcome is not guaranteed) *Advantages:* Prevents pregnancy permanently *Disadvantages:* Requires informed consent; rare complications	Teach couple alternative methods if permanent sterility is not desired. Caution that pregnancy is still possible for a short period of time following vasectomy.

Plan/Implementation

- Assess client's learning needs.
- Provide information as needed (see Table 4.2).

Evaluation: Client describes family planning options; asks questions about them; uses chosen method consistently according to directions; lists potential problems with specific method; reports problems associated with use.

Goal 3: Client will understand the importance of periodic examinations in reproductive health maintenance.

Table 4.3 Interpretation of Pap Test Results

Class I	No abnormal cells
Class II	Atypical cells (rule out inflammation)
Class III	Suspicious abnormal cells
Class IV	Malignant cells may be in situ
Class V	Invasive cancer

Plan/Implementation

- Explain the need for periodic Papanicolaou (Pap) smears (cells taken from cells of squamo-columnar junction) to detect cancer of the uterus and abnormalities of cervical, vaginal cells (frequency varies according to sexual activity, age, risk).
- Explain importance of regular self-breast examination after cessation of menstrual period (days 5–7 of menstrual cycle) or after menopause on regular monthly basis.
- Demonstrate self-breast examination (palpation and inspection of breasts and nipples while standing and reclining); ask client for return demonstration; emphasize reporting any changes or suspicious findings immediately.
- Tell client to see physician for regular breast examination.
- Explain value of mammography.
- Discuss meaning, purposes, and interpretation of various tests.
- Provide supplemental reading materials to increase client's knowledge.

Evaluation: Client performs self-breast examination regularly at end of each menstrual cycle; schedules appointments for periodic checkups and Pap smears.

Goal 4: Client will be physically and psychologically prepared for menopause; will make informed choices and comply with treatment.

Plan/Implementation

- Allow client to voice feelings about menopause.
- Teach client how to maintain and promote health and prevent osteoporosis (see Table 4.4).
- Discuss normal developmental changes that occur with menopause.
- Dispel "myths" concerning menopause.
- Discuss sexuality needs, family planning until ovulation ceases.
- Provide emotional support, anticipatory guidance.

Evaluation: Client lists the signs and symptoms of menopause; participates in decisions about treatment as an informed consumer.

References

Davis, B., Holtz, N. & Davis, J. (1985). *Conceptual Human Physiology*. Columbus: Merrill.

Jensen, M. & Bobak, I. (1985). *Maternity and Gynecologic Care*. St. Louis: Mosby.

Kjervik, D. & Martinson, I. (1986). *Women in Health and Illness*. Philadelphia: Saunders.

Sloane, E. (1985). *Biology of Women*. New York: Wiley.

Special Touch: A Personal Plan of Action for Breast Health. (1987). American Cancer Society. IMMN 2095 LE.

Peterkin, B. (1985). Dietary Guidelines. *Journal of Nutrition Education*. 17 (5), 188–9.

Sandelowski, M. (1984). *Women, Health and Choice*. Englewood Cliffs: Prentice-Hall.

Table 4.4 Health Teaching to Reduce Risk of Osteoporosis

All adult women should

- Eat a balanced diet to ensure adequate vitamin and mineral intake.
- Increase daily food sources of calcium (dairy products, seafood, yogurt, greens) to prevent or compensate for bone loss.
- Decrease excess phosphorous intake (animal proteins, dairy products, diet soda) to prevent calcium excretion. (Aluminum antacids may be suggested as phosphorous binders.)
- Maintain adequate vitamin D intake (sunlight, fortified milk products) to balance calcium and phosphorous.
- Exercise regularly to strengthen bones.

Menopausal and postmenopausal women should

- Take calcium carbonate or calcium gluconate supplements as prescribed by a physician.
- Avoid calcium preparations purchased in health food stores that contain lead, bone meal, and dolomite.
- Follow physician recommendations on estrogen replacement therapy to prevent further bone loss.

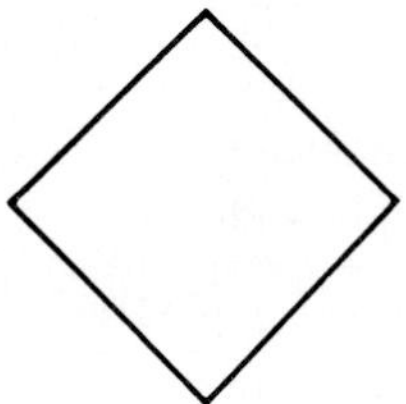

Antepartal Care

General Concepts

☐ Normal Childbearing

1. Definition: care provided to a woman and her family during pregnancy
2. Normal adaptations: changes that occur in body systems of childbearing women due to the influence of hormones and growth on the embryo/fetus
   a. Integumentary system
      1) changes in skin pigmentation stimulated by elevated levels of melanocyte-stimulating hormone
         a) chloasma (mask of pregnancy): brown blotches that appear on face and neck, often visible in 2nd trimester; usually fade after delivery
         b) linea nigra: a dark line that extends from umbilicus to mons veneris; will lighten after delivery
      2) striae gravidarum: pink or slightly reddish streaks on abdomen, thighs, or breasts, resulting from stretching of underlying connective tissue due to adrenal cortex hypertropy; grow lighter after delivery but never disappear completely
      3) vascular spider nevi and palmar erythema
   b. Reproductive system
      1) changes in the uterus
         a) size: increases in length (6–32 cm), width (4–24 cm), and depth (2.5–22 cm)
         b) weight increase: 60–1,000 gm
         c) shape: from globular to oval; wall thickens and then becomes thin at term
         d) location: rises out of pelvis at 12th week; near xiphoid process at term
         e) structure
            ■ body of uterus
              – three distinct uterine segments in pregnancy
              – vascularity increases
              – muscle fiber changes, mainly enlargement of pre-existing fibers
                * longitudinal fibers will shorten with contraction of labor to cause effacement
                * middle layer fibers constrict blood vessels in labor; add to force of labor
                * inner fibers exert pressure on blood vessels in lower uterus; prevent hemorrhage
              – new fibroelastic tissue develops and strengthens uterine wall
            ■ softening of the lower uterine segment (*Hegar's sign*)
            ■ cervix: softens (*Goodell's sign*) and increases in vascularity
            ■ formation of mucus plug (prevents bacterial contamination)
         f) contractility: *Braxton Hicks' contractions* occur intermittently throughout pregnancy
      2) changes in the vagina
         a) increased vascularization, which results in purplish discoloration (*Chadwick's sign*) beginning 6th week of pregnancy
         b) thickening of mucosa
         c) loosening of connective tissue
         d) increased vaginal discharge (thick, whitish) without signs of itching or burning
      3) changes in the breasts
         a) enlargement and prominence of superficial veins
         b) increase in size and firmness
         c) Montgomery's glands in aerola enlarge
         d) nipples become more prominent, aerolae darken and increase in diameter
         e) colostrum may be secreted in 4th or 5th month (16–20 weeks) and subsequently in small amounts until delivery
         f) alveoli and duct system enlarge
      4) changes in joints and ligaments

a) relaxation of pelvic joints and ligaments
b) hypertrophy and elongation of
- broad, round ligaments (stabilize uterus)
- uterosacral ligaments (support cervix)

5) changes in abdomen: occur to accommodate progressive growth in uterine size
a) at end of 12th week the uterus is at level of symphysis pubis
b) by 22–24 weeks uterus is at level of umbilicus
c) by the 38th week the uterus is at level of xiphoid process until lightening occurs
d) decrease in fundal height after lightening in primiparous women

c. Endocrine system (placenta)
1) function of placenta
a) secretes hormones from early weeks of pregnancy: estrogen, progesterone, human chorionic gonadotropin (HCG), and human placental lactogen (HPL), also called human chorionic somatomammotropin
b) acts as a barrier to some substances and organisms, e.g., heparin in large doses does not cross; bacteria are less likely to cross placenta than a virus (barrier not effective for nicotine, alcohol, depressants, stimulants, antibiotics, etc.)
c) nutrition: transports nutrients and water-soluble vitamins to fetus and eliminates wastes
d) exchanges: fluid/gas transport
- diffusion, e.g., O_2 and CO_2, water, electrolytes (low molecular weight)
- facilitated transport, e.g., glucose
- active transport: amino acids, calcium, iron (high molecular weight)
- pinocytosis, e.g., gamma globulin, albumin, fats-particles
- leakage due to slight placental defects, allows fetal and maternal blood cells to mix slightly

2) dimensions
a) 15 × 3 cm
b) discoid
c) 400–600 gm at term
d) covers quarter of uterine wall
e) fetal-placental weight ratio at term is 6:1

3) structure and development
a) fully developed by 12th week from the decidua basalis and chorion of the embryo; functions most effectively through 40–41 weeks; may be dysfunctional in postmaturity
b) normally develops in the posterior surface of the upper uterine segment
c) two surfaces
- fetal (amniotic) surface: chorionic villi and their circulation; membranes: amnion (inner), chorion (outer) fused
- maternal surface: decidua basalis (hypertrophied endometrium of pregnancy) and its circulation; cotyledons present
d) umbilical cord: 55 cm at term; most commonly is centrally inserted into fetal surface of placenta; contains one vein to oxygenate fetus and two arteries to carry deoxygenated blood from fetus to placenta to mother

4) hormones
a) estrogen and progesterone: after 1st 2 months of gestation, placenta is major source of production; responsible for growth of uterus and development of breasts
b) human chorionic gonadotropin (HCG): secreted by 3rd week after fertilization, detected in urine 10 days after missed period (basis for simple pregnancy tests); HCG prolongs life of corpus luteum; radioimmunoassay (RIA) for HCG will be positive the 2nd day after implantation
c) human chorionic somatomammotropin (human placental lactogen): secreted by 3rd week after ovulation; prepares breasts for lactation, influences somatic cell growth of fetus; antagonist to insulin, considered principal maternal diabetogenic factor

d. Musculoskeletal system
1) relaxation and increased mobility of pelvic joints result in a waddling gait and instability
2) increase in normal lumbosacral curve due to enlarging uterus, poor posture may increase problem
3) stress on ligaments and muscles of mid and lower spine

4) backache and leg cramps may occur

e. Cardiovascular system
1) heart and vessels
a) heart rate increases 10–15 beats/minute in 2nd trimester; persists to term
b) blood pressure should remain constant during pregnancy with a decrease in the 2nd trimester
c) increase in vasculature: dilation of pelvic veins, varicose veins, varicosities of the vulva, hemorrhoids
2) cardiac output increases 20%–30% during 1st and 2nd trimesters to meet increased tissue demands
3) blood volume altered in pregnancy; total increase approximately 20%–30% peaking in 3rd trimester; increases immediately after delivery due to fluid shift
a) plasma volume increases out of proportion to the red cell increase resulting in hemodilution; this causes normal physiologic anemia
b) hemoglobin range 10–16 gm/100 ml; may decrease; problem if it falls below 10
c) hemotocrit range 35%–42%; may decrease approximately 10% in 2nd and 3rd trimesters; anemia if it falls below 35
d) average white count 5,000–11,000/mm^3 (higher than normal)
4) palpitations: common in early and late pregnancy because of sympathetic nervous system disturbance and increased intra-abdominal pressure

f. Renal system
1) elimination/fluid transport greatly increased due to circulatory changes and need to excrete fetal waste products
2) glomerular filtration rate increases 50%
3) renal functioning is compromised in standing or sitting position; lateral recumbent position enhances kidney function
4) reduced renal threshold for sugar, glycosuria may occur; reflection of kidneys' inability to absorb glucose; appears to have little relationship to serum glucose
5) increased amount of urine; decreased specific gravity
6) dilatation of ureters, especially on the right, may lead to urinary stasis
7) decreased bladder tone, caused by progesterone effect
8) increased pressure on bladder by enlarging uterus (1st and 3rd trimesters), therefore decreased capacity and frequency

g. Respiratory system
1) diaphragm rises as much as 1 inch; dyspnea may occur until lightening (60% of pregnant women)
2) thoracic cage is pushed upward and widens
3) increased vital capacity, tidal volume, respiratory minute volume to supply maternal, fetal needs
4) increased vascularization due to elevated estrogen can cause nasal stuffiness; nosebleed, voice changes, eustachian tube blockage

h. Digestive system
1) gastrointestinal motility and digestion slowed, because of progesterone effects
2) delayed emptying time of stomach; reflux of food
3) upward displacement and compression of stomach
4) displacement of intestines as fetus develops
5) decreased secretion of HCl
6) slower emptying of gallbladder may lead to gallstone formation
7) common problems
a) nausea and vomiting (morning sickness, 50%–75% of pregnant women)
b) pica/food/substance cravings (e.g., laundry starch, clay)
c) acid indigestion or heartburn
d) constipation
e) hemorrhoids
f) bleeding, swollen gums due to estrogen

i. Psychosocial adaptations in pregnancy
1) factors influencing a woman's response to pregnancy (varies with developmental stage)
a) memories of her own childhood
b) cultural background
c) existing support systems
d) socioeconomic conditions
e) perceptions of maternal role
f) impact of mass media
g) coping mechanisms
2) maternal adaptations to pregnancy
a) 1st trimester: initial ambivalence about pregnancy; pregnant woman places

main focus upon self, i.e., physical changes associated with pregnancy and emotional reactions to pregnancy
   - **b)** 2nd trimester: relatively tranquil period; acceptance of reality of pregnancy; increased awareness and interest in fetus; introversion and feeling of well-being
   - **c)** 3rd trimester: anticipation of labor and delivery and assuming mothering role, viewing infant as reality vs fantasy; fears and fantasies and dreams about labor are common; "nesting" behaviors (e.g., preparing layette)
- **3)** psychologic tasks of pregnancy (Rubin, 1961)
   - **a)** acceptance of pregnancy as a reality and incorporation of fetus into body image
   - **b)** preparation for physical separation from fetus (birth)
   - **c)** attainment of maternal role
- **4)** developmental tasks of pregnancy
   - **a)** accept the biologic fact of pregnancy (i.e., "I am pregnant.")
   - **b)** accept the growing fetus as distinct from self and as a person to care for (i.e., "I am going to have a baby.")
   - **c)** prepare realistically for the birth and parenting of the child, (i.e., "I am going to be a mother.")
- **5)** paternal reactions to pregnancy
   - **a)** vary with developmental stage, sociocultural factors (as with woman) and involvement
   - **b)** 1st trimester: ambivalence and anxiety about role change; concern or identification with mother's discomforts
   - **c)** 2nd trimester: increased confidence and interest in mother's care; difficulty relating to fetus; "jealousy"
   - **d)** 3rd trimester: changing self-concept; active involvement common; fears about delivery, mutilation/death of partner/fetus
- **6)** sibling reactions to pregnancy
   - **a)** normal rivalry dependent on developmental stage
   - **b)** may need increased affection and attention
   - **c)** regression in behavior (may appear in bed-wetting and thumb sucking)

3. Signs and symptoms of pregnancy (see Table 4.5)

a. Presumptive symptoms (subjective)

Table 4.5 Signs and Symptoms of Pregnancy

Symptoms	Signs
Presumptive	
Amenorrhea	Chadwick's sign
Breast sensitivity	Breast enlargement
Nausea, vomiting	Skin pigmentation, striae
Urinary frequency	
Fatigue	
Quickening	
Probable	
Enlarged abdomen	Ballottement
Hegar's sign	Braxton Hicks' contractions
Goodell's sign	Positive pregnancy tests
Positive	
	By examiner • fetal movements • fetal outline—sonography x-ray • fetal heart tones

- **1)** amenorrhea (approximately 2 weeks after conception)
- **2)** breast sensitivity and fullness (as early as fourth week)
- **3)** nausea and vomiting (primarily 5–12 weeks)
- **4)** urinary frequency (6–12 weeks)
- **5)** fatigue (first trimester)
- **6)** quickening: maternal perception of fetal movement 18–20 weeks in primipara, 16 weeks in multipara

b. Presumptive signs (objective)
- **1)** dark blue discoloration of the vaginal mucosa (Chadwick's sign) (8–12 weeks)
- **2)** skin pigmentation and striae

c. Probable signs (objective)
- **1)** enlargement of abdomen
- **2)** changes in the uterus: size, shape, and consistency (Hegar's sign) (5–7 weeks)
- **3)** softening of the cervical tip (Goodell's sign) (6th week)
- **4)** ballottement: movement of the fetus in the pregnant uterus by the examiner (16–32 weeks)
- **5)** Braxton Hicks' contractions (early as 8 weeks throughout pregnancy)
- **6)** positive pregnancy test: biologic and immunologic tests based on secretion of HCG in maternal urine or in serum (7–14 days)

d. Positive signs (objective)

1) fetal outline and movements felt by examiner (about 20 weeks)
2) presence of fetal heart sounds detected by fetoscope at 16 weeks (Doppler, 10 weeks)
3) confirmation of pregnancy by ultrasonography
4) x-ray outline of fetal skeleton (rarely used)

4. Fetal development
   a. During 1st lunar month (1 lunar month = 4 weeks)
      1) following fertilization, the ovum (zygote) begins a process of rapid cell division (mitosis or cleavage) leading to formation of *blastomers*, which eventually become a ball-like structure called the morula
      2) the *morula* changes into a *blastocyst* after entering the uterus
      3) implantation occurs within 1–2 days, when the exposed cells of the trophoblast (cellular walls of the blastocyst) implant in the anterior or posterior fundal portion of the uterus
      4) the cells of the embryo will differentiate into three main groups: an outer covering (ectoderm), a middle layer (mesoderm), and an internal layer (entoderm)
         a) ectoderm: later differentiates into epithelium of skin, hair, nails, nasal and oral passages, sebaceous and sweat glands, mucous membranes of mouth and nose, salivary glands, the nervous system
         b) mesoderm: later differentiates into muscles; bones; circulatory, renal, and reproductive organs; connective tissue
         c) entoderm: differentiates into epithelium of gastrointestinal and respiratory tracts, the bladder, thyroid
   b. Subsequent lunar months
      1) end of 1st lunar month (4 weeks): heart functions; beginning formation of eyes, nose, digestive tract; arm and leg buds
      2) end of 2nd lunar month (8 weeks): recognizable human face, rapid brain development, appearance of external genitalia
      3) end of 3rd lunar month (12 weeks): placenta fully formed and functioning; sex determination apparent; bones begin to ossify; less danger of teratogenic effects after this time; length: 3½ in (9 cm), weight: ½ oz (2 gm)
      4) end of 4th lunar month (16 weeks): external genitalia obvious; meconium present in intestinal tract; eye, ear, and nose formed; fetal heart beat heard with fetoscope; length: 6½ in, weight: 4 oz
      5) end of 5th lunar month (20th week): lanugo present; fetus sucks and swallows amniotic fluid; quickening (mother can feel movement); length: 10 in, weight: 8 oz
      6) end of 6th lunar month (24th week): vernix present; skin reddish and wrinkled; considered viable, but usually doesn't survive if born now; length: 12 in, weight: 1 lb 5 oz
      7) end of 7th lunar month (28th week): iron stored; surfactant production begins; nails appear; better chance of survival if delivered than in earlier gestation; length: 15 in, weight: 2 lb 8 oz (1,000 gm)
      8) end of 8th lunar month (32 weeks): iron, calcium stored; more reflexes present; if delivered preterm, good chance of survival
      9) end of 9th lunar month (36 weeks): well padded with subcutaneous fat; survival same as term
      10) end of 10th lunar month (39–40 weeks or full term): lanugo shed, nails firm, testes fully descended; length: 18–22 in (45–55 cm), weight: average 7½ lb (3,400 gm)
   c. Fetal circulation
      1) fetus receives oxygen via placenta (see Figure 4.19, page 459)
      2) oxygenated blood enters fetal circulation through umbilical vein of cord to the ductus venosus and liver; ductus venosus attaches to inferior vena cava and allows blood to bypass liver
      3) from inferior vena cava, blood flows into right atrium and goes directly on to the left atrium through the foramen ovale
      4) blood enters right atrium through superior vena cava, flows to right ventricle, to pulmonary artery (small amount enters lungs for nourishment); the ductus arteriosus shunts blood from pulmonary artery into the aorta, allows bypass of fetal lungs
      5) two umbilical arteries return deoxygenated blood from fetus to placenta
   d. Amniotic fluid
      1) multiple origins; composition changes in pregnancy; from maternal serum to fetal urine towards term
      2) appearance: clear, pale, straw colored, with faint characteristic odor; neutral to

slightly alkaline (pH 7.0–7.25) while vaginal secretions are normally acidic

3) volume: about 30 ml at 10 weeks, 350 ml at 20 weeks, approximately 1,000 ml at term; specific gravity 1.007 to 1.025
   a) *oligohydramnios* is less than 300–500 ml of fluid
   b) *polyhydramnios* is greater than 1,500–2,000 ml of fluid
4) contains albumin, urea, uric acid, creatinine, lecithin, sphingomyelin, bilirubin, epithelial cells, fat, fructose, leukocytes, enzymes, lanugo
5) functions
   a) protects fetus from injury
   b) separates fetus from fetal membrane
   c) allows fetus freedom of movement
   d) provides source of oral fluids
   e) serves as excretion-collection system
   f) exchanges at rate of 500 ml/hour (at term)
   g) regulates fetal body temperature

☐ Overview of Management

1. Interdisciplinary health team: nurses, nurse practitioners, midwives, physicians, social workers, dietitians, and other health care providers
2. Schedule of visits
   a. Routine if no complications
      1) every 4 weeks, up to 32 weeks
      2) every 2 weeks from 32–36 weeks (more frequently if problems exist)
      3) every week from 36–40 weeks
   b Initial visit
      1) obtain family and obstetric history
         a) personal/social profile of childbearing family, including cultural patterns, education, economic level, support systems, coping methods
         b) maternal factors affecting course of pregnancy: smoking, use of alcohol and/or drugs, past and current medical problems, activities of daily living, sleep patterns, nutrition, bowel habits
         c) family planning measures; health history during pregnancies; history of infertility
         d) attitudes toward present pregnancy
         e) history of preceding pregnancies and perinatal outcomes (TPAL)
            - T: number of term births (i.e., born at 37 weeks gestation or beyond)
            - P: number of premature births
            - A: number of abortions (spontaneous or induced)
            - L: number of living children
            - *gravida*: all pregnancies regardless of duration or outcome, including present pregnancy
            - *parity*: past pregnancies resulting in viable fetus (20–24 weeks), whether born dead or alive (twins considered as one)
         f) past personal and family medical history
      2) calculate expected date of delivery (confinement) (EDC) using Naegele's rule: count back three calendar months from the 1st day of the last regular menstrual period (LMP) and add seven days (see Table 4.6)
   c. Initial and subsequent visits
      1) assess vital signs and blood pressure for normal range/baseline
      2) check urine for albumin and glucose: ideally not more than 1+ sugar with protein negative
      3) monitor weight gain: a total gain of 25–30 lb is recommended, depending on prepregnant nutritional state
         a) 2–4 lb in the 1st trimester
         b) 11–14 lb in the 2nd trimester
         c) 8–11 lb in the 3rd trimester (i.e., 0.5 lb weekly)
      4) assess fetal growth and development over duration of pregnancy
         a) fetal heart rate
         b) abdominal palpation
         c) fundal height
      5) allow time for client to express concerns, problems or discomfort, and learning needs
      6) document accurately

Application of the Nursing Process to Normal Childbearing, Antepartal Care

1. **Assessment/Analysis**
   a. Refer to "Initial and Subsequent Visits"

Table 4.6 Naegele's Rule

If first day of last menstrual period was
June 17, 1989
substract 3 months
+
add 7 days
Estimated date of delivery is March 24, 1990

b. Refer to "Initial and Subsequent Visits"

2. Plans, Implementation, and Evaluation

Goal 1: Client will maintain optimal health through preventive health measures and regular antepartal/prenatal care; fetus will be well oxygenated and nourished throughout gestation.

Plan/Implementation

- Measure vital signs, including temperature, blood pressure, pulse, respiration.
- Assess client: general physical assessment including height and weight (initial visit).
- Assist with physical examination and bimanual pelvic examination
  - prepare and arrange necessary equipment (gloves, lubricant [for digital exam], vaginal speculum, materials for Pap smear [no lubricant used], light, pelvimeter)
  - prepare client for procedure by providing explanation, instructing her to empty bladder, and placing her in lithotomy position, position hands across chest
  - provide emotional support and maintain comfort of client before and during examination (using relaxation, breathing, and focusing techniques)
- Measure fundal height using McDonald's rule (in 2nd and 3rd trimester): symphysis pubis to fundus (see Table 4.7)
- Estimate fetal weight (EFW): rump-to-crown length in utero in cm × 100 = EFW in gm.
- Check for fetal heart beat, detectable as early as 16th week with fetoscope, and by 10–12 weeks with Doppler device.
- Assist in obtaining samples for laboratory studies
  - clean catch urine for urinalysis, albumin, glucose, and asymptomatic bacteriuria
  - blood for hemoglobin, hematocrit, type, Rh, rubella titer (greater than 1:8 shows immunity)
  - sickle cell disease or trait in black women
  - standard tests for sexually transmitted diseases (serology for syphilis; smears for gonorrhea, herpes)

Table 4.7 McDonald's Rule

Height of fundus (in cm)
- × 2/7 = duration of pregnancy in *lunar months*
- × 8/7 = duration of pregnancy in *weeks*

  - schedule glucose tolerance test during 24–28 weeks
- Encourage regular antepartal care
  - explain need for continuity
  - describe "*danger signals*" (e.g., vaginal bleeding, dizziness or visual spots, swelling of face or fingers, epigastric pain, physical trauma) or reportable signs that require immediate medical care
- Promote health through anticipatory guidance: rest and exercise, personal hygiene, sexual activity, dental care, clothing, travel, immunizations, smoking, alcohol use, substance abuse
  - tell couple to expect an increased need for sleep during entire pregnancy, with fatigue common in first trimester; needs vary among individuals; plan rest times during day
  - teach relaxation methods in preparing for sleep
  - advise to continue usual exercise regimen; avoid introduction of strenuous sports; avoid exercise leading to fatigue, exhaustion, overheating, dehydration
  - explain exercise limitations related to the changing center of gravity (e.g., high impact aerobics, jogging)
  - avoid sauna/whirlpool activities
  - suggest that client may continue to work except if exposed to toxic chemicals, radiation, biologic or safety hazards (if job requires sitting for long period of time, encourage frequent position changes)
  - teach hygiene and skin care; daily baths if desired (caution on safety getting into and out of bathtub); avoid soap on nipples; towel-dry breasts; for vaginal discharge: daily bathing, wear cotton underwear (douching not recommended)
  - suggest that changes in sexual desire/response may occur, related to discomforts or anxieties of pregnancy; encourage couple to share their concerns and feelings; alternative coital positions may be helpful, as may be other methods of satisfying sexual needs; coitus may be continued throughout pregnancy unless premature labor, rupture of membranes, or bleeding occur
  - encourage dental checkup early in pregnancy and delay extensive dental work and x-ray examinations when possible; hypertrophy and tenderness of gums is a common problem
  - recommend comfortable, nonrestricting maternity clothing, well-fitting bra, and low-heeled, supportive shoes

- advise client to stop or reduce cigarette consumption; *maternal smoking is associated with low birth weight*
- advise client to *avoid alcohol consumption* during pregnancy as alcohol, even in minimal-to-moderate amounts, is harmful to fetus; linked to fetal alcohol syndrome
- warn client to avoid medication, particularly in the 1st trimester (over-the-counter and prescription drugs may cross placental barrier); physicians must weigh advantages versus risks of medications for individual clients
- suggest that while travelling long distances by auto, walk frequently; use seatbelts for safety
- teach couple that attenuated, live vaccines (e.g., mumps, rubella) are contraindicated for immunizations during pregnancy

Evaluation: Client receives initial and regular antepartal care to prevent/detect any early complications; avoids substances that may potentially harm the fetus; fetus maintains a growth and development pattern appropriate for gestational age as evidenced by maternal weight gain, fundal height, activity level, and other antenatal screening techniques; is protected from environmental hazards and stresses (e.g., alcohol, nicotine).

Goal 2: Client will be aware of common discomforts of pregnancy and know how to relieve them.

Plan/Implementation

- Teach health maintenance: relief of common discomforts
  - *morning sickness*: eat dry crackers or toast before slowly arising; eat small frequent meals; avoid greasy, highly seasoned food; take adequate fluids between meals
  - *breast tenderness*: wear a well-fitted, supportive bra with wide, adjustable straps
  - *heartburn and indigestion*: avoid overeating, ingesting fatty or fried food; take small, frequent meals; avoid taking sodium bicarbonate; remain upright 3–4 hours after eating
  - *backache*: maintain proper body alignment (pelvic tilt) and use good body mechanics; use maternity girdle in selected situations; wear comfortable shoes; use proper mattress; rest frequently; do pelvic-rock exercise, tailor sitting
  - *leg cramps*: stretch involved muscles, i.e., extension of leg with dorsiflexion of the foot (may be related to alterations in calcium, phosphorus)
  - *varicose veins*: elevate legs frequently when sitting or lying down in bed; avoid sitting or standing for prolonged periods of time or crossing legs at the knees; avoid tight or constricting hosiery or garters (physican may suggest wearing supportive hose)
  - *hemorrhoids*: apply warm compresses; upon recommendation of physician, reinsert hemorrhoids (place client in a side-lying or knee-chest position; use gentle pressure and a lubricant), avoid constipation; take sitz baths
  - *constipation*: increase fluid intake (ideal is 6–8 glasses/day), roughage; develop good daily bowel movement habits, exercise
  - *urinary frequency*: empty bladder regularly; report any burning, dysuria, cloudiness, blood in urine
  - *ankle edema*: change position, lie on left side; rest with legs and hips elevated (report any edema in face and in hands)
  - *uterine contractions* (Braxton Hicks'): normal during late pregnancy; report if they progressively increase and are accompanied by signs of labor
  - *faintness*: avoid staying in one position over a long period of time; arise from bed from a lateral position (to prevent supine hypotension)
  - *shortness of breath*: use proper posture when erect; sleep with head elevated by several pillows (left lateral position preferred)

Evaluation: Client identifies own basic discomforts of pregnancy and appropriately relieves them.

Goal 3: Client will have adequate knowledge of nutrition to meet her own developmental needs, the physical requirements of pregnancy and lactation, and fetal growth and development.

Plan/Implementation

- Obtain complete nutritional profile (suggest client use 24-hour recall)
  - prepregnant and current nutritional status (e.g., overweight, underweight, anemic)
  - physical symptoms possibly indicative of poor nutrition (e.g., dry scaly skin, lack of skin turgor, fatigue)
  - socioeconomic status: available finances for a balanced diet; customs and cultural/religious restrictions
  - dietary habits: regularity of meals, junk food intake, pica, peer pressure

- knowledge of nutritional needs, basic four food groups, recommended allowances during pregnancy
- Assess for nutritional risk factors at the onset of pregnancy
  - adolescence
  - frequent pregnancies
  - poor reproductive history
  - economic deprivation
  - bizarre food patterns
  - vegetarian diet
  - smoking, drug addiction, alcoholism
  - chronic systemic disease
  - prepregnant weight: overweight, underweight including anorexia and bulimia
- Assess for nutritional risk factors during pregnancy
  - anemia of pregnancy
  - pregnancy-induced hypertension
  - inadequate/excessive weight gain
  - demands of lactation
- Teach based on consideration of mother's age, routine activity, developmental needs, cultural dietary patterns, and risk factors.
- Encourage good nutritional practices; see Tables 4.4, 4.8, and 4.9, 4.10
  - discuss well-balanced diet including basic 4 groups as adapted during pregnancy
  - recommend that pregnant adolescents take in additional calories, protein, and calcium for own developmental needs
  - suggest a minimum fluid intake of 6–8 glasses of fluids or water/day
  - discuss possible vitamin and mineral supplements (e.g., iron, folic acid)
  - caution against overdose of vitamins A and D (may cause fetal deformities)
  - monitor weight gain each antepartal visit; a total weight gain of 25–30 lb is usually recommended
  - recognize when restrictions in salt may be indicated (e.g., high sodium foods: carrots, spinach, celery, carbonated beverages, canned soup, bacon, ham, monosodium gluconate, pickles, olives)
  - refer to nutritionist for additional teaching/ counseling as needed

Evaluation: Client identifies the basic four food groups and their components; knows the nutrients/ calories needed each day; follows a balanced diet; gradually and steadily gains 25–30 lb during the pregnancy; fetus maintains a growth and

Table 4.8 Recommended Dietary Allowances for Females Aged 11–50[1]

	Non-pregnant Girls and Women (Age in Years)		(Mean Weight in Lb)			
Nutrients	**11–14 (101)**	**15–18 (120)**	**19–22 (120)**	**23–50 (120)**	**Pregnant Women**	**Lactating Women**
Energy (kcal) (mean)	2,200	2,100	2,100	2,000	+300	+500
Protein (gm)	46	46	44	44	+ 30	+ 20
Vitamin A (mcg)	800	800	800	800	+200	+400
Vitamin D (mcg)	10	10	7.5	5	+ 5	+ 5
Vitamin E (mg)	8	8	8	8	+ 2	+ 3
Vitamin C (mg)	50	60	60	60	+ 20	+ 40
Thiamin (mg)	1.1	1.1	1.1	1.0	+ .04	+ 0.5
Riboflavin (mg)	1.3	1.3	1.3	1.2	+ 0.3	+ 0.5
Niacin (mg)	15	14	14	13	+ 2	+ 5
Vitamin B_6 (mg)	1.8	2.0	2.0	2.0	+ 0.6	+ 0.5
Folacin (mcg)	400	400	400	400	+400	+100
Vitamin B_{12} (mcg)	3	3	3	3	+ 1	+ 1
Calcium (mg)	1,200	1,200	800	800	+400	+400
Phosphorus (mg)	1,200	1,200	800	800	+400	+400
Magnesium (mg)	300	300	300	300	+150	+150
Iron (mg)	18	18	18	18	Suppl[2]	[2]
Zinc (mg)	15	15	15	15	+ 5	+ 10
Iodine (mg)	150	150	150	150	+ 25	+ 50

[1]Note: From *Recommended Dietary Allowances* by the Committee on Dietary Allowances, Food and Nutrition Board, Division of Biological Sciences; Assembly of Life Sciences, National Research Council, 9th rev. ed., 1980, Washington, DC: National Academy of Sciences.
[2]Recommendation: Iron supplement of 30–60 mg during pregnancy and for 2–3 months postpartum. Iron needs during lactation do not differ substantially from those of nonpregnant women. The supplement is to replenish stores depleted by pregnancy.

Table 4.9 Selected Nutrients Essential for Health in Pregnancy and Lactation

Nutrient	Food Source
Iron	Liver, meat, eggs, whole enriched grains, leafy vegetables, nuts, legumes, dried fruits, oysters, clams
Calcium	Milk, cheese, ice cream, whole grains, leafy vegetables, egg yolks, dried beans
Vitamin C	Citrus fruits, tomatoes, cantaloupe, strawberries, potatoes, broccoli, leafy greens
Protein	Milk, pudding, custard, yogurt, cheese, meat, poultry, fish, eggs, legumes, nuts

development pattern appropriate for gestational age.

Goal 4: Client/family will verbalize a familiarity with the relaxation techniques and exercises that are part of childbirth education; will experience reduced anxiety about childbirth and parenting.

Plan/Implementation

- Explain the purpose and scope of childbirth education (decrease fear and anxiety through knowledge, effective use of relaxation techniques to reduce pain perception during labor/delivery.
- Discuss various methods (see Table 4.11).
- Offer direct instructions (Le Boyer) or referral to appropriate resources (e.g., La Leche League or International Childbirth Education Association).

Evaluation: Couple expresses a positive attitude toward pregnancy and is adequately prepared for birth experience; openly expresses their concerns and provides emotional support to each other; begins the role transition to parenthood.

Table 4.10 Pregnant Woman's Daily Food Intake

Food Group	Recommended Daily Amount
Dairy products	Three to four 8-oz cups
Meat group	Two 3–4 oz servings; 1 egg
Grain products, whole grain or enriched	4–5 servings
Fruits/fruit juices	3–4 servings; include 4 oz of orange or grapefruit juice
Vegetables/ vegetable juices	3–4 servings (1 or 2 servings raw; 1 serving of dark green or deep yellow)
Fluids	4–6 glasses (8 oz) water plus other fluids to equal 8–10 cups/day

Note: From *Obstetric Nursing* by S. Olds, et al., 1984, Menio Park, CA: Addison-Wesley.

☐ High-risk Childbearing

1. Definition: any existing or developing condition or factor that prevents or impedes the normal progress of pregnancy to the delivery of a viable, healthy, term infant.
2. Assessment of risk factors (some that already exist cannot be altered)
   a. Age: under 17 or over 35 (greater risk over 40)
      1) pregnant adolescents: have a higher incidence of prematurity, pregnancy-induced hypertension, cephalopelvic disproportion, poor nutrition, and inadequate antepartal care
      2) women over 35: have an increased risk of chromosomal disorders in infants (e.g., Down syndrome), pregnancy-induced hypertension, and cesarean delivery
   b. Parity
      1) multiparity: two or more pregnancies (may not be significant)
      2) grand multiparity: six or more pregnancies
      3) interval between pregnancies
   c. Past health history
      1) diabetes
      2) heart disease
      3) renal conditions
      4) essential hypertension
      5) anemia
      6) thyroid disorder
      7) physical abuse
   d. Past obstetrical history
      1) lack of antepartal care/poor compliance with visit schedule (may be a factor in late detection of health problems); contributes to high infant mortality rate in this country
      2) abortions: spontaneous
      3) ruptured ectopic pregnancy
      4) premature deliveries or intrauterine-growth retardation
      5) congenital malformations: result of genetic disorders
      6) cesarean births
      7) previous fetal death

Table 4.11 Childbirth Preparation

Method	Chief Focus	Breathing/Relaxation Techniques
G.D. Read	Earliest modern physician to identify fear-tension-pain cycle Avoidance of medication; removed childbirth from illness orientation	
Gamper	Based on Read; use of uterus as focal point	Abdominal/natural breathing
Bradley	Based on Read/Gamper Focus on individual relaxation methods Mother–centered; coached by husband Emphasis on consumer decision-making	Diaphragmatic breathing
Lamaze (psychoprophylactic)	Conscious application of conditioned responses to stimuli Use of focal point outside mother's body	Chest breathing in early labor Increasing rate as labor progresses Cleansing breaths

8) pregnancy-induced hypertension
9) diabetes
10) vaginal bleeding in pregnancy
11) isoimmunization
12) multiple gestation

e. Current obstetric history
1) pregnancy-induced hypertension (21% of maternal deaths)
2) infections (18% of maternal deaths)
a) sexually transmitted diseases
b) TORCH syndrome
c) other viral diseases e.g., hepatitis or AIDS
d) bacterial infections e.g., tuberculosis
3) hemorrhage (14% of maternal deaths)
4) exposure to toxic environmental agents
5) use of drugs
6) multiple gestation
7) abnormal presentation
8) premature rupture of membranes
9) chronic health problems, e.g., diabetes, cardiac disease, anemia
10) co-existing medical problems
11) abnormal antenatal test results (e.g., on amniotic-fluid analysis, ultrasound)

f. Socioeconomic-cultural status
1) low socioeconomic status: often associated with
a) inadequate nutrition
b) lack of general knowledge about health care needs
2) incidence of small-for-gestational-age babies is common in some Asian and black women and adolescents

g. Malnutrition or deprivation: less than 4 kg weight gain by 30th week of gestation; may be related to eating disorders

h. Drug or alcohol addiction: associated with congenital anomalies, intrauterine-growth retardation, and numerous other problems

i. Smoking: associated with low-birth-weight infants

3. Diagnostic tests, biophysical and biochemical, to evaluate fetal-placental function or fetal maturity; critical in high-risk pregnancy

a. Daily fetal movement count (DFMC)
1) definition: periodic recording of fetal movements to assess active and passive fetal states in normal pregnancies, as well as in those with complications
2) procedure: a noninvasive test that may be done directly by pregnant woman
3) interpretation (optimal number of fetal movements varies with source)
a) normally 3 or more movements felt in an hour when lying down, although fetal states normally vary (cyclic periods of rest and activity)
b) marked decrease in fetal activity (unrelated to sleep) of 2 or less movements/hour should be reported and NST may be scheduled
4) reassure client there are fetal rest-sleep states with minimal or no fetal movement

b. Nonstress testing (NST)
1) definition: observation of fetal heart rate (FHR) related to fetal movement (acclerations suggest fetal well-being with good prognosis)
2) procedure
a) performed in an ambulatory setting or in the hospital obstetrical unit by nurse trained in test administration
b) requires external electronic monitoring (indirect) using ultrasound transducer to measure FHR and tokodynamometer

to trace fetal activity and/or spontaneous uterine activity

   c) pregnant woman placed in semi-Folwer's or left lateral position, may be turned slightly to the left
   d) maternal BP recorded initially
   e) requires 30–50 minutes to administer test (10- to 12-minute tracing obtained)
   f) client must activate "mark button" with each fetal movement

3) interpretation
   a) reactive (normal): 2 FHR accelerations (greater than 15 bpm) above baseline—lasting 15 seconds or more—occur with fetal movement in a 10- to 20-minute period
   b) nonreactive (abnormal): failure to meet the reactive criteria indicates the need for additional evaluation, perhaps using contraction stress test or oxytocin challenge test
   c) unsatisfactory result: uninterpretable FHR or fetal activity recording; additional testing performed in 24 hours or OCT done

c. Contraction stress test (CST) or oxytocin challenge test (OCT)
   1) definition: the response of the fetus (e.g., FHR pattern) to induced uterine contractions is observed as an indicator of uteroplacental and fetal physiologic integrity
   2) indications: pregnancies at risk for placental insufficiency or fetal compromise
   3) procedure
      a) performed on an outpatient basis in or near the labor and delivery unit
      b) requires external electronic monitoring (indirect) using ultrasound tansducer to measure FHR and tokodynamometer to trace uterine activity
      c) pregnant woman placed in semi-Fowler's or left lateral position
      d) maternal blood pressure recorded initially and at intervals during test
      e) requires 60 minutes to 3 hours to complete test
      f) increasing doses of oxytocin are administered as a dilute intravenous infusion according to hospital protocol or physician's orders until uterine contractions occur
   4) interpretation
      a) negative (normal): the absence of late decelerations of FHR with each of three contractions during a 10-minute interval; known as "negative window"
      b) positive (abnormal): the presence of late decelerations of FHR with three contractions during a 10-minute interval; known as "positive window"
      c) equivocal or suspicious: the absence of a positive or negative window, i.e., criterion of three contractions in a 10-minute interval is not achieved
      d) unsatisfactory tests occur when interpretable tracings are not obtained or adequate uterine contractions are not achieved
      e) high-risk pregnancies are usually allowed to continue if a negative OCT is obtained; test is repeated weekly for these clients

d. Nipple-stimulation contraction test
   1) baseline data obtained through monitoring as in CST procedure
   2) breast stimulated by warm towel application or nipple rolling
   3) interpretation: as with CST, uterine contraction with absence of late decelerations is the desired result

e. Ultrasonography
   1) definition: a noninvasive procedure involving the passage of high-frequency sound waves through the uterus in order to obtain an outline of the fetus, placenta, uterine cavity, or any other area under examination
   2) purposes
      a) confirm pregnancy (1st trimester)
      b) determine fetal viability
      c) estimate fetal age through measurement of the biparietal diameter of the fetal head; most accurate at 12–24 weeks
      d) monitor fetal growth
      e) determine fetal position
      f) locate placenta
      g) detect fetal abnormalities
      h) identify multiple gestation
      i) confirm fetal death
   3) procedure
      a) advise pregnant woman to consume one quart of water 2 hours prior to procedure and avoid emptying bladder; scanning is done when the bladder is full (exception: prior to amniocentesis)
      b) transmission gel spread over maternal abdomen
      c) sonographer scans vertically and

horizontally in sections across abdomen

4) possible risk
   a) none known with brief, infrequent exposure to high intensity sound
   b) couple and physician should discuss indications, benefits, and potential risks

f. Chorionic villi sampling
1) definition: removal of a small sample of chorionic villi for examination
2) purposes
   a) detect chromosomal defects
   b) detect biochemical abnormalities
3) procedure
   a) done at 8–10 weeks gestation
   b) catheter passed through cervix into the uterus (guided by sonography)
   c) sample aspirated under negative pressure
4) advantages
   a) early detection of abnormalities allowing for first trimester termination of the pregnancy if desired
   b) results available within 2–10 days
5) disadvantages
   a) risk of abortion
   b) infection

g. Amniocentesis
1) definition: an invasive procedure for amniotic fluid analysis to assess fetal health and maturity; done from the 14th week of gestation
2) procedure
   a) ultrasonography is first performed to locate the placenta
   b) pregnant woman must empty bladder before procedure, if greater than 20 weeks gestation
   c) baseline vital signs and FHR are assessed; monitor every 15 minutes
   d) pregnant woman is placed in supine position and given an abdominal prep
   e) a needle is passed through the abdominal and uterine walls into the amniotic sac and a small amount of amniotic fluid is withdrawn
3) possible risks: overall less than 1%
   a) maternal: hemorrhage, infection, Rh isoimmunization, abruptio placentae, labor
   b) fetal: death, infection, hemorrhage, abortion, premature labor, injury from needle
4) observe client closely for 30–40 minutes following procedure; instruct client to report any side effects (e.g., unusual fetal activity, vaginal discharge, uterine contractions, fever, or chills)

h. Laboratory studies
1) urinary or serum estriol determination: to assess placental functioning
   a) steroid precursor produced by the adrenals of the fetus is synthesized into estriols in the placenta and is excreted by the maternal kidneys; mother's levels normally rise during pregnancy
   b) serial estriol determinations are obtained with repeat blood samples or 24-hour urine collections after 20th week of gestation (preferably after 32 weeks); instruct re 24° urine collection (i.e., discard first specimen, then save all urine; refrigerate)
   c) a sudden drop in estriol level is associated with fetal hypoxia; continuous low levels associated with compromise of fetus
2) Serum placental lactogen
   a) hormone produced by placenta; levels rise through 36 weeks gestation then stabilize
   b) low values indicate possible fetal distress, values low in threatened abortion, toxemia, intrauterine growth retardation, postmaturity
3) analysis of amniotic fluid (see Table 4.12)
   a) chromosomal studies to assess genetic disorders (e.g., Down syndrome, cell culture for karyotype)
   b) determination of sex chromatin in fetal cells to assess sex-linked disorders
   c) biochemical analysis of fetal-cell enzymes to assess inborn errors of metabolism
   d) determination of lecithin to sphingomyelin ratios (L/S ratios) to assess fetal lung maturity (most reliable)
      - lecithin and sphingomyelin are important components of surfactant, a phosphoprotein that lowers surface tension in the fetal lungs and facilitates extrauterine expiration
      - an L/S ratio of 2:1 or greater is generally associated with fetal lung maturity except for selected high-risk neonates (e.g., infants of diabetic mothers)

Table 4.12 Laboratory Studies of Fetal Well-Being

Study	Purpose/Indication	Interpretation
Urinary/serum estriol	Asess placental functioning	Sudden drop = fetal hypoxia Continuous low levels = fetal compromise
Amniotic fluid analysis	Chromosomal studies	Detection of genetic disorders
	Determination of sex chromatin	Detection of sex-linked disorders
	Biochemical analysis of fetal cell enzymes	Detection of inborn errors of metabolism
	Fetal lung maturity (licithin/sphingomyelin ratios)	L/S ratio of 2:1 or greater = fetal lung maturity
	Alpha-fetoprotein (AFP) levels	High levels = neural-tube defects
	Creatinine levels	More than 2.0 mg = fetal age greater than 36 weeks
	Identification and evaluation of Rh incompatibility	Increased bilirubin = evaluate for intrauterine transfusion and/or delivery
	Lipid cells (Nile blue stain)	20% cells stained orange = fetal weight at least 2,500 gm
	Meconium presence	Fetal hypoxia (except with breech)

- **e)** evaluation of phospholipids (PG) (Nile blue stain); useful if membranes have ruptured prematurely
- **f)** determination of creatinine level: 2.0 mg or greater suggests fetal age greater than 36 weeks
- **g)** identification and evaluation of isoimmune disease; usually done after 24th week to assess bilirubin levels and optical density
- **h)** determination of alpha-fetoprotein (AFP) levels to assess neural-tube defects such as anencephaly, spina bifida, congenital nephrosis, esophageal atresia, fetal demise (blood or amniotic fluid may be tested)
- **i)** identification of meconium (often indicative of fetal hypoxia)

Application of the Nursing Process to the High-Risk Pregnant Client

1. Assessment
- **a.** Risk factors (see page 399)
- **b.** Results of diagnostic tests

2. Analysis
- **a.** Safe, effective care environment
  - **1)** potential for trauma
  - **2)** potential for infection
- **b.** Physiological integrity
  - **1)** ineffective airway clearance/potential for aspiration
  - **2)** actual/potential fluid volume deficit
- **c.** Psychological integrity
  - **1)** anxiety
  - **2)** anticipatory grieving
- **d.** Health promotion/maintenance
  - **1)** altered family processes
  - **2)** actual/potential altered parenting
  - **3)** knowledge deficit

3. Plan, Implementation, and Evaluation

Goal: The pregnant woman and partner will verbalize an understanding of symptoms (danger signals) of high-risk conditions to be reported immediately.

Plan/Implementation
- ■ Teach woman/partner to immediately report any of the following danger signals
  - – infection
  - – vaginal bleeding
  - – generalized edema
  - – trauma
  - – leaking amniotic fluid
  - – elevated temperature
  - – headache
  - – visual changes, e.g., spotting before eyes
  - – abdominal, epigastric pain
  - – projectile vomiting
  - – decreased fetal activity
- ■ Reinforce the importance of keeping appointments as scheduled and of complying with therapeutic regimen.
- ■ Provide emotional support.
- ■ Assess client and fetal heart rate at each subsequent visit for potential/actual problems.
- ■ Document accurately.

Evaluation: The pregnant woman or partner reports danger signals immediately upon detection.

Selected Health Problems in the Antepartal Period

☐ Abortion

1. General Information

a. Definition: one of the bleeding disorders of pregnancy, it is termination of pregnancy before viability (less than 20 weeks gestation or less than 500 gm fetus) as a result of elective procedures or reproductive failure. Approximately 75% of all spontaneous abortions occur during the 2nd and 3rd month of gestation.

b. Types
- **1)** *therapeutic* (or induced): pregnancy that has been purposely terminated
- **2)** *spontaneous:* natural termination of pregnancy without therapeutic intervention
- **3)** *threatened:* possible loss of the products of conception; slight bleeding, mild uterine cramping, cervical os closed, no passage of tissue
- **4)** *inevitable:* threatened loss of the products of conception that cannot be prevented or stopped; moderate bleeding, cramping; open cervical os; no passage of tissue
- **5)** *incomplete:* the expulsion of part of the products of conception and the retention of other parts in utero; heavy bleeding, severe cramping, open os, passage of tissue
- **6)** *complete:* the expulsion of all the products of conception, slight bleeding, mild cramping, closed os, passage of tissue
- **7)** *missed:* retention of the products of conception in utero after the fetus dies, slight bleeding, no cramping, closed os, no passage of tissue
- **8)** *habitual:* spontaneous abortion in three or more successive pregnancies

c. Predisposing factors (spontaneous abortion): often unknown (20%–25%), may be associated with
- **1)** embryonic/fetal problems (50%–60%): disorganization of germ plasma, ovular defects, chromosomal aberration, faulty placental development
- **2)** maternal problems (15%–20%): systemic infections, severe nutritional deprivation, abnormal pathologic conditions of the reproductive tract, endocrine dysfunction, trauma, medical diseases

2. Nursing Process

a. Assessment/Analysis
- **1)** identify symptoms (spontaneous vaginal bleeding, uterine cramping, contractions)
- **2)** evaluate blood loss: save pads; assess saturation, frequency of change
- **3)** recognize signs and symptoms of shock (e.g., rapid, thready pulse; pallor; decreased BP; restlessness; clammy skin)

b. Plan, Implementation, and Evaluation

Goal: Client will be free from complications.

Plan/Implementation
- Note and record blood and tissue loss.
- Institute nursing measures to treat shock if necessary (see "Shock" page 170).
- Monitor I&O.
- Replace fluids as ordered.
- Prepare for dilatation and curettage (D&C) as necessary (incomplete abortion).
- Provide emotional support of grieving process (refer to *Loss, Death and Dying* page 30).

Evaluation: Client is free from excessive blood loss, fluid imbalance, infection.

☐ Incompetent Cervical Os

1. General Information

a. Definition: mechanical defect in the cervix, often a cause of habitual 2nd trimester abortions or preterm labor (premature cervical dilation)

b. Predisposing factors: anatomical deviation of the cervix, cervical trauma from D&C, conization, cauterization, or cervical lacerations with previous pregnancies

c. Medical treatment: physician determines preferred surgical intervention, suturing of cervix during the 14th–18th weeks of gestation, or prior to next pregnancy
- **1)** permanent suture (Shirodkar procedure); subsequent delivery by cesarean section
- **2)** temporary purse string (McDonald procedure); suture removed at term, with vaginal delivery

2. Nursing Process

a. Assessment/Analysis
- **1)** history of miscarriages/abortions
- **2)** relaxed cervical os on pelvic examination

b. Plan, Implementation, and Evaluation

Goal: Client with an incompetent cervical os will report problems, seek treatment, and comply with restricted activity; will maintain gestation to term.

Plan/Implementation (post-op)
- Suggest limited activity for 2 or more weeks following this procedure.
- Tell client to report signs of labor.
- Monitor fetal growth to term and continue routine prenatal assessment and care.
- Observe for signs of labor, infection, and premature rupture of the membranes.

Evaluation: Client complies with activity restrictions after treatment; carries fetus to term.

☐ Ectopic Pregnancy

1. General Information

a. Definition: an *extrauterine* pregnancy, implantation occurring most often in ampulla of the fallopian tubes

b. Incidence: 1 in 80 to 1 in 200 live births, 7th cause of maternal mortality (from rupture of tube leading to hemorrhage, infection, and shock)

c. Predisposing factors: any condition that causes constriction of the fallopian tube (e.g., pelvic inflammatory disease, puerperal and postabortion sepsis, developmental defects, prolonged use of an IUD)

d. Medical treatment: diagnosis, ultrasound, surgical intervention (laparoscopy, laparotomy with salpingectomy)

2. Nursing Process

a. Assessment/Analysis

1) signs and symptoms
- **a)** lower unilateral abdominal tenderness, cramps related to stretching of the tube
- **b)** knifelike pain in lower quadrant (only when tube has ruptured)
- **c)** profound shock, if ruptured
- **d)** vaginal spotting

Figure 4.4 Common Site of Ectopic Pregnancy

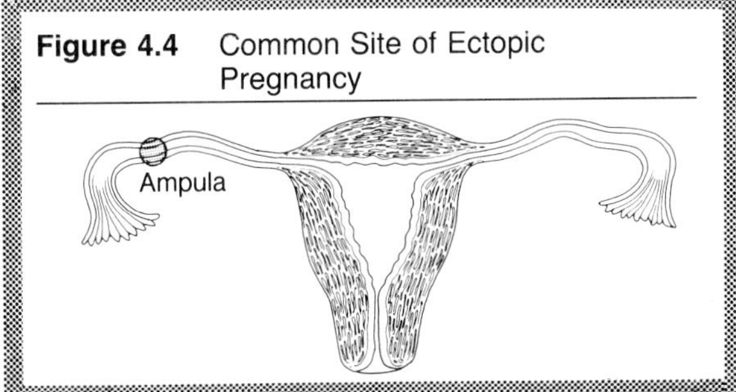

2) history: last menstrual period

3) prior history of infection, IUD use

b. Plan, Implementation, and Evaluation

Goal: Client will report early signs of ectopic pregnancy; will be free from complications following surgery; will return to a homeostatic state.

Plan/Implementation
- Monitor vital signs; carry out an ongoing assessment for shock.
- Maintain intravenous infusion for administration of plasma/blood, antibiotics, or other required medication.
- Prepare client for surgery, physically and emotionally.
- Post-op, continue to monitor vital signs, I&O; have client cough and deep breathe q2h.
- Support grieving process.

Evaluation: Client seeks treatment before rupture of tube, is free from other complications; regains post-op homeostasis.

☐ Hydatidiform Mole

1. General Information

a. Definition: a developmental anomaly of the chorion causing degeneration of the villi and formation of grapelike vesicles; fertilized ovum is initially present but usually no embryo develops

b. Incidence: 1 in 1,500 pregnancies

c. Predisposing factors: unknown; however, it is associated with induction of ovulation by clomiphene therapy and increased maternal age

Figure 4.5 Hydatidiform Mole

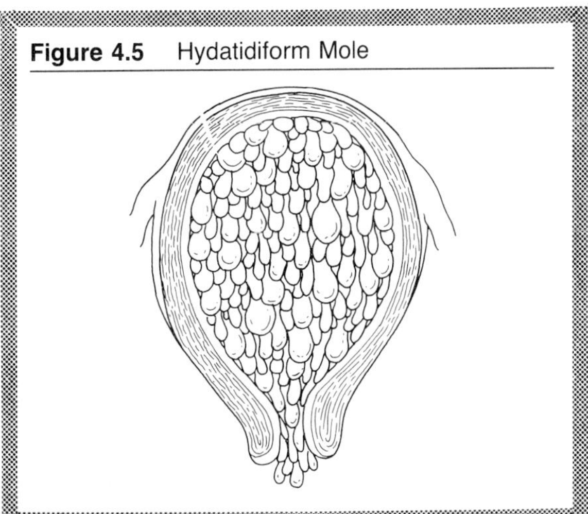

d. Medical treatment

1) surgical intervention (D&C or, in women over 45 or with profuse bleeding, hysterectomy)
2) medical intervention: monitor HCG levels; chemotherapy, if indicated
3) close supervision for one year

2. Nursing Process

a. Assessment/Analysis

1) signs and symptoms
   a) initially appears as a normal pregnancy
   b) uterus larger than expected for reported gestational age
   c) lower uterine segment soft and full upon palpation
   d) excessive nausea and vomiting (hyperemesis gravidarum)
   e) brownish discharge or vaginal spotting; onset around 12th week of gestation
   f) hypertension and other symptoms of preeclampsia (e.g., proteinuria)
2) pregnancy test: HCG often very high

b. Plan, Implementation, and Evaluation

Goal: Client will report abnormal signs, seek treatment; will comply with physician's plan for supervision for one year to detect signs of choriocarcinoma; will delay subsequent pregnancy.

Plan/Implementation

- Administer plasma/blood replacement as ordered.
- Maintain fluid and electrolyte balance through replacement.
- Emphasize need for follow-up supervision for 1 year with HCG measurement, examination to detect choriocarcinoma, chemotherapy if indicated.
- Emphasize that pregnancy should be avoided for at least 1 year.
- Provide emotional support.

Evaluation: Client has hydatidiform mole removed; complies with regular schedule of visits following therapy; avoids pregnancy until cleared by physician.

☐ Placenta Previa

1. General Information

a. Definition: abnormal implantation of placenta in lower uterine segment

b. Incidence: 1 in 170 pregnancies; most common cause of bleeding in late pregnancy

c. Predisposing factors: decreased vascularity of upper uterine segment, multiparity, scarring from prior surgery

d. Degrees of placenta previa

1) *partial*: placenta partially covers the internal os
2) *complete*: placenta totally covers the cervical os (cesarean birth necessary)

Figure 4.6 Placenta Previa

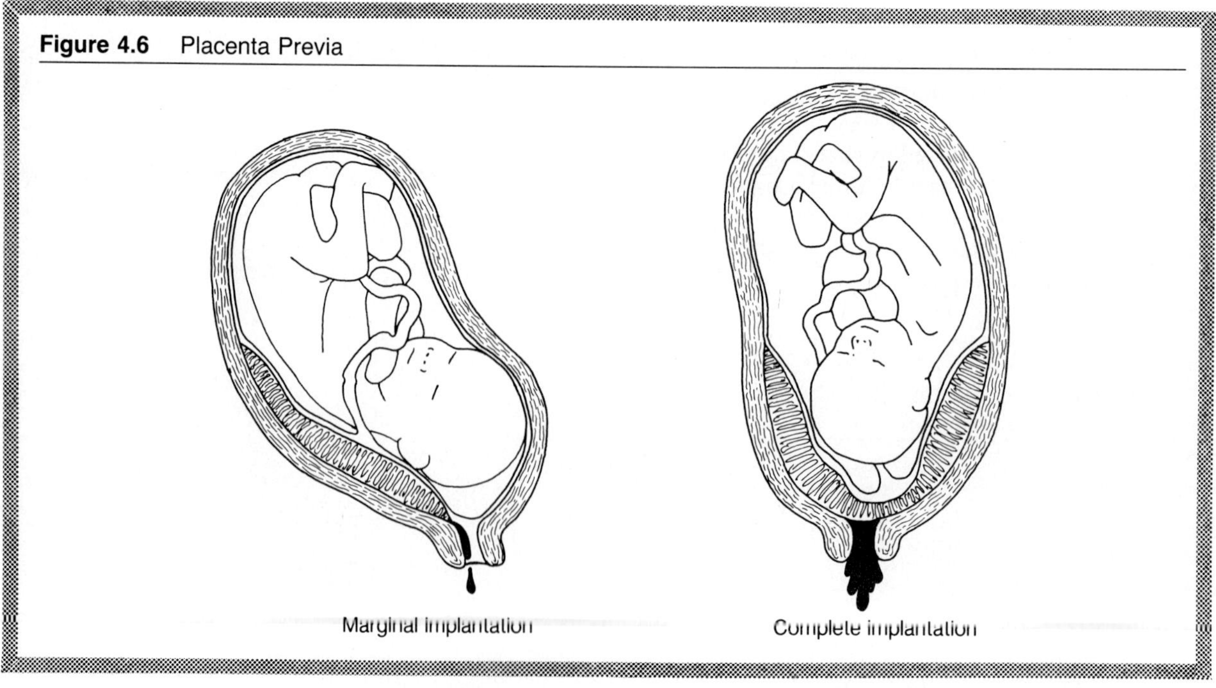

3) *low-lying or marginal*: placenta encroaches on margin of internal os

e. Placental abnormalities in formation or implantation: associated with maternal bleeding during the 3rd trimester or intrapartum period; hemorrhage is the leading cause of maternal mortality

f. Medical intervention: diagnosis; blood and fluid replacement and cesarean birth if placental placement prevents vaginal birth of fetus

2. Nursing Process

a. Assessment/Analysis

1) signs and symptoms
   a) painless, bright red, vaginal bleeding in the 3rd trimester (often begins in 7th month); early episodes may have small amount of bleeding; several episodes of profuse bleeding may occur
   b) soft uterus
   c) manifestations of hemorrhage, shock
2) diagnosis is confirmed by ultrasound

b. Plan, Implementation, and Evaluation

Goal: Client will report signs of bleeding from abnormal placental implantation; will maintain fluid balance, experience minimal blood loss; will understand need for cesarean birth for total placenta previa; will deliver healthy newborn.

Plan/Implementation

- Maintain bedrest, avoid vaginal examinations, and observe carefully (conservative management).
- Monitor blood loss closely.
- Assess maternal vital signs and FHR frequently.
- Institute appropriate nursing measures if shock develops (i.e., administer fluids, transfusions).
- Give physical and emotional preparation for possible cesarean birth; physician may perform "double setup."
- Observe for associated problems (e.g., prematurity of newborn, DIC).

Evaluation: Couple is adequately prepared for possible cesarean birth; client is free from frank hemorrhage, shock; delivers a healthy newborn at or near term.

☐ Abruptio Placentae

1. General Information

a. Definition: premature partial or complete separation of normally implanted placenta; also known as accidental hemorrhage or ablatio placentae

b. Incidence: 1 in 80 to 1 in 200 pregnancies

c. Predisposing factors: pregnancy-induced hypertension, fibrin defects; associated with older multigravidas

d. Types
   1) *marginal* (overt): evident external bleeding; placenta separates at margin

Figure 4.7 Abruptio Placentae

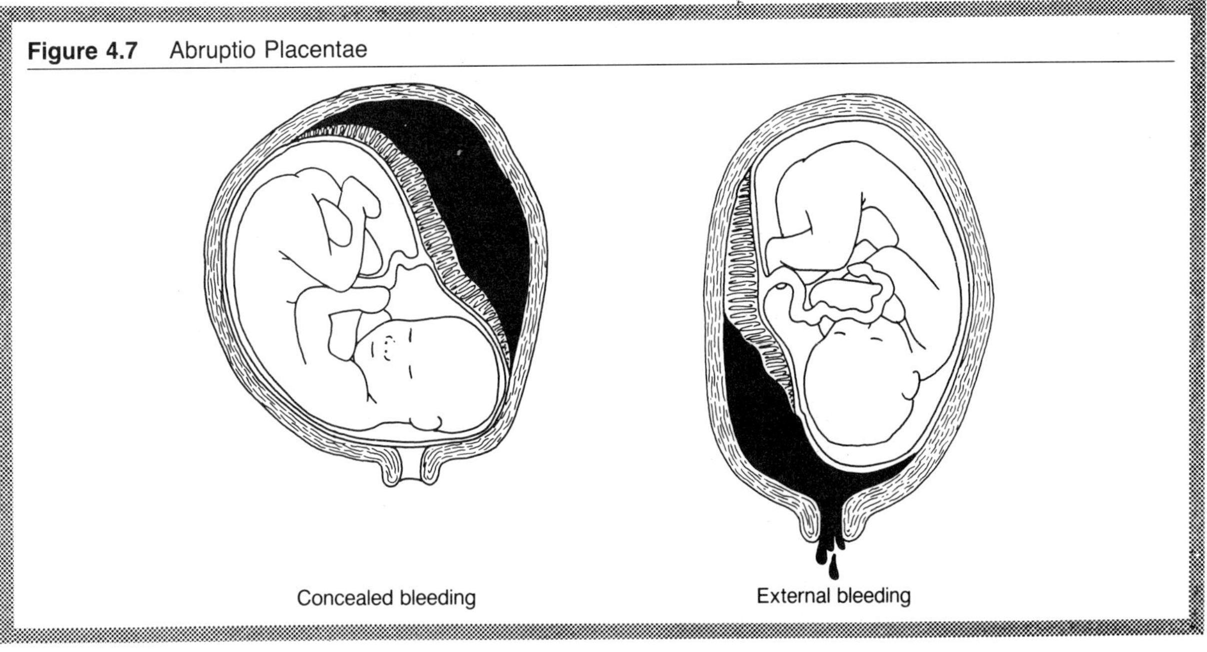

2) *concealed* (covert): bleeding not evident or inconsistent with extent of shock observed; placenta separates at the center

e. Medical intervention: diagnosis; blood and fluids replacement; cesarean birth as necessary to save fetal or maternal lives

2. Nursing Process

a. Assessment/Analysis

1) signs and symptoms
   a) bleeding: 3rd trimester, amount of bleeding is not an accurate indicator of degree of separation
   b) severe abdominal pain
   c) rigid distended uterus
   d) enlarged uterus
   e) shock
   f) associated problems, e.g., renal failure, hypofibrinogenemia
2) diagnosis: ultrasound

b. Plan, Implementation, and Evaluation

Goal: Client will maintain homeostasis despite signs of placental separation; will maintain fluid balance, have blood loss replaced; couple will understand the need for emergency surgery or vaginal delivery as indicated; will deliver a viable, well-oxygenated newborn.

Plan/Implementation

- Maintain bedrest.
- Monitor FHR and maternal vital signs.
- Assess blood loss and uterine pain.
- Administer blood replacement as ordered by physician.
- Institute nursing measures for shock (e.g., flat in bed, monitor vital signs frequently, keep warm, increase IV fluids); see also "Shock" page 170.
- Provide emotional support; explain what is happening and all procedures; encourage expression of feelings.
- Prepare (physical and emotional) for emergency cesarean birth or prompt delivery.
- Observe for associated problems after delivery, e.g., DIC, poorly contracted uterus, fetal neonatal hypoxia.

Evaluation: Couple is prepared for emergency birth; client delivers a viable newborn; has blood loss controlled; maintains fluid balance.

☐ Pregnancy-Induced Hypertension (Hypertensive Disorders)

1. General Information

a. Definition: a group of disorders characterized by presence of hypertension, with onset during last 10 weeks of pregnancy or in preceding pregnancy

b. Incidence: 6%–7% of all gravidae; one of three major causes of maternal mortality and a significant cause of fetal/neonatal deaths

c. Common types
   1) pregnancy-induced hypertension (toxemia)
      a) preeclampsia
      b) eclampsia
   2) chronic essential hypertension
      a) antecedent to pregnancy
      b) with superimposed preeclampsia (coincidental with pregnancy)

d. Predisposing factors: age (less than 17 or over 35 years), primiparity, low socioeconomic class, inadequate protein intake, diabetes, previous history of hypertension; absence of early/regular antepartal care is a factor in late detection and treatment

e. Etiology: unknown
   1) vasospasm and ischemia believed to be underlying mechanism
   2) impaired placental function may result from vasospasm
   3) development of uteroplacental changes leading to decreased oxygen and nutrition to fetus
   4) may lead to degenerative changes in renal, endocrine, hematologic systems and the brain

f. Medical interventions: bedrest, increased protein in diet, possible salt reduction, medications to prevent convulsions and reduce blood pressure, early delivery

2. Nursing Process

a. Assessment/Analysis

1) 3rd trimester onset of hypertension, edema, rapid weight gain, and proteinuria
2) classification (see Table 4.13)
   a) mild preeclampsia: symptoms generally appear after 24th week of pregnancy
      - BP elevation: systolic increases 15–30 mm Hg and diastolic increases 10–15 mm Hg over baseline on 2 occasions 6 hours apart (or pressures are over 140/90 mm Hg and below 160/100 mm Hg)

Table 4.13 Classification of Pregnancy-Induced Hypertension

Mild Preeclampsia	
Elevated BP	An increase of 15–30 mm Hg or more above base × 2 at least 6 hours apart
Weight gain	More than 1 lb/week in 3rd trimester
Edema	Generalized, slight
Proteinuria	1 gm/liter (1+)
Hyperreflexia	3+
Severe Preeclampsia	
All changes associated with mild eclampsia, plus	
Elevated BP	160–110 mm Hg or more with clients on bedrest × 2, 6 hours apart
Edema	Massive weight gain, swelling, puffiness of face, hands, fingers
Proteinuria	5 gm/liter/hour or more (4+)
Oliguria	400 ml or less/24 hours
Hyperreflexia	4+
Other	Severe headache, dizziness, blurred vision, retinal arteriolar spasm, spots before eyes, nausea and vomiting, epigastric pain, irritability, hyperreflexia
Eclampsia	
All changes associated with preeclampsia, plus	
Tonic and clonic convulsions or coma	
Hypertensive shock or crisis	

- weight gain of more than 1 lb/week in 3rd trimester
- edema of hands and feet
- urine protein is less than 1 gm/liter in 24 hours (1+ or 2+ proteinuria)
- urine output is greater than 500 ml in 24 hours
- hyperreflexia

b) severe preeclampsia
- BP rises above 160/110 or has risen 60/30 mm Hg or more above prepregnancy or early pregnancy level
- massive generalized or pulmonary edema
- urine protein is 5 gm or more per 24 hours
- urine output is 500 ml or less in 24 hours
- late symptoms include severe headache, dizziness, visual problems (blurred vision, retinal arteriolar spasm), nausea and vomiting; epigastric pain, irritability
- hyperreflexia
- the only cure for preeclampsia is delivery of the all of the products of conception

c) eclampsia: the onset of clonic or tonic convulsions or coma in a woman with preeclampsia

b. Plans, Implementation, and Evaluation

Goal 1: Client will comply with schedule for care; will verbalize an understanding of a balanced diet and other care; will not develop marked BP changes; will report potential/actual problems immediately; will maintain a stable BP after delivery; will deliver a well-oxygenated newborn.

Plan/Implementation
- Detect preeclampsia through early and regular antepartal care.
- Prevent severe preeclampsia/eclampsia by promoting regular antepartal care and good nutrition (with adequate protein).
- Monitor BP, weight, edema, urine, and reflexes (each antepartal visit).
- Instruct to take daily weight at home.
- Provide bedrest, if signs of pregnancy-induced or preexisting hypertension occur (at home for milder forms of preeclampsia; hospitalization for severe preeclampsia).
- Provide specific dietary information; may include reduced sodium.
- Monitor I&O, BP, weight, urine for protein, FHR for hospitalized client.
- Monitor administration of magnesium sulfate (anticonvulsant and sedative) if ordered, see Table 4.14; assess for *signs* of *toxicity*

Table 4.14 Anticonvulsion Agents

Drug Name	Action	Side Effects	Nursing Implications
Magnesium sulfate	Anticovulsant that decreases amount of acetylcholine (IV or IM) liberated with nerve impulse, relaxes smooth muscle, depresses CNS, lowers BP. Especially valuable in lowering seizure threshold in women with pregnancy–induced hypertension; may be used in preterm labor to decrease uterine activity (no FDA approval for this use at this time)	*Maternal:* severe CNS depression hyporeflexia, flushing, confusion *Fetal:* tachycardia, hypoglycemia, hypocalcemia, hypomagnesemia	Monitor for seizures. Observe for signs of CNS depression. Monitor fetal heart rate. Have calcium gluconate available to counteract magnesium sulfate. Discontinue infusion if respirations are below 12, reflexes are severely hypotonic, output is below 20–30 ml/hour, or in event of mental confusion or lethargy or fetal distress.

- symptoms of CNS depression (anxiety followed by drowsiness, lethargy)
- respirations less than 12/minute
- reduced BP
- deep tendon reflexes absent or less than 1+
- signs of paralysis
- DO NOT continue $MgSO_4$ if signs of toxicity or if urinary output less than 30 ml/hour; antidote is calcium gluconate (10%) solution

■ Administer sedatives, antihypertensives, and anticonvulsants, e.g., phenobarbital, diazepam (Valium), hydralazine (Apresoline), as ordered by physician to control symptoms and to prevent eclampsia and CVAs.
■ Monitor progress of labor.
■ Provide emotional support to couple.

Evaluation: Client complies with prenatal teaching; maintains pregnancy as long as possible without compromising self or fetus; is safely delivered of a healthy newborn; has blood pressure controlled prior to and after delivery.

Goal 2: Client will be free from physical injury in the event of seizure; will regain homeostasis; will maintain fetal oxygenation.

Plan/Implementation (if convulsion occurs)
■ Maintain patent airway.
■ Suction to prevent aspiration.
■ Protect mother from injury.
■ Note nature, onset, and progression of seizure.
■ Monitor for signs of abruptio placentae.
■ Administer O_2.
■ Monitor FHR.
■ Administer medications as ordered.

Evaluation: Client recovers from convulsion(s) without physical injury; remains stable; fetal heart rate is within normal limits.

□ Diabetes

1. General Information

a. Definition: an inherited metabolic disorder characterized by a deficiency in insulin production from the beta cells of the islets of Langerhans in the pancreas (see also page 225)
b. Incidence: 1 in 100 pregnancies; the condition may be a concurrent disease in pregnancy or have its first onset during gestation
c. Predisposing factors
  1) family history of diabetes
  2) glucosuria
  3) obesity
  4) history of repeated spontaneous abortions or fetal loss (stillbirth)
  5) history of delivery of infants over 10 lb
d. Classes (White's Classification, currently used in high-risk OB management): according to age at onset and pathologic changes; varies from type I, II classification
  1) Class A: diabetes that can often be controlled by diet; includes gestational diabetes (90% of all pregnant diabetics)
    a) onset or first recognition during pregnancy
    b) often a family history
    c) insulin may be needed; severity of symptoms varies
  2) Class B: onset after age 20; duration 0–9 yeras; no vascular involvement
  3) Class C: onset age 10–19; duration 10–19 years; no vascular involvement
  4) Class D: onset before age 10; duration 20

or more years; calcification present in legs; retinitis

5) Class E: presence of calcified pelvic vessels
6) Class F: presence of nephritis

e. Effects of diabetes: maternal risk and fetal loss increase as classes change from A to E
   1) effects of maternal diabetes on the fetus/infant
      a) overall perinatal mortality increases when mother has diabetes
      b) as classes change from A to E, increased incidence of ketoacidosis for mother (high risk for fetus)
      c) greater risk (3–4 times) of congenital abnormalities that may result in neonatal death
      d) hypoxia and fetal death more common
      e) infants large-for-gestational-age (classes A, B, C)
      f) neonatal hypoglycemia common as a result of fetal response to hyperglycemia of mother
   2) effects of diabetes on the mother
      a) uteroplacental insufficiency often complicates pregnancy
      b) higher incidence of dystocia
      c) susceptibility to infections

f. Effects of pregnancy on diabetes
   1) insulin resistance progressively increases in most pregnant diabetics
   2) blood sugar less easily controlled
   3) insulin shock common

g. Medical treatment (physicians' recommendation is for routine screening of all pregnant women by the 24th–28th week to identify gestational diabetes; reducing possible fetal risk)
   1) diagnostic tests (with *criteria* for *high risk* as seen in gestational diabetes or insulin-dependent diabetes)
      a) 2-hour postprandial blood sugar: >120 mg
      b) 100 gm oral glucose tolerance test (highly sensitive)
         - fasting blood sugar: >105 mg/dl
         - 1 hour: >190 mg/dl
         - 2 hours: >165 mg/dl
         - 3 hours: >145 mg/dl
      c) mean blood glucose test (HgbAlc [glycosolated hemoglobin]): at risk over 8.8%; indicates recent hyperglycemia
      d) chem strip blood glucose testing may be advised
      e) urine glucose monitoring inaccurate during pregnancy
   2) nutritional counseling with calories and sucrose ingestion altered
   3) insulin therapy as indicated based on blood glucose; use of oral hypoglycemics is contraindicated
   4) hospitalization to stabilize condition if necessary
   5) monitoring of fetal/placental oxygenation with nonstress testing, CST, ultrasound, L/S ratio, estriol levels
   6) cesarean birth or induction at 36–37 weeks if evidence of fetal compromise; attempt made to maintain pregnancy until fetal lungs are mature

2. Nursing Process

a. Assessment/Analysis

1) signs and symptoms of hypoglycemia and hyperglycemia (refer to Table 3.31, page 230)
2) indications of hydramnios, preeclampsia, infection
3) history of large-for-gestational-age (LGA) newborn/s
4) insulin requirements

b. Plan, Implementation, and Evaluation

Goal: Client will follow prescribed diet/insulin; will detect problems and report them immediately; will carry gestation to near-term; will adequately oxygenate fetus.

Plan/Implementation

- Stress importance of onging, regular, more frequent antepartal care.
- Assist in performance of diagnostic tests.
- Demonstrate accurate glucose-testing technique; have client return demonstration.
- Educate client regarding nutritional needs: strict adherence to prescribed dietary regimen.
- Teach to give own insulin (regular insulin preferred); observe for accuracy and correct as necessary.
- Regulate insulin dose as prescribed by blood glucose levels, not by urine tests, due to lowered renal threshold; expect altered requirements in intrapartal and postpartal periods.
- Recognize and share with client changes in her diabetic state
  – as pregnancy develops, insulin need increases
  – insulin need will decrease postpartum

- Promote good personal hygiene to prevent infection
- Monitor for early signs of infection.
- Assure mother that she will be able to breast-feed her infant, if she wishes.
- Initiate ophthalmologic referral.

Evaluation: Client complies with diet and insulin regimen during pregnancy; prevents complications of diabetes during pregnancy and the puerperium; carries pregnancy as close to term as possible; delivers a newborn with minimal problems.

☐ Cardiac Disorders

1. General Information

a. Definition: includes a number of heart diseases/defects, which include both congenital and acquired conditions. Pregnant women with heart disease are seen more frequently today because of better care, screening and surgical correction of defects. Refer also to "Congestive Heart Failure" page 178.

b. Effects of pregnancy on heart disease: alters heart rate, blood pressure, and volume of cardiac output

c. Incidence: 0.5%–2% of all pregnant women

d. Predisposing factors: syphilis, arteriosclerosis, renal and pulmonary disease, rheumatic fever, congenital defects of the heart, surgical repair of defects

e. Types: New York Heart Association's functional classification system for clients with heart disease (based on client history of past and present disability and uninfluenced by presence or absence of physical signs); used in current obstetrical management

1) Class 1: no limitation of activity; no symptoms of cardiac insufficiency
2) Class 2: slight limitation of activity; asymptomatic at rest; ordinary activities cause fatigue, palpitations, dyspnea, or angina
3) Class 3: marked limitation of activities; comfortable at rest; less than ordinary activities cause discomfort
4) Class 4: unable to perform any physical activity without discomfort; may have symptoms even at rest

f. Prognosis depends on

1) functional capacity of heart
2) complications that further increase cardiac load
3) quality of health care provided
4) maternal and fetal risk (increases from Classes 1 to 4; women in Classes 3, 4 will have serious problems in pregnancy)
   - a) maternal heart failure
   - b) spontaneous abortion or premature labor, caused by maternal hypoxia
   - c) maternal dysrhythmias
   - d) intrauterine-growth retardation

g. Medical treatment

1) confirm diagnosis
   - a) difficult to differentiate heart disease, because of normal cardiac changes that occur with pregnancy
     - functional systolic murmurs common
     - edema and some dyspnea frequently present in last trimester
     - changes in position of heart suggest cardiac enlargement
   - b) criteria for establishment of diagnosis of heart disease
     - continuous diastolic or presystolic heart murmur
     - a loud, harsh systolic murmur, especially if associated with a thrill
     - unequivocal cardiac enlargement
     - severe dysrhythmia
2) hospitalization: may be necessary 1–4 weeks before delivery
3) prophylactic antibiotic treatment to prevent subacute bacterial endocarditis
4) vaginal delivery (method of choice, using regional anesthesia and forceps)

2. Nursing Process

a. Assessment/Analysis

1) fetal heart rate; maternal vital signs
2) compliance with prescribed therapeutic regimen
3) cardiac and respiratory status at rest/with activity

b. Plan, Implementation, and Evaluation

Goal: Client will comply with treatment and will notify physician of problems; will be free from complications; will regain homeostasis after delivery; will maintain optimal fetal oxygenation.

Plan/Implementation

- Encourage early and regular antepartal care; monitor vital signs, FHR; weight.
- Promote compliance with therapeutic regimen.
- Teach proper nutrition with adequate iron intake to prevent anemia.
- Stress need for additional rest

- Classes 1 and 2: some limits on strenuous activity
- Classes 3 and 4: bedrest with expert medical supervision
- Semi-Fowler's position in bed if helpful for breathing; left lateral preferred

■ Prevent exposure to persons with upper respiratory tract infections; provide early treatment of URIs.

■ Observe the subtle changes in condition indicative of congestive heart failure (e.g., rales with cough, decreased ability to carry out household tasks, increased dyspnea on exertion, hemoptysis, tachycardia, progressive edema).

■ Administer medications as ordered by physician (e.g., diuretics, digitalis); explain actions, side effects to woman and significant other.

■ Maintain continuous maternal and fetal monitoring during the intrapartum period; advise client to avoid pushing, position in semi-Fowler's.

■ Postpartum, assess for signs of hemorrhage, puerperal infection, thromboembolism, congestive heart failure; avoid giving ergonovine and other oxytocics.

Evaluation: Client complies with regimen of rest, exercise, and care; is free from complications of cardiac disease during pregnancy/puerperium; delivers a healthy newborn.

☐ Anemia

1. General Information

a. Definition: decrease in the oxygen-carrying capacity of the blood

b. Cause: often because of low iron stores and reduced dietary intake

c. Incidence: 20% of all pregnant women; 90% of anemias are caused by iron deficiency; it is the most frequently encountered complication of pregnancy

d. Predisposing factors: heredity, malnutrition

e. Prognosis: maternal and fetal mortality and morbidity rates are increased; specifically

1) anemia aggravates existing problems such as cardiac disease during pregnancy

2) anemic women have increased incidence of abortion, premature labor, infection, pregnancy-induced hypertension, and postpartum hemorrhage

3) maternal anemia is associated with intrauterine-growth retardation

4) severe anemia may cause heart failure

f. Types of disorders

1) iron deficiency: most common

2) folic acid deficiency (megaloblastic anemia): less than 3% of all gravidae; caused by poor diet and malabsorption

3) hemoglobinopathies, e.g., sickle cell anemia (higher mortality in pregnancy; crises common) (refer to *Nursing Care of the Child* page 580), thalassemia

2. Nursing Process

a. Assessment/Analysis

1) signs and symptoms are usually absent in mild to moderate iron-deficiency anemia

2) diagnosis based upon

a) Hgb < than 11 gm/dl or Hct < 37%

b) Hgb < 10.5 gm/dl or Hct < 35% in 2nd trimester

c) Hgb < 10 gm/dl or Hct < 33% in 3rd trimester

3) nutritional intake

b. Plan, Implementation, and Evaluation

Goal: Client will maintain an optimal Hgb and Hct; will be free from severe anemia; will comply with diet and treatments/medication; will maintain adequate fetal oxygenation.

Plan/Implementation

■ Monitor Hgb or Hct levels at initial antepartal visit and in later pregnancy.

■ Provide dietary counseling regarding importance of iron-rich diet (minimum of 18 mg/day).

■ Instruct to take oral iron compounds ferrous sulfate or gluconate) as daily supplement as ordered; teach regarding side effects

- change in color of stools (become black)
- take with a source of vitamin C to facilitate absorption
- take with food only if gastric distress occurs (better absorbed between meals)

■ Provide folic acid supplement of 5 mg/24 hours orally for folate deficiency, as ordered.

■ Observe for symptoms of hemolytic crisis (e.g., chills, fever, pain in back and abdomen, prostration, shock) with hemoglobinopathies.

■ Refer for genetic counseling (women with inherited disorders).

Evaluation: Client eats a balanced, adequate, iron-rich diet during pregnancy; takes prescribed iron medications; maintains health; delivers newborn of appropriate size for gestational age.

☐ Hyperemesis Gravidarum (Pernicious Vomiting of Pregnancy)

1. General Information

a. Definition: excessive vomiting during pregnancy, leading to dehydration, starvation, electrolyte imbalance

b. Cause: not always clear; may be psychologic, or due to multiple pregnancy, hormonal abnormalities, or hydatidiform mole

c. Prognosis: severe cases may lead to dehydration and fluid-electrolyte complications

2. Nursing Process

a. **Assessment/Analysis** (signs and symptoms are related to severity)

1) mild: slight dehydration and weight loss

2) severe: metabolic acidoses, hypoproteinemia, hypovitaminosis, jaundice, hemorrhage

b. **Plan, Implementation, and Evalaution**

Goal: Client will retain food/fluids; will maintain hydration.

Plan/Implementation hospitalization may be necessary)

- Administer parenteral fluids.
- Promote a quiet environment.
- Provide frequent, small meals when oral feedings are tolerated.
- Refer to psychologic consult if necessary.

Evaluation: Client is free from vomiting; maintains fluid and electrolyte balance; eats adequate diet; begins to gain weight.

☐ Infections

1. General Information

a. Definition: a variety of infectious agents can affect maternal and fetal health, leading to increased morbidity and mortality. Maternal disease that is mild or even asymptomatic can cause severe anomalies or death in the embryo/fetus/neonate.

b. Types of infectious diseases

1) the TORCH complex (*T*oxoplasmosis, *O*ther, *R*ubella, *C*ytomegalovirus infection, *H*erpes)

a) *toxoplasmosis* (protozoa)

- transmitted through ingestion of raw or undercooked meat; through improper hand washing after handling cat litter that has been contaminated with infected cat's feces
- maternal symptoms may be absent or nonspecific
- possible to detect by serologic screening
- organism readily crosses placenta
- fetal effects include hydrocephaly, chorioretinitis, mental retardation, neurologic damage

b) *other*

- *B-hemolytic streptococcal* infection: streptococci estimated to be present in genital tract of approximately 15% of women of childbearing age; associated with urinary tract infection; may cross placenta and cause septic abortion, puerperal sepsis, stillbirth, neonatal sepsis; sensory impairment, retardation
- *syphilis*: prenatal serologic screening test is important for prevention of congenital syphilis; associated with late abortion, stillbirth, prematurity, severe anemia, and congenital syphilis
- *gonorrhea*: may cause postpartum infection, pelvic inflammatory disease, sterility; danger to newborn is ophthalmia neonatorum, sepsis, pneumonia; refer to "Sexually Transmitted Diseases" page 541
- *acquired immune deficiency syndrome* (AIDS): viral infection with severe depression of immune system; perinatal transmission from infected mother to fetus; high mortality rate; precautions as for Hepatitis B (see also "Newborn Care" page 454)
- *nongonococcal urethritis* (NGU)
  - mild; may be asymptomatic
  - increasingly common STD
  - organism: chlamydia
  - partner should be treated; erythromycin often used for pregnant client
  - may cause stillbirth, pneumonia, conjunctivitis in newborn

c) *rubella*: extremely teratogenic in 1st trimester

- transmitted transplacentally
- congenital rubella syndrome in the neonate includes cataracts, hemolytic anemia, heart defects,

mental retardation, deafness (1st trimester exposure)
- exposure after the 1st trimester can lead to intra-uterine growth retardation, sepsis
- infected infant can shed live viruses for many months after birth
- women with low titers should receive vaccine in early postpartum period and avoid pregnancy for at least 2 months

d) *cytomegalovirus* (CMV); also called cytomegalic inclusion disease (CMID): member of herpes virus group
- adult usually asymptomatic or has mononucleosis-like symptoms; very common
- transmission in adults is respiratory, possibly venereal
- transmission to fetus is transplacental; occasionally may be transmitted during passage through birth canal
- no effective treatment
- effects on neonate include mental retardation, intrauterine-growth retardation, congenital heart defects, deafness, microcephaly

e) *herpes simplex virus* (HSV II)
- sexually transmitted, painful vesicles present on cervix, vaginal wall, vulva, and thighs; last 10 days to 2 weeks; remissions, exacerbations
- usual mode of transmission to neonate is passage through birth canal; may occur transplacentally in rare cases
- infection results in high infant mortality, preterm births
- cesarean birth, if pregnant woman has active herpes virus, type 2

2) tuberculosis
- **a)** rarely transmitted to fetus
- **b)** may be asymptomatic
- **c)** disease must be arrested by usual methods of care for client with Tb
- **d)** infant usually kept from close contact with mother, if active, to protect from infection

3) urinary tract infections
- **a)** affect approximately 10% of gravidae, generally due to *E. coli*; may be asymptomatic
- **b)** predisposing factors: urinary stasis, related to anatomic changes during pregnancy; poor hygiene
- **c)** increased incidence of pyelonephritis if bacteria present
- **d)** associated with increased incidence of premature labor
- **e)** treated with appropriate antibiotic after culture

4) condylomata (genital warts)
- **a)** viral transmission
- **b)** may be transmitted to fetus at birth
- **c)** should be treated with laser beam, antibiotics, cautery, cryosurgery
- **d)** biopsy indicated for large warts (potential malignancy)

5) monilial infections
- **a)** caused by fungus *Candida albicans*
- **b)** present in about 20% of pregnant women
- **c)** fetus may contract thrush if infection not cured prior to delivery

6) trichomonas vaginalis
- **a)** protozoan
- **b)** treated with metronidazole (Flagyl), which may possibly be teratogenic and should not be used during first half of pregnancy

7) hepatitis
- **a)** may cause abortion, preterm birth, fetal or newborn hepatitis
- **b)** precautions depending on type A or B; refer to ''Hepatitis'' page 212

2. Nursing Process

a. Assessment/Analysis

1) routine smears, cultures, serologic studies for sexually transmitted disease; selected laboratory tests as indicated
2) signs and symptoms of infectious diseases

b. Plan, Implemenation, and Evaluation

Goal: Client will be free from infection in pregnancy; will seek medical care and will comply with treatment if exposed to infection; when indicated, partner will comply with treatment; fetal effects will be minimized.

Plan/Implementation
- Review precautions in order to minimize exposure to infection.
- Teach client to report any symptoms (e.g., vesicles, discharge, rash, elevated temperature).
- Administer drugs as ordered for sexually

transmitted diseases (e.g., penicillin for syphilis).
- Promote compliance of partner.
- Instruct to take drugs as ordered (e.g., isoniazid [INH], streptomycin, PAS); explain expected actions, side effects; avoid self-medication.

Evaluation: Client is free from infectious disease; maternal or fetal risks are minimized; client/partner comply with therapeutic regimen.

☐ Multiple Gestation

1. General Information

a. Definition: gestation of two or more fetuses. Twins may be produced from a single ovum (monozygotic or identical twins) or from separate ova (dizygotic or fraternal). Fraternal twinning is an inherited autosomal recessive trait and is more common (70%) than identical twins (30%). Triplets result from one, two, or three separate ova.

b. Incidence: 2%–3% of all viable births

c. Predisposing factors
- **1)** blacks have higher incidence of multiple pregnancies, compared with whites
- **2)** family history of dizygotic twins

d. Prognosis
- **1)** increased risk of premature labor, pregnancy-induced hypertension (25%), hemorrhage, placenta previa
- **2)** increased risk of delivery of low-birth-weight infants, often premature (50%)
- **3)** increased risk of maternal anemia (40%–50%)
- **4)** increased risk of uterine inertia (10%), hydramnios (5%–10%), intrauterine asphyxia (5%)
- **5)** increased risk of secondary cessation or weakening of effective uterine contractions
- **6)** monozygotic twins have higher mortality and morbidity rates than dizygotic twins, because of increased congenital anomalies, twin-to-twin transfusion syndrome, and intrauterine-growth retardation

2. Nursing Process

a. Assessment/Analysis
- **1)** early identification of multiple pregnancy based upon
  - **a)** history
  - **b)** weight gain
  - **c)** abdominal palpation
  - **d)** asynchronous fetal heart beats
  - **e)** ultrasonography
- **2)** maternal and fetal status: prenatal visits every 2 weeks
- **3)** nutritional status

b. Plan, Implementation, and Evaluation

Goal: Client with a multiple pregnancy will report early signs of health problems; will comply with health regimen and keep regular antepartal appointments; will deliver as close to term as possible.

Plan/Implementation
- Advise frequent rest periods; left lateral position provides oxygenation for fetal/placental unit.
- Teach balanced diet, with adequate protein; iron and vitamin supplements as ordered.
- Monitor FHR carefully for indication of fetal distress.
- Prepare for vaginal delivery unless complications arise (e.g., fetal distress, cephalopelvic disproportion)
- Administer oxytocic agent as ordered immediately following birth to prevent postpartum hemorrhage (very important because of overdistention of the uterus).

Evaluation: Client is free from complications (e.g., anemia); carries multiple pregnancy to term (or close to term), with delivery of health newborns.

☐ Adolescent Pregnancy

1. General Information

a. Definition: pregnancy in a female under 17 years of age (see also "The Healthy Child" page 517)

b. Incidence: worldwide, ⅓ of all births are to girls under 17 years of age; one million teenage pregnancies per year (10% of all teenagers) (World Health Organization 1977)

c. Predisposing factors: teenage pregnancies are associated with
- **1)** earlier onset of menarche
- **2)** changing sexual behavior
- **3)** poor family relationships
- **4)** poverty

d. Prognosis
- **1)** for pregnant girls under 15 years, a high risk of stillbirths, low-birth-weight infants, neonatal mortality, and cephalopelvic disproportion
- **2)** increased maternal risk of pregnancy-induced hypertension, prolonged labor, iron-deficiency anemia, and urinary tract infections

2. Nursing Process

a. Assessment/Analysis

1) nutrition status
2) knowledge of physiology of pregnancy
3) emotional status
4) support systems

b. Plan, Implementation, and Evaluation

Goal: The pregnant teen will maintain good health; will eat a balanced diet with adequate protein; will prepare for birth and care of newborn; will achieve developmental tasks of adolescence and pregnancy; fetus will develop appropriately for gestation.

Plan/Implementation

- Assist pregnant teen to achieve developmental tasks of adolescence (in addition to those of pregnancy)
  - develop sense of identity
  - accept changing body image
  - develop close, mature relations with peers (male and female)
  - socialize into appropriate gender role
  - establish an independent and satisfying life-style
- Provide dietary counseling regarding
  - importance of well-balanced meals
  - selection of nutritionally valuable, yet acceptable food
  - increased protein, calcium, and iron intake
- Prepare for childbirth; arrange for coaching assistance.
- Refer to social service for
  - career and educational counseling
  - options regarding child care/adoption
  - support services in community, i.e., parenting classes, supplemental food programs
- Instruct in child care.
- Teach family planning.

Evaluation: Client is free from preventable complications; has a positive birth experience; delivers a healthy newborn; cares safely for newborn or arranges for alternate placement; achieves appropriate developmental tasks.

References

Butnarescu, G., & Tillotson, D. (1983). *Maternity nursing theory to practice*. New York: Wiley

Cataldo, C., & Whitney, E. (1986). *Nutrition and diet therapy*. St. Paul: West Publishing.

*Devore, N., & Baldwin, K. (1986). Ectopic pregnancy on the rise. *American Journal of Nursing*. *86*, 674–678.

†Devore, N., Jackson, V., & Piening, S. (1983). TORCH infections. *American Journal of Nursing*, *83*, 1661–1665.

Diabetes Association issues statement on gestational diabetes. (1986). *NAACOG Newsletter*, *13*(9), 7–8.

Elsea, S. (1985). Ethics in maternal child nursing. *MCN: American Journal of Maternal/Child Nursing*, *85*(10), 303.

Ferguson, H. (1988). Biophysical profile scoring: The fetal Apgar. *AJN*. *88*(5), 662–663.

Hammer, R., Bower, E., & Messina, L. (1984). The prenatal use of Rh D immune globulin. *MCN: American Journal of Maternal/Child Nursing*, *9*, 29–31.

Hammer, R., & Tufts, M. (1986). Chorionic villi sampling. *MCN: American Journal of Maternal/Child Nursing*, *11*, 29–31.

*Hoffmaster, F. (1983). Detecting and treating pregnancy-induced hypertension. *MCN: American Journal of Maternal/Child Nursing*, *8*, 398–405.

Jensen, M., & Bobak, I. (1985). *Maternity and gynecologic care*. St. Louis: Mosby.

Ketter, D., & Shelton, B. (1984). Pregnant and physically fit, too. *MCN: American Journal of Maternal/Child Nursing*, *9*, 120–122.

Knuppel, R., & Drukker, J. (1986). *High risk pregnancy*. Philadelphia: Saunders.

Leonard, L. (1984). Pregnancy and the underweight woman. *MCN: American Journal of Maternal/Child Nursing*, *9*, 331.

Mayberry, L., & Forte, A. (1985). Pregnancy-related DIC. *MCN: The American Journal of Maternal/Child Nursing*, *10*(3), 168–173.

Mercer, R. (1983). Assessing and counseling teenage mothers during the perinatal period. *Nursing Clinics of North America*, *18*(2), 293–296.

Moore, M. (1983). *Realities in chilbearing*. Philadelphia: Saunders.

Mueller, L. (1985). Pregnancy and sexuality. *Journal of Obstetric, Gynecologic, and Neonatal Nursing*, *14*(4), 289–294.

Neeson, J., & May, K. (1986). *Comprehensive maternity nursing*. Philadelphia: Lippincott.

Olds, S., London, M., & Ladewig, P. (1986). *Maternal-newborn nursing*. Menlo Park, CA: Addison-Wesley.

Osborne, N., & Pratson, L. (1984). Sexually transmitted diseases and pregnancy. *Journal of Obstetric, Gynecologic and Neonatal Nursing*, *13*(7), 9–12.

Perley, N., & Bills, B. (1983). Herpes genitalis and the childbearing cycle. *MCN: American Journal of Maternal/Child Nursing*, *8*, 213–217.

Pritchard, J., MacDonald, P., & Gant, N. (1985). *Williams Obstetrics* (17 ed.). Norwalk, CT: Appleton-Century-Crofts.

Reeder, S., Martin, L. (1987). *Maternity nursing*. Philadelphia: Lippincott.

Richardson, E., & Milne, L. (1983). Sickle cell disease and the childbearing family—An update. *MCN: American Journal of Maternal/Child Nursing*, *8*, 417.

Rubin, R. (1961). Basic maternal behavior. *Nursing Outlook*, *9*, 683–686.

Smith, J. (1988). The dangers of prenatal cocaine use.

MCN: The American Journal of Maternal/Child Nursing, *13*(3), 174–179.

Stolte, K. (1986). Nursing diagnosis and the childbearing woman. *MCN: American Journal of Maternal/Child Nursing*, *11*(1), 1, 13–15.

Wallace, A. (1987). The effects of aerobic exercise on the pregnant woman, fetus and pregnancy outcome. A review. *Journal of Nurse Midwifery*, *32*(5), 277–290.

Wiener, M., & Pepper, G. (1985). *Clinical pharmacology and therapeutics in nursing* (2nd ed.). New York: McGraw-Hill.

Zacharias, J. (1983). A rational approach to drug use in pregnancy. *Journal of Obstetric, Gynecologic and Neonatal Nursing*, *12*(3), 183–187.

*See reprint section

†Highly recommended

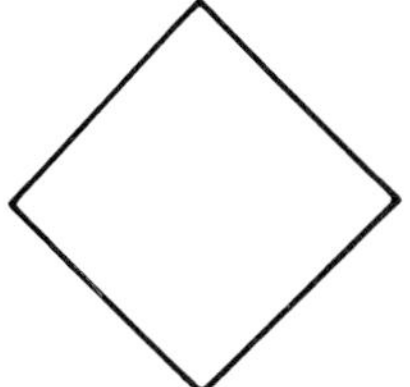

Intrapartal Care

General Concepts

Normal Childbearing

1. Definitions
   a. Labor: a series of processes by which the products of conception are expelled from the maternal body
   b. Delivery: the actual event of birth
2. Essential factors in labor: the four Ps
   a. *Powers*: uterine contractions, voluntary bearing down, abdominal muscle contractions, contractions of levator ani muscle
   b. *Passsageway:* bones, tissues, ligaments
      1) type of pelvis: gynecoid, android, anthropoid and platypelloid; refer to "The Structure of the Female Pelvis" page 383
      2) adequacy of planes of true pelvis
         a) true pelvis forms the birth canal through which fetus must pass
         b) three distinct levels
            - plane of inlet
            - midplane (plane of least dimensions)
            - plane of outlet
      3) condition of soft tissues (lower uterine segment, cervix, and vaginal canal)
   c. *Passenger*: the fetus
      1) attitude (habitus or posture): the relation of the fetal parts to its own trunk; normal attitude of the fetus in utero is complete flexion
      2) engagement: the entrance of the greatest diameter of the presenting part through the plane of inlet and the beginning of the descent through the pelvic canal (biparietal diameter of head is fixed in pelvis)
      3) lie: the relation of the long axis of the fetus to the long axis of the mother; it is either transverse, longitudinal, or oblique
         a) transverse lie: long axis of fetus is at right angle to mother's long axis; it is a pathologic lie if present at term
         b) longitudinal lie: long axis of the fetus is parallel to mother's long axis; it has two alternatives
            - cephalic presentation (head first)
            - breech presentation (buttocks first)
      4) presentation and presenting part: that part of the fetal body that enters the true pelvis and presents itself at the internal os for delivery; the presentation is dependent upon the attitude of the fetal extremities to its body and the fetal lie
         a) in cephalic presentations (95% of term deliveries), the fetal head is the presenting part: the head may be
            - completely flexed upon the fetal chest (vertex presentation)
            - moderately flexed (sinciput presentation)
            - partially extended (brow presentation)
            - hyperextended with chin presenting (face presentation)
         b) in breech presentations (3% of term births)
            - the fetal knees and hips both may be flexed, positioning the thighs on the abdomen and calves on the posterior thighs (complete breech)
            - the hips may be flexed and the knees extended (frank breech)
            - extension of the knees and hips (footling breech)
            - shoulder presentation is commonly known as a transverse lie
      5) position: the relationship of a specific established point (i.e., occiput, sacrum, shoulder, chin, brow, mentum or face) of the fetus to one of the quadrants of the mother's pelvis
         a) breech presenation: sacrum (S)
         b) cephalic presentation: occiput (O)
         c) shoulder presentation: scapula (Sc)
         d) 6 different positions are thus possible for each of the above by relating the established point to the right or left side of the mother's pelvis and to the anterior or posterior aspect

Figure 4.8 Selected Categories of Presentation

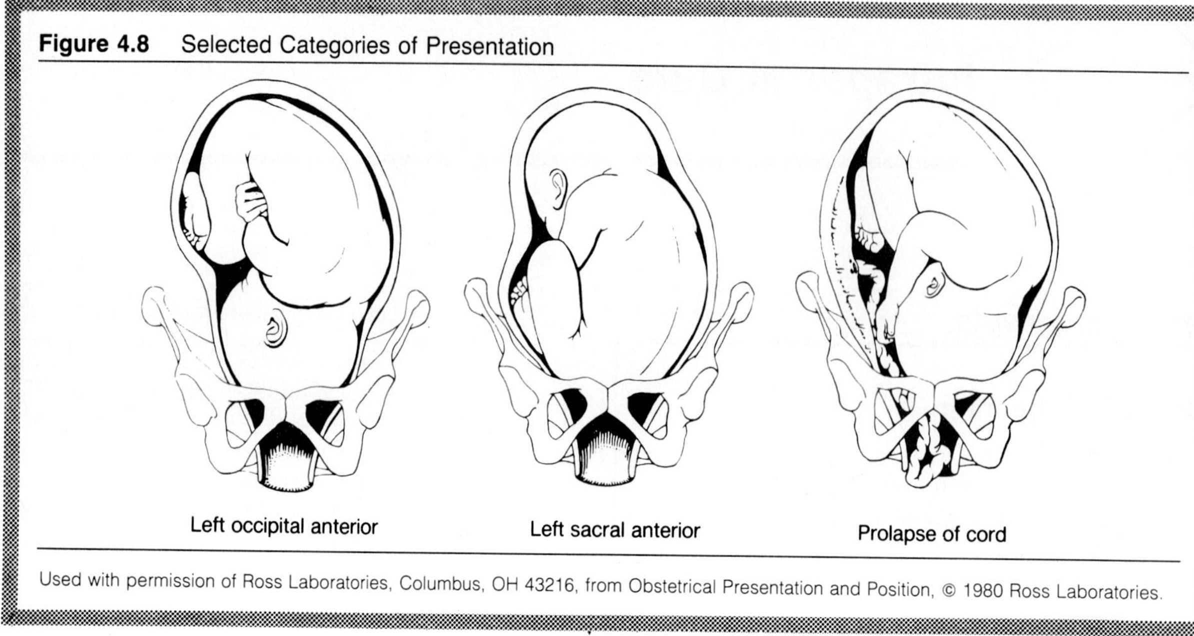

Used with permission of Ross Laboratories, Columbus, OH 43216, from Obstetrical Presentation and Position, © 1980 Ross Laboratories.

6) station: the relationship of the presenting part of the fetus to the ischial spines of the mother (i.e., the degree of engagement); measured in centimeters above or below the pelvic midplane from the presenting part to the ischial spines
   a) station 0 is at the ischial spines
   b) minus station is above the spines
   c) plus station is below the spines

d. *Person*: pregnant woman's general behavior and influences upon her (psyche)
   1) maternal response to uterine contractions
   2) cultural influences and perceptions about labor and delivery
   3) antepartal and/or childbirth education
   4) ability to communicate feelings to significant other(s) and staff
   5) support system

3. Signs of labor
   a. Premonitory signs of labor: changes indicative that labor will shortly be approaching
      1) increased Braxton Hicks' contractions: intermittent contractions of the uterus occurring throughout pregnancy; generally painless but may cause discomfort in late pregnancy
      2) lightening or engagement: the descent of the fetus into the pelvic cavity; generally occurs 2–3 weeks before the onset of labor in primigravidas; causes increased bladder pressure and reduced diaphragm pressure
      3) show: blood-tinged mucus discharged from cervix shortly before or during labor
      4) sudden burst of energy
      5) weight loss resulting from fluid loss and electrolyte shifts
      6) increased backache and sacroiliac pressure due to fetal pressure
      7) spontaneous rupture of membranes may occur; woman will be advised to enter hospital immediately
   b. True versus false labor
      1) true labor
         a) contractions increase progressively in strength, duration, and frequency
         b) regular pattern, not relieved by walking (walking may increase the strength of the contractions)
         c) felt in back or radiating towards front
         d) *effacement and dilation of the cervix*
         e) fetal membranes
            - intact: generally in early labor, indicated by negative Nitrazine paper test (yellow to yellow-olive paper) or negative ferning
            - ruptured: generally in active labor, indicated by positive Nitrazine paper test (blue green to blue paper or positive ferning); false readings may be obtained if contaminated by blood; meconium staining may indicate fetal distress, except in breech presentation
      2) false labor
         a) an exaggeration of the periodic uterine contractions normally occurring during pregnancy

b) does not produce progressive dilation, effacement, or descent
c) contractions are irregular and do not increase in frequency, duration, or intensity
d) walking has no effect on contractions
e) discomfort felt in lower abdomen and groin
f) absence of bloody show

4. Labor onset theories
   a. Oxytocin stimulation: alone or in combination with other factors
   b. Progesterone withdrawal: allowing uterine contractions to progress
   c. Estrogen stimulation: causing hypertrophy of myometrium and increased production of contractile proteins
   d. Prostaglandin secretion: effect on uterine muscle (increased uterine irritability)
   e. Fetal endocrine secretion of cortical steroids
   f. Distention of uterus: with subsequent pressure on nerve endings stimulating contractions and increased irritability of uterine musculature
5. Physiologic alterations occurring during labor
   a. Dilation to 10 cm: the process by which the cervix opens
   b. Effacement: thinning, shortening, and obliteration of cervix
   c. Physiologic retraction ring: the separation of the upper (active, thicker) and lower (passive, thinner) uterine segments in labor
6. Fetal positional response to labor (mechanisms of labor)
   a. Engagement: descent of fetus into true pelvis
   b. Descent: the passage of the presenting part through the pelvis
   c. Flexion: further flexion of the fetal head when it meets resistance from the pelvic floor
   d. Internal rotation: the process by which the long axis of the fetal skull changes from the transverse diameter to an anteroposterior diameter at the outlet
   e. Extension of the head as it leaves the outlet
   f. External rotation of the head (restitution): in order to rotate the shoulders and leave the outlet
   g. Expulsion of the total baby
7. Fetal heart rate during labor
   a. Baseline fetal heart rate (FHR): fetal heart rate when there are no contractions or in between contractions; normally between 120–160/minute; see Figure 4.9 and Table 4.15
   b. Baseline variability: normal irregularities of FHR caused by autonomic nervous system stimuli (may be altered in normal fetal sleep, prematurity, medications) (*NOTE*: true beat-to-beat variability can be determined only by direct fetal or internal monitoring); see Figure 4.9
   c. Periodic changes: FHR changes during contractions

Figure 4.9 Tracing of Normal Fetal Heart Rate

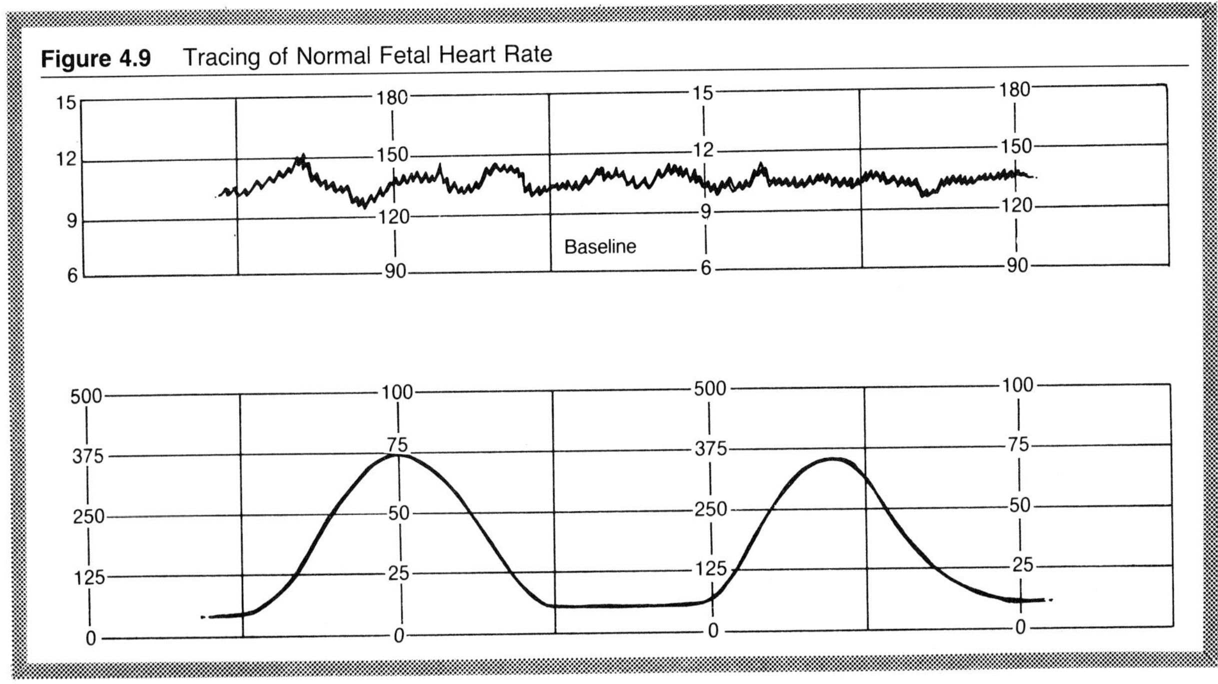

Table 4.15 Baseline Fetal Heart Rate (Normal range: 120–160 beats/minute)

	Tachycardia	Bradycardia
Mild	161–180 bpm	100–119 bpm
Marked	Greater than 180 bpm	Less than 100 bpm
Causes	Maternal fever Early fetal hypoxia Drugs Amnionitis	Maternal hypotension Late fetal hypoxia Drugs

1) accelerations: transient rise in FHR greater than 15 beats/minute for more than 15 seconds related to uterine contractions; see Figure 4.10
2) decelerations: transient decrease in FHR related to uterine contractions; see classifications in Table 4.16

☐ Ongoing Management and Nursing Care

1. Fetal monitoring: monitor FHR by either
   a. Periodic ausculation: count for 1 full minute during and immediately after uterine contractions
   b. Electronic fetal monitor
      1) external or indirect electronic monitoring: applied when membranes intact
         a) *tokodynamometer*: disk attached over fundus and secured with belt; provides continuous record of external pressure created by contractions, allows measurement of frequency and duration of contractions
         b) *ultrasonic transducer*: applied at site of loudest fetal heart beat, secured with belt (conducting gel is spread over transducer); provides continuous FHR recording, which is interpreted in

Figure 4.10 Acceleration of Fetal Heart Rate in Response to Uterine Activity

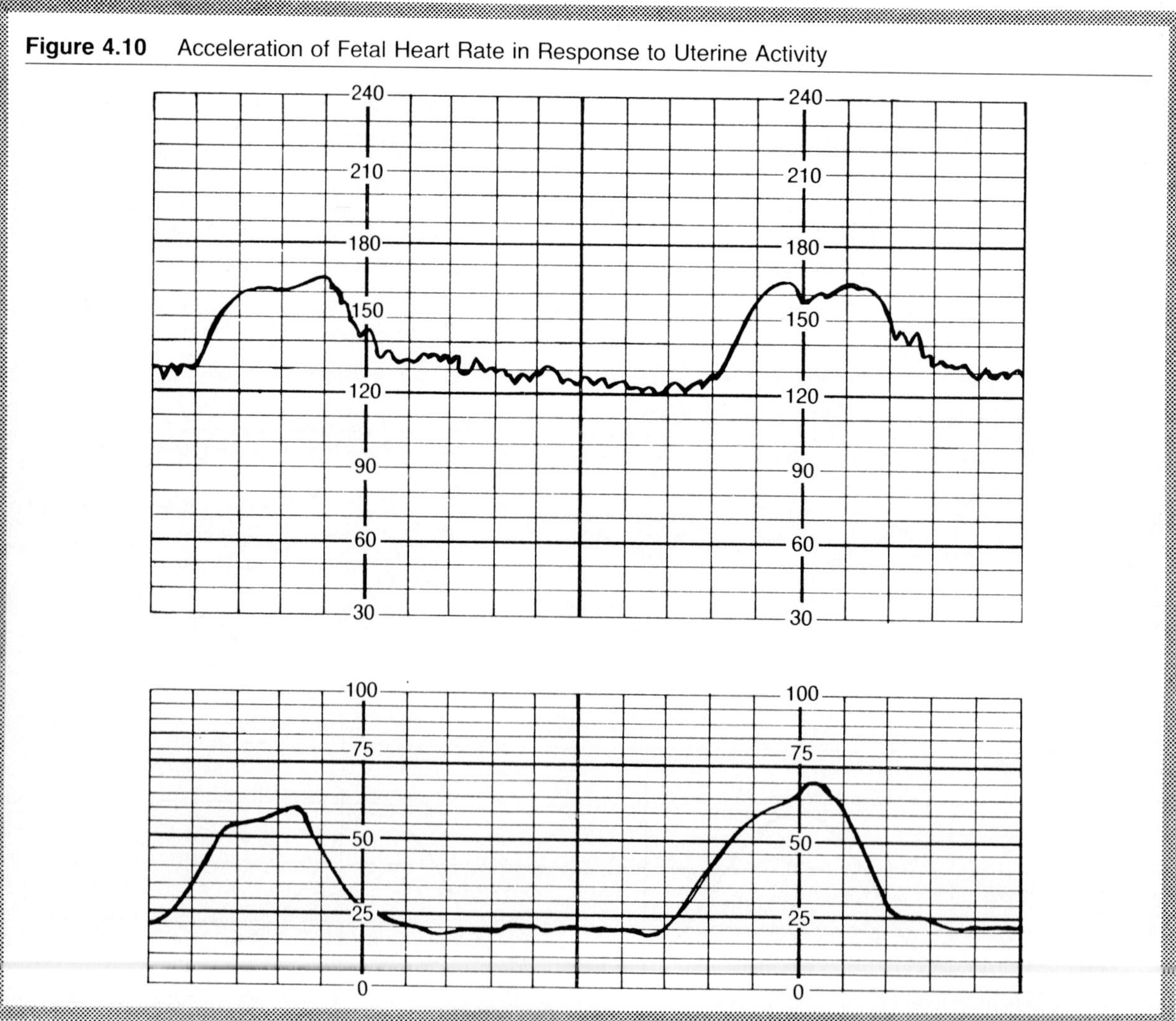

Figure 4.11 Types of Deceleration in Fetal Heart Rate

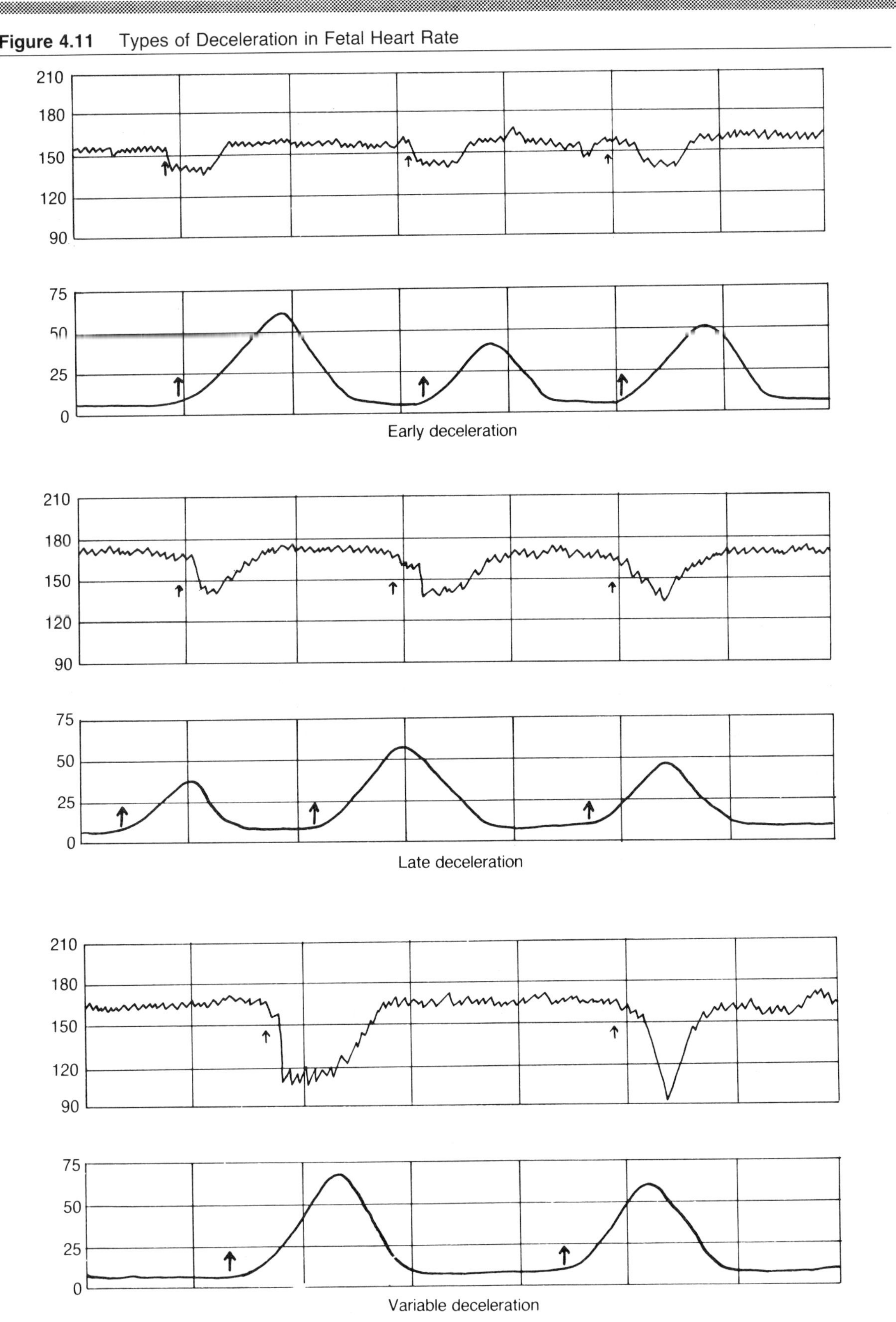

Table 4.16 Deceleration in Fetal Heart Rate

Type 1 (early decelerations)

- Cause: fetal head compression
- FHR decreases with onset of contraction and mirrors the pattern of contractions
- FHR returns to baseline as the contraction ends
- Range of drop in FHR within normal parameters
- Has a uniform shape
- Innocuous
- Nursing implications: continue observation.

Type 2 (late decelerations)

- Cause: uteroplacental insufficiency causing fetal hypoxia
- FHR decreases *after* the onset of contraction
- FHR deceleration persists beyond completion of contraction
- Range of drop in FHR within normal
- Has a uniform shape
- Ominous
- Nursing implications: turn client to left side, give O_2, summon physician.

Type 3 (variable decelerations)

- Cause: umbilical cord compression
- FHR decreases at any point *during* or *between* contractions
- Decelerations may be jagged V- or U-shape
- Range of drop in FHR is large and extends below normal
- Not uniform in shape
- Ominous
- Nursing implications: turn woman to left side, give O_2, summon physician.

relation to uterine activity; phonocardiography may also be used for indirect fetal electrocardiography

2) internal or direct monitoring: applied when membranes have ruptured and cervix has dilated 2–3 cm
   a) *pressure transducer*: an intrauterine catheter filled with water is inserted beyond presenting part; allows measurement of frequency, duration, intensity of contractions
   b) *internal spiral electrode*: applied to fetal scalp; provides continuous measurement of FHR, baseline variability, and periodic changes

c. Fetal blood sampling: a small volume of fetal blood is taken (from a small puncture into the fetal scalp) to assess fetal hypoxia during labor
   1) procedure
      a) an invasive technique requiring rupture of the fetal membranes and cervical dilation (3–4 cm); performed when fetus is in jeopardy
      b) pregnant woman generally placed in a lithotomy position
      c) an amnioscope (plastic or metal truncated cone) is employed for visualization of presenting part of fetus during the procedure
      d) electronic fetal monitoring is desirable during the procedure
      e) after procedure, observe for vaginal bleeding (of fetal origin) and fetal tachycardia
   2) laboratory analysis of fetal pH, pO_2, and pCO_2 is done from blood sample (normal pH: 7.25–7.35; pH of 7.20 is associated with hypoxia)

2. Uterine contractions: refer to Table 4.17 and Figure 4.12; monitor
   a. Frequency: timed from beginning of one to beginning of next contraction
   b. Duration: timed from beginning to end of one contraction
   c. Intensity: degree of muscle contraction; may be mild, moderate, strong (50–100 mm Hg)
   d. Tonus: pressure within the uterus in between contractions; only measurable with an intrauterine catheter (10–12 mm Hg)

3. Analgesics: drugs that relieve pain or alter its perception may alter level of consciousness and reflex activity; administer as ordered and monitor effects; common obstetric analgesics include
   a. Narcotics (e.g., meperidine [Demerol])
      1) may initially slow labor, have depressive effect on neonatal respirations
      2) administered when client in active labor (4–5 cm)

Table 4.17 Stages and Phases of Labor

First Stage (onset of regular contractions to complete dilatation)			
	Latent: Phase I	***Active: Phase II***	***Transition: Phase III***
Time			
Primipara	8½ hours	4 hours	1 hour
Multipara	5½ hours	2 hours	10–15 minutes
Cervix			
Effacement	0–50%	Completed	
Dilatation	0–3 cm	4–7 cm	8–10 cm
Contractions			
Frequency	More than 10 minutes apart	3–5 minutes	2–3 minutes
Duration	30 seconds	45 seconds	60–90 seconds
Intensity	Mild: less than 50 mm Hg	Moderate: 50–75 mm Hg	Hard 75–100 mm Hg
Manifestations	Abdominal cramps, backache, client generally excited, alert, talkative, in control, may rupture membranes	Show; moderate increase in pain; client more apprehensive; fear of losing control; focusing on self; skin warm and flushed	Client may be irritable and panicky; may lose control; amnesic between contractions; perspiring, nausea and vomiting common; trembling of legs, pressure on bladder and rectum, backache, increased show, circumoral pallor.
Second Stage (complete dilatation to birth of newborn)			
Time			
Primipara	30–50 minutes		
Multipara	20 minutes		
Contractions			
Frequency	2–3 minutes		
Duration	60–90 seconds		
Intensity	Very hard: 100 mm Hg		
Manifestations	Decrease in pain from transitional level, increased bloody show, pressure on rectum, urge to bear down, bulging perineum, client excited and eager, in control		
Third Stage (delivery of newborn to delivery of placenta)			
Time	5–30 minutes		
Contractions	Strong; uterus changing to globular shape		
Manifestations	Gush of blood, apparent lengthening of cord, client focuses on newborn, excited about birth, feeling of relief		
Fourth Stage (delivery of placenta to homeostasis)			
Time	Usually defined as 1st hour postpartum		
Uterus	Firm, at midline, 2 finger breadths above umbilicus		
Manifestations	Lochia rubra, exploration of newborn, parent-infant bonding begins, newborn alert and responsive: first period of reactivity		

b. Tranquilizers
  1) produce sedation and relaxation; often given with narcotics because of potentiating effects; when given alone, there may be little or no analgesia; may cause excitement and disorientation in presence of pain
  2) examples: promethazine HCl (Phenergan), hydroxyzine pamoate (Vistaril), promazine HCl (Sparine) and diazepam (Valium)
  3) effects
    a) peak action within 60 minutes
    b) may last 6–8 hours depending on stage of labor and activity of client

c. Amnesics (rarely used today)
  1) produce sedation and alter memory
  2) example: scopolamine (belladonna alkaloid)
  3) may cause dysrhythmias and fetal tachycardia

d. Sedatives
  1) produce sedation; may depress fetus

Figure 4.12 Assessment of Uterine Contractions

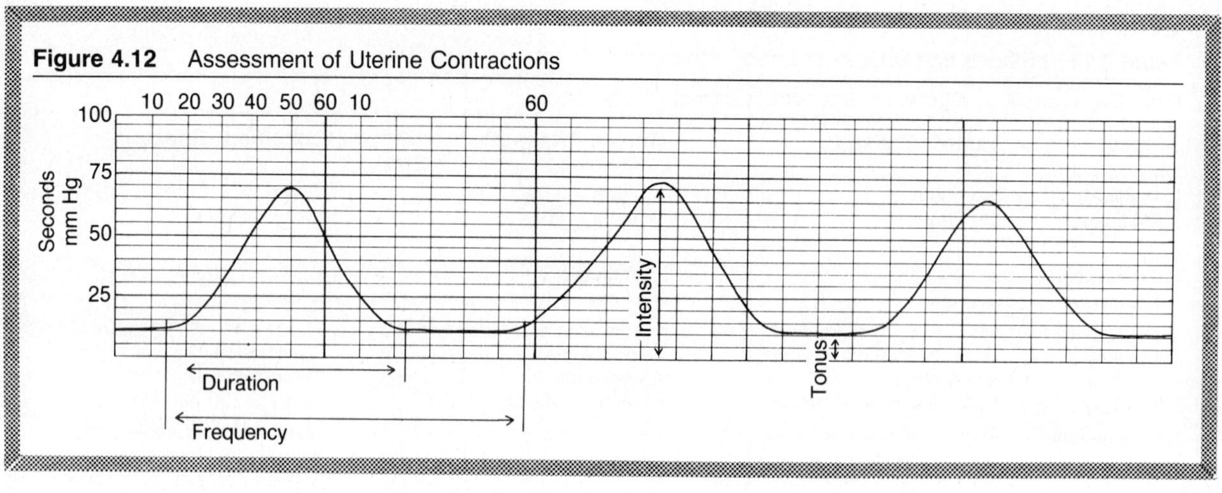

2) examples: secobarbital sodium (Seconal) and pentobarbital sodium (Nembutal) may be given in early labor

4. Anesthetics: produce a local or generalized loss of sensation
   a. General
      1) induce sleep
      2) examples: nitrous oxide, halothane (Fluothane), thiopental (Pentothal sodium), cyclopropane)
      3) may depress fetus
      4) danger of pulmonary aspiration of gastric contents
      5) uterine atony
   b. Local
      1) used for pain relief during episiotomy and perineal repair
      2) example: lidocaine (Xylocaine)
      3) any agent may cause an allergic response
   c. Regional
      1) for relief of perineal and uterine pain
      2) usually safe for infant unless maternal hypotension occurs
      3) types
         a) *paracervical block*: given in 1st stage active phase; rapid relief of uterine pain; relieves pain of contractions; no effect on perineal area; does not interfere with bearing-down reflex; fetal bradycardia may occur
         b) *peridural block*: given in 1st stage active phase or 2nd stage of labor; produces rapid relief of uterine and perineal pain; may be given in single doses or continuously
            - epidural: may cause maternal hypotension
            - caudal: same side effects as epidural
         c) *intradural blocks*: given in 2nd stage
            - spinal block: rapid onset; relieves uterine and perineal pain; may cause maternal hypotension; client must remain flat for 8–12 hours
            - saddle block (low spinal): rapid onset of pain relief; used for forceps delivery; client must remain flat for 8–12 hours
         d) *pudendal block*: given in 2nd stage of labor; affects perineum for about ½ hour; safe for newborn; no effect on contractions
         e) *local anesthesia*: blocks primary nerve pathways in 2nd stage; for delivery, episiotomy; short-term inhibition of pain perception

Application of the Nursing Process to Normal Childbearing, Intrapartal Care

1. Assessment/Analysis
   a. Premonitory signs of labor
   b. Labor status: true labor; stage and phase of labor (refer to Table 4.17)
   c. Uterine contractions
   d. Due date
   e. Membranes intact or ruptured
   f. Fetal response to labor
   g. Psychological factors: preparation for childbirth; support systems; culture/religious beliefs
   h. Newborn adaptation at birth
   i. Maternal homeostasis after delivery

2. Plans, Implementation, and Evaluation

Goal 1: The client will experience minimal anxiety on admission to the labor and delivery unit; will be knowledgeable about the birth process and procedures performed.

Plan/Implementation

- Orient client to physical setting and review basic procedures to be performed.
- Determine onset, duration, and frequency of contractions.
- Determine client's knowledge of the labor and delivery process, childbirth preparation.
- Obtain baseline vital signs and BP
- Perform Leopold's maneuver (see Figure 4.13): have client empty bladder and flex knees for abdominal relaxation; warm hands, then proceed with
  - fundus palpation: note breech or cephalic presentation
  - lateral palpation: note back and small parts of fetus
  - just above symphysis pubis, note position and mobility of fetal head
  - midline about 2 inches above Poupart's ligaments, note position and descent of head, location of back

Figure 4.13 Leopold's Maneuvers

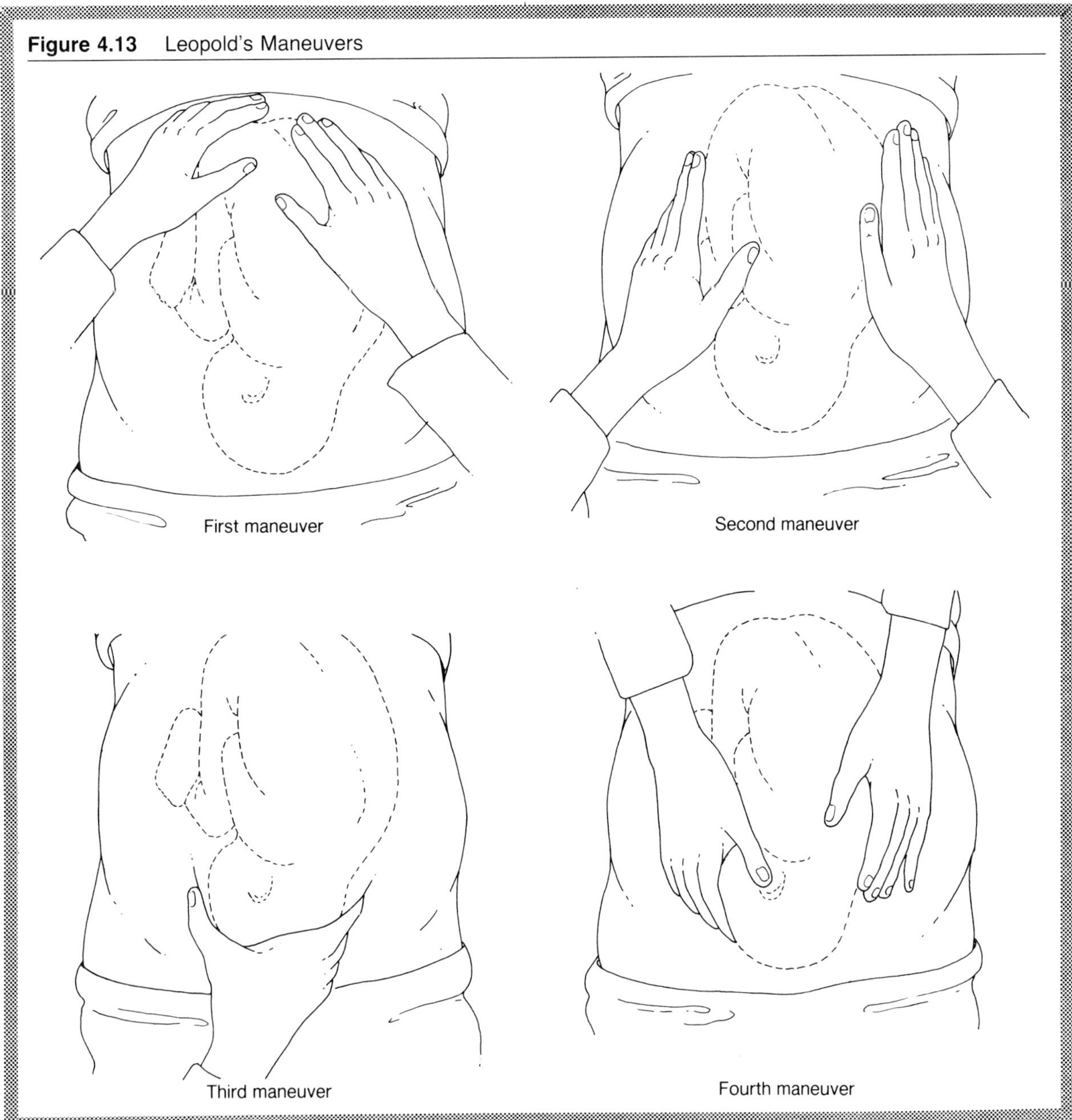

- Observe FHR and pattern changes in relation to contractions (*NOTE*: the use of electronic fetal monitoring for every woman is determined by hospital policy/physician. Obtain consent to use an internal electrode.
- Prepare and position client appropriately for initial vaginal exam and reinforce the rationale for exam; explain the results of exam.
- Note color, consistency, amount, and gross appearance of amniotic fluid.
- Obtain laboratory specimens: urine for protein (normally neg), glucose (normally neg), and ketones (normally neg); blood for Hgb (normal range 12–16 gm/100 ml), Hct (normal range 38%–45%), WBC (normal range 4,500–11,000 ml), VDRL.
- Determine time of last food ingestion.
- Document all assessments.
- Review process of labor.
- Provide emotional support to client and coach.
- Perform vulvar and/or perineal preparation as ordered.
- Administer cleansing enema if ordered by physician; check FHR after procedure.

Evaluation: Client is admitted to labor and delivery unit; verbalizes an understanding of status; displays minimal anxiety.

Goal 2: Client will be comfortable and safe during the 1st stage of labor; will be supported by coach; will maintain optimal fetal oxygenation.

Plan/Implementation

- Take maternal vital signs qh, if stable and within normal limits.
- Monitor temperature q2h if membranes ruptured more than 24 hours previously or if temperature is greater than 37.5°C (may indicate infection or dehydration).
- Observe blood pressure between contractions q1–2h.
- Watch for supine-hypotensive syndrome caused by pressure of enlarged uterus on vena cava (decreased BP, pulse, pallor, clammy skin); condition may be prevented or corrected by placing client in left lateral position.

Monitor fetal status
  - auscultate FHR using a stethoscope q30min (early labor) to q5min (transition) (see Figure 4.14); count rate for 1 full minute (normal is 120–160/minute) or observe FHR tracing from electronic monitor for baseline changes, variability, and periodic changes related to contractions
  - check FHR immediately after rupture of membranes
  - check for prolapse of cord; client may feel cord slither down vagina, nurse may see cord outside vagina or palpate cord on vaginal examination; if cord is prolapsed, place in Trendelenburg's or knee-chest position (to minimize pressure of presenting part on cord), give O_2, notify physician immediately; grave danger of fetal hypoxia because of cord compression; prepare for immediate delivery

- Monitor uterine contractions through abdominal palpations q30min (in early labor) to q5min (in transition); note regularity, frequency, intensity, and duration or observe uterine tracings from electronic monitor for tonus, frequency, duration, and intensity of contractions.
- Document all assessments.
- Assist with or perform periodic vaginal examination to assess dilatation and effacement of cervix, fetal descent, presentation, lie.
- Monitor fluid and electrolyte balance
  - record I&O
  - encourage voiding q2h; catheterize for bladder distention
  - observe for signs of dehydration
  - note diaphoresis
  - monitor parenteral therapy; specific use determined by medical regimen and duration of labor
- Provide sufficient nourishment according to medical policy and client need
  - NPO routine in many hospitals, especially if client is receiving medication; observe for signs of hypoglycemia
  - ice chips or liquid diet may be given in some settings (*NOTE*: GI absorption and motility are decreased during labor)
  - observe for nausea and vomiting during transition (common)
- Maintain a safe environment
  - client may ambulate in early labor if desired, unless there are contraindications (e.g., membranes ruptured, medications, IV infusion)
  - Keep side rails up as necessary to prevent injury during active labor
  - advise client and coach not to smoke
- Administer basic comfort measures: pillows to support body; frequent position change; bathe face and body as necessary; backrubs; effleurage for abdominal discomfort; change linen and pads frequently.
- Assist client with breathing techniques or provide direct coaching as necessary

Figure 4.14 Site of Auscultation of FHR with Fetus in ROA Position

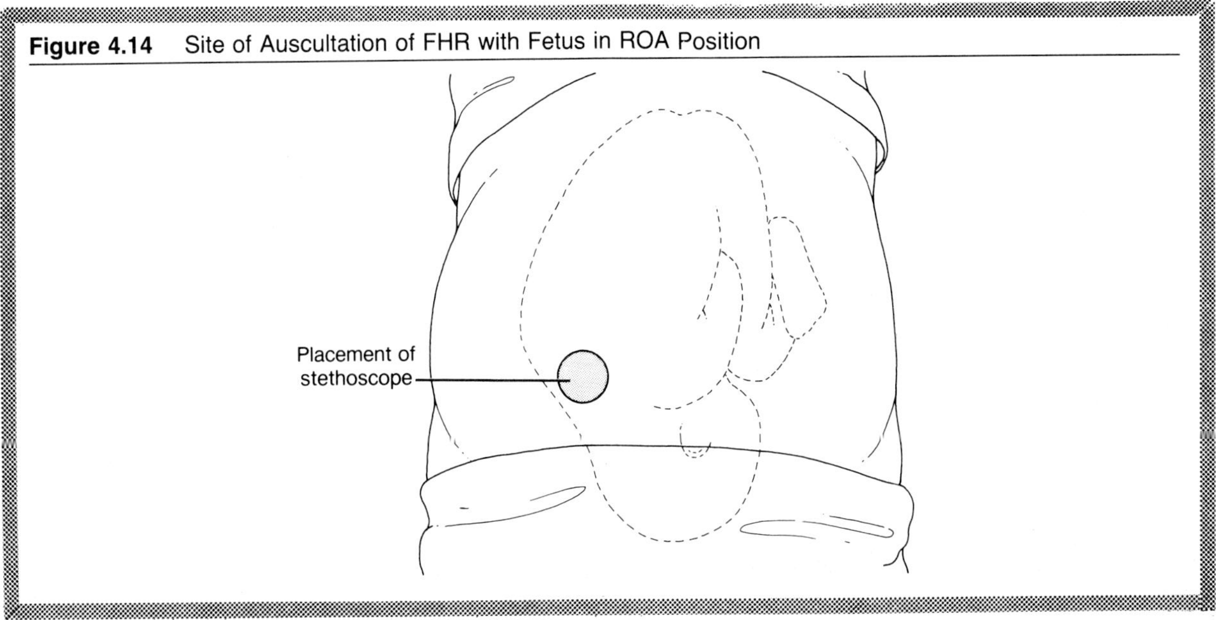

- utilize appropriate techniques taught in antepartal or childbirth classes or instruct as necessary (e.g., abdominal breathing, shallow chest breathing, panting)
- advise client to rest between contractions but wake client and begin breathing techniques at onset of next contraction
- observe for symptoms of hyperventilation (light-headedness, dizziness, tingling and numbness of lips); if it occurs, slow down breathing, breathe into paper bag or cupped hands
- support coach by giving periodic relief for a break and nourishment
- praise efforts and keep client and significant other informed about progress in labor

■ Assess ability to manage pain, desire for medications.

■ Administer analgesics (or assist with anesthetic administration) as ordered by physician, in accordance with client's preference/decision
- provide relaxing environment by maintaining calm manner and reducing external stimuli
- administer and record administration of medications ordered
- note client and fetal response to medication; report any undesired side effects
- monitor client's vital signs and FHR q5–15min, depending on drug given
- place client in appropriate position for administration of anesthetic
- place client in lateral position, increase IV fluids if hypotension develops
- administer 6–8 liters of O_2/minute for maternal hypotension or late decelerations in FHR

Evaluation: During the 1st stage of labor, the client maintains homeostasis, is as comfortable as possible; is supported effectively by coach/nurse; fetal heart rate is normal in response to contractions.

Goal 3: Client will be maintained during the 2nd stage of labor; will assist with birth by effective pushing, supported by coach; a healthy newborn will be delivered with minimal trauma.

Plan/Implementation

■ Maintain a safe environment
- if transfer to delivery room is required, plan move between uterine contractions (multiparas may be transported at 8–9 cm dilation, primiparas at full dilation with perineal bulging)
- wear appropriate apparel and assist significant other in proper hand washing and obtaining appropriate scrub attire for delivery room; birthing room regulations may be flexible
- place client in optimal position on delivery table for birth of newborn
  - * for lithotomy position: pad stirrups; maintain equal height of legs; ensure no pressure on popliteal space
  - * alternate positions may include semi-Fowler's on birthing table, side lying, squatting

- Prep vulvar and perineal area wearing sterile gloves.
- Palpate fundus for uterine contractions, or assess electronically.
- Monitor FHR by either ausculation with a fetoscope or electronically.
- Monitor BP at intervals.
- Encourage strong pushing with contractions
  - instruct client to begin by taking 2 short breaths, then hold and bear down; legs should be spread with knees slightly flexed
  - show the client which muscles are to be used by showing or touching those muscles in the pelvic floor
  - use blow-blow breathing pattern to prevent pushing between contractions
- Assist physician/midwife as necessary.
- Promote emotional well-being of client and coach
  - inform them about progress and all procedures
  - position mirror so delivery may be viewed
  - encourage rest and relaxation between contractions
  - praise frequently for efforts

Evaluation: Client is positioned appropriately and safely for delivery; pushes and bears down effectively; is supported by coach; delivers fetus with minimum trauma.

Goal 4: Client will remain stable during the 3rd stage; will expel placenta intact; will be free from excessive bleeding; newborn will remain stable and have early contact with mother.

Plan/Implementation

- Note time of delivery of infant.
- Provide immediate newborn care; refer to page 454.
- Place newborn close to client, on uncovered abdomen if possible.
- Allow client to touch and explore infant after cord is cut.
- Assess for signs that placenta has separated
  - uterus rises up in abdomen
  - uterus changes to globular shape
  - sudden trickle of blood appears
  - umbilical cord lengthens
- Observe time and mechanism of placental delivery; chart on delivery record
  - Duncan mechanism: maternal surface of the placenta presents upon delivery; appears dark and rough; increased risk of retained placental fragments
  - Schultze mechanism: fetal surface of the placenta presents upon delivery; appears shiny, smooth
- Inspect placenta for intactness and 3 blood vessels.
- Palpate uterus to check for muscle tone at frequent intervals (firm and contracted).
- Administer and document oxytocic agents as ordered (see Tables 4.18, 4.20)
  - drug and dose determined by individual need and physician's order; may be given IM or added to existing IV
  - used to prevent/control postpartum hemorrhage by stimulating uterine contractility
  - very important with overdistention or poor muscle tone
- Measure BP at q5–15min intervals (decreases in BP are often associated with blood loss and administration of oxytocic drugs).
- Give antilactation agents (see Table 4.25)
- Send cord blood to lab if client is Rh negative or O positive (for direct Coombs' test).
- Allow client (and significant other if present) opportunity to see and directly touch newborn (promotes bonding) after initial stabilization.
- Initiate breast-feeding (hospital policies may vary).

Evaluation: Client remains stable during the 3rd stage of labor; delivers placenta intact; experiences good uterine contractions; has minimal bleeding; parent-infant bonding is fostered.

Goal 5: Client will remain stable in birthing room or during transfer to recovery room; will be free from complications; will maintain homeostasis; will bond with newborn.

Plan/Implementation

- Take vital signs q15min until stable (temperature upon admission and subsequently as indicated
- Check height of fundus
  - palpate q15min during 1st hour
  - note position in relation to umbilicus (at or just above umbilicus, 1–2 finger breadths)
  - note consistency: should be firmly contracted; if boggy, massage until firm (avoid overmassaging)
- Palpate bladder for distention; measure initial voiding; catheterize if necessary (full bladder displaces the uterus).
- Observe lochia q15min during 1st hour; note amount (small, moderate, or heavy), color (rubra), consistency; presence of large clots

Table 4.18 Uterine Smooth Muscle Stimulants

Drug Name	Action	Side Effects	Nursing Implications
Ergonovine maleate (Erogtrate)	Reduces risk of or treats postpartum hemorrhage by stimulating uterine contraction	Nausea, vomiting, dizziness, hypotension, hypertension	Monitor BP before and during administration. Palpate fundus and note lochia.
Methylergonovine maleate (Methergine)	Stimulates uterine contraction, increases uterine muscle tone, prevents/controls postpartum hemorrhage	Nausea, vomiting, dizziness, slight changes in BP (less likely than with Erogtrate), headaches	Monitor contractions, lochia.

may indicate retained placental fragments; flow is considered excessive if bleeding saturates pad within 15 minutes (flow may increase as oxytocics wear off).

- Check perineum: note general appearance, any swelling, redness, bruising, drainage, condition of episiotomy; assess for pain.
- Assess for afterpains.
- Promote general comfort
  - cover client with warm blanket if chilling or shivering occur; may be caused by sudden release of intra-abdominal pressure, excitement, rapid decrease of hormones, fetal blood cells in maternal circulation
  - position for maximum comfort; encourage rest
  - give partial bath
- Provide contact with newborn, if not possible in delivery room
- Assist with breast feeding if desired.
- Perform and teach peri care (see page 443); reinforce that pad should be applied from front to back.
- Maintain adequate fluid intake; state specific amounts of fluids to be taken in 8-hour period.
- If transfer to recovery room required, ensure that both client and baby are stabilized
  - monitor client's vital signs q15min until stable
  - palpate position, firmness, and consistency of fundus
  - observe lochia for quantity, color, and consistency
- Transfer to postpartum unit when condition stable (usually within 1–2 hours) or may remain in birthing room).

Evaluation: Client is physiologically and psychologically stable; couple gazes at, holds, touches, and cuddles newborn.

Application of the Nursing Process to the High-risk Intrapartal Client

1. **Assessment**
   a. Risk factors in pregnancy
   b. Problems identified in the intrapartal period
   c. Alterations of labor progress
2. **Analysis**
   a. Safe, effective care environment
      1) potential for infection
      2) potential for injury
   b. Physiological integrity
      1) pain
      2) impaired gas exchange
   c. Psychological integrity
      1) anxiety
      2) ineffective individual coping
   d. Health promotion/maintenance
      1) knowledge deficit
3. **Plan, Implementation, and Evaluation**

Goal: Client and fetus will experience no undetected complications; will receive immediate treatment for problems; will have a safe birth experience. Newborn and mother will maintain physiological and psychological integrity.

Plan/Implementation

- Observe for potential/actual problems in labor and delivery.
- Act immediately to maintain fetal/maternal well-being.
- Report problems to physician.
- Administer therapy/medications as ordered.
- Document assessments and care.
- Support couple in difficult birth situation.

Evaluation: Client/fetus at risk have problems detected and treated immediately; return to a homeostatic state following a safe delivery.

Selected Health Problems in the Intrapartal Period

☐ Dystocia

1. General Information

- **a.** Definition: difficult, painful labor and/or delivery characterized by abnormally slow progress as a result of abnormalities in the mechanics involved
- **b.** Incidence: approximately 5% of intrapartum women (largely primigravidae) experience some type of dystocia
- **c.** Types: fall into four categories, which may exist alone or in combination
  - **1)** the *powers* (or forces): the main ones are
    - **a)** hypertonic uterine dysfunction (primary inertia); see Table 4.19
      - the uterine muscle is in a state of greater than normal muscle tension; contractions are of poor quality, and the force of the contraction is distorted
      - increased tonus
      - no cervical changes
      - is a problem in the latent phase of labor
      - treatment: sedation
    - **b)** hypotonic uterine dysfunction (secondary inertia)
      - the tone or tension of the muscle is defective or inadequate, synchronous but not adequate
      - during active phase, uterine contractions reduce in intensity and get farther apart
      - treatment: stimulation of labor (e.g., ruptured membranes, give oxytocin)
  - **2)** the *passageway*: abnormalities in the size or character of the birth canal that form an obstacle to the descent of the fetus
    - **a)** cephalopelvic disproportion (CPD): disproportion between the size of the fetal head and that of the birth canal
      - most frequently caused by a contracted pelvis: slight irregularities in the structure of the pelvis may delay the progress of labor; marked deformities often make delivery through the natural passages impossible
    - **b)** types of pelvic contractions
      - contraction of the inlet
      - contraction of the midpelvis
      - contraction of the outlet
      - a combination
  - **3)** the *passenger*: variations in position, presentation, or development of the fetus; includes a variety of conditions that are associated with prolonged labor, failure to progress, lack of engagement
    - **a)** abnormal position: persistent occiput posterior position (25% of pregnancies)
    - **b)** faulty presentation
      - shoulder, face presentation
      - breech presentation
    - **c)** excessive size of fetus
      - a fetus over 4,000 gm (8 lb 13½ oz) may be too large to pass through the birth canal of some pregnant women; the fetal head also becomes less malleable when fetal weight increases
      - hydrocephalus (internus): excessive accumulation of cerebrospinal fluid in the ventricles of the brain with consequent enlargement of the cranium; incidence: 1 in 2,000 births
      - enlargement of the body of the fetus, e.g., abdominal distention, tumors
  - **4)** the *person*: maternal factors (e.g., anxiety, lack of education, fear) can lengthen labor

Table 4.19 Uterine Dysfunction in Labor

	Hypertonic	Hypotonic
Phase of labor	Latent	Active
Contractions	Intense, high tonus	Weak, ineffective
Symptoms	Painful	Painless
Fetal distress	Fetal hypoxia	Tendency for sepsis
Treatment	Sedation	Stimulation of labor

2. Nursing Process

a. Assessment/Analysis

- **1)** vaginal exam, pelvimetry, or ultrasound to establish diagnosis
- **2)** false labor vs true labor
- **3)** fetal status
- **4)** cause of dystocia
- **5)** complications of uterine dysfunction
  - **a)** maternal exhaustion
  - **b)** intrapartum infection
  - **c)** traumatic operative delivery

Table 4.20 Oxytocin

Drug Name	Action	Side Effects	Nursing Implications
Pitocin	Stimulates uterine smooth muscle to contract; increases intracellular calcium. Used in dilute concentrations IV (10 units in 500 or 1000 ml normal saline); infusion rate gradually increased to induce or augment labor contractions and stimulate cervical effacement and dilatation before delivery. After delivery acts to stimulate uterine contraction and prevent hemorrhage due to atony.	***In labor*** Maternal: overstimulation of uterus resulting in rapid labor, delivery; tetany and uterine rupture; abruptio placenta; water intoxication Fetal: hypoxia, distress, trauma with precipitous delivery ***Following Delivery*** Water intoxication, uterine atony (if overused)	Monitor/record vital signs and contractions (frequency, duration, strength). Discontinue infusion if contractions exceed 70–90 seconds, for signs of tetany or abruptio placenta. Record I&O. Monitor FHR; discontinue infusion if distress; turn client to left side. Report problems immediately to responsible physician. Monitor BP, uterine contraction, lochia, output.

d) fetal death and injury

6) presentation of fetus by palpation (Leopold's maneuver)

7) meconium staining of amniotic fluid (normal when associated with breech presentation)

8) anxiety

b. Plans, Implementation, and Evaluation

Goal 1: Client will have dystocia detected; the client with a dystocia will remain stable during the intrapartal period; will deliver a healthy, stable newborn.

Plan/Implementation

- Assess uterine contractions/pattern.
- Plot individual labor pattern, compare to Friedman curve (average labor curve of cervical dilatation and hours in labor, Figure 4.15)
- Assist with ultrasonographic or radiographic studies for laboring woman who has previously suspected CPD.
- Assess immediately when physician artificially ruptures fetal membranes for prolapsed cord and FHR; if cord prolapsed, see page 439.
- Monitor IV therapy and electrolyte replacement.
- Administer broad-spectrum antibiotics as ordered for treatment of intrauterine infection.
- Promote rest.
- Support family.

Evaluation: Abnormalities in the powers, passageway, or passenger are identified during the antepartal or early intrapartal period; client with dystocia is promptly treated; client/fetus remain stable during difficult labor; healthy newborn is delivered.

Goal 2: Client will have effective uterine contractions with oxytocin augmentation; will maintain adequate fetal oxygenation.

Plan/Implementation

- Administer oxytocin (Pitocin) according to physician's order or hospital's protocol and client's condition (see Table 4.20); the physician must consider the following criteria before administration
  - there must be true hypotonic dysfunction; oxytocin ABSOLUTELY CONTRAINDICATED for *hypertonic* uterine dysfunction
  - the client must be in true labor (progressed to at least 3 cm dilation and cervix thinning
  - no mechanical obstructions to safe delivery exist (e.g., cephalopelvic disproportion)
  - the condition of the fetus must be good: regular fetal heart rate, no meconium staining
  - the client usually must be less than 35 years old and less than a para 5 (greater age and parity increase the risk of uterine rupture)
  - the uterus must not be overdistended because of a large infant (weighing 4,000 gm or more) or multiple gestation
  - no previous history of cesarean births
- monitor administration of oxytocin
  - increase infusion rate as ordered
  - use infusion pump
  - monitor vital signs, infusion rate frequently
  - continue electronic fetal monitoring; observe and document fetal heart rate pattern with contractions (duration, intensity, tonus, and frequency)

Figure 4.15 Friedman Curve

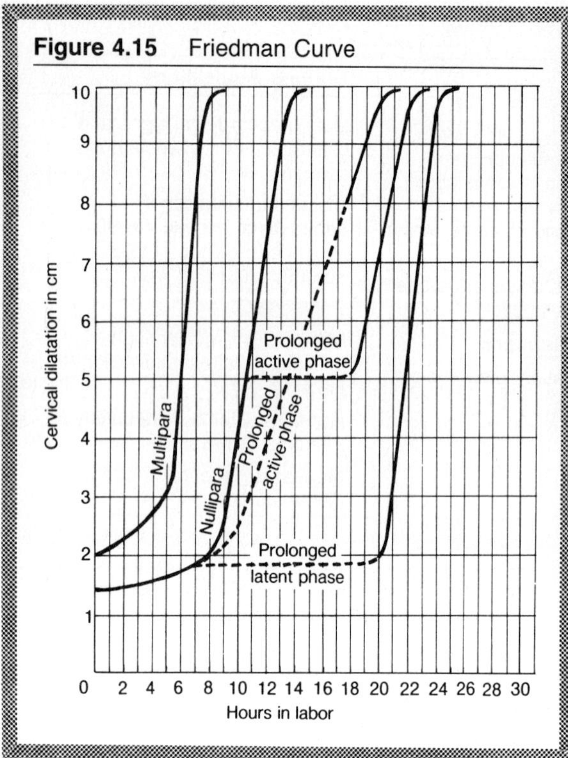

- place client in a left lateral position to maximize uterine blood flow by reducing pressure on vena cava and aorta
- never leave client unattended (physician must be available)
- assess for problems (e.g., rigid abdomen, intense pain)
- if uterine tetany occurs, or contractions exceed 70–90 seconds duration, or there is fetal distress or bradycardia, discontinue oxytocin
- give O_2 for signs of fetal distress
- monitor for abruptio placentae

Evaluation: Client is free from complications related to oxytocin administration; has effective uterine contractions; maintains optimal fetal status.

Goal 3: Client will experience minimal anxiety; will be supported and comforted during labor.

Plan/Implementation

- Inform client about her status and measures taken to help her.
- Provide basic comfort measures as in normal labor.
- Assess level of fatigue and ability to cope with pain.
- Provide emotional support to client and significant other.
- Assist with administration of local anesthetic to interrupt peripheral neurohormonal mechanisms (hypertonic uterine contractions).
- Assist with administration of anesthesia to relax uterus (hyperactive uterine contractions).
- Discuss rationale and expected outcomes with client and partner if cesarean birth indicated.

Evaluation: Client experiences minimal anxiety; knows the status of labor and the fetus; rests comfortably between contractions, treatments; is supported by coach/nurse.

Goal 4: Client with an abnormal fetal position or presentation will be safely delivered and free from complications; will deliver a newborn in stable condition.

Plan/Implementation

- Assist with vaginal or rectal exam to determine fetal presenting part.
- Explain and prepare client for ultrasonic or radiographic studies to confirm previously unsuspected malpositions (anomalies often undetected before intrapartum period).
- Assess effectiveness of labor and fetal well-being by continuous electronic monitoring.
- Encourage left lateral position.
- Provide emotional support and coaching as indicated (labors are often prolonged).
- Support significant other.
- Apply sacral pressure and frequent backrubs to keep pressure of fetal occiput off client's sacrum (occiput posterior presentation).
- Observe for cord prolapse (occurs in 1 in every 400 births) when membranes rupture (see page 433).
- Assist with vaginal delivery or cesarean birth as indicated by fetal presentation, labor progression, and maternal well-being.

Evaluation: Client delivers a healthy newborn safely free from complications, despite dystocia.

☐ Premature Labor

1. General Information

a. Definition: onset of labor before completion of 37 weeks gestation

b. Predisposing factors and complications necessitating delivery of preterm infant

1) maternal

- **a)** diabetes
- **b)** cardiovascular and/or renal disease
- **c)** pregnancy-induced or chronic hypertension
- **d)** infection: chorio amnionitis
- **e)** uncontrolled hemorrhage associated

with placenta previa or abruptio placentae
f) prematurely ruptured membranes
g) incompetent cervix
h) smoking
i) severe isoimmunization
2) fetal
a) multiple pregnancy
b) hydramnios
c) infection

c. Prognosis: fetal/neonatal mortality is less than 5% in pregnancies when gestation has lasted 35 or more weeks and the fetus is larger than 2,000 gm

2. Nursing Process

a. Assessment/Analysis

1) identify women at risk
2) assess for true labor (contractions of increased frequency and duration, effacement and dilation of cervix)
3) estimate gestation

b. Plan, Implementation, and Evaluation

Goal: Client in preterm labor will experience a cessation of labor; will progress to a safe delivery.

Plan/Implementation

- Maintain bed rest, lateral recumbent position in a quiet environment.
- Administer selected tokolytic agents to suppress labor as prescribed by physician (e.g., isoxuprine [Vasodilan], ritodrine, terbutaline, magnesium sulfate)
  - assess the effects of drugs upon the pattern of labor (uterine contractions) and fetal well-being via electronic monitoring system
  - avoid these drugs for control of premature labor if contraindicated (e.g., client has a cardiac condition, gestation less than 20 weeks)
  - if administering ritodrine: assess for specific cardiovascular side effects (see Table 4.21)
  - if administering magnesium sulfate: assess BP, reflexes, respirations, and urinary output before and during administration (see Table 4.14)
- Document response to therapy; alter dose as ordered.
- Maintain adequate hydration through oral or parenteral intake.
- Monitor I&O.
- Monitor client's vital signs.
- Provide emotional support to client and significant other.
- Administer glucocorticoid therapy (betamethasone) if indicated to prevent respiratory distress syndrome in newborn
  - drug is effective if delivery can be delayed 48 or more hours
  - avoid use if delivery is imminent or if maternal hypertensive or cardiovascular disorders exist
  - observe for signs of pulmonary edema (reported in rare cases when ritodrine and corticosteroids are used together)
- Administer minimal analgesics for pain during labor and delivery.
- Prepare for preterm delivery if maternal complications are present (e.g., diabetes, hemorrhage, eclampsia) or dilation progresses.

Evaluation: Client carries the pregnancy to term or safely delivers the newborn.

☐ Emergency Birth (unassisted by physician or midwife)

1. General Information

a. May occur in a hospital or community setting
b. Predisposing factors: precipitate labor, environmental problems, absence of physician/midwife
c. Prognosis: increased maternal and fetal risk associated with possible
1) intrauterine hypoxia (precipitate labor or delivery)
2) laceration of the perineum
3) infection

2. Nursing Process

a. Assessment/Analysis

1) fetal status
2) stage and phase of labor

b. Plan, Implementation, and Evaluation

Goal: Client will deliver newborn, free from complications, despite an emergency situation.

Plan/Implementation

- Remain with client; have another adult (if present) call for assistance; remain calm.
- Provide as clean an environment as possible.
- Instruct client to pant when head crowns.
- Rupture amniotic sac (if intact) when fetal head crowns.
- Apply gentle pressure on fetal head to prevent head from "popping out," damaging fetal head, and causing maternal lacerations.

Table 4.21 Tocolytic Agent

Drug Name	Action	Side Effects	Nursing Implications
Ritodrine Hydrochloride IV (Yutopar—oral) (only drug with current FDA approval for preterm labor)	Relaxes arterioles in uterine muscle; vasodilator. As a beta sympathetic agent, stops uterine contractions in preterm labor of at least 20 weeks (membranes should be intact). IV solution (150 mg to 500 ml fluid) is given at increasing rates until desired effect is achieved.	Maternal: tachycardia, tremors, palpitations, PVCs; pulmonary edema, widening pulse pressure, headache, hyperglycemia hypokalemia, anxiety, diarrhea (contraindicated if history of CV, thyroid disease; asthma) Fetal: tachycardia, hypoxia, acidosis	Maintain infusion rate; increase as ordered. Monitor apical pulse; report and document pulse above 120; check BP frequently. Record I&O; observe for side effects. Monitor glucose and potassium levels. Teach client expected responses such as nervousness. Explain that the value of therapy is to allow time for fetal lung development (glucocorticoids may be ordered to stimulate surfactant). Monitor for signs of pulmonary edema. Have antidote (propranolol) available. Monitor and document FHR.

- Deliver fetal head between contractions.
- Check for cord around neck; if wrapped around neck, slip cord over infant's head.
- Clear airway and facilitate mucus drainage; do not hold upside down by feet or ankles.
- Dry newborn rapidly (maintain at level of uterus).
- Cover infant with blanket or towel to prevent heat loss.
- Clamp cord in 2 places and cut between the 2 clamps; use sterile or clean scissors or knife; leave intact if medical assistance will be available shortly.
- Observe for placental separation
  - do not pull on cord
  - instruct client to gently push out placenta
- Place newborn on client's abdomen or to breast to stimulate uterine contractions.
- Assess client following birth.

Evaluation: Client is safely delivered of a healthy newborn; is free from complications.

(*NOTE*: The next four selected health problems are classified as "Operative Obstetrics.")

☐ Episiotomy

1. General Information

a. Definition: an incision made into the perineum to facilitate delivery

b. Indications: any condition that places the woman at risk for perineal tearing, e.g.
  1) rapid labor
  2) large baby
  3) malposition of the fetus

c. Prognosis: generally heals within 2–4 weeks following delivery; may cause mild to moderate discomfort in the postpartum period

d. Types (see Figure 4.16)
  1) median (midline)
    a) advantages: easily repaired; generally less painful; minimal blood loss
    b) disadvantages: increased risk of 3rd or 4th degree extension
  2) mediolateral (right or left)
    a) advantage: minimal risk of extension into rectum
    b) disadvantages: greater blood loss; repair more difficult; area more painful during healing; possible damage to pubococcygeal muscle

2. Nursing Process: see *Postpartal Care*, Nursing Goal 1 page 443.

☐ Forceps

1. General Information

a. Definition: obstetric instruments that are used

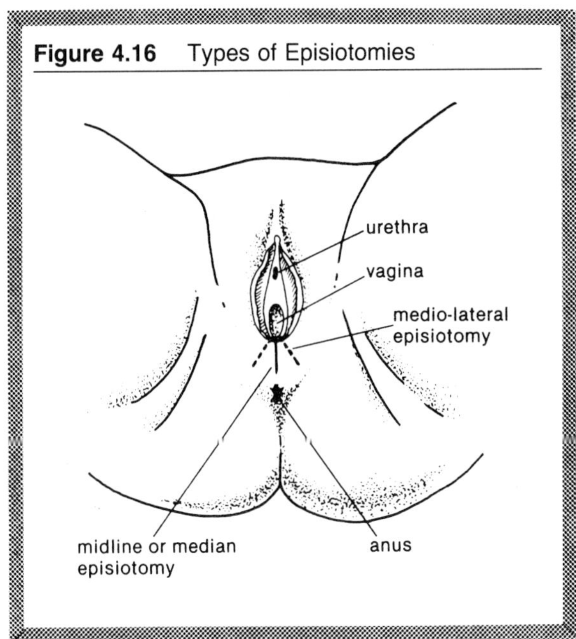

Figure 4.16 Types of Episiotomies

to extract the fetal head during delivery. Each consists of a blade, shank, handle, and lock.

b. Predisposing factors
   1) maternal
      a) to shorten 2nd stage of labor in dystocia
      b) expulsive efforts that are ineffective or deficient
      c) if pushing is contraindicated because of a chronic disease or cardiac problem
   2) fetal
      a) premature labor (to protect fetal head)
      b) fetal distress
      c) arrested descent
      d) abnormal presentation

c. Prognosis
   1) perineal lacerations may occur with a difficult forceps delivery or may follow a precipitate delivery
      a) 1st degree laceration involves fourchette, perineal skin, and vaginal mucosa
      b) 2nd degree laceration involves skin, mucous membrane, muscles of perineal body
      c) 3rd degree laceration involves skin, mucous membranes, muscles of perineal body, and rectal sphincter
      d) 4th degree laceration involves all features of 3rd degree lacerations plus tearing into the lumen of the rectum
   2) pressure by forceps on fetus's facial nerve may cause temporary paralysis of one side of the face
   3) perinatal morbidity and mortality increased, particularly with midforceps delivery
   4) increased risk of postpartum hemorrhage with midforceps delivery
   5) maternal complications following forceps or other traumatic delivery may include cystocele, rectocele, or uterine prolapse later in life

d. Types of forceps deliveries
   1) outlet or low forceps: fetal head on perineal floor
   2) midforceps: fetal head at the level of ischial spines

2. Nursing Process

a. Assessment/Analysis
   1) cervix fully dilated prior to use of forceps
   2) head engaged
   3) fetus in vertex presentation (or face with mentum anterior)
   4) membranes ruptured
   5) no cephalopelvic disproportion
   6) bowel and bladder empty

b. Plan, Implementation, and Evaluation

Goal: Client and fetus will experience minimal trauma, despite forceps delivery.

Plan/Implementation
- Explain procedure to client and significant other.
- Provide physician with selected forceps.
- Monitor fetal heart rate continuously during procedure.
- Assess newborn for forceps bruises.

Evaluation: Client is free from complications of forceps delivery; delivers a healthy newborn with minimal trauma.

☐ Vacuum Extraction (used infrequently in current practice)

1. General Information

a. Definition: the use of an obstetric instrument consisting of a suction cup attached to a suction pump for extraction of the fetal head; it employs negative pressure and traction

b. Predisposing factors
   1) prolonged labor
   2) fetal distress
   3) fetal malposition
   4) chronic maternal disease or complications that contraindicate pushing

c. Prognosis
   1) increased risk of tissue necrosis of the fetal head, cephalhematoma, and cerebral trauma
   2) increased risk of trauma to vagina and cervix
   3) increased risk of postpartum hemorrhage

2. Nursing Process

a. **Assessment/Analysis**
   1) fetal status
   2) fetal position

b. **Plan, Implementation, and Evaluation**

Goal: Client will verbalize understanding of the procedure; will deliver fetus safely.

Plan/Implementation
- Clarify procedure following physician's explanation.
- Assemble and set up necessary equipment.
- Monitor fetal heart rate continuously.
- Assist the physician with the suction apparatus.
- Assess newborn for caput and cerebral swelling.

Evaluation: Newborn is delivered safely, using the vacuum extractor.

☐ Cesarean Birth

1. General Information

a. Definition: delivery of a newborn through abdominal wall and uterine incisions. The procedure may be prearranged and performed prior to the onset of labor (elective) or unplanned and initiated after the onset of labor (emergency).

b. Indications
   1) cephalopelvic disproportion
   2) weakened or defective uterine scar, caused by previous cesarean birth or other uterine surgery (VBAC or vaginal birth after cesarean may be an option for selected women): refer to page 435
   3) severe preeclampsia, eclampsia, or poorly controlled diabetes
   4) placenta previa or premature separation
   5) dystocia
   6) pelvic tumors
   7) maternal vaginal infection (e.g., herpes virus type 2 or gonorrhea)
   8) fetal distress
   9) prolapsed cord
   10) fetal abnormalities (e.g., hydrocephalus)
   11) abnormal presentations (e.g., breech)
   12) multiple birth

c. Prognosis
   1) related to the reasons the cesarean delivery was performed, the type of procedure used, length of time membranes were ruptured, and the nature of complications occurring
   2) perinatal mortality increases with fetal immaturity and complications compromising uteroplacental blood exchange

d. Types (see Figure 4.17)
   1) classical: vertical incision is made through the visceral peritoneum and into the full body of the uterus above the bladder; performed infrequently
      a) advantages: simple and rapid to perform, useful when there is an anterior placenta previa
      b) disadvantages
         - potential for rupture of the scar with subsequent pregnancy
         - increased risk of small bowel adhesion to the suture line
   2) lower segment: incision made into the lower segment of the uterus
   3) extraperitoneal: incision is made into the lower uterine segment without entering the peritoneal cavity

2. Nursing Process

a. **Assessment/Analysis**
   1) indications
   2) maternal and fetal well-being
   3) pain and anxiety

b. **Plans, Implementation and Evaluation**

Figure 4.17 Types of Cesarean Incisions

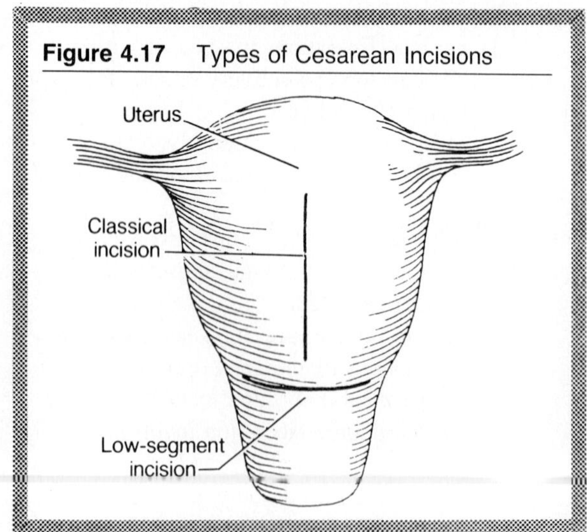

Goal 1: Preoperatively, client and fetus will be free from problems; client will be physically and emotionally prepared for the cesarean birth.

Plan/Implementation

- Provide care as for any surgical procedure: refer to "Perioperative Period" page 157 (preop care will vary with an elective versus an emergency cesarean birth).
- Perform or request laboratory studies: type and crossmatch, CBC, Hgb, and Hct, Rh.
- Insert Foley catheter.
- Monitor fetal heart rate.
- Administer atropine or antacid as ordered.
- Prepare emergency equipment for resuscitation of mother and newborn.

Evaluation: Client and fetus are in no distress; couple is prepared for cesarean birth.

Goal 2: Client will tolerate surgery; will achive post-op homeostasis; will initiate maternal-infant bonding; newborn will be free from preventable complications.

Plan/Implementation

- Refer to "Perioperative Period" page 157, Goal 5 page 160, and "Postpartum Care" page 441.
- Assist physician with surgical procedure as necessary
- Monitor maternal-fetus status.
- Assess for signs and symptoms of hemorrhage
- Administer oxytocic agents as ordered by physician.
- Provide assistance as necessary during mother-infant interactions.
- Monitor recovery from anesthesia.
- Anticipate possible feelings of failure.
- Provide emotional support to help mother and significant other integrate the experience.

Evaluation: Client is free from complications; remains stable and comfortable during the post-op period; initiates bonding; newborn is in good condition.

☐ Vaginal Birth After Cesarean Delivery (VBAC)

1. General Information

a. Incidence: VBAC is increasing; 60%–65% of women who attempt vaginal deliveries after cesarean delivers do so

b. Contraindications
   1) upper segment uterine incision
   2) other contraindications for vaginal deliver (e.g., CPD)

2. Nursing Process

a. **Assessment/Analysis**
   1) maternal status
   2) fetal responses to contractions

b. **Plan, Implementation, and Evaluation**

Goal: Client will be free of complications with labor, vaginal delivery after previous cesarean birth; will deliver newborn in good condition.

Plan/Implementation

- Monitor uterine contractions very frequently.
- Monitor fetal status continuously.
- Assess for threatened rupture or rupture of uterus (see "Rupture of the Uterus" below).

Evaluation: Client experiences normal labor free from complications; client and newborn are in satisfactory condition.

☐ Rupture of the Uterus

1. General Information

a. Definition: the uterus ruptures from the stress of labor; rupture may be complete or partial

b. Occurrence: rare, 1 in every 2,000 births

c. Predisposing factors
   1) previous surgery of myometrium or cesarean birth
   2) oxytocin (Pitocin) induction (2nd most common cause)
   3) nonprogressive labor
   4) very intense contractions
   5) faulty position or fetal abnormalities
   6) injudicious use of forceps
   7) trauma

d. Prognosis
   1) maternal mortality 5%–10%
   2) fetal mortality is high: 50%–75%

2. Nursing Process

a. **Assessment/Analysis**
   1) sharp abdominal pain (during contractions); onset sudden
   2) tachypnea, tachycardia, anxiety, cool and clammy skin, confusion (shock); rapid change in condition
   3) sudden absence of uterine contractions (with complete rupture)
   4) uterus palpated as a hard mass adjacent to fetus
   5) hemorrhage into the abdominal cavity and/or vagina
   6) abdominal tenderness

b. Plan, Implementation, and Evaluation

Goal: Client will be free from hemorrhage or uterine rupture; will maintain fluid and electrolyte balance; will verbalize an understanding of the need for emergency surgery; will maintain oxygenation of fetus.

Plan/Implementation

- Assess carefully during labor; report any signs of an impending rupture.
- Monitor fetal status.
- Implement appropriate measures for failure to progress.
- Provide immediate treatment for shock.
- Prepare client/significant other for possible emergency cesarean birth or hysterectomy.
- Provide emotional support to couple.

Evaluation: Client delivers newborn in stable condition before rupture of uterus; has hemorrhage controlled; is in good condition following emergency surgery.

□ Amniotic Fluid Embolism

1. General Information

a. Definition: the entrance of amniotic fluid into the maternal circulation through the placental site and venous sinuses

b. Occurrence: extremely rare complication that occurs in the intrapartum or early postpartum period

c. Predisposing factors: rapid, intense contractions from oxytocin infusion; multiparity with large fetus

d. Prognosis

1) fetal death will result if delivery is not implemented immediately

2) maternal death may occur within 1–2 hours if emergency interventions are ineffective

3) presence of meconium and/or mucus in amniotic fluid is indicative of increased lethality, graver outlook

2. Nursing Process

Refer to "Pulmonary Embolus" page 448.

References

Aukamp, V. (1984). *Nursing care plans for the childbearing family*. Norwalk, CT: Appleton-Century-Crofts.

Austin, S. (1986). Childbirth classes for couples desiring VBAC. *MCN: American Journal of Maternal/Child Nursing*, *11*, 250.

Brengman, S., & Burns, M. (1983). Ritodrine HCl and preterm labor. *American Journal of Nursing*, *83*, 537–540.

Burroughs, A. (1986). *Bleier's maternity nursing*. Philadelphia: Saunders.

Glazer, G., & Hulme, M. (1987). Prostaglandin gel for cervical ripening. *MCN*. *12*, 28–31.

McKay, S. (1984). Squatting: An alternate position for the second stage of labor. *MCN: American Journal of Maternal/Child Nursing*, *9*, 181–183.

Murray, M. (1986). Nipple stimulation contraction stress test for the high risk patient. *MCN: The American Journal of Maternal/Child Nursing*, *11*, 331–335.

Shortridge, L. (1983). Using ritodrine HCL to inhibit preterm labor. *MCN: American Journal of Maternal/Child Nursing*, *8*, 58.

Young, Y. & Poppe, C. (1987). Breast pump stimulation to promote labor. *MCN*. *12*, 124–126.

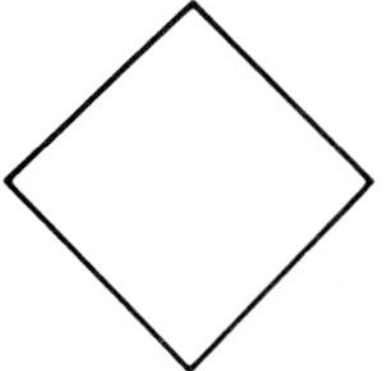

Postpartal Care

General Concepts

☐ Normal Childbearing

1. Definition: the postpartum period (puerperium) starts immediately after delivery and is completed when the reproductive tract has returned to the nearly pre-pregnant state and family readjustment has occurred (usually defined as 6 weeks)
2. Restoration to pregravid status
   a. Uterine involution
      1) process of involution takes 4–6 weeks to complete
         a) weight of uterus decreases from 2 lb to 2 oz
         b) hormones decrease
         c) autolysis occurs (enzyme action)
         d) contractions increase muscle tone
         e) vasoconstriction occurs at placental site
         f) endometrium regenerates
         g) fundus steadily descends into true pelvis; fundal height decreases about 1 finger breadth (1 cm) per day; by 10 days postpartum, cannot be palpated abdominally
      2) factors delaying involution
         a) multiparity
         b) conditions causing overdistention of uterus
         c) infection
         d) retained placenta or membranes
         e) hormonal deficiencies
      3) cervical involution
         a) after one week, muscle begins to regenerate
         b) small lacerations may heal or need cauterization
         c) external os remains wider than in a nonparous woman
         d) internal os closed after one week
      4) lochia (see Table 4.22)
         a) constituents: blood, mucus, particles of decidua, cellular debris, leukocytes, RBCs
         b) changes from rubra (delivery day to day 3: bright red) to serosa (days 4–10: brownish pink) to alba (days 10–14: white, due to increased leukocytes); normally has fleshy odor; decreases daily in amount; increases with ambulation, c.o.; lochia disappearance coincides with healed internal reproductive tract
         c) signs of abnormal lochia
            - foul smell
            - excessive amount (any stage)
            - scant (during rubra stage)
            - return to rubra after serosa and/or alba
      5) after-birth pains due to contraction of uterus are reported primarily in multiparas as well as in mothers who
         a) have a history of blood clots
         b) were treated with oxytocic drugs
         c) breast-feed their infant
         d) had an overdistended uterus during pregnancy (large baby, multiple gestation, polyhydramnios)
   b. Perineal healing
      1) vaginal distention decreases although muscle tone is never restored completely to its pregravid state
      2) vaginal rugae begin to reappear around 3rd week
      3) lacerations or episiotomy suture line gradually heal
      4) hemorrhoids common, generally subside
   c. Bladder and bowel function: physiologic adaptations include
      1) increased urinary output due to normal diuresis
      2) increased bladder capacity; trauma to the bladder during delivery may diminish urge to void
      3) urine may show increased acetone, nitrogen, albumin, and lactose
      4) edema of the urethra and vulva
      5) GI tract motility sluggish because of

Table 4.22 Lochia Changes

Time Postpartum	Characteristics
Delivery—day 3	Lochia rubra (red)
4–10 days	Lochia serosa (brownish to pink)
10–14 days	Lochia alba (white)

a) relaxed abdominal and intestinal muscles
b) decreased intra-abdominal pressure because of distention of the abdominal wall

d. Restoration of abdominal wall
1) abdomen may be soft and flabby, usually returns to normal state by 6–8 weeks
2) striae fade to silvery white; linea nigra fades

e. Breast changes: condition of breasts during pregnancy maintained for first 2 days postpartum; physiologic adapatations include
1) establishment of lactation
a) colostrum secreted during 1st 2–3 days postpartum
b) prolactin released from anterior pituitary gland
c) oxytocin (released from posterior pituitary) causes let-down reflex
2) engorgement
a) onset usually day 3
b) lasts 24–48 hours
c) caused by venous and lymphatic stasis of the breasts
3) mechanism of lactation: sucking activates nerve impulses from nipple to spinal cord to pituitary gland
a) anterior pituitary gland produces prolactin only if breasts are emptied; seems to inhibit FSH and LH
b) posterior pituitary gland secretes oxytocin, causing let-down reflex when milk is ejected from ducts
4) effect on mother
a) increased metabolic-system stress
b) loss of large amounts of stored protein and fats
c) increased need for calcium, phosphorus, and all nutrients, and fluids; see Table 4.8 (note the increased need of the lactating woman)
d) hastens involution of uterus, may decrease incidence of breast cancer
e) enhances physical closeness with infant (usually pleasurable)
5) infant's sucking stimulates milk production of 200–300 ml (6–10 oz) by day 4; by end of 6 weeks; about 600 ml/day

f. General physiologic status
1) restoration of energy reserves
a) immediate need for sleep
b) subsequent need for sleep and rest increased
2) blood
a) decreased in volume
b) moderate anemia if excessive blood loss at delivery
c) leukocytosis immediately after delivery
d) elevated fibrinogen levels during 1st week postpartum; may contribute to thrombophlebitis
3) weight loss
a) usually 11–15 lb immediately because of baby, placenta, amniotic fluid, and diuresis
b) 5 lb in following week
4) vital signs
a) temperature: 1st day may be 38°C (100.4°F)
b) pulse: initially decreases postpartum, range 50–70
c) blood pressure: normal limits

3. Maternal psychologic adaptation (see Table 4.23)
a. Adaptive responses to parental role (Rubin, 1961)
1) taking-in phase: 1st 2–3 days postpartum
a) passive and dependent behavior
b) mother focuses upon own needs rather than baby's, e.g., sleeping and eating
c) verbalizations center on reactions to delivery (help integrate experience)
d) beginning to recognize child as an individual
2) taking-hold phase: 3rd to 10th day postpartum
a) mother strives for independence; wants to care for self and child
b) strong element of anxiety
- unsure of mothering role (primipara)
- unsure of own ability to physically care for child
c) stage of maximum readiness for learning
d) interested in learning baby care
e) may show mood swings
3) letting-go phase: 10 days to 6 weeks
a) achieves independent, realistic role transition

Table 4.23 Maternal Psychological Adaptation (Rubin)

Phase	Characteristics	Nursing Implications
Taking in (1–2 days postpartum)	Mother passive, dependent, concerned with own needs; verbalizes delivery experience	Assist mother in meeting physical needs; structure day for her. Allow time for verbalization.
Taking hold (3rd–10th day postpartum)	Mother strives for independence; strong anxiety element; maximal stage of learning readiness; mood swings may occur	Teach infant care, stay with parents during care and activities. Provide positive reinforcement of parenting abilities.
Letting go (10 days to 6 weeks postpartum)	Mother achieves interdependence; realistic regarding role transition; accepts baby as separate person; new norms established for self	Assist mother in providing for her increased energy requirements; provide positive reinforcement as she identifies her roles with her support system. Allow her to verbalize her new role.

b) learns to accept baby as separate person and establishes new norms for self

b. Postpartum blues (see Table 4.23 and "Postpartum Depression" page 451).

Application of the Nursing Process to Normal Childbearing, Postpartal Care

1. Assessment/Analysis

a. Degree of homeostasis achieved
b. Vital signs
c. Fundus: height, consistency, and position
d. Lochia: amount, color, consistency, and odor
e. Perineum: REEDA, comfort, hemorrhoids
f. Bladder: distention and displacement
g. Bowel: constipation
h. Breasts/nipples: secretions, engorgement; nipple variations/condition; color, support
i. Psychological status
j. Homan's sign: thrombophlebitis
k. Costovertebral angle (CVA) tenderness: kidney infection

2. Plans, Implementation, and Evaluation

Goal 1: Client will achieve homeostasis; will be comfortable; will be knowledgeable about self-care.

Plan/Implementation

- Review antepartum and intrapartum records for history
  - antepartal care, labor and delivery, chronic conditions
  - lab values: Hgb, Hct, VDRL, blood type, RH factor, rubella titre
- Monitor vital signs on admission to postpartum unit, then q4–8 hours
  - BP may drop initially after birth, then returns to normal
  - bradycardia (50–70/minute) common 1st 6–10 days postpartum
  - temperature may be elevated within 1st 24 hours because of dehydration
  - temperature of 38°C (100.4°F) or above on any 2 consecutive days is considered febrile (excluding 1st 24 hours); possible causes: endometritis, urinary tract infection
- Monitor ongoing postpartal progress by daily assessment.
- Promote perineal healing and relief of perineal and hemorrhoidal discomfort
  - inspect episiotomy daily for normal healing; observe for redness, edema, ecchymosis, discharge, approximation (REEDA), and hematoma
  - apply ice pack during 1st 24 hours to prevent edema (as ordered)
  - encourage use of sitz baths, cool astringent compresses, topical anesthetic creams as ordered
  - use heat lamp treatments for 20 minutes, 3 times/day, 10–20 inches from perineum (if ordered)
  - teach proper technique for frequent peri care, e.g., dry perineal area from front to back, blot rather than wipe; apply perineal pad carefully; cleanse area front to back in shower daily
  - reinforce teaching of peri-care and comfort measures
- Treat after-birth pains
  - encourage frequent voiding
  - advise mother to lie on her abdomen
  - give analgesics as ordered
- Administer RhoGAM if ordered; indicated for unsensitized (negative Coombs' test) RH negative women bearing an Rh-positive child; given within 72 hours of delivery (antepartal

RhoGAM is used on a research basis for selected clients) (see Table 4.24).
- Observe abdomen for muscle tone, diastasis recti abdominis; measure degree of any diastasis; teach exercise to correct.
- Promote bowel and bladder function
  - encourage usual voiding patterns
  - recognize signs of bladder distention and catheterize if necessary
  - ambulate to bathroom
  - measure initial voidings
  - check for signs of urinary infection (e.g., frequency, burning)
  - encourage adequate fluid intake and a balanced diet, high in fiber to avoid constipation
  - use stool softeners, cathartics, and enemas as ordered by physician
- Document accurately.

Evaluation: Client has stable vital signs, adequate intake and output; experiences no more than minimal pain and discomfort; performs self-care.

Goal 2: Client will verbalize and demonstrate knowledge of breast changes, breast care, lactation, or suppression of lactation.

Plan/Implementation
- Teach daily cleansing of breast; breast-feeding mother should wash nipples with clear water only (nipples are cleansed by natural antiseptic lysozyme).
- Encourage air drying of nipples for 15–30 minutes after breast-feeding.
- Apply bland cream or ointment (e.g., lanolin, A&D ointment) to sore nipples after feeding.
- Explain mechanisms of lactation.
- Help mother place infant to breast; demonstrate proper positioning.
- Teach lactating mother to relieve breast engorgement (e.g., frequent emptying of breasts by nursing, manual expression, breast pump).
- Apply warm packs prior to feeding for discomfort; ice packs may be used in between feedings for engorgement (varies with physician's suggestions).
- Promote comfort with use of supportive nursing bra.
- Give analgesics as ordered.
- Observe breasts for
  - colostrum secretion
  - engorgement
  - nipple inversion or cracking
  - inflammation and/or pain
- Promote comfort of nonlactating client with use of supportive bra, ice packs, limited fluids; do not express milk or pump breasts; give medication if prescribed (see Table 4.25).

Evaluation: Lactating client demonstrates correct care of breasts, wears a supportive bra; feeds newborn comfortably, knows how to express milk (manually and via pump); non-nursing client lists measures to suppress lactation.

Goal 3: Client will verbalize knowledge of nutrition to meet own needs and supply calories/nutrients for lactation.

Plan/Implementation
- Review basic 4 food groups.
- Encourage nutritious snacks and increased fluids.

Table 4.24 Rh O (D) Human Immune Globulin

Drug Name	Action	Side Effects	Nursing Implications
RhoGAM	Provides transient passive immunity by preparing RBCs containing Rh positive antigens for lysis by phagocytes.	Transfusion reaction	Explain protection is for next pregnancy. Teach to carry identification card and to inform physician of Rho-GAM history.
Anti Rh O (D) gamma globulin	Prevents antibody formation in unsensitized Rh negative women, with negative newborn cord blood Coombs' test (these antibodies cause hemolysis of fetal RBCs). Effective if administered to woman during pregnancy or within 72 hours of abortion or miscarriage or delivery of each Rh positive infant.	Contraindicated if antibodies are present	Instruct that woman will need additional dose following each miscarriage/abortion or delivery of Rh positive infant if antibodies remain negative (Coombs' test).

Table 4.25 Lactation Suppressant Drugs

Drug Name	Action	Side Effects	Nursing Implications
Deladumone OB	Suppresses lactation as a combined estrogen/testosterone	Thromboembolism due to high estrogen (rarely used today)	Obtain informed consent. Teach about risks of estrogens.
Tace(chlorotrianisene)	Synthetic estrogen, prevents postpartum breast engorgement	Thromboembolism	Obtain informed consent. Teach risks versus benefits.
Parlodel (bromocriptine mesylate)	Ergot derivative; reduces prolactin level and inhibits lactation	Hypotension, nausea, dizziness, vomiting, vasospasm, GI bleeding	Stabilize BP before administering. Teach to continue use for 14 days. Observe for drowsiness; dizziness.

- Teach lactating client to increase amount of protein, calcium, iron, phosphorus, and vitamins (see Table 4.8).
- Advise avoidance of drugs that affect breast milk.

Evaluation: Client verbalizes understanding of dietary recommendations; selects foods from the basic four food groups to meet postpartal needs.

Goal 4: Client will be knowledgeable about rest and exercise in the immediate postpartal period.

Plan/Implementation

- Encourage early ambulation to prevent thrombophlebitis and constipation. *NOTE*: if client had conduction anesthesia, have her maintain recumbent position for 10–12 hours.
- Restrict dangling of feet for long periods while sitting on side of bed (constricts popliteal arteries and veins).
- Encourage frequent rest periods during day with minimal interruptions.
- Teach postpartum exercises to strengthen muscles of back, pelvic floor, and abdomen; Kegel or pelvic-floor exercises increase vaginal tone.

Evaluation: Client takes several rest periods during the day; performs postpartum exercises correctly.

Goal 5: Parents will continue to bond/attach to the newborn.

Plan/Implementation

- Encourage physical closeness between newborn and parents; teach them to use eye-to-eye contact and an en face position.
- Encourage physical examination: exploration with fingertips/palms, touching and stroking.
- Compare newborn's likeness to and differences from other family members.
- Encourage addressing newborn by name.
- Explain how normal newborn appears.
- Allow parents to verbalize their positive feelings, concerns and questions about newborn.
- Stay with parents during feeding and care activities as needed.
- Suggest newborn behavioral cues.
- Teach newborn care.
- Provide positive reinforcement of parenting abilities.

Evaluation: Parents exhibit bonding/attachment behaviors (e.g., gaze at, cuddle, fondle, talk to newborn); make positive statements about newborn.

Goal 6: Client will verbalize an understanding of common maternal role conflicts.

Plan/Implementation

- Explain that
  - independence vs dependence
  - idealized vs realistic role
  - love and resentment of newborn
  - self-fulfillment and motherhood
  - love for significant other and newborn
- Promote maternal psychologic adaptation
  - listen to and assist mother to interpret events of labor and delivery
  - clarify any misconceptions about the birth experience
  - encourage rooming-in or extended feeding periods with baby
  - obtain information for evaluating the future parent-child relationship, i.e., plans for newborn, naming

- act as a role model in assisting the mother with maternal tasks

Evaluation: Client states own conflicts about maternal role; asks questions about own feelings, caring for baby.

Goal 7: Parents will be knowledgeable about home care of mother, newborn, and siblings.

Plan/Implementation

- Provide discharge planning and teaching information about
  - normal physiologic changes
  - expected weight loss
  - lochia: may last up to 3–6 weeks
  - changes in abdominal wall
  - perineal healing: episiotomy sutures absorb in about 3 weeks
  - diaphoresis common in 1st 2–3 weeks (“night sweats”)
  - maintaining lactation
  - return of menses and ovulation (if mother not nursing, menses return within 6–12 weeks; in nursing mother, menses return within 4–18 months)
- Teach maternal self-care, needs (e.g., rest, sleep, balanced diet, increased fluids if nursing); proceed slowly with activities.
- Instruct to report any of the following
  - increased temperature
  - increased lochia or reverse in trend in lochia characteristics
  - signs of bladder infection (e.g., frequency, burning)
  - pain in calf
- Discuss/demonstrate newborn care (see page 454)
- Provide opportunity for client to bathe newborn in hospital, if possible.
- Review feeding technique.
- Discuss concerns and questions about newborn care, behavior, and basic needs.
- Review approaches to manage sibling rivalry: extra attention and special times needed for other children.
- Discuss family planning
  - review of methods (see Table 4.2)
  - discuss methods previously used
  - emphasize that breast-feeding is not a form of contraception
- Discuss sexual adjustment; encourage open communication between partners
  - sexual intercourse may be resumed after cessation of lochia and when comfort permits (except if hematoma or infection); physician may suggest delay until postpartal examination in 2–3 weeks
  - breast-feeding mothers may experience decreased vaginal lubrication or breasts leaking/spurting milk during orgasm
  - fatigue and hormonal changes may influence desires
  - altered body image may affect satisfaction
  - birth control measures should be used as soon as coitus is resumed
  - consult physician before resuming use of birth control pills, diaphragm
- Review need for follow-up medical care to
  - assess involution
  - determine family planning needs
  - provide early treatment of problems

Evaluation: Parents demonstrate knowledge and skills for maternal self-care, newborn care; describe plans to set aside separate and special times for newborn’s siblings; have an appointment for follow-up care.

Application of the Nursing Process to the High-risk Postpartal Client

1. **Assessment**
   - **a.** Risk factors in pregnancy, labor, and delivery
   - **b.** Potential/actual problems following delivery
2. **Analysis**
   - **a.** Safe, effective care environment
     - **1)** potential for injury
     - **2)** potential for infection
     - **3)** knowledge deficit
   - **b.** Physiological integrity
     - **1)** altered tissue perfusion
     - **2)** potential fluid volume deficit
     - **3)** pain
   - **c.** Psychological integrity
     - **1)** anxiety
     - **2)** powerlessness
     - **3)** altered role performance
   - **d.** Health promotion/maintenance
     - **1)** potential altered parenting
     - **2)** altered health maintenance
     - **3)** impaired adjustment
3. **Plan, Implementation, and Evaluation**

Goal: Client will be free from undetected problems; will maintain physiological and psychological integrity.

Plan/Implementation

- Teach client normal postpartal adaptation.
- Observe for actual/potential problems in

immediate postpartal period (e.g., signs of developing hemorrhage/hematoma, infection).

- Instruct on reportable signs at discharge.
- Discuss possible problems of delayed involution.
- Administer treatment/medication as ordered.
- Reinforce importance of complying with postpartal check-up.

Evaluation: Client has problems assessed, reported to physician and is treated; has homeostasis restored.

Selected Health Problems in the Postpartal Period

☐ Postpartum Hemorrhage

1. General Information

a. Definition: postpartum *bleeding of more than 500 ml* after delivery

b. Incidence: 3rd highest cause of maternal mortality

c. Predisposing factors

1) *uterine atony:* most common cause, often associated with

a) conditions that overdistend the uterus
- delivery of a large infant
- multiple gestation
- hydramnios

b) multiparity

c) use of deep general anesthesia

d) premature separation of the placenta

e) obstetrical trauma

f) abnormal labor pattern (e.g., prolonged labor)

g) oxytocin stimulation or augmentation during labor

h) overmassage of an already contracted uterus

2) *lacerations:* more common after operative obstetrics

a) perineum

b) vagina

c) cervix

3) *retained placenta fragments*: predicted by Duncan mechanism or manual removal by physician; associated with

a) entrapment by uterine constriction ring

b) premature uterine contraction by massage or ergot administration

c) abnormal adherence of all or part of placenta to uterine wall (e.g., placenta accreta)

d. Prognosis: leading cause of maternal mortality, 14% of all maternal deaths are from hemorrhagic complications

e. Types

1) *early* postpartum hemorrhage occurs within the 1st 24 hours after birth; incidence is 1 in 200 births

2) *late* postpartum hemorrhage occurs between the 2nd day and 6th week postpartum; incidence is 1 in 1,000 births; more common in women with history of abortions or uterine bleeding during pregnancy

2. Nursing Process

a. Assessment/Analysis

1) Inspection of placenta to determine intactness

2) evaluation of vaginal bleeding postdelivery

a) may be slow and continuous (most common) or rapid and profuse

b) blood may escape from the vagina or accumulate in the uterus or maternal tissues

c) bleeding from a laceration appears often as bright red vaginal bleeding in presence of a well-contracted uterus

3) palpate fundus for firmness, height, and position

4) recognize signs of shock; see "Shock" page 170

5) assess bladder distention

b. Plan, Implementation, and Evaluation

Goal: Client will be free from undetected hemorrhage and shock; will have blood volume restored; will regain homeostasis; will comply with discharge teaching.

Plan/Implementation

- Remain with the client.
- Massage boggy fundus gently but firmly, cupping uterus between 2 hands; avoid overmassage.
- Administer oxytocic agents in 4th stage of labor as prescribed by physician (see Table 4.18 and 4.20).
- Monitor closely during acute phase of hemorrhage (e.g., vital signs, intake, output, level of consciousness, fundal firmness, bleeding, CVP).
- Encourage frequent voiding.
- Replace fluid and blood as ordered.
- Administer O_2 per face mask at 4–7 liters
- Maintain asepsis, since hemorrhage predisposes to infection.

- Give prophylactic antibiotics as ordered.
- Support significant other.
- Assist with pre-op preparation (for surgical removal of retained placental fragments), suturing as indicated.
- Teach prior to discharge signs of possible late hemorrhage (critical because of increasingly early discharge).
- Counsel client to increase iron in diet; iron supplements; administer Imferon if ordered.
- Arrange for follow-up care.

Evaluation: Client is free from hemorrhage; regains homeostasis; lists signs and symptoms of late hemorrhage; selects foods high in iron with daily diet.

☐ Hematoma

1. General Information

a. Definition: a collection of blood, often on the external genitalia, as a result of injury to a blood vessel during spontaneous or forceps delivery; occurs once in every 500–1,000 deliveries; most common site of a genital tract hematoma is the lateral wall in the area of the ischeal spines

b. Predisposing factors: prolonged pressure of fetal head on vaginal mucosa; forceps delivery

2. Nursing Process

a. Assessment/Analysis

1) complaints of *severe perineal pain or rectal pressure* (very important)
2) visible large mass at the introitus or labia majora
3) bruising, ecchymosis
4) pain upon palpation
5) inability to void owing to pressure of hematoma on the urethra
6) signs and symptoms of shock in presence of well-contracted uterus and no visible vaginal bleeding

b. Plan, Implementation, and Evaluation

Goal: Client will experience minimal discomfort while the hematoma is treated/absorbed.

Plan/Implementation

- Monitor changes/enlargement of hematoma.
- Notify physician of condition.
- Promote general comfort
  - apply cold to site
  - administer analgesics as ordered
- Prepare woman for surgery, if indicated, to evacuate the hematoma.
- Assess for further vaginal bleeding.

Evaluation: Client's hematoma does not enlarge; client experiences only minimal discomfort.

☐ Pulmonary Embolus

1. General Information

a. Definition: the passage of a thrombus, often originating in one of the uterine or other pelvic veins, into a lung, where it obstructs the circulation of blood; usually occurs at end of 1st week postpartum

b. Predisposing factors
1) infection
2) hemorrhage
3) thrombosis

c. Prognosis: maternal mortality high with large and undetected clots (Refer to ''Pulmonary Embolus'' page 192)

☐ Puerperal Infection

1. General Information

a. Definition: any inflammatory process in the genital tract within 28 days following abortion or delivery of a newborn

b. Incidence: 2nd highest risk of maternal mortality (18%)

c. Criterion: an elevation in temperature of 38°C (100.4°F) for two consecutive days, with the onset after the 1st 24 hours postpartum

d. Origin
1) *endogenous*: infection from within or other preexisting infection
2) *exogenous*: infection introduced by others and/or poor technique

e. Predisposing factors
1) debilitating antepartal conditions
   a) anemia
   b) malnutrition
2) debilitating conditions related to labor and delivery
   a) invasive procedures, e.g., multiple vaginal examinations
   b) operative obstetrical procedures, e.g., cesarean delivery, forceps delivery
   c) soft-tissue trauma and/or hemorrhage
   d) prolonged labor after membranes rupture
   e) prolonged labor resulting in weak, exhausted mother
3) retention of placental fragments

f. Prognosis
1) one of three leading causes of maternal mortality
2) outcome improved with early detection

and appropriate medical and nursing management

g. Types of infection
   1) localized lesions of perineum, vulva, and vagina
   2) endometritis: localized infection of lining of uterus, usually beginning at placental site
   3) local infection may extend through venous circulation, resulting in
      a) infectious thrombophlebitis
      b) septicemia
   4) local infection may extend through lymphatics to cause
      a) peritonitis
      b) parametritis
      c) salpingitis

h. Bacterial causative agents
   1) *Streptococcus hemolyticus*: very virulent, early onset and rapid progression; less common today
   2) *E. coli*
   3) mixed aerobic-anaerobic infection: low virulence, two or more species of bacteria present; tends to be contained locally (abscess)

2. Nursing Process

a. Assessment/Analysis

1) temperature greater than 38°C (100.4°F)
2) lochia is abnormal
   a) remains rubra longer or becomes brown
   b) may have foul odor
   c) scant or profuse in amount
3) tachycardia (may be 100–120/minute)
4) delayed involution
   a) fundal height does not descend as rapidly
   b) uterus may feel larger and softer
   c) woman may have pain and/or tenderness over the uterus
5) pain, tenderness, or inflammation of perineum
6) malaise
7) fatigue
8) chills
9) abnormal lab results: leukocytosis, increased sedimentation rate
10) calf tenderness, positive Homans' sign

b. Plan, Implementation, and Evaluation

Goal: Client will be free from local or systemic infection; will have infection treated early, with complications; will have homeostasis restored.

Plan/Implementation

- Determine source of infection and take measures to prevent further problems.
- Obtain specimens for culture and sensitivity as ordered.
- Take vital signs frequently.
- Isolate woman, if indicated.
- Encourage semi-Fowler's position to facilitate lochia drainage.
- Change peri pads frequently.
- Reinforce perineal hygiene techniques; encourage hand washing.
- Provide comfort measures (e.g., sitz baths to promote perineal healing).
- Administer analgesics as ordered.
- Maintain adequate hydration with oral or intravenous fluids (2,000–4,000 ml/day).
- Administer antibiotic therapy as prescribed by physician.
- Administer oxytocic medications as prescribed by physician.
- Maintain bed rest.
- Encourage high caloric fluid intake; high protein diet.
- Inform client about condition of newborn if separated.
- Maintain bed rest with leg elevated for suspected thrombophlebitis; give anticoagulants if prescribed.

Evaluation: Client responds to treatment for infection (e.g., falling temperature, negative cultures, relief of symptoms, increasing energy).

☐ Mastitis

1. General Information

a. Definition: an inflammation of the breast as a result of an infection, usually caused by *Staphylococcus aureus or Streptococcus hemolyticus*; mainly seen in breast-feeding mothers
b. Predisposing factors: nipple fissure, erosion of the aerola; overdistention, milk stasis
c. Prognosis: condition is generally preventable; prompt and appropriate treatment with antibiotic therapy significantly decreases maternal morbidity

2. Nursing Process

a. Assessment/Analysis

1) blocked milk duct: hard, warm, reddened, and tender site; often in the outer, upper quadrant of the breast

2) mastitis
- fever
- breast may have red area, be warm to touch and tender; lump may be visible
- pain, chills
- engorgement
- axillary adenopathy
- tachycardia often present (usual time of occurrence is 2–4 weeks after delivery)
- headache

b. Plan, Implementation, and Evaluation

Goal: Client will be free from undetected mastitis; will comply with treatment to prevent further complications; will maintain lactation, if desired.

Plan/Implementation
- Administer antibiotics as ordered by physician.
- Promote comfort
  - suggest supportive bra
  - apply local heat or cold
  - administer analgesics as prescribed by physician
- Maintain lactation in breast-feeding mothers
  - regular nursing of infant (controversial, will vary with physician)
  - manual expression of breast milk
  - use of a breast pump
- Encourage good handwashing and breast hygiene.
- Offer emotional support.
- Prepare client for incision and drainage of abscess if necessary.

Evaluation: Client is free from symptoms of mastitis; maintains milk supply.

☐ Postpartum Cystitis

1. General Information

a. Definition: an infection of the bladder occurring in about 5% of postpartum women; usually caused by coliform bacteria

b. Predisposing factors: trauma to the bladder during vaginal delivery or cesarean birth; catheterization during and/or after labor

2. Nursing Process

a. Assessment/Analysis

1) frequency
2) dysuria
3) nocturia
4) urgency
5) hematuria
6) slight elevation of temperature
7) abnormal lab values

b. Plan, Implementation, and Evaluation

Goal: Client will report early symptoms of cystitis; will comply with treatments; will maintain adequate fluid intake and output.

Plan/Implementation
- Obtain specimen for culture and sensitivity.
- Administer antibiotic therapy and analgesics as prescribed by physician.
- Increase fluid intake; monitor I&O.
- Teach prevention of cystitis
  - good perineal hygiene in labor, delivery, postpartum
  - frequent and complete emptying of bladder

Evaluation: Client experiences decreasing signs and symptoms of cystitis (e.g., no burning on urination, no urgency); maintains adequate intake and output.

☐ Psychological Maladaptions

1. General Information:
Postpartum depression occurs in some new mothers; physical as well as psychological symptoms may be evident; usually benign and self-limiting, but can last for years in most severe form

a. Defintions on continuum (see Table 4.26)

1) *postpartum blues*: mild and brief; originates 2–10 days after birth; affects up to 80% of new mothers
2) *atypical depression*: moderate and longer lasting; more disabling; affects 10%+ of new mothers
3) *psychosis*: severe and long-term risks of suicide and infanticide; affects 0.5%–3.0% of new mothers

b. Manifestations (see also *Elated-Depressive Behavior* page 50)

1) feelings of sadness, guilt, irritation
2) tearfulness, crying
3) decreased energy, decision-making ability
4) insomnia
5) decreased appetite, anorexia

c. Theories of etiology

1) hormonal changes
2) fatigue, discomfort
3) immaturity
4) sensory deprivation or overload
5) nonsupportive environment

2. Nursing Process

a. Assessment/Analysis

1) behavioral and psychologic responses, e.g., depression, anger, blues that persist

Table 4.26 Postpartum Depression

Type	Characteristics	Incidence
Blues	Mild, brief; originates 2–10 days after birth	80%
Atypical	Moderate, longer lasting; physical as well as psychological symptoms	10%
Psychosis	Severe; may be long-term risks of suicide, infanticide	0.5–3.0%

2) maladaptations in attachment
3) delusions, hallucinations

b. Plan/Implementation, and Evaluation

Goal: Client will be free from psychologic maladaptation or psychosis postpartum; will seek medical care and will comply with treatment; will function adequately as a parent.

Plan/Implementation
- Recognize early signs of problems.
- Refer client to obstetrician to evaluate physiologic status.
- Support positive parenting behaviors.
- Refer client to resource: psychiatrist, nurse psychotherapist, pediatrician, support group, public health nurse.

Evaluation: Client receives prompt treatment and support for maladaptive responses or psychosis; shows signs of attachment to newborn and increased feelings of self-worth.

Selected Long-term Problems Associated with Childbearing

☐ Uterine Prolapse With or Without Cystocele or Rectocele

1. General Information

a. Definitions
1) *prolapse*: downward displacement
2) *cystocele*: relaxation of the anterior vaginal wall with prolapse of the bladder
3) *rectocele*: relaxation of the posterior vaginal wall with prolapse of the rectum

b. Predisposing factors
1) multiparity
2) pelvic tearing during childbirth
3) inappropriate bearing down during labor
4) congenital weakness
5) vaginal-muscle weakness associated with aging
6) less common in ethnic women of color

c. Medical treatment
1) preventive
a) correctly performed episiotomy
b) postpartum perineal exercises
c) spaced pregnancies
2) surgical intervention
a) vaginal hysterectomy
b) anterior and/or posterior vaginal repair (colporrhaphy)
3) post-op care
a) no hormones needed
b) evaluate success of repair

2. Nursing Process

a. Assessment/Analysis
1) uterine prolapse
a) dysmenorrhea
b) cervical ulceration
c) pelvic pain
d) dragging sensation in pelvis and back
2) cystocele
a) incontinence or dribbling with cough, sneeze, or any activity that increases intra-abdominal pressure
b) retention
c) cystitis
3) rectocele
a) constipation
b) hemorrhoids
c) sensation of pressure

b. Plans, Implementation, and Evaluation

Goal 1: Client will remian free from undetected complications following vaginal hysterectomy and/or an anterior and posterior colporrhaphy.

Plan/Implementation
- Give general pre-and post-op care (see page 157).
- Administer cleansing douche and enema preop as ordered.
- Instruct client to refrain from coughing, sneezing, or straining.
- Promote perineal healing as in postpartal care (page 441).
- Note amount and character of vaginal drainage (differs from postpartal bleeding).
- Avoid rectal temps or tubes.

- Apply vaginal creams as ordered.
- Check Homans's sign.

Evaluation: Client has minimal vaginal drainage; heals incision well.

Goal 2: Client will regain normal urinary and bowel control and muscle tone.

Plan/Implementation

- Monitor urinary output.
- Provide Foley (urethral) catheter care.
- Perform perineal (Kegel) exercises qh and gradual bladder training: i.e., when urinating stop the stream and then let it resume; performed with every voiding and hourly.
- Observe for abdominal distention.
- Ambulate as soon as possible.
- Instruct on gradual increase of residue in diet.
- Administer stool softeners and mineral oil prior to 1st bowel movement.
- Provide emotional support.

Evaluation: Client has normal bladder/bowel control.

☐ Uterine Fibroids

1. General Information

a. Definition: benign uterine tumors of connective tissue and muscle

b. Incidence

  1) 20%–25% of women over 30 have myomas

  2) higher incidence in blacks

c. Predisposing factors

  1) infertility

  2) hormone usage

  3) age (often disappear with menopause)

d. Medical treatment: depends on symptoms such as bleeding, pressure, and client's age and reproductive status

  1) medical intervention

    a) close supervision

    b) no hormone administration

    c) reassess after menopause

  2) surgical intervention

    a) simple myomectomy (subsequent pregnancies may require delivery by cesarean section)

    b) hysterectomy

      - vaginal approach
      - abdominal approach

2. Nursing Process

a. Assessment/Analysis

  1) menorrhagia

  2) dysmenorrhea

  3) low back and pelvic pain

  4) constipation

  5) uterine enlargement

  6) history of infertility or miscarriage

  7) presence of predisposing factors

b. Plans, Implementation, and Evaluation

Goal: Client will be free from problems while being managed conservatively until pregnancy and birth are achieved.

Plan/Implementation

- Discourage hormone usage.
- Support client's decision for immediate pregnancy.
- Monitor for increased severity of symptoms.

Evaluation: Client experiences no increase in symptoms.

References

Affonso, D., & Domino, G. (1984). Postpartum depression: A review. *Birth*, *11*(4), 231–235.

Balkam, J. Guidelines for drug therapy during lactation. *Journal of Obstetric, Gynecologic, and Neonatal Nursing*, *15*(1), 65–70.

Blakemore, K. (1986). Lactation suppression is a matter of choice. *Contemporary OB/GYN*, *28*(11), 39–40, 45, 48, 50, 54, 59.

Dilts, C. (1985). Nursing management of mastitis due to breastfeeding. *Journal of Obstetric, Gynecologic, and Neonatal Nursing*, *14*(4), 286–288.

Fishman, S., Rankin, E., Soeken, K., & Lenz, E. Changes in sexual relationships in postpartum couples. *Journal of Obstetric, Gynecologic, and Neonatal Nursing*, *15*(1), 58–63.

*Fullar, S. (1986). Care of postpartum adolescents. *MCN: American Journal of Maternal/Child Nursing*, *11*(6), 398–403.

Gorrie, T. (1986). Postpartal nursing diagnosis. *Journal of Obstetric, Gynecologic, and Neonatal Nursing*, *15*(1), 52–56.

Hawkins, J., & Govin, B. (1985). *Postpartum Nursing: Health Care of Women*. New York: Springer Publishing.

Konrad, C. (1987). Helping mothers integrate the birth experience. *MCN: American Journal of Maternal/Child Nursing*, *12*(4), 268–269.

McKay, S., & Mahan, C. (1985). Ways to upgrade postpartal care. *Contemporary OB/GYN*, *26*, 63–65, 68–69, 73, 76.

Malinowski, J. (1978). Bladder assessment in the postpartum patient. *Journal of Obstetric, Gynecologic, and Neonatal Nursing*, *7*(4), 14–16.

Martell, L., & Mitchell, S. (1984). Rubin's "puerperal change" reconsidered. *Journal of Obstetric, Gynecologic, and Neonatal Nursing*, *13*(3), 145–149.

Montgomery, E. (1986). Pelvic power. *Community Outlook*, *10*, 33–34.

Mozley, P. (1985). Predicting postpartum depression. *Contemporary OB/GYN*, *25*(5), 173–176, 179.

Ramler, D. (1986). A comparison of cold and warm sitz baths for relief of postpartum perineal pain. *Journal of Obstetric, Gynecologic, and Neonatal Nursing*, *15*(1), 471–474.

*See Reprint Section

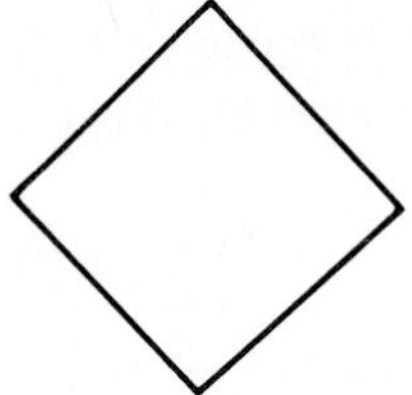

Newborn Care

The Normal Newborn

1. Definition: full-term newborn
2. Gestational age: 38–41 weeks; between 10th and 90th percentiles on growth curves
3. A newborn may have higher than normal risk of morbidity and mortality because of a maternal condition during the antepartal or intrapartal period, e.g., bleeding, poor nutritional status; maternal drug, smoking, alcohol history; hypertension, infection (refer to "High-risk Childbearing" page 399).
4. Risk factors may be increased because of events/problems at birth or in the immediate newborn period.

General Characteristics

1. Transition period
   a. Phase one: first period of reactivity
      1) birth through first 30 minutes
      2) awake, alert, active
      3) strong sucking reflex
      4) rapid and irregular respirations and heart rate
      5) falling body temperature
   b. Sleep period
   c. Phase two: second period of reactivity
      1) onset 4–8 hours after birth; variable duration in first 24 hours
      2) awakens; alert; mild cyanosis may occur
      3) frequent gagging with mucus regurgitation
      4) frequently passes first meconium stool
2. Stabilization with wakeful periods about every 3–4 hours
3. Behavior
   a. Sleeping and waking (Brazelton, 1973)
      1) individuality from birth: each normal newborn has unique, *usually predictable* behavioral responses in the first days of life
      2) state patterns
         a) pattern is a predictor of newborn's receptivity and cognitive response to stimuli
         b) sleep-wake states (alternate periods of physiologic state and behavior)
            - deep or light sleep states
            - awake states
            - drowsiness
            - quiet alert (best for learning)
            - active alert (high activity level)
            - crying
      3) unique ability to "comfort" self by finger or thumb sucking (self-quieting) and to shut out stimuli (habituation)
   b. Sensory responses to environmental stimuli
      1) sight (response to visual stimulation)
         a) pupillary and blink reflexes present
         b) vision present; can focus 8–12 inches
         c) some degree of color and pattern discrimination: prefers complex stimuli
         d) can fixate and track for short distance to midline
         e) focuses on human face
         f) prefers colors to black/white
      2) hearing (response to auditory stimulation)
         a) *in utero*: responds to music and to sound of mother's voice
         b) *in newborn*: within hours of birth, responds to sound by generalized activity depending on reactive state
            - loud sounds elicit Moro's reflex
            - prefers appealing sound
      3) *taste*: response to feeding
         a) differentiates between sweet and bitter
         b) vigor of sucking may vary with arousal
      4) *smell*: response to olfactory stimulation
         a) present as soon as nose is cleared of mucus and amniotic fluid
         b) sensitive, discriminates, e.g., odor of mother's breast milk
      5) *touch*: response to tactile stimulation
         a) well developed
         b) reacts to painful and soothing stimuli
4. Posture
   a. May assume prenatal position
   b. Assumes partially flexed position
   c. Resists having extremities extended

5. Size (compared for length, weight, weeks of gestation on growth curves)
   a. Length
      1) normal ranges 45–55 cm (18–22 in)
      2) average: 50 cm (20 in)
      3) rapid growth in 1st 6 months
   b. Weight
      1) normal range 2,500–4,000 gm (5 lb 8 oz to 8 lb 13 oz)
      2) average weight 3,400 gm (7 lb 8 oz)
      3) 5%–10% of birth weight may be lost in 1st few days of life because of
         a) minimal intake of nutrients
         b) fluid shift
         c) loss of excess fluid (70% of newborn's body weight is fluid)
         d) passage of meconium
      4) regains birth weight within first 2 weeks
   c. Head circumference
      1) normal range 33–35 cm (13–14 inches)
      2) approximately 1–2 cm more than chest circumference
      3) essential assessment for suspected hydrocephalus
   d. Chest circumference
      1) normal range 30–32 cm (12–13 in)
      2) shape and measurements change as newborn grows
   e. Symmetry
      1) face symmetrical
      2) ears symmetrical; placed opposite outer canthus of eyes
      3) bilateral asynchronous movements of extremities
6. Vital signs
   a. Blood pressure: normal range 60–80/40–50 mm Hg
   b. Pulse: normal range 120–150/minute (apical) if newborn is quiet
   c. Respirations
      1) normal range 30–50/minute
      2) irregular and shallow
      3) diaphragmatic and abdominal breathing normal
   d. Temperature
      1) normal axillary range 36.5°–37°C (97.6°–98.6°F)
      2) temperature should stabilize within several hours of birth

☐ Specific Body Parts: usual findings and common variations

1. Skin
   a. Texture: smooth, elastic
   b. Color
      1) pinkish or ruddy color over face and most of body
      2) color varies with ethnic background
   c. Erythema toxicum (newborn rash)
      1) pink papular rash anywhere on the body, appearing within 24–48 hours of birth
      2) harmless and disappears within a few days
      3) must be differentiated from rashes found in infections
   d. Localized cyanosis of extremities (acrocyanosis): peripheral circulation not well established
   e. Mottling (irregular discoloration of skin): due to vasoconstriction and lack of fat, hypoxia
   f. Birthmarks (e.g., port-wine stain, strawberry) may or may not disappear with age, depending on type and location
   g. Vernix caseosa
      1) white, odorless, cheese-like substance on skin, usually found in folds of axillae, groin
      2) produced in utero; diminishes close to term
      3) gradually absorbed or washed off after birth
   h. Lanugo
      1) fine, downy hair on shoulders, back, upper arms, forehead, and cheeks
      2) gradually disappears close to term
   i. Desquamation
      1) dry peeling of the skin, particularly on palms and soles
      2) requires no treatment
      3) more pronounced in postmature newborn
   j. Milia
      1) pinpoint white papules on cheeks, across bridge of nose, or on chin; caused by blocked sebaceous glands
      2) require no treatment
      3) disappear in a few weeks
   k. Nevi (stork bite): red spots found on back of neck and eyelids; usually disappear spontaneously before end of 1st year
   l. Mongolian spots: areas of grayish-blue pigmentation most often found on buttocks and sacrum; increased frequency in specific racial groups; may disappear by school age
   m. Physiologic jaundice (icterus neonatorum)
      1) yellowish discoloration of newborn skin/sclera often appearing 48–72 hours after birth (refer to "Neonatal Jaundice" page 467)

2) is common and appears in 50%–70% of newborns
3) disappears in 7–10 days

2. Head
   a. Appears round and symmetrical; full movement to right and left, up and down; may be covered by silky hair in varying amounts
   b. Molding: the shaping of the fetal head to accommodate passage through the birth canal as a result of overriding of the cranial bones; the head will return to its normal shape in about 2–3 days
   c. Cephalohematoma: a collection of blood between the periosteum and the bone of the skull
      1) caused by rupture of periosteum capillaries from pressure during the birth process
      2) swelling usually severe but does not cross suture lines
      3) spontaneously resolves in 3–6 weeks
   d. Caput succedaneum
      1) localized, edematous area of the scalp, usually caused by birth process
      2) extends across suture lines
      3) is absorbed and disappears by 3rd–4th day of life
   e. Fontanels (soft spots)
      1) anterior
         a) diamond shaped, palpable
         b) 3–4 cm long, 2–3 cm wide
         c) found between frontal and parietal bones
         d) closes within 18 months
      2) posterior
         a) triangular shaped, usually palpable
         b) 1–2 cm
         c) found between occipital and parietal bones
         d) closes within 3 months

3. Eyes
   a. Appearance
      1) blue or grey-blue
      2) bright and clear
      3) pupils equal in size
      4) eyes evenly placed on face
      5) lacrimination in 50% of neonates not evident until 2–4 weeks old
   b. Movement
      1) to all directions
      2) poor neuromuscular control
   c. Common variations
      1) subconjunctival hemorrhage: red spot on sclera, rupture of small capillaries during delivery; will be absorbed in about 2 weeks
      2) chemical conjunctivitis: inflammation with discharge, resulting from reaction of silver nitrate or other chemical agents (must be differentiated from infectious process)

Figure 4.18 Bones, Fontanels, and Sutures of Newborn's Skull

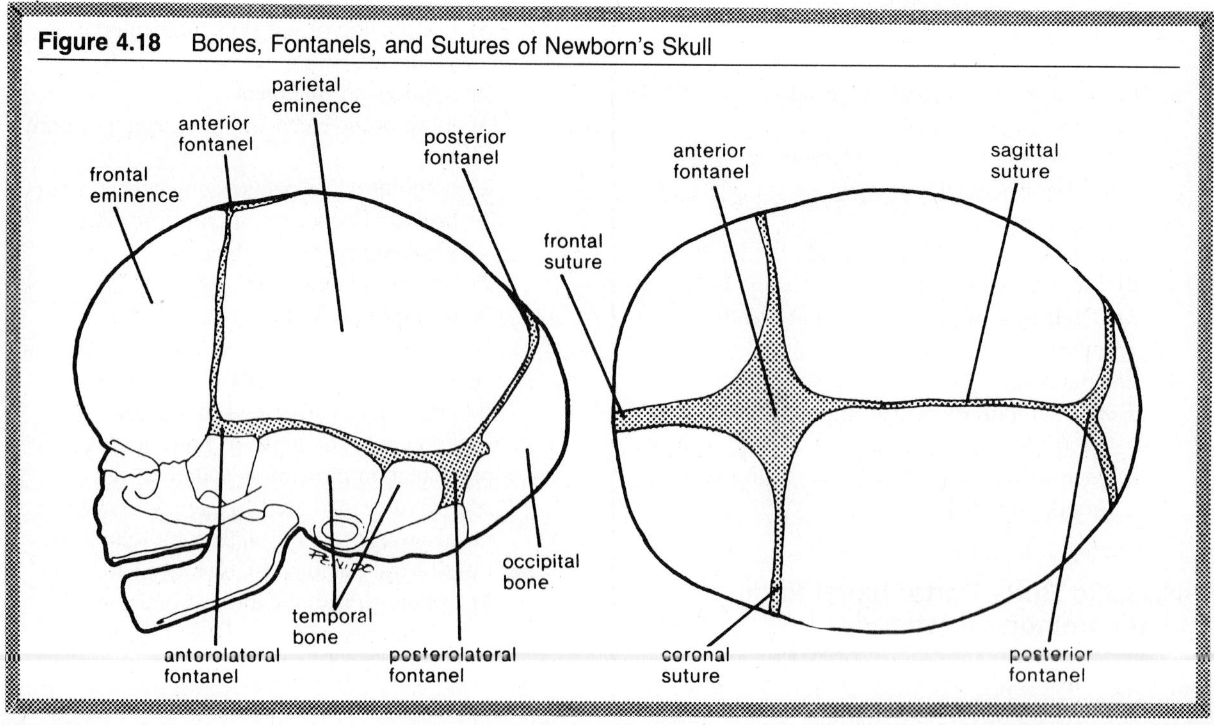

d. Vision (refer to Sensory Responses page 454)
4. Mouth
   a. Lips: appear equal on both sides of facial midline; symmetry of movement
   b. Tongue
      1) in midline; moves freely in all directions
      2) size proportional to mouth
      3) color pink (varies with ethnic group); white, cheesy coating may indicate thrush (related to maternal monilial vaginal infection)
   c. Palate: intact
   d. Epstein's pearls: small epithelial cysts on hard palate or gums; will disappear at 1–2 weeks
   e. Saliva: small quantity present
5. Ears
   a. Well-formed cartilage by term; recoil rapidly; may be flattened against skull because of pressure during birth
   b. Placement: same level and position on both sides of head (low set ears are associated with trisomy 13 or 18 and renal agenesis)
   c. Hearing: refer to Sensory Responses page 454
6. Nose
   a. Shape: varies; may appear flattened because of delivery process
   b. Placement: evenly placed in relation to eyes and mouth
   c. Nares: bilateral patency; newborns are nose breathers
   d. Sneezing common
7. Neck
   a. Appears short; head moves freely
   b. Skin folds present; no webbing
8. Chest
   a. Shoulders: sloping; width greater than length
   b. Chest movements: bilateral expansion equal with respiration; no retractions
   c. Breath sounds: loud and equal bilaterally; clear on crying
   d. Cough reflex: absent; appears by 2nd or 3rd day of life
   e. Heart: rhythm regular, normal rate; usually heard to left of midclavicular space at 3rd or 4th interspace; may have functional murmurs (refer to page 455 for normal vital-sign values)
   f. Breasts
      1) flat; nipples symmetrical; breast-tissue diameter greater than 5 mm
      2) breast engorgement common in both sexes; occurs by 3rd day of life and may last up to 2 weeks; may have some nipple discharge due to maternal hormonal influence in utero and subsequent withdrawal after birth
9. Abdomen
   a. Prominent: cylindrical shaped; movements synchronous with respirations
   b. Umbilical cord stump
      1) two arteries and one vein apparent at birth, surrounded by Wharton's jelly
      2) cord begins drying within 1–2 hours after birth, shed by 7–10 days after birth
      3) protrusion of umbilicus often apparent in black newborns; assess for umbilical hernia
   c. Diastasis recti (separation of recti muscles): common in black or preterm neonates
   d. Bowel sounds: audible
   e. Femoral pulses: palpable and equal bilaterally
10. Genitalia
   a. Female
      1) labia majora cover labia minora; symmetrical, slightly edematous
      2) clitoris enlarged
      3) vaginal tag (hymen) may be evident
      4) a mucoid, vaginal discharge is common
      5) pseudomenstruation: blood-tinged discharge is normal
      6) some vernix caseosa may be between labia
   b. Male
      1) urethral meatus evident at tip of penis
      2) foreskin covers glans; prepuce not easily retractable
      3) extensive rugae on scrotum
      4) testes descended and palpable bilaterally in scrotal sac; if not, check inguinal, femoral, or abdominal areas for undescended testes
11. Buttocks and anus
   a. Buttocks: symmetrical; anus patent
   b. Gluteal folds: symmetrical
12. Extremities and trunk
   a. Muscle tone: good
   b. Position: extremities slightly flexed
   c. Arms and legs: arms equal in length; legs equal in length; legs shorter than arms
   d. Five digits on each hand and foot; freely movable, nails present
   e. Normal palmar crease (simian line indicative of Down syndrome)
   f. Spine: straight and flat (prone position)
   g. Fat pads and creases covering soles of infant's feet

☐ Systems Adaptations

1. Neuromuscular: normal neonatal reflexes
   a. Sucking: newborn's tendency to suck any object that comes in contact with lips; essential for nutritional intake, oral satisfaction; begins to disappear at 12 months
   b. Rooting: newborn's tendency to turn head in direction of stimulus and open lips to suck when object touches cheek or mouth; disappears at 7 months
   c. Spontaneous reflexes
      1) swallowing: usually follows sucking
      2) gagging: lifelong reflex
      3) yawning
      4) stretching
      5) sneezing
      6) hiccoughing
   d. Moro: newborn's tendency to symmetrically extend both arms and legs and then draw them up in normal flexed position in response to sudden movement or loud noise; most significant reflex indicative of CNS status; disappears at 1–4 months
   e. Grasp
      1) palmar grasp; newborn's tendency to grasp an examiner's finger when palm is stimulated; lessens at 3–4 months
      2) plantar grasp: newborn's tendency to curl toes downward when sole of foot is stimulated; lessens at 8 months
   f. Tonic neck: newborn's tendency to assume a fencer's position when head is turned to one side; the extremities on the same side extend, while flexion occurs on opposite side; response sometimes more dominant in leg than arm; disappears at 3–4 months
   g. Stepping or walking: newborn's tendency when held upright to take steps in response to feet touching a hard surface; disappears at 4 weeks
   h. Babinski's: newborn's tendency to hyperextend toes with dorsiflexion of big toe when one side of sole is stimulated from heel upward across ball of foot; disappears at 1 year
   i. Motor function: head may be maintained erect for short periods of time; head lag less than 45°; movement of extremities may be jerky
2. Cardiorespiratory
   a. Circulatory adaptations occurring after birth and ligation of umbilical cord
      1) closure of ductus arteriosus, foramen ovale, and ductus venosus
         a) caused by changes in pressure in the 1st days of life
         b) allows oxygenation of all body systems
      2) closure of umbilical vessels after clamping of cord
   b. Pulses (reflect systemic circulation)
      1) femoral, brachial; easily palpable
      2) radial, temporal; more difficult to palpate
   c. Respirations
      1) initiation of respirations
         a) 1st breath: inflation of lungs in response to increased pCO_2 and lower pH
         b) reduction of pulmonary vascular resistance
         c) increased pulmonary blood flow
         d) recoil of chest causing replacement of fluids
         e) surfactant reduces alveolar surface tension
      2) respiratory secretions may be abundant
      3) may be irregular with short periods of apnea
   d. Blood pressure
      1) highest immediately after birth; at lowest level at 3 hours
      2) crying and moving cause changes in BP (up to 20 mm Hg)
3. Hematologic
   a. Blood values (venous samples): average ranges for a normal, full-term newborn
      1) hemoglobin: 14–20 gm/100 ml (reflects oxygenation of tissues); broken down to bilirubin
      2) hematocrit: 42%–61%
      3) RBC: 5–7.5 million/mm^3
      4) WBC: approximately 20,000/mm^3 (10,000–30,000/mm^3)
      5) platelets: 100,000–280,000
      6) blood volume: 78–98 ml/kg depending on cord clamping
   b. Leukocytosis: normal; related to birth trauma
   c. Fetal RBCs: have short life (80–100 days); hemolyzed RBCs deposit bilirubin in body tissues
   d. Neonatal jaundice (physiologic jaundice): common in 50% of newborns on 2nd or 3rd day of life because of deposits of bilirubin
   e. Coagulation
      1) inability to synthesize vitamin K because of absence of intestinal flora normal in older people
      2) supplementary injection of vitamin K, e.g., AquaMEPHYTON, given prophylactically to promote normal clotting

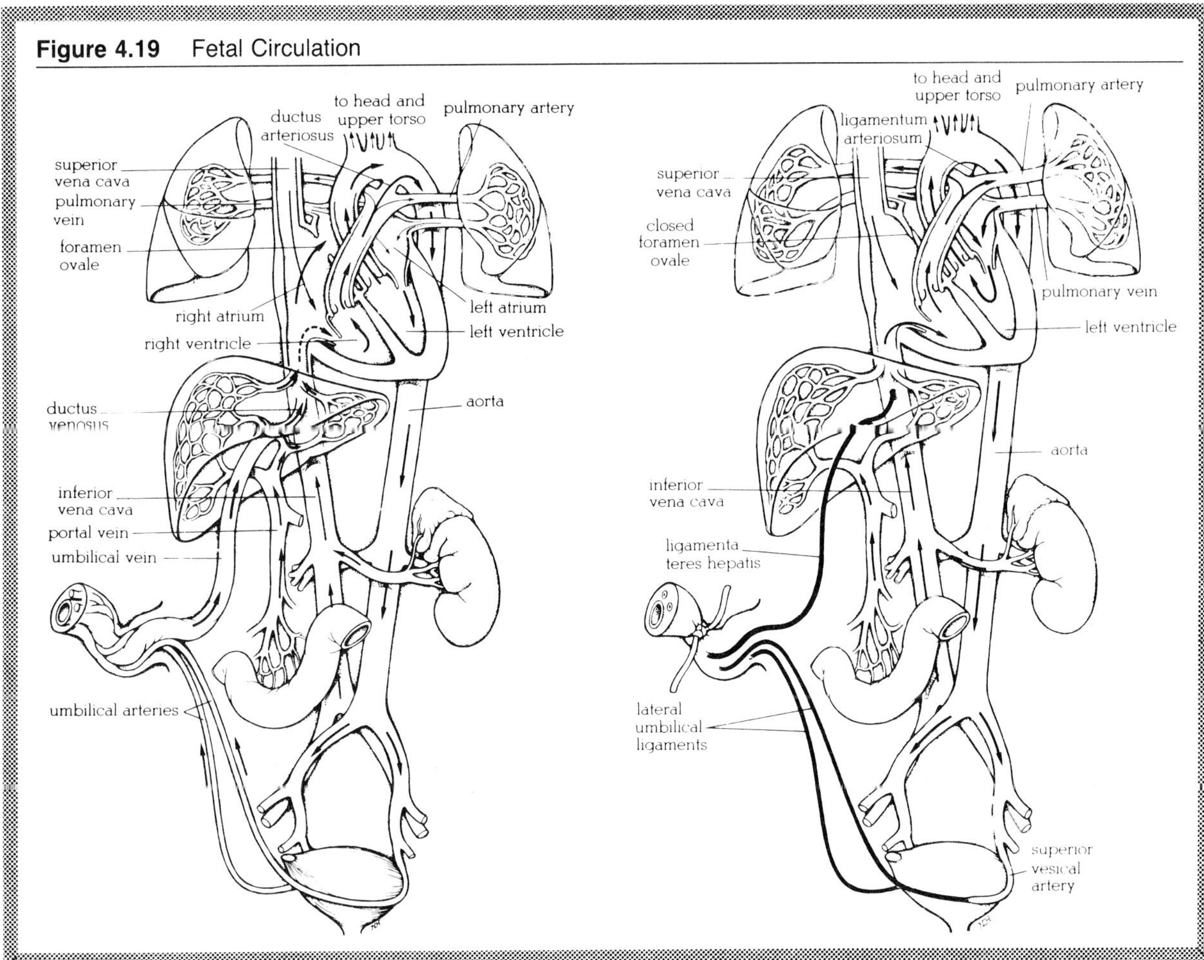

Figure 4.19 Fetal Circulation

4. Thermoregulation (temperature regulation)

a. Adaptive factors

1) newborn responds to cold with increased motor activity and restlessness

2) increased metabolism compensates for cold stress, since newborn does not shiver

3) brown fat (or brown adipose tissue) is the newborn's major source of thermogenesis (2%–6% of body weight) (located between scapulae, around kidneys, sternum, adrenals, and in the axillae); reserves are rapidly depleted with cold stress

b. Heat loss: disproportionate to adult because of large skin surface to body mass; mechanisms of heat loss include

1) *convection*: loss of heat from body surface to cooler surrounding air, e.g., newborn placed in cool incubator

2) *evapoartion*: loss of heat from body occurring when fluid converts to vapor, e.g., wet newborn loses heat immediately after birth in delivery room

3) *conduction*: transfer of heat from warm object to a cooler surface, e.g., newborn placed on a cold object

4) *radiation*: indirect transfer of heat from a warmer object to a cooler one, e.g., newborn loses heat to cool wall of incubator

5. Elimination (gastrointestinal and renal)

a. Stools: change according to feeding

1) meconium stool: viscous, dark green or black; formed of mucus, vernix, lanugo, hormones, carbohydrates; 1st one usually passed within 24–48 hours (if no stool passed, assess for imperforate anus, intestinal obstruction)

2) 2nd–6th day, transition stools: loose, green-brown, seedy

3) breast-fed newborns: golden yellow, mushy stools, often after each feeding

4) bottle-fed newborns: soft, yellow-brown stools; more formed; 4–6/day

b. Stomach capacity: 50–60 ml; empties in about 3 hours

c. Urination: newborn usually urinates in 1st 24

hours; if newborn unable to void, assess for fluid intake and distention
   1) frequency: initially 6–10/day, then up to 20/day
   2) color: pale yellow (immature kidneys cannot concentrate); may appear cloudy if decreased fluid intake
   3) uric acid excretion is high; appears as red spots on diaper ("brick spots")

6. Immunologic
   a. In utero: full-term fetus has had IgG (immunoglobulins) transferred; maternal antibodies may be present (depending on mother's immunity) for tetanus, diphtheria, pertussis, measles, mumps, rubella
   b. At birth: immunologic system immature
      1) capable of some antibody response to immunizing agents
      2) phagocytosis ineffective
      3) cannot localize infection or respond with a well-defined recognizable inflammatory response, as can older child
      4) breast milk: contains IgA; gives immunologic protection from some infections
      5) elevated temperature may not reflect infection in newborn

7. Nutrition
   a. Sucks, swallows, and digests feedings; these reflexes may be weak in prematures
   b. Digestion
      1) unable to digest complete carbohydrates because of insufficient quantities of amylase
      2) can absorb simple CHO and protein
      3) fat absorption poor because of insufficient lipase
   c. Regurgitation is common
      1) cardiac sphincter is immature, nervous control of stomach incomplete
      2) newborns often spit up mucus in 1st 24 hours after birth
   d. Blood sugar normally 30–50 mg/100 ml (full term)
   e. Benefits from immunoglobulins, enzymes, and lactobacilli in breast milk
   f. Psychologic factors
      1) both bottle- and breast-feeding can be satisfying
      2) attachment facilitated by breast-feeding
      3) stress can inhibit successful breast-feeding
   g. Initial feedings: breast milk or sterile water given 4–6 hours after birth to assess sucking reflex and absence of structural anomalies
   h. Subsequent feedings
      1) bottle-fed newborns: q3–4h or on demand
      2) breast-fed newborns: q2–3h or on demand
   i. Fluid needs vary with age and size of newborn; average intake of 17½ oz/day for 7-lb baby
   j. Calories: 80–120 cal/kg/day (birth to 5 months); most commercial formulas contain 20 calories/oz (see Table 4.27)

☐ Gestational Age Variations Based on Neuromuscular Responses and External Physical Characteristics

(Dubowitz, Ballard, see Figure 4.20)

1. Premature newborn
   a. Definition: born before 38 weeks gestation, regardless of birth weight
   b. Etiology: associated with chronic hypertensive disease, toxemia, placenta previa, abruptio placentae, incompetent cervix, infections, smoking, multiple gestation, inadequate maternal nutrition, maternal age under 20; premature rupture of membranes
   c. General appearance: will vary with gestational age
      1) head large in proportion to body

Table 4.27 Nutritional Comparison of Human and Cow's Milk

	Amounts per Liter		
Nutrients	**Human Milk (Breast)**	**Cow's Milk[1] (Whole)**	**Common Formulas[2]**
Protein (gm)	10.12	32[3]	15
CHO (gm)	67.82[4]	45.4	72
Lipid	43.12	35.7	36
Calories	684.00	626.0	640

[1]Not given to newborns.
[2]Examples are Similac, Enfamil.
[3]Because of the higher percentage of protein, cow's milk must be diluted to avoid kidney overload.
[4]Breast milk is higher in lactose, which limits pathogenic growth.

Figure 4.20 Newborn Maturity Rating and Classification

Estimation of Gestational Age by Maturity Rating

Symbols: X - 1st Exam O - 2nd Exam

Neuromuscular Maturity

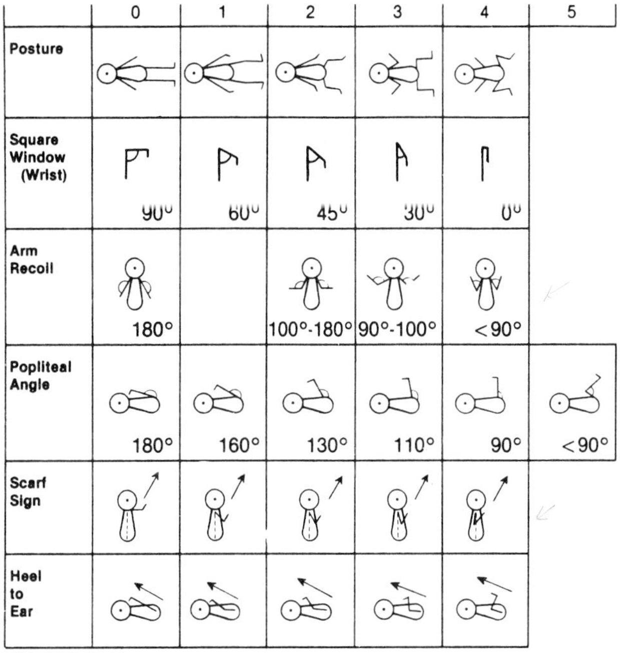

	0	1	2	3	4	5
Posture						
Square Window (Wrist)	90°	60°	45°	30°	0°	
Arm Recoil	180°		100°-180°	90°-100°	<90°	
Popliteal Angle	180°	160°	130°	110°	90°	<90°
Scarf Sign						
Heel to Ear						

Physical Maturity

	0	1	2	3	4	5
Skin	gelatinous red, trans-parent	smooth pink, visible veins	superficial peeling &/or rash, few veins	cracking pale area, rare veins	parchment, deep cracking, no vessels	leathery, cracked, wrinkled
Lanugo	none	abundant	thinning	bald areas	mostly bald	
Plantar Creases	no crease	faint red marks	anterior transverse crease only	creases ant. 2/3	creases cover entire sole	
Breast	barely percept.	flat areola, no bud	stippled areola, 1-2 mm bud	raised areola, 3-4 mm bud	full areola 5-10 mm bud	
Ear	pinna flat, stays folded	sl. curved pinna, soft with slow recoil	well-curv. pinna, soft but ready recoil	formed & firm with instant recoil	thick cartilage, ear stiff	
Genitals *Male*	scrotum empty, no rugae		testes descend-ing, few rugae	testes down, good rugae	testes pendulous, deep rugae	
Genitals *Female*	prominent clitoris & labia minora		majora & minora equally prominent	majora large, minora small	clitoris & minora completely covered	

Gestation by Dates ______________ wks

Birth Date __________ Hour __________ am/pm

APGAR __________ 1 min __________ 5 min

Weight __________ Length __________

Head __________ Chest __________

Maturity Rating

Score	Wks
5	26
10	28
15	30
20	32
25	34
30	36
35	38
40	40
45	42
50	44

Scoring Section

	1st Exam = X	2nd Exam = O
Estimating Gest. Age by Maturity Rating	_____ Weeks	_____ Weeks
Time of Exam	Date _____ Hour _____ am/pm	Date _____ Hour _____ am/pm
Age at Exam	_____ Hours	_____ Hours
Signature of Examiner	_____ M.D.	_____ M.D.

Scoring system: Ballard, J. et al. "A Simplified Assessment of Gestational Age." *Pediatric Research*. April 1977:374. Assessment of gestational age: Sweet, A. "Classification of the Low-Birth-Weight Infant" in *Care of the High Risk Neonate*, Klaus, M. and Fanaroff, A., Eds. Philadelphia: Saunders, 1979. Reprinted with permission.

Table 4.28 High-Risk Conditions for Newborns by Gestational Age and Growth Classifications

	Gestational Age		
Growth Class	**SGA**	**Average**	**LGA**
Preterm			
Apnea of prematurity	X	X	X
Brain damage	X		
Congenital abnormalities	X	X	X
Hyperbilirubinemia	X	X	X
Hypoglycemia	X	X	X
Infection	X	X	X
Intracranial hemorrhage	X	X	X
Meconium aspiration	X		
Neonatal asphyxia	X		
Polycythemia	X		X
Pulmonary hemorrhage	X		
Respiratory distress syndrome	X	X	X
Temperature instability	X	X	X
Term			
Brain damage	X		
Birth injuries			X
Congenital abnormalities	X		X
Hypoglycemia	X		X
Polycythemia	X		X
Infection	X		
Meconium aspiration	X		
Neonatal asphyxia	X		
Pulmonary hemorrhage	X		
Temperature instability	X		
Post-term			
Brain damage	X	X	X
Congenital abnormalities	X		X
Hypoglycemia	X		X
Infection	X		
Meconium aspiration	X	X	X
Neonatal asphyxia	X	X	X
Polycythemia	X	X	X
Pulmonary hemorrhage	X		
Temperature instability	X		

2) transparent appearance to skin
3) lack of subcutaneous fat
4) excessive lanugo
5) immature neurologic system
6) minimal flexion of extremities
7) fontanels large; sutures prominent

d. Associated problems
1) *high mortality rate*
2) *respiratory distress syndrome* (RDS), related to immaturity of lungs and deficiency of surfactant (*NOTE*: L/S ratio determined by amniocentesis is helpful prior to delivery to determine lung maturity)
3) *infection*: low WBC count, increased polymorphonuclear cells
4) *feeding problems*
   a) regurgitates food easily
   b) may aspirate because of weak or absent suck-swallow reflexes
   c) may require gavage feedings
   d) breast milk or 24-calorie/ml formula advised
5) *hypoglycemia* (glucose less than 20 mg/100 ml), caused by decreased glycogen and fat stores, decreased glyconeogenesis
6) *hypothermia* and cold stress, owing to poor temperature control, increased surface area for cooling, extension of extremities, lack of brown fat
7) *jaundice* because of impaired bilirubin conjugation in liver
8) *intracranial hemorrhage*, related to birth trauma or hypoxia after birth
9) *apnea*, related to fatigue or immaturity of respiratory mechanism
10) *oxygen therapy complications*: retrolental fibroplasia, bronchopulmonary dysplasia (alveolar-bronchial necrosis)

2. Postmature newborn

a. Definition: born after 42 weeks of gestation (specific reference to potential intrauterine growth retardation)
b. General appearance: related to advanced gestational age and placental insufficiency
   1) thin, long newborn
   2) dry, parchmentlike skin
   3) decreased or absent vernix
   4) little subcutaneous tissue; loose skin
   5) meconium staining of amniotic fluid (nails and skin stained yellow) related to hypoxia
   6) lanugo absent
   7) alert, wide-eyed (sign of hypoxia)
   8) nails lengthened
c. Associated problems: higher morbidity and mortality
   1) *hypoxia*: may be related to placental insufficiency
   2) *hypoglycemia*: caused by decreased glycogen stores
   3) *postmaturity syndrome* with intrauterine asphyxia and fetal distress
   4) *polycythemia*: response to hypoxia
   5) *seizure disorders*: related to hypoxia (chronic)
   6) *cold stress* related to minimal subcutaneous fat
   7) *meconium aspiration*

3. Small-for-gestational-age (SGA) newborn
   a. Definition: significantly underweight for gestational age (i.e., birth weight at or below the 10th percentile on intrauterine growth Denver curve); also known as intrauterine-growth-retardation or small-for-dates newborn
   b. Etiology: associated with maternal malnutrition, pregnancy-induced hypertension, diabetes, drug addiction, alcoholism, smoking, maternal viral infections, prescribed or over-the-counter drugs, placental abnormalities or acute hypoxia, and other conditions affecting uteroplacental sufficiency
   c. General appearance
      1) little subcutaneous tissue
      2) loose, dry skin
      3) loss of muscle mass in trunk and extremities
      4) desquamation
      5) length often normal yet weight decreased
      6) polycythemia: may be related to intrauterine hypoxia
      7) meconium staining of nails, skin
      8) appears alert because of hypoxia
   d. Associated problems
      1) *intrauterine infection* if exposed to organisms while in utero
      2) *asphyxia at birth*: associated with intrauterine hypoxia
      3) *hypoglycemia*: caused by decreased glycogen stores and decreased glyconeogenesis (increased metabolic rate due to heat loss)
      4) *hypothermia*: related to decreased subcutaneous tissue and fat and poor thermal regulation
      5) *congenital anomalies* (10–20 times more frequent)
      6) *respiratory distress*: often follows perinatal asphyxia
      7) *hypocalcemia*: may be related to asphyxia and respiratory diseases
      8) *meconium aspiration*: subsequent possible minimal brain dysfunction

4. Large-for-gestational age (LGA) newborn
   a. Definition: significantly overweight for gestational age (birth weight at or above 90th percentile on intrauterine growth curve; usually over 9 lb 15 oz)
   b. Etiology: unclear; may be genetic predisposition associated with multiparity and maternal diabetes
   c. General appearance
      1) fat and puffy
      2) may be edematous
      3) poor muscle tone
   d. Associated problems
      1) *birth trauma* because of CPD
      2) *hypoglycemia* related to lack of maternal glucose (after birth)
      3) *hypocalcemia*
      4) *polycythemia*
      5) *congenital birth defects*

Application of the Nursing Process to the Normal Newborn

1. **Assessment/Analysis**
   a. Immediate (in delivery room; birthing room or other setting)
      1) airway
         a) patency
         b) secretions: may contain mucus, blood, and amniotic fluid
      2) Apgar score: provides index of infant's initial condition and baseline for subsequent assessments at 1 and 5 minutes; the five-minute score is the better indicator of adaptation (see Table 4.29)
         a) 0–2: severe asphyxia, extremely poor condition
         b) 3–6: mild to moderate asphyxia, fair condition

Table 4.29 Apgar Scoring Chart

Sign	Score 0	Score 1	Score 2
Heart rate	Absent	Slow (below 100)	Over 100
Respiratory effort	Absent	Slow, irregular, weak cry	Good strong cry
Muscle tone	Flaccid	Some flexion of extremities	Well flexed
Reflex irritability			
• catheter in nostril	No response	Grimace	Cough or sneeze
• slap to sole of foot	No response	Grimace	Cry and withdrawal of foot
Color	Blue, pale	Body pink, extremities blue	Completely pink

c) 7–10: very mild or no distress, good condition

3) gross appearance: appears to be free from obvious birth defects

4) umbilical cord

a) early clamping: less possibility of placental transfusion

b) late clamping: expansion of newborn's blood volume, high systolic BP, higher Hgb

c) blood vessels: two arteries, one vein

b. Ongoing

1) vital signs

2) passage of meconium and/or urine

3) umbilical cord

4) tracheoesophageal fistula or esophageal atresia, manifested by

a) cyanosis during feeding

b) immediate regurgitation

c) inability to swallow feeding

5) parent-infant bonding

2. Plans, Implementation, and Evaluation

Goal 1: Newborn will adapt successfully to extrauterine life during the immediate period following birth; will have early contact with mother/father.

Plan/Implementation

- Facilitate the immediate establishment of respiration
  - clear air passages before onset of respirations (suction with DeLee or bulb syringe)
  - provide gentle tactile stimulation that aids breathing
  - assist physician with resuscitation as necessary (heart beat to respiratory ventilation rate is 5:1)
- Prevent hypothermia: maintain newborn's body temperature and minimize heat loss; metabolic rate and O_2 consumption are minimized
  - dry rapidly
  - place on mother's skin, in warmed Isolette, under radiant heater or in warm blanket
  - LeBoyer or admission bath may be given when temperature stable
- Provide prophylactic treatment of eyes with a 1% silver nitrate or other antibacterial agent such as erythromycin (0.5%) for protection against ophthalmia neonatorum, which may be caused by gonococcal or chlamydial infection.
- Promote bonding/attachment.
- Place appropriate identification bands on newborn and mother; footprint may be taken.
- Weigh and measure newborn.
- Administer a single dose of vitamin K IM, as ordered to prevent hypoprothrombinemia.
- Send cord blood to lab as ordered.

Evaluation: Newborn maintains adequate oxygenation, breathes normally; maintains body temperature; is held by parent.

Goal 2: Newborn will continue to maintain homeostasis free from problems (e.g., respiratory, feeding, elimination difficulties).

Plan/Implementation

- Check identification on admission to nursery.
- Monitor newborn's condition (frequency of assessment determined by condition)
  - assess apical pulse and respiration for 1 full minute
  - note periods of apnea (should not exceed 20 seconds)
  - suction if mucus is excessive
  - position on side to promote drainage, especially after feedings
  - observe skin, sclera, mucosa color (jaundice or cyanosis)
  - observe for respiratory changes or fatigue during feedings
  - maintain adequate nutrition by assisting new mother with bottle- or breast-feeding

- Note time of 1st urination and passage of meconium; then monitor elimination.
- Weigh daily or every other day and record on chart; newborn may take up to 10 days to regain birth weight after initial 5%–10% loss.
- Obtain blood sample for phenylketonuria (PKU) (Guthrie test)
  - a recessive hereditary disorder characterized by deficiency in the liver enzyme phenylalanine hydroxylase that is needed for conversion of phenylalanine into tyrosine
  - leads to mental retardation if undetected
  - newborn must have protein feedings 24–48 hours prior to test; with early discharge, parents must bring newborn back to lab for blood test in 2 days

  NOTE: in some states screening for hypothyroidism and other metabolic tests may be required.

Evaluation: Newborn has vital signs within normal range; ingests nutritional fluids appropriate for size; voids and passes meconium.

Goal 3: Newborn will remain infection free.

Plan/Implementation

- Prevent infections from developing in newborn and spreading within nursery/mother-baby unit
  - use proper hand-washing/scrub technique to prevent staff-to-newborn and newborn-to-newborn infection
  - exclude personnel with known infections from caring for newborns
  - instruct parents about importance of hand-washing and proper technique
  - isolate newborns with any signs of infection or risk
  - assess/clean newborn's cord daily with alcohol and a designated antibacterial agent (e.g., Triple Dye)
- Bathe and maintain personal hygiene of the newborn
  - use plain water on face and mild soap on body for daily care
  - proceed from clean to dirty areas, i.e., eyes to face, to genitals
- Assess condition of circumcised penis: keep clean and observe for bleeding; a sterile petroleum jelly or antibiotic ointment may be applied during 1st 24 hours; check for voiding (*NOTE*: currently, pediatricians discourage routine circumcision for health/medical reasons; cultural/religious practices should be considered in decision making.

Evaluation: Newborn has normal temperature; no signs of infection; is protected from exposure to infectious agents.

Goal 4: Parents will verbalize an understanding of principles and techniques of newborn care; will demonstrate proper, safe care feeding.

Plan/Implementation

- Assess parents' knowledge and past experience with child care
- Offer modified or complete rooming-in.
- Encourage new parent's involvement in newborn care (to foster bonding/attachment).
- Demonstrate techniques of bathing and daily care
  - emphasize safety and asepsis
  - suggest timing of care (prior to feeding)
  - teach cord care
  - emphasize frequent cleansing of diaper area to prevent rash
- Allow mother to give care in hospital.
- Reinforce knowledge of care-giving.
- Discuss the importance of touch and stimulation in developing trust.
- Reinforce knowledge of feeding.
  - benefits of breast- vs bottle-feeding (should be discussed in antepartal classes)
  - frequency of nursing (every 2–3 hours on demand)
  - length of nursing time (newborn obtains greatest quantity in 20–25 minutes)
  - importance of emptying breasts
  - position of newborn for nursing
  - common feeding problems (e.g., burping, regurgitation, constipation, hiccups)
  - position on side or abdomen after feeding

Evaluation: Parents demonstrate correct feeding, bathing, holding of newborn.

Goal 5: Parents will know what to expect at home regarding newborn's behavior, sleep patterns, stools, weight gain, feeding; will verbalize an understanding of reportable problems; will discuss adjustments of siblings.

Plan/Implementation

NOTE: criteria for discharge teaching vary with gestational age, weight, early discharge, general health status of newborn and mother, home environment, ages of siblings, and available resources.

- Counsel on breast-feeding or formula preparation at home

- discuss common concerns (sore nipples, supplementary feedings, expression of milk)
- review methods of formula preparation, care of bottles and nipples (aseptic and terminal methods, dishwashing)
- discuss bottle-fed newborn's daily needs: intake approximately 3 oz, 6 times/day initially
- delay solids until 6 months
- avoid cow's milk until 12 months

■ Discuss expected weight gain (birth weight doubles by 5–6 months, triples by 1 year).
■ Counsel on sibling adjustments to newborn.
■ Discuss newborn behavior and development in discharge teaching
- sleep needs: average 20 hours/day with wide variations; intermittent altertness
- crying: newborn's method of communicating basic needs
- discuss plans for health care follow-up of newborn (clinic, physician, nurse practitioner)
- refer to resource such as the community health nurse for assistance
- teach *reportable signs* of problems, e.g., constipation, diarrhea, fever, vomiting, behavioral changes

Evaluation: Parents demonstrate knowledge of correct newborn care; describe adequate equipment for home care; express confidence in ability to care for newborn; list reportable signs; discuss plans for dealing with sibling adjustments.

Application of the Nursing Process to the Newborn at Risk

1. **Assessment**
   a. Maternal risk factors
   b. Actual/potential problems identified during fetal life
   c. Immediate adaptation to extrauterine life
   d. Actual/potential problems noted after birth
2. **Analysis**
   a. Safe, effective care environment
      1) potential for injury
      2) potential for infection
   b. Physiological integrity
      1) impaired gas exchange
      2) ineffective airway clearance
      3) potential altered nutrition: less than body requirements
   c. Psychological integrity
      1) anxiety (parental)
      2) altered role performance
   d. Health promotion/maintenance
      1) potential ineffective family coping
      2) knowledge deficit
3. **Plan, Implementation, and Evaluation**

Goal: Newborn will be free from undetected problems; will have problems treated immediately and will maintain physiological integrity. Family will comply with teaching for health maintenance and promotion.

Plan/Implementation
■ Perform ongoing assessments.
■ Notify physician of problems/changes in status.
■ Document altered condition.
■ Implement specific therapy as ordered.
■ Share information with family.
■ Maintain a safe environment.
■ Promote asepsis.
■ Teach parents care specific for problem.

Evaluation: Newborn has problems detected and treated immediately; has homeostasis maintained. Family complies with recommended follow-up care.

Selected Health Problems in the Newborn

☐ Hypothermia

1. General Information

a. Definition: a drop in the newborn's body temperature below 36.5°C (97.7°F), produced by rapid heat loss to the environment. All newborns are at risk for heat loss because of their limited subcutaneous fat and large surface area in relation to body weight
b. Predisposing factors
   1) newborns with reduced stores of subcutaneous fat, e.g., premature, postmature, SGA newborns
   2) newborns with reduced glycogen reserves, e.g., premature, nutritionally deprived, SGA newborns

2. Nursing Process

a. **Assessment/Analysis**
   1) newborn's body temperature
   2) signs of cold stress
      a) increased activity level
      b) crying
      c) increased respiratory rate
      d) cyanosis
      e) mottling of skin

b. Plan, Implementation, and Evaluation

Goal: Newborn will expend a minimum amount of extra energy in the production of heat; will be free from periods of hypothermia.

Plan/Implementation

- Prevent heat loss in delivery room (refer to Goal 1 page 464).
- Administer warmed air or O_2 to newborn prn.
- Monitor newborn's temperature frequently; maintain axillary temp at 36.5°C (97.8°F), abdominal skin temperature at 36.1°–36.7°C (97°–98°F).
- Place crib or incubator away from draft and windows.
- Keep portholes of incubator/Isolette closed.

Evaluation: Newborn maintains a skin temperature of 36.1°–36.7°C.

☐ Neonatal Jaundice

1. General Information

a. Definition: excessive levels of bilirubin in the blood and tissues of the newborn (bilirubin is a product derived from the breakdown of erythrocytes and hemoglobin)

b. Expected levels of serum bilirubin (in mg/dl)

1) *full term*

a) 1st 24 hrs: 2–6

b) day 2: 6–7

c) days 3–5: 4–12

2) *premature*

a) 1st 24 hrs: 1–6

b) day 2: 6–8

c) days 3–5: 10–15

c. Predisposing factors

1) prematurity

2) isoimmunizations: maternal red blood cell-destroying antibodies are transferred to the fetus, resulting in fetal erythrocyte destruction; after initial maternal sensitization occurs, the effects upon subsequent pregnancies with blood incompatibilities increase in severity

a) Rh negative mother and Rh positive father may produce an Rh positive fetus; this leads to antigen-antibody response affecting subsequent fetus

b) mother with type O blood and father with type A, B, or AB produce a fetus with type A, B, or AB (generally results in less severe disease than Rh incompatibility)

3) polycythemia

4) exposure to drugs in utero

Figure 4.21 Rh Sensitization

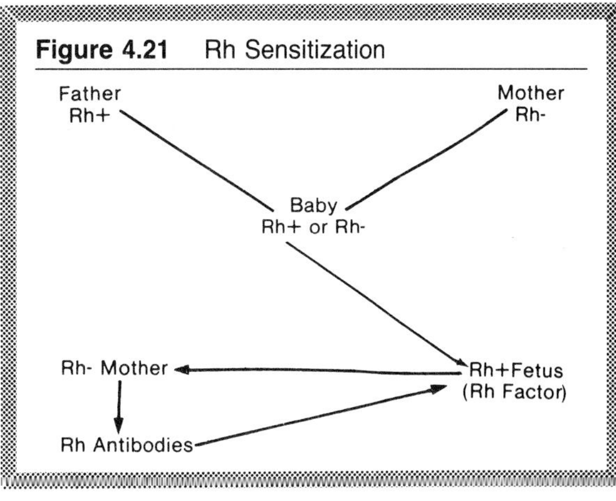

5) sepsis

d. Common forms

1) physiologic jaundice

a) onset

- full-term newborn: jaundice appears after 24 hours and disappears by end of 7th day
- preterm newborn: jaundice appears after 48 hours and disappears by 9th or 10th day

b) lab values

- bilirubin is unconjugated (indirect); below 6 mg/100 ml, and newborn is without evidence of hemolytic disease or infection
- RBCs and WBCs are normal

2) pathologic jaundice (hyperbilirubinemia)

a) onset: occurs within 1st 24 hours after birth

b) lab values: characterized by rising bilirubin level in excess of normal

- in full-term newborn: rises 6 mg/100 ml in 24 hours or value exceeds 12 mg/100 ml or persists beyond 7 days
- in premature newborn: exceeds 15 mg/100 ml; persists beyond 10 days
- direct bilirubin greater than 1.0 mg/100 ml

c) severe sequela is kernicterus (deposit of unconjugated bilirubin in basal ganglia of brain) when bilirubin levels rise over 20 mg/100 ml in full-term newborns and over 9–10 mg/100 ml in preterm newborns; signs and symptoms include

- lack of interest in feeding
- sluggish Moro's reflex with incomplete flexion of extremities

- opisthotonic posturing
- vomiting
- bulging fontanels
- twitching convulsions (late symptom)

3) breast-milk jaundice: yellowing of newborn's skin caused by high concentration of enzyme lipoprotein lipase, which breaks down lipids to form free fatty acids and glycerol; increasing the amount of free fatty acids is thought to inhibit conjugation of bilirubin; may affect 1%–2% of breast-fed newborns
   a) onset: after mature milk is secreted; 48–96 hours after delivery
   b) lab values: bilirubin level begins to rise about 4th day, peaks at 10–15 days of age, returning to normal between 3rd and 12th weeks of age

e. Associated problems
1) hydrops fetalis (erythroblastosis fetalis) related to Rh or ABO incompatibility: generalized edema, pleural and pericardial effusions, ascites
2) hepatosplenomegaly
3) progressive hemolytic anemia

2. Nursing Process

a. Assessment/Analysis

1) prenatal history
   a) positive hemantigen test (maternal blood serum)
   b) positive indirect Coombs' (maternal blood serum)
   c) no prior history of RhoGAM use
2) early identification of newborns at risk; includes those with
   a) predisposing factors (e.g., prematurity, birth trauma)
   b) delayed passage of meconium
   c) placental enlargment (may weigh ½–¾ of newborn's weight)
   d) visible jaundice of skin (bilirubin greater than 7 mg/100 ml): blanch bridge of nose or chest
   e) abnormal bleeding (e.g., extensive bruising or cephalohematoma)
   f) positive direct Coombs' test (neonatal cord blood)
   g) yellow-stained vernix on cord
3) signs and symptoms of polycythemia, especially in large-for-gestational-age newborns
   a) decrease in peripheral pulses
   b) redness of hands and feet
   c) tachycardia
   d) respiratory distress
4) newborn pallor with jaundice, appearing within 24–36 hours after birth
5) increased optical density of amniotic fluid

b. Plan, Implementation, and Evaluation

Goal: Newborn will not develop undetected neonatal jaundice; will be free from kernicterus.

Plan/Implementation

- Interpret laboratory values and recognize deviations from normal (i.e., rise in serum bilirubin, Hgb decrease, rapid decrease in hematocrit, positive Coombs').
- Offer early feedings (prevent reabsorption of bilirubin).
- Give appropriate dose of vitamin K as ordered (decreases prothrombin time).
- Give appropriate care to newborn undergoing phototherapy (method of treatment in which bilirubin is transported from skin to blood to bile and excreted)
  - remove clothing
  - protect eyes with eye patches (to prevent retinal damage)
  - turn every 2 hours for maximum skin exposure
  - provide adequate fluids
  - feed q2–3h to prevent metabolic disorders (may be removed from light for feedings)
  - assess for signs of dehydration (e.g., sunken fontanels)
  - maintain lights 16 inches away
  - monitor temperature every 2 hours
  - monitor weight gain and loss
  - observe for side effects (e.g., bronze skin, peripheral vasodilatation, temperature and metabolic disturbances, diminished activity, loose stools)
- Assist with exchange transfusion as indicated (newborn receives negative blood if problem related to Rh incompatibility since no A, B, or Rh antigens are present in negative blood. Antibodies remaining are gradually removed; no further hemolysis occurs).
  - observe for signs of transfusion reaction
  - educate parents about procedure

Evaluation: Newborn shows signs of decreasing jaundice (e.g., falling serum bilirubin level, decreasing yellowing of skin); is free from kernicterus.

☐ Respiratory Distress

1. General Information

a. Definition: difficulty in maintaining respiratory function adequate to meet oxygen needs; caused by a variety of problems

b. Predisposing factors

1) dysmaturity (SGA newborns)
2) prematurity
3) postmaturity
4) maternal diabetes
5) maternal bleeding
6) fetal asphyxia
7) birth asphyxia
8) pregnancy-induced hypertension
9) prolonged labor after rupture of the amniotic membranes
10) meconium-stained amniotic fluid
11) low Apgar score
12) cesarean birth

c. Common respiratory disorders

1) respiratory distress syndrome (RDS), also known as hyaline membrane disease (HMD)
   a) definition: deficiency of surfactant activity leading to atelectasis, which prevents adequate gas exchange
   b) characterized by collapse of the alveoli
   c) most frequently affects preterm newborns, especially those weighing between 1,000 and 1,500 gm; it is also observed in newborns of diabetic mothers, and newborns of mothers whose pregnancies were complicated by antepartum vaginal bleeding
2) meconium-aspiration syndrome
   a) aspiration of meconium-stained amniotic fluid into the lungs may occur with asphyxic or placental disturbances in utero
   b) associated with intrauterine-growth-retardation (SGA newborns) and postmaturity (post-term newborns)

d. Associated problems

1) hypoxia
2) atelectasis
3) bronchopulmonary dysplasia, retrolental fibroplasia (complications of O_2 administration)

2. Nursing Process

a. Assessment/Analysis

1) use *Silverman-Andersen scale*: index of respiratory distress (scores of 0 are indication of good respiratory function)
   a) grunting: sound of air pushing past partially closed glottis, heard during expiration
   b) retractions: sternal and intercostal; due to use of accessory muscles to aid in breathing
   c) flaring nares: due to newborn's effort to lessen resistance in narrow nasal passages
   d) seesaw respirations: flattening of chest with inspiration and bulging of abdomen, caused by utilization of abdominal muscles during prolonged, forced respirations
2) cyanosis
3) alterations in respiratory rate, rhythm, and depth
   a) tachypnea: respiratory rate greater than 60/minute or greater than 15/minute over baseline
   b) bradypnea: respiratory rate less than 30/minute
   c) apneic spells: absence of respiration for 20 seconds or more
4) falling body temperature

b. Plan, Implementation, and Evaluation

Goal: Newborn will maintain adequate oxygen levels to meet physiologic demands; will be free from undetected respiratory distress or further complications.

Plan/Implementation

- Collect blood gas samples and pH via umbilical line; interpret results of studies.
- Administer prescribed oxygen (dependent on results of blood-gas study)
  - give warmed and humidified oxygen
  - monitor concentration and pressure of oxygen
- Monitor oxygen concentration through oximeter, blood gas and pH studies, and transcutaneous oxygen tension.
- Maintain newborn in supine position, with head slightly extended to improve respiratory function or leave newborn flat.
- Evaluate skin color
  - pallor
  - plethora
  - cyanosis: circumoral, generalized, at rest or with activity
- Maintain thermoneutral environment.
- Minimize energy expenditure by keeping newborn warm.
- Facilitate newborn's respiratory efforts

Figure 4.22 Silverman-Andersen Scale

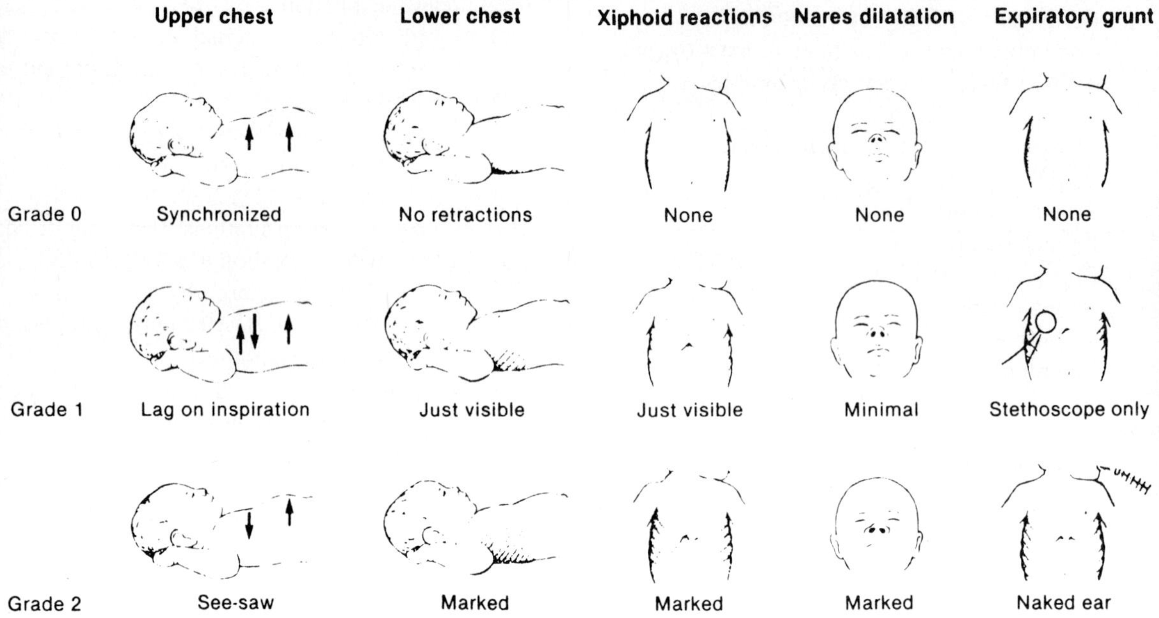

	Upper chest	Lower chest	Xiphoid reactions	Nares dilatation	Expiratory grunt
Grade 0	Synchronized	No retractions	None	None	None
Grade 1	Lag on inspiration	Just visible	Just visible	Minimal	Stethoscope only
Grade 2	See-saw	Marked	Marked	Marked	Naked ear

SOURCE. Ross Laboratories, Nursing Inservice Aid #2, Columbus, OH; Reprinted with permission. W. Silverman and D. Andersen, *Pediatrics* 17:1, 1956, American Academy of Pediatrics.

- continuous positive airway pressure (CPAP): controlled pressure exerted upon expiration to prevent collapse of alveoli
- oxygen hood (to provide controlled oxygen and humidity)

■ Suction endotracheal tube q1–2h as needed; protect from extubation.
■ Protect skin on nasal septum from breakdown and undue pressure from endotracheal tube.
■ Provide for nutritional needs (IV, gavage, hyperalimentation) with minimal energy expenditure.
■ Prevent/detect complications.
■ Give supportive care to parents.

Evaluation: Newborn adequately meets oxygen needs of body; maintains respiratory rate between 30 and 60 without dyspnea; is free from complications from therapy.

☐ Neonatal Necrotizing Enterocolitis (NEC)

1. General Information

a. Definition: a disorder of vascular ischemia, affecting the gastrointestinal mucosa, often associated with perforation

b. Incidence: approximately 5% of all newborns in intensive care nurseries; morbidity and mortality can be reduced by early detection and treatment of asphyxia (within 30 min of birth)

c. Predisposing factors
  1) neonatal asphyxia and hypoxia
  2) pregnancy-induced hypertension
  3) maternal vaginal bleeding
  4) excessive amounts of feeding
  5) immature immunologic system
  6) prematurity

d. Associated problem: sepsis

2. Nursing Process

a. Assessment/Analysis
  1) abdominal distention
  2) pallor
  3) poor feeding
  4) gastric residuals (2 ml or more) before feedings
  5) occult blood in stool (positive guaiac test)
  6) increased apneic periods

b. Plan, Implementation, and Evaluation

Goal: Newborn will be free from necrotizing enterocolitis, or complications from NEC.

Plan/Implementation

■ Check bowel sounds.
■ Monitor stools and gastric secretions for blood.

- Monitor abdominal distention.
- Record I&O, nature and type of gastric secretion.
- Administer parenteral therapy or hyperalimentation as ordered.
- Monitor for signs of dehydration.
- Maintain nasogastric suction on low, intermittent suction.
- Test urine for glucose to monitor tolerance for hyperalimentation solution.
- Administer antibiotic therapy as indicated.
- Provide appropriate pre- and post-op care when surgery is required (resection or colostomy).

Evaluation: Newborn receives prompt and appropriate treatment of any abnormalities (e.g., asphyxia, feeding problems); is free from sepsis and other complications of NEC.

☐ Hypoglycemia

1. General Information

a. Definition: decreased blood glucose level: less than 30 mg/100 dl (full-term) in first 72 hours of life or 45 mg/dl thereafter; less than 20 mg/dl in prematures (*NOTE*: Dextrostix below 45 in term newborn, at 1 hour, warrants further testing)

b. Etiology: the beta cells in the fetal pancreas become overstimulated in utero because of high levels of circulating maternal glucose; after birth, insulin production remains higher than circulating glucose

c. Predisposing factors
- **1)** malnourished newborns
  - **a)** prematurity
  - **b)** intrauterine-growth-retardation
  - **c)** postmaturity
  - **d)** twin pregnancy (smaller newborn affected)
- **2)** newborns of diabetic mothers (usually LGA)
- **3)** large-for-gestational age newborns (i.e., greater than 8.8 lb)
- **4)** newborns of mothers with pregnancy-induced hypertension
- **5)** severe Rh incompatibility
- **6)** severely stressed newborns, e.g., newborns with cold stress, infections, respiratory distress

d. Associated problems
- **1)** jaundice
- **2)** hypocalcemia (serum calcium less than 7–7.5 mg/dl); those at risk include prematures, newborns of diabetic mothers, newborns with birth trauma and perinatal asphyxia

2. Nursing Process

a. Assessment/Analysis
- **1)** note if any of predisposing factors are present
- **2)** signs and symptoms of hypoglycemia
  - **a)** apnea
  - **b)** lethargy
  - **c)** irregular respiration
  - **d)** feeding difficulties
  - **e)** jitteriness
  - **f)** twitching
  - **g)** weak, high-pitched cry
- **3)** signs and symptoms of hypocalcemia
  - **a)** neonatal tetany
  - **b)** twithing from central nervous system irritability
  - **c)** jerking tremors
  - **d)** seizures
  - **e)** cyanosis
  - **f)** high-pitched cry
  - **g)** respiratory distress
  - **h)** poor feeding
- **4)** laboratory values for deviations from normal
- **5)** behavior and reflexes
  - **a)** daily weight
  - **b)** note frequency and amount of urination and stools

b. Plan, Implementation, and Evaluation

Goal: Newborn will maintain normal blood glucose level for gestational age; will have hypoglycemic reactions detected before complications develop; will maintain adequate nutrition and fluid and electrolyte balance.

Plan/Implementation
- Perform Dextrostix or laboratory blood glucose on admission to nursery, and for newborns at risk for hypoglycemia, q30min 6 times, then qh 3 times, then q2h 6 times until stable; notify physician if Dextrostix result is less than 45 mg (full-term) and less than 20 mg (preterm).
- Provide adequate calories for all newborns.
- Feed newborns at risk for hypoglycemia sterile water within 1st hour of life, followed with glucose water, formula (oral or tube feeding as indicated), or breast milk.
- Administer 10%–25% glucose, IV or orally, as ordered
- Minimize handling of newborn.
- Observe carefully for signs of seizure related to low blood sugar.
- Recommend regular pediatric care throughout childhood.

Evaluation: Newborn maintains normal blood sugar level; has hypoglycemic reactions detected early; ingests calories appropriate for size; maintains fluid and electrolyte balance (e.g., moist mucous membranes, good skin turgor).

☐ Newborn Infection

1. General Information

a. Definition: an invasion of the fetus or newborn by bacterial or viral microorganisms during pregnancy, during or following birth

b. Predisposing factors
  1) poor maternal nutrition
  2) TORCH (toxoplasmosis, other, rubella, cytomegalovirus, herpes) syndrome
  3) intrauterine growth retardation (SGA)
  4) prematurity, especially gestational age less than 34 weeks
  5) prolonged labor after rupture of membranes

c. Modes of transmission
  1) chronic transplacental infection, acquired in utero through the placenta
    a) usually due to viruses; others include bacteria, protozoa
    b) onset early in gestation
    c) may lead to growth retardation
  2) ascending intrauterine infection, acquired through the cervix after rupture of membranes
    a) onset late in gestation
    b) usually due to bacteria, often *E. coli*; herpes virus
    c) may lead to premature labor and subsequent premature birth
  3) newborn infection, acquired after birth from organisms in the environment or via transmission from another person or newborn (sepsis is most common infection seen in newborn)
    a) often due to staphylococcus, streptococcus, or *E. coli*
    b) preterm newborns at greatest risk for this type of infection because of lower immunologic defenses
    c) more common in boys than girls

d. Associated problems
  1) generalized sepsis
  2) septic shock (evidenced by fall in BP and tachypnea)
  3) hyperbilirubinemia
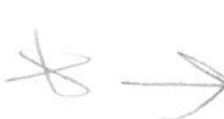
  4) meningitis (evidenced by bulging anterior fontanel)
  5) increased mortality rate, especially in premature newborns

2. Nursing Process

a. Assessment/Analysis
  1) antenatal and intrapartal history to identify newborns at risk
  2) septic workup if infection suspected (blood culture, lumbar puncture, gastric aspiration, umbilical-stump culture, stool culture, amniotic-membrane culture)
  3) signs and symptoms
    a) lethargy
    b) newborn does not "look right"
    c) poor feeding and sucking
    d) increased respiratory rate
    e) jaundice
    f) WBC increase
    g) loss of weight
    h) restlessness; tremors; convulsions
    i) diarrhea and vomiting
    j) abdominal distention
    k) skin rashes and/or skin lesions
    l) hypo- or hyperthermia

b. Plan, Implementation, and Evaluation

Goal: Newborn will be free from undetected infection; will not experience complications or generalized sepsis.

Plan/Implementation
- Treat immediately by administering antibiotics as ordered (e.g., penicillin, kanamycin, polymyxin); observe for side effects.
- Prevent spread of infection by isolating septic newborns.
- Monitor thermal environment.
- Monitor body temperature (temperature rise is *not* an early sign of sepsis); in later stages, observe for severe hyper- or hypothermia.
- Take daily weight.
- Monitor I&O; observe for dehydration.
- Provide adequate nutrition.
- Promote respiratory function.
- Observe for central nervous system involvement (lethargy, apnea, seizures, tremors).

Evaluation: Newborn shows signs of decreasing infection (e.g., decreasing respirations, skin temperature between 36.1° and 36.7°C); does not develop generalized sepsis.

☐ Neonatal Drug and Alcohol Addiction

1. General Information

a. Drug addiction
  1) definition: drug dependence evident in the newborn as a result of maternal substance

abuse (see *Substance Use Disorders* page 81)

2) associated problems
   a) convulsions
   b) hypothermia

b. Fetal alcohol syndrome
   1) definition: a group of disorders characterized by teratogenesis as a result of chronic maternal alcoholism during pregnancy; high incidence in female newborns
   2) associated problems
      a) intrauterine-growth-retardation; microcephaly
      b) ocular structural defects
      c) limb anomalies
      d) cardiovascular disturbances and anomalies (e.g., atrial and ventricular septal defects)
      e) mental retardation
      f) fine-motor dysfunction
      g) prematurity
      h) convulsions

2. Nursing Process

a. Assessment/Analysis

1) signs and symptoms: onset according to time of last maternal use, type or combinations of drug taken, amount of drug taken, and length of addiction (onset of withdrawal generally occurs within 24 hours in alcohol addiction; can be up to 72 hours with some drugs)
   a) CNS signs
      - restlessness
      - jittery and hyperactive reflexes (e.g., constant sucking)
      - high-pitched, shrill cry
      - convulsions
   b) GI system signs
      - feeds poorly
      - vomiting
      - diarrhea
      - dehydration
   c) respiratory system signs
      - nasal stuffiness
      - yawning and sneezing
      - apnea
      - tachypnea
      - excessive secretions
2) fluid-balance status

b. Plans, Implementation, and Evaluation

Goal: Newborn will not injure self; will experience or will have controlled severe symptoms associated with withdrawal or seizures; parents will understand the need for follow-up care.

Plan/Implementation
- Reduce stimuli in environment and minimize handling.
- Protect from injury (swaddle newborn in snug-fitting blanket).
- Promote bonding/attachment.
- Ensure newborn receives required fluid and caloric intake; use pacifier between feeding.
- Feed on demand; give small amounts at frequent intervals.
- Use pacifier between feedings.
- Administer IV therapy as ordered.
- Position on side to avoid aspiration.
- Measure I&O; watch for signs of dehydration due to vomiting, loose stools, poor feeding.
- Weigh frequently.
- Give skin care with special attention to body folds; expose to air.
- Protect skin from injury (mittens on hands, sheepskin on crib, pads on sides of crib).
- Give medications as ordered
  - phenobarbital (6 mg/kg/24 hours, IM, or 2 mg PO qid)
  - paregoric (2–4 gtts/kg orally q4–6h; dose may increase to 20–30 gtts/kg q4–6h)
- Maintain patent airway if seizure occurs.
- Maintain adequate warmth.
- Document accurately.
- Teach parents the importance of long-term follow-up health care.

Evaluation: Newborn is comfortable and free from seizures, complications of withdrawal; has homeostasis restored; parents have an appointment with physician/clinic for follow-up care.

☐ Acquired Immune Deficiency Syndrome (AIDS)

1. General Information

a. Definition: a disease that affects the immune system (T-cells) and renders one unable to fight disease or infection. High mortality rate in the first three years of life; no known cure. Currently 50% of infants born to HIV-positive women will be infected.

b. Modes of transmission to newborn
   1) transplacental
   2) through breast milk
   3) contact with body fluids

2. Nursing Process

a. Assessment/Analysis

1) often small-for-gestational-age (SGA)
2) hepatosplenomegaly
3) neurologic abnormalities (e.g., microcephaly
4) prominent, box-like forehead
5) increased distance between inner canthi; flattened nasal bridge
6) recurrent infections, e.g., interstitial penumonia
7) evidence of Epstein-Barr viral infection

b. Plan, Implementation, and Evaluation

Goal: The newborn will be isolated from others to prevent the spread of the disease; will be free from complications of AIDS; parents will understand need for referral and follow-up care.

Plan/Implementation

- Assess infants of mothers at risk (e.g., IV drug users, prostitutes, positive HIV test) for signs/symptoms of AIDS.
- Promote bonding/attachment.
- Isolate to prevent spread of disease.
- Use Universal Precautions for blood and body fluids.
- Educate parents about disease process, transmission, current treatment, follow-up care.
- Provide emotional support to family.

Evaluation: Newborn is free from complications; parents keep follow-up care appointments.

☐ Birth Injuries/Congenital Anomalies

1. General Information

a. Birth injuries
   1) definition: physical trauma to the newborn resulting from the birth process
   2) predisposing factors: large-for-gestational-age newborn, dystocia
   3) common types of injuries
      a) brachial plexus injuries
      b) cephalohematomas
      c) fractures
      d) intracranial hemorrhage

b. Congenital anomalies
   1) definition: a variety of defects or disorders, which may be evident or concealed at birth; the physical and developmental consequences will vary with selected problem(s)
   2) incidence: 6 in 1,000 total births
   3) predisposing factors
      a) past personal or family history of congenital anomalies, genetic factors (e.g., chromosomal aberrations)
      b) exposure to toxic agents, viruses, or drugs during pregnancy
      c) genetic-environmental interaction

2. Nursing Process

a. Assessment/Analysis

1) Birth injuries
   a) decreased mobility of arm, abnormal positioning (brachial-plexus injuries)
   b) swelling of head caused by rupture of the blood vessels between a cranial bone and the periosteum (cephalohematoma)
   c) swelling, irritability associated with pain, decreased mobility of affected extremity, abnormal positioning at rest (fractures)
   d) respiratory irregularities with cyanosis, reduced responsiveness, high-pitched cry, tense fontanel, or convulsions (intracranial hemorrhage due to hypoxia and hypovolemia seen mainly in prematures)
2) Congenital anomalies
   a) antepartum/intrapartum high-risk factors, including maternal history of
      - chronic alcoholism or drug addiction
      - family members born with cogenital defects
      - exposure to toxic agents in environment
      - infections (e.g., TORCH)
      - high altitude resident
   b) hydramnios: associated with
      - neurologic defects such as hydrocephalus, anencephalus, and spina bifida
      - gastrointestinal malformation such as esophageal atresia, cleft palate, pyloric stenosis
      - Down syndrome
      - congenital heart disease
      - maternal diabetes
      - prematurity
   c) oligohydramnios, associated with anomalies of the renal system

b. Plans, Implementation, and Evaluation

Goal 1: Newborn will not develop undetected complications of birth injury.

Plan/Implementation

- Assess for asymmetrical movements by placing

newborn on back and observing movements of arms and legs.

- Screen all LGA newborns for birth injuries; listen for high-pitched, weak cry; observe muscle tone (poor), hypertonicity, hyperactivity, flaccidity.
- Palpate fontanels for bulging, tenseness.
- Observe pupillary response.
- Position head higher than hips (for intracranial hemorrhage); minimal handling; provide warmth; maintain adequate nutrition.
- Implement specific treatment, which varies with nature and extent of insult.
- Document observations.

Evaluation: Newborn receives early treatment of birth injury; is free from long-term sequelae (e.g., mental retardation) when possible.

Goal 2: Newborn will have anomalies recognized and treated early; will be free from complications; will maintain homeostasis; parents will understand need for referral.

Plan/Implementation

- Screen for apparent and hidden congenital anomalies (often done upon admission to nursery).
- Implement appropriate therapeutic measures (interdisciplinary health care team approach essential).
- Refer family for care and genetic counseling.

Evaluation: Newborn adapts successfully to extrauterine life; receives appropriate treatment for defect; parents have an appointment for appropriate referral.

☐ Parental Reaction to a Sick, Disabled, or Malformed Newborn

1. General Information

a. The grief and mourning process: initiated by birth (parents grieve over the loss of normality in their newborn)

b. Stages of grief and mourning (refer to *Loss, Death and Dying* page 30)

1) 1st stage
- **a)** initial sadness
- **b)** guilt feelings ("What did I do to cause this? What happened?")
- **c)** shock over reality of situation
- **d)** denial
- **e)** general anger at situation; overprotectiveness of the newborn
- **f)** neglect of other family members
- **g)** isolation/loneliness (increases after mother's discharge from hospital)

2) 2nd stage: developing awareness of reality of situation

3) restitution: coming to terms with situation

2. Nursing Process

a. Assessment/Analysis

1) stage of grief and mourning

2) parental behavior: adaptive or maladaptive

b. Plan, Implementation, and Evaluation

Goal: Parents will accept support in their grief over the ill, disabled, or malformed newborn.

Plan/Implementation

- Allow parents to express grief (may be shown as anger, denial, depression, crying); be supportive.
- Modify hospital policies when possible to allow early contact with newborn and frequent visitation; encourage parents to see newborn, to touch and hold newborn in neonatal intensive care unit.
- Point out normal characteristics of their newborn to parents.
- Encourage parental participation in care (e.g., providing breast milk, bathing, feeding).
- Recognize signs of maladaptive responses
  - possibility of abuse or neglect
  - overwhelming guilt
- Expect repeated periods of sadness.
- Provide simple explanations for procedures.
- Refer parents to social worker for follow-up while newborn is in hospital, according to family need.
- Encourage parents who are unable to visit to call nursery for progress reports.
- Refer to public health nurse (official agency or visiting nurse) for health supervision upon discharge of newborn.
- Plan for follow-up or institutionalization as necessary.

Evaluation: Parents grieve for their newborn's condition; express feelings of sadness, anger; allow nursing staff/family/friends to support them.

References

Avery, M.E., & Taeusch, H.W. (Eds). (1984). *Schaeffer's Diseases of the Newborn*. Philadelphia: Saunders.

Bobak, I., & Jensen, M. (1987). *Essentials of maternity nursing*. St. Louis: Mosby.

Brazelton, T. (1973). *Neonatal behavioral assessment scale*. Philadelphia: Lippincott.

Brooten, D., Brown, L., Hollingsworth, A., Tanis, J., & Bakewell-Sachs, S. (1985). Breast-milk jaundice. *JOGNN*. *14*(3), 220–3.

Cohen, M.A. (1984). Transcutaneous oxygen monitoring for sick neonates. *MCN*. *9*(5), 324–30.

Fantazia, D. (1984). Neonatal hypoglycemia. *JOGNN*. *13*(15), 297–301.

Korones, S.B. (1986). *High risk infants: The basis for intensive care nursing*. (4th ed) St. Louis: Mosby.

Lacamera, D. (1985). The acquired immunodeficiency syndrome. *Nursing Clinics of North America*. *20*(1), 241–256.

Locklin, M. (1987). Assessing jaundice in full term newborns. *Pediatric Nursing*, *13*(1), 15–19.

Mitchell, C., & Rutherford, P.A. (1987). The fragile survivor. *AJN*. *87*(5), 603–606.

Phototherapy and nursing care of the newborn with hyperbilirubinemia. (1986). *NAACOG OGN Nursing Practice Resource*, *15*, 2–8.

Whaley, L., & Wong, D. (1987). *Nursing care of newborns and children* (3rd ed.). St. Louis: Mosby.

*Whitaker, C. (1986). Death before birth. *American Journal of Nursing*, *86*(2), 157–158.

Wilkerson, N. (1988). A comprehensive look at hyperbilirubinemia. *MCN: The American Journal of Maternal/Child Nursing*. *13*(5), 360–364.

Withers, J., & Bradshaw, E. (1986). Preventing neonatal hepatitis. *MCN: American Journal of Maternal/Child Nursing*, *11*, 270–272.

*See Reprint Section

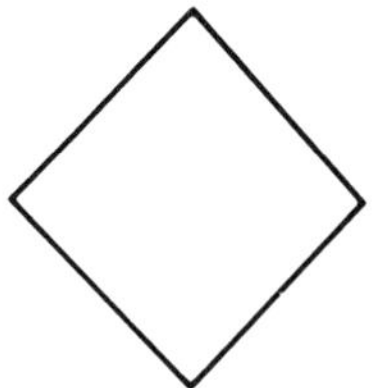

Reprints

Nursing Care of the Childbearing Family

Devore, N., & Baldwin, K. "Ectopic Pregnancy on the Rise" 439
Smith, J. "The Dangers of Prenatal Cocaine Use" 479
Hoffmaster, J. "Detecting and Treating Pregnancy-induced Hypertension" 444
Whitaker, C. "Death Before Birth" 457
Fullar, S. "Care of Postpartum Adolescents" 500
Wilkerson, N. "A Comprehensive Look at Hyperbilirubinemia" 506

AMERICAN JOURNAL OF NURSING

ECTOPIC PREGNANCY ON THE RISE

BY NANCY DEVORE/KAREN BALDWIN

Pelvic inflammatory disease is increasing, too—and that's just one reason why ectopic pregnancy remains a devastating problem.

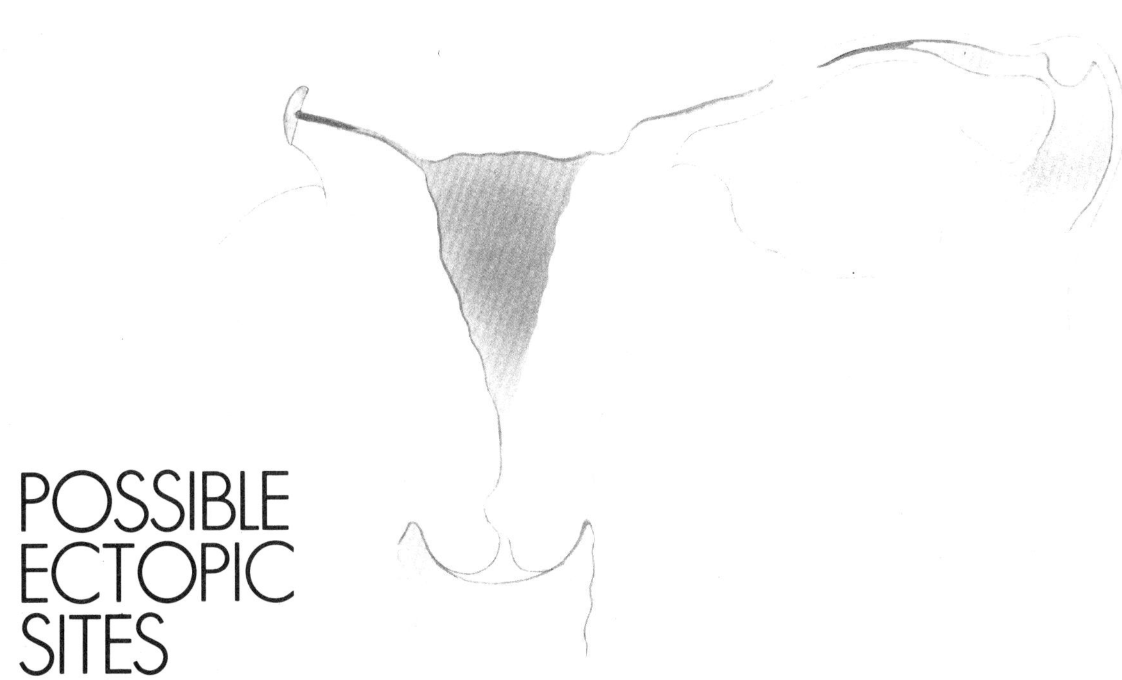

CAROL DONNER

Reprinted from American Journal of Nursing, June 1986.

The actual incidence of ectopic pregnancy (EP) is difficult to calculate since it is likely that many EPs abort spontaneously, remain asymptomatic, or reabsorb without diagnosis or treatment. Yet an undiagnosed ectopic pregnancy can not only endanger a woman's fertility, it can endanger her life. The number of reported EPs tripled between 1970 and 1980—to one EP for every 100 to 200 deliveries in 1982(1). Although 95 percent of ectopic pregnancies implant in the fallopian tubes, other sites include the ovary, cervix, cornua, or elsewhere in the abdominal or peritoneal cavity.

The mortality and morbidity of ectopic pregnancy is often related to delay in diagnosis and treatment. As the pregnancy grows, the trophoblast invades surrounding tissues and erodes vessels, increasing the risk of rupture of the organ with subsequent hemorrhage.

Although improved diagnostic and surgical techniques and greater availability of blood for transfusion have lowered mortality, EP is still responsible for six to 10 percent of all maternal deaths. The risk of death from an EP is 10 times higher than from childbirth and 50 times more likely than from a legal abortion(2). About one third of such deaths can be prevented by prompt treatment(3).

Moreover, following an EP, 38 to 70 percent of women become infertile, and those who do become pregnant have a four to 27 percent risk of another EP(4). The physical, emotional, and financial costs can be overwhelming.

THWARTED IMPLANTATION

Although EP has been strongly associated with a number of factors, the lack of well-controlled prospective studies has precluded the establishment of a firm etiology.

An ectopic pregnancy may be caused by factors that increase a fertilized ovum's tendency to implant in an aberrant site—such as endometriosis. Or an EP may be caused by factors that block the ovum's passage into the uterus—such as previous inflammation, abdominal or pelvic surgery, structural anomalies (from DES exposure or other embryological accidents), use of progesterone-only contraceptive methods (oral contraceptives, progesterone-impregnated IUDs, or the newer long-acting progesterone implants). Or an EP may be caused by migration of an ovum or zygote from one ovary across the peritoneal cavity to the opposite tube(1).

Debate continues over whether prior or current use of an intrauterine device, drug therapy to induce ovulation, and embryo transfer predispose a woman to EP.

Thirteen to 31 percent of women with EP have had pelvic inflammatory disease (PID)(1). Studies from Sweden and Great Britain suggest that 60 percent of all PID may be caused by *Chlamydia trachomatis*(5). In the United States, an estimated 20 percent of women with PID have cultures positive for chlamydia(5). Because chlamydia tends to cause more tubal scarring than gonorrhea, this increasingly prevalent organism may result in an even higher incidence of EP and sterility.

Women who have had abdominal or pelvic surgery for ruptured appendix, ovarian cysts, leiomyomata—or even tubal ligation, tuboplasty, or hysterectomy—are at risk for EP. If a tubal ligation or hysterectomy was not performed during the proliferative phase of the menstrual cycle, fertilization and implantation may have taken place.

The link between EP and the IUD is uncertain: Dorfman reports that a current user of an IUD is 0.8 times more likely and a past user 1.4 times more likely to have an EP than a woman who has never used an IUD(2). Ory suggests that the risk may be threefold in a woman who has used an IUD for more than 25 months and that the susceptibility to EP continues for a year after the IUD is removed(6). This risk may be related to the greater incidence of salpingitis and PID in IUD users.

Finally, the use of progesterone-only contraceptives, including long-acting implants, has been associated with

Nancy DeVore, CNM, MS, MSN, is director of the Nurse Midwifery Practice, Albert Einstein College of Medicine/Bronx Municipal Hospital Center, The Bronx, NY. Karen Baldwin, CNM, MS, is a nurse-midwife at Bronx Municipal.

COUNSELING: WHAT TO SAY

To begin:
"It can be frightening when surgery is needed so quickly. What do you remember thinking or feeling at the time?" This acknowledges fear and encourages discussion.

OR

"Losing a pregnancy at any point can be sad—especially after you tried to become pregnant for so long. What sort of thoughts did you have about the baby?" This acknowledges the couple's past infertility problem, gives permission to the patient to fantasize about the pregnancy, and promotes discussion.

OR

(If the patient has not given any clues about wanting the pregnancy) "Losing a pregnancy at any point brings up many feelings. Sometimes people feel relieved, other times they feel sad, angry, or frightened. What sort of feelings have you had?" This acknowledges the possibility of ambivalence and stimulates discussion.

When your patient asks:
"With only one tube, are my chances of conceiving cut in half?" "They are smaller, but not by half. The remaining tube can function as a passageway for an egg released from the opposite ovary."

OR

"Will I have another ectopic pregnancy?" "Your risk is greater, but most subsequent pregnancies are normal. Now that you've had an EP, we will watch you closely, and if you do have another, you may need less drastic surgery next time."

OR

"When can I become pregnant again?" "You will probably ovulate again in four to six weeks, but it's a good idea to wait at least until you've had a menstrual period so that we'll be able to date any new pregnancy. If you've had major surgery, you need to allow time for healing, building up your iron stores, and reestablishing a good nutritional state. Emotionally, you might want to wait about six months so that you and your partner can work through your grief over this pregnancy, and be ready to welcome a new one in its own right."

OR

"What can I use for birth control until I'm ready for another pregnancy?" "Barrier methods—diaphragm, condom—are best, because they have no side effects. If you don't plan on becoming pregnant again for a long time, you might want to consider oral contraceptives. An IUD is not a good idea, because it may interfere further with future fertility."

higher rates of EP. Chavkin reports a twofold to fivefold increase of EP among women taking such oral contraceptives, possibly from the progesterone-induced slowed peristalsis in the fallopian tubes(7). More work is needed to substantiate these theories.

ZEROING IN ON EP

Although diagnosis of EP prior to rupture is the key to reducing mortality and morbidity and preserving fertility, its varied clinical signs and the lack of easy and definitive laboratory tests make early diagnosis difficult. Thus the best diagnostic aid is a high index of suspicion for EP in any woman of reproductive age.

A comprehensive history is the first step. It includes:

- ☐ Age: Well over half of women with EP are 20 to 30 years old, although EP can occur anytime from menarche to menopause(1).
- ☐ Parity: 10 to 35 percent are nulliparous(1).
- ☐ Past health history: abdominal or pelvic surgery, in-utero exposure to DES, genital tract anomalies, leiomyo mata, endometriosis.
- ☐ Menstrual history: usual cycle, any amenorrhea, oligomenorrhea, intermenstrual bleeding.
- ☐ Contraception: past or present use of an IUD, use of progesterone contraceptives, prior tubal ligation or hysterectomy.
- ☐ Obstetric history: Primary or secondary infertility is common. A woman who has had an EP is 30 to 50 times as likely to have a subsequent one(1). It is probable that the factors that caused the first EP occurred bilaterally and thus predispose the patient to another EP, as do a previous puerperal or postabortive infection or sequelae from surgery for the first EP. Uncomplicated legal abortion as performed in the United States does not seem to increase rates of EP(8).

The classic clinical presentation—amenorrhea or abnormal vaginal bleeding, abdominal and pelvic pain, and a palpable adnexal mass—occurs in only about a third of women with EP.

Most women with EP report changes in menstrual pattern: Some report amenorrhea but many describe spotting or other irregular bleeding that may be misinterpreted as menses. Since cervicitis or bleeding from implantation often look identical, the significance of menstrual changes may be overlooked.

Also, if a woman has an IUD, irregular bleeding and discomfort may be incorrectly attributed to the device. It is important to remember that 20 to 40 percent of women with an EP have normal bleeding patterns.

Pain is the most likely indicator. Nine out of 10 women with EP have abdominal or pelvic pain, ranging from dull localized discomfort to diffuse excruciating pain. The pain is thought to be caused by distension of the tube from bleeding within the lumen or by irritation of the peritoneum from bleeding into the cavity. Shoulder pain—referred pain from intraperitoneal hemorrhage that irritates the diaphragm—is reported by up to 15 percent.

Other symptoms include nausea, vomiting, syncope, and urinary or rectal pressure or tenderness—all signs of early pregnancy.

On physical examination, vital signs show wide variation. Although eight to 18 percent of women with EP are admitted in shock with rapid pulse and hypotension, most are seen before hemorrhage begins(1). To prevent rupture and hemorrhage, it is essential to avoid applying excessive pressure during the pelvic exam. The abdomen may be normal or may be tender with rebound pain, guarding, distension, or reduced or absent bowel sounds. Pelvic findings may be negative or may include tenderness on cervical motion (from bleeding into the peritoneal cavity), slight uterine enlargement (from a buildup of the endometrial lining), or adnexal fullness, masses, or tenderness. Hayes notes that adnexal masses are palpable in only 50 percent of women(9).

Given the less-than-specific clinical picture, it is easy to understand why in two studies 42 to 50 percent of women later shown to have an EP had been seen by a physician and had been sent home before a correct diagnosis was made(10).

Diagnostic tests include hormone levels, ultrasound, culdocentesis, and laparoscopy. Such exams detect trophoblastic tissue and identify the ectopic site.

Biochemical tests of pregnancy are based on the amounts of various hormones produced by trophoblastic tissue. To be useful they must not only detect pregnancy but must distinguish ectopic from intrauterine pregnancy. The most commonly analyzed hormone is human chorionic gonadotropin (HCG).

HCG, a glycoprotein produced by the trophoblast, has two subunits. The alpha subunit is identical to that for FSH, LH, and TSH, while the beta subunit is specific for HCG. (See chart.) HCG can be detected a few days after implantation (8 days after conception, 22 days from the last menstrual period). HCG increases in concentration until 12 to 13 weeks after the LMP.

The major advantages of the slide or tube agglutination of the HCG radioreceptor assay tests are that the screens can be performed easily and that the results are quickly available (within two minutes to two hours).

Since these methods screen for the alpha subunit, which cross-reacts with

WHAT MIMICS ECTOPIC PREGNANCY?

Inflammatory or obstructive disorders

Appendicitis	Urinary tract infection
Pancreatitis	Renal calculi
Cholecystitis	Inflammatory bowel disease

Hemoperitoneum

Anticoagulant therapy
Erosion of cystic or appendiceal artery
Rupture of spleen, liver; small bowel tumor; aneurysm; varicose vein

GYN pathology

PID	Torsion or rupture of ovarian cyst
Mittelschmerz	Degenerating leiomyomata
Endometriosis	Dysfunctional uterine bleeding

Obstetrical entities

Intrauterine pregnancy with corpus luteum cyst
Hemorrhagic corpus luteum cyst
Threatened or incomplete spontaneous abortion
Heterotopic pregnancy
Psychiatric problems, personality disorders

LH, the sensitivity must be high to avoid contamination of the results. Unfortunately this means that an EP may well grow to the size where it will rupture before a pregnancy confirmation is obtained. The beta subunit HCG radioimmunoassay is much more sensitive for a gestation, but requires special laboratory procedures which may take four to 24 hours.

At first, an EP may produce HCG at rates that mimic normal gestation, but as the trophoblast is sheared off the tubal wall, there is less functioning tissue and thus the HCG level plateaus or diminishes. Because spontaneous abortion presents a similar picture, differentiation is difficult without sonography.

Ultrasound is the next step. When a pregnancy test is positive, absence of intrauterine gestation five to six weeks after the last menstrual period and absence of a pulsating fetal heart rate within the gestational sac two weeks later indicate an EP. Because of the possibility of a heterotopic pregnancy (that is, coexistent intrauterine and extrauterine pregnancies), however, even the presence of an intrauterine pregnancy does not rule out EP. Ultrasonography has a 70 to 90 percent success rate in diagnosing EP. Eventually, as equipment and techniques improve, visualization of an EP will become likely.

Both HCG and ultrasound can be repeated serially to clarify uncertain results. In a normal pregnancy, the mean doubling time of HCG is 1.98 days and the lower limit of normal increase in 48 hours is 66 percent(11). Therefore, quantitative HCG tests drawn 48 hours apart should show a 66- to 200-percent increase in level.

A normal intrauterine gestational sac doubles in size between four and six weeks after the last menstrual period(12). A pseudogestational sac will not grow. A pseudogestational sac, which occurs in 10 to 20 percent of EPs, is endometrium that is hyperplastic decidua. It resembles a gestational sac on sonogram, but usually lacks symmetry and has no fetal echoes(13).

The most reliable diagnosis of EP depends on a combined biochemical and biophysical approach. Although HCG levels can be ascertained much earlier than sonographic results, when HCG reaches 6000-6500 mIU/ml, an intrauterine gestation, if it exists, should be visible on ultrasound(13).

Neither HCG nor ultrasound may be available in an emergency. Surgical examination—either culdocentesis or laparoscopy—are the options. Culdocentesis (aspiration of peritoneal fluid through a needle inserted into the cul-de-sac) is the most rapid means to confirm hemoperitoneum. Although the woman may have some discomfort, anesthesia is not usually required for the procedure. If it yields more than 3 cc of unclotted blood, culdocentesis is considered positive.

Positive in 85 percent of ruptured

HCG ASSAYS

Test	Time requirement	Level of sensitivity / When obtained	%Sensitivity	Subunit measured	Positive features	Limitations
Urinary HCG latex agglutination-inhibition slide test	2 minutes	800-1500 MIU / 21-24 days after contraception (35-38d from LMP)	30-83%	Alpha	Easily performed Rapid results	Cross reactivity with LH False pos. with tubo-ovarian abscess, 2 or 3+ albumin 31% false negative False negative with very dilute urine
Urinary HCG latex agglutination-inhibition tube test	1½ hours	250 MIU / 14 days after contraception (28d from LMP)	80%	Alpha	Easily performed Rapid results	Same as above
Serum HCG Radioreceptor assay (RRA)	1 hour	200 MIU / 14 days after contraception (28d from LMP)	85-94%	Alpha	Rapid results	Invasive venipuncture Cross reactivity with LH False pos. with tubo-ovarian abscess 6% false negative Requires laboratory facilities
Serum HCG B-subunit Radioimmunoassay (B-HCG-RIA)	3-24 hours	5-15 MIU / 7 days after contraception (21d from LMP)	89-100%	Beta	Pos. results prior to first missed menses Highly accurate	Invasive venipuncture Difficult to obtain: requires special laboratory procedures Expensive Lengthy performance time
Urine HCG immunoenzymetric assay (Monoclonal antibodies)	1 hour	50 MIU / 14 days after contraception (28d from LMP)	100%	Beta	Easily performed Rapid results	False neg. with very dilute urine

and 65 percent of unruptured EPs, culdocentesis does not differentiate a ruptured ectopic pregnancy from a ruptured hemorrhagic corpus luteum. However, the approach is the same for both—immediate exploratory laparotomy to find and control the source of bleeding. A culdocentesis that yields clear fluid or none at all may signal technical problems or the absence of any active bleeding. Still, it does not rule out EP.

Laparoscopy (endoscopy performed under local anesthesia through a small abdominal incision) can confirm a suspected unruptured EP and provide access for some less radical surgical procedures, such as tubal aspiration or salpingotomy. But when rupture is presumed and the patient is unstable, laparotomy is preferable.

SURGERY FOR EP

Ectopic pregnancy was almost always fatal until a century ago, when surgery was first used to correct the problem. Today, a woman is immediately treated for hypovolemia, followed by laparotomy with salpingectomy (if the tube has ruptured).

If a woman's history is suspicious but her BP and pulse are normal, there is time to make a more definite diagnosis. A rapid urine pregnancy test is done, CBC, type and crossmatch are drawn, and an IV is started. If the urine pregnancy test is negative but clinical suspicion for EP is high, a beta HCG is drawn and, if time permits, ultrasound and culdocentesis can be done.

Surgery is usually the treatment of choice. Debate continues as to whether the surgery should be radical—removal of the fallopian tube and possibly the ovary on the affected side (salpingo-oophorectomy)—or conservative.

Conservative treatment aims to preserve all or most of the structure and function of the affected fallopian tube. Some clinicians advise the conservative approach for all women with EP who want to remain fertile.

If the tube has not ruptured, several types of conservative surgery can be done, depending on the site of the EP and the degree of tubal involvement:

The *milking technique* (squeezing the tube to express the EP), is successful only if the EP is in the fimbriated section of the tube. One drawback: trophoblastic tissue may remain in the affected tube, predisposing the woman to adhesions, complications in later pregnancies, and further surgery.

In *linear salpingostomy* the products of conception are suctioned out and the remaining trophoblastic tissue is gently removed through an incision on the anterior portion of the tube over the pregnancy site. One study revealed an 80-percent rate of successful pregnancy following this surgery(14).

When an EP develops in the midsegment or isthmic section of the tube, the portion of the tube involved is removed and two ends are sutured together.

Complications of conservative surgery include residual trophoblastic tissue and delayed hemorrhage, both of which may mandate subsequent surgery. If the tube has ruptured, tubal restoration is unlikely.

In addition to the usual postop care, be sure that any Rh-negative woman who has had an EP is offered RhoGAM prophylaxis.

HOW TO HELP

Although gonorrhea is the culprit in most tubal infection in the United States, most infected women have no symptoms of pelvic infection(15). Therefore, cultures should always be taken with any gynecological infection or dysuria, before an endometrial biopsy, hysterosalpingogram, or IUD insertion, and at annual examinations.

Obviously, contraception prevents EP. The pill is the most effective contraceptive, protecting against both extrauterine as well as intrauterine pregnancy. It may reduce the risk of PID from gonorrhea(16). Be sure that any woman considering an IUD is aware of increased risk of PID and of the association between PID and EP.

The nurse must suspect EP in any woman of reproductive age presenting gynecological complaints. If the patient is stable, much of the nurse's role may be explanation of diagnostic findings. Such a presentation must be done in an empathic manner, to help the woman and her partner to realize the potential seriousness of the problem, without generating fear. If rupture has occurred, the nurse assists with emergency procedures to stabilize vital signs, to diagnose hemoperitoneum, and to prepare the patient for surgery.

Psychological support of such a woman and family in crisis is of utmost importance. The couple may need counseling to help them to work through any fears of death or disfigurement, the loss of the pregnancy, and their concerns about future pregnancies. Fantasies about the baby begin very early for some couples. Thus, even when the earliest embryo is lost, the couple may feel sadness and grief.

Be especially sensitive to any ideas that the EP was "punishment" for prior sexual behavior or abortions. Peer support, available through bereavement groups, may help the couple resolve their loss.

Through nonjudgmental listening, reiteration of facts, and helping the couple express their sadness about the loss, you can help the woman and her partner work through their feelings about the pregnancy and its thwarted beginnings.

REFERENCES

1. Patrick, J. D. Ectopic pregnancy—A brief review. *Ann.Emerg.Med.* 11:576-581, Oct. 1982.
2. Dorfman, S. F. Ectopic pregnancy. Thinking ectopic: key to diagnosis. *Postgrad.Med.* 76:65-68, Aug. 1984.
3. Dorfman, S. F., and others. Ectopic pregnancy mortality, United States, 1979-1980: clinical aspects. *Obstet.Gynecol.* 64:386-390, Sept. 1984.
4. Strathy, J. H., and others. Incidence of ectopic pregnancy in Rochester, Minnesota, 1950-1981. *Obstet.Gynecol.* 64:37-43, July 1984.
5. Holmes, K. K. The chlamydia epidemic. (interview) *JAMA* 245:1718-1723, May 1, 1981.
6. Ory, H. W. Ectopic pregnancy and intrauterine contraceptive devices: new perspectives. The women's health study. *Obstet.Gynecol.* 57:137-144, Feb. 1981.
7. Chavkin, W. The rise in ectopic pregnancy—exploration of possible reasons. *Int.J.Gynecol.Obstet.* 20:341-350, Aug. 1982.
8. Daling, J. R., and others. Ectopic pregnancy in relation to previous induced abortion. *JAMA* 253:1005-1008, Feb. 15, 1985.
9. Hayes, H. R., and Hayley, E. C. Intrauterine and ruptured tubal ectopic pregnancy: a diagnostic challenge. *Ann.Emerg.Med.* 13:355-358, May 1984.
10. Berry, C. M., and others. The radioreceptor assay for HCG in ectopic pregnancy. *Obstet.Gynecol.* 54:43-46, July 1979.
11. Kadar, N., and others. A method of screening for ectopic pregnancy and its indications. *Obstet.Gynecol.* 58:162-165, Aug. 1981.
12. Wexler, S., and others. Pseudogestational sac in ectopic pregnancy. *Acta.Obstet.Gynecol.Scand.* 63(1):63-65, 1984.
13. Kadar, N., and others. Discriminatory HCG zone, its use in the sonographic evaluation for ectopic pregnancy. *Obstet.Gynecol.* 58:156-161, Aug. 1981.
14. Langer, R., and others. Conservative surgery for tubal pregnancy. *Fertil.Steril.* 38:427-430, Oct. 1982.
15. DeCherney, A. H., and Maheux, R. Modern management of tubal pregnancy. *Curr.Problems Obstet.Gynecol.* 6:1-38, May 1983.
16. Ory, H.W. The noncontraceptive health benefits from oral contraceptive use. *Family Planning Perspectives* 1982: 14:182-184.

The Dangers Of Prenatal Cocaine Use

Because of the dramatic effects cocaine can have on both mother and fetus, prevention, early detection, and intervention are essential.

JUDY SMITH

On several different occasions, Beth, a 24-year-old, middle-class, married woman, had snorted small amounts of cocaine. She had used cocaine when she was with close friends, while alone with her husband, and a few times by herself. She was convinced that she could take it or leave it at will; addiction, she was sure, was not a problem for her.

When she found out she was six weeks pregnant, she discontinued her cocaine use entirely, and her pregnancy progressed without any observable problems. She used cocaine once at about 28 weeks' gestation without any complications.

At 34 weeks' gestation, she snorted an unspecified quantity of cocaine at 8:00 P.M. Shortly afterward, she felt strong contractions begin. She was admitted to the labor unit at 9:15 P.M. with contractions every 2 to 3 minutes and fetal tachycardia. Tocolysis was attempted with magnesium sulfate per protocol. An hour later, late decelerations appeared on the fetal monitor and Beth was quickly prepared for a cesarean birth. She delivered a viable, 4-pound 10-ounce girl with Apgars of 5 and 7 and no noticeable congenital anomalies.

Beth typifies the difficulties the health care system confronts when coping with cocaine abuse during pregnancy. There has been a marked increase in cocaine use in the United States during the past few years and cocaine has become more socially acceptable and more widely available to both the affluent and the poor of the nation. Thousands of women from middle and upper socioeconomic classes are addicted to what many see as the glamour drug of the 1980s.

Approximately 20 million people in the United States have used cocaine on one occasion, and 5 million use it regularly (1). The National Institute on Drug Abuse reports that among street drugs, U.S. high school students favor cocaine second only to marijuana (2). There is a lack of national data on maternal cocaine abuse, but indications that the problem is growing are unmistakable. One New York City hospital recently reported that 10 percent of all newborns born there had a positive urine screen for cocaine (1).

In addition to the physiologic dangers cocaine use during pregnancy produces, it also raises difficult legal and ethical questions. How do we balance the rights of the mother with the rights of her unborn child? Should the mother be held legally accountable for endangering her fetus, or are both the mother and the baby considered victims of a disease? Was the mother aware of the harmful effects cocaine can have on a growing fetus? Was she in need of preconceptional education? If a mother is identified as a cocaine user, should her infant be sent home with her to a potentially drug-using environment?

The legal obligations and responsibilities of caregivers are equally clouded. Does the caregiver have a legal responsibility to the fetus to report the mother's cocaine use? What impact will the caregiver's report have on the issues of patient confidentiality and the mother's right to privacy?

Lately, the national trend is to protect child welfare, health, and safety through enforcement of the child abuse and neglect reporting laws rather than to maintain maternal confidentiality (3). Keeping this trend in mind when determining legal obligation and responsibility to report suspected child abuse or neglect resulting from perinatal use of illicit drugs can be beneficial.

Pharmacology of Prenatal Cocaine Use

The rapidly growing number of cocaine-affected pregnancies has caught health care providers by surprise. Data related to the effects of cocaine on the developing fetus are now appearing in the literature and represent intense, ongoing investigation of cocaine's cause and effect relationships.

There are many common misconceptions about cocaine use (see Cocaine Misconceptions). For pregnant women, the most profound misconception is that the placenta protects the unborn baby from toxic substances taken during pregnancy.

JUDY E. SMITH, R.N.P., M.N., *is a certified ob/gyn nurse practitioner and an associate professor of maternal-child nursing at California State University, Long Beach, California. For reprints of this article, see the classified section.*

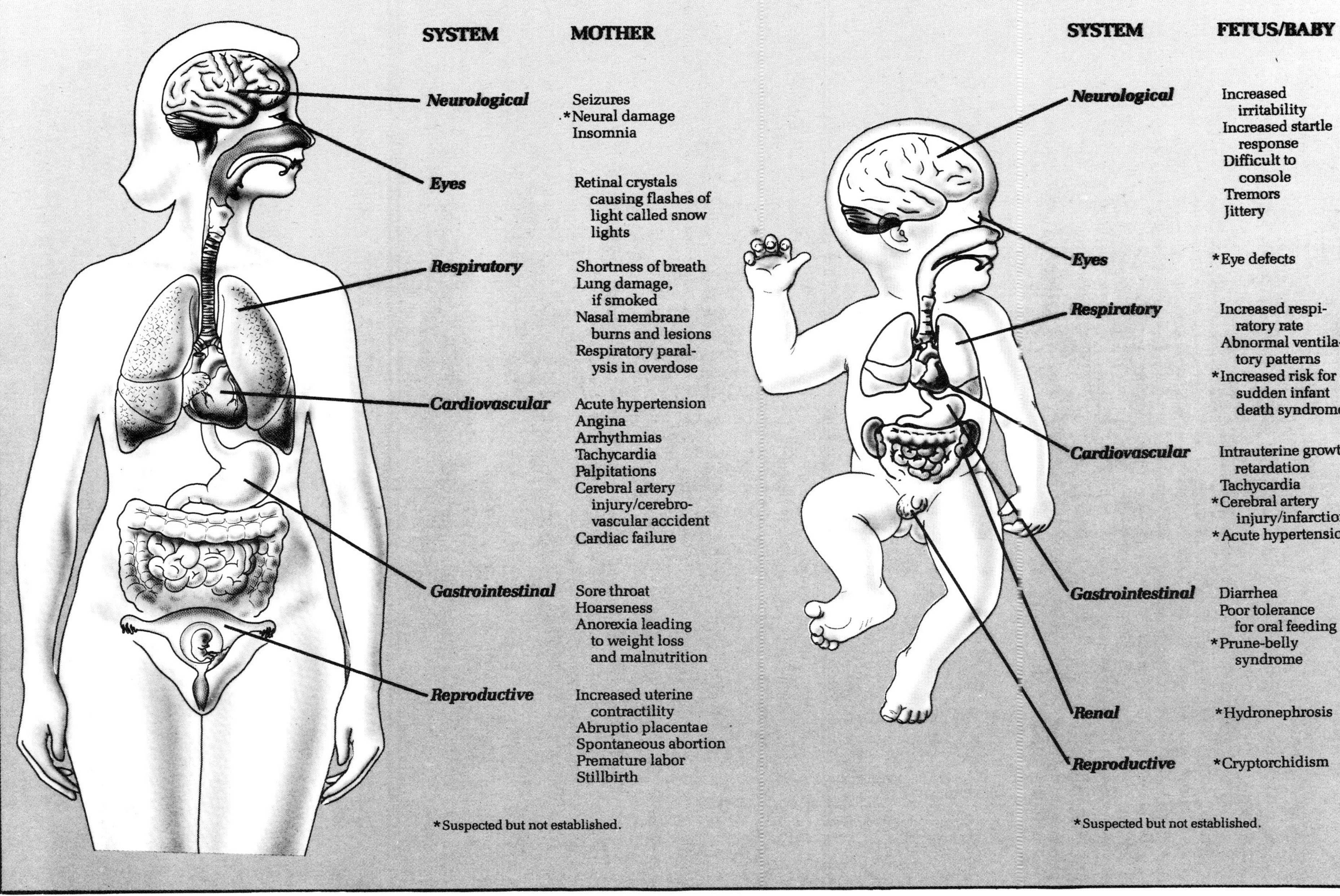
EFFECTS OF MATERNAL COCAINE USE ON MOTHERS AND FETUSES/BABIES
SYSTEM
MOTHER
Neurological
Seizures
*Neural damage
Insomnia
Eyes
Retinal crystals causing flashes of light called snow lights
Respiratory
Shortness of breath
Lung damage, if smoked
Nasal membrane burns and lesions
Respiratory paralysis in overdose
Cardiovascular
Acute hypertension
Angina
Arrhythmias
Tachycardia
Palpitations
Cerebral artery injury/cerebrovascular accident
Cardiac failure
Gastrointestinal
Sore throat
Hoarseness
Anorexia leading to weight loss and malnutrition
Reproductive
Increased uterine contractility
Abruptio placentae
Spontaneous abortion
Premature labor
Stillbirth
*Suspected but not established.
SYSTEM
FETUS/BABY
Neurological
Increased irritability
Increased startle response
Difficult to console
Tremors
Jittery
Eyes
*Eye defects
Respiratory
Increased respiratory rate
Abnormal ventilatory patterns
*Increased risk for sudden infant death syndrome
Cardiovascular
Intrauterine growth retardation
Tachycardia
*Cerebral artery injury/infarction
*Acute hypertension
Gastrointestinal
Diarrhea
Poor tolerance for oral feeding
*Prune-belly syndrome
Renal
*Hydronephrosis
Reproductive
*Cryptorchidism
*Suspected but not established.

Many drugs freely cross the placenta. Drugs such as cocaine that act upon the central nervous system are often lipophilic and of relatively low molecular weight, characteristics that make it easier for the substance to cross the placenta and the fetal blood-brain barrier (1).

Animal studies documenting the pharmacologic effects of cocaine on physiology are consistent in their findings (see Effects of Maternal Cocaine Use on Mothers and Fetuses/Babies). Cocaine stimulates the central nervous system much as amphetamines do. It has a half-life in plasma of about one hour following administration, making it a stimulant of short duration. Additionally, cocaine stimulates the peripheral nervous system and prevents norepinephrine reuptake at the nerve terminals (4). The result is a high circulating level of norepinephrine, which causes vasoconstriction, tachycardia, acute hypertension, and uterine contractions. In pregnancy, placental vasoconstriction results, restricting blood flow to the fetus (1).

There has also been a recent and dramatic increase in the use of alkaloidal cocaine, better known as crack. Crack is often smoked because it vaporizes at relatively low temperatures. As it is absorbed by the pulmonary vasculature, it produces a rapid euphoria, which diminishes in 30 minutes. Crack is used repeatedly to regain the euphoric state, a pattern that can lead to high levels of fetal exposure in pregnant women (5).

COCAINE MISCONCEPTIONS

Cocaine is a harmless drug. The cocaine epidemic and all the talk about the hazards of using the drug are scare tactics and media hype. Cocaine is one of the most insidious drugs on the illicit market today. It can exacerbate psychiatric problems and cause severe physical problems, even death. Its use has wrecked innumerable families and careers. In some cities, cocaine deaths are becoming more common than heroin deaths.

Even if cocaine is harmful, it harms only the user. Cocaine abuse can hurt not only its users, but those around them—families, friends, co-workers, employers, employees. Treating drug abuse drives up health care costs, which affects everyone. Cocaine is the most expensive drug dependence to treat, perhaps because relapses and retreatment are common. The annual cost of cocaine abuse to American society is estimated at $25–$35 billion.

Cocaine is nonaddictive. Cocaine is the most powerful psychological reinforcer of any of the illicit drugs, allowing for profound dependence. The biochemical mechanisms of cocaine dependence are not understood and why some casual users become addicted while others don't is unclear.

Cocaine is only habit-forming if it is smoked or injected. Although the most serious dependencies are generally found among those who freebase (smoke cocaine) or use the drug intravenously, a significant number of people in treatment for cocaine-related problems have only inhaled it.

People who only use the drug once a week, or once a month, don't become dependent on it. Dependency and abuse can't be thought of only in terms of frequency. Some people who use cocaine once a month do so in binges during which they may ingest huge quantities. Any use at all, but particularly daily or binge use, puts a person at risk for addiction.

Based on "Cocaine Use In America," *Prevention Networks*, National Institute on Drug Abuse. (DHHS publ. No. ADM 86-1433) Washington, D.C., U.S. Government Printing Office, Apr. 1986.

Pregnancy Complications

Women who use cocaine during pregnancy are more likely than nonusers to have spontaneous first-trimester abortions, a finding consistent with the implication of placental vasoconstriction induced by cocaine use (1). The incidence of abruptio placentae, usually occurring within an hour of cocaine administration, is higher than in the nonusing population (1,5,7). This finding is attributed to the acute hypertension caused by cocaine and the well-established relationship between hypertension and abruptio placentae.

Third trimester use of cocaine by pregnant women has been reported to induce a sudden onset of uterine contractions, fetal tachycardia, and excessive fetal activity within hours or even minutes of ingestion (1,6). The premature labor and abnormal fetal heart rate patterns experienced by Beth are not unusual.

In the general population, cocaine has been associated with palpitations, angina, and arrythmias. Even small amounts of cocaine found in sensitive individuals have been linked to deaths resulting from cardiac failure (8). For pregnant women, cocaine-induced tachycardia further strains the already overworked maternal heart.

The teratogenic effect of cocaine on the developing fetus is relatively unknown at this time. Cocaine's profound impact on cardiovascular function can potentially place the exposed fetus in jeopardy for both short- and long-term adverse effects (5). There have been only isolated reports and small-sample pilot studies that suggest cocaine might be responsible for congenital anomalies. One infant studied by Ira Chasnoff exhibited cryptorchidism, prune-belly syndrome, and hydronephrosis that may have been associated with maternal cocaine use (6). The effects of cocaine as a human teratogen must be studied more extensively before conclusions can be derived.

Effects on the Newborn

The consequences of cocaine exposure to the fetus are ambiguous. Unlike opiate-exposed neonates, cocaine-exposed infants do not seem to experience the classic neonatal abstinence syndrome. Infants born to mothers who have used cocaine during pregnancy tend to be shorter, lower in birthweight, and have smaller head circumferences as compared to infants of women who were drug-free during pregnancy (1).

Cocaine-exposed infants may show mild to

moderate tremulousness and increased irritability, muscular rigidity, and startle response. They are difficult to console and state lability is pronounced (5,6). In addition, elevated respiratory and heart rates, poor tolerance for oral feedings, diarrhea, and disturbed sleep patterns have been linked to cocaine exposure in utero (9,10). Newborns exhibiting these symptoms are evaluated for cocaine exposure in utero (see the section on postpartum care).

Maternal prenatal cocaine use also places the infant at potentially increased risk for sudden infant death syndrome (SIDS). Abnormal sleeping ventilatory patterns implicated in SIDS have been reported in cocaine-exposed neonates (10). The rate of SIDS in cocaine-exposed neonates may be as high as 15 percent, more than three times the rate in heroin-exposed neonates (1).

Perinatal cerebral infarction in infants exposed to cocaine just prior to birth has also been reported (1,11). The finding of perinatal cerebral infarction in cocaine-exposed neonates tends to parallel reports of acute cerebral and myocardial infarction in young adults shortly after cocaine use (1).

Caring for Cocaine Users

Planning appropriate nursing interventions for cocaine using women can be a difficult and intricate task. Assessment can be exceptionally complex due to the lack of clear physical signs that indicate cocaine use. Cocaine addiction can be concealed by demeanors from shy and secretive to outgoing and witty. Consequently, nurses may find it difficult to identify the cocaine abusing woman.

Prevention, undoubtedly, is the most effective and ideal nursing intervention. Many women, like Beth, are unaware of the potential dangers inherent in cocaine use. The key to any successful prevention effort is getting accurate information to those at greatest risk.

A substantial proportion of cocaine users are young, well-paid, well-educated, upwardly mobile professionals in their 20s and 30s (2). Anne, a 32-year-old advertising executive, visited her private obstetrician-gynecologist for a preconceptional consultation and evaluation. The office nurse asked her about any history of cocaine use, which Anne immediately denied. The nurse used a well-planned, nonjudgmental, natural-appearing pause at this point. Anne qualified her answer with, "Well, very, very rarely and not enough to cause any harm or alarm." The pause gave Anne a moment to think about the question. The nurse's nonjudgmental manner and nonthreatening attitude invited Anne's honest disclosure, paving the way for preconceptional education about the dangers of cocaine use in pregnancy.

Young professionals tend to be fairly sophisticated. Many grew up in the 1960s and early 1970s, when scare-tactic approaches to prevention destroyed the credibility of the information presented. For this reason, nurses must make special efforts to deliver information straightforwardly and unemotionally (2). The nurse in Anne's obstetrician-gynecologist's office gave Anne factual information about cocaine use and corrected her misconceptions (1).

Prevention efforts targeted to the teenaged population require a different approach than those designed for adult professionals. Teenagers are not apt to perceive health hazards as real and immediate dangers. Effective interventions for teens center around dispelling the popular idea that cocaine use is normal, acceptable, and that everybody uses drugs. Pairing the well-documented health hazards of cocaine use with those of amphetamines or heroin, which have been more widely studied and publicized, allows nurses to draw on teenagers' background knowledge to construct meaningful parallels. Enlisting the aid of teen peers to impart information to teen groups enhances the effectiveness of prevention efforts and can be accomplished cost effectively via a videotaped presentation shown in a clinic waiting room.

Educational efforts must rely on current preliminary data and will need to be updated as new information becomes available. Widespread knowledge is the best means to the long-term end—prevention.

Early detection of cocaine use in pregnancy complemented by appropriate intervention and follow-up affords the best outcome for both mother and infant. In order to identify maternal cocaine use, the nurse must be tactfully inquisitive. During the initial contact, assessing the woman's mood, attention to personal grooming, and affect may provide subtle or overt clues to the possibility of cocaine or other substance use.

As the nurse compiles a nursing and medical history, the ideal opportunity for questioning substance abuse presents itself. Standard history forms include questions about smoking practices, alcohol use, and over-the-counter drug use. Altering the form to guide the questioning toward ascertainment of illicit drug use is a simple task (see Drug Use Assessment).

Selecting nonjudgmental, sensitively-constructed questions and delivering them at the same speed and in the same tone of voice and matter-of-fact manner as nonsensitive questions maximize the likelihood that the woman will answer truthfully. A woman is more likely to respond honestly if the nurse has conveyed that she will not react with shock, accusations, or a guilt-laden lecture. The development of trust and rapport are prerequisites for helping substance-abusing pregnant women confront their drug problems.

Identifying cocaine use during pregnancy can be concurrently challenging and frustrating. Often the woman will deny that she uses cocaine and fails to realize how she has incorporated the drug into her life. The woman may believe she has control over her cocaine use. Showing her the connection between cocaine use and related health problems may enable her to more realistically face the impact of cocaine use on her pregnancy. Counseling, education, and careful prenatal health care management can help forestall continued maternal cocaine use, limiting adverse fetal effects from cocaine exposure and reducing the risk of related maternal complications (1).

Ellen, a 28-year-old woman pregnant with her second child, came to the clinic for her first prenatal visit at 21 weeks' gestation. She was underweight, appeared quite nervous, and was in a hurry to leave. Ellen denied use of any drugs or alcohol. She was referred to the clinic's nutritionist as intervention for her inadequate weight gain. She missed her next prenatal appointment.

At her next visit, Ellen still hadn't gained any weight, and complained of her heart racing at times, of having headaches, and of having insomnia. The nurse suspected drug use and used the fact that Ellen hadn't followed nutritional guidelines to build a trusting, nonjudgmental rapport. She then sensitively asked her about drug use.

Ellen admitted that she had used cocaine but had stopped when she suspected she was pregnant. As the nurse related her concerns about cocaine use in pregnancy in general terms, Ellen interjected that her current use of cocaine was quite regular. She appeared to be relieved at having revealed the problem. Her nurse identified the short-term goals of Ellen's care: correcting Ellen's nutritional deficit and helping her give up her use of cocaine.

The nurse referred Ellen to a local cocaine treatment program; her prenatal care continued to be provided at the clinic. She began to follow her nutrition program and gained adequate weight during the remainder of the pregnancy. At the clinic, Ellen received a great deal of support and encouragement for her weight gain, for her continued involvement in the treatment program, and for abstaining from cocaine. She gave birth to a normal appearing, 40-week gestation boy weighing 7 pounds 4 ounces; his Apgars were 9 and 9. Ellen continued to attend her treatment program's support group and abstained from cocaine use even after she delivered a healthy son.

Recognizing intrapartum cocaine effects is as difficult as antepartum detection. Many signs are subtle and can appear unrelated. Fetal tachycardia, excessive fetal activity, and a sudden onset of unusually strong uterine contractions at the beginning of labor alert the nurse to inquire about recent cocaine use. Fetal meconium passage and a precipitous labor and delivery can also be related to use of cocaine (1).

Toxicologic urine screening will detect cocaine ingestion within the past 24 hours. Cocaine reaches the brain and neurons of the sympathetic nervous system in 3 minutes when it is inhaled, in 15 seconds when it is injected, and in 7 seconds when it is smoked. In the latter, it is rapidly metabolized by the liver, which makes it difficult to screen anything other than current use (2). Toxicologic blood screening also renders information regarding the quantity of cocaine in the blood.

The goal when treating a woman in labor who has recently ingested cocaine is to stabilize both mother and fetus. Placing the patient in a lateral recumbent position and administering oxygen via face mask may improve fetal oxygenation and bradycardia. Monitoring of the fetus and of maternal blood pressure and pulse provides valuable, continuous, assessment data. Seizure precautions and neurologic assessments are critical if the woman is in a transient, acute, cocaine-induced hypertensive episode. Assessment of respiratory rate and rhythm will enable the nurse to detect respiratory impairment and paralysis associated with cocaine overdose (2). Given the short half-life of cocaine in plasma, maternal stabilization usually occurs within an hour.

After the mother and fetus are stable, the mother must be carefully observed for the signs of

DRUG USE ASSESSMENT

Drug History	No	Yes	Type	Amount	Frequency of Use	Last Time Used	How Taken	Comments
A. Alcohol								
B. Nicotine								
C. Medications								
Vitamins								
Laxatives								
Antacids								
Cold Remedies								
Caffeine								
Aspirin								
Pain Relievers								
Sleeping Aids								
Sedatives								
Tranquilizers								
Marijuana								
Cocaine								
Heroin								
Hallucinogens								
D. Drug Allergies								

abruptio placentae: headache, constant abdominal pain, and excessive vaginal bleeding. The potential for catastrophic abruptio placentae is high and must be anticipated.

Postpartum Care

Cocaine use by a pregnant woman may go unnoticed during prenatal and intrapartum care. Detection may first occur during the assessment of the infant in the nursery. If a nurse suspects neonatal cocaine exposure, she must initiate both treatment of the infant and maternal psychosocial interventions without delay.

Toxicologic urine screening will detect neonatal cocaine exposure within the past six to nine days. Most drugs persist longer in fetuses and newborns than they do in adults because immature neonatal livers take longer to metabolize the drug. Fetuses and infants have a relative deficiency of plasma cholinesterases, the enzymes that break down cocaine. Cocaine and cocaine metabolites can persist in the newborn's urine for several days after delivery (13).

If the neonate is being breast-fed and begins to demonstrate signs of cocaine exposure, evaluate the mother for current cocaine use. Cocaine can be transferred from mother to infant through breast milk (2).

The mother whose cocaine use has gone undetected until after delivery must be postpartally evaluated to determine the degree of her substance abuse. The mother's nurse does this by eliciting from the mother information about the magnitude of her drug use, whether her significant others use drugs, her treatment history, and her expectations for future cocaine use. With this information, nurses can plan appropriate interventions, including health education about cocaine use, referral to a local treatment program, and arranging close follow-up care that ensures a safe environment for the baby (12). In all cases, an approach individualized for each woman's situation is most likely to succeed.

Follow-up discussion with Beth after the birth of her daughter revealed that she was unaware of the risks she had imposed on her unborn baby and herself by using cocaine during her pregnancy. She explained her beliefs about the drug, saying that although cocaine use is illegal, she had thought her use of the drug was safe because she only inhaled small amounts. She had thought of her cocaine use as recreational because she had only taken the drug occasionally, usually in social settings. Many people across the nation share her view that small, recreational use of cocaine is harmless (8).

Beth had discontinued her cocaine use when she discovered she was pregnant because she wanted a healthy baby and knew she shouldn't take any kind of drug unless it was prescribed for her. Later in the pregnancy, on the two occasions when she used cocaine, Beth said that she had been influenced and pressured by her friends to try just a small amount. Because she had no adverse effects at 28 weeks' gestation, she had thought it would be safe to use cocaine again. Throughout the discussion, Beth cried, expressed a great deal of guilt and regret, and reached out for someone to help her cope with her overwhelming feelings.

Beth's nurses chose crisis intervention for her care plan because of Beth's overwhelming feelings of guilt and regret regarding the premature birth of her daughter. After coping with the immediate crisis, Beth was able to concentrate on learning about cocaine use. Once she became aware of the harmful effects of cocaine, she was able to discontinue further use of the drug. She was discharged from the hospital with written material about cocaine and a resource telephone number.

Who's At Risk?

The magnitude of the maternal cocaine abuse problem is just beginning to surface. Attempts to organize approaches to meet this new challenge are now emerging. One is a national drug treatment referral hotline (800-662-HELP), which was established so that people can call for information about treatment facilities within their communities. No one, regardless of their competence or success in other areas of life, is immune from the dangers of cocaine.

REFERENCES

1. CHASNOFF, I. J. Perinatal effects of cocaine. *Contemp.OB/GYN* 29:163–179, May 1987.
2. NATIONAL INSTITUTE ON DRUG ABUSE. Cocaine use in America. IN *Prevention Networks.* (DHHS Publ. No. ADM 86-1433) Washington, D.C., U.S. Government Printing Office, Apr. 1986, pp. 1–14.
3. CHASNOFF, I. J., ED. *Drug Use In Pregnancy.* Norwell, MA, MTP Press Ltd., 1986, pp. 147–155.
4. HOLLAND, D. J. Cocaine use and toxicity. *JEN* 8:166–169, July–Aug. 1982.
5. LEBLANC, P. E., AND OTHERS. Effects of intrauterine exposure to alkaloidal cocaine. *Am.J.Dis.Child.* 141:937–938, Sept. 1987.
6. CHASNOFF, I. J., AND OTHERS. Cocaine use in pregnancy. *N.Engl.J.Med.* 313:666–669, Sept. 12, 1985.
7. ACKER, D., AND OTHERS. Abruptio placentae associated with cocaine use. *Am.J.Obstet.Gynecol.* 146:220–221, May 15, 1983.
8. NATIONAL INSTITUTE ON DRUG ABUSE. *Cocaine Addiction.* (DHHS Publ. No. ADM 85-1427) Washington, D.C., U.S. Government Printing Office, 1985.
9. NEWALD, J. Cocaine infants: a new arrival at hospitals' steps? *Hospitals* 60:96, Apr. 5, 1986.
10. WARD, S. L., AND OTHERS. Abnormal sleeping ventilatory patterns in infants of substance-abusing mothers. *Am.J.Dis.Child.* 140:1015–1020, Oct. 1986.
11. CHASNOFF, I. J., AND OTHERS. Perinatal cerebral infarction and maternal cocaine use. *J.Pediatr.* 108:456–459, Mar. 1986.
12. CHYCHULA, N. M. Screening for substance abuse in a primary care setting. *Nurse Pract.* 9:15–24, July 1984.
13. CHASNOFF, I. J. Cocaine and pregnancy. *Childbirth Educator* 37–42, Winter 1986–1987.

Detecting And Treating Pregnancy-Induced Hypertensio

Reprinted from MCN: The American Journal of Maternal/Child Nursing, November/December 1983.

Although the etiology of pregnancy-induced hypertension remains unclear, women who are at risk of developing it can be identified and helped.

JOAN E. HOFFMASTER

Hypertensive disorders of pregnancy, variously called preeclampsia, eclampsia, eclamptogenic toxemia, gestational hypertension, and EPH (edema, proteinuria, hypertension) gestosis, are leading causes of maternal deaths. They contribute significantly to perinatal death rates also. Yet the causes of these disorders remain obscure.

Preeclampsia, which occurs primarily during first pregnancies, is characterized by the development of proteinuria and/or edema in conjunction with hypertension. It affects between 1.5 and 12 percent of expectant mothers. Women who are members of groups that have a high predisposition for hypertension, such as blacks, are at greater risk.

Generally, preeclampsia arises after 20 weeks' gestation and in the absence of preexisting hypertensive vascular or renal disease. With trophoblastic disease, signs of preeclampsia may develop prior to 20 weeks' gestation (1–3). When preeclampsia progresses to the occurrence of convulsions that are not caused by other cerebral conditions, it is called *eclampsia*. (For more information on the classification, definitions, and characteristics of pregnancy-induced hypertension, see "Pregnancy-Induced Hypertension: Prenatal

JOAN E. HOFFMASTER, R.N., M.S., *is the coordinator of the Improved Pregnancy Outcome and Improved Child Health Projects, Public Health Region 2, Texas Department of Health. She helped establish a special program for adolescent pregnancy care at Texas Tech University Health Sciences Center/R. E. Thomason General Hospital in El Paso, Texas. She is a certified nurse midwife.*

ASSOCIATIONS WITH PREGNAN

Clinical Criteria	*Early Indicators*
Blood pressure	Persistent creeping-upward trend in diastolic blood pressure while still in normal range. Midtrimester blood pressur of 125/75 to 130/80 mmHg or greater; midtrimester arterial pressure of 82 mmHg or greater.
Proteinuria Quantitative (per liter) Qualitative/dipstick	
Edema	
Weight gain	2 pounds or more per week (no other signs).
Gastric/epigastric	
Central nervous system	
Extremities/reflexes	
Pulmonary	
Renal	
Placenta	
Fetus	
Laboratory findings: Plasma creatinine Hematocrit Blood viscosity Platelets Serum uric acid	
Prenatal, predictive blood pressure screening	Supine pressor test between 20 and 32 weeks' gestation, mean arterial pressure test (midtrimester).

A Review

INDUCED HYPERTENSION

Mild to Moderate Preeclampsia	*Severe Preeclampsia*
Persistent diastolic pressure of 90 mmHg. At least 140/90 mmHg but less than 160/110 mmHg or 30 mmHg or more rise in systolic pressure over baseline or 15 mmHg or more rise in diastolic pressure over baseline.	160/110 mmHg or higher.
(Proteinuria may be absent.) 0.3 gm to 2 gm per liter in 24 hours. 1+ to 2+ qualitatively.	(Proteinuria may be absent.) 5 gm or more per liter in 24 hours 3+ to 4+ qualitatively.
Possibly present.	Probably present; face edema.
2 pounds or more per week or 6 pounds or more per month.	2 pounds or more per week.
	Possible nausea and/or vomiting. Epigastric pain.
	Scotoma (blind spots). Photophobia, blurred vision. Headache.
Possible hyperreflexia (not present earlier).	Hyperreflexia; clonus.
	Pulmonary edema; cyanosis.
Normal to decreased renal function.	Decreased renal function. Oliguria (less than 500 ml/24 hours). Anuria possible.
	Decreased blood flow.
	Decreased fetal movement.
	Rising level. Rises. Elevated. Reduced. Level exceeding 7 mg/100 ml.

Potential Adverse Outcomes	*Factors Associated with Risk*
Maternal death.	**First pregnancy.**
Fetal death.	**Under age 20 or over age 35.**
Premature labor.	**Malnutrition.**
Fetal growth retardation.	**Chronic hypertension or other vascular disease.**
Mental retardation.	**Diabetes mellitus.**
Abruptio placentae.	**Multiple pregnancy.**
Intravascular coagulation fibrinolysis (ICF) syndrome.	**Polyhydramnios.**
Massive intracranial hemorrhage.	**Trophoblastic disease.**
Grand mal seizure (eclampsia).	**Chronic renal disease.**
Bilateral cortical necrosis of the kidney or tubular necrosis.	**Hydrops fetalis.**
	Previous preeclampsia, eclampsia, or hypertension.
	Poor health care.
	Family history of preeclampsia, eclampsi or hypertension.
	Inadequate prenatal care.

Nursing Concerns" by Lois Sonstegard, *MCN* 4:90–95, March/April 1979.)

Dietary, endocrine, genetic, toxic, hemodynamic, stress, uterine stretch reflex, and immunologic mechanisms have all been cited as possible causes of pregnancy-induced hypertension. Researchers also have suggested that preeclampsia may involve a partial breakdown of mechanisms that ensure that the fetoplacental unit is not rejected as an allograft. The possible association of circulating antigen-antibody complexes with the development of pregnancy-induced hypertension continues to be investigated (2,3).

Judith Lueck and her colleagues more recently have observed multiple forms of a helminth-like organism, *Hydatoxi lualba*, in association with the trophoblast of hydatidiform mole and placentas from toxemic women (4). However, the exact mechanisms involved in the progressive development of toxemia remain to be determined (5). Uteroplacental ischemia is believed to play a key role in the genesis of pregnancy-induced hypertension, although it is not known whether it is a primary event or is secondary to hypertension-related vasospasm (6).

Associated Pathologic Changes

Various pathologic changes in many of the body's systems, particularly the vascular system, are associated with pregnancy-induced hypertension.(See table "Associations with Pregnancy-Induced Hypertension.") One of the most notable changes in the vascular system, vasospasm, causes arterial hypertension. Vasospasm and hypertension are in some way related to the presence of chorionic villi (with or without a fetus); these conditions are more likely to develop when there is an overabundance of trophoblastic tissue, which occurs in cases of multiple fetuses, hydatidiform mole, erythroblastosis fetalis, and maternal diabetes (2).

Other changes associated with pregnancy-induced hypertension include a lessening or absence of the normal rise in blood volume, resulting in hemoconcentration, coagulopathy, and hemolysis (7). Plasma levels of renin, angiotensin II, and aldosterone decrease, while vascular sensitivity to pressor hormones increases. Reduced maternal perfusion of the placenta, with increased uterine activity both spontaneously and in response to oxytocin, contributes to greater risk of uterine hyperstimulation with oxytocin. Decreased placental function, in turn, retards fetal growth. (See "Placental Function and Its Role in Toxemia" by Anna M. Tichy and Dianne Chong, *MCN* 4:84–89, March/April 1979.)

Renal blood flow and glomerular filtration are reduced as pregnancy-induced hypertension develops. The concentration of uric acid in blood plasma commonly is elevated because of decreased clearance by the kidney. Fluid changes often occur, with an accumulation of extracellular fluid above normal pregnancy levels. However, the presence of such edema by itself does not indicate a poor pregnancy outcome. Similarly, a lack of appreciable edema in instances of preeclampsia or eclampsia does not signal a more favorable pregnancy outcome (2).

Early Nursing Focus

Monitoring early for the potential or signs of preeclampsia helps to protect both mother and baby. Since the disease may be influenced by characteristics of the individual woman as well as the environment, the nurse must assess a number of variables, including the expectant mother's blood pressure, weight, and diet as well as the development of proteinuria and edema (8).

Blood pressure. Generally, hypertension is diagnosed when blood pressure is greater than 140/90 mmHg. It also is indicated if systolic pressure rises by at least 30 mmHg or diastolic pressure rises by at least 15 mmHg on at least two occasions six or more hours apart.

During pregnancy, however, certain variations in blood pressure are normal. For example, an older primigravida tends to have higher blood pressure than her younger counterpart, although blood pressure usually falls with succeeding pregnancies up to a parity of five. In addition, late in the first trimester until near term, systolic pressure often decreases by 20 to 30 mmHg and diastolic pressure by 10 to 15 mmHg. During this period, blood pressure greater than 120/80 mmHg may be considered elevated (6).

Of course, blood pressure measurements tend to vary according to the individuals recording them; the size of the arm cuff being used (narrow or short cuffs may cause readings to be 5 to 10 mmHg above their actual values); the position of the individual being examined; and the selection of the end point for recording diastolic pressure (9). Most American authorities use the fifth phase of Korotkoff, or disappearance of sound, to represent true diastolic pressure (3).

A persisting diastolic pressure of 90 mmHg or more is considered abnormal. Nearly 25 percent of all cases of eclampsia occur when blood pressure is considered to be borderline, while about 50 percent occur when blood pressure is less than 160/110 mmHg (10).

One study of blood pressure during and following the first pregnancies of adolescents suggests that gestational hypertension may simply be unmasking latent hypertension. When compared

RECORD OF FINDINGS AT PRENATAL VISITS

Neg – Pos + Date	Headaches	Dizziness/Visual Problem	Nausea/Vomiting	Edema—Face or Hands	Bleeding/Discharge	Abdominal Pain/Cramping	Constipation	Urinary Complaints	Fetal Movements Daily by History	Weeks of Gestation	Fundal Heights (cms)	Fetal Heart Rate Doppler (D) Fetoscope (F)	Presentation/Lie	Weight	Blood Pressure	Albumin	Sugar	Ketones	Allergies: Remarks/Signed
eb 11	–	Dizz +	–/–	–	–/–	–	–	–	–	10	–	(D) + 156	–	133	116/64	–	–	–	urine pregnancy test Positive on Feb 5
eb 20	–	–	+/+	–	–/–	–	–	+	–	11	–	(D)+ 152	–	132	102/60	+ Trace	–	–	Urinary complaints
eb 28	Mild +	–	N+/V-	–	–/–	–	–	–	–	12	–	(D) + 148	–	132½	100/60	–	–	–	Pregnancy classes recommended
ar 15	+	–	N+/V-	–	–/–	–	–	–	–	14	6	(D)+ 156	–	134	100/58	–	–	–	Attending "early pregnancy" classes
ar 29	Mild +	–	–/–	–	–/–	–	–	–	–	16	13	(D)+ 148	–	135½	98/56	–	–	–	Prenatal Vitamins
pr 11	–	–	–/–	–	–/–	–	–	–	–	18	16	(D)+ 152	–	137½	98/58	–	–	–	Individual counseling c̄ social workers
pr 22	–	–	–/–	–	–/–	–	–	–	+	20	18	(F) + 144	–	139	100/58	–	–	–	FHT + c̄ fetoscope Quickening 1 wk ago
ay 6	–	–	–/–	–	–/–	–	+	–	+	22	20	(F)+ 152	–	141½	96/54	–	–	–	Attending "mid-pregnancy" classes
ay 28	–	–	–/–	–	–/–	–	–	–	+	25	23	(F)+ 140	–	144	96/56	–	–	–	Low Hgb & Hct 11 gm 33.5%
un 18	–	–	–/–	–	/	Pain LLQ	–	–	+	28	27	(F)+ 156	Br	146½	96/54	–	–	–	Ⓛ Round Ligament pain- Body mechanics Demonstrated
ul 1	–	–	–/–	–	–/–	–	–	–	+	30	28	(F)+ 144	Ceph	148	98/56	–	Trace	–	Individual Counseling re: Plans Rollover test positive
ul 15	–	–	–/–	–	–/–	–	–	–	+	32	30	(F)+ 136	Ceph	149¾	102/58	–	–	–	Attending "Childbirth prep" classes. Rollover ⊕
ul 30	–	–	–/–	p.m. feet	–/–	–	–	–	+	34	32	(F) + 152	Ceph	152	106/62	–	–	–	Low Back discomfort – exercises practiced
ug 6	–	–	–/–	p.m feet	–/–	–	–	–	+	35	33	(F) + 138	Ceph	152½	112/66	–	–	–	Upward trend in B.P. – watch closely
ug 9	–	–	–/–	p.m. feet	–/–	–	–	–	+	35½	33	(D) + 156	Vtx	153	116/64	–	–	–	Hgb & Hct improved 12 gm 38%
ug 12	–	–	–/–	Hands Face Feet	–/–	–	–	–	+	36	34	(F)+ 148	Vtx	159	126/82	Trace	–	–	Rapid wt & B.P. rise Admitted - High risk unit

with women in a matched control group six and nine years after giving birth, the women who had a history of hypertension during pregnancy still had higher blood pressure. Also, the blood pressure of these women correlated with the high blood pressure of their children and their own mothers (11).

Weight. Among primigravidas, the development of hypertension has been associated with obesity (12). After a woman's first pregnancy, obesity or increased weight gain above 30 pounds apparently does not predispose the expectant mother to hypertension. However, a pattern of weight gain of more than two pounds per week or six pounds per month should be suspect for impending pregnancy-induced hypertension (10). For some women, sudden and excessive weight gain is the first sign of preeclampsia.

Diet. Evidence suggests that diet has an influence on the etiology of preeclampsia. Thomas Brewer has shown that adequate nutrition reduces the incidence of hypovolemia and hypoperfusion during pregnancy (13). Expectant mothers need a sufficient amount of protein as well as adequate caloric intake, especially if they are predisposed to pregnancy-induced hypertension (14). (See "The Community Health Nurse's Nutrition Guidelines"

NURSING PROCESS RECORD

Date	Problem Identification	Nursing Diagnoses	Action/Intervention	Evaluation*
Feb. 11	Fifteen-year-old nullipara (Janet). Unplanned pregnancy. No continuing relationship or contact with father of baby; does not wish to see him. Requested prenatal care, expressing desire for provider staff assistance throughout pregnancy.	Health status altered; at risk in pregnancy (psychosocial and biophysical). Developmental adolescent tasks compromised by superimposed pregnancy developmental tasks. Relationship with significant other altered. Vulnerability in personal relationships and own self-concept. Sexuality development conflicts.	Ongoing assessment of family and other support units. Lend staff support as indicated. Encourage Janet to attend special adolescent group education and counseling (early-, mid-, and late-pregnancy groups) and to take responsibility for participating in her own health maintenance. Multidisciplinary team care by nurse, physician, social worker nutritionist, and others as indicated. Plan for postpartum follow-up counseling in regard to her feelings about sexual relationships and future decision making about her sexuality.	*__Maintain frequent schedule of prenatal visits with close involvement of family.__* (Janet and family kept all appointments; mother and father visited periodically to request information and to contribute to planning Janet's care.) *__Everything that is done is to become part of the teaching process.__* *__Participates in group educational sessions with multidisciplinary team and in her own assessments at each visit.__* (Checks her own weight and urine with supervision. Later in pregnancy, assists in measuring uterine growth and in palpating for fetal movements and position.) Assists in recording of these for her own health record.
Feb. 20	Occasional mild nausea and vomiting (morning only). Weight loss. Sometimes skips breakfast.	Alterations in hormonal and gastrointestinal functioning during first trimester. Nutritional sufficiency compromised for meeting pregnancy needs.	Suggestions given for diet changes to reduce nausea in morning, following assessment of present nutrition pattern. Encouraged to take along for morning snacks and eating en route to school: fruit, boiled eggs, raw vegetables, peanut butter, crackers, and so forth.	*__Acceptance and use of information.__* *__Nausea decreased__* in one week, and weight gain resumed.
Feb. 20	"Burning" sensation while urinating and "hurting low" in abdomen. (Medical diagnosis: urinary tract infection.)	Urinary elimination altered by pregnancy; dysuria present. Health management: preventive self-care needed. Risk of urinary tract infection increased during pregnancy.	Instructed Janet about preventive care to follow throughout pregnancy to prevent bacteriuria and/or urinary symptoms; will recheck urinary status each visit. (Medical prescription of antibiotic for urinary tract infection.)	Janet reports increased intake of water (decreased soft drinks) and use of perineal washes after elimination. *__Monthly urine cultures remained negative; no further urinary symptoms.__*
Feb. 20	Missing school and feels tired and nauseated; asks why she feels this way.	Lacks information about normal and abnormal pregnancy changes.	Encouraged to begin pregnancy classes; to write down questions to bring to each visit; and to go to school.	*__Further questions stimulated and exploration of feelings and concerns precipitated__* as a result of classes. *Continued school.*
April 22	Concerned about getting heavier and hips and breasts becoming larger.	Altered body image because of pregnancy is intensified during adolescence.	Talked about body changes occurring, what they mean, and how she feels about them.	*__Continued to gain weight__* appropriate for her.
April 22	Doesn't know what friends at school and others will think about her being pregnant; feels ashamed. Not going out with friends [illegible]	Fear of rejection or reaction by others. Self-esteem diminished; expressions of shame. Social isolation; less social contact with peers.	Special individual counseling, allowing Janet to explore her feelings and to help sort out her own decisions and their possible short-term and long-term consequences. Encouraged parents' involvement in Janet's	*__Able to talk about concerns.__* *__Openly verbalized feelings and conflicts.__* Maintained peer relationships throughout pregnancy and *__successfully completed the school year__* in which pregnancy and de-

	Thinking about quitting school and getting a job; doesn't want parents' help.	Independence-dependence conflict; expresses anger and conflicting actions.	a family.	*Family support and consistency to facilitate growth in identity development and conflict resolution.* Both parents participated in counseling/planning sessions.
May 6	Constipation problem.	Altered bowel elimination because of pregnancy.	Suggested changes in diet: adding more fiber foods, fresh vegetables, fresh fruits, and fluids.	*Relief from constipation* after trial adjustments to diet and fluid intake.
May 28	Low hemoglobin (11 gm) and hematocrit (33.5%)	Altered nutritional-metabolic requirements during pregnancy. Fluid volume physiologic increase (hemodilutional effect).	Reassessment of nutritional pattern, counseling, and meal planning to supply identified deficiencies; emphasis on adequate protein and caloric content plus vitamin and mineral supplements.	*Appropriate weight gain pattern and rise in hemoglobin and hematocrit* indicated improved dietary pattern (goal for weight gain of about one pound per week during latter half of pregnancy).
June 18	Wanted to talk about adoption for baby; tears in eyes. Father expressed concern about her feelings; mother put arm around her.	Family coping/stress tolerance alteration. Coping growth potential indicated by expressions and actions. Feelings of conflict and indecision expressed. Grieving/anticipatory sadness expressed about coming loss of baby.	Family came together with provider staff and Janet to evaluate and work out problems through family mechanisms. Special counseling provided to assist in decision making about adoption.	*Evidence of strength* of family shown by mutual support and by taking responsibility. *Janet made decision* to have baby adopted. Anxious to return to school after delivery. Shows growth in making decisions and taking responsibility.
July 1	Supine pressor test is positive.	Indicator of risk for pregnancy-induced hypertension. High activity and low rest pattern.	Recommended daily rest periods in lateral recumbent position.	
Aug. 6	Complaints about not sleeping well; low backaches; and baby moving so much. Expressed fear of labor and delivery; wishes it was over.	Sleep pattern disturbance and discomforts of late pregnancy. Fears expressed (usual to late pregnancy). Vulnerable to embarrassment or being hurt physically or emotionally.	Normalcy of her fears explained; reassured her. Prepared in advance in as concrete terms as possible for what to expect and how to help; gentleness applied in all situations. Toured high-risk unit and labor and delivery area to familiarize Janet with setting.	*Able to express her concerns and verbalize fears.* Able to be dependent when needed. *Care administered by specially prepared staff* (antepartum, intrapartum, and later follow-up) and familiar persons throughout.
Aug. 6	Upward trend in blood pressure.	Indicator of risk for preeclampsia.	Bed rest at home; daily checks by community health nurse. On "homebound" school program.	*Close observation for early recognition of danger signs* for preeclampsia.
Aug. 12	Rapid increase of blood pressure and weight. (Medical diagnosis: preeclampsia.)	Potential alteration in fetal-placental circulation as well as compromise of fetal and/or maternal welfare.	Admitted to high-risk (limited ambulation) unit; accompanied to unit and introduced to the area by familiar staff persons. Family members were able to visit Janet daily. Main focus of care was ambulation as desired and a diet consisting of a minimum of 2,400 calories per day and one gram of protein per each kilogram of weight plus supplemental foods from home. Assessments of fetal and maternal well-being included laboratory tests (renal function, serial urinary protein and estriol levels), daily weight measurements, nonstress tests, frequent blood pressure tests, and elicitation of symptoms.	*Delivered seven-pound girl spontaneously at 40 weeks without major problems.*

*Based on stated outcome criteria (underlined).

by Barbara B. Deskins and Mary Fucile Laska, *MCN* 7:202-205, May/June 1982.)

Proteinuria. An increase in perinatal mortality is associated with proteinuria during pregnancy, regardless of blood pressure levels. Proteinuria accompanied by hypertension further increases the chance of perinatal death. Studies indicate that the dipstick method of testing urine for the presence of protein is reliable when using clean midstream or catheter specimens of urine. A 2+ or more reading of proteinuria is considered significant, a 1+ reading is questionable, and a trace is negligible (9).

Proteinuria frequently develops later than excessive weight gain and nearly always later than hypertension (2). Although 41 percent of eclamptics do not manifest proteinuria, it may be the most ominous sign of preeclampsia when it does develop (3,10).

Edema. By itself, edema is a common physiologic occurrence of pregnancy. However, in association with hypertension and proteinuria, edema is linked to a poor pregnancy outcome (9). Eclampsia may occur in 60 percent of women with only slight to moderate edema and in about 20 percent of women without edema (10). Since only about 15 percent of women with generalized edema develop preeclampsia, it is a very rough clinical parameter (3).

Determining Who Is at Risk

Two clinical tests, mean arterial pressure and the supine pressor (rollover) test, are useful in predicting a woman's chances of developing pregnancy-induced hypertension. Mean arterial pressure reflects the resistance against which the heart works and thus is an indicator of cardiac work. It is calculated by adding the diastolic pressure to one-third of the pulse pressure. For example, a blood pressure of 140/90 mmHg would equal a mean arterial pressure of 107 mmHg. (Note that blood pressures of 134/68 mmHg, 110/80 mmHg, and 130/70 mmHg all yield a mean arterial pressure of 90 mmHg.)

An increase of 20 mmHg in mean arterial pressure is considered ominous, as is blood pressure as low as 125/75 mmHg if it occurs before the thirty-second week of pregnancy. Perinatal morbidity and mortality have been shown to increase when midpregnancy mean arterial pressure is greater than 95 mmHg or when blood pressure rises above 130/80 mmHg (3,6,8). Additionally, in the absence of proteinuria or edema, a trend toward increased perinatal deaths has been noted when mean arterial pressure exceeds 92 mmHg by the beginning of the third trimester (8).

The supine pressor test, developed by Norman Gant and his colleagues, is based on the supine hypertensive response (15). For this test, done between 28 and 32 weeks' gestation, blood pressure is measured in the superior arm in the lateral recumbent position until stable. The woman then rolls over to the supine position, and blood pressure is measured immediately and again five minutes later. An increase of 20 mmHg or more in diastolic blood pressure while in the supine position is considered a positive indicator of potential development of pregnancy-induced hypertension (6,15).

A negative supine pressor test generally is accepted as sound evidence that pregnancy-induced hypertension will not develop (6). A single positive supine pressor test is accurate in predicting the development of pregnancy-induced hypertension in about 25 to 75 percent of all cases. One study showed that women who had two positive supine pressor tests and an average mean arterial pressure during the second trimester greater than 85 mmHg had an 88 percent chance of developing pregnancy-induced hypertension (16).

> *Evidence suggests that diet can influence the etiology of preeclampsia. Thomas Brewer has shown that adequate nutrition reduces the incidence of hypovolemia and hyperfusion during pregnancy. Expectant mothers need both a sufficient amount of protein and calories.*

Intervention Measures

When risk factors such as borderline elevations in blood pressure or rapid weight gain are present, prenatal assessments need to be made at weekly or biweekly intervals. Once the signs of preeclampsia are clearly recognized, hospitalization is indicated, with activities and care appropriate to the severity of the case. In instances of lesser severity, limited ambulation on a high-risk pregnancy unit may be appropriate. Bed rest in the lateral recumbent position is necessary for a large portion of the day, and a diet ample in protein and coloric content is essential.

Frequent surveillance for visual disturbance, epigastric pain, headaches, rapid weight gain, and proteinuria is required. Plasma creatinine is measured often. The precise age of the fetus is determined, and fetal growth, welfare, and size are evaluated regularly. The expectant mother can assess fetal movements by making a daily count (14).

The expectant mother's sodium and fluid intake is neither restricted nor encouraged. However, diuretics, especially thiazides, must be avoided. Diuretics are ineffective in deterring the course of preeclampsia/eclampsia, and they may further compromise intravascular volume as well as deplete sodium and potassium stores. For the infant, diuretics may cause decreased placental perfusion, thrombocytopenia, hyperbilirubinemia, and altered carbohydrate metabolism.

Antihypertensives also must be avoided unless diastolic pressure reaches 110 mmHg or more. Note that sodium restriction, antihypertensives, and diuretics have all been shown to decrease the placental clearance of dehydroepiandrosterone sulfate to estradiol and may thereby decrease uteroplacental perfusion (2,14,17).

A Case in Point

The following case example illustrates the kinds of basic care needed by women who are at risk of developing pregnancy-induced hypertension. It demonstrates how nursing care for an underlying medical problem is integrated with nursing care to meet other needs of the patient.

After a positive pregnancy test and early examination confirmed pregnancy, 15-year-old Janet received counseling and requested to continue being seen for prenatal care during her pregnancy. It was her first pregnancy. The health history for her family revealed that, for the previous two years, Janet's mother had regularly taken medication for high blood pressure. However, Janet had no previous health problems of significance.

Throughout her pregnancy, Janet was seen by a multidisciplinary team that worked closely with Janet's parents and a girl friend, her major support system. Because of her young age, the fact that she never had been pregnant before, a family history of hypertension, and positive supine pressor tests on two occasions, Janet was assessed at frequent intervals. When she experienced rapid weight gain and rising blood pressure, she was hospitalized.

Janet's care included limited ambulation, adequate diet, and close surveillance during the last weeks of pregnancy. (The findings for each prenatal visit are summarized in the accompanying charts.) As a result of this care, Janet's pregnancy culminated in an uncomplicated, vaginal birth.

A Better Chance

Expectant mothers who are at risk of developing pregnancy-induced hypertension need to be identified as early as possible. For the woman who has a hypertensive disorder, frequent monitoring of her condition throughout pregnancy and appropriate care measures can improve her chances of having a successful pregnancy outcome.

REFERENCES

1. BEER, A. E. Possible immunologic bases of preeclampsia/eclampsia. *Semin.Perinatol.* 2:39–56, Jan. 1978.
2. PRITCHARD, J. A. AND MACDONALD, P. C. *Williams Obstetrics.* 16th ed. New York, Appleton-Century-Crofts, 1980, pp. 665–697.
3. CAVANAGH, DENIS, AND KNUPPEL, R. A. Preeclampsia and eclampsia. IN *Principles and Practice of Obstetrics and Perinatology*, ed. by Leslie Iffy and H. A. Kaminetzky. New York, John Wiley & Sons, 1981, pp. 1271–1290.
4. LUECK, JUDITH, AND OTHERS. Observation of an organism found in patients with gestational trophoblastic disease and in patients with toxemia of pregnancy. *Am.J.Obstet.Gynecol.* 145:15–26, Jan. 1, 1983.
5. ALADJEM, SILVIO, AND OTHERS. Experimental induction of a toxemia-like syndrome in the pregnant beagle. *Am.J.Obstet.Gynecol.* 145:27–38, Jan. 1, 1983.
6. O'SHANUGHNESSY, RICHARD, AND ZUSPAN, F. P. Managing acute pregnancy hypertension. *Contemp.OB/GYN* 18:85–98, Nov. 1981.
7. CUNNINGHAM, F. G., AND PRITCHARD, J. A. Hematologic considerations of pregnancy-induced hypertension. *Semin.Perinatol.* 2:29–38, Jan. 1978.
8. WELT, S. I., AND CRENSHAW, M. C., JR. Concurrent hypertension and pregnancy. *Clin.Obstet.Gynecol.* 21:619–648, Sept. 1978.
9. DAVIES, A. M. Epidemiology of the hypertensive disorders of pregnancy. *Bull.WHO* 57(3):373–386, 1979.
10. HALVERSON, G. M. Toxemia in pregnancy. *Wis.Med.J.* 79:27–28, July 1979.
11. KOTCHEN, J. M., AND OTHERS. Blood pressure of young mothers and their children after hypertension in adolescent pregnancy: six-to-nine year follow-up. *Am.J.Epidemiol.* 115:861–867, June 1982.
12. FRIEDMAN, E. A., AND NEFF, R. K. *Pregnancy Hypertension: A Systematic Evaluation of Clinical Diagnosis Critera.* Littleton, Mass., John Wright—PSG, 1977, pp. 204–212.
13. BREWER, T. Role of malnutrition in pre-eclampsia and eclampsia. *Am.J.Obstet.Gynecol.* 125:281–282, May 15, 1976.
14. GILSTRAP, L. C., III, AND OTHERS. Management of pregnancy-induced hypertension in the nulliparous patient remote from term. *Semin.Perinatol.* 2:73–81, Jan. 1978.
15. GANT, N. F., AND OTHERS. A clinical test useful for predicting the development of acute hypertension in pregnancy. *Am.J.Obstet.Gynecol.* 120:1–7, Sept. 1, 1974.
16. PHELAN, J. P. Enhanced prediction of pregnancy-induced hypertension by combining supine pressor test with mean arterial pressure of middle trimester. *Am.J.Obstet.Gynecol.* 129:397–400, Oct. 15, 1977.
17. MATHEWS, D. D., AND OTHERS. A randomized controlled trial of complete bed rest versus ambulation in the management of proteinuric hypertension during pregnancy. *Obstet.Gynecol.Surv.* 38:94–95, Feb. 1983.

BIBLIOGRAPHY

GANT, N. F., AND OTHERS. Clinical management of pregnancy-induced hypertension. *Clin.Obstet.Gyneol.* 21:397–409, June 1978.

KELLEY, MAUREEN. Maternal position and blood pressure during pregnancy and delivery. *Am.J.Nurs.* 82:809, May 1982.

_____., AND MONGIELLO, ROSANNE. Labor, delivery, and postpartum. *Am.J.Nurs.* 82:813, May 1982.

WILLIS, S. E. Hypertension in pregnancy, pathophysiology. *Am.J.Nurs.* 82:791–792, May 1982.

_____., AND SHARP, E. S. Prenatal detection and management. *Am.J.Nurs.* 82:798, May 1982.

DEATH BEFORE BIRTH

BY CONNIE M. WHITAKER

Sad personal experience taught this perinatal nurse what should be done for a mother whose baby dies in utero.

Reprinted from American Journal of Nursing, February 1986.

Perinatal nursing is usually rewarding: Daily, we see parents overjoyed with tiny new additions to their families. But when a baby dies, whether in utero or in the neonatal period, parents need a great deal of support. I know, because it happened to me.

The mother is usually the first to suspect that the baby has died. She slowly realizes that her baby has stopped moving. She may push on her abdomen, hoping to feel the familiar little kick in response to her touch. Anxiety and doubt creep in. The mother vacillates: She expects the baby to move, yet she knows that it will not. She rationalizes: "The baby is tired—he needs rest," or "The baby is just in a quiet phase."

I suspected that something was wrong when I noticed that my baby had not moved since early in the day. The next morning, the baby was still not moving—and morning was usually an active time for him. I kept thinking that this could not happen to me, that I wanted my baby too much to lose him.

Later in the day I called my obstetrician and went in to have the fetal heart tones checked. My fears were confirmed: We could not hear the fetal heart.

Even as I denied and rationalized, I knew that the baby had died. All night I reviewed obsessively the events leading up to the death of my baby.

The next day I was admitted to the labor and delivery unit where I worked. It was a great comfort to me to see my friends and co-workers. Later, I thought of all the women in my position who saw only strangers, just when they most needed warmth, comfort, and support. As I reflected on my feelings and those of my husband, I jotted down the following reminders for my future nursing care of grieving parents:

A woman whose baby has died in utero needs to be in a room where she may be alone with her partner or support person—without unnecessary noises or interruptions. Imagine trying to cope with grief while hearing cheerful banter from the nurse's station.

Allow the partner to stay with the patient until delivery. Inform hospital staff of a diagnosis of fetal death before they enter the patient's room. That way, upsetting remarks can be avoided. If possible, alert the admitting clerk before the patient arrives so that no unnecessary questions are asked.

Usually, the patient is admitted for external monitoring of the fetal heart and for a sonogram. Be sure an experienced nurse listens for heart tones so that the process is not prolonged, especially if fetal death is not yet confirmed. It was very difficult for me to lie there and listen and hope, only to hear the Doppler's cathedral silence. Once fetal death is confirmed, avoid listening "one more time" for the heartbeat.

If at all possible, have the same nurse care for the patient from admission until after delivery. Having someone with her who is at least a little familiar helps a great deal.

Sonogram is usually the next step. Be sure to explain what ultrasound is, that it is painless, and why it is important to have a full bladder before the test is done. Other indications that may also confirm fetal death are: the presence of gas in the abdominal cavity and abdominal arteries on x-ray; Spalding's sign, the collapse and overlapping of cranial bones; and levels of chorionic gonadotropin, maternal urinary estriol, and maternal alpha-fetoprotein.

Although each patient reacts to fetal death in her own way, I doubt that I could have withstood the emotional trauma of going home to wait for labor to begin spontaneously. I felt that delivery of the fetus would help me to accept the death and begin to grieve.

The next morning, I had an amniocentesis. The fluid return was brown, a final indication of fetal demise. Within a few hours of prostaglandin injection I was in labor, and that evening I delivered a male infant who had no apparent abnormalities. Seeing the baby and holding it, I began to accept that the baby had died. I asked myself why: Why did this perfect little baby, who was wanted so badly, die? What had I done to cause the death of the baby? I guess every mother of a stillborn asks these questions and, like me, finds no answers.

Patients with stillborns need to be

At the time this article was written, Connie M. Whitaker, RN, BSN, was perinatal supervisor at Greene Memorial Hospital, Xenia, OH.

PETER FIORE

'DID WE DO ALL WE COULD?'

BY JOELLEN W. HAWKINS

In the maternal-child area, healthy babies and women are the rule rather than the exception, unless of course, the population is skewed in the high-risk category. Maternal mortality is low and only about 2 percent of all infants are born with severe anomalies(1). Maternal-child staff seem lulled into the security of the general cheer that pervades most units. Tragedy—a stillbirth, for example—tends to catch even the most experienced staff off guard.

Working as a staff nurse and as clinical instructor in maternal-child nursing for several years, I have witnessed many heartbreaking situations. On one unusual four-month clinical rotation with undergraduate nursing students, I saw several tragedies, one after another.

The spontaneous delivery of an 18- to 20-week stillborn fetus to a woman with a poor reproductive history began the series. The nurses seemed to need to talk about the birth as though seeking reassurance that they had done all they could. Together we looked at the perfectly formed fetus and the small, infarcted placenta. We vacillated between clinical discussion and expressions of anger, grief, and sorrow.

The next day, a staff nurse lost her much-wanted infant in a spontaneous abortion. The rest of us reacted strongly, some with anger, others with tears, as we tried both to rationalize the event and to support each other.

The cesarean birth of an anencephalic infant to a couple who had previously had a spontaneous abortion all but devastated the staff. The physician's decision not to feed the baby brought the nursery staff to me seeking support for their need to care for and nurture the infant. We shared feelings, tears, and the sorrow we felt for the parents and for the tiny anomalous infant who lived for several days. With the physician's acquiescence, we fed the baby, and stroked and cuddled him.

An abruptio placentae and subsequent loss of a baby was next. The cumulative effect of these tragedies was beginning to show. Tempers flared, and staff seemed less attentive to women with problems.

The event that nearly precipitated a crisis for the staff was a rare complication—acute fatty liver of pregnancy. The young woman who was affected was carrying her third child. She was jaundiced and in acute distress. She had felt no fetal movement for two days. After a few hours in our labor unit, she was transferred to a large women's hospital in town. For days, the nurses followed her progress through the loss of her baby, her critical phase, and her slow recovery. They were as distressed by the possibility of the mother's death as by the baby's.

The staff felt each of these tragedies deeply, identifying closely with the women whose babies were lost. Most of these women had been in childbirth classes and, with their partners, were anticipating the joyful sharing of the birth after their nine months of waiting.

Women who have high-risk deliveries need to fill in any missing data about their labor and delivery experiences, to understand the events and share them with others who were there(2). So, too, it seems, do nurses who witness a tragedy on the maternal-child unit. They have to go over what happened, to review whether everything was tried that could have been, and to identify the role each person played. Moreover, just as the woman needs assurance that the crisis with her infant is not her fault, so do her nurses.

Mercer has described the tasks of a mother of a defective child(3). Some apply equally well to nurses caring for families who have lost a baby. Appraisal of self as a mother and as a person parallels the nurse's reassessment of herself as a care provider. It is also common for the nurse to find herself the target of the aggressive feelings of a parent who has lost a child. A nurse who is under attack needs support to be able to continue caring for a woman in crisis.

Clinicians, supervisors, head nurses, primary nurses, clinical faculty, and staff nurses are all in a position to assess stress in a co-worker and to provide support. Small group discussions, informal sharing sessions, and one-to-one talks can all help. Touching and feeding an infant with a fatal anomaly may be easier if two staff members work together. Newer staff members can benefit most when more experienced staff are there to lend a hand. It is important to recognize that the feelings and responses of nurses to tragic human experiences are those of caring men and women as well as of professionals.

Joellen W. Hawkins, RN, PhD, is professor and coordinator, maternal-child health graduate nursing program, Boston College, Chestnut Hill, MA.

REFERENCES

1. Vaughn, V. C., and others, eds. *Nelson's Textbook of Pediatrics.* 12th ed. Philadelphia, W. B. Saunders Co., 1983, p. 311.
2. Affonso, D. D. "Missing pieces"—a study of postpartum feelings. *Birth Fam.J.* 4:159-164, Winter 1977.
3. Mercer, R. T. Responses of mothers to the birth of an infant with a defect. IN *ANA Clinical Sessions, American Nurses' Association 1974, San Francisco.* New York, Appleton-Century-Crofts, 1975, p. 341.

allowed to decide whether to be sedated during labor and delivery or to remain awake. I chose to be sedated, fearing the baby might be anencephalic. I also saw no reason for going through the discomfort of labor without the reward.

Some physicians and nurses advise against showing the patient and her partner the dead baby. I guess they feel that they are protecting the parents. Before having a stillborn, I agreed, but I don't believe that I fully accepted the death of my baby until I saw him for myself. I consider the few moments that I had with my son very important: The memories of those moments are all that I have left of my second child.

If the parents decide to see the baby, prepare them. Tell them that the baby will be cold and discolored. Explain any abnormalities or maceration. Be sure the baby is clean and wrapped in a blanket. If the parents wish, leave them alone with the baby, but assure them that you will be close by. Grandparents and other family members may be allowed to see the baby, if they and the parents wish.

When we grieve, we are accepting that someone very important to us is gone. Never assume that because a baby is immature, or because he is yet unborn, the mother has not formed a close bond with him. Long before the baby is moving, he has become a very important person to his mother.

Obvious mourning is usually a positive sign. Being able to break down and cry and talk about the baby may help the mother. I wanted to talk to anyone who came near me. I needed to talk about the delivery. Remember that manifestations of grief vary considerably from person to person.

After delivery, let the patient decide whether to stay on the postpartum unit. Ask the staff to assure the patient that they have the time to listen. Let the patient know that you are upset about her loss. Be honest and open. It is all right to cry with the patient, to touch her, and to let her know that you really care.

Above all, be sensitive. Do not put a patient with a stillborn in the same room with a mother of a live baby, and try not to put her into a room where she might hear other babies crying. Never assume that remarks like, "You can always have another baby," "The baby was premature anyway," or "You have other children" can *ever* provide any comfort at all. Quite the contrary. □

Care of Postpartum Adolescents

An effective relationship with adolescent mothers is built on understanding their unique cognitive and emotional needs.

SUZANNE A. FULLAR

Today in the United States approximately 16 percent of all births and 28 percent of all first births are to women less than 20 years of age (1). Of adolescent women who deliver, 96 percent choose to keep and rear their children (2). As a result, many postpartum nurses will find themselves caring for newly delivered adolescent mothers—often a very different experience than caring for an adult woman.

Adolescent pregnancy and motherhood superimpose a situational crisis upon the ongoing developmental crisis of adolescence. While the adolescent is physically mature, she may not have achieved a parallel degree of cognitive and emotional development. Behavior that would not be tolerated in an adult woman may be normal for an adolescent patient. Teaching strategies and assessment tools designed for adults may be ineffective or inappropriate for adolescents.

The accompanying Adolescent Postpartum Care Plan is part of a larger plan developed for use by nurses who care for postpartum adolescents delivering through the Rochester Adolescent Maternity Program at the University of Rochester Medical Center. A series of generic Kardex have been created by nurses at the medical center to organize data collection, provide measurable goals for nursing care, and reduce documentation time. The care plan becomes a part of the patient's permanent record following delivery.

The plan is based on the developmental knowledge that adolescence is a time of great physical, social, and cognitive change. Physical growth is second only to that of infancy. As secondary sex characteristics develop, these changes must be integrated into a sense of self as male or female. The adolescent must also move from dependence on the family of origin to independence—economic, geographic, and emotional. Peer relationships aid in this task as well as in the formation of a separate identity. A growing ability to think abstractly enables the adolescent to anticipate future events, consider complex moral questions, and appreciate the needs and feelings of others.

SUZANNE A. FULLAR, R.N., M.S., *is a pediatric nurse practitioner and project nurse with the Rochester Adolescent Maternity Program at the University of Rochester Medical Center in Rochester, New York.*

The period may be divided into three stages to better understand what the teen may be like at a particular age and how to most effectively care for her. Because each adolescent is different from her peers and develops at her own rate, however, it is important to view the given ages as guidelines rather than fixed limits. The table Stages of Adolescence shows how each one brings about changes in the adolescent's life that not only affect how she sees and deals with her world, but also how others view and react to her.

Establishing a Relationship

Understanding normal adolescent behavior will help the postpartum nurse establish realistic expectations for the adolescent mother. This in turn will facilitate development of a positive nurse-patient relationship, which is the key to supportive nursing care and effective patient teaching.

In order to establish such a relationship, however, the nurse needs to be aware of her own feelings about these patients and about her own adolescent years. Teenage sexuality, pregnancy, and motherhood are all highly emotional issues, and most professionals are justifiably concerned and apprehensive about adolescent parenting. Infants of adolescent mothers experience more accidents and more developmental delays (3–6). The teen mother herself is often disadvantaged educationally, vocationally, and socially (7,8). While preliminary data indicate that adolescents interact differently with their infants than do adult women, a lack of research controlling for socioeconomic status makes these findings tentative (8,9).

But developing a relationship with the younger mother is not always easy. Teenagers are often awkward in social situations and mistrust authority figures, particularly those of a different race or social class. Remaining nonjudgmental is the most important rule in gaining an adolescent's trust. This may mean that the nurse must get beyond her own feelings about teen pregnancy, overlook the younger mother's preoccupation with her appearance, and focus instead on positive aspects, such as how she holds and talks to her infant.

The nurse can also make an effort to get to know the young woman as an individual. Ask her about herself, and not just about the baby. Although she is proud of her newborn, the teen's normal egocentrism demands that she be the center of attention. Start with her most immediate concerns. What was labor like? Who was with her? How is she feeling now? What does she need? Often an adolescent who was not very communicative during the prenatal course will suddenly begin to talk following delivery, as if a giant weight of fear and apprehension had been lifted. Having someone listen emphathically will help her work through the labor and delivery experience, correct misconceptions, and develop trust in her nurse.

Many teens find it difficult to talk spontaneously and need help from a sensitive nurse to express their feelings. While open-ended questions or long silences may only increase their anxiety, gentle inquiries may help them feel at ease. It is sometimes useful to suggest that young mothers often "feel like this" or "wonder about this," thus assuring the patient that her feelings are normal and making it easier for her to discuss her concerns. Questioning her checklist-style, on the other hand, will produce a minimum of information and create distrust, particularly if the teen senses that the nurse is interested less in her than in completing a hospital form.

Assessing the Family

In addition to asking about her labor, delivery, and postpartum experiences, the nurse needs to learn about the young mother's life at home. Who are the other members of her household? What preparations have been made for the baby? Who will be helping her, and for how long? This is especially important for a younger teen or for one who plans to return to school. It is also advisable to find out whether the young woman has any problems with her family. As the teen talks about her home life, her plans, and her expectations regarding motherhood, the nurse can begin to place her in one of the three developmental stages. This will help determine whether her plans are realistic and whether the family is sufficiently involved.

When family members visit, ask how they view the young mother. Do they think she is capable of parenting? Are they concerned but eager to help, or do they see the baby as "her problem"? Will they provide the assistance she expects? She may anticipate more support than they can give, but she may also say there is no one to help although several relatives have offered. How does the teen respond to members of her family when they visit? These interactions will indicate fairly clearly the state of family relationships and the amount of support that can be expected following discharge. Many parents who reacted with hurt or anger to the pregnancy become enthusiastic at the birth of a grandchild and supportive of a daughter in need. The adolescent may also be more willing to accept her family's support at this time.

It is important as well to find out about the father of the baby. Few adolescent mothers will be married; many others will not be in touch with the baby's father and may be involved in an entirely new relationship. This can be a very sensitive area and should be approached with care. The nurse can ask the teen if the father knows about the delivery and if he is planning to visit. Then she can gently determine what the relationship is at present and how the adolescent would like it to

STAGES OF ADOLESCENCE

Area	*Early Adolescent* 11–14	*Mid-Adolescent* 15–17	*Late Adolescent* 18–20
Body	Rapid changes leading to discomfort and self-consciousness; body image in flux	Growing comfort with body	Acceptance of adult body
Family	Strong but ambivalent ties to family	Struggle for independence and autonomy; constant testing of limits	Reestablishment of ties with family
Peers	Same-sex friends most common	Strong peer influence assists in separation from family	Individual relationships sought and valued
Sexuality	Undifferentiated relationships with same and opposite sex; fantasy common but actual activity infrequent	Sexual experimentation and risk taking; need to feel grown-up; tendency to be easily influenced	Intimate, committed relationships sought
Cognition	Concrete, here-and-now thinking; inability to appreciate long-term consequences of actions; denial as major defense	Impulsive and unpredictable behavior; variable ability to think abstractly	Abstract thinking achieved by most but not all
Identity	Self-concept changing from child to adult; awkward and shy in social situations; authority figures looked to for guidance	Preoccupation with self and own concerns; moodiness; limited social skills; authority figures viewed as threats to autonomy	Ability to appreciate others' needs and feelings; authority figures viewed as equals

be. Often teens who have ended a relationship months ago with few regrets will become tearful when their baby is born without a father present or involved. Some may also have expected the delivery to bring back an estranged boyfriend.

Finally, the nurse must assess the adolescent and her infant. Who does she feel the baby looks like? Does he meet her expectations? Is she enthusiastic about holding him and showing him off, or does she keep him in his bassinette and hold him only when she is encouraged to do so? Her apparent disinterest may be the result of a number of factors—inexperience, exhaustion following delivery, anxiety about being in the hospital, disappointment with the real versus the expected baby, or fears about the child's normalcy—to name just a few.

Most adolescents have little idea how a normal newborn looks and behaves, nor will they talk about things that worry them, such as moulding of the head or forceps marks. Cord care may be frightening to the teen, but instead of asking for help she may simply do nothing. The young mother may believe that a normal newborn's lack of interest in feeding during the first 24 hours is a reflection on her ("he doesn't like me") or on the infant ("he's a bad baby and won't eat"). Many adolescent mothers are afraid that they will spoil their baby by holding it, and few understand the newborn's visual and auditory abilities. The nurse can reassure the young mother and facilitate bonding by explaining normal newborn appearance and behavior and helping her identify her infant's cues.

It is also important to observe the young mother with her infant and try to understand her interaction with him in the context of the developmental stage she has reached. How does she respond when the baby cries? Does she try to figure out why he is unhappy and attempt different strategies until he is quieted? Or does she try to feed him and then hand him over to the nurse or to her mother if she is not immediately successful, or even worse, give up and lay him in the bassinette? The older adolescent is most able to identify a problem, think of alternative solutions, appraise the possible benefits and drawbacks of each, and try them one by one. These problem-solving skills will enable her to respond appropriately to most of her child's needs. Unfortunately, the early or mid-adolescent usually lacks this cognitive maturity and needs adult supervision, guidance, and support to parent effectively.

Teaching the Teenager

The intellectual and cognitive abilities of an adolescent are not always easy to assess, but these limitations must be considered if patient teaching is to be effective. Some adolescents have failed in school, and others may be mentally retarded or in special education classes. The nurse can often identify a teen's learning problems by asking her about school—the last grade she completed, classes she liked and disliked, and any special education classes she may have taken.

As a result of such negative school experiences, some teens may dislike attending formal hospital classes. A young mother who does not have the self-control or attention span required to sit through an hour-long class on infant care may enjoy a hands-on, one-to-one teaching session with her nurse. Such teaching with a live infant is particularly effective with younger mothers, whose thinking is still fairly concrete and focused on the "here-and-now."

Forming a small group class is another useful technique. Teens feel more at ease with their peers, and in this atmosphere they can also learn from each other—an approach that is particularly useful when teaching about birth control. Those who have used contraception in the past can talk about their positive and negative experiences with each method, and then the group can discuss how to use contraceptives effectively.

Many adolescent mothers have spent years caring for younger siblings, so it is wise to find out how much each patient knows before beginning to teach. This shows respect for the teen's past experience and avoids alienating her from the start. Positively reinforcing even small parts of desirable behaviors is the most effective way to encourage change. Many teens are rarely told they are doing something right and respond well to such praise,

Many teens find it difficult to talk spontaneously and need help from a sensitive nurse to express their feelings.

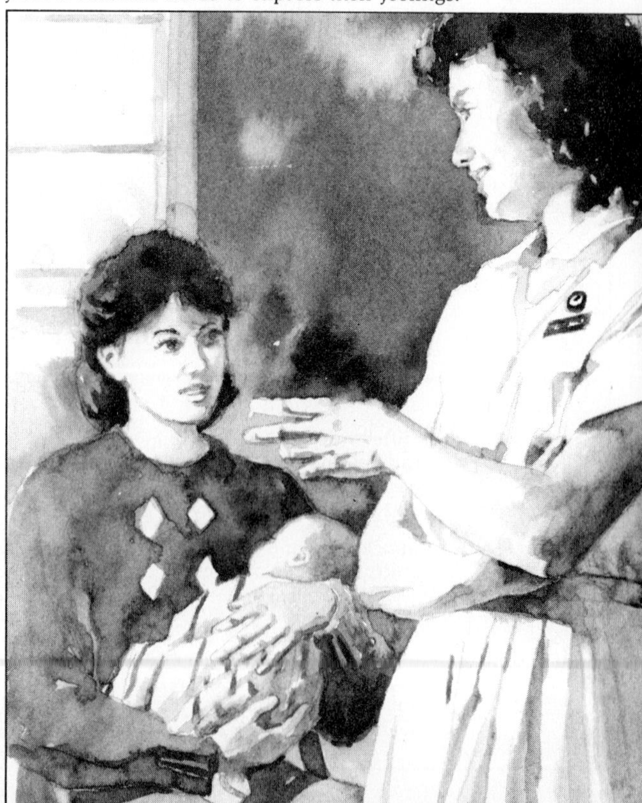

but they are likely to ignore continued criticism.

In addition to individual and small group teaching, media presentations can be very effective. Teens are media-hungry and often respond enthusiastically to films, videos, or slides. Supplementary written materials can also be used, but they must be at a reading level the patient can understand. Most of the available postpartum pamphlets are either inappropriate or too difficult for many adolescents, so nurses may need to design their own (11) (see "Written Reinforcement for Teaching" in *MCN*, September/October 1986).

Effective teaching can be measured by observing the adolescent and her infant or by having her explain in her own words what she has learned about a particular topic. Staff must also be consistent in terms of what they teach and what they expect of a patient. The younger teen will become confused and the mid-adolescent will rebel if each person who works with her has different expectations. By using materials at an appropriate educational level and in a format acceptable to the young, adolescent mother, the nurse can be certain she has done everything possible to maximize her teaching efforts.

Developmentally Based Nursing Care

Knowing how far the adolescent has progressed in her own development is the key to delivering both effective teaching and effective nursing care. The late adolescent can often be treated like an adult in terms of how she is expected to care for her infant and respond to patient teaching. The early and mid-adolescent may behave differently, necessitating different expectations and a different teaching style.

The early adolescent tends to cling and demand attention. She may be afraid to initiate any activity with her infant and may instead wait passively for help from the nurse or from her mother. The nurse who understands that this is normal behavior will be able to relate to her in a more patient and caring way. She can also help to decrease the teen's anxiety by modeling expected behavior and then praising her for carrying it out. Because family members will probably be involved in child care once the infant is discharged, teaching should be directed to them as well as to the adolescent.

Staff members often find the mid-adolescent the most frustrating, because she cannot admit her own fears or acknowledge that she needs help. She may act as if she knows everything about infant care and appear bored and disinterested during teaching sessions. It is important to remember that the adolescent's own insecurity makes it difficult for her to depend on adults while she is striving to become one herself.

Although the nurse needs to avoid power struggles with the mid-adolescent, she must nevertheless set and enforce reasonable limits. She should communicate her expectations matter-of-factly and in a nonauthoritarian manner, and whenever possible offer several choices so that the teen feels she has some control. Like other postpartum patients, the teen can be expected to get out of bed at the appropriate hour, care for her infant, and give a return bath demonstration.

The nurse should try to develop a supportive relationship with her adolescent patients, but if this seems impossible, remember that they often absorb more of what is taught than is apparent. Remember, too, that a little positive reinforcement goes a long way. Teens have a vested interest in downgrading the importance of the nurse and her suggestions in order to feel in control. The patient who acted sullen or disinterested during her hospital teaching sessions may enjoy showing her family the "right way" to do things once she is back home again.

If the adolescent develops behavioral problems or has trouble making plans for herself and her infant, other health care professionals may be helpful. A nurse or social worker who knew her while she was pregnant may be a valuable source of information about the teen's coping abilities, family problems, and educational history. The community health nurse is another excellent resource if she began visiting during the prenatal period.

When there has been no previous professional involvement, the hospital social worker can be an important ally in determining the adequacy of discharge planning and can help the teen to obtain needed material resources. If an early or mid-adolescent is without visible family support and has not made appropriate plans, the social worker may need to initiate a referral to child protective services. She will also need to refer any adolescent who has a history of drug or alcohol abuse at delivery or whose behavior in the hospital is clearly a danger to her infant.

Fortunately, few young mothers have such serious problems. It is usually not until several months later, when family support wanes and her emotional resources are exhausted, that the burdens of parenthood may become overwhelming to the young mother. For this reason it is important that the teen and her infant continue to receive professional support and guidance.

Plans for the baby's ongoing medical care should be initiated prior to discharge, and if possible, the adolescent should meet with one of the pediatric providers. A community health nursing referral will help to ensure continued surveillance and teaching. In addition, many communities now have programs that offer teens support and parenting education. A referral or even an informational

ADOLESCENT POSTPARTUM CARE

OB/GYN NURSING
PATIENT CARE PLAN

DATE	INT.	PROB. #	NURSING DIAGNOSIS/ PATIENT PROBLEM	EXPECTED OUTCOMES/ GOALS	NURSING INTERVENTION	PROBLEM STATU Revised/Resolved/Respor
		1	Potential for disturbance of normal adolescent tasks. **1.** Independence **2.** Intimacy **3.** Identity	By discharge pt. will identify one adult support person and describe his/her role in child care. The pt. will have clothing and formula for the infant and a place to live with the infant after discharge.	**1.** Review prenatal chart for pertinent social, emotional and educational information. **2.** Assess family support re: birth and infant care. **3.** Refer to Social Work, CHN or Child Protective as needed. **4.** Assess FOB involvement and teen's feelings about him. **5.** Assess future plans for work, school, infant care. **6.** Accept importance of visitors (peers and family) *BUT* set limits when necessary.	
		2	Potential for inadequate parenting due to normal adolescence: **1.** Egocentrism (self involvement). **2.** "Now" orientation.	By discharge pt. will demonstrate initiation of bonding process including enface behavior and positive statements about the infant.	**1.** Describe and demonstrate unique aspects of infant and infant cues. **2.** Provide positive reinforcement to mother for caretaking effort. Focus attention on mother as well as infant. **3.** Encourage verbalization of reactions toward L&D experience and anticipated versus actual appearance and behavior of newborn. **4.** Assess influence pts. family and cultural beliefs may have on infant care, receptivity to teaching, etc. **5.** Assess bonding—see Section XI. **6.** Assure that baby has pediatric provider and patient understands how to reach him/her.	
		3	Potential for inadequate infant nutrition.	By time of discharge pt. will demonstrate adequate feeding technique as evidenced by appropriate timing, intake and positioning.	**1.** Assess knowledge re: different feeding methods and give information as needed. **2.** *Breastfeeding* **a.** Reinforce decision, give extra support and guidance, especially at feeding times. **b.** Anticipatory guidance teaching re: common problems of early breastfeeding. **c.** Alert CHN that patient is breastfeeding *before* discharge so early home visit can be made.	
		4	Potential for inadequate learning due to normal adolescent development: **1.** Concrete thinking **2.** Minimum literacy **3.** Apparent lack of interest (i.e., over confident behavior or non-attentiveness). **4.** Resistance to authority figures.	By discharge pt. will demonstrate minimal safe infant care including appropriate positioning, diapering, feeding and dressing techniques.	**1.** Assess current knowledge of and experience with infant care. **2.** Assess developmental level, intellectual ability and gear teaching to this level. **3.** Provide info through multiple modalities (1:1, groups, visual, written). *CAUTION:* Written material must be at patient's reading level. **4.** Direct teaching to mother and other significant caregivers. **5.** Positively reinforce even small parts of desired behaviors. **6.** Offer choices or options where possible.	
		5	Potential for repeat pregnancy.	By time of discharge pt. will choose a contraceptive method and be able to describe its use—will identify a health care provider for own GYN care.	**1.** Assess past contraceptive history. If used, reason method stopped, myths about method. **2.** Teach regarding methods available and necessity of ongoing contraception. **3.** Stress need to call provider for problems with method. **4.** Assess and encourage plans for continuing GYN and personal health care.	

INT.	FULL SIGNATURE	TITLE	INT.	FULL SIGNATURE	TITLE	INT.	FULL SIGNATURE	TITLE

Used with permission of Strong Memorial hospital, University of Rochester, Rochester, NY.

pamphlet about such a program could make the difference between parenting success or failure.

Adolescent mothers are very likely to become pregnant again. Their repeat pregnancy rate has been as high as 40 percent within the first year after delivery and 70 percent by the third year (8). These rates are particularly disturbing because nearly all postpartum women are discharged with a contraceptive method. Simply handing out a prescription for pills, however, will not prevent an unwanted pregnancy.

Discussing Contraception

The nurse should begin to discuss contraceptive planning with the young mother as soon after delivery as possible. Shorter hospital stays make it increasingly difficult to cover all the required topics, but contraception cannot be taught in the last few minutes before discharge. With the labor experience fresh in their minds, most postpartum adolescents are highly receptive to information on how to prevent another pregnancy.

It is best to begin by asking the teen what she knows about contraception and what experience she has had with the various methods. Does she have any idea how her female organs work? Many adolescents barely understand their bodies or realize that they remain fertile and can become pregnant again very soon. A diagram of the female reproductive system will help to correct any misconceptions and clarify the abstract concepts involved. This can be as elaborate as a flip chart or as simple as a sketch.

Many teens have very definite ideas about what contraceptive methods they will or will not use, as well as what methods are acceptable to their boyfriend. The nurse can save valuable teaching time and hold the patient's interest by focusing on the preferred method. Then she can discuss a backup technique and briefly mention the others.

More adolescents use an oral contraceptive than any other method, and many used it before becoming pregnant. If this is the case with the patient, find out about her experience with the pill, why she stopped taking it, and what problems she anticipates if she begins taking it again. If she refuses to take a certain kind of pill because she associates it, however incorrectly, with a variety of physical ailments, asking the physician to prescribe another brand may mean the difference between compliance and noncompliance.

Whether or not they have ever used it, teens often believe a number of myths about the pill—for example, that it causes cancer, sterility, or obesity. Normal side effects are also very disturbing to the young teen, who is extremely sensitive to any change in her body functioning. She needs to know that severe headaches or abdominal, chest, or leg pains may be the first signs of serious complications, but that these are rare in women her age and that pregnancy poses greater dangers. Common side effects such as nausea and breakthrough bleeding should also be explained. They are annoying, but will usually disappear after several months. Reassure her that even if they do not, there are many kinds of oral contraceptives and the right one for her can be found.

No matter what method of contraception the teen selects, a number of questions must be discussed. How will she obtain it? Does she have enough money or insurance to pay for it? Does she understand how it is used? How do her family and boyfriend feel about her choice and will their feelings influence whether she uses it regularly? Who will she call about problems? Does she know checkups are necessary, and who she will see?

Sometimes it helps to follow up birth control teaching with a simple handout that describes how to use a particular contraceptive method and explains the danger signals, the side effects and how to minimize them, and where to call if there are problems. This "help line" number is perhaps the most important piece of information the nurse can provide. Too many teens are sent home with a method, stop using it for some minor reason, and never call until they are pregnant again.

Caring for the adolescent mother can offer a unique challenge to the postpartum nurse. These patients demand sensitive, innovative, and developmentally based nursing care, but their enthusiasum and openness can amply reward the nurse who takes time to win their trust. With adequate support and education, adolescents can become competent and loving mothers whose parenting abilities often seem far beyond their years.

REFERENCES

1. U.S. NATIONAL CENTER FOR HEALTH STATISTICS. *Final Natality Statistics, 1978.* Monthly Vital Statistics Report (Suppl.) 29(1) (DHHS Publ. No. (PHS) 80-1120), Washington, D.C., U.S. Government Printing Office, 1980.
2. ALAN GUTTMACHER INSTITUTE. *11 Million Teenagers: What Can Be Done About the Epidemic of Adolescent Pregnancies in the United States.* New York, Planned Parenthood Federation of America, 1976.
3. TAYLOR, B., AND OTHERS. Teenage mothering, admission to hospital, and accidents during the first 5 years. *Arch.Dis.Child.* 58:6–11, Jan. 1983.
4. ROTHENBERG, P. B., AND VARGA, P. E. The relationship between age of mother and child health and development. *Am.J.Public Health* 71:810–817, Aug. 1981.
5. BALDWIN, W., AND CAIN, V. S. The children of teenage parents. *Fam.Plann.Perspect.* 12:34–43, Jan.–Feb. 1980.
6. CAMP, B. W., AND OTHERS. Infants of adolescent mothers: maternal characteristics and developmental status at 1 year of age. *Am.J.Dis.Child.* 138:243–246, Mar. 1984.
7. HARDY, J. B., AND OTHERS. Long-range outcome of adolescent pregnancy. *Clin.Obstet.Gynecol.* 21:1215–1232, Dec. 1978.
8. ELSTER, A. B., AND OTHERS. Parental behavior of adolescent mothers. *Pediatrics* 71:494–503, Apr. 1983.
9. MERCER, R. T., AND OTHERS. Adolescent motherhood: comparison of outcome with older mothers. *J.Adolesc.Health Care* 5:7–13, Jan. 1984.
10. AMBROSE, L. Misinforming pregnant teenagers. *Fam.Plann.Perspect.* 10: 51–57, Jan.–Feb. 1978.

A Comprehensive Look At Hyperbilirubinemia

Jaundice, although common, is not well-understood. This article, the first of two, explains its development, relevant research, and preventive measures.

NORMA NEAHR WILKERSON

Hyperbilirubinemia, although common among normal infants, is poorly understood and of uncertain clinical significance. Approximately 80 percent of all newborns become clinically jaundiced (1). Fifty percent of full-term newborns become visibly jaundiced in the first week of life (2). This article, the first of two, describes the natural history of neonatal jaundice in healthy, full-term infants, provides an overview of current literature on hyperbilirubinemia, distinguishes the various etiologic categories, and discusses preventive measures. The second article, to be published in *MCN*'s January–February issue, describes methods of treating hyperbilirubinemia.

How Bilirubin Metabolizes

Bilirubin metabolism is a function of both the liver and the intestinal tract. Infants are born with relative polycythemia, a surplus of red blood cells. The excess compensates for the relative hypoxia of intrauterine life. As fetal red blood cells mature, die, and are catabolyzed, bilirubin, a breakdown product, is formed. One molecule of hemoglobin produces four molecules of bilirubin (1). In utero, the mother's hepatic and intestinal function clear the fetus's blood of excess bilirubin.

In normal, full-term infants, excess red blood cells deteriorate in neonatal circulation, causing a rise in serum bilirubin to between 3 and 5 mg/dl. The bilirubin molecules, which are insoluble in water, then bind to albumin, a carrier protein, for transport through the bloodstream to the liver (see Bilirubin Metabolism). Hepatocytes, with the assistance of a ligand, are able to conjugate (attach) albumin-bound bilirubin molecules with molecules of glucuronide, a product of liver glycogen. Conjugated bilirubin is water soluble and can thus be cleared from the bloodstream.

Conjugated bilirubin is excreted from the liver into bile. Via the gallbladder, it passes into the intestine. Meconium, which has accumulated in the fetus's bowel, is loaded with bilirubin. After birth, when the sterile fetal bowel is colonized with normal flora, bacterial enzymes convert bilirubin into urobilinogen, most of which is eliminated from the body when the infant defecates. If stool remains in the newborn's bowel for a prolonged period of time, bilirubin is reabsorbed by the bloodstream and must then be recirculated.

There are many opportunities for neonatal bilirubin metabolism to be disrupted in otherwise healthy, full-term infants. Such disruption causes hyperbilirubinemia. Prenatal or intrapartum hypoxia, associated with increased fetal blood volume, increased fetal-placental blood volume, and increased neonatal blood volume can ultimately result in increased bilirubin production (see Proposed Pathogenesis of Polycythemia). Delayed cord clamping at birth can also cause a large placental transfusion, predisposing the newborn to polycythemia and hyperbilirubinemia as well (3). Normal, full-term infants who experience bruising, hematomas, or trauma from long, difficult, or forcep deliveries are at risk for increased and more rapid breakdown of red blood cells, leading to elevated bilirubin levels. Or, increased bilirubin can result if the mother has been mildy sensitized to Rh, A, or B antigens and has produced antibodies that break down fetal/neonatal red blood cells into bilirubin products.

In addition, the immaturity of a newborn's liver inhibits the physiology of bilirubin transport. Because a newborn's bowel is sterile, the lack of normal bacterial enzymes can interrupt bilirubin excretion, resulting in reabsorption.

Relating Bilirubin to Jaundice

Thus, some degree of physiologic jaundice (PJ) is a normal finding as the infant matures. Visible jaundice occurs as insoluble bilirubin, at serum

NORMA NEAHR WILKERSON, R.N., PH.D., *is associate professor of nursing, University of Wyoming School of Nursing, Laramie, Wyoming. This article is based on the presentation she made at the 1987 second national MCN Convention. For reprints, see the classified section.*

levels greater than 5 mg/dl, is deposited in fatty, subcutaneous tissue. Sclera, mucous membranes, and urine can also become yellow in color as hyperbilirubinemia progresses. But what does jaundice actually indicate?

Researchers first began to investigate hyperbilirubinemia in the 1950s by studying the importance of conjugated and unconjugated bilirubin, abnormalities of bilirubin excretion, and Rh isoimmunization (4). Studies supported the association between high serum bilirubin levels (unconjugated hyperbilirubinemia) and kernicterus in infants with hemolytic disease. Kernicterus rarely occurs with serum bilirubin levels less than 20 mg/dl, yet controversy over the potential neurological deficits that can occur with serum bilirubin levels less than 20 mg/dl persists (5).

Barbara Foerder retrospectively studied 175 children who had been normal, full-term infants (6). She found no differences in development, as measured by Brazelton and Bayley scales at 3 months, 10 months, and 24 months of age, between infants who were jaundiced as newborns (serum bilirubin levels of less than 20 mg/dl) and those who were not.

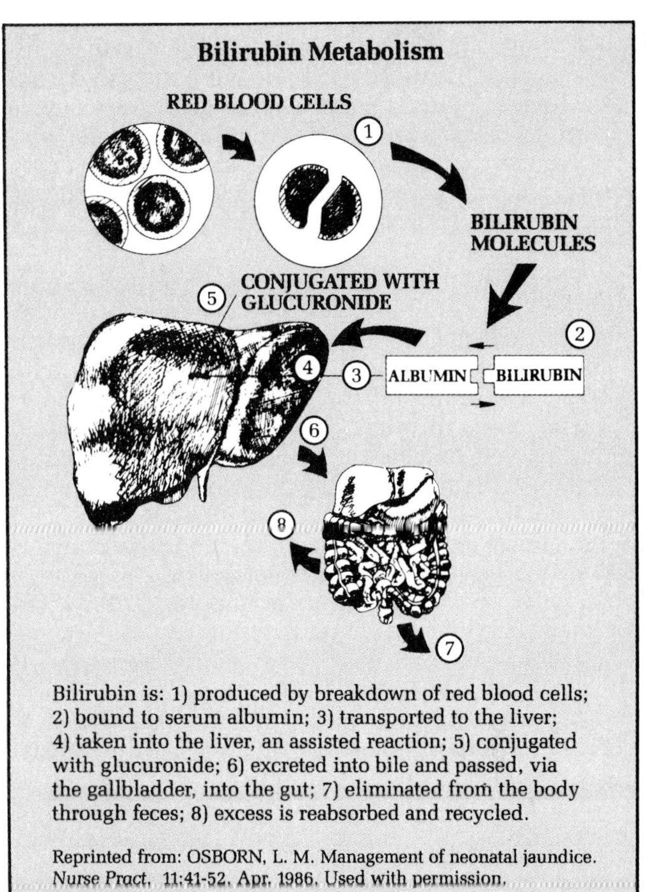

Bilirubin is: 1) produced by breakdown of red blood cells; 2) bound to serum albumin; 3) transported to the liver; 4) taken into the liver, an assisted reaction; 5) conjugated with glucuronide; 6) excreted into bile and passed, via the gallbladder, into the gut; 7) eliminated from the body through feces; 8) excess is reabsorbed and recycled.

Reprinted from: OSBORN, L. M. Management of neonatal jaundice. *Nurse Pract.* 11:41-52, Apr. 1986. Used with permission.

How Is Breast-Feeding Involved?

In the 1960s, researchers documented reports of breast-fed infants with prolonged jaundice (7–9). As the infants described in these reports had elevated serum bilirubin levels that continued for longer than normal periods of time, the syndrome was dubbed breast milk jaundice (BMJ) and received much attention. The condition was described as unconjugated hyperbilirubinemia in otherwise healthy, breast-feeding infants. The diagnosis is usually made after the infant's first two weeks of life. If the mother continues to breastfeed, BMJ can last for as long as four months.

Early theorists associated BMJ with pregnane-3 alpha, 20 beta-diol, a maternal steroid present in breast milk of mothers whose infants had BMJ (10,11). The steroid inhibits glucuronide formation. Later studies suggested that breast milk's glucuronide inhibiting property is related to elevated lipase activity in the milk (12). Breast milk in which lipase activity is abnormally high develops abnormally elevated concentrations of free fatty acids, which then inhibit glucuronyl transferase, the enzyme that allows unconjugated bilirubin to attach to glucuronide. The normal newborn's limited ability to absorb and digest fat may also affect bilirubin metabolism (13–15).

Most recently, researchers have arrived at another hypothesis. BMJ develops, they propose, because increased presence of beta-glucuronidase in breast milk leads to increased neonatal intestinal absorption of bilirubin; increased levels of beta-glucuronidase were found in the feces of breast-fed infants (15,16). Breast-fed infants, as compared to formula-fed newborns, have more acidic feces, less output of stool, and have distinctive intestinal bacterial flora, all of which may account for the differences in fecal beta-glucuronidase activity and bilirubin levels between breast-fed and formula-fed newborns.

The rate at which the newborn evacuates stool directly relates to the amount of bilirubin reabsorbed. Frequent sucking shortens gut transit time and promotes greater output of stool. Studies to compare frequency of feeding with bilirubin levels in breast-fed and formula-fed infants are now being designed (17).

There is a difference, however, between BMJ and breast-feeding associated jaundice (BFAJ). Jaundice that presents within the first few days of life has been documented to occur with greater frequency in breast-fed infants than in formula-fed infants. This form of hyperbilirubinemia is not *caused* by breast milk, but may be correlated with the infant's success at breast-feeding. Lucy Osborne's research correlates BFAJ with lighter weight and poor weight recovery (1). She speculates that "the increased weight loss reflects the quality of nursing. Infants with good functional nursing stimulate an early adequate milk supply. Those who are not breast-feeding well may suffer a relative caloric deprivation, which can then lead to decreased hepatic clearance of bilirubin and subsequent indirect hyperbilirubinemia" (18).

Her findings can be compared with those of Manoel DeCarvalho (17). He demonstrated that feeding frequency and serum bilirubin levels were reliably correlated (r = −.361). Infants who nursed more than eight times per day had average serum bilirubin levels of 6.5 mg/dl as compared to an average of 9.3 mg/dl for babies who breast-fed less frequently.

Their findings are consistent with those of a population study of 498 full-term, appropriate for gestational age infants conducted by J. E. Clarkson and colleagues (19). They found that infants who first passed meconium less than 12 hours following delivery were less jaundiced than those who first passed meconium more than 12 hours after delivery. Babies who by four days of age had gained weight tended to be much less jaundiced than those who had lost more than 5 percent of their birth weight in their first four days of life.

Living at a high altitude is another factor associated with increased incidence of neonatal hyperbilirubinemia (20). In a retrospective study of all infants born during a 14-month period in Leadville, Colorado (elevation 3,100 meters), the incidence of hyperbilirubinemia (total serum bilirubin levels greater than 12 mg/dl) was more than twice that of infants born in Denver (elevation 1,600 meters); the incidence was four times that of infants born at sea level.

Jaundice Related to Obstetric Interventions

The incidence of physiologic jaundice not associated with pathophysiologic factors seems to have increased through the 1970s and 1980s. Four specific obstetric interventions are associated with the higher incidence: labor induction, epidural anesthesia, the use of intravenous fluids during labor, and delayed or limited feeding during the infant's first 24 hours of life (21).

Findings of studies investigating the use of oxytocin and prostaglandin for induction of labor are inconsistent. One multifactorial survey of 981 infants reports that elevated bilirubin levels occurred reliably more often when medium or high doses of oxytocin had been used during labor (22). In addition, artificial rupture of membranes and use of oxytocin to induce labor were associated with increased bilirubin levels. When oxytocin was used only to enhance labor (augmentation), it was not found to be related (23).

However, in J. E. Clarkson's population study, the effects of artificial membrane rupture, epidurals, and oxytocin for induction were not found to be significantly related to hyperbilirubinemia in the newborn (19). A Danish prospective study failed to substantiate relationships between hyperbilirubinemia and induction after premature rupture of membranes (N = 250), artificial membrane rupture (N = 270), or induction with oxytocin without amniotomy (N = 219) (24).

N. B. Knepp and colleagues investigated another intervention. They observed elevated bilirubin levels in infants of mothers receiving intravenous 5 percent dextrose (25). The researchers hypothesized a relationship between hydration and increased fetal insulin production. A study of 51 Jamaican women who received no intravenous fluids and 43 who received fluids in varying amounts yielded similar results (26). Serum bilirubin levels were above 10 mg/dl in 15 percent of the infants whose mothers received intravenous fluids; levels above 10 mg/dl were recorded in 4 percent of infants of mothers who did not.

Because well-controlled studies that eliminate potential maternal, fetal, or neonatal complications that increase the incidence of infant jaundice are difficult to design, the influence of obstetric interventions on time of the newborn's first feeding, the quality of the infant's suckling, the frequency of feedings, and gut transit time is difficult to measure. Further efforts to investigate the various hypotheses related to neonatal hyperbilirubinemia are necessary. It is vital to determine whether hospital routines, management, and structured interactions between mother and infant are related to the physiology of hyperbilirubinemia in breast-fed infants.

Proposed Pathogenesis of Polycythemia

Prenatal Hypoxia → ↑ Erythropoietin Production → ↑ Erythropoiesis
↓
↑ Fetal-Placental Blood Volume
↓
Intrapartum Hypoxia → Shifting of Blood From Placenta to Fetus → ↑ Fetal Blood Volume
↓
Delayed Cord Clamping At Birth → Postnatal Placental Transfusion → ↑ Neonatal Blood Volume
(Vaginal Delivery)

Reprinted from: OH, W. Neonatal polycythemia and hyperviscosity. *Pediatr. Clin. North Am.* 33:523-532, June 1986. Used with permission.

Applying Research to Practice

Given the well-documented relationships between normal neonatal physiology, infant feeding practices, and hyperbilirubinemia, it is obvious that rigid feeding schedules contribute to increased neonatal jaundice. Instead, mothers need to be encouraged to breast-feed their infants as soon after birth as possible and as frequently as possible thereafter. Based on the literature and my clinical experience, I recommend a two-hour interval between feedings during the first week,

Variables and Prevention of Nonpathologically-Induced Hyperbilirubinemia

Relevant Variables	*Physiologic Jaundice (PJ)*	*Breast Milk Jaundice (BMJ)*	*Breast-Feeding Associated Jaundice (BFAJ)*
Incidence	20 percent of all neonates have bilirubin levels of 5.0 mg/dl.	1–2 percent of breast-fed neonates have bilirubin levels of 15–25 mg/dl.	10 percent of breast-fed infants have bilirubin levels of 9.0–19.0 mg/dl.
Appearance of Jaundice	Usually in the second to third day of life.	After first week of life when physiologic jaundice is waning.	Usually in second to third day of life.
Clinical Progression	Bilirubin peaks at 5–10 mg/dl by third to fifth day of life; decreases to below 2 mg/dl by day seven. Rate of accumulation below 5 mg/dl/24 hours.	Bilirubin peaks at 10–15 days of life. Infants may remain jaundiced for weeks, rarely months. Diagnosis confirmed if level drops with cessation of breast-feeding for 24–48 hours. Levels usually rise slowly, but not to previous level with resumption of breast feeding.	Bilirubin peaks by second to third day of life. Rate of accumulation below 5 mg/dl/24 hours. Typically, breast-feeding is not well-established. Bilirubin level may go as high as 15–19 mg/dl.
Etiology and Associated Factors	Excess of fetal red blood cells in neonatal circulation. Load can be increased by perinatal hypoxia, trauma, or passage of maternal serum antibodies to Rh, A, or B antigens during transition from fetal to neonatal circulation after birth. Mean peak serum conjugated bilirubin levels increase at higher elevations and in Chinese, Japanese, Korean, and American Indian populations.	Controversy still exists over cause. Current explanations are: increase in intestinal absorption of bilirubin due to beta-glucuronidase (present in feces of breast-fed infants); and less frequent stooling of breast-fed infants.	Smaller, less vigorous infants who do not nurse well. Caloric deprivation then leads to decreased hepatic transport and clearance of bilirubin. Poor intake of milk is the cause, not factors related to breast milk.
Primary Prevention	All neonates experience some degree of hyperbilirubinemia. It can be exacerbated by delayed passage of meconium, limited caloric intake, and higher elevations. Identify infants at risk, increase feedings, and decrease gut transit time.	Breast-fed infants should be monitored. If history of BMJ in previous sibling, promote early, frequent feedings and exposure to sunlight, and provide parental anticipatory guidance.	Infants at risk require early and frequent feedings. If breast-feeding is not well-established in first 24 hours, caloric supplementation may be useful.
Secondary Prevention	Increased feedings, exposure to sunlight, phototherapy if bilirubin approaches 18–20 mg/dl.	Interrupt nursing for 24–48 hours to confirm diagnosis. Follow-up required to support and reestablish breast-feeding.	Increase feedings to provide calories; phototherapy may be instituted if levels approach 18–20 mg/dl.
Tertiary Prevention	Usually no complications if infant is monitored and treated to keep level below 20 mg/dl. Risk of kernicterus increases as levels rise above 18–20 mg/dl.	Usually self-limiting and benign. No reported cases of kernicterus caused by BMJ.	Same as tertiary prevention of physiologic jaundice.

particularly if the infant's bilirubin level is rising. Frequent breast-feeding sessions that begin soon after birth stimulate maternal milk productivity, stimulate the infant's intestinal motility, and can help keep bilirubin levels low.

I also recommend rooming-in in order to keep mother and infant in close proximity. Mothers can be encouraged to nurse their infants whenever the infants begin to awaken, root, and suck on their fists, early signs of the stimulus to feed. If the infant is offered the breast at this time, rather than after crying has begun, breast-feeding sessions are more likely to be successful and mutually beneficial. Studies that investigate these variables in relation to nipple soreness have shown that limiting suckling time is not a proven technique for preventing or treating sore nipples (27–29).

Mothers can also be encouraged to expose their infants to natural sunlight. Feeding and caring for the infant in front of a window and giving the infant sun baths in warm daylight are primary prevention strategies. On the other hand, parents must be warned to avoid exposing the infant to excessive amounts of sun. With the trend toward early discharge, the need for outpatient monitoring of jaundiced infants cannot be overlooked.

When to Begin Treatment

Even if an otherwise healthy infant's serum indirect bilirubin concentration rises, the mother can continue breast-feeding. Generally, a healthy full-term infant with a bilirubin level greater than 12 mg/dl is examined to exclude pathophysiologic conditions such as blood incompatibilities, hypothyroidism, inherited glucuronyl transferase deficiency, or biliary atresia. Whether the infant is experiencing normal physiologic jaundice or breast milk jaundice, treatment (phototherapy) is not required unless serum bilirubin nears 12–15 mg/dl by the second day of life or reaches 15–18 mg/dl thereafter. Kernicterus has never been reported in an infant with BMJ (30).

Some caregivers accept 15–16 mg/dl as the level at which to initiate phototherapy. However, Barbara Foerder's findings support a higher cutoff (6). She found no significant differences in developmental outcomes between hyperbilirubinemic infants (levels ranged from 5 to 19 mg/dl) and controls. Furthermore, she found that hyperbilirubinemic children who were breast-fed scored better than formula-fed hyperbilirubinemics at 3, 10, and 24 months, findings that also support continuation of breast-feeding for hyperbilirubinemic infants. If the infant's serum bilirubin level approaches 20 mg/dl, diagnosis of BMJ must be made. If the mother stops breast-feeding for 24 to 48 hours and the infant's serum bilirubin level decreases, the diagnosis of BMJ is confirmed and no further tests are required (5). Interrupting breast-feeding if the infant's serum bilirubin level is below 15–16 mg/dl may unnecessarily impede breast-feeding.

Mothers who must interrupt breast-feeding in order to confirm BMJ diagnosis need supervision and support from nursing staff with well-prepared lactation skills. Nurses can teach these mothers to pump their breasts in order to maintain their milk supply until they resume breast-feeding. Nurses can also minimize stress mothers may feel if they believe that they have caused their infants to become ill. Discussions in which the mother can express her fears and concerns will alleviate some maternal stress. Assuring parents that their infant's jaundice is transitional also reduces parental distress.

Infants who must remain hospitalized for phototherapy and their parents require special intervention. (Specifics about phototherapy, its mechanism of action, side effects, and use at home are discussed in my second article on hyperbilirubinemia, to be published in the January–February *MCN*. Transcutaneous bilirubinometry and exchange transfusions are covered as well.) These infants will benefit from frequent contact with their parents and must be accessible to parents for feeding, holding, and comforting. Nurses can also teach parents to care for their infant even while the infant is receiving phototherapy.

However, it is important to remember that physiologic jaundice and breast milk jaundice have no long-term harmful effects if properly monitored and judiciously treated. Aggressive, early treatment with phototherapy or substitution of formula for breast milk is not generally justified for healthy, full-term infants diagnosed with physiologic hyperbilirubinemia (31).

REFERENCES

1. OSBORN, L. M. Management of neonatal jaundice. *Nurse Pract.* 11:41–52, Apr. 1986.
2. MAISELS, M. J. Jaundice in the newborn. *Pediatr.Rev.* 3:305–319, 1982.
3. OH, W. Neonatal polycythemia and hyperviscosity. *Pediatr.Clin.North Am.* 33:523–532, June 1986.
4. KIVLAHAN, C., AND JAMES, E. J. The natural history of neonatal jaundice. *Pediatrics* 74:364–370, Sept. 1984.
5. MAISELS, M. J. Hyperbilirubinemia. In *Current Therapy in Neonatal Perinatal Medicine 1984-1985*, ed. by N. M. Nelson. St. Louis, C. V. Mosby Co., 1985.
6. FOERDER, B. A. Neonatal jaundice: effects on development to age two years. *Commun.Nurs.Res.* 20:38, 1987.
7. NEWMAN, A. J., AND GROSS, S. Hyperbilirubinemia in breast-fed infants. *Pediatrics* 32:995–1001, Dec. 1963.
8. ARIAS, I. M., AND OTHERS. Prolonged neonatal unconjugated hyperbilirubinemia associated with breast feeding and a steroid, pregnane-3 (alpha), 20 (beta)-diol, in maternal milk that inhibits glucuronide formation in vitro. *J.Clin. Invest.* 43:2037–2047, Nov. 1964.
9. STIEHM, E. R., AND RYAN, J. Breast milk jaundice. Report of eight cases and effect of breast feeding on incidence and severity of unexplained hyperbilirubinemia. *Am.J.Dis.Child.* 109:212–216, Mar. 1965.
10. BROOTEN, D., AND OTHERS. Breast-milk jaundice. *JOGNN* 14:220–223, May–June 1985.
11. ARIAS, I. M., AND OTHERS. Neonatal conjugated hyperbilirubinemia associated with breastfeeding and a factor in milk that inhibits glucuronide formation in vitro. *J.Clin.Invest.* 42:913–918, June 1963.
12. HARGREAVES, T. Effect of fatty acids on bilirubin conjugation. *Arch.Dis.Child.* 48:446–449, June 1973.
13. DeANGELIS, C., AND OTHERS. Breast milk jaundice. *Wis.Med.J.* 79:40–42, Feb. 1980.
14. POLAND, R. L. Breast-milk jaundice. *J.Pediatr.* 999:86–88, July 1981.
15. DeCARVALHO, M. D., AND OTHERS. Fecal bilirubin excretion and serum bilirubin concentrations in breast-fed and bottle-fed infants. *J.Pediatr.* 107:786–790, Nov. 1985.
16. GOURLEY, G. R., AND AREND, R. A. Beta-glucuronidase and hyperbilirubinaemia in breast-fed and formula-fed babies. *Lancet* 22:644–646, Mar. 1986.
17. DeCARVALHO, M. D., AND OTHERS. Frequency of breastfeeding and serum bilirubin concentration. *Am.J.Dis.Child.* 136:737-738, Aug. 1982.
18. OSBORNE, L. M. Op. cit., p. 49.
19. CLARKSON, J. E., AND OTHERS. Jaundice in full term healthy neonates—a population study. *Aust.Paediatr.J.* 20:303–308, Nov. 1984.
20. MOORE, L. G., AND OTHERS. Increased incidence of neonatal hyperbilirubinemia at 3,100 m in Colorado. *Am.J.Dis.Child.* 138:157–161, Feb. 1984.
21. COGAN, R., AND HINZ, R. The etiology of "physiological" neonatal jaundice: the role of interventions. *ICEA Review* 7(1):1–7, 1983.
22. JEFFARIES, M. J. A multifactorial survey of neonatal jaundice. *Br.J.Obstet.Gynaecol.* 84:452–455, June 1977.
23. CHEW, W. C., AND SWANN, I. L. Influence of simultaneous low amniotomy and oxytocin infusion and other maternal factors on neonatal jaundice: a prospective study. *Br.Med.J.* 1:72–73, Jan. 8, 1977.
24. LANGE, A. P., AND OTHERS. Neonatal jaundice after labour induced or stimulated by prostaglandin E2 or oxytocin. *Lancet* 1:991–994, May 1982.
25. KNEPP, N. B., AND OTHERS. Fetal and neonatal hazards of maternal hydration with 5% dextrose before cesarean section. *Lancet* 1:1150–1152, 1982.
26. SINGHI, S., AND OTHERS. Hazards of maternal hydration with 5% dextrose. *Lancet* 2:335–336, Aug. 7, 1982.
27. DeCARVALHO, M. D., AND OTHERS. Does the duration and the frequency of early breastfeeding affect nipple pain? *Birth* 11:81–84, Summer 1984.
28. L'ESPERANCE, C., AND FRANTZ, K. Time limitation for early breastfeeding. *JOGNN* 14:114–118, Mar.–Apr. 1985.
29. BOROVIES, D. L. Assessing and managing pain in breast-feeding mothers. *MCN* 9:272–276, July–Aug. 1984.
30. LASCARI, A. D. "Early" breast-feeding jaundice: clinical significance. *J.Pediatr.* 108:156–158, Jan. 1986.
31. PALUDETTO, R., AND OTHERS. Moderate hyperbilirubinemia does not influence the behavior of jaundiced infants. *Biol.Neonate* 50:43–47, July 1986.

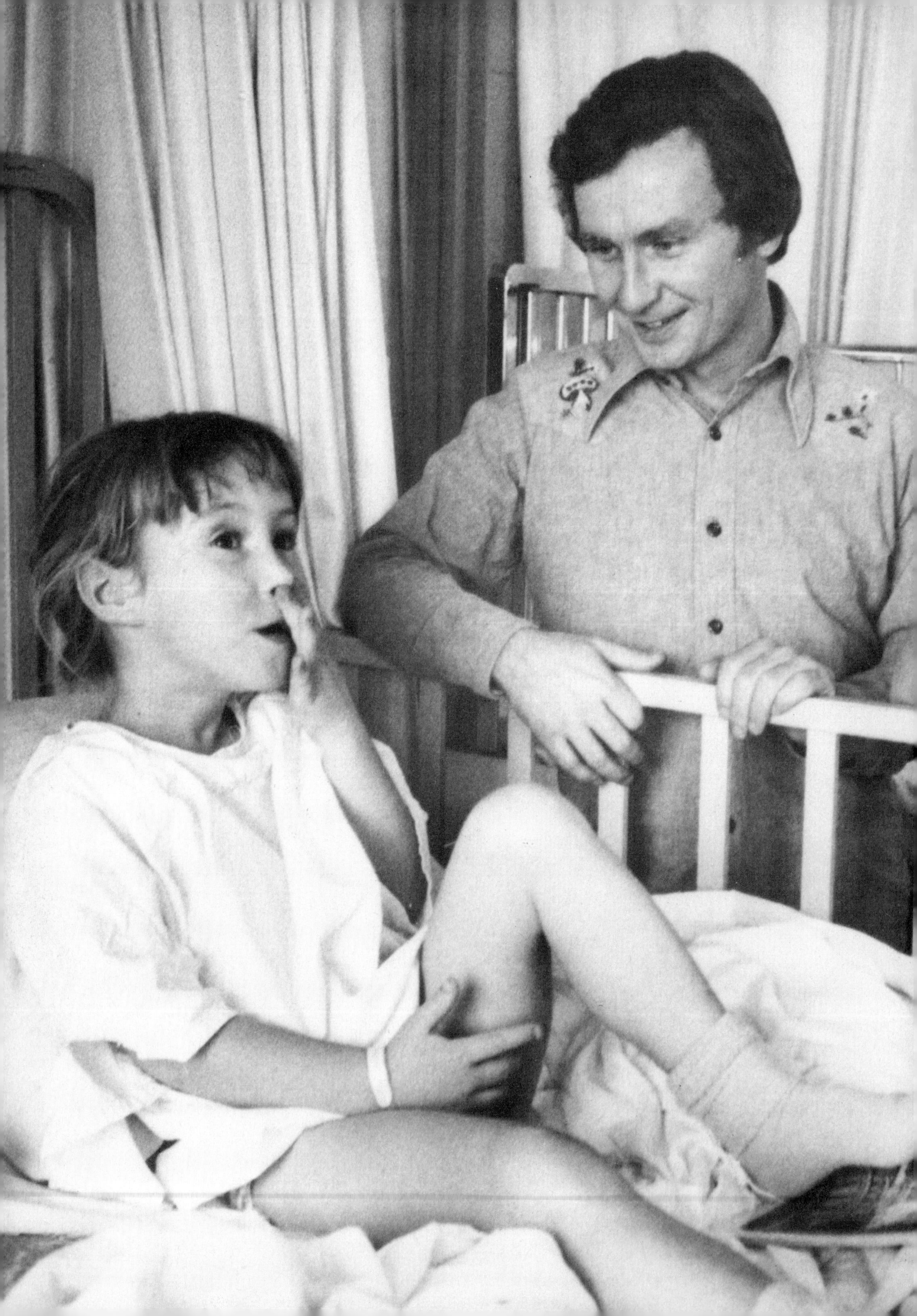

Nursing Care of the Child

Coordinator

Susan Droske, MN, RN

Contributors

Karen S. Bernardy, MSN, RNC
Stephen Jones, MSN, RNC
Judith K. Leavitt, MEd, RN
Mariann C. Lovell, MS, RN
Michele A. Michael, PhD, RN
Tamra Parsons, MSN, RN
Bernadette Mazurek Vulcan, MSN, RNC, PNP

Section 5: Nursing Care of the Child

THE HEALTHY CHILD 517

General Concepts 517

Infant 517

Toddler 520

Preschooler 522

School Age 523

Adolescent 524

Application of the Nursing Process to the Healthy Child 525

THE ILL AND HOSPITALIZED CHILD 529

Overview 529

Application of the Nursing Process to the Ill and Hospitalized Child 530

SENSATION, PERCEPTION, AND PROTECTION 535

General Concepts 535

Overview/Physiology 535

Application of the Nursing Process to the Child with a Sensory Problem 535

Selected Health Problems: Interference with Sensation 535

Otitis Media 535

Tonsillectomy and Adenoidectomy 537

Strabismus 537

Application of the Nursing Process to the Child with an Interference with Protection: Communicable Disease 538

Selected Health Problems: Communicable Diseases, Skin Problems, Infestations 538

Communicable Diseases 538

Sexually Transmitted Diseases 541

Common Skin Problems and Infestations 543

Pinworms 543

Application of the Nursing Process to the Child with an Interference with Protection: Safety 545

Selected Health Problems Resulting in an Interference with Protection: Safety 545

Poisonous Ingestions 545

Burns 548

Application of the Nursing Process to the Child with Developmental or Neurologic Disabilities 553

Selected Health Problems: Developmental or Neurologic Disabilities 555

Mental Retardation 555

Attention Deficit Disorder 556

Down Syndrome 556

Cerebral Palsy 557

Hydrocephalus 558

Spina Bifida 559

Seizure Disorders 560

Meningitis 563

OXYGENATION 565

General Concepts 565

Overview/Physiology 565

Application of the Nursing Process to the Child with Respiratory Problems 565

Selected Health Problems Resulting in an Interference with Respiration 565

Sudden Infant Death Syndrome 567

Acute Spasmodic Laryngitis (Spasmodic Croup) 568

Acute Epiglottis 568

Laryngotracheobronchitis 568

Bronchiolitis 568

Bronchopulmonary Dysplasia 568

Bronchial Asthma 569

Application of the Nursing Process to the Child with Cardiovascular Dysfunction 571

Selected Health Problems Resulting in an Interference with Cardiac Functioning 572

Congenital Heart Disease 572

Rheumatic Fever and Rheumatic Heart Disease 578

Application of the Nursing Process to the Child with Hematologic Problems 579

Selected Health Problems Resulting in an Interference with Formed Elements of the Blood 579

Iron-Deficiency Anemia 579

Sickle Cell Anemia 580

Hemophilia 582

NUTRITION AND METABOLISM 584

General Concepts 584

Overview/Physiology 584

Application of the Nursing Process to the Child with Problems of Nutrition and Metabolism 584

Selected Health Problems Resulting in an Interference with Nutrition and Metabolism 585

Vomiting and Diarrhea 585

Nonorganic Failure to Thrive 587

Pyloric Stenosis 588

Celiac Disease 589

Cleft Lip and Palate 590

Congenital Hypothyroidism 592

Insulin-Dependent Diabetes Mellitus 593

Cystic Fibrosis 595

ELIMINATION 598

General Concepts 598

Overview/Physiology 598

Application of the Nursing Process to the Child with Elimination Problems 598

Selected Health Problems Resulting in an Interference with Urinary or Bowel Elimination 598

Hypospadias 598

Urinary Tract Infection 599

Vesicourethral Reflux 600

Nephritis 601

Nephrosis 602

Lower GI Tract Obstruction 603

MOBILITY 605

General Concepts 605

Overview/Physiology 605

Application of the Nursing Process to the Child with an Interference with Mobility 605

Selected Health Problems Resulting in an Interference with Mobility 609

Congenital Clubfoot 609

Congenital Hip Dysplasia 609

Legg-Calvé-Perthes Disease 610

Scoliosis 610

Osteomyelitis 611

CELLULAR ABERRATION 613

General Concepts 613

Overview/Physiology 613

Application of the Nursing Process to the Child with Cancer 613

Selected Health Problems Resulting from CellularAberration 618

Leukemia 618

Solid Tumors 619

REPRINTS 621

Section 5 Tables

5.1 Vital Sign Ranges in Children 518
5.2 Average Daily Caloric Needs of Infants and Children 519
5.3 American Academy of Pediatrics Recommended Immunization Schedule 520
5.4 Commonly Used Pediatric Restraints 532
5.5 Medication and Temperature Guide 532
5.6 Medication Administration for Young Children 533
5.7 Estimating Pediatric Drug Doses 534
5.8 Types of Isolation 540
5.9 Sexually Transmitted Diseases 542
5.10 Common Skin Problems and Infestations 544
5.11 Commonly Ingested Poisonous Substances 546
5.12 Systemic Responses to Burn Injury 549

5.13 Levels of Retardation 555
5.14 Signs and Symptoms of Increased Intracranial Pressure in Infants and Children 559
5.15 Medications Used to Treat Seizure Disorders 562
5.16 Hematology Values in Children 566
5.17 Comparison of Croup and Bronchiolitis 568
5.18 Medications Used to Treat Bronchial Asthma 569
5.19 Cardiac Catherization in Children: Nursing Considerations 571
5.20 Comparison of Type 1 (insulin dependant) and Type 2 (non-insulin dependant) Diabetes Mellitus 593
5.21 Types of Traction 606
5.22 Commonly Used Chemotherapeutic Agents 614
5.23 Child's Conception of Death 617
5.24 Common Solid Tumors in Children 620

Section 5 Figures

5.1 Estimation of Burn Surface Area 550
5.2 Normal and Abnormal Hearts 573
5.3 Common Modes of Genetic Transmission 581
5.4 Types of Traction 607
5.5 Petaled Cast Edges 609

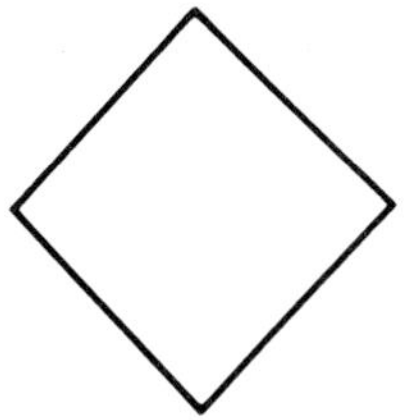

The Healthy Child

General Concepts

☐ Infant (1 month to 1 year)

1. Normal growth and development
   a. Psychosocial development—Erikson: trust vs mistrust (see Table 2.1)
      1) trust: infant's needs are met consistently, resulting in feelings of physical comfort and emotional security; learns to love and be loved
      2) depends on the quality of the primary care giver-infant relationship
   b. Physical growth and development
      1) physical growth should follow standard growth curves
      2) length: 50% increase by 1 year (grows from average 20 inches at birth to 30 inches at 1 year)
      3) weight
         a) gains about 1½ lb/month during the first 6 months; ¾ lb/month the second 6 months
         b) doubles at 5–6 months
         c) triples by 1 year (18–25 lb at 1 year)
      4) head circumference greater than chest circumference until age 2
      5) vital signs (see Table 5.1)
         a) pulse 80–150; average 100
         b) respirations 20–50
      6) developmental characteristics
         a) cephalocaudal (head to tail): gross motor skills
            - 5 months: turns over, no head lag when in sitting position
            - 6 months: sits alone with hands held forward for support
            - 8 months: sits steadily without support, pulls to a standing position
            - 9 months: able to "crawl," able to regain balance when sitting
            - 1 year: stands upright, able to "cruise" about a room by holding onto objects; may take first "solo" steps
         b) proximal to distal (central axis of body outward) and general to specific (differentiate): fine motor skills
            - 3–4 months: arm control; supports upper body weight; scoops objects with hands
            - 6 months: transfers objects from one hand to the other
            - 10 months: pincer (thumb-index finger) grasp
         c) fontanels
            - anterior: closes at 12–18 months
            - posterior: closes at 2 months (may be closed at birth)
         d) teeth: development begins in utero
            - 4–8 months: central mandibular incisors
            - 1 year: 8 teeth (average)
   c. Cognitive development—Piaget: sensorimotor stage (birth to 2 years)
      1) 1 month: reflexive
      2) 1–4 months
         a) visually follows objects 180°
         b) recognizes familiar faces and objects
         c) turns head to locate sounds
         d) discovers parts of own body (hands, feet)
      3) 4–8 months: beginning object permanence
         a) searches for objects that have fallen
         b) imitates expressions and gestures of others
         c) smiles at self in mirror (mirror-image play)
         d) begins development of depth and space
      4) 9–12 months: searches for hidden objects
   d. Socialization
      1) 1 month: differentiates between face and object
      2) 2 months: social smile
      3) 4 months: recognizes primary care giver
      4) 7–8 months: shy with strangers
      5) 9–10 months: separation anxiety
   e. Vocalization (language development)
      1) 2 months: differentiated cry
      2) 3 months: squeals with pleasure

Table 5.1 Vital Sign Ranges in Children (Averages)

Pulse[a]	1 month–1 year	80–150/bpm
	1 year–5 years	80–120/bpm
	5 years–10 years	70–110/bpm
	10 years–16 years	60–100/bpm
Respiration[a]	1 month–1 year	20–50/min
	1 year–5 years	20–40/min
	5 years–10 years	18–30/min
	10 years–16 years	14–26/min
Blood Pressure	1 month–1 year	80/50 mm Hg
	1 year–5 years	90/60 mm Hg
	5 years–10 years	100–110/60–70 mm Hg
	10 years–16 years	110–120/70–80 mm Hg

[a]Lower numbers in range represent values with child asleep.

3) 5 months: simple vocal sounds (ooh, aah), turns to voice
4) 6 months: begins to imitate sounds
5) 9 months: first word (dada, baba); says ''dada,'' ''mama'' specifically
6) 12 months: two words besides mama and dada; uses gesture language, e.g., ''up'' (points) or ''bye'' (waves)

f. Play (solitary)
1) purposes: to stimulate sensorimotor development
2) toys
a) washable
b) easily handled
c) bright colors
d) safe, no sharp points or small removable parts
e) nonlead paint
3) types of toys
a) mobiles (black and white, bright colors)
b) rattles, musical toys
c) squeeze toys, sponge toys
d) activity box for crib or playpen
e) balls, blocks
f) pots and pans (9–10 months)
4) games: peek-a-boo and patty-cake

2. Nutrition
a. Caloric needs: approximately 400 (newborn) to 1,200 (1-year-old) kcal/day (see Table 5.2 for recommended averages); actual caloric requirements depend on baby's activity and rate of growth.
b. Introduction of solid foods
1) when to start solids: variety of opinions; some evidence that early feeding of solids is linked to food allergies and overweight
2) does not need solids first 4–6 months
a) salivary enzymes and intestinal antibodies to aid digestion not present until 4–6 months
b) extrusion reflex lasts until 3–4 months
c) chewing movements begin at 6–7 months
3) introduce foods one at a time; continue 3 or 4 days before introducing another
4) give small quantities (start with 1 tsp)
c. Types of foods: each introduced one at a time, each for 2–3 days
1) cooked cereals are introduced first at 5–6 months; rice cereal is preferable (high iron content, easily digested, less likely to cause allergic reaction)
2) strained/cooked vegetables are introduced next at 6–7 months (before fruits, which have lower iron content)
3) strained/mashed fruits are introduced at 7–8 months (bananas are preferable first fruit)
4) ground/pureed meats are introduced at 8–9 months, egg yolks at 10 months (delay egg whites until 12 months)
5) chewable and finger foods are introduced when teething begins (6–9 months): zwieback, toast, crackers
6) avoid nuts, raisins, popcorn, gum, candy (can be aspirated)
d. Self-feeding: at 6 months infant begins handling spoon, finger foods; by 1 year, most infants are able to use a spoon well; weaning—ready for introduction of a cup at 6–8 months, should be weaned gradually from breast or bottle; offer juice in a cup; drink independently from a cup at 1 year (may still want bottle or breast for security)
e. Food allergies (a common health problem in infancy)
1) common foods causing allergic responses

Table 5.2 Average Daily Caloric Needs of Infants and Children*

Age	Calories
Birth–6 months	53 × weight in pounds = kcal/day (400–800 kcal/day)
6 months–1 year	48 × weight in pounds = kcal/day (800–1,200 kcal/day)
1–3 years	1,300 kcal/day
4–6 years	1,700 kcal/day
7–10 years	2,400 kcal/day
11–16 years	
Boys	2,700 kcal/day
Girls	2,200 kcal/day

*These daily averages may vary considerably for an individual child, depending on the child's activity level, length (height), and body build.
Source: Food and Nutrition Board of the National Research Council, National Academy of Sciences.

include
- **a)** milk
- **b)** foods containing wheat, corn, or soy (protein gluten)
- **c)** egg white (albumin)
- **d)** chocolate
- **e)** citrus foods

2) indications of hypersensitivity to food
- **a)** urticaria
- **b)** abdominal pain, vomiting, and diarrhea
- **c)** respiratory symptoms

3) diagnosis
- **a)** singular addition of food
- **b)** food diary or history
- **c)** skin testing not useful (because of immature immune system)

4) treatment
- **a)** removal of causative food
- **b)** change to soy formula (if milk allergy)
- **c)** elimination diet

3. Sleep

a. Most infants have nocturnal sleep pattern by 3 months

b. 6 months: sleep through night

c. 8–9 months: two naps during day, sleep 10–12 hours at night

d. Anticipatory guidance for parents

1) each infant's sleep patterns are unique

2) best indicators of adequate sleep are normal activity during waking hours and normal physical growth

3) sleeping arrangements are influenced by family's cultural beliefs and customs

4. Health care

a. Immunizations

1) see Table 5.3 for recommended schedule of the American Academy of Pediatrics

2) contraindications
- **a)** febrile illness
- **b)** previous severe reaction to toxoid
- **c)** presence of skin rash
- **d)** malignancy
- **e)** pregnancy
- **f)** poor immunologic response
- **g)** administration of gamma globulin, plasma, or blood in previous 6–8 weeks
- **h)** give measles vaccine only after Tb test has been found to be negative (Tb fulminates in presence of measles virus)

3) common side effects
- **a)** mild fever
- **b)** malaise
- **c)** soreness and swelling at injection site (DPT)
- **d)** mild rash (measles, rubella)

4) advise parents of possible side effects; use of acetaminophen for fever (aspirin is contraindicated because of possible link between viral illness, aspirin, and Reye's syndrome)

b. Accident prevention: accidents are the second leading cause of death in this age group

1) aspiration/suffocation
- **a)** avoid propping bottles
- **b)** keep small objects out of reach
- **c)** check toys for small parts or sharp edges
- **d)** close pins when changing diaper
- **e)** keep plastic bags away

2) falls
- **a)** never leave on elevated surface unattended
- **b)** keep crib rails up

3) auto accidents: use infant car seats (crash-tested, rear-facing)

Table 5.3 American Academy of Pediatrics Recommended Immunization Schedule (1988)

Age	Immunization
2 months	Diphtheria/tetanus toxoid/pertussis (DPT) Trivalent oral poliovirus (TOPV)
4 months	DPT #2 TOPV #2
6 months	DPT #3 TOPV #3 (optional in US)
12 months	Tuberculin test (may be done at 15 month visit)
15 months	Measles, mumps, rubella (MMR)
18 months	DPT #4 TOPV #4 PRP-D (*Haemophilus* b diphtheria toxoid conjugate)
4–6 years	DPT #5 TOPV #5
14–16 years	Tetanus and diphtheria toxoids (adult-type)—Td; repeat every 10 years

Primary Immunization for Children* Not *Immunized in First Year of Life

Age	Immunization
Under 7 Years	
First visit	DPT, TOPV, Tb test, MMR
Interval after first visit:	
• 1 month	PRP-D
• 2 months	DPT, TOPV
• 4 months	DPT
10–16 months or preschool	DPT, TOPV
7 Years and Over	
First visit	Td, TOPV, Tb test, MMR
Interval after first visit:	
• 2 months	Td, TOPV
• 8–14 months	Td, TOPV
10 years later	Td; repeat every 10 years

4) burns: check water temperature before immersing infant; keep hot substances away from infant (cigarette ashes, coffee, etc.); check temperature of foods/formulas; expose to sun gradually

☐ Toddler (1 year to 3 years)

1. Normal growth and development
  a. Psychosocial development—Erikson: autonomy vs shame and doubt
    1) all activities move toward independence; expands independence by exploring environment and extending its limits
    2) verbally negative ("No!") even when agreeable to request
  b. Physical growth and development
    1) vital signs: pulse and respirations decrease, blood pressure increases with increasing size and age (see Table 5.1)
    2) teeth: all 20 deciduous present by 2½–3 years
    3) general appearance: potbellied, exaggerated lumbar curve, wide-based gait
    4) practices and increases muscle coordination and physical abilities
      a) climbs; goes up steps, cannot get down, and won't accept help
      b) jumps in place
      c) pushes and pulls toys
      d) scribbles spontaneously
      e) builds a tower of cubes
  c. Cognitive development—Piaget: sensorimotor and preconceptual stages
    1) 13–18 months
      a) very curious
      b) identifies geometric shapes
      c) opens doors and drawers
      d) points to body parts

e) puts objects into holes, smaller objects into each other
2) 19–24 months
a) egocentric thinking and behavior
b) beginning sense of time; waits in response to "just a minute"
3) 24–36 months
a) beginning magical thinking
b) understands prepositions (e.g., over, under, behind, up, etc.)
c) animism (attributes lifelike characteristics to inanimate objects)
d) understanding of cause and effect relationships is determined by proximity of two events; therefore, should be disciplined immediately
e) increasing attention span

d. Socialization
1) 15 months
a) resistant to sitting in laps
b) wants to move independently
2) 18 months to 2½ years: imitates parent behaviors (e.g., housework)
3) dawdling and ritualistic behavior
4) temper tantrums may be used to assert independence and gain control, especially when desires are thwarted
5) 18–24 months: learns to undress self
6) 24–36 months: able to dress self with minimal help
7) may be attached to transitional objects, such as a favorite blanket or stuffed animal
8) territorial: possessive of own toys and body

e. Vocalization
1) understands simple commands
2) 18 months: 20 words, names 1 body part
3) 2 years: makes simple 2- or 3-word sentences; uses pronouns, plurals; knows full name

f. Play (parallel)
1) purpose: to help child make transition from solitary to cooperative play
2) child will play beside, not with another child
3) types of toys
a) cars and trucks
b) push-pull toys
c) blocks, building toys, balls
d) telephone
e) stuffed toys and dolls
f) large crayons, coloring and hardboard books
g) clay, finger paints
h) wood puzzles
4) games: likes to throw and retrieve objects, prefers "rough and tumble" play

2. Nutrition and dental care
a. Growth slows, appetite smaller; "physiologic anorexia" (may eat a great deal one day and little the next); needs an average of 1,300 calories/day (see Table 5.2)
1) ritualistic food preferences
2) likes finger foods (crackers, celery, carrot sticks)
3) drinks from cup
4) self-feeds by 18 months
5) prone to iron-deficiency anemia, especially if milk intake is high

b. Anticipatory guidance for parents
1) serve small portions
2) recommended daily milk intake 24–32 oz
3) do not give bottle as a substitute for solid foods; give solids before or with milk
4) do not use food as a reward
5) recognize ritualistic needs (e.g., same dishes, utensils, chair)
6) do not force child to eat

c. Dental care guidelines
1) brush and floss twice daily with help from parents
2) first visit to dentist as soon as all primary teeth have erupted (2½–3 years)
3) use fluoridated water or oral fluoride supplement (0.25–0.5 mg/day)
4) limit concentrated sweets
5) do not allow child to take a bottle containing juice or milk to bed since "bottle mouth caries" may result

3. Elimination: toileting practices
a. Learning bowel and bladder control is one of the major tasks of toddlerhood and is dependent on physiologic and cognitive factors
b. Myelinization of nerve tracts occurs around 15–18 months of age (physiologic readiness)
c. Toddler uses toileting activities to control self and others
d. Independent toileting depends on
1) physiologic readiness
2) ability to verbally communicate need to defecate or urinate
3) ability to get to toilet and manage clothing
4) psychologic readiness

e. Ages
1) 18 months: bowel control
2) 2–3 years: daytime bladder control
3) 3–4 years: nighttime bladder control

4. Limit setting and discipline help child learn self-

control and socially appropriate behavior, promote security
   a. Enforcement of limits should be consistent and firm
   b. Discipline should occur immediately after wrongdoing
   c. Positive approach is best
   d. Disapprove of the behavior, *not* the child
   e. Types of discipline
      1) redirecting child's attention
      2) ignoring the behavior
      3) time-out
      4) reasoning and reprimanding, loss of privileges (for older children)
      5) corporal punishment (controversial)
5. Accident prevention: accidents are leading cause of death from 1–15 years of age.
   a. Falls
      1) Motor development is far ahead of judgment and perceptions
      2) climbs over side rails; change to regular bed
      3) climbs stairs; use safety gates
      4) supervise at playgrounds
   b. Poisonous ingestions (leading cause of injury and death): keep poisons and sharp objects locked up and out of reach
   c. Supervise when near cars; use car safety seats
   d. Burns: cover electrical outlets; do not leave unattended in bathtub, near hot stove, fireplace, etc.; teach child what "hot" means
   e. Drowning: supervise near water (e.g., bathtub, toilet, pools, lakes)

☐ Preschooler (3–6 years)

1. Normal growth and development
   a. Psychosocial development—Erikson: initiative vs guilt
      1) learns how to do things, derives satisfaction from activities
      2) needs exposure to variety of experiences and play materials
      3) imitates role models
      4) imaginative
         a) reality vs fantasy blurred
         b) may have imaginary friends
      5) exaggerated fears, e.g., fear of mutilation, monsters
   b. Physical growth and development
      1) body contours change: thinner and taller
      2) blood pressure 100/60 mg Hg
      3) motor skills: better control of fine and gross ones; posture more erect
         a) uses scissors and simple tools
         b) draws a person
            ■ 4 years: 3 parts
            ■ 5 years: 6 or 7 parts
         c) rides a tricycle or "big wheel"
         d) skips and hops, throws and catches a ball well (5 years)
         e) walks downstairs as well as upstairs alternating feet on steps
   c. Cognitive development—Piaget: preconceptual and intuitive thought stages
      1) increased sense of time and space (tomorrow, afternoon, next week)
      2) less egocentric
      3) beginning social awareness
      4) centration
         a) thinks of one idea at a time
         b) unable to think of all parts in terms of whole
         c) conclusions based on immediate visual perceptions
      5) increased ability to think without acting out; anticipates events
   d. Socialization
      1) capable of sharing; begins to have "best friends"
      2) dresses self completely
      3) may be physically aggressive
      4) boasts and tattles
      5) learns appropriate social manners
      6) separates easily from mother
   e. Vocalization
      1) 3-year-old: constantly asks how-and-why questions; vocabulary 300–900 words
      2) 5-year-old: uses sentences of adult length
      3) knows colors, numbers, alphabet
      4) understands analogies ("If fire is hot, ice is [cold].")
      5) stuttering (dysfluency) is fairly common among toddlers and preschoolers; normal variation of language development; parents should ignore stuttering so child does not become anxious; persistent stuttering beyond age 5 may require speech therapy
   f. Play (cooperative)
      1) purpose: to learn to share and play in small groups, to learn simple games and rules, language concepts, social roles
      2) play may be dramatic, imitative, or creative; expresses self through play
      3) types of toys
         a) housekeeping toys
         b) playground equipment
         c) wagons
         d) tricycles; big-wheel cycles
         e) water colors
         f) materials for cutting and pasting

g) simple jigsaw puzzles
h) picture books
i) dolls
j) TV (controversial but a contemporary reality)

2. Nutrition: a slow-growth period; needs an average of 1,700 calories/day (see Table 5.2)
   a. Appetite remains decreased; has definite food preferences; less picky
   b. Self-feeding: 4-year-old uses fork, can use knife to spread; able to get snacks for self
   c. Sets the table; learns table manners
   d. Able to pour from a pitcher
3. Sleep
   a. Sleep problems are most common in this age group
   b. Requires 9–12 hours/night
   c. May or may not take one nap during day
   d. May have fears of the dark, or may awaken with nightmares
   e. Guidelines for care givers
      1) provide quiet time before bedtime
      2) use a nightlight
      3) adhere to a consistent bedtime pattern
4. Sexuality
   a. Knows sex differences by 3 years
   b. Imitates masculine or feminine behaviors; gender identity well established by 6 years
   c. Sexual curiosity and exploration
      1) masturbation is normal; especially common in preschoolers, may increase in frequency when child is under stress
      2) curious about anatomical differences and seeks to "investigate" them
   d. Guidelines for care givers
      1) assess what child already knows when child asks a question
      2) answer questions simply, honestly, and matter-of-factly (avoid detailed explanations), using correct terminology
      3) masturbation: redirect child's attention without punishing or verbally reprimanding; teach child that touching genitals is not appropriate in public
5. Accident prevention
   a. Motor vehicle accidents (leading cause of injury and death)
      1) street safety: teach to wait at curb until told to cross; avoid riding cycles near street or driveways
      2) wear seat belt
   b. Drownings: teach to swim; supervise near pools, lakes, etc.
   c. Burns: teach not to play with matches or lights; supervise near fireplace; teach how to escape from burning home
   d. General safety: teach not to talk to strangers; child should know own name, address, telephone number, and how to seek help if lost

☐ School Age (6–12 years)

1. Normal growth and development
   a. Psychosocial development—Erikson: industry vs inferiority
      1) develops a sense of competency and esteem academically, physically, and socially
      2) school phobias may occur as a result of increased competition, desire to succeed, fear of failure
      3) desire for accomplishment so strong that young school-age child may try to change rules of game to win
      4) gains competence in mastering new skills and tasks; assumes more responsibilities
      5) desires to get along socially; more responsive to peers
      6) still needs reassurance and support from family and trusted adults
   b. Physical growth and development
      1) growth is slow and regular (1–2 inches gain in height per year, 3–6 lb weight gain per year), prepubertal females are usually taller than males
      2) motor skills: increases strength and physical ability, refines coordination
         a) 6 years: jumps, skips, hops well; ties shoelaces easily, prints
         b) 7 years: vision fully developed, can read regular-size print; can swim and ride a bicycle
         c) 8 years: writes rather than prints; increased smoothness and speed
         d) 9 years: fully developed hand-eye coordination; individual capabilities/ talents emerge
         e) 10 years: increased strength, stamina, coordination
         f) 11 years: awkward; nervous energy (drumming fingers, etc.)
   c. Cognitive development—Piaget: concrete operations stage (7–11 years)
      1) decentering: can consider more than one characteristic at a time; leads to ability to emphathize and sympathize
      2) reversibility: able to imagine a process in reverse
      3) conservation: able to conserve (mentally

retain) physical properties of matter even when form is changed
4) able to classify objects and verbalize concepts involved in doing so
5) reasons logically
6) able to think through a situation and anticipate the consequences; may then alter course of action

d. Socialization
1) prefers friends to family; life is centered around school and friends
2) relationships with peers and adults other than parents of increasing importance
3) increasing social sensitivity
4) more cooperative; improved manners
5) school phobia: difficulty coping with the academic or social demands of school may result in psychosomatic complaints (stomachache, headache) and refusal to attend school; best managed by rewarding school attendance, withdrawing privileges and attention for school avoidance
6) by 10 years enjoys privacy (e.g., own room, box that locks)

e. Vocalization
1) curious about meaning of different words; rapidly expanding vocabulary
2) likes name-calling, word games (e.g., rhymes)
3) develops a sense of humor; giggles and laughs a great deal; silly
4) knows clock and calendar time

f. Play (cooperative, team, rule-governed, same sex together)
1) purposes: to learn to bargain, cooperate and compromise; to develop logical reasoning abilities; to increase social skills
2) types of toys, entertainment
a) play figures, trains, model kits
b) games, jigsaw puzzles, magic tricks
c) books: joke and comic books, storybooks, adventure, mystery
d) TV, Nintendo games, tapes, radio
e) riding a bicycle
f) organized activities (sports, Scouts, music and dancing lessons, camping, slumber parties)

g. "collecting" age: stamps, cards, rocks, etc.

2. Nutrition and dental health
a. Appetite increases; needs an average of 2,400 calories/day (see Table 5.2); breakfast is important for school performance
b. More influenced by mass media; more likely to eat junk food because of increased time away from home
c. Nutrition education
1) teach basic four food groups
2) teach basic cooking skills, meal planning
3) nutritious snacks
d. Dental health
1) loss of deciduous teeth (begins 5–7 years of age); eruption of permanent ones, including 1st and 2nd molars
2) many schoolage children will wear braces
a) good oral hygiene is important
b) reassure re appearance
3) dental caries are a major health problem
a) caused by poor nutrition, influence of TV advertising contributing to increased intake of carbohydrates and concentrated sweets, inadequate dental hygiene
b) prevention: good brushing and flossing techniques, regular dental checkups, fluoridated water, good nutrition

3. Accident prevention
a. Accepts increasing responsibility for own safety; safety education is essential
b. Motor vehicle accidents
1) teach how to cross street
2) bike safety
3) use car safety belts
c. Drowning
1) learn to swim
2) teach water safety
d. Burns
1) teach safety around fires (e.g., fireplaces, camp fires), safe use of candles, matches
2) teach not to play with explosives or guns
e. Sports injuries: teach re appropriate protective equipment

☐ Adolescent (12–20 years)

1. Normal growth and development
a. Psychosocial development—Erikson: identity vs identity diffusion
1) "Who am I?"
2) "What do I want to do with my life?"
3) accepts changes in body image
4) experiences mood swings; vacillates between maturity and childlike behavior
5) continually reassesses values and beliefs
6) begins to consider career possibilities
7) gains independence from parents
b. Physical growth and development: puberty (onset in males occurs two years later than females on the average)
1) males: development of secondary sex characteristics
a) increase in size of genitalia

b) swelling of breasts
c) growth of pubic, axillary, facial, and chest hair
d) voice changes
e) increase in shoulder breadth
f) production of spermatozoa; nocturnal emissions

2) females: development of secondary sex characteristics
a) increase in transverse diameter of pelvis
b) development of breasts
c) change in vaginal secretions
d) growth of pubic and axillary hair
e) menstruation: 12 years (average)

3) both sexes
a) acne
b) perspiration
c) blushing
d) rapid increase in height and weight
e) fatigue (since heart and lungs grow at slower rate)

c. Cognitive development—Piaget: formal operations (11 years and older); attained at different ages and depends on formal education, experience, cultural background
1) abstract thinking
2) forms hypotheses, analytical thinking
3) can consider more than two categories at same time
4) generalizes findings
5) thinks about thinking; philosophical; concerned with social and moral issues

d. Socialization
1) with adults
a) may resent authority
b) wishes to be different from parents: may ridicule them
c) has need for parent figures
d) develops crushes on adults outside the family, "hero worship"
2) with peers
a) overidentifies with group: same dress, same ethical codes
b) has close friendships with members of same sex
c) develops heterosexual relationships, sexual experimentation (may be sexually active)

e. Recreation, leisure activity: expanding variety
1) parties, dances
2) Nintendo games, television, movies, music (radio, tapes)
3) telephone conversations, daydreaming
4) sports, games, hobbies
5) reading and writing
6) part time jobs (especially babysitting) to earn extra money

f. Sexual activity
1) 50% of adolescents have engaged in sexual activity
2) educate re birth control methods, pregnancy, sexually transmitted disease

2. Nutrition
a. Appetite increases with rapid growth; puberty changes nutritional requirements; needs basic four food groups
b. Caloric needs vary with activity level, sex, body build (see Table 5.2)
1) girls need approximately 2,200 calories/day
2) boys need an average of 2,700 calories/day
c. Increased need for protein, calcium, iron, and zinc
d. Sports activity may increase nutritional requirements
e. Eating habits are easily influenced by peer group
1) intake of junk food
2) fad diets and dieting: can lead to health problems, including anorexia nervosa
3) overeating or inactivity: may result in obesity

3. Accident prevention
a. Motor vehicle accidents: enroll in driver-training programs, wear seat belts
b. Drownings: teach water safety, first aid, CPR
c. Sports injuries: educate for prevention
d. Alcohol and drug abuse: education
e. Suicide: be alert for signs of depression

Application of the Nursing Process to the Healthy Child

1. Assessment
a. Health history
1) general health status: incidence of illnesses in past year, visits to health provider, immunization history, current medications
2) developmental history: parents' health status, mother's obstetric history with this child, child's neonatal history, achievement of developmental milestones, self-care abilities, behavior, and temperament
3) parents' perceptions and concerns
4) parents' knowledge of development, child care, safety, nutrition, etc.
5) child's home and school environments:

safety, appropriate stimulation, barriers to development

6) nutrition: daily food and fluid intake, child's preferences and dislikes, self-feeding abilities, special needs (cultural/religious practices, allergies), eating patterns
7) dental care: number of teeth, tooth eruption (discomfort, management), daily oral hygiene, self-brushing and flossing, fluoride (water or daily supplement), dental visits
8) elimination: daily routine, toilet trained or diapers, problems (e.g., diarrhea, constipation, enuresis; how managed)
9) activity/sleep: exercise and activity patterns; sleep habits: sleep environment, daily total, special needs, problems
10) sexuality: gender knowledge and identity, sexual curiosity and exploration, sexual knowledge, primary and secondary sex characteristics; adolescent: knowledge, sexual activity, contraception, pregnancy, sexually transmitted disease

b. Clinical appraisal

1) development
   a) observation of age-appropriate developmental behavior and abilities
   b) administration of developmental screening tools when indicated to screen for delays, e.g., Denver Developmental Screening Test (a screening tool to detect developmental problems in four areas: personal-social, fine motor-adaptive, language, gross motor; *not* an intelligence test; does not predict future developmental potential)
   c) home environment: visit to appraise for support of or barriers to development
2) general physical appraisal
   a) growth: length, weight, head circumference; percentiles on standard growth curves
   b) vital signs: annual BP screening over age 3 (especially in high-risk children) (see Table 5.1)
   c) general health: skin, activity, attention span, ability to communicate, etc.
   d) vision/hearing screening
      - vision testing
        - binocularity tests for strabismus; if strabismus is not detected and corrected by age 6 years, amblyopia (dimness of vision, even blindness) may result
          * corneal light reflex test
          * cover test
        - visual acuity tests; Snellen E (preschoolers or illiterate children) or Snellen alphabet chart
        - head tilting or squinting may indicate visual impairment
        - ophthalmoscopic exam
        - referral criteria
          * 3 years: vision in one or both eyes 20/50 or worse
          * 4–6 years: vision in one or both eyes 20/40 or worse
          * 7 years and older: vision in one or both eyes 20/30 or worse
          * children with one-line or more difference between both eyes (example: 20/30 in left eye, 20/40 in right)
          * abnormal findings from cover test or corneal light reflex test
      - hearing testing
        - otoscopic exam
        - conduction tests
          * Rinne test (comparison of bone and air conduction)
          * Weber's test (bone conduction)
        - pure tone audiometry (audiogram) to test for conductive or sensorineural hearing impairments

2. Analysis

a. Safe, effective care environment
1) potential for injury
2) sensory-perceptual alteration: visual, auditory, kinesthetic, tactile, olfactory
3) knowledge deficit

b. Physiological integrity
1) potential activity intolerance
2) altered nutrition: potential for less/more than body requirements
3) fatigue

c. Psychological integrity
1) decisional conflict
2) altered role performance
3) body image disturbance, self esteem disturbance

d. Health promotion/maintenance
1) ineffective family coping: potential for growth
2) altered growth and development
3) health seeking behaviors

3. General Nursing Plans, Implementation, and Evaluation

Goal 1: Child will achieve optimum development.

Plan/Implementation

- Provide information to parents on normal growth and development
  - what to expect (skills, behavior)
  - age-appropriate play activities and materials
  - ways to stimulate development
- Discuss child-rearing methods and styles, limit-setting, and ways to cope with child-rearing problems.
- Administer screening tools during well-child visits to detect developmental delays (e.g., language, speech, gross and fine motor, social, self-help).
- Refer for further evaluation or to early intervention services if developmental delay detected.

Evaluation: Child grows and develops within expected range; is free from delays in development; parents cope effectively with child-rearing concerns and problems.

Goal 2: Child will experience a safe environment and will be free from accidental injury.

Plan/Implementation

- Provide anticipatory guidance to parents concerning age-related safety hazards, and ways to prevent accidental injury (safety-proofing the home, auto safety restraints, swimming and bicycling safety, safe toys, driver education).

Evaluation: Child is free from accidental injury.

Goal 3: Child will receive optimal nutrition and dental care.

Plan/Implementation

- Provide teaching and counseling to parents concerning child's nutritional requirements, feeding techniques, dental hygiene, tooth eruption, food allergies, and feeding abilities.

Evaluation: Child's physical growth follows growth curve; child receives daily nutritional requirements (calories, protein, CHO, fats, vitamins/minerals); feeds self in accordance with developmental abilities; receives appropriate dental hygiene and care and is free from dental caries; child's food allergies are detected and diet is adjusted as needed.

Goal 4: Child will get adequate rest and sleep.

Plan/Implementation

- Provide anticipatory guidance to parents concerning child's sleep needs, patterns of sleep in childhood, and ways to cope with sleep problems.

Evaluation: Child gets amount of sleep required for optimal growth and development; parents cope with child's sleep problems.

Goal 5: Child will develop healthy sexuality.

Plan/Implementation

- Provide anticipatory guidance to parents concerning child's developing sexuality
  - what to expect (questions, behaviors)
  - answer child's questions matter-of-factly, honestly, accurately
- Teach child about sex and sexuality appropriate to child's age and expressed interest

Evaluation: Child develops gender-appropriate sexual identity and healthy sexuality.

Goal 6: Child will be free from preventable communicable diseases.

Plan/Implementation

- Reinforce to parents the importance of childhood immunizations.
- Administer immunizations according to recommended schedule.

Evaluation: Child receives immunizations according to recommended schedule; is free from preventable communicable diseases.

References

Biro, P. & Thompson, M. (1984). Screening young children for communication disorders. *MCN: American Journal of Maternal/Child Nursing, 9*, 410–413.

Castiglia, R. & Petrini, M. Selecting a developmental screening tool. *Pediatric Nursing, 11*(1), 8–17.

Dickey, S. (1987). *A guide to the nursing of children.* Baltimore: Williams and Wilkins.

Lee, J. & Fowler, M. (1986). Merely child's play? Developmental work and playthings. *Journal of Pediatric Nursing, 1*, 260–270.

Nachem, B. & Bass, R. (1984). Children still aren't being buckled up. *MCN: American Journal of Maternal/Child Nursing, 9*, 320–323.

Pediatric Nutrition Handbook. (1985). American Academy of Pediatrics: Committee on Nutrition. (2nd ed.)

Pillitteri, A. (1987). *Child health nursing: Care of the growing family.* (3rd ed.) Boston: Little, Brown and Company.

Pipes, P. (1985). *Nutrition in infancy and childhood* (3rd ed.). St. Louis: Mosby.

Rimar, J. (1986). Haemophilus influenzae type b polysaccharide. *MCN: American Journal of Maternal/ Child Nursing, 11*, 8–17.

Report of the Committee on Infectious Diseases (21st ed.) (1988). American Academy of Pediatrics.

Scipien, G. et al. (1986). *Comprehensive pediatric nursing* (3rd ed.). New York: McGraw-Hill.

Selekman, J. (1980). Immunization: What's it all about? *American Journal of Nursing, 80*, 1440–1443.

Servonsky, J. & Opas, S. (1987). *Nursing Management of Children*. Boston: Jones and Bartlett.

Verzemnieks, I. (1984). Developmental stimulation for infants and toddlers. *American Journal of Nursing, 84*, 749–752.

Whaley, L. and Wong, D. (1986). *Nursing care of infants and children* (3rd ed.). St. Louis: Mosby.

Wishon, O. and Kinnick, V. (1986). Helping infants overcome the problem of obesity. *MCN: American Journal of Maternal/Child Nursing, 11*, 118–121.

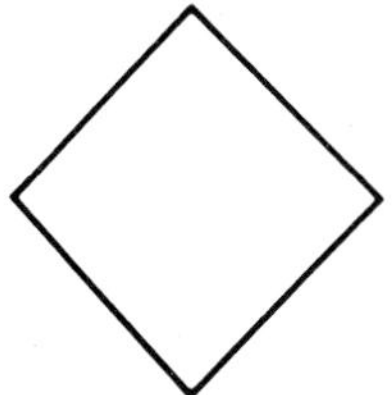

The Ill and Hospitalized Child

General Concepts

Overview

1. Hospitalization and illness are stressful for children
   - **a.** Difficulty changing routines
   - **b.** Limited coping mechanisms
   - **c.** Reason for hospitalization is often less significant than consequences (e.g., separation from familiar persons and surroundings, painful procedures, restricted mobility)
2. Major stressors for the child
   - **a.** Separation
   - **b.** Loss of control
   - **c.** Body injury
   - **d.** Pain
   - **e.** Immobility
3. Factors that affect responses to illness and hospitalization
   - **a.** Developmental level (see below, ''Developmental Responses to Hospitalization'')
   - **b.** Past experiences, especially with hospitalization and surgery
   - **c.** Level of anxiety: child and parents
   - **d.** Relationship between parents and child
   - **e.** Nature and seriousness of illness or injury; circumstances of hospitalization
   - **f.** Family background: education, culture, support systems
4. Developmental responses to hospitalization
   - **a.** Infant
     - **1)** separation: before attachment (under 4–6 months) not as significant; older infant's response is significant with crying, rage, protest; stranger anxiety
     - **2)** loss of control
       - **a)** expects that crying will bring immediate response from care giver (changed, fed, held); may interfere with development of trust
       - **b)** in hospital
         - ■ immediate response may not occur
         - ■ need may be met by unfamiliar person
         - ■ unable to express needs or understand explanations
     - **3)** immobility: restrictions and restraints interfere with activity and sucking (see Table 5.4)
     - **4)** pain: procedures cause discomfort; responds by crying and withdrawal
   - **b.** Toddler
     - **1)** separation
       - **a)** fear of unknown and abandonment
       - **b)** separation anxiety is similar to grief; so encourage protest behaviors as healthy response
         - ■ protest: cries loudly, rejects attentions of nurses, wants parent
         - ■ despair: cries in monotonous tone, state of mourning, ''settling in''
         - ■ denial: renewed interest in surroundings; seems adjusted to loss, but actually repressing feelings for parent
       - **c)** disruption in routines (eating, sleep, toileting) decreases security and control
       - **d)** regression: attempts to seek comfort by returning to earlier, dependent behaviors
         - ■ clinging, whining
         - ■ wetting
         - ■ wanting bottle, pacifier
     - **2)** loss of control: special concern because major task is to gain autonomy
     - **3)** body injury: fears intrusive procedures (e.g., rectal temperature, injections) and reacts intensely
     - **4)** immobility: cannot freely explore environment; may interfere with motor, language development
     - **5)** pain: becomes emotionally distraught and physically resistant to painful procedures
   - **c.** Preschooler
     - **1)** separation
       - **a)** may view as punishment for something thought or done
       - **b)** more subtle responses than toddler

(quiet crying, sleep problems, loss of appetite)
2) loss of control: their active imagination may lead to exaggeration or misinterpretations of hospital experiences; fears and fantasies may get the best of them
3) body injury/body integrity
a) confusion between reality and fantasy
b) casts and bandages are particular problems, since child is not assured that all body parts that were there before are there now; much worry over body integrity
4) pain
a) recognizes cues that signal an impending painful experience
b) able to anticipate pain: may try to escape, may become physically combative
5) immobility: prevents mastery of fears; preschooler often feels helpless

d. School-age child
1) separation
a) from family and friends
b) easier than other age groups because of cognitive level and better time concept
2) fear of loss of control
a) through immobility
b) enforced dependence
c) fear of injury and death; death anxiety peaks
d) does not want others to see loss of control (e.g., crying), tries to appear brave
3) pain: responses are influenced by cultural variables; usually uses passive coping strategies (lies rigidly still, shuts eyes, clenches teeth and fists)
4) immobility: affects sense of physical achievement and need for competition

e. Adolescent: loss of control/enforced dependence when the need is to move toward own identity and independence

Application of the Nursing Process to the Ill and Hospitalized Child

1. Assessment

a. Child's development level and major fear associated with age group
1) infant: separation
2) toddler: separation, intrusive procedures
3) preschooler: body mutilation, pain
4) school-age: loss of control, separation from peers
5) adolescent: change in body image and self-identity, loss of esteem

b. Child's perceptions/understanding of illness and hospitalization

c. Family responses to child's hospitalization
1) parents may react with denial, disbelief, guilt, fear, anxiety, frustration, and depression
2) alterations in family routines and life-style
3) parents' coping mechanisms
a) support systems for parents, e.g., friends, extended family members
b) financial resources
c) family's ability to cope with the child's illness
d) ability to express reaction to child's illness

d. Child's responses to pain: unable to express verbally; often results in underutilization of pain-relief methods
1) through observation
a) verbally: younger child often uses incorrect words, e.g., "bad," "funny," "hot"; older child often reluctant to complain because of fear of "shots"
b) behaviorally: pulling at area (ear), irritable, loss of appetite, lying or moving in unusual position
c) physiologically: vomiting, change in vital signs, flushed skin, increased sleep time, sleep disruptions
2) asking child to rate the pain, e.g., using happy/unhappy faces, or scale of 0–10

2. Analysis

a. Safe, effective care environment
1) potential for infection
2) potential for injury
3) sensory-perceptual alteration

b. Physiological integrity
1) ineffective airway clearance/potential for aspiration
2) pain
3) fluid volume deficit

c. Psychological integrity
1) ineffective individual coping
2) anxiety/fear
3) body image disturbance

d. Health promotion/maintenance
1) altered growth and development
2) knowledge deficit
3) altered family processes

3. Plans, Implementation, and Evaluation

Goal 1: Child will be prepared psychologically for hospitalization.

Plan/Implementation

- Encourage preadmission preparation
  - *before 2 years*: explanation is ineffective; allow to take favorite toy and objects
  - *2–7 years*: usually tell child ahead in days equal to years of age, e.g., 2 years = 2 days ahead, 6 years = 6 days ahead
  - *over 7 years*: tell child when parent knows (use judgment)
- Orient child and family to surroundings.
- Anticipate and alleviate age-related needs and fears

  to develop trust in infant
  - arrange for rooming-in
  - ensure consistency of care giver
  - provide security objects (e.g., toy, blanket)
  - make routine patterns as similar as possible to home
  - hold, cuddle, stroke

  to help toddler maintain control
  - use familiar words (e.g., child's word for toileting)
  - ask parents to leave familiar objects with child (e.g., toy, blanket)
  - encourage rooming-in and parental participation in care
  - accept regressive needs but avoid promoting them (e.g., don't put toilet-trained child back in diapers)
  - provide explanations immediately prior to any procedure with use of simple, concrete words
  - use time orientation in relation to familiar activities (e.g., "after naptime")
  - prepare parents to recognize and accept regressive behavior following discharge
  - maintain limit setting to provide consistency for child
  - don't offer choices when there are none

  to help preschooler relieve body-mutilation anxiety
  - allow child to wear underwear
  - provide reassurance regarding invasive procedures
  - encourage play that incorporates equipment/treatments
  - concept of time is related to routine activities (e.g., when you wake up, after lunch, etc.)
  - allow some choices to promote feelings of control and mastery (choice of fluids, play activities)

  to help school-age child maintain a degree of control
  - provide explanations of illness, treatment with pictures, simple anatomic diagrams, dolls (call them models or teaching models with older child), books, step-by-step illustrations
  - maintain educational level during long-term hospitalization to help meet need for accomplishment
    - * homework; contact with own schoolteacher
    - * in-hospital teacher
  - allow to participate in planning care by choosing food, times for bath or treatments

  to help adolescent maintain esteem and identity
  - maintain peer contacts
    - * visiting should be open to adolescents
    - * place in adolescent unit or room
  - encourage participation in decision making regarding own body
- Provide *honest* explanations, information, and support
  - determine level of understanding based on cognitive development and preexisting knowledge
  - use age-appropriate language, terminology, and timing prior to instruction
- Foster a sense of safety and security
  - encourage rooming-in, security objects for younger children
  - determine child's routine, rituals, nickname
  - implement age-appropriate safety measures, e.g., bubble top (covered) cribs, raised crib rails (see Table 5.4)

Evaluation: Child maintains developmental level; expresses feelings/desires about hospital (e.g., wants to go home); maintains attachments (family, favorite objects, friends).

Goal 2: Parents will feel in control.

Plan/Implementation

- Allow and encourage parents to participate in child's care; provide 24-hour open visiting and rooming-in facilities.
- Foster family relationships between ill child and family members; include siblings.
- Provide support; help family identify persons or community resources who can help.
- Provide information about child's illness, treatment, and care at rate that parents are able to accept and cope with.

Evaluation: Parents express satisfaction with care givers and information provided; child and parents maintain/regain supportive relationships.

Table 5.4 Commonly Used Pediatric Restraints

Type	Indications	Precautions
Jacket	In crib (alternative to crib net) In high chair. To maintain horizontal position in crib	Tie in back. Secure ties underneath crib or high chair.
Crib net	To prevent infant or toddler from climbing over side rails	Avoid nets with tears or large gaps. Tie to bedsprings, not to crib sides.
Crib cover	To prevent toddler from climbing out of crib	Ensure all latches are locked.
Mummy	For infant or small toddler needing short-term restraint • venipuncture • gavage feedings • eye, ear, nose, throat exams	Keep top of mummy sheet level with shoulder. Maintain arms and legs in anatomical position. Expose needed extremity only.
Clove hitch or commercial ties	For arm/leg restraints to limit motion for venipunctures	Observe for adequacy of circulation. Pad under restraint. Tie ends to crib springs. Remove q2h for ROM exercise.
Elbow	To prevent touching of head or face • scalp vein infusions • post-op, repair of cleft lip, palate	Pad stiff material. Use pins or ties to prevent slippage. Remove one at a time q2h for ROM exercise.

Goal 3: Child undergoing hospital procedures and surgery will be prepared.

Plan/Implementation

- Refer to "Perioperative Period" in *Surgery* page 157.
- Measure child's height and weight (used for calculating medications and IV fluids).
- Explain procedure, recovery room, and post-op care to child (appropriate for age) and to parents
  - use concrete words and visual aids
  - use neutral words, e.g., "fixed" instead of "cut"
  - emphasize body part involved and any change in function
  - use drawings and storytelling to evaluate child's understanding
  - take child and parent to see equipment and rooms, if possible

Day of surgery

- Keep NPO (shorter duration for a child compared with an adult).
- Check for loose teeth and inform anesthesiology.
- Allow favorite toy to accompany child to OR.
- Encourage parents to remain with child as long as possible.
- Clothe child for OR: diaper for non-toilet trained child; permit older child to wear underwear under hospital gown, if possible.
- Administer pre-op medications as ordered; oral or parenteral form is influenced by type, amount, age, accessibility; see Tables 5.5 and 5.6.

Table 5.5 Medication and Temperature Guide

Age Group	Usual Form of Oral Medication	Available Injection Sites	Usual Route for Temperature
Infant	L	VL	A R
Toddler	L P (crush)	VL	A R
Preschooler	L P (crush or chew)	VL VG GM D for immunizations	A R O (older child)
School-age child	L P	VL VG GM D	O A
Adolescent	L P C	VL VG GM D	O A
	P—pills L—liquid C—capsules	VL—vastus lateralis GM—gluteus medius VG—ventro gluteal D—deltoid	O—oral A—axillary R—rectal

Table 5.6 Medication Administration for Young Children

Age	Developmental Considerations	Nursing Implications
1–3 months	Strong sucking reflex Extrusion reflex	Allow sucking for oral meds, e.g., nipples, syringes. Give meds in small amounts to allow for swallowing. Keep head upright. Place liquid in center or side of mouth, toward back.
	Reaches randomly	Control child's hands when giving oral meds.
	Whole body reacts to painful stimuli	Use own body to control infant's arms and legs for parenteral meds.
3–12 months	Extrusion reflex disappears Drinks from cup Can finger feed Can spit out medication	Use medicine cup/syringe rather than spoon. Offer physical comforting more than verbal.
12–30 months	Development of large motor skills Can spit out meds or clamp jaw shut Can use medicine cup Auditory canal is not straight Autonomy vs shame/doubt Ritualistic Takes pride in tasks	Never leave meds where child can reach or throw. May need two adults to give injections (one to restrain). Give ear drops by pulling pinna down and back. Be honest about taste/pain, use distractions. Be firm, ignore resistive behavior Give choices when possible.
2½–3½ years	Has eating likes and dislikes Little sense of time Tries to coerce, manipulate Has fantasies Body boundaries are unclear	Disguise med taste. Use chewable meds. Use concrete and immediate rewards (stickers, badges). Give choices when possible, but do not offer if there are none. Be consistent. Give simple explanations; assure medicine is not for a punichmont. Use Band-Aids for covering injection sites.
3½–6 years	Develops proficiency at tasks Refining senses Has loose teeth Can make decisions Has a sense of time Takes pride in accomplishment Developing a conscience Fears mutilation, punishment May master pill swallowing	Allow child to handle equipment (e.g., syringes). Unable to disguise tastes and smells. Consider teeth when deciding route. Allow choice about route, if possible. Allow participation in choice of administration time when possible (e.g., before or after meals). Explain in simple terms reason for meds. Avoid prolonged reasoning. Use simple command by trusted adult that med is to be given. Allow control when possible. Praise after med is given.

Evaluation: Child is NPO; is prepared correctly for surgery; child and family know what to expect postoperatively.

Goal 4: Postoperatively, child will maintain adequate pulmonary ventilation and circulation, fluid and electrolyte balance.

Plan/Implementation

- Turn, position, and get child to cough at least q2h.
- Allow some crying in infants to achieve deep breathing.
- Use inspirometer, straw games with older child to ensure deep breathing.
- Monitor IV closely
  - if microdrip (60 gtts/ml used), gtts/min = ml/hour
  - check for fluid overload
- Exercise restrained limbs q2h; fasten restraint ties to crib or bed.

Evaluation: Child has adequate ventilation and circulation, normal color, no evidence of cyanosis, adequate fluid intake and output.

Goal 5: Child will be free from pain.

Plan/Implementation

- Be alert to nonverbal messages in a very young child or child who may fear injections and not wish to communicate discomfort.
- Medicate for nausea and pain as ordered (often analgesics such as acetaminophen are used).
- Determine correct medication dosage (see Table 5.7).

Table 5.7 Estimating Pediatric Drug Doses

Pediatric medication dosages may be estimated using one of several formulas. Three of the most common formulas are:

1. *Body surface area (BSA)*: most reliable method; must plot child's height and weight on a nomogram (available in reference texts)

$$\frac{\text{body surface area of child (m}^2\text{)}}{1.7\ (\text{m}^2)} \times \text{adult dose} = \text{estimated pediatric dose}$$

Example: Child's BSA is .34; usual adult dose is 500 mg. What is the child's estimated dosage?

$$\frac{.34}{1.7} \times 500\ \text{mg} = 100\ \text{mg}$$

2. *Clark's rule*: based on child's body weight; may be used with infants and young children

$$\frac{\text{child's weight (lb)}}{150\ \text{lb}} \times \text{adult dose} = \text{estimated pediatric dose}$$

Example: Child weighs 75 lb; usual adult dose is 1 gram. What is the child's estimated dosage?

$$\frac{75\ \text{lb}}{150\ \text{lb}} \times 1000\ \text{mg} = 500\ \text{mg}$$

3. *Young's rule*: used for children over age 2 years

$$\frac{\text{child's age in years}}{\text{child's age in years} + 12} \times \text{adult dose} = \text{estimated pediatric dose}$$

Example: Child is 6 years old; usual adult dose is 300 mg. What is the child's estimated dosage?

$$\frac{6}{6 + 12} \times 300\ \text{mg} = 100\ \text{mg}$$

- Assess for response to medications.

Evaluation: Child experiences minimal pain.

Goal 6: Child will use diversional activity and play to cope with the stress of hospitalization.

Plan/Implementation

- Refer to *Healthy Child* page 517.
- Help child participate in nursing activities, e.g., tea party for fluid intake, inspirometer for deep breathing, bean bags for range of motion.
- Use drawings, storytelling, puppets to help child express feelings about illness.
- Allow child to use syringes, needles with supervision.

Evaluation: Child expresses fears and feelings during play; adapts to hospital routine with minimal distress.

Goal 7: Child and family will receive appropriate discharge teaching.

Plan/Implementation

- Provide oral and written instructions regarding
  - activities and restrictions
  - diet
  - procedures
  - medications: schedule, administration, storage, side effects
- Teach parents procedures that must be performed at home.
- Contact appropriate outside resources as needed, e.g., homebound teacher, Visiting Nurse Association.

Evaluation: Child (as appropriate) and parent describe medical regimen that must be carried on at home (e.g., medications, diet, restrictions); demonstrate how to do procedures or give medications, know how to obtain refills, arrange for follow-up appointments.

References

Hazinski, M. F. (1985). Nursing care of the critically ill child: A seven point check. *Pediatric Nursing, 11*, 453–461.

Landier, W., Barrell, M., & Styffe, E. (1987). How to administer blood components to children. *MCN: American Journal of Maternal/Child Nursing, 12*, 178–184.

*Reynolds, E., & Ramenofsky, M. (1988). The emotional impact of trauma on toddlers. *MCN: American Journal of Maternal/Child Nursing, 13*, 106–109.

Rimar, J. (1987). Guidelines for the IV administration of medications used in pediatrics. *MCN: American Journal of Maternal/Child Nursing, 12*, 322–340.

*Rimar, J. (1988). Recognizing shock syndromes in infants and children. *MCN: American Journal of Maternal/Child Nursing, 13*, 32–37.

Rushton, C. (1986). Promoting normal growth and development in the hospital environment. *Neonatal Network, 4*, 21–30.

Whaley, L., & Wong, D. (1986). *Nursing care of infants and children* (3rd ed.). St. Louis: Mosby.

Zurlinden, J. (1985). Minimizing the impact of hospitalization for children and their families. *MCN: American Journal of Maternal/Child Nursing, 10*(3), 178–182.

Zweig, C. (1986). Reducing stress when a child is admitted to the hospital. *MCN: American Journal of Maternal/Child Nursing, 11*(1), 24–26.

*See Reprint Section

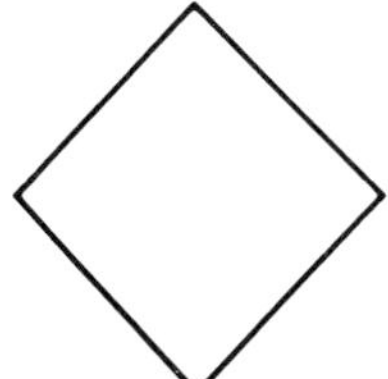

Sensation, Perception, and Protection

General Concepts

Overview/Physiology

1. Immunologic differences in children
   a. Newborn receives passive immunity from mother for most major childhood communicable diseases (assuming mother is immune)
   b. The young infant's immune system is not fully developed; therefore, the infant is more prone to infectious disease
   c. The eustachian tube in infants and young toddlers is shorter and straighter than in older children and adults, leading to increased risk of middle ear infections.
   d. Increasing exposure of preschoolers and school-age children to infectious disease and the immaturity of their immune system leads to increased incidence of infections
2. Integumentary (skin) differences in children
   a. The skin is less thick during infancy
   b. The epidermis is fragile and more prone to irritation
   c. The infant's skin is more sensitive to changes in temperature (especially extremes of heat and cold) and is more susceptible to invasion by bacteria and other infectious organisms
3. Neurologic differences in children
   a. The greatest neurologic changes occur during the first year of life
   b. The brain reaches 75% of adult size by age 2, 90% by age 4
   c. Cortical development is usually complete by age 4
   d. Primitive neonatal reflexes disappear as higher centers of the brain take over; most neonatal reflexes disappear or diminish by 3–4 months of age; their persistence may indicate a neurologic problem

Application of the Nursing Process to the Child with a Sensory Problem

1. **Assessment**
   a. Nursing history
      1) Frequent earaches or sore throats, persistent nosebleeds or sinus problems, allergies
      2) Eye crosses, deviates outward or inward, tears excessively; history of other vision problems
      3) Parental concerns re child's vision or hearing
   b. Clinical appraisal
      1) Otoscopic exam, ear pain or "fullness", hearing loss
      2) Ophthalmoscopic exam, head tilting or squinting
      3) Hypertrophy of tonsils, sore throat
   c. Diagnostic tests
      1) Vision and hearing testing (refer to "The Healthy Child" page 526)
2. **Analysis**
   a. Safe, effective care environment
      1) sensory-perceptual alteration: visual, auditory, tactile
      2) potential for injury
      3) potential for infection
   b. Physiological integrity
      1) pain
      2) actual/potential impaired skin integrity
   c. Psychological integrity
      1) body image disturbance
      2) anxiety
   d. Health promotion/maintenance
      1) knowledge deficit
      2) self-care deficit
      3) altered growth and development
3. **Nursing Plans, Implementation, and Evaluation**

Selected Health Problems: Interference with Sensation

☐ Otitis Media

1. General Information

   a. Definition: middle ear infection; two types:
      1) *serous otitis media*: nonpurulent effusion of middle ear

2) *suppurative otitis media (acute or chronic)*: accumulation of viral or bacterial purulent exudate in middle ear

b. Cause
   1) serous: unknown but there appears to be a relationship with allergies
   2) suppurative: pneumococci, *H. influenzae*, streptococci

c. Incidence: one of the most common illnesses of infancy and early childhood

d. Medical treatment
   1) diagnosis
      a) otoscopic exam
         - inflamed, bulging tympanic membrane (acute) or dull gray membrane (serous)
         - no visible landmarks or light reflex
      b) tympanometry (measures air pressure in auditory canal): decreased membrane mobility
   2) antibiotic therapy: ampicillin (may cause diarrhea; given q6h) or amoxicillin (more expensive but fewer side effects; given TID) 10–14 days
   3) surgical intervention: incision of membrane (myringotomy) and insertion of myringotomy tubes in cases of recurrent, chronic otitis media

2. Nursing Process

a. Assessment/Analysis
   1) *suppurative otitis*
      a) pain (infants may pull or hold ears)
      b) irritability
      c) high fever
      d) lymphadenopathy
      e) purulent discharge (indicates rupture of membrane)
      f) nasal congestion, cough
      g) anorexia, vomiting
      h) diarrhea
   2) *serous otitis*
      a) ear "fullness"
      b) popping senstion when swallowing
      c) conductive hearing loss

b. Plans, Implementation, and Evaluation

Goal 1: Child will be free from infecting organism and recurrence of infection.

Plan/Implementation
- Teach parents to administer antibiotics as prescribed.
- Educate parents concerning importance of adhering to medication regimen for full course of therapy.
- Clean drainage from ear with cotton balls and water.

Evaluation: Child shows no signs or symptoms of continuing infection (e.g., pulling at ears, fever); no discharge from ears; disease does not recur.

Goal 2: Child will receive comfort measures and be free from pain and fever.

Plan/Implementation
- Monitor body temperature.
- Teach parents to administer antipyretic analgesics (acetaminophen or aspirin).
- Control fever with tepid baths or sponging.
- Avoid foods that require chewing.
- Apply external heat (warm water bottle or heating pad).

Evaluation: Child is free from pain, able to play and sleep comfortably; child's temperature returns to normal.

Goal 3: Child will have no permanent hearing impairment.

Plan/Implementation
- Monitor for signs of hearing loss (decreased attention and responsiveness).
- Conduct audiometry screening at routine intervals.
- Refer child to appropriate resources if results are abnormal.

Evaluation: Child has normal hearing.

Goal 4: Child/family will receive appropriate information concerning home care following a myringotomy and insertion of tubes.

Plan/Implementation
- Tell parents to expect some drainage from the ear for several days post-op; obvious bleeding is not normal and the physician should be notified.
- Keep ear dry; avoid activities that require submerging the head in water (e.g., swimming).
- Before bathing, place cotton balls in the external canal to keep the ear dry (some physicians recommend dipping them in Vaseline first).
- Advise parents that if the child develops fever, headache and nausea/vomiting (meningitis) to notify physician.
- Check the ears periodically in case the PE

tubes become dislodged (they normally remain in approximately 6 months and then fall out spontaneously).

Evaluation: Child has uneventful recovery; family implements home care without problems/complications.

□ Tonsillectomy and Adenoidectomy

1. General Information

a. Definition: surgical excision of the tonsils and adenoids; usually done after three years of age because of the danger of excessive bleeding and tonsillar regrowth

b. Indications for surgery: controversy exists regarding the value of surgery; most widely accepted reasons are chronic tonsillitis (most common cause is beta strep, group A) and airway obstruction.

2. Nursing Process

a. **Assessment/Analysis**

1) airway obstruction: noisy or increased respiration; restless/change in behavior; diaphoretic; pale/cyanotic
2) active infection: fever, sore throat, enlarged lymph nodes; elevated WBCs
3) bleeding disorders: bleeding and coagulation time: PT, PTT
4) pre-op anxiety: child/family's knowledge concerning surgery

b. **Plans, Implementation, and Evaluation**

Goal 1: Preoperatively, the child and family will be prepared psychologically for hospitalization and surgery (refer to "The Ill and Hospitalized Child" page 529).

Goal 2: Postoperatively, the child will remain free from excessive bleeding or hemorrhage; maintain a patent airway.

Plan/Implementation

- Position child on side with knee on upper side flexed until alert and recovered from surgery.
- Monitor vital signs frequently.
- Observe for excessive swallowing, vomiting of fresh blood, restlessness, frequent clearing of throat.
- Inspect surgical site for signs of oozing.
- Discourage child from coughing, sneezing, crying, sucking on straw (puts tension on suture line).
- Employ comfort measures
  - ice collar to promote vasoconstriction and reduce pain
  - analgesics prn (avoid aspirin)
  - nonirritating, cool liquids (ice chips, Popsicles, Jell-O); avoid milk products
  - mouth care (no gargling or toothbrush)

Evaluation: Child maintains patent airway free from hemorrhage; experiences minimal pain/discomfort.

Goal 3: Child/family will receive appropriate information concerning home care.

Plan/Implementation

- Observe for delayed hemorrhage (5–10 days post-op) caused by infection or tissue sloughing during healing process.
- Limit child's activities for 1–2 weeks.
- Provide daily rest periods.
- Keep child away from anyone with an active infection (e.g., URI).
- Provide nonirritating foods to child for 1–2 weeks; no hot, citrus, spicy, or rough foods; encourage clear liquids.
- Have child refrain from coughing, clearing throat, or gargling (sore throat usually last 7 10 days).

Evaluation: Child's surgical site heals with no complications; child resumes normal diet/activities 1–2 weeks postoperatively.

□ Strabismus

1. General Information

a. Definition: neuromuscular defect of the eye that can cause visual impairment, either diplopia (double vision) or amblyopia (suppression of vision in one eye)

b. Incidence: normal in young infants; considered abnormal after 4 months of age, requiring evaluation and treatment

c. Medical treatment (done before age 6 to preserve or restore vision in affected eye)

1) eye muscle exercises (orthoptics)
2) corrective lenses
3) patching unaffected eye to strengthen muscles of affected eye
4) surgical correction

2. Nursing Process

a. **Assessment/Analysis**

1) eye crosses or deviates outward; may be unilateral or bilateral
2) squinting; head tilting
3) cover test: unaffected eye is covered while child focuses on an object, cover is removed, affected eye deviates

4) corneal light reflex test: shine penlight on bridge of child's nose while child fixates on a distant object, light reflects from a different point on each pupil, indicating an imbalance

b. Plans, Implementation, and Evaluation

Goal 1: Child and parents will implement treatment plan (exercises, patching, or corrective lenses).

Plan/Implementation

- Teach child and parents how to carry out prescribed treatment measures.
- Emphasize importance of adhering to treatment plan.

Evaluation: Child cooperates with and adheres to corrective measures; has vision restored; experiences no worsening of visual impairment.

Goal 2: Child will be prepared for eye surgery; complications will be prevented.

Plan/Implementation

- Assist child in becoming familiar with post-op environment (e.g., call light, bedside table).
- Minimize changes in child's post-op environment.
- Speak to child in normal voice tones; identify self and purpose *before* proceeding with care.
- Maintain eye patches or shields as prescribed.
- Keep side rails up, pad as necessary.
- Teach child to avoid straining, coughing, sudden movement, rubbing eyes (use elbow restraints if necessary).
- Observe and report ocular redness, discharge, itching, or pain.
- Instill eye ointments or drops as prescribed (inner to outer canthus).
- Provide auditory and tactile play activities (music, reading to child, story tapes, favorite attachment objects).

Evaluation: Child's eye heals without injury or infection; child copes with sensory deprivation and cooperates with care.

Application of the Nursing Process to the Child with an Interference with Protection: Communicable Disease

1. Assessment

a. Nursing history
- **1)** immunization history
- **2)** history of exposure to disease
- **3)** previous communicable diseases, how treated
- **4)** signs and symptoms of current illness
  - **a)** alterations in skin sensation
  - **b)** skin lesions
  - **c)** pain or tenderness
  - **d)** itching
  - **e)** fever

b. Clinical appraisal
- **1)** skin lesions: size, color, distribution (general, localized), configuration (single, clustered, diffuse, linear), type of lesion (macule, papule, visicle, pustule, crust)
- **2)** description of infestation (lice, scabies, ringworm, pinworms)

c. Diagnostic tests
- **1)** microscopic exam of lesions
- **2)** culture of organism

2. Analysis

a. Safe, effective care environment
- **1)** potential for poisoning
- **2)** potential for infection

b. Physiological integrity
- **1)** pain
- **2)** fluid volume deficit
- **3)** impaired skin integrity

c. Psychological integrity
- **1)** body image disturbance
- **2)** social isolation
- **3)** anxiety

d. Health promotion/maintenance
- **1)** knowledge deficit
- **2)** self-care deficit
- **3)** altered health maintenance

3. General Nursing Plan, Implementation, and Evaluation

Goal: Child will be free from communicable disease (infection, infestation) and will not spread communicable diseases to others.

Plan/Implementation

- Ensure immunizations remain up to date.
- Explain prescribed treatment to parents/child and encourage them to comply with therapy.
- Prevent child's exposure to others during communicable period.
- Identify contacts who may also require treatment.

Evaluation: Child is free from communicable disease; does not transmit disease to others.

Selected Health Problems: Communicable Diseases, Skin Problems, Infestations

☐ Communicable Diseases

1. General Information

a. Definition: a disease caused by a specific agent or its toxic products, transmitted by direct contact or indirectly through contaminated articles; the incidence of communicable disease has significantly decreased with availability and widespread use of immunizations

b. Types of immunity
- **1)** active: antibodies formed by the body as a result of having had the disease or through immunization
- **2)** passive: introduction of antibodies formed outside the body, such as by placental transfer, breast milk, or gamma globulin injection

c. Medical treatment
- **1)** prevent through immunization (refer to Table 5.3)
- **2)** antibiotic therapy for scarlet fever (penicillin/erythromycin) and Rocky Mountain Spotted Fever (tetracycline/chloramphenicol)
- **3)** rubella titer before pregnancy or during 1st trimester

2. Nursing Process

a. Assessment/Analysis
- **1)** prodromal period
  - **a)** malaise
  - **b)** anorexia
  - **c)** coryza
  - **d)** sore throat
  - **e)** fever
  - **f)** lymphadenopathy
  - **g)** headache
- **2)** specific characteristics
  - **a)** *chickenpox (varicella zoster)*: rash begins as macule, progresses to papule and vesicle which breaks open and crusts over; all stages present in varying degrees at same time; rash begins on trunk and spreads to extremities and face; intense pruritus; child communicable until all lesions crusted
  - **b)** *mumps (parotitis)*: after puberty, sterility in males is major complication; encephalitis is frequent complication of mumps for any age group
  - **c)** *German measles (rubella)*: greatest concern is teratogenic effect on fetus during 1st trimester of pregnancy; rubella titer on women of child-bearing age highly recommended
  - **d)** *Rocky Mountain Spotted Fever (RMSF)*: transmitted by ticks; found primarily along Atlantic coast and Rocky Mountain region; high fever and rash beginning on ankles, wrists, soles of feet; may see edema and CNS problems; methods for tick removal include applying nail polish, Vaseline, or heated needle to tick and withdrawing tick gently with tweezers
  - **e)** *roseola (exanthema subitum)*: seen in children age 6 months to 2 years; high fever for 3–4 days; temperature returns to normal with onset of rosy-pink, macular rash; rash fades with pressure and lasts 1–2 days; febrile convulsions
  - **f)** *scarlet fever:* caused by beta hemolytic *Streptococcus* group A; high fever, strawberry tongue, and red pinpoint rash, especially in skin folds; rheumatic fever or acute glomerulonephritis may follow
  - **g)** *Reye's Syndrome*: while not communicable, is a serious complication that may occur after a viral infection (e.g., chickenpox, flu); child appears to have recovered from viral infection and then usually begins to vomit; may see changes in LOC; increased ICP and seizures; increased risk in children who received aspirin during viral illness; acetaminophen is drug of choice for this reason

b. Plans, Implementation, and Evaluation

Goal 1: Child will be prepared for isolation, will not spread disease.

Plan/Implementation
- Explain reason for isolation to child and parents.
- Provide age-appropriate play
  - diversion
  - plan time to play with child
  - TV in room (except if photophobic)
- Accept expressions of fear, anger, restlessness, boredom
- If child is hospitalized, use appropriate isolation procedures (see Table 5.8)
- Discontinue isolation as soon as period of communicability is over.

Evaluation: Child accepts restrictions of isolation

Table 5.8 Types of Isolation

Mode of Transmission	Isolation	Nursing Responsibilities
Direct contact airborn (droplets)	Strict	Private room Handwashing Gown, gloves, mask Double bag linen and trash Sterilize all reusable equipment Lab specimen precautions
Airborn (droplets)	Respiratory	Private room Handwashing Mask Double bag respiratory trash Lab specimen precautions
Direct/indirect contact with feces	Enteric	Private room Handwashing Gowns and gloves when in contact with feces or materials contaminated with feces Double bag contaminated articles Lab specimen precautions
Direct/indirect contact with purulent material or drainage from infected body sites	Drainage/secretion precautions	Handwashing Gown and gloves when in contact with contaminated linen, dressings, etc. Double bag linen/trash
Direct/indirect contact with infected blood or body fluids	Universal Precautions	Handwashing Gowns and gloves when in contact with body fluids soiled linens, clothes, dressings, etc. Protective eyewear when splashing of body fluids can be expected Double-bag contaminated articles Avoid needle-stick injuries Dispose of used needles correctly Keep emergency ventilation devices at bedside if indicated Health care personnel with open skin lesions should avoid all direct patient care
	Severely compromised client (reverse)	Private room with positive pressure air flow Handwashing Gowns, gloves, mask Sterilize linen, clothing, etc.

(stays in room); engages in age-appropriate activities; other cases of disease do not occur.

Goal 2: Child will be free from complications and long-term sequelae.

Plan/Implementation

- Observe and report signs of encephalitis: headache, bizarre behavior changes, seizures, fever, muscle weakness.
- Observe and report signs of vision or hearing loss.
- Observe and report signs of respiratory or cardiac complications: pneumonia, laryngotracheitis, otitis media, rheumatic fever.
- Observe and report signs of orchitis (mumps).

Evaluation: Child is free from complications and long-term sequelae (e.g., neurologic disability, sensory impairment, sterility, cardiac damage).

Goal 3: Child will ingest adequate food and fluids to meet nutritional needs.

Plan/Implementation

- Avoid rough or acidic foods; offer bland foods.
- Use colorful glasses, straws, liquids to enhance appetite.
- Offer favorite foods and fluids (ice cream, pudding, gelatin).
- Advance from liquids to regular diet as tolerated.

Evaluation: Child ingests adequate daily intake; is free from dehydration; eats a soft diet of sufficient caloric content.

Goal 4: Child will experience minimal discomfort.

Plan/Implementation

- Give antipyretics for fever or discomfort (dose: 1 grain/year up to 10 years q4h prn).
- Bedrest until fever subsides.
- Change bed linen and clothing daily.
- Provide humidifier as needed.
- Use tepid baths to relieve fever and itching; keep skin clean; observe for signs of secondary skin infection.
- Apply calamine lotion for itching (wash off completely once a day to prevent maceration of skin); administer antihistamines or antipruritic medications.
- Keep fingernails short and clean; apply mittens if needed.
- Dim lights if photophobia present.
- Warm compresses/irrigations of saline to eyes (measles).
- Local applications of heat or cold to relieve parotid discomfort (mumps).

Evaluation: Child rests and sleeps comfortably; has only minimal fever and itching.

☐ Sexually Transmitted Diseases (STDs)

1. General Information

a. Definition: a communicable disease transmitted by direct genital contact or sexual activity; STDs are the most prevalent communicable diseases in the US; majority of cases occur in adolescents and young adults; some STDs are contracted by newborn (*Candida* [thrush], herpes, gonorrheal conjunctivitis); STDs in infants and children usually indicate sexual abuse and should be investigated

b. Cause (see Table 5.9)

c. Medical treatment (see Table 5.9)

2. Nursing Process

a. Assessment/Analysis (see Table 5.9)

b. Plans, Implementation, and Evaluation

Goal 1: Client will participate in treatment of STD; will not transmit the disease to others.

Plan Implementation

- Use a straightforward, nonjudgmental approach when taking nursing history.
- Reassure client of confidentiality of information and exam.
- Teach signs, symptoms, and transmission mode of STD.
- Avoid sexual contact with partner while infected.
- Provide clear, specific, written and oral explanations of medical treatment.
- Counsel women of childbearing age concerning transmission of STD to newborn
  - gonorrheal conjunctivitis (may cause blindness)
  - neonatal herpes infection (may cause blindness, deafness, mental retardation, or may be fatal)
  - congenital syphilis (passively transmitted through placenta)
  - oral candidiasis (thrush)
- Assist with identification and treatment of sexual contacts.
- Report cases of gonorrhea, syphilis to health department.
- Teach how to reduce risk of reinfection.

Evaluation: Client participates in treatment plan; is free from disease recurrence; does not transmit disease to others.

Goal 2: Client will resolve feelings of embarrassment, shame, guilt, and negative self-worth resulting from diagnosis.

Plan/Implementation

- Treat with respect, dignity.
- Ensure confidentiality.
- Provide sexuality education to dispel myths and misinformation.
- Encourage to express any feelings of shame, embarrassment, guilt, loss of esteem.
- Refer to self-help groups (herpes) in community as appropriate.

Evaluation: Client resolves negative feelings about diagnosis; utilizes support group (when appropriate); client's confidentiality is protected.

Goal 3: Client will be aware of sexual practices that will reduce the chances of acquiring a STD.

Plan/Implementation

- Avoid sex with individuals who have multiple partners.
- Follow strict personal hygiene habits (e.g., bathing, diet, etc.).
- Use only water-soluble lubricants.
- Use condoms lubricated with nonoxynol-9.
- Avoid douching before and after sex (increases the risk of infections because the body's normal defenses are reduced/destroyed).
- Be aware of symptoms of STD (fever, weight loss, persistent diarrhea, enlarged lymph nodes, unusual discharge, dysuria, bruising).

Evaluation: Client enjoys a healthy sex life; remains free from STD.

Table 5.9 Sexually Transmitted Diseases

Causative Agent	Incidence	Assessment	Medical Treatment
Gonorrhea *Neisseria gonorrheae*	Most commonly reported communicable disease	Males: dysuria, frequency, purulent urethral discharge Females: purulent vaginal discharge; 60% asymptomatic Diagnosis: by gram stain or culture (Thayer-Martin medium) Complications if untreated: Males: prostatitis and epididymitis Females: pelvic inflammatory disease, infertility, arthritis	Penicillin or other antibiotics Probenicid may be given to delay excretion of penicillin
Herpes *Herpesvirus hominus* type 2	300,000–500,000 new cases/year	Active lesions: painful vesicular lesions that ulcerate Signs and symptoms of systemic illness: fever, headache, and/or general adenopathy Diagnosis: isolation of virus in tissue culture; demonstration of multinucleated giant cells on microscopic exam	Viscous lidocaine to ease pain Keep lesions clean and dry • apply cornstarch • use warm air blower • wear loose clothing Females: dysuria may be eased by voiding in warm water Acyclovir (Zovirax) may decrease duration of the initial or subsequent episodes, but doesn't prevent recurrences
Syphilis *Treponema pallidum*	Third most commonly reported communicable disease	Primary (3 weeks postexposure): classic chancre (painless, red, eroded lesions with indurated border at point of entry) Secondary (1–3 months postexposure): cutaneous, nonpruritic, diffuse lesions on face, trunk, and/or extremities Tertiary (10–30 years postexposure): cardiac and neurologic destruction Diagnosis: positive darkfield slide of organism; VDRL, RPR, or FTA	Penicillin
Trichomoniasis *Trichomonas vaginalis*	May be the most frequently acquired sexually transmitted disease in the U.S.	Symptoms range from none to frothy, greenish-grey vaginal discharge Diagnosis: microscopic identification of motile protozoan	Metronidazole (Flagyl)
Candidiasis *Candida albicans*	Overall incidence in U.S. is unknown	Erythematous, edematous, pruritic vulva Thick, white, "cottage-cheese"-like discharge	Nystatin (Mycostatin) vaginal suppositories or cream; if this fails, clotrimazole 1% (Lotrimin)
Scabies *Sarcoptes scabiei*	Epidemic in U.S.	Intense, nocturnal genital itching Diagnosis: microscopic examination of shave excision of lesion	1% gamma benzene hexachloride lotion (Kwell) A-200 Pyrinate, RID in children under 5

(continued)

Table 5.9 Continued

Causative Agent	Incidence	Assessment	Medical Treatment
Chlamydia *Chlamydia trachomatis*	More prevalent than gonorrhea Affects approximately 3 million Americans a year	Major cause of nongonococcal urethritis in men (frequency, dysuria) Accounts for 20%–30% of all pelvic inflammatory diseases May be transmitted to the newborn during delivery and result in conjunctivitis and pneumonia Many women are asymptomatic; others may complain of frequency, dysuria, urgency, abnormal vaginal discharge, even bleeding Diagnosis: identification of organism through culture	Tetracycline/erythromycin; should take medication at least 7–10 days; sexual partners should also be treated
Acquired immune deficiency syndrome (AIDS) *Human immunodeficiency virus (HIV)*	Pandemic; over 62,000 reported cases world wide, 70% in U.S.	Individuals at risk: Homosexual/bisexual Intravenous drug users Hemophiliacs Anyone receiving blood transfusions Sexual partners of individuals at risk Children via intrauterine placental or perinatal transmission Early symptoms: lymphadenopathy, weight loss, fever, diarrhea; symptoms disappear in 4–6 weeks and patient enters asymptomatic carrier state (AIDS related complex or ARC) Late symptoms: opportunistic infections (pneumocystis carinii), cancer (Kaposi's sarcoma)	Limited success with chemotherapy Antibiotics, antifungals Investigational antiviral drugs

☐ Common Skin Problems and Infestations

1. General Information

a. Definition: inflammatory responses, bacterial infections, or insect infestation of the skin, hair, or scalp; common in preschoolers and school-age children whose close contact increases their susceptibility

b. Cause (see Table 5.10)

c. Medical treatment (see Table 5.10)

2. Nursing Process (see Table 5.10)

☐ Pinworms (Helminths)

1. General Information

a. Definition: parasitic infestation primarily of the intestinal tract; worms deposit eggs in anal area causing severe itching; eggs attach to child's fingers causing reinfection when fingers are put in mouth

b. Incidence: approximately half of all school-age children will have pinworms at some time

c. Medical treatment

1) stool for ova and parasites (not a reliable test for pinworms)

2) cellophane-tape test; child should be rechecked 2–3 times because of "false" negative findings; tape test should be done in early morning (i.e., 5:00 AM to 6:00 AM)

3) antihelminth

a) pyrvinium pamoate (Povan), single dose 5 mg/kg; stools turn red; tablets should not be chewed because they stain teeth

b) piperazine citrate 65 mg/kg daily for 3 days; contraindicated in children with impaired renal/hepatic function or seizure disorders

2. Nursing Process

a. Assessment/Analysis

1) intense anal itching (worsens at night)/ vaginitis

2) enuresis

Table 5.10 Common Skin Problems and Infestations

Cause	Assessment	Medical Treatment	Plan/Implementation
Acne Vulgaris: skin lesions (comedos) caused by increased sebaceous secretions during puberty and adolescence; more than ¾ of all adolescents are affected			
Corynebacterium acnes Dietary factors (chocolate, iodine) have not been substantiated Exaggerated by menstruation, stress, oil-based cosmetics, oral contraceptives	Sebum blocks skin pores, resulting in local inflammation Blackheads, papules, cysts, or nodules appear on face, back, chest arms, neck	Topical antibiotics. Tetracycline or prednisone for severe cases. Ultraviolet light.	Teach adolescent to avoid picking or squeezing lesions (may cause infection and scarring). Encourage regular cleansing of skin, especially when sweaty (hot weather, after exercise). Avoid using caps, headbands. Recommend over-the-counter anti-acne cleansers and cover creams (contain alcohol and benzoyl peroxide, a peeling and drying agent) to help keep skin dry. Encourage a healthy life-style: balanced diet, exercise, rest; minimize stress.
Atopic Dermatitis (Eczema): allergic reaction to foods, environmental inhalants and pollen			
Unknown	Disease of remissions and exacerbations Lesions appear as papules, vesicles, and crusts; begin on cheeks and spread to face, flexor surfaces of body Intense itching that may lead to secondary skin infection Some consider eczema a precursor to asthma	Elimination diet. Topical steroids. Nonsoap preparations (Cetaphil). Wet soaks with Burow's solution. Antihistamines for itching.	Teach parents the importance of adhering to the diet. Teach administration of meds • steroids may mask infections; may see rebound effect when ointment discontinued • antihistamines may cause drowsiness Control itching by • administering meds as ordered • avoiding soap preparations • keeping nails cut; covering hands with mittens; may need to use elbow restraints • cotton clothing • avoiding overheating • exposure to ultraviolet light (irritates and dries the lesions) • wet soaks with Burow's PRN (e.g., nap time)
Impetigo Contagiosa: superficial bacterial skin infection			
Staphylococcus, streptococcus	Vesicles that rupture to form honey-colored crusts; erupt most often on face, axillae, and extremities; itches; highly contagious	Removal of crusts with Burow's solution. Topical bacteriocidal ointment (Neosporin). Penicillin in severe cases.	Teach child/parent how to soften and remove crusts, apply antibiotic ointment. Teach administration of oral antibiotics (penicillin/ erythromycin). Prevent scratching by keeping nails clipped, using mitts or elbow restraints as necessary. Teach child to use own towels, washcloths until lesions heal.

(continued)

Table 5.10 Continued

Cause	Assessment	Medical Treatment	Plan/Implementation
Lice (pediculosis): parasitic infestation of head (capitis), body (corporis), or pubic area (pubis)			
Pediculus humanus	Ova (nits) on hair shafts Itching, skin excoriation Enlarged lymph nodes	Kwell (gamma benzene) shampoo or lotion. (Not recommended for children younger than 5) A-200 Pyrinate. RID.	Teach parents how to apply prescribed shampoo or lotion; caution against Kwell overuse (neurotoxicity); should repeat treatment in 7–10 days. May need to cut long hair. Use fine-tooth comb dipped in vinegar to remove nits. Discard contaminated combs and brushes. Teach children not to exchange such personal items as towels, combs and brushes, hats. Launder bed linens, towels. Use gamma benzene spray on upholstered furniture.
Ringworm (tinea): superficial fungal infection of head (capitis), body (corporis), "jock itch" (cruris), "athlete's foot" (pedis)			
Various fungi	Scaly, *Capitis* circumscribed patches Areas of patchy hair loss Itching Green concentric ring under Wood's light (ultraviolet) illumination Positive culture	Oral griseofulvin: 20 mg/kg/day for 7–14 days. Local antifungal preparations • Whitfield's ointment • tolnaftate (Tinactin).	Teach parents how to administer oral and local antifungal agents. Shampoo frequently using clean towels, combs, brushes. Keep child's hair short. *Corporis and cruris* Avoid wearing nylon underwear and tight-fitting clothes. Keep affected areas clean and dry. Identify and treat source (often from household pets). *Pedis* Wear clean, light, cotton socks. Wear well-ventilated shoes. Apply topical antifungal powder containing tolnaftate. Avoid bare feet in public places (such as school gym) until infection has cleared.

3) irritability/restlessness
4) night walking/insomnia

b. Plan, Implementation, and Evaluation

Goal: Child will be free from infestation, will not reinfest self.

Plan/Implementation

- Identify other family members and close contacts who may also need treatment.
- Teach good handwashing and personal hygiene (after toileting and before eating).
- Wear tight-fitting diapers or panties.
- Change and launder underwear, pajamas, and bed linens daily.
- Have child sleep alone.
- Wear mitts or socks to prevent scratching.
- Carry out proper disposal of feces.
- Ensure parents understand importance of carrying out these measures.

Evaluation: Child is free from infestation; does not reinfest self or transmit it to others; parent establishes adequate sanitation.

Application of the Nursing Process to the Child with an Interference with Protection: Safety

See Selected Health Problems

Selected Health Problems Resulting in an Interference with Protection: Safety

☐ Poisonous Ingestions

1. General Information

a. Definition: the swallowing of common non-nutritive materials that can cause health problems and/or poisoning. Common ingested substances: lead, corrosives, hydrocarbons, aspirin, acetaminophen, sedatives/hypnotics
b. Incidence: poisonous ingestions are the 5th leading cause of death between 1 and 4 years of age; peak incidence is toddler years
c. Cause: developmental curiosity; incorrect storage of potentially toxic substances
d. Aim of treatment is to remove ingested toxic substance from body or to neutralize its effects as quickly as possible
e. Vomiting, or use of an emetic, is contraindicated when
   1) child is comatose, convulsing, or in severe shock (increases risk of aspiration)
   2) substance is a hydrocarbon (aspiration may cause a chemical pneumonia)
   3) substance is a corrosive (acid or alkali) (emesis may further damage or perforate esophageal muscosa); see Table 5.11 for general information, treatment, and assessment of specific ingestions

2. Nursing Process

a. **Assessment/Analysis** (see Table 5.11)

b. **Plans, Implementation, and Evaluation (for all ingestions)**

Goal 1: Child will receive emergency treatment for acute poisonous ingestion.

Plan/Implementation
- Instruct parent to contact poison control center (provide telephone number) or take child to nearest emergency facility.
- Instruct to induce vomiting (if appropriate) by stimulating gag reflex and giving syrup of ipecac; do not use salt water as an emetic.
- Position child to avoid aspiration when vomiting; give physical support while child is vomiting.

Table 5.11 Commonly Ingested Poisonous Substances

General Information	Nursing Assessment	Medical Treatment
Aspirin (salicylate poisoning)		
Most common cause of childhood poisoning Toxic dose: 2 grains/lb body weight Lethal dose: 3–4 grains/lb Effects: stimulates respiratory center → respiratory alkalosis; increases metabolism → fever, metabolic acidosis (from high level of ketones)	GI effects • vomiting • thirst CNS effects • hyperventilation • confusion, dizziness • staggered gait • coma Hematopoietic effects • bleeding tendencies Metabolic effects • sweating • hyponatremia • hypokalemia • dehydration • hypoglycemia	Induce vomiting with syrup of ipecac • 6–12 months of age: 10 ml (2 tsp) and as much water as possible • over 1 year: 15 ml (1 tbsp) and 2–3 glasses of water. Gastric lavage. IV fluids, sodium bicarbonate (enhances excretion), electrolytes. Vitamin K for hypoprothrombinemia. Glucose for hypoglycemia. Diuretics: acetazolamide (Diamox). Dialysis when potentially lethal doses have been ingested.
Acetaminophen (Tylenol)		
Toxic dose: uncertain, do not exceed recommended levels Effects: cellular necrosis of the liver resulting in liver dysfunction and, in some cases, hepatic failure	First stage (first 24 hours) • nausea • vomiting • sweating • pallor or cyanosis • weakness Second stage (24–48 hours) • SGOT, SGPT elevated • liver tenderness (RUQ) • prolonged prothrombin time Third stage (1 week) • liver necrosis • hepatic failure • possible death	Induce vomiting or gastric lavage (see aspirin). Acetylcysteine (Mucomyst) as an antidote, given PO with fruit juice or Cola, or via NG tube (offensive odor). IV fluids. Sodium-restricted, high-calorie, high-protein diet.

(continued)

Table 5.11 Continued

General Information	Nursing Assessment	Medical Treatment
Corrosives (lye, bleach, ammonia)		
Extent of damage depends on the causticity of the substance and the amount ingested	Grossly visible whitish burns of mouth and pharynx; color darkens as ulcerations form Edema Respiratory distress Difficulty swallowing Excess drooling Severe pain Shock	*DO NOT INDUCE VOMITING; DO NOT LAVAGE.* Activated charcoal may be given. Dilute with small amounts of water. Tracheostomy if respiratory distress is severe. IV fluids while child is NPO. Analgesics, steroids, antibiotics, antacids. Possible gastrostomy. Possible esophageal dilations to prevent strictures (or maintain patency of esophagus). Colon transplant if esophageal damage is severe (done when child is older).
Hydrocarbons (gasoline, kerosene, turpentine, mineral seal oil)		
Immediate concern is aspiration, which can cause severe (or fatal) chemical pneumonitis. Systemic effects from GI absorption of hydrocarbons are relatively mild.	Burning sensation in mouth and throat Characteristic breath odor Nausea, anorexia, vomiting Lethargy Fever	*DO NOT INDUCE VOMITING.* Supportive measures for respiratory effects, pneumonitis (O_2, antibiotics, IV fluids).
Lead (chronic poisoning)		
Approximately 4% of children under age 6 years have excessive lead levels in their blood; peak age is 2–3 years; black children have 6 times greater risk.	Hematopoietic effects • anemia CNS effects • irritability • lethargy • hyperactivity • developmental delays • clumsiness • seizures • disorientation • coma, possible death GI effects • anorexia • nausea, vomiting • constipation • lead line along gums Skeletal effects • increased density of long bones • lead lines in long bones Renal effects • glycosuria • proteinuria • possible acute or chronic renal failure	Remove child from lead source, hospitalize. Chelating agents: EDTA usually used in combination with BAL; given IM q4h for 5 days (causes lead to be deposited in bone and excreted via kidneys); monitor kidney function because EDTA is nephrotoxic; monitor calcium levels because EDTA enhances excretion of calcium. Calcium, phosphorus, vitamin D to aid lead excretion. Anticonvulsants for seizure control. Oral or IM iron for anemia. Follow-up lead levels to monitor progress (lead is excreted more slowly than it accumulates in the body).

- Tell parent to keep original container label for determining antidote.
- Analyze ingested substance, child's output
  - bring in container and any remaining substance
  - bring in any vomitus or urine output since ingestion
- Make appropriate referrals, e.g., social service.

Evaluation: Parent institutes correct emergency care of child; child receives appropriate follow-up care.

Goal 2: Child will maintain adequate oxygenation.

Plan/Implementation

- Monitor vital and neuro signs at least q15min until stable and as indicated.
- Administer O_2 therapy as ordered.
- Assess color of skin, nail beds, and mucous membranes.
- Report difficulty breathing or swallowing *STAT*; may require a tracheotomy; keep

laryngoscope, endotracheal tube, and tracheotomy tray at bedside.
- Observe for seizure activity.
- If breathing is labored, stay with child to reduce fear and anxiety.

Evaluation: Child remains free from respiratory distress; maintains normal respiratory rate, color.

Goal 3: Child's ingestion will be recognized and treated early to prevent complications; child will be kept safe during treatment regimen.

Plan/Implementation
- Institute seizure precautions.
- Check vital signs frequently until stable; if temperature elevated, sponge with tepid water; may need to use cooling blanket; observe for febrile seizures.
- If child confused, provide safety measures as appropriate.
- Record I&O accurately.
- Monitor urine output (EDTA is potentially toxic to kidneys).
- Prepare child for painful injections (EDTA and BAL); mix with local anesthetic (Procaine HCl); rotate injection sites.
- Increase fluid intake to 1–2 times maintenance (aspirin).

Evaluation: Child returns to normal activities with no residual effects; is free from acquired injuries.

Goal 4: Child will regain fluid and electrolyte balance; will rest comfortably.

Plan/Implementation
- Observe and report signs of respiratory alkalosis (deep and rapid breathing, lightheadedness, tetany, convulsions, coma).
- Observe and report signs of metabolic acidosis (deep breathing, short of breath, disorientation, coma).
- Observe and report signs of metabolic alkalosis (depressed respirations, hypertonicity, tetany).
- Observe and report signs of hypokalemia: malaise, thirst, polyuria, cardiac dysrhythmias, decreased BP, thready pulse, depressed reflexes.
- Observe and report signs of hypo-/ hyperglycemia.
- Administer analgesics as ordered.
- Soothe child with gentle touching and soft voice.
- Monitor vital signs frequently until stable.
- Offer clear liquids in small amounts (if child is able to swallow); observe for nausea, ability to swallow.
- Evaluate hydration status frequently.

Evaluation: Child's fluid and electrolyte balance remains stable; child experiences minimal or no pain.

Goal 5: Parents will receive appropriate information to prevent or reduce recurrences.

Plan/Implementation
- Provide anticipatory guidance concerning developmental issues and accidents.
- Teach the essentials of prevention (child-proofing environment).
  - do not place substances in unmarked containers
  - keep harmful substances out of child's reach, in locked cabinets
  - teach child that medication is not candy
  - emphasize poisonous quality of abused over-the-counter drugs
- Provide appropriate supervision of the child.
- Provide love and attention to the child.
- Observe child for pica.
- Obtained continued medical care as appropriate.
- Support parents/child in dealing with feelings about ingestion (guilt and anger).

Evaluation: Parent modifies home environment to prevent recurrence of ingestion.

☐ Burns

1. General Information

a. Definition: tissue damage that results from thermal, chemical, electrical, or radioactive agents (see Table 5.12)

b. Incidence
   1) third leading cause of accidental injury and death in children
   2) over 50% of burns occur in children 5 years of age or younger
   3) thermal burns are most common

c. Classification
   1) percentage of body surface burned
      a) rule of nines (adults) (see Figure 5.1)
      b) modified rule of nines (children) (see Figure 5.1)
   2) degree of damage (depth of burn injury)
      a) 1st degree: superficial partial thickness; pain, redness, no tissue or nerve damage, superficial epidermis affected
      b) 2nd degree: deep-dermal partial thickness; pain, pale-to-red edematous

Table 5.12 Systemic Responses to Burn Injury

Alterations in fluid volume	Altered capillary permeability results in shifts of water, protein, and electrolytes from the intravascular to interstitial spaces which reduces the circulating blood volume The body adapts through vasoconstriction, tachycardia, and conservation of fluid volume by renal reabsorption. However, this is temporary and unless the deficit is corrected, burn shock will result • fluid losses continue for 3–4 days with major losses in the first 12 hours • severe edema of burned tissue occurs with mild to moderate edema to the rest of the body; once fluid begins to shift back to intravascular spaces, diuresis occurs (within 48 hours) and the edema subsides • sodium and potassium are exchanged with sodium entering the cell and potassium entering intravascular spaces; one diuresis occurs, potassium is excreted, child becomes hypokalemic and replacement therapy essential • fluid volume deficit results in decreased renal blood flow which impairs glomerular filtration; acute renal failure may develop if fluid replacement not adequate • hemolysis of RBCs may lead to anemia and renal tubular obstruction
Alterations in metabolism	Increased metabolic rate and oxygen consumption are the body's usual responses to major burns • the stress of a burn injury causes –glycogen breakdown leading to depletion of energy stores within 24 hours postburn, followed by glyconeogenesis (breakdown of protein stores) –negative nitrogen balance (elevated BUN and urine urea nitrogen) –increased blood glucose levels • elevated aldosterone and antidiuretic hormone (ADH) levels • metabolic acidosis (often compensated for by respiratory alkalosis)
Potential complications related to burn injury	The body's response to a burn is systemic in nature and carries the potential of affecting every system of the body • respiratory problems: inhalation injury, aspiration, bacterial pneumonia, pulmonary edema • wound infection (usually occurs within 3–5 days postburn; most often caused by gram-negative organisms, especially *Pseudomonas*) • Curling's ulcer (gastric or duodenal stress ulcer) • paralytic ileus (most common when burned surface is greater than 20%) • arterial hypertension • CNS disturbances: disorientation, personality changes, seizures (especially in burned children), coma

skin, vesicles, entire affected area of epidermis and varying amounts of dermis affected

c) 3rd degree: full thickness; painless; skin white, red, or black; edematous; bullae; nerves, epidermis, dermis destroyed; subcutaneous adipose tissue, fascia, muscle and bone may also be destroyed or damaged

d. Medical treatment (moderate to severe burns)

1) medical intervention

a) immediate emergency care

- extinguish burn (teach children to "Stop, Drop, and Roll")
- slowly immerse burn injury in cool water if possible (relieves pain, inhibits edema formation, slows tissue damage)
- do *not* use ice water, ice packs, or topical ointments
- cover burn with clean cloth (e.g., clean bed sheet)
- cover with blankets (uninvolved areas) if child is hypothermic
- remove constrictive clothing and jewelry before swelling occurs
- if child is alert and oriented, provide warm liquids
- transport to nearest medical facility if burn is extensive

b) admission care

- establish airway (O_2, intubation if laryngeal edema is a risk)
- *frequently* assess blood gases
- initiate fluid and electrolyte therapy based on body weight and percent of surface area burned
  - one-half of total estimated fluid requirements for the first 24 hours

Figure 5.1 Estimation of Burn Surface Area

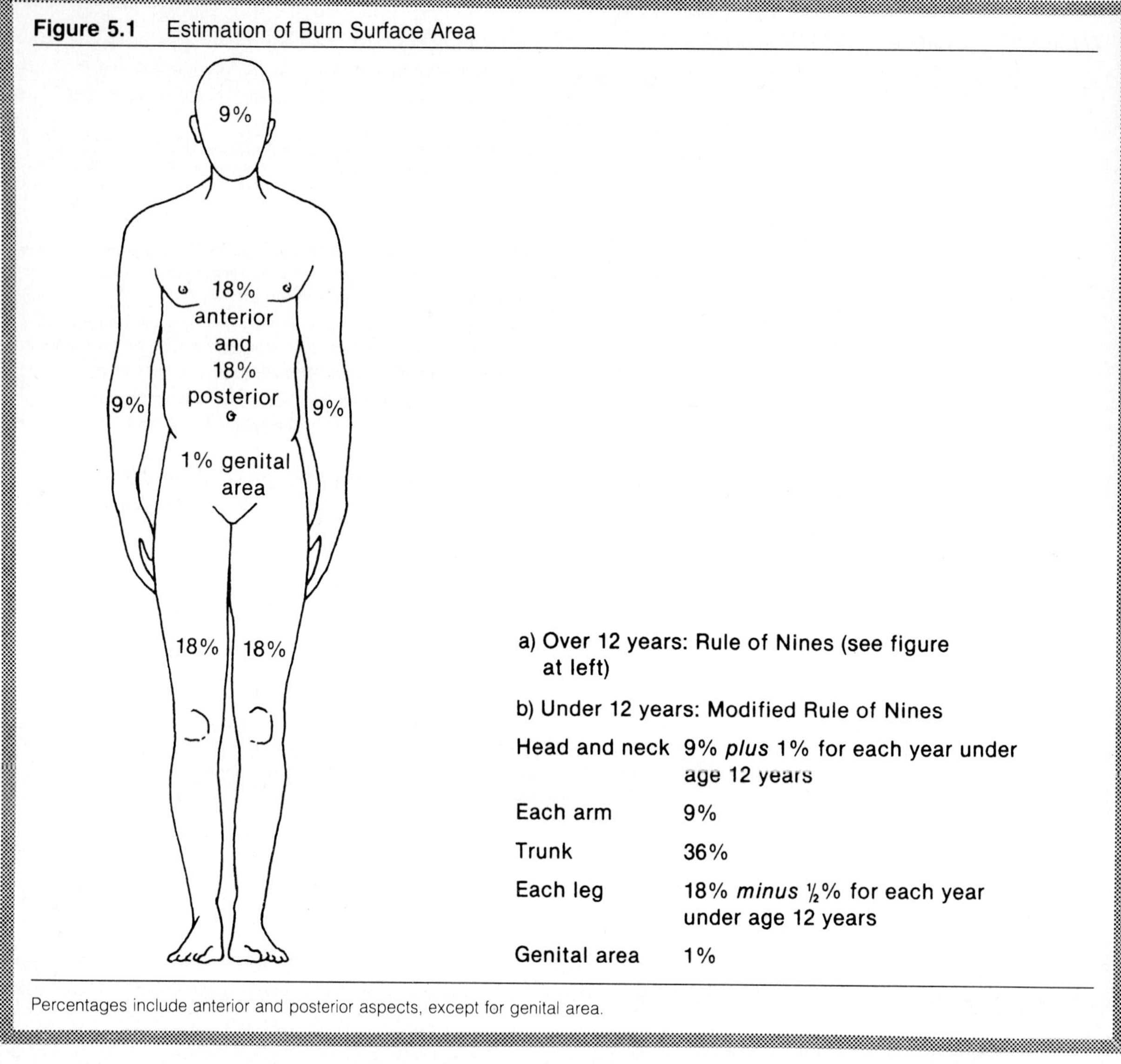

a) Over 12 years: Rule of Nines (see figure at left)

b) Under 12 years: Modified Rule of Nines

Head and neck	9% *plus* 1% for each year under age 12 years
Each arm	9%
Trunk	36%
Each leg	18% *minus* ½% for each year under age 12 years
Genital area	1%

Percentages include anterior and posterior aspects, except for genital area.

is usually replaced in the first 8 hours following the burn injury
- types of solutions used may vary
  * first 24 hours: crystalloid solutions, such as normal saline or Ringer's lactate
  * following diuresis, colloid solutions such as albumin or plasma
- ■ assess other injuries
- ■ insert urinary indwelling catheter for accurate assessment of urinary output
- ■ insert NG tube to prevent vomiting, abdominal distention, or gastric aspiration
- ■ administer IV pain medication as ordered
- ■ administer antibiotics (penicillin or erythromycin) to prevent infection (broad-spectrum antibiotics are not used because of possibility of superimposed infections)
- ■ immunized with tetanus toxoid (according to recommended schedule)

c) care of burn wounds
- ■ open method: reverse isolation
  - burn exposed to air; crust or eschar forms a protective barrier
  - topical medication
    * mafenide acetate (Sulfamylon): penetrates wound rapidly, is painful, causes mild acidosis
    * silver sulfadiazine (Silvadene): penetrates wound slowly; is

soothing, causes no acid-base complications, keeps eschar soft; debridement easier

- closed method
  - burn covered with nonadherent fine-mesh gauze and fluffed-gauze outer layer covered by stretch gauze bandages
  - topical medication
    * nitrofurazone (Furacin): acts by interfering with bacterial enzymes; most frequent problem is allergic contact dermatitis; may see superinfections
    * betadine: painful, effective against variety of infectious organisms; may cause toughening of eschar and difficult debridement
- primary surgical excision: immediate surgical excision of burned tissue with grafting; reduces risk of infection; blood loss may be significant
- debridement and hydrotherapy (Hubbard whirlpool tank): done regardless of the method of treatment utilized
- grafting and reconstructive surgery: long-term treatment; to improve function and cosmetic appearance

2. Nursing Process

a. Assessment/Analysis

1) respiratory status: patency of airway (burns of head, neck, and chest areas predispose child to respiratory distress)
2) extent and depth of burn, location of burn injury
3) observe for early signs of shock (behavioral changes, tachycardia, alterations in BP, diminished output)
4) presence of pain (frequently manifested as irritability, depression, hostility, or aggression)
5) observe for signs of hemorrhage (decreased BP; rapid, thready pulse; diaphoresis; pallor; decreased body temperature)
6) monitor laboratory findings
   a) hematocrit, arterial blood gases
   b) sodium, chloride, potassium, CO_2
   c) BUN, creatinine
   d) serum protein
   e) urine pH, specific gravity
7) child's and parent's emotional responses to burn injury

b. Plans, Implementation, and Evaluation

Goal 1: Child will maintain adequate oxygenation.

Plan/Implementation

- Observe for respiratory distress (wheezing, rales, dyspnea, increased rate, nasal flaring, stridor, air hunger).
- Monitor arterial blood gases.
- Carefully monitor intubated child who is assisted by a respirator; humidified O_2 as ordered.
- Suction qh or prn.
- Prevent aspiration: maintain patency of nasogastric tube.
- Turn, cough, deep breathe; use inspirometer (to prevent hypostatic pneumonia); provide humidified air.
- Check eschar on neck and chest for constriction; assist with escharotomy as needed.

Evaluation: Child is free from respiratory distress; maintains adequate oxygenation.

Goal 2: Child will maintain adequate hydration and electrolyte balance.

Plan/Implementation

- Monitor vital signs qh and prn; CVP line if appropriate.
- Monitor I&O hourly (10–20 ml/hour for child under 2 years; 20–50 ml/hour for child over 2 years; 30–50 ml/hour for adult); check urine gravity and pH (may need to catheterize).
- Observe for signs of hemorrhage (bleeding; decreased BP; decreased body temperature; rapid, thready pulse).
- Observe for signs of dehydration (thirst, dry tongue, decreased urinary output, decreased BP, tachycardia, poor skin turgor).
- Monitor IV therapy (*NOTE*: check for adequate renal function prior to adding potassium to IV).
- Observe for signs of fluid overload (venous distention, increased BP, short of breath, rales, behavioral changes).
- Observe for signs of electrolyte imbalance (cardiac dysrhythmias, tingling of fingers, abdominal cramps, convulsions, spasms).

Evaluation: Child is free from shock, maintains adequate circulatory volume and electrolyte balance.

Goal 3: Child will be free from infection and have optimal wound healing.

Plan/Implementation

- Maintain reverse (protective) isolation as ordered.
- Administer antibiotics and tetanus prophylaxis as ordered.
- Utilize sterile technique with wound care; handle wound carefully to prevent damage to healing tissues.
- Encourage self-care to increase child's sense of control and autonomy; encourage child (when possible) to participate in dressing changes.
- Observe for and report signs of wound infection (temperature elevation, redness at wound edge, purulent or green-grey drainage, offensive odor).
- Observe for and report signs of systemic infection (increased body temperature, chills, tachycardia, hyperemic).
- Observe for and report signs of respiratory infection (increased body temperature, signs of respiratory distress).

Evaluation: Child's wounds heal without complications; child assumes an active role in the healing process.

Goal 4: Child will have minimal pain/discomfort.

Plan/Implementation

- Administer analgesics as ordered; observe for response.
- Utilize comfort measures (e.g., pillows).
- Teach child to change focus to music, TV, friends; use imaging when appropriate.

Evaluation: Child experiences no more than minimal pain or discomfort; develops coping strategies that reduce/modify painful experiences (e.g., dressing changes).

Goal 5: Child will maintain adequate nutritional intake to prevent nitrogen loss and GI complications.

Plan/Implementation

- Provide a high-protein, high-calorie diet; determine special likes/dislikes.
- Offer small frequent meals; encourage family to bring food from home.
- Assess bowel sounds for possible paralytic ileus (early postburn period).
- Observe for signs of Curling's ulcer (coffee ground emesis, abdominal distention, anemia); usually occurs during the 3rd–4th week postburn in children (first week postburn in adults).
- Give supplemental vitamins and minerals (vitamins A, B, and C; iron and zinc), antacids as ordered.

Evaluation: Child ingests therapeutic diet as ordered; is free from gastrointestinal complications.

Goal 6: Child will achieve functional use of burned area and successful cosmetic results.

Plan/Implementation

- Protect graft site from injury; if grafted area exposed, child may need to be immobilized.
- When pockets of fluid accumulate under graft site, gently "roll" the fluid out at the graft edges with a sterile cotton-tipped swab.
- Do not change dressing on donor site (prevents tearing of underlying delicate epithelium).
- Observe for signs of infection at graft sites.
- Minimize scar formation by maintaining affected areas in a functional position; use splints when appropriate.
- Assist with range-of-motion (ROM) exercises as ordered.
- Encourage ambulation when appropriate.
- Encouarge child's participation in self-care and activities of daily living.
- Provide explanations to child and family for positioning requirements.

Evaluation: Child has full (or increasing) ROM of affected/nonaffected joints; has no footdrop, contractures; heals graft sites without complications.

Goal 7: Child will verbalize concerns and feelings about altered body image.

Plan/Implementation

- Assess child's/parent's adjustment to altered body image (child's verbalizations and nonverbal behavior).
- Spend time listening to concerns and feelings.
- Utilize play therapy.
- Offer preprocedure preparation according to age.
- Utilize visual, auditory, and tactile stimulation.
- Problem solve with use of elastic bandages, camouflage clothes, and use of makeup to enhance appearance.
- Refer to support groups.

Evaluation: Child talks about effect of burns on body; asks questions about what others will think of his/her body; participates in activities appropriate for age and personal interest.

Goal 8: Child/family will receive appropriate information concerning home care of burns.

Plan/Implementation
- Teach family how to change the burn dressing utilizing clean technique; have family return demonstration; remember to adapt dressing change to family needs.
- Instruct family to observe for signs of wound infection.
- Review importance of vitamin C and protein in the healing process and discuss ways to increase these nutrients in the child's diet.
- Teach family appropriate care of a healed burn
  - wash with mild soap and apply lubricating cream or jelly (nonperfumed)
  - avoid direct sun
  - use meds prn for pruritus
  - observe for signs of infection
  - integrate ROM into daily routine
- Discuss developmental aspects of disfiguring injuries; include extended family, peers, school teachers, etc. in rehabilitation; return child to school as soon as possible.
- Stress importance of self-care activities to strengthen sense of self.

Evaluation: Child's burns heal with minimal contractures; child participates in routine ADLs; returns to school.

Application of the Nursing Process to the Child with Developmental or Neurologic Disabilities

1. **Assessment:** developmental and neurologic disabilities include any serious, chronic disability caused by an impairment of physical or mental functioning, or both, that occurs in childhood, is likely to persist throughout life, and results in limitations in daily functioning; it may cause significant and permanent interruptions in the child's physical, emotional, and social growth and development; early detection and appropriate intervention are essential to promote optimum development; approximately 10% of all children and adolescents have some type of developmental disability
   a. Nursing history
      1) achievement of developmental milestones; child's self-care abilities
      2) developmental delays: motor, language, social, cognitive, such as persistent head lag, failure to roll over, delayed speech, impaired social functioning
      3) perceptual problems: vision, hearing
      4) perinatal history (refer to *Newborn Care* page 454)
      5) family history: congenital anomalies, hereditary factors, infections
      6) child's health history: illnesses, allergies, medications, immunizations
      7) communication, memory, attention problems, school performance
      8) current health problem(s): signs and symptoms, medical treatment, home management, concerns or problems
      9) parents'/family's perception of health problem
         a) child's adaptation to disability
         b) family's ability to cope with loss of "perfect child" (refer to *Loss, Death and Dying* page 31)
         c) stressors: economic, marital, lack of time and energy
         d) threats to self-esteem and control
         e) overprotectiveness or rejection of child
   b. Clinical appraisal
      1) general: level of consciousness, affect, attention span; head and circumferences, cranial sutures and fontanels; vital signs, including BP
      2) persistent or absent neonatal reflexes
      3) posture: persistent extension/flexion of extremities, scissoring, frog-leg position, opisthotonos
      4) motor function: muscle size and tone; symmetrical, spontaneous movements of all extremities; involuntary movements such as tremors, spasticity, athetosis
      5) developmental skills: assess for developmental progress (e.g., Denver Developmental Screening Test), gross and fine motor development, language, self-help skills (dressing, feeding, toileting)
      6) vision: infant's ability to focus on small objects; vision screening tests for older children (refer to "Healthy Child" page 526)
      7) hearing: startle reflex is a rough estimate of sound perception in infants; audiometry is unreliable with infants, toddlers, and mentally retarded children
   c. Diagnostic tests (refer to *Nursing Care of the Adult* page 272)

2. **Analysis**
   a. Safe, effective care environment
      1) potential for injury
      2) sensory-perceptual alteration: tactile, visual
      3) impaired home maintenance management

b. Physiological integrity
   1) impaired physical mobility
   2) activity intolerance
   3) altered nutrition: more/less than body requirements

c. Psychological integrity
   1) anticipatory grieving
   2) body image disturbance
   3) altered thought processes

d. Health promotion/maintenance
   1) altered growth and development
   2) self-care deficit
   3) altered family processes

3. General Nursing Plans, Implementation, and Evaluation

Goal 1: Child will achieve optimum level of growth and development.

Plan/Implementation
- Screen children at risk for developmental disabilities so problems are detected and treated early to minimize developmental delays.
- Keep child's activities in the mainstream as much as possible to promote self-sufficiency, adjustment, and mental development
  - refer family to infant stimulation, developmental, and special education programs
  - maintain open communication between family and all members of interdisciplinary team
- Treat child according to developmental (not chronologic) age.
- Provide guidance for learning acceptable social behaviors.
- Identify parenting concerns and ways to handle them (e.g., discipline: consistency; nurturance: needs are identical to any other child).
- Include activities that enhance child's self-esteem and self-worth.
- Provide a variety of stimuli; help child pay attention to distinct stimuli.
- Break tasks into small components; use positive reinforcement (verbal praise, hugs, stickers).
- Provide visual and auditory cues, and opportunities for practice (repetition enhances learning).
- Teach self-care skills for activities of daily living (e.g., hygiene, feeding, dressing)
  - allow child as much independence as possible, even if activities take longer (remember to stress that child is a family member too)
  - acknowledge and positively reinforce parents' care of child and child's progress
  - help parents provide a stimulating, healthful environment for the child (mainstreaming)

Evaluation: Child achieves and maintains optimum developmental potential; performs ADL as independently as possible; is maintained in a community setting.

Goal 2: Adolescent/young adult will receive appropriate education regarding sexuality.

Plan/Implementation
- Emphasize that adolescent may understand more than he/she can communicate.
- Provide appropriate information concerning developmental changes, menstruation, birth control.
- Provide explanations at level adolescent can understand.

Evaluation: Adolescent/young adult receives information regarding sexuality at age-appropriate levels.

Goal 3: Parents/family members will express feelings about having a child with a developmental disability, and their ability to cope.

Plan/Implementation
- Allow parents/family members opportunities to express their grief; be supportive and anticipate repeated periods of sadness, anger; acknowledge this is usually a lifetime process.
- Help parents identify and reinforce child's capabilities and normal characteristics (this is *first* a child, and then a child with a disability).
- Encourage family discussion and coping with changes that may occur in the family system as a result of caring for the child.
- Refer the family to appropriate community resources.

Evaluation: Parents/family express feelings/concerns regarding child's limitations; develop realistic plans to care for the child at home; include child as a member of the family constellation; involve all family members in child's care; utilize appropriate community resources, e.g., parent-support groups, available programs.

Goal 4: The family will remain cohesive and function at its optimal level.

Plan/Implementation
- Identify families at risk for adapting poorly to disability and chronic illness

  - recognize that certain family types (e.g., single-parent families, teen parents) may require more support and guidance in care of child
  - consider the availability of extended-family members and their ability and willingness to participate in care of child
- Determine the family's perception of the child's disability and encourage realistic discussion about the child's capabilities and limitations.
- Identify support systems within the family and community (e.g., home health care).
- Encourage activities that enhance individual and family development for *all* family members.
- Provide respite care to family when necessary.

Evaluation: Family discusses realistic perceptions about the child; utilizes available support systems; participates in activities outside the home; families at risk for poor adaptation are identified and receive the necessary support or referral for counseling and assistance.

Selected Health Problems: Developmental or Neurologic Disabilities

☐ Mental Retardation (MR)

1. General Information

a. Definition: below average intellectual functioning that becomes apparent during childhood development and is associated with impairment in adaptive behavior; manifestations include impaired learning, inadequate social adjustment, and delayed or lowered potential capacity for achievement; see Table 5.13 for classification levels

b. Causes

1) *prenatal*: chromosomal/genetic variations (Down syndrome, PKU, Tay-Sachs), German measles or infection in mother during pregnancy, incompatible blood between mother and child (Rh or ABO), glandular disorders, toxic chemicals, nutritional deficiencies, excessive maternal drug or alcohol use

2) *perinatal*: birth injury such as anoxia or intracranial hemorrhage

3) *postnatal*: encephalitis, head trauma, glandular disturbances, inadequate developmental stimulation in early childhood, post-cardiac arrest, poisoning

c. Incidence: 3% of the US population; 1 in 10 American families has an MR member; 70%–80% are in the borderline or mild (EMR) category (see Table 5.13); 20%–30% are moderately, severely, or profoundly retarded (the latter are most often cared for in residential institutions)

2. Nursing Process

a. Assessment/Analysis

1) developmental lags in motor and adaptive behaviors

Table 5.13 Levels of Retardation (Classification System of American Association on Mental Deficiency)

Level	IQ Range	Potential Mental Age	Rehabilitation Potential
Level 0: Borderline	68–83	Close to normal	Usually capable of marriage, being *self-supporting* (probable low socioeconomic living standard).
Level 1: Mild or educable	52–67	8–12 years	Can usually be maintained in community. *Can work but needs supervision in financial affairs*; 4th- or 5th-grade academic possibilities (special classes for educable mentally retarded [EMR]) and vocational skills, but often has difficulty holding a job in a competitive market.
Level 2: Moderate	36–51	3–7 years	1st- to 3rd-grade academic potential (special classes for trainable mentally retarded [TMR]) or *vocational training in sheltered workshop in neighborhood job*.
Level 3: Severe	20–35	Toddler	*Minimal self-help skills* and independent behavior (toilet training, dressing self). School placement in handicapped or TMR program. Some are able to work in a sheltered workshop.
Level 4: Profound	Less than 20	Young infant	May require *total care*; may have CNS damage.

2) persistence of neonatal reflexes
3) perceptual deficits
4) level of functioning (see Table 5.13)

b. Plan Implementation, and Evaluation (see General Nursing Plans page 554)

Goal: When hospitalized, the mentally retarded child will adapt to hospitalization, will maintain independence in ADL, will ingest adequate food and fluids.

Plan/Implementation

- Adapt hospital routines to child's as much as possible.
- Explain all procedures and treatments carefully, at level child can understand.
- Maintain consistency to promote security within child's environment.
- Encourage parent/family participation in care.
- Assist with feeding as necessary; bring special cups, feeding utensils from home.
- Be sure to follow through on what you tell child (e.g., if you say you will return at a certain time, be sure to do it).
- Use positive reinforcement.

Evaluation: Child accepts staff members' explanations and cooperates in care; feeds and dresses self; takes prescribed diet and fluids.

☐ Attention Deficit Disorder (ADD)

1. General Information

a. Definition: syndrome of behaviorally related problems that include inattention and impulsivity. DSM-III-R classification differentiates ADD with and without hyperactivity. Previously known as minimal brain dysfunction or hyperkinesis.

b. Causes: No definite pathophysiologic basis has been determined; possible causes include neurotransmitter imbalances, lead poisoning, allergies, and genetic factors.

c. Incidence: 5%–10% of school-age children, boys affected 4–6 times more frequently

d. Medical Treatment

1) diagnosis: parent and teacher report of behavior, objective home and classroom observation, psychologic evaluation; results compared with DSM-III-R criteria
2) treatment
   a) behavioral management
   b) medication: methylphenidate (Ritalin)
      - dosage: 0.3–1.0 mg/kg/day adjusted according to child's behavior
      - side effects: anorexia, upper abdominal pain, insomnia, growth suppression, tachycardia
      - nursing implications
        - administer with or after meals to minimize appetite suppression
        - do not administer after 4:00 PM to minimize insomnia

2. Nursing Process

a. Assessment/Analysis

1) distractability
2) impulsiveness
3) emotional lability
4) low frustration tolerance
5) high incidence of learning disabilities
6) hyperactivity (may or may not be present)

b. Plan Implementation, and Evaluation

Goal: Child/parent will be prepared for home management.

Plan/Implementation

- Assist parents to
  - provide a very structured environment with regular routines.
  - establish clear, simple rules and firm limits.
  - prevent overstimulation and fatigue in the child.
  - provide daily rest or quiet times.
  - reward any partially successful efforts at self-control.
- Teach parents/child administration, action, and side effects of medication.
- Reinforce importance of regular, routine administration of medications.
- Refer for family or individual counselling as necessary.
- Encourage parents to work closely with school personnel to minimize impact of ADD on learning.

Evaluation: Child learns/effectively; parents are satisfied with child's behavior pattern.

☐ Down Syndrome (Trisomy 21)

1. General Information

a. Definition: extra chromosome 21 (trisomy 21), due to a failure of the chromosome to split during gametogenesis; mental capacity varies from level 1 (educable) to level 3 (severely retarded); one of the most common causes of mental retardation

b. Cause: associated with increased maternal or paternal age

c. Incidence: 1 in 600–650 live births

d. Medical treatment: diagnosis is usually based on clinical manifestations; chromosome studies may be done

2. Nursing Process

a. Assessment/Analysis

1) physical manifestations
   a) small round head, flat nose, protruding tongue, high arched palate
   b) slanted eyelids, Brushfield spots (speckles in iris)
   c) muscle hypotonia, hyperflexible joints
   d) simian crease, short fingers, clinodactyly
   e) congenital heart malformations in 40% of cases
   f) weak respiratory accessory muscles
   g) increased incidence of leukemia and GI anomalies
2) mastery of development tasks
3) intellectual functioning
4) child's routine for ADL

b. Plans, Implementation, and Evaluation

Goal 1: Child will be free from respiratory infection.

Plan/Implementation
- Teach parents (and child as appropriate) preventive health measures
  - prevent exposure to individuals with URIs
  - encourage optimal nutrition, adequate rest
  - keep immunizations up-to-date
- Obtain medical care at onset of infection (may need antibiotics).

Evaluation: Child has no more than a minimal number of URIs.

Goal 2: Child will ingest adequate food and fluids and will experience minimal feeding difficulties.

Plan/Implementation
- Teach parents appropriate feeding techniques
  - use bulb syringe to clear nasal passages before feedings
  - use a long-handled, infant spoon (rubber-coated) to place food to side and back of mouth
- Reassure parents that infant's tongue thrust does not mean dislike of food.
- When hospitalized or in school, encourage foods from home if child not ingesting adequate amounts.
- Adjust caloric requirements based on child's size and activity level to prevent child from becoming overweight.
- Provide high roughage and liberal fluids to prevent constipation.

Evaluation: Child experiences minimal feeding difficulties (airway remains clear during feeding, child ingests food sufficient for growth); maintains weight within expected limits for height as child grows older; remains free from constipation.

☐ Cerebral Palsy

1. General Information

a. Definition: nonprogressive muscular impairment resulting in abnormal muscle tone and incoordination; spastic type most common (upper motor neuron involvement), dyskinetic (athetoid) type second-most common; may be mild to severe

b. Associated defects: mental retardation (may have normal or superior intelligence), seizures, minimal brain dysfunction; speech, hearing, oculomotor impairment

c. Incidence
1) 25,000 babies with cerebral palsy born annually (5:1,000 live births)
2) most common developmental disability of childhood
3) higher incidence in low-birth-weight babies or from birth with other complications, especially during the perinatal period, that result in cerebral anoxia

d. Medical treatment
1) braces, ambulation devices (crutches, walker)
2) surgical correction of extremity deformities (especially lengthening of heel cord to improve stability and function)
3) medications: muscle relaxants, anticonvulsants, tranquilizers

2. Nursing Process

a. Assessment/Analysis

1) spasticity
   a) hypertonicity of muscles (continuous reflexive contraction of muscles leading to tightening and shortening)
   b) persistence of neonatal reflexes
   c) scissoring
   d) poor posturing
   e) delayed gross and fine motor development

f) uneven muscle tone
g) intellectual functioning may be impaired
2) dyskinesis (athetosis)
a) continuous uncontrollable, wormlike movements of arms, legs, torso, face and tongue
■ intensified by stress
■ absent during sleep
b) drooling
c) poor speech articulation

b. Plans, Implementation, and Evaluation

Goal 1: Child will ingest adequate nutrition.

Plan/Implementation
- Provide adequate calories to meet additional energy demands of constant muscle activity (athetoid).
- Feed slowly; provide calm, peaceful environment.
- Modify feeding technique to deal with extrusion reflex.
- Ensure adequate fluid intake.
- Use special silverware and dishes as needed (e.g., padded spoon, nonskid dishes).
- Teach importance of daily dental hygiene; routine dental care.

Evaluation: Child ingests calories and other nutrients needed for adequate growth; chews and swallows food adequately; has optimal dental hygiene and care; is free from dental caries or gum problems.

Goal 2: Child will develop maximum mobility and self-help skills.

Plan/Implementation
- Teach parents appropriate stretching and range-of-motion exercises.
- Teach use of braces or splints, special support chairs, or wheelchairs as needed.
- Encourage participation in programs of physical and occupational therapy, speech therapy as needed.
- Avoid movement that triggers abnormal reflexes.
- Teach self-help skills, beginning with simplest ones first; teach only 1 skill at a time until it is learned.
- Provide needed adaptive devices (special utensils, Velcro fastenings).

Evaluation: Child is free from contractures; demonstrates maximum mobility (with assistance as needed); participates in self-care tasks (e.g., feed self, dress self).

Goal 3: Child will be free from skin breakdown.

Plan/Implementation
- Reposition frequently and gently massage pressure points with lotion.
- Check braces, splints for tightness and pressure; adjust as needed.
- Utilize special equipment (''egg-crate'' mattress, sheepskin).
- Keep linens and clothes dry; if wet with urine/stool, change as soon as possible.

Evaluation: Child's skin is intact, free from pressure sores.

☐ Hydrocephalus

1. General Information

a. Definition: excessive accumulation of cerebral spinal fluid (CSF) within the ventricles of the brain; three common types
1) excess secretion of CSF
2) obstructive (noncommunicating): results from an obstruction in the ventricular pathway
3) communicating: results when the CSF is not absorbed from the subarachnoid space

b. Causes: developmental malformation (congenital), tumors, infections, head injury

c. Medical treatment
1) diagnosis: lumbar puncture, CAT scan (refer to *Nursing Care of the Adult* page 272)
2) surgical insertion of shunt to bypass obstruction or drain excess fluid
a) atrioventricular (AV) shunt: lateral ventricle to right atrium of heart
b) ventriculoperitoneal (VP) shunt: lateral ventricle to peritoneal cavity
c) one-way valves are used in both cases to prevent backflow of blood or peritoneal secretions
3) rehospitalization is common for blocked/infected shunt, or for lengthening of shunt as child grows

2. Nursing Process

a. Assessment/Analysis
1) for signs and symptoms of increased intracranial pressure to prevent/minimize brain damage (see Table 5.14)
2) shiny scalp with dilated veins (congenital hydrocephalus)
3) sunset eyes (congenital hydrocephalus)

b. Plans, Implementation, and Evaluation

Table 5.14 Signs and Symptoms of Increased Intracranial Pressure in Infants and Children*

Causes	Hydrocephalus Intracranial tumors Cerebral trauma Meningitis, encephalitis
Manifestations Infants	Bulging fontanels High-pitched cry Vomiting, feeding difficulty (poor suck) Seizures Opisthotonos Rapid increase in head circumference (especially occipital-frontal diameter)
Older children (same as adults)	Headache Nausea, vomiting Change in level of consciousness Papilledema Diplopia Motor dysfunction (grasp, gait) Behavior changes, irritability Change in vital signs (elevated systolic PB, wide pulse pressure, decreased pulse and respirations) Seizures

*Review *Nursing Care of the Adult* page 275 for content on head injury.

Goal 1: Child will maintain adequate nutrition and hydration.

Plan/Implementation

- Offer small frequent feedings; do not overfeed.
- Burp often.
- After feeding, position on side with head elevated.
- Provide rest period after feedings.
- Assess for dehydration.

Evaluation: Child ingests food and fluid given; has elastic skin turgor, moist mucous membranes.

Goal 2: Postoperatively, child will be free from complications.

Plan/Implementation

- Measure head circumference daily.
- Position on unoperative side relative to appearance of fontanel: if fontanel normal, elevate head; if fontanel depressed, position child flat in bed.
- Observe for signs of redness, skin breakdown on scalp; use sheepskin or water mattress.
- Turn at least q2h.
- Do frequent neuro checks (LOC, PERLA).
- Observe for signs of infection.
- *Pump shunt only with a physician's order*, to maintain patency (usually done when shunt valve is a bubble type).

Evaluation: Child's fontanels remain flat (no bulging or depression) with no further increase in head circumference; has no signs of infection or pneumonia (e.g., elevated temperature, increased pulse rate, reddened area around operative site); suffers no brain damage.

☐ Spina Bifida

1. General Information

a. Definition: congenital defect involving incomplete formation of vertebrae, often accompanied by herniation of parts of the central nervous system

1) meningocele: herniation of sac containing spinal fluid and meninges

2) meningomyelocele: herniated sac containing CSF, meninges and malformed portion of spinal cord and nerve roots (most serious type); sac may be covered by skin or a very thin, transparent tissue layer that tears easily and permits leakage of CSF

b. Motor and sensory impairment: relative to level and extent of defect; usually involves sensorimotor deficits of lower extremities, bowel and bladder dysfunction, associated orthopedic anomalies, and often hydrocephalus

c. Medical treatment

1) prenatal diagnosis: amniocentesis shows increased alpha-fetoprotein; done when mother has a history of having a child with a neural tube defect

2) surgical intervention to close defect within 24–48 hours to decrease chance of infection and minimize nerve damage

2. Nursing Process

a. Assessment/Analysis

1) condition of sac
2) motor and sensory impairment: flaccid or spastic paralysis, response to painful stimuli, lower-extremity movement
3) bladder and bowel function: dribbling of urine, leakage of stool
4) associated orthopedic anomalies: clubfoot, congenital dislocated hip
5) signs of infection (fever, irritability, lethargy)
6) signs of increased intracranial pressure (see Table 5.14), increased head circumference (especially following surgery)

b. Plans, Implementation, and Evaluation

Goal 1: Child will be free from rupture of sac and infection; postoperatively, incision will heal without complications.

Plan/Implementation
- Position on side or prone.
- Use Bradford frame.
- Protect sac with sponge doughnut when holding infant.
- Apply moist sterile dressings as ordered.
- Observe for leakage of CSF from sac.
- Observe for signs of meningitis (e.g., fever, irritability, nuchal rigidity).
- Meticulously cleanse diaper area to prevent contamination of sac or post-op wound site with urine/stool; check incision frequently for signs of infection.
- Postoperatively, observe for signs of hydrocephalus or shunt malfunction; daily head circumference; neuro checks.

Evaluation: Child is free from local or systemic infection (e.g., reddened skin around site, elevated temperature); has intact sac (preoperatively); has optimal wound healing postoperatively.

Goal 2: Child will maintain skin integrity (lifelong goal).

Plan/Implementation
- Observe for reddened areas, breaks in skin.
- Change position frequently.
- Use sheepskin or water mattress.
- Massage pressure areas to promote circulation.
- Teach self-help skills concerning skin care.

Evaluation: Child's skin is intact, free from reddened areas or pressure sores.

Goal 3: Child will experience love and physical contact.

Plan/Implementation
- Talk to infant (use face to face position).
- Touch, stroke child.
- Encourage parents to caress, stroke, and talk to infant (cannot be held pre-op or early post-op) to promote parent-infant attachment.

Evaluation: Child receives physical and voice contact from staff and parents/family; parents caress and talk to infant.

Goal 4: Child will gain optimal bowel and bladder function (long-term goal).

Plan/Implementation
- Empty bladder manually by applying gentle downward pressure (Credé method).
- Provide diet with adequate fluids (those that acidify urine such as apple and cranberry juice) and fiber (as child grows older).
- Teach parent (and child when older) to care for
  - intermittent catheterizations (self-catheterization)
  - indwelling Foley catheter
  - ileal conduit
- Administer urinary antiseptics, stool softeners as prescribed.

Evaluation: Child has adequate urinary output and an established bowel routine; is free from urinary tract infection.

Goal 5: Child will be from lower extremity deformity.

Plan/Implementation
- Provide passive ROM exercises.
- Keep hips abducted using blanket rolls.
- Provide physical therapy; fitting with braces (usually long leg braces) and crutches for ambulation as child grows older.

Evaluation: Child maintains full ROM of joints; has no contractures of hip or lower extremity.

☐ Seizure Disorders

1. General Information

a. Definition: episode of uncontrolled, electrical activity in the brain; neuronal discharges become excessive and irregular resulting in loss of consciousness, convulsive body movements, or disturbances in sensations or behavior

b. Incidence: occur in 0.5% of all children; it has been estimated that 4%–6% of all children will experience one or more seizures by the time they reach adolescence

c. Cause: possible causes include infection, tumors, trauma, acid-base imbalances, epilepsy, allergies, anoxia, and hypoglycemia

d. *Epilepsy:* chronic brain dysfunction manifested by recurrent seizures; unknown etiology; higher incidence in children; may see *status epilepticus*: recurrent seizures occurring at such frequency that full consciousness is not regained between seizures.

e. Types of seizures and manifestations
   1) generalized seizures
      a) *grand mal*: sudden loss of consciousness followed by tonic phase (stiffening of body) and clonic phase (jerky movements of trunk and extremities); periods of depressed or apneic breathing may occur; child may fall asleep after the seizure or be confused and irritable.
      b) *petit mal* (absence seizures): child appears to be daydreaming; all verbal and motor behavior stops; may occur 10 or more times/day; usually lasts 10–30 seconds; child usually alert after the seizures; no memory episode
      c) *akinetic*: child experiences a sudden loss of body tone accompanied by loss of consciousness; lasts a few seconds; resumes ADL afterwards
      d) *infantile spasms*: similar to a startle reflex; involves jerking of the head and clonic movements of the extremities; usually disappear by 2–3 years of age; may develop into more generalized seizures; usually accompanied by other problems (e.g., mental retardation)
   2) partial seizures
      a) *Jacksonian*: twitching begins at distal end of extremity, eventually involving entire extremity and possibly entire side of body; no loss of consciousness; not commonly seen in children
      b) *psychomotor*: characterized by altered state of consciousness (e.g., dreamlike); may chew, smack lips, mumble; lasts several minutes; child has no memory of behavior
   3) febrile seizures: transient disorder usually the result of an extracranial infection (e.g., otitis media); peak incidence between 6 months and 3 years of age; resemble grand mal seizures
   4) breathholding: usually benign; child begins to cry, holds his breath and experiences brief cyanosis with loss of consciousness; precipitating factors may be anger or frustration

f. Diagnosis: complete and accurate history and physical; thorough description of the seizure including onset, time of day, type of seizure, precipitating factors; EEG necessary for evaluating the seizure disorder

g. Medical treatment: anticonvulsants to elevate the child's excitability threshold and prevent seizures (refer to Table 5.15)

2. Nursing Process

a. Assessment/Analysis

1) history of seizure activity, recent episodes, management
   a) preseizure behavior: aura, loss of consciousness
   b) seizure activity: tonic/clonic phase; inappropriate behavior; fecal or urinary incontinence during the seizure
   c) postseizure behavior: memory lapse, headache, instability, loss of consciousness, lethargy
2) use of anticonvulsant medications, side effects

b. Plans, Implementation, and Evaluation

Goal 1: Child will maintain adequate respiratory function and be free from injuries during a seizure (primary concern with status epilepticus).

Plan/Implementation

- Gently lower the standing or sitting child to the floor (supine position).
- Maintain a patent airway by hyperextending the neck and pulling the jaw slightly forward; turn the head to the side to facilitate drainage of mucus and saliva.
- Have O_2 and suction available (if possible).
- *Do not place anything in the child's mouth*; in the past it was believed that a padded tongue blade prevented the child from "swallowing" or biting tongue; simply turning the child's head to the side accomplishes the same effect and diminishes trauma.
- Do not restrain child.
- Remove any toys or dangerous objects that might injure the child during a seizure; pad side rails if possible.

Table 5.15 Medications Used to Treat Seizure Disorders

Drug	Route	Side Effects	Nursing Implications
Carbamazepine (Tegretol)	PO	Drowsiness Ataxia Vertigo Anorexia Aplastic anemia	Periodic CBC and liver enzymes. Avoid excessive sunlight because of photophobia. Administer with food.
Clonazepam (Clonopin)	PO	Nausea and vomiting Rash Nystagmus Drowsiness Anemia	Monitor behavioral changes. Frequent respiratory assessment because bronchial secretions are increased.
Diazepam (Valium)	IV push over 1–2 min; may repeat q15 min × 2	Drowsiness Dry mouth Constipation Anorexia	Used for status epilepticus. Only inject 5 mg/min. Monitor BP (hypotension) and respirations (respiratory depression). Do not dilute with IV solutions.
Ethosoximide (Zarontin)	PO	Drowsiness Ataxia Blurred vision Anorexia GI upset	Monitor liver and kidney function. Administer with food.
Phenobarbital	PO	Nausea and vomiting Drowsiness Rash Irritability Mild ataxia	Monitor BP and respiration during IV administration. Paradoxical reaction in children. Taper medication when discontinuing.
Phenytoin (Dilantin)	PO, IV	Gingival hypertrophy Dermatitis Ataxia Drowsiness Nystagmus Bone-marrow suppression	Meticulous oral hygiene. Administer with food to reduce GI upset. Monitor liver enzymes.
Primidone (Mysoline)	PO	Nausea and vomiting Drowsiness Ataxia Headache Gum pain	Observe for folic acid deficiency. Taper medicine when discontinuing. Hemorrhage in newborns whose mothers are taking this med.
Sodium valproate (DepaKene)	PO	GI upset Nausea and vomiting Drowsiness Leukopenia; thrombocytopenia	Administer with meals. Potentiates dilantin/phenobarb. Monitor liver enzymes Periodic CBC, bleeding time.

- Loosen tight or restrictive clothing.
- Observe the seizure carefully
  - preseizure activity; aura, incontinence
  - seizure activity: include onset and initial focus of seizure, duration, change in respirations, progression of movement through body, changes in neurologic status
  - postseizure activity: duration, status, behavior
- Administer anticonvulsant medication as ordered.
- Monitor blood gases.

Evaluation: Child maintains adequate respiratory function; is free from injuries; experiences cessation of seizure activity.

Goal 2: Child and family will learn how to cope with the long-term problems associated with seizure disorders.

Plan/Implementation

- Encourage good health practices including adequate sleep, good nutritional habits, and exercise.
- Provide appropriate explanations concerning cause of seizure activity, actions of medications, importance of periodic reevaluation.
- Teach the importance of adhering to medication routine, common side effects, importance of period blood and urine studies, behavior

changes that may occur as a result of anticonvulsant medication.
- Stress the importance of never discontinuing anticonvulsant medication abruptly.
- Instruct family concerning care of child during a seizure.
- Encourage child/family to discuss fears, anxieties concerning seizure disorder.
- Inform child/family about situations that might precipitate seizures
  - illness, fever stress
  - occur more frequently during menses or as a result of alcohol ingestion
- Ensure child wears a Medic Alert bracelet
- Provide information concerning vocational guidance and federal and state laws regarding limitations that might be imposed on the younger child or adolescent.
- Provide information concerning support groups in the community.

Evaluation: Child functions independently regarding ADL; adheres to medical regimen; child and family discuss fears and anxieties concerning seizure disorder; become involved in support groups.

☐ Meningitis

1. General Information

a. Definition: a syndrome caused by inflammation of the meninges of the brain and spinal cord; two basic types
  1) *bacterial*: *H. influenzae, Streptococcus pneumoniae*, or *Neisseria meningitidis* (meningococcus)
  2) *aseptic*: viruses, parasites, fungi

b. Cause: may be preceded by otitis media, tonsillitis, or other URI

c. Incidence: occurs more often in boys; peak incidence is late infancy and toddlerhood; *Haemophilus b* diphtheria toxoid conjugate vaccine given at 18 months of age will protect child from meningitis caused by *H. influenzae*

d. Characteristics
  1) generally determined by age of child
    a) newborn presents with nonspecific symptoms such as poor sucking and feeding, apnea, weak cry, diarrhea, jaundice; tense anterior fontanel does not occur until late
    b) infant may present with fever, poor feeding, nausea and vomiting, increased irritability, high-pitched cry, and seizures
    c) child and adolescent present with classic signs of fever, headache, nuchal rigidity, seizures, altered sensorium, projectile vomiting
  2) petechial or purpural rash due to extravasation of RBCs usually seen in meningococcal meningitis
  3) long-term complications include blindness, deafness, mental retardation, hydrocephalus, cerebral palsy, and seizures

c. Medical treatment
  1) diagnosis: lumbar puncture to examine CSF; usual findings
    a) elevated WBC
    b) decreased glucose
    c) elevated protein
    d) positive culture
  2) medications
    a) antibiotics (large doses given IV)
    b) anticonvulsants
    c) antipyretics

2. Nursing Process

a. Assessment/Analysis
  1) neurologic status (may see increased ICP [Table 5.14] secondary to cerebral edema resulting from inappropriate ADH secretion)
    a) neuro check (LOC, PERLA, motor activity, vital signs)
    b) Brudzinski's sign (pain on flexion of neck)
    c) Kernig's sign (pain on knee extension while lifting knee from a supine position)
    d) opisthotonus
  2) meningeal irritation (e.g., high-pitched cry, nuchal rigidity, irritability)
  3) seizure activity (see page 560)
  4) hydration (e.g., output, specific gravity, signs and symptoms of dehydration)

b. Plans, Implementation, and Evaluation

Goal 1: Others will be free from infecting organism; disease will not spread.

Plan/Implementation
- Place in strict isolation (for at least 24 hours after initiation of antibiotic therapy)
- Teach parents, others isolation procedures.
- Assist with lumbar puncture to determine causative organism.
- Administer antibiotics as prescribed, observe side effects.

Evaluation: Disease does not spread to others; family adheres to isolation procedures.

Goal 2: Child will remain free from neurologic complications and long-term sequelae.

Plan/Implementation

- Implement seizure and safety precautions, e.g., side rails up (padded), oxygen and suction available.
- Do frequent neuro checks with vital signs.
- Minimize environmental stimuli (lights, noise) and movement to lessen possibility of seizures.
- Elevate head of bed slightly (to decrease intracranial pressure).
- Administer anticonvulsants as ordered.
- Monitor fluid intake to prevent dilutional hyponatremia (due to inappropriate ADH secretion).
- Monitor for long-term sequelae: seizures, hydrocephalus, mental retardation, ataxia, hemiparesis, deafness.
- Provide parental support and reassurance concerning recovery.

Evaluation: Child shows no signs of complications (e.g., seizure activity); resumes normal activities.

Goal 3: Child will maintain adequate hydration and nutrition.

Plan/Implementation

- Maintain NPO during acute phase of illness.
- Administer IV fluids as ordered; restrain as needed to maintain infusion site.
- Carefully monitor I&O to prevent fluid overload (can increase intracranial pressure), specific gravity, weight.
- Advance diet as tolerated as child recovers.

Evaluation: Child is adequately hydrated; is free from signs of fluid overload; receives adequate nourishment.

References

Berry, R. (1988). Home care of the child with AIDS. *Pediatric Nursing, 14*, 341–344.

Burn care. (1985). *American Journal of Nursing, 85*, 30–50.

Ellis, J. (1988). Using pain scales to prevent undermedication. *MCN: The American Journal of Maternal/Child Nursing, 13*, 180–182.

Henley, M., & Sears, J. (1985). Pinworms: A persistent pediatric problem. *MCN: American Journal of Maternal/Child Nursing, 10*, 111–114.

Holaday, B. (1984). Challenges of rearing a chronically ill child: Caring and coping. *Nursing Clinics of North America, 19*(2), 361–368.

Hurley, A. & Whelan, E. (1988). Cognitive development and children's perception of pain. *Pediatric Nursing, 14*, 21–24.

Jackson, P. (1985). When the baby isn't perfect. *American Journal of Nursing, 85*(4), 396–400.

Kosowski, M., & Sopcyk, J. (1985). Feeding hospitalized children with developmental disabilities. *MCN: American Journal of Maternal/Child Nursing, 10*(3), 190–194.

McLaury, P. (1983). Head lice: Pediatric social disease. *American Journal of Nursing, 83*, 1300–1303.

*Meier, E. (1983). Evaluating head trauma in infants and children, *MCN: American Journal of Maternal/Child Nursing, 8*(1), 54–57.

Mott, S., Fazekas, N., & James, S. (1985). *Nursing care of children and families: A holistic approach*. Menlo Park, CA: Addison-Wesley.

Nurses Drug Alert. (1984). Tetanus prophylaxis. *American Journal of Nursing, 84*, 493–494.

Scipien, G., et al. (1986). *Comprehensive pediatric nursing* (3rd ed.). New York: McGraw-Hill.

Servonsky, J., & Opas, S. (1987). *Nursing management of children*. Boston: Jones & Bartlett.

Waechter, E., Phillips, J., & Holaday, B. (1985). *Nursing care of children* (10th ed.). Philadelphia: Lippincott.

Whaley, L., & Wong, D. (1986). *Nursing care of infants and children* (3rd ed.). St. Louis: Mosby.

White, J. (1983). Special needs of hospitalized children with learning disabilities. *MCN: American Journal of Maternal/Child Nursing, 8*(6), 209–212.

Young, R. (1977). Chronic sorrow: Parent's response to the birth of a child with a defect. *MCN: American Journal of Maternal/Child Nursing, 2*(1), 38–42.

*See Reprint Section.

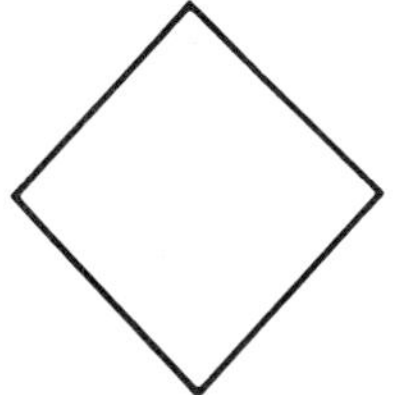

Oxygenation

General Concepts

Overview/Physiology

1. Respiratory system
   - **a.** Chest configuration (AP diameter) changes from round to more flattened as child grows
   - **b.** Steady increase in number and surface area of alveoli from birth to age 12; infants and young children have less alveolar surface for gas exchange
   - **c.** Cricoid cartilage is at the level of the 4th cervical vertebra in infants, 5th cervical vertebra in children (important when positioning children for resuscitation, intubation, or tracheostomy)
   - **d.** More susceptible to respiratory obstruction and atelectasis because of narrow tracheal and bronchiolar pathways
   - **e.** More susceptible to infections because of immature immune system and frequent contacts with infectious organisms
   - **f.** In infancy, nasal passages are narrow and infants are obligatory nose breathers (important to remember when feeding infants—mucus accumulation and mucosal swelling may hamper feeding)
2. Cardiovascular system
   - **a.** Changes during transition from fetal to postnatal circulation
     - **1)** lungs inflate, resulting in increased pressure in left side of heart
     - **2)** foramen ovale closes
     - **3)** ductus arteriosus closes
     - **4)** obliteration of ductus venosus and umbilical vessels
   - **b.** Blood pressure gradually increases, and pulse and respiratory rates gradually decrease as child grows
3. Hematologic system
   - **a.** All components necessary for normal hematologic functioning are present at birth except vitamin K, which is administered intramuscularly to the newborn (refer to *Nursing Care of the Childbearing Family* page 458); see Table 5.16
   - **b.** *All* bones are engaged in blood cell production until growth ceases in late adolescence

Application of the Nursing Process to the Child with Respiratory Problems

1. **Assessment**
   - **a.** Nursing history
     - **1)** any known breathing problems, respiratory allergies, activity intolerance (does child have problems keeping up with other children during play?), incidence of respiratory illnesses, treatment, home management
     - **2)** environmental factors: dust or pollen in home, play or school environments; do parents or child smoke?
   - **b.** Clinical appraisal
     - **1)** general appearance: color (pallor, cyanosis), respiratory effort (dyspnea, stridor, grunting, prolonged expirations), restlessness, irritability, fatigue, prostration, clubbing of fingers and toes
     - **2)** respiratory rate, depth, character; presence of respiratory signs (cough: character, productive or nonproductive; rhinitis; retractions; nasal flaring)
     - **3)** fever
     - **4)** breath sounds: upper respiratory tract, all lobes of lungs; presence of wheezing, rales, rhonchi
   - **c.** Diagnostic tests (refer to *Nursing Care of the Adult* page 166)
2. **Analysis**
   - **a.** Safe, effective care environment
     - **1)** knowledge deficit
     - **2)** potential for infection
   - **b.** Physiological integrity
     - **1)** ineffective breathing pattern
     - **2)** impaired gas exchange
     - **3)** ineffective airway clearance
   - **c.** Psychological integrity
     - **1)** anxiety
     - **2)** social isolation

Table 5.16 Hematology Values in Children

Hematocrit	35%–47%
Hemoglobin	10.5–16 g/dl
Red blood cell count (RBC)	3.9–5.1 million/mm³
White blood cell count (WBC)	5,500–13,500/mm³ (between 2–13 years) 5,000–20,000/mm³ (under age 2)
Platelets	150,000–400,000/mm³
Arterial blood gases	
pO_2	83–108 mm Hg (65–80 mm Hg newborn)
pCO_2	35–45 mm Hg (27–40 mm Hg newborn)
pH	7.35–7.45 (7.27–7.47 newborn)

d. Health promotion/maintenance
   1) diversional activity deficit
   2) altered growth and development

3. General Nursing Plans, Implementation, and Evaluation

Goal 1: Child will maintain adequate oxygenation and a patent airway.

Plan/Implementation
- Monitor respiratory status
  - vital signs (respirations, pulse, temperature)
  - skin and nail-bed color, dyspnea, cough, nasal flaring, retractions
  - lung sounds
  - use of sternal and thoracic muscles
  - behavioral changes (restlessness, irritability, disruptions in patterns)
- Be alert for signs of airway obstruction
  - rapidly rising heart rate and increased respiratory rate, diaphoresis
  - restlessness, anxiety, agitation (indicate hypoxia)
  - increased stridor, retractions
  - pallor or cyanosis
- Position to ease respiratory effort (semi- to high-Fowler's); loosen clothing to allow maximum chest expansion.
- Avoid sedatives that depress respirations and cough reflex (e.g., narcotics).
- Keep endotracheal tubes, laryngoscope, and tracheostomy tray at bedside for emergency use.
- Never leave child unattended if in respiratory distress (changes in condition can occur very rapidly).
- Initiate CPR when necessary

  Infant (age 1 and younger)
  - position on back on a flat, firm surface (move child as a single unit)
  - clear airway of foreign matter/mucus
  - open airway by placing head in a neutral position, lift chin (avoid over-extension)
  - look, listen, feel for breaths
  - give 2 breaths of 1–1½ second each, mouth-to-mouth and nose
  - check brachial pulse to assess circulation
  - perform chest compressions if necessary
    * compress lower sternum with 2–3 fingers ½–1 inch at a rate of at least 100 compressions/minute
    * give 5 compressions to 1 breath
  - reassess after 10 cycles and every few minutes thereafter

  Child (ages 1–8)
  - position on back on a flat, firm surface (move child as a single unit)
  - clear airway of foreign matter/mucus
  - open airway with head-tilt/chin-lift maneuver (avoid over-extension)
  - look, listen, feel for breaths
  - give two breaths of 1–1½ second each, mouth-to-mouth
  - check carotid pulse to assess circulation
  - perform chest compressions if necessary
    * compress lower sternum with heel of one hand 1–1½ inches at a rate of 80–100 compressions/minute
    * give 5 compressions to 1 breath
  - reassess after 10 cycles and every few minutes thereafter
- Provide care for child with an endotracheal (ET) tube or tracheostomy
  - perform ET tube/trach care and suctioning
  - restrain child as needed
  - provide reassurance to child and parents
  - change position q2h
  - anticipate needs since child cannot verbalize
  - inform child about inability to speak
  - devise alternate means of communication; reassure that voice will return when able to breathe normally again

Evaluation: Child maintains a patent airway; exhibits signs of adequate oxygenation (normal skin color, quiet breathing, alert and oriented, clear lung sounds).

Goal 2: Child will be free from respiratory distress.

Plan/Implementation
- Provide care for child in mist tent with cool

mist and O_2 as ordered (periodically analyze O_2 level)
- plan care to minimize opening of tent
- tuck sides of tent tightly to prevent loss of O_2 and mist
- maintain ice chamber or cooling mechanism
- monitor tent-chamber temperature
- keep child as warm and dry as possible to prevent chilling (change clothing and bed linens frequently)
- provide diversion and comfort measures to minimize child's fear and anxiety
  * reassure that child won't be left alone; encourage parent to stay with child
  * provide favorite toy or object (no furry or mechanical toys)

■ Assist with chest percussion, vibration, and postural drainage as needed; position child so gravity facilitates drainage from specific lobes.

Evaluation: Child cooperates with mist tent therapy; is free from respiratory distress.

Goal 3: Child will be adequately hydrated.

Plan/Implementation

■ Provide humidified atmosphere to help loosen secretions.

■ Ensure adequate fluid intake
- withhold oral fluids until respiratory distress subsides
- monitor IV fluids to prevent dehydration or fluid overload

Evaluation: Child has elastic skin turgor, normal urine output, adequate fluid intake; is free from signs of dehydration or fluid overload.

Goal 4: Child will conserve energy and remain physically comfortable.

Plan/Implementation

■ Administer sedatives (e.g., phenobarbital) as ordered (no narcotic sedatives, no cough suppressants).

■ Administer antipyretics, tepid sponge bath for fever.

■ Schedule treatments and nursing activities to allow uninterrupted periods for maximum rest/sleep.

■ Monitor child's response to care (feeding, chest physical therapy) to prevent tiring.

■ Provide quiet age-appropriate play activities.

Evaluation: Child conserves energy; cooperates with care and treatments; approximates normal rest/sleep patterns; engages in quiet play activities.

Selected Health Problems Resulting in an Interference with Respiration

□ Sudden Infant Death Syndrome (SIDS) or "Crib Death"

1. General Information

a. Definition: sudden unexpected death of an infant or young child, in which an adequate cause cannot be determined

b. Incidence: higher incidence in boys, infants with low birth weight or low Apgar scores, infants with CNS disturbances; greater incidence in siblings

c. Etiology: unknown; evidence supports theory of relationship between periodic apnea and chronic hypoxemia

d. Peak occurrence: winter or early spring; between ages of 2 and 4 months

2. Nursing Process

a. Assessment/Analysis

1) parents' knowledge of SIDS

2) availability of support systems, e.g., family, friends, SIDS organization, mental health center

3) apnea monitoring of high-risk infants (premies, subsequent siblings) or "near-miss" infants

a) parents' knowledge of and adjustment to home apnea monitoring

b) infant's apnea patterns

b. Plans, Implementation and Evaluation

Goal 1: Parents will receive information and support to help them adjust to loss.

Plan/Implementation

■ Explain that they are not responsible for infant's death (parents feel guilty).

■ Provide information about SIDS.

■ Allow expression of feelings; provide support as parents cope with loss, grief, and mourning.

■ Refer to local SIDS organization/support group: Foundation for Sudden Infant Death.

■ Refer to other community supports, e.g., church, community mental health centers.

Evaluation: Parents ventilate feelings about loss of infant; have a referral for counseling.

Goal 2: Parents will maintain and cope with home apnea monitoring.

Plan/Implementation

■ Teach parents mechanics of home monitoring equipment.

- Teach parents infant CPR.
- Provide emotional support to parents.
- Help parents identify and utilize resources for relief (e.g., qualified sitters).

Evaluation: Parents demonstrate ability to implement home monitoring, demonstrate correct infant CPR, adjust to home apnea monitoring.

☐ Acute Spasmodic Laryngitis (Spasmodic Croup)

☐ Acute Epiglottitis

☐ Laryngotracheobronchitis (LTB)

☐ Bronchiolitis

Refer to Table 5.17

☐ Bronchopulmonary Dysplasia

1. General Information

a. Definition: a chronic obstructive pulmonary disease characterized by thickening of the alveolar walls and bronchiolar epithelium; most surviving infants recover by 1 year of age

b. Occurrence: primarily in low birth weight infants with hyaline membrane disease who

Table 5.17 Comparison of Croup and Bronchiolitis

	Acute Spasmodic Laryngitis (Spasmodic Croup)	Acute Epiglottitis	Acute Laryngotracheobronchitis (LTB)	Bronchiolitis
Definition	Acute spasm of larynx, resulting in partial upper airway obstruction	Severe inflammation of the epiglottis that progresses rapidly	Inflammation of larynx, to a lesser extent of trachea and bronchii, resulting in spasm and partial airway obstruction	Inflammation of the bronchioles with accumulation of mucus and exudate, resulting in lung hyperinflation, dyspnea, and cyanosis Lower airway disease
Peak age of occurrence	1- to 3-year olds	3- to 8-year-olds	Infants and toddlers (most common form of croup)	2- to 12-month-olds (3rd leading cause of death in this age group)
Cause	Viral	Bacterial (usually H influenza, type B)	Usually viral, but may be bacterial	Viral (especially RSV*)
Assessment	Awakens with barklike, metallic cough Hoarseness Inspiratory stridor Usually occurs at night No fever May be preceded by URI Attack may recur for several nights	Sore throat Inflamed, cherry-red epiglottis Dysphagia, drooling Muffled voice Tripod posturing Suprasternal and substernal retractions High fever Restlessness Sudden onset, rapid progression	Preceded by URI Harsh, brassy cough Inspiratory stridor Substernal and suprasternal retractions, rales, and rhonchi Labored, prolonged expirations Low-grade fever	Paroxysmal cough Flaring nares Intercostal and subcostal retractions Rales with prolonged expirations, wheezing, grunting Diminished breath sounds, areas of consolidation Irritability, fatigue
Specific medications and treatment, additional nursing plan/ implementation (see also General Nursing Plans page 566)	Usually treated at home. Teach emergency home care • steam inhalation • subemetic dose of ipecac • cool mist humidifier Insure adequate fluid intake (clear liquids). Prepare parents for possible recurrence for several nights.	Emergency hospitalization: intubation or tracheostomy IV antibiotics (ampicillin, chloramphenicol) Antipyretics *Do not try to visualize child's throat* (may precipitate laryngospasm and death). Be alert for signs of airway obstruction.	Hospitalization (intubation if needed) Racemic epinephrine in severe cases IV fluids until respiratory distress subsides	Home care; hospitalization in severe cases Epinephrine or aminophylline in severe cases Percussion, vibration, and postural drainage If RSV, practice good handwashing

*Respiratory syncytial virus.

have been mechanically ventilated with high concentrations of oxygen for prolonged periods of time

c. Cause: etiology unknown, but apparently related to hyaline membrane disease, prolonged exposure to high oxygen concentration, and use of positive pressure ventilation

d. Medical treatment
  1) oxygen
  2) medications: bronchodilators, diuretics (when complicated by congestive heart failure), antibiotics for respiratory infection

2. Nursing Process

a. Assessment/Analysis (refer also to "General Nursing Goal 2" page 566)
  1) tachypnea
  2) cyanosis with feeding or crying
  3) signs of pulmonary hypertension and right-sided heart failure (e.g., fluid retention, rales, wheezing, retractions)

b. Plans, Implementation, and Evaluation (see General Nursing Plans page 566)

☐ Bronchial Asthma

1. General Information

a. Definition: an obstructive reversible condition of the small bronchioles of the lower respiratory tract; a complex health problem that involves biochemical, immunologic, endocrine, and psychologic factors leading to
  1) edema of mucous membranes
  2) congestion of airways with tenacious mucus
  3) spasm of smooth muscle of bronchi and bronchioles causing narrowed airway and trapping of air in alveoli

b. Cause: believed to be an allergic hypersensitivity to foreign substances, such as plant pollens, mold, dust, smoke, animal hair, or foods; other contributing factors are changes in environmental temperatures (especially cold air), emotional distress, fatigue, physical exertion, and infections

c. Medical treatment: acute asthma is a medical emergency
  1) during acute episodes, treatment is directed toward relieving bronchial spasm, obstruction and edema, and expectoration of secretions (see Table 5.18)
    a) rapid-acting bronchodilators
    b) corticosteroids
    c) expectorants (no suppressants)
    d) antibiotics (to treat any concurrent infection)
  2) supportive measures
    a) cool, humidified environment
    b) IV fluids to ensure adequate hydration

Table 5.18 Medications Used to Treat Bronchial Asthma*

Drug	Dose and Route	Nursing Implications
Bronchodiliators		
Epinephrine	0.01 ml/kg of body weight/dose (no more than 0.5 ml total) in 1:1,000 aqueous solution SC	Short acting; dose may be repeated in 20 minutes × 3–4 doses. Do not use solution if discolored. Observe for tachycardia, elevated BP, weakness, tremors, nausea, pallor. Metabolized more rapidly in children than adults.
Theophylline Aminophylline	5 mg/kg of body weight/q6h • IV during acute attacks • PO during home management	Observe for nause, vomiting ("coffee grounds"), hypotension, restlessness, fever, convulsions.
Corticosteroids		
Hydrocortisone (Solu-Cortef) or methylprednisolone (Solu-Medrol)	20–240 mg/day depending on severity of attack IV during acute attack	Anti-inflammatory action relieves airway obstruction by reducing edema.
Expectorants		
SSKI (saturated solution of potassium iodide)	1 drop/year of age, tid, PO, in juice	These preparations liquify secretions to aid expectoration.
Guaifenesin (Robitussin)	5 ml tid, PO	
Syrup of ipecac	Subemetic dose PO prn	

*Refer to *Nursing Care of the Adult* Tables 3.18, 3.19 for additional drug information.

c) sedatives to control anxiety

3) status asthmaticus: continued severe respiratory distress in spite of medical intervention; child is in imminent danger of respiratory arrest and requires immediate hospitalization (to treat dehydration and acidosis and improve ventilation)
   a) NPO or sips of clear liquids
   b) IV fluids for hydration and medication administration
   c) sodium bicarbonate (IV) to correct acidosis
   d) humidified O_2
   e) mechanical ventilation in severe cases
   f) corticosteroids (hydrocortisone or methylprednisolone IV)
   g) aminophylline
   h) isoproterenol via intermittent positive pressure breathing
4) long-term therapy includes removing the offending allergens, desensitization to allergens, normalization of respiratory function, and development of a personalized and effective therapeutic regimen

2. Nursing Process

a. Assessment/Analysis

1) prolonged expiratory wheezing
2) hacking, paroxysmal coughing, nonproductive at first, cough becomes rattling with thick, clear mucus
3) deep red lips
4) diaphoresis
5) child sits in upright position
6) intercostal and suprasternal retractions
7) coarse breath sounds
8) shallow irregular respirations with sudden increase in rate and ineffective coughing may signal impending asphyxia (status asthmaticus)
9) barrel chest and hunched shoulders (chronic asthma)

b. Plans, Implementation, and Evaluation

Goal 1: Child will resume normal breathing pattern, will maintain a patent airway, and will liquify and raise secretions.

Plan/Implementation

- Monitor frequency, amount, and appearance of expectorated mucus.
- Position in high-Fowler's or in a chair; administer O_2 to relieve cyanosis and anoxia (cyanosis appears in children with a pO_2 less than 55–65 mm Hg).
- Teach child to use diaphragm rather than just lungs, to pull in and expel deep breaths of air when first feeling a tightening sensation in chest.
- Administer prescribed medications, including nebulizers; know the action, dose ranges, side effects, and contraindications for all medications administered.

Evaluation: Child resumes normal breathing pattern (no wheezing, rales, cyanosis), maintains patent airway, liquifies and raises secretions.

Goal 2: Child will control anxiety during acute attacks.

Plan/Implementation

- *Never* leave child alone during an acute attack; if parental anxiety is too high, it is better for child if someone who is calm and supportive stays with child; work with parent until parent can be a calming influence.
- Hold child in an upright position and rock (as effective as bedrest if a relaxed, confident approach is used).
- Reduce the level of nonproductive stimuli by keeping room quiet, with dimmed lighting; use touch, soft music, and controlled noise levels to induce relaxation and rest.
- Teach child and parent panic control, i.e., to imagine how to stay calm (what works best) in stressful situations

Evaluation: Child remains calm and copes with asthma attack.

Goal 3: Child will avoid and/or eliminate allergens or precipitating factors in environment.

Plan/Implementation

- Identify possible precipitating factors with child and family; teach child and parent to avoid stressful experiences, extremes of temperature, unnecessary fatigue, and exposure to infections.
- Modify environment as indicated (no furry pets, damp dusting, nonallergic pillows and bedding, elimination of allergenic foods from diet, air filters).
- Assist with immune therapy (hyposensitization for allergens such as dust, molds, and pollens).
- Administer prophylactic antibiotics during periods of high susceptibility (e.g., winter, pollen or flu season).
- Guide parents in planning a total program that promotes rest, moderate exercise, appropriate

activities (swimming, baseball, skiing), balanced nutrition, controlled levels of emotional stress.

- Remind and urge child/parent to see physician regularly and at the first indication of a respiratory infection or attack.
- Refer family to psychologic/mental health services when indicated.

Evaluation: Child/parent describes the importance of good nutrition and rest in preventing respiratory infections; identifies situations or agents that precipitate an asthmatic attack and conscientiously tries to modify or avoid these; recognizes signs of an impending attack (cough, wheezing, fever, N&V, increased anxiety or tension) and the steps to take to minimize distress (position, rest, medications, fluids).

Application of the Nursing Process to the Child with Cardiovascular Dysfunction

1. **Assessment/Analysis**
   a. Nursing history
      1) delayed growth patterns
      2) frequent respiratory infections
      3) activity intolerance, weakness, fatigue
      4) anorexia, weight loss, fatigue during feedings
      5) chest pain, dyspnea, pallor or cyanosis, clubbing of fingers and toes
      6) medications: parent knowledge of side effects
      7) family and obstetric history
   b. Clinical appraisal
      1) general appearance: pallor, cyanosis, clubbing of fingers and toes, cold extremities, mottling, edema, distended neck veins
      2) vital signs: apical pulse rate and character, presence of murmurs, gallops, friction rubs; blood pressure in upper and lower extremities; rate, depth, and character of respirations; rate, quality, and symmetry of peripheral pulses especially of lower extremities
   c. Diagnostic tests (refer to *Nursing Care of the Adult* page 167)
      1) cardiac catheterization in infants and children: aids in diagnosis of congenital anomalies, and abnormalities in oxygen saturation, pressure, and cardiac output; right-sided (venous) catheterization is usually done in children (see Table 5.19)
      2) blood gas determination (see Table 5.16)
2. **Analysis**
   a. Safe, effective care environment
      1) potential for infection
      2) sensory-perceptual alteration
   b. Physiological integrity

Table 5.19 Cardiac Catheterization in Children: Nursing Considerations

Preprocedural	Postprocedural
Psychologic preparation (see *Ill and Hospitalized Child* for developmental considerations) • explain in simple terms what child will experience and what it will feel like (e.g., skin prep: "cold"; catheter insertion: "pressure"; injection of contrast medium: "warm all over" [do not use the word "dye"]; darkness of room, and sounds of "picture-taking"); do not explain too far in advance of procedure. • allow child to play with and manipulate equipment (e.g., gown and mask, syringes, sandbag). • arrange for child and parent to visit catheterization room the day before to see the equipment and meet staff. Physical preparation • NPO 4–6 hours before the procedure (give 5% DW orally as prescribed 2–3 hours before the procedure for infants with cyanotic heart disease and polycythemia); use pacifier for infants. • obtain baseline vital signs, including brachial and pedal pulses. • Administer pre-op meds as ordered (child is not anesthetized).	Maintain bed rest with frequent checks on vital signs until stable. Do not take blood pressure in affected extremity. Monitor skin color and warmth, especially distal to catheter-insertion site. Palpate brachial or pedal pulses distal to catheter insertion for presence, strength, symmetry. Observe operative site for bleeding, edema, hematoma formation. Maintain sandbag or pressure dressing on operative site as ordered. Notify physician of any signs of complications (e.g., poor circulation, unstable vital signs, fever, bleeding). Apply direct pressure over site if bleeding occurs.

1) activity intolerance
2) decreased cardiac output
3) impaired gas exchange

c. Psychological integrity
1) anxiety
2) fear

d. Health promotion/maintenance
1) diversional activity deficit
2) ineffective family coping: compromised

3. **General Nursing Plans, Implementation, and Evaluation**

Goal 1: Child will have adequate oxygenation and decreased workload of heart.

Plan/Implementation
- Monitor vital signs frequently
  - apical pulse one full minute while sleeping
  - peripheral pulses
  - BP
  - respiratory status
  - body temperature
- Schedule treatments and nursing care to prevent tiring and promote adequate rest/sleep.
- Maintain bedrest as ordered.
- Provide age-appropriate diversional activities to prevent boredom and help child maintain bedrest.
- Avoid restrictive clothing and tight diapers.
- Minimize crying and emotional distress (pre-op)
  - encourage parent to room-in or visit frequently
  - provide pacifier or favorite attachment object
  - hold and cuddle child
- Relieve anoxic spells (congenital heart disease)
  - place child in knee-chest (squatting) position
  - administer O_2 as ordered
  - administer sedatives, analgesics as ordered
- Avoid extremes of environmental temperature.

Evaluation: Child is free from signs of respiratory or cardiac distress (e.g., no dyspnea, tachycardia); cooperates with bedrest, rests comfortably, plays quietly.

Goal 2: Child will be free from infections.

Plan/Implementation
- Protect child from exposure to others with respiratory infections.
- Immunize child according to AAP recommended schedule (see Table 5.3)
- Observe for signs of endocarditis (fever, malaise, anorexia) and pneumonitis (dyspnea, tachycardia, fever).
- Teach child and parents importance of antibiotic prophylaxis (long-term therapy or short-term course for dental work, surgery, childbirth).

Evaluation: Child remains free from upper respiratory infections; is immunized on schedule; child and parents comply with antibiotic prophylaxis.

Selected Health Problems Resulting in an Interference with Cardiac Functioning

☐ Congenital Heart Disease

1. **General Information**

a. Hemodynamics: related to 3 principles
1) pressure gradients: blood flows from higher to lower; normally left side of heart is higher pressure
2) resistance: the higher the resistance the less the flow; normally the systemic circulation has higher resistance than pulmonary vasculature; larger vessels have less resistance than smaller, narrow ones
3) quality of pumping action of heart effects the flow

b. Physical consequences of cardiac problems
1) increased workload of the heart (causes changes in systolic and diastolic pressures)
2) pulmonary hypertension (from increased pulmonary resistance)
3) inadequate systemic output from recirculated blood flow
4) cyanotic defects: no pure oxygenated blood, tissue hypoxia and hypoxemia, stimulates erythropoesis, resulting in polycythemia

c. Cause: not known exactly; predisposing factors include
1) certain chromosome disorders (e.g., Down syndrome)
2) maternal and fetal infections (e.g., rubella in first trimester)
3) maternal alcoholism, undernutrition, diabetes, age over 40 years

d. Types of defects
1) acyanotic defects: blood flows from the arterial (left, oxygenated) side of the heart to the venous (right, deoxygenated) side; there is no mixing of unoxygenated blood with oxygenated blood in the systemic circulation (see Figure 5.2)

a) *atrial septal defect* (ASD)
- flow of blood is from left atrium to right atrium (normal flow resistance)

Figure 5.2 Normal and Abnormal Hearts

a. Superior Vena Cava **b.** Inferior Vena Cava **c.** Right Atrium **d.** Right Ventricle **e.** Pulmonary Artery **f.** Pulmonary Vein **g.** Left Atrium **h.** Left Ventricle **i.** Aorta

I. THE NORMAL HEART

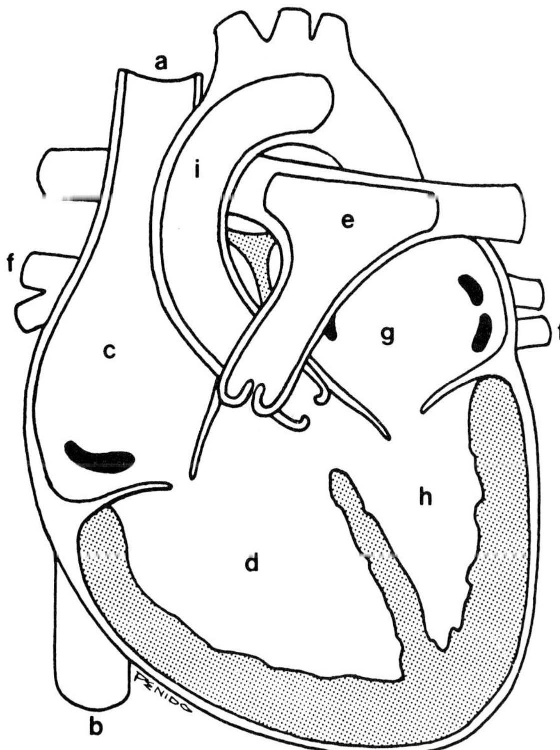

II. ACYANOTIC DEFECTS

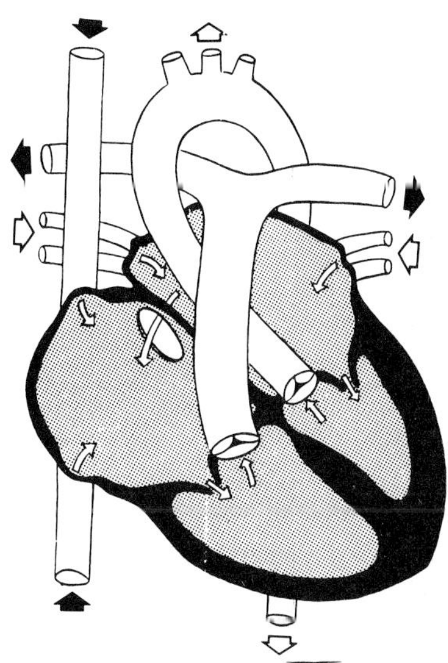

Atrial Septal Defect (Left to Right Shunt)

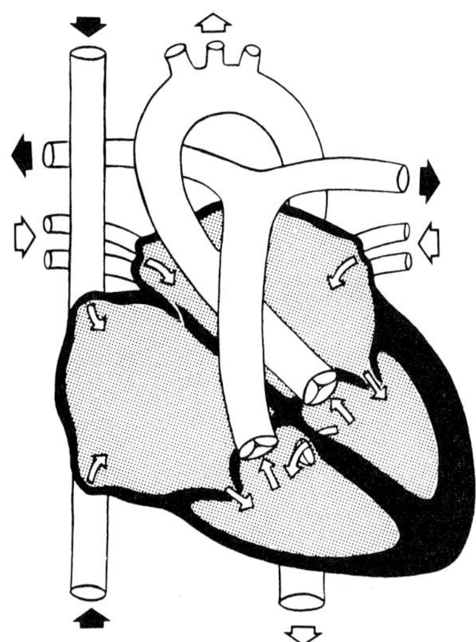

Ventricular Septal Defect (Left to Right Shunt)

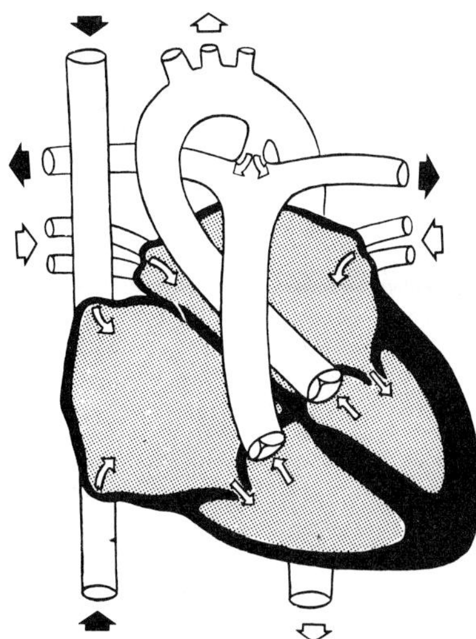

Patent Ductus Arteriosus

(continued)

Figure 5.2 Continued

(II. ACYANOTIC DEFECTS, Cont.)

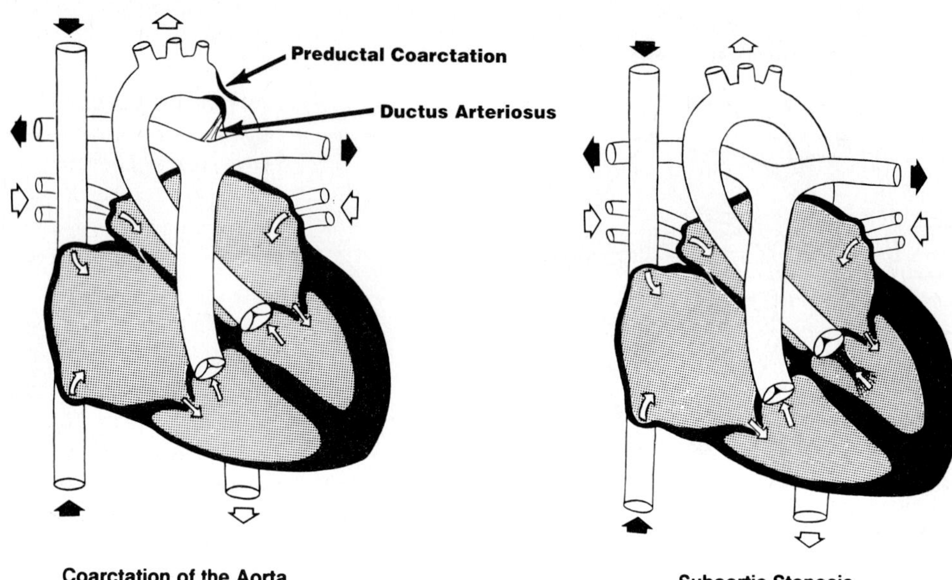

Coarctation of the Aorta

Subaortic Stenosis

III. CYANOTIC DEFECTS

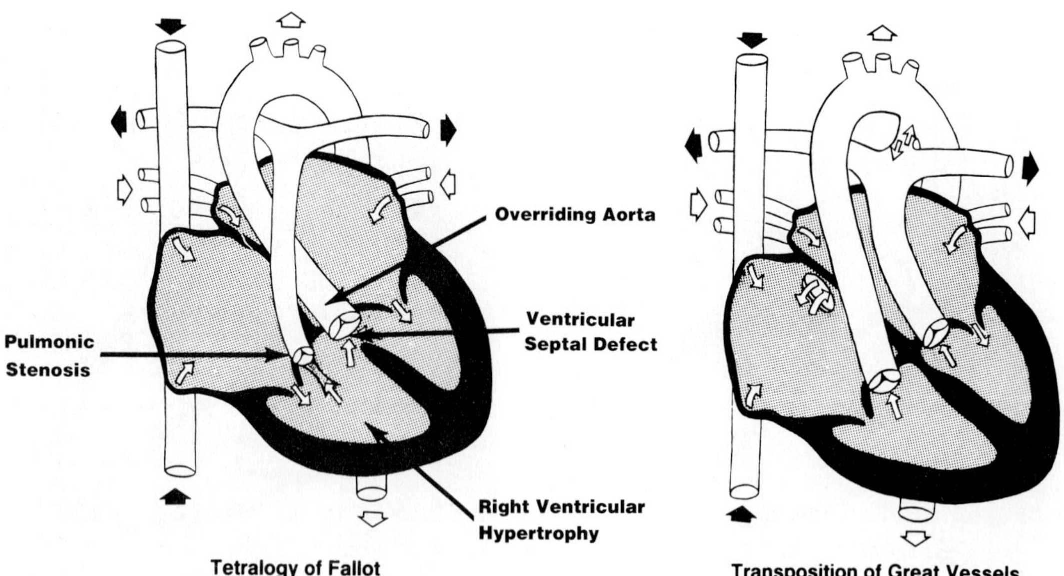

Tetralogy of Fallot

Transposition of Great Vessels

SOURCE: Nursing Inservice Aid #2, Congenital Heart Abnormalities Aid, Ross Laboratories, Columbus, OH 43216. Used with permission.

- increased blood flow to right side of heart
- treatment: surgical closure or patch graft of defect; 99% survival rate

b) *ventricular septal defect* (VSD)
- most common cardiac defect
- flow of blood is from left ventricle (higher pressure) to right ventricle where oxygenated blood mixes with venous blood
- may cause right ventricular hypertrophy and increased pulmonary vascular resistance
- 50% close spontaneously within 1–3 years of age
- often associated with other cardiac defects (tetralogy of Fallot, transposition of great vessels, patent ductus arteriosus [PDA], pulmonic stenosis)
- infants with severe VSD may develop congestive heart failure and eventually right-to-left shunting
- treatment: surgical closure or patch graft of defect
- complications include conduction disturbances, CHF, or endocarditis

c) *patent ductus arteriosus* (PDA)
- ductus arteriosus (normal in fetus) fails to close: some blood is shunted by higher pressure in aorta to pulmonary artery
- leads to recirculation through lungs and return to left atrium and ventricle; effect is increased workload on left side of heart, increased pulmonary congestion
- pulse pressure is wide; left ventricular hypertrophy and congestive heart failure may develop
- characteristic machinery-like murmur
- treatment: surgical ligation (closed-heart surgery) at 1–2 years of age; 99% survival rate
- in very ill newborns, medical closure of the ductus with the prostaglandin inhibitor, indomethacin, may be tried

d) *coarctation of the aorta*
- a narrowing of the aorta
  - preductal: narrowing proximal to ductus arteriosus
  - postductal: distal to the ductus arteriosus; effect is increased pressure proximal to defect and decreased pressure distal to defect
- blood pressure is higher in upper extremities (BP may be unequal in arms if defect is between inominant and left subclavian arteries)
- bounding upper-extremity pulses, weak or absent femoral and popliteal pulses
- lower extremities may be cool, pale
- cramps (claudication)
- headaches, dizziness, epistaxis
- treatment: surgical resection and end-to-end anastomosis (or graft) at about age 4 (to allow for growth of aorta)

e) *pulmonic/aortic stenosis*
- pulmonic stenosis interferes with flow of blood from right ventricle to pulmonary artery
- aortic stenosis interferes with blood flow from left ventricle to aorta
- both pulmonic and aortic stenosis
  - may be asymptomatic
  - are usually of the valves
  - increased resistance can cause right ventricular hypertrophy with pulmonary stenosis, left ventricular hypertrophy with aortic stenosis
  - aortic stenosis may result in sudden death after strenuous exercise or activity because of increased sudden oxygen demand and resultant myocardial ischemia
- treatment: valvulotomy or valve replacement

2) cyanotic defects: those defects in which unoxygenated blood from right side of heart mixes with oxygenated blood on left side causing the unoxygenated blood to be circulated through the systemic circulation (right-to-left shunt); results in cyanosis

a) *tetralogy of Fallot*
- most common cyanotic heart defect in children
- severe VSD
- severe pulmonic stenosis: right-to-left shunting of blood through ventricular septal defect because of pulmonic stenosis and increased pulmonary resistance; results in desaturated blood entering systemic circulation
- right ventricular hypertrophy

- overriding aorta: because the aorta overrides the septal defect, much of the systemic flow is venous and, therefore, unoxygenated
- treatment
  - palliative surgical correction in infancy to increase pulmonary blood flow (Blalock-Taussig anastomosis of right or left subclavian artery and corresponding pulmonary artery)
  - corrective surgical repair; closure of VSD (corrects overriding aorta) and pulmonary valvulotomy or valve replacement

b) *transposition of the great vessels*

- the aorta arises out of the right ventricle so that venous blood enters directly into the systemic circulation, bypassing the lungs; the pulmonary artery arises out of the left ventricle and goes through the lungs; once the foramen ovale and ductus arteriosus close, the situation is incompatible with life (unless ASD or VSD is present)
- treatment
  - palliative surgical correction to prevent CHF and reduce pulmonary vascular resistance
    * surgical creation of an ASD
    * balloon atrial septostomy during cardiac catheterization to enlarge existing ASD
    * pulmonary artery banding
  - corrective surgical repair: creation of a new atrial septum that tunnels blood to the correct ventricle

e. Additional medical management: digoxin, potassium, diuretics (if in congestive heart failure), antibiotics

2. Nursing Process

a. Assessment/Analysis

1) infant or child with acyanotic heart defect

a) poor weight gain, small stature
b) increased incidence of respiratory infections
c) exercise intolerance
d) tachycardia, tachypnea, dyspnea
e) *not* cyanotic

2) infant or child with cyanotic heart defect

a) usually cyanotic at time of birth
b) babies have difficulty eating because of inability to breathe and suck at same time
c) delayed physical growth because of chronic hypoxia
d) frequent and severe respiratory infections
e) moderate to severe exercise intolerance
f) chest pain that becomes severe with O_2 demand
g) hypoxic spell may occur during periods of high O_2 demand (feeding, crying, physical exertion during play)

- severe shortness of breath
- increased cyanosis and chest pain
- squats with arms thrown over knees, and knees on chest to relieve respiratory distress

h) chronic hypoxia causes erythropoietin to be released from kidneys to stimulate bone marrow to produce more red blood cells; also causes clubbing of fingers and toes

- Hgb may rise 20–30 gm or more with a hematocrit as high as 60% 80%
- increased RBC results in increased blood viscosity (polycythemia)

i) polycythemia and sluggish circulation may cause cerebral thrombosis (stroke) and paralysis, sometimes occurring at a very young age

3) pre-op assessment

a) baseline vital signs, including apical pulse; existence and quality of peripheral pulses, especially of lower extremities; compare pulses
b) educational needs of child and parents for preoperative teaching and postoperative experience
c) laboratory values to assess potential problems

4) post-op assessment

a) respiratory status, chest tubes, chest-tube drainage, breath sounds
b) vital signs, including apical and femoral pulses, arterial and venous pressures, cardiac rhythm
c) hydration status and output
d) signs and symptoms of congestive heart failure
e) color of skin, mucous membranes, nail beds, and earlobes
f) level of discomfort and anxiety
g) surgical incisions (suture line)

b. Plans, Implementation, and Evaluation

Goal 1: Child will maintain adequate oxygenation and a patent airway.

Plan/Implementation

Pre-op and post-op

- Count respirations and apical pulse 1 full minute.
- Pin diapers loosely, use loose-fitting pajamas.
- Feed slowly with frequent rest periods; burp frequently.
- Position at 45° after feeding.
- Suction nose and throat if cough is inadequate.
- Give O_2 as ordered and necessary.
- Administer digoxin as prescribed
  - give at regular intervals
  - do not mix with other foods or fluids
  - hold drug and notify physician if apical pulse rate is below 100 in infants, below 90 in toddlers, or below 70 in older children
  - give 1 hour before or 2 hours after meals/feedings
  - observe for signs of toxicity (bradycardia, nausea, anorexia, vomiting, disorientation)
- Administer diuretics as prescribed
  - monitor I&O closely
  - ensure fluid intake within prescribed restrictions
  - encourage high potassium foods or administer prescribed potassium supplements

Post-op (palliative or corrective surgery)

- Monitor constantly.
- Take precautions in care of closed chest drainage (bottles below level of bed, no kinks in tubing, do NOT empty bottles, monitor fluid level and fluctuation in tube, character of drainage).
- Avoid elevating foot of bed (causes intestines to put pressure on diaphragm).
- Administer O_2 as ordered.
- Establish and follow coughing routine; allow crying post-op in infant and young child to facilitate lung expansion; use inspirometer (incentive spirometry) with older children.
- When child has recovered from anesthesia, elevate head of bed to reduce pressure on diaphragm.
- Use nasogastric suction to reduce gastric distention.
- Be alert to signs of CHF, hypovolemic shock, pneumonia, hemothorax (dyspnea), atelectasis (dyspnea, increased pulse), cerebral thrombosis

Evaluation: Child has normal skin color, a patent airway, breathes freely; no signs of complications.

Goal 2: Child will maintain adequate hydration and electrolyte balance.

Plan/Implementation

- Encourage fluid intake within fluid restrictions for child; monitor I&O *very* accurately (be especially alert to thoracotomy drainage, fluid used to administer IV medications or flush CVP or arterial lines).
- Monitor daily weights.
- Check urine specific gravity and pH.
- Be alert to early signs and symptoms of pulmonary edema, cardiac overload, and congestive heart failure (e.g., tachycardia, dyspnea, tachypnea, moist respirations, rales, rhonchi, sweating [in infants], edema).
- Be aware that dehydration with cyanotic heart disease increases blood viscosity, and therefore risk of thrombosis.
- Observe for signs of hypokalemia (altered lab values, cardiac dysrhythmias).

Evaluation: Child has adequate I&O; no signs or symptoms of fluid or electrolyte imbalance, stroke, or congestive heart failure.

Goal 3: Child and parents will experience no more than moderate anxiety.

Plan/Implementation

- Encourage child and parents to disclose their feelings about the surgery, hospitalization, treatments (use projective techniques with child); answer their questions.
- Prepare child and parents for treatments, surgical routine, and discharge; consider developmental age, environment, culture and ethnicity, timing needs, ability to understand.
- Help parents and others understand the importance of treating child as normally as possible (to provide for optimal emotional-social development and to avoid overprotecting and sheltering).

Evaluation: Child and parents describe realistic expectations about child's illness and hospitalization; establish and adhere to age-appropriate limits; demonstrate knowledge about procedures, medications.

Goal 4: Child and parents will be adequately prepared for discharge and home care.

Plan/Implementation

- Encourage and support parents in their attempts to allow child age-appropriate independence and responsibilities.
- Teach parents safe administration of

medications, side effects, signs of complications, when to seek medical attention.
- Refer parents to community health nursing agency for home follow-up if indicated.

Evaluation: Child gradually assumes self-care responsibilities and age-appropriate independence; parents state signs of complications and when to seek attention; administer medications correctly.

☐ Rheumatic Fever and Rheumatic Heart Disease

1. General Information

a. Definition: an inflammatory disease caused by group A beta hemolytic streptococcal infection; affects collagen (connective) tissue such as heart, joints, central nervous system, and subcutaneous tissue

b. Occurrence: primarily affects school-age children; higher incidence in cold or humid climates, crowded living environments, and with strong family history of rheumatic fever

c. Medical treatment

1) antibiotics (penicillin or erythromycin)

a) to eradicate any lingering infection

b) for long-term prophylactic treatment

2) salicylates to control joint inflammation, fever, pain

2. Nursing Process

a. Assessment/Analysis: revised Jones criteria (American Heart Association)

1) major manifestations

a) carditis: mitral and aortic valves most commonly affected with symptoms of tachycardia, cardiomegaly, pericarditis, murmurs, congestive heart failure; carditis is the only manifestation that may cause permanent damage

b) painful migratory polyarthritis in large joints with manifestations of acute pain, warmth, redness, edema; permanent deformities do not follow

c) chorea (Saint Vitus' dance or Sydenham's chorea): purposeless, irregular movements of the extremities, muscular weakness, emotional lability, facial grimacing

- follows the acute febrile phase
- may last for months, but is self-limiting
- relieved by rest and sleep

d) erythema marginatum rheumaticum: macular rash with wavy, well-defined border on trunk

e) subcutaneous nodules: small, nontender swellings in groups over bony prominences

2) minor manifestations

a) arthralgia

b) fever

c) elevated erythrocyte sedimentation rate (ESR)

d) elevated C-reactive protein

e) leukocytosis

f) anemia

g) prolonged PR and QT intervals on ECG

3) other

a) positive throat culture

b) elevated ASO titer

b. Plans, Implementation, and Evaluation

Goal 1: Child will be free from pain and will rest comfortably.

Plan/Implementation
- Administer salicylates as ordered.
- Use cradles to keep bed linen off painful joints.
- Position joints on pillows; handle gently.

Evaluation: Child does not complain of pain, rests and sleeps comfortably.

Goal 2: Child with chorea will be protected from injury.

Plan/Implementation
- Utilize side rails and pad sides of bed.
- Provide understanding and emotional support; reassure child and family that chorea will resolve spontaneously.
- Provide with alternative means to do written work, e.g., typewriter, personal computer, oral reports.
- Assist child in self-care to promote independence and positive self-concept.

Evaluation: Child ambulates without falling, does not sustain injury.

Goal 3: Child/family will be prepared for home care and long-term management.

Plan/Implementation
- Emphasize importance of compliance with long-term antibiotic therapy for prevention of serious heart damage
  - prepare child for monthly injections of penicillin
  - stress seriousness of recurrence and possible

consequences (death or severe disability from heart disease)

- Plan for continuation of schoolwork, realistic career goals.
- Refer to community health nurse for follow-up as needed.
- Instruct parents to take vital signs, administer medications, ensure restrictions.

Evaluation: Child returns to full activity with no residual cardiac involvement.

Application of the Nursing Process to the Child with Hematologic Problems

1. **Assessment**
   a. Nursing history
      1) dietary intake, especially dietary iron
      2) history of bleeding tendencies (easy bruising, gum bleeding, epistaxis), response to injury or trauma
      3) general symptoms: fatigue, irritability, anorexia, pain, edema
      4) recent stressful situations: exposure to temperature extremes, emotional stress
      5) family history of hematologic disorders
      6) current treatment, home management, general health
   b. Clinical appraisal
      1) general appearance: pallor, lethargy, bruising, physical growth (over or underweight for age)
      2) vital signs: tachycardia, tachypnea, hypotension
   c. Diagnostic tests (refer to *Nursing Care of the Adult* page 163)
2. **Analysis**
   a. Safe, effective care environment
      1) potential for injury
      2) potential for infection
      3) knowledge deficit
   b. Physiological integrity
      1) impaired gas exchange
      2) fatigue
      3) altered cerebral tissue perfusion
   c. Psychological integrity
      1) anxiety
      2) altered role performance
      3) body image disturbance
   d. Health promotion/maintenance
      1) ineffective family coping: compromised
      2) diversional activity deficit
      3) altered growth and development
3. **General Nursing Plans, Implementation, and Evaluation**

Goal 1: Child will be free from pain.

Plan/Implementation

- Administer prescribed analgesics (no aspirin).
- Handle and move child gently.
- Provide bedrest with covers off affected areas.
- Provide age-appropriate diversional activities.

Evaluation: Child is free from pain; rests comfortably.

Goal 2: Child will conserve energy.

Plan/Implementation

- Schedule nursing care and treatment to prevent tiring and to provide uninterrupted periods of rest.
- Provide quiet age-appropriate play activities.
- Counsel parents concerning plan for activity and rest at home.

Evaluation: Child engages in activities of daily living without tiring, has age-appropriate rest and sleep periods.

Selected Health Problems Resulting in an Interference with Formed Elements of the Blood

☐ Iron-Deficiency Anemia

1. **General Information**
   a. Definition: a decrease in the number of erythrocytes and/or a decreased Hgb level: less than 10 gm/dl
   b. Occurrence: most common nutritional disorder in US resulting in reduced oxygen-carrying capacity of blood; most common childhood anemia
      1) primarily in children 6–24 months of age who have a diet low in iron
      2) in premature infants (inadequate iron stores)
      3) in adolescent girls, with increased growth and menstruation
      4) in adolescent boys, with androgen-related increase in hemoglobin concentration
   c. Cause: impaired production of red blood cells, resulting from deficient iron stores
      1) inadequate dietary intake
      2) impaired absorption
      3) blood loss
      4) excessive demand (prematurity, puberty, pregnancy)
   d. Medical treatment
      1) oral iron supplements (ferrous iron), 10–15 mg/day for 3 months

2) parenteral iron therapy (iron dextran [Imferon]) IM or IV
3) blood transfusions with packed red cells (if Hgb is less than 4 gm/dl)

2. Nursing Process

a. Assessment/Analysis

1) nutritional history (daily intake)
2) pallor (porcelain-like skin)
3) poor muscle development
4) may be overweight (''milk baby'')
5) exercise intolerance, lethargy
6) susceptible to infection

b. Plan, Implementation, and Evaluation

Goal: Child will ingest diet and medications to maintain adequate Hgb level.

Plan/Implementation

- Explain the necessity for a proper diet to parents
  - provide adequate sources of iron and teach parent/child what they are
  - for infants: iron-fortified formula and cereal, iron supplements
  - for older children: foods high in iron, e.g., meat, vegetables, fruit
  - give solids before milk
- Teach parents correct administration of oral iron preparations as ordered
  - give ferrous sulfate (Fer-In-Sol) in 3 divided doses/day, between meals with citrus juice
  - continue for 4–6 weeks after red blood cell count returns to normal
  - liquid iron temporarily stains teeth (use straw, or dropper to back of mouth, brush child's teeth)
  - oral iron causes stools to become dark green
- If oral preparations ineffective, administer parenteral iron as prescribed using IM Z-track method: painful and stains subcutaneous tissue; do not use deltoid; no more than 1 ml/site; use air bubble, don't massage over injection site, avoid tight clothing over injection site.
- Limit milk intake to 1 quart/day or less.

Evaluation: Child takes diet and medications as ordered; child's Hgb level returns to normal.

☐ Sickle Cell Anemia

1. General Information

a. Definition: autosomal recessive defect (see Figure 5.3) found primarily in blacks, resulting in production of abnormal hemoglobin (hemoglobin S) and characterized by intermittent episodes of crisis

b. Occurrence 1:400 black Americans, or 75,000 people in US

1) sickle cell trait: heterozygous form (carrier); 1 in 12 black persons is a carrier
2) sickle cell disease: homozygous form (has the disease); may have vaso-occlusive crisis: painful, acute occurrence usually precipitated by decreased O_2 tension, which causes cells to become viscous and assume a sickle shape, obstruct blood vessels, and cause tissue ischemia, infarction, and necrosis

c. Cause: defective form of hemoglobin (hemoglobin S), inherited by autosomal recessive genetic transmission

d. Medical treatment: symptomatic treatment of crisis

1) bedrest to decrease O_2 expenditure
2) adequate hydration: oral and IV fluids to increase blood volume and mobilize sickled cells
3) electrolyte replacement (hypoxia causes metabolic acidosis)
4) relief of pain
   a) acetaminophen
   b) codeine
   c) meperidine (Demerol)
5) blood transfusions
6) O_2 for severe hypoxia (on a short-term basis)
7) antibiotics to treat concurrent infection

2. Nursing Process

a. Assessment/Analysis

1) parents with sickle cell trait
2) signs and symptoms (depend on organ involved); not evident until after 6 months of age
   a) chronic hemolytic anemia
   b) frequent infections, related to decreased ability of spleen to filter bacteria
   c) organ deterioration (spleen, liver, kidney, heart, CNS)
   d) chronic pain: joints, abdomen, back
   e) bone deterioration (osteoporosis, skeletal deformities) from increase in marrow
   f) leg ulcers in adolescents
3) manifestations of vaso-occlusive crisis
   a) severe abdominal pain: caused by organ hypoxia

Figure 5.3 Common Modes of Genetic Transmission

A. Autosomal Dominant Diseases

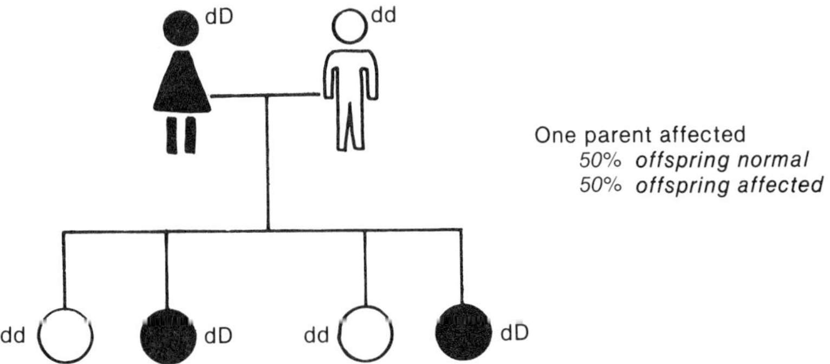

One parent affected
50% offspring normal
50% offspring affected

Key: d = normal gene; D = abnormal, *dominant* gene

Examples: Huntington's disease, osteogenesis imperfecta, polydactyly

B. Autosomal Recessive Diseases

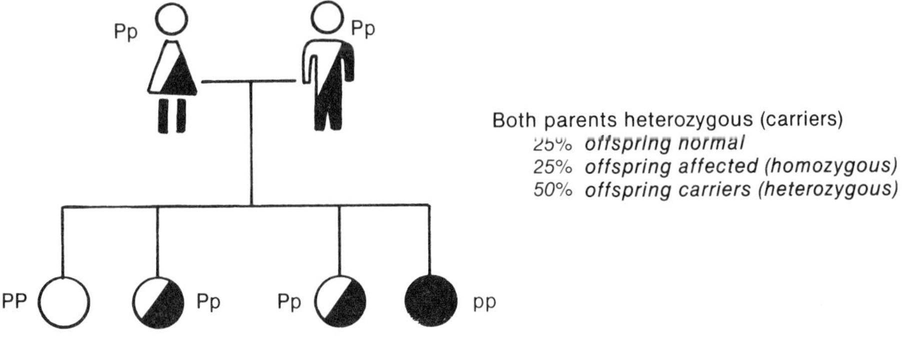

Both parents heterozygous (carriers)
25% offspring normal
25% offspring affected (homozygous)
50% offspring carriers (heterozygous)

Key: P = normal gene; p = abnormal, *recessive* gene

Examples: phenylketonuria, cystic fibrosis, sickle cell disease, galactosemia, Tay-Sachs disease, thalassemia

C. Sex-Linked Recessive Diseases (X-Linked)

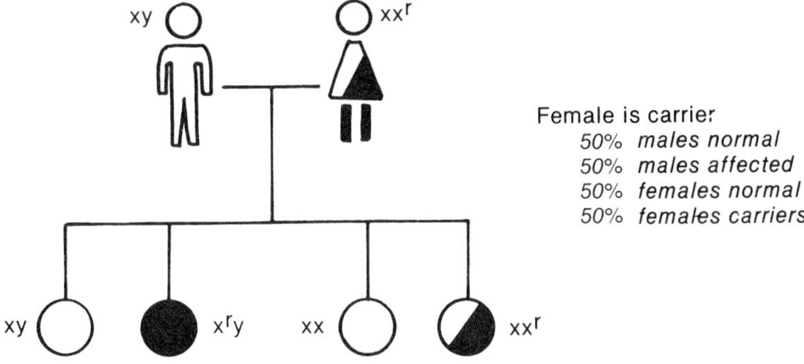

Female is carrier
50% males normal
50% males affected
50% females normal
50% females carriers

Key: xy = normal *male* sex chromosome pattern; xx = normal *female* sex chromosome pattern; r = sex-linked *recessive* gene

Examples: hemophilia, color blindness, agammaglobulinemia, G6PD deficiency, X-linked Duchenne's muscular dystrophy

b) hand-foot syndrome: swelling of hands and feet
c) fever: due to dehydration or possible concurrent infection
d) arthralgia

b. Plans, Implementation, and Evaluation

Goal 1: Child's episodes of vaso-occlusive crisis will be prevented or minimized.

Plan/Implementation

- Teach crisis-prevention methods to child/parent
  - avoid situations resulting in decreased O_2 concentration such as high altitudes, constrictive clothing, extreme physical exertion, exposure to cold
  - avoid emotional distress
  - maintain adequate hydration (child should receive at least *minimum* daily fluid requirement)
  - protect from infection
    * prevent exposure to persons with infections
    * promote adequate nutrition
    * obtain medical care at onset of infection (may need antibiotics)
    * keep immunizations current

Evaluation: Parent/child adheres to plan for crisis prevention; child's crisis episodes are minimized.

Goal 2: Child will receive appropriate supportive care during crisis.

Plan/Implementation

- Relieve pain
  - administer analgesics
  - handle gently
  - use heating pad on painful areas
- Monitor hydration/electrolyte status
  - monitor I&O; offer liquids frequently
  - regulate IV fluids, blood transfusion
  - observe for fluid or electrolyte imbalance
- Assess for signs of infection; protect from exposure to infectious sources during crisis.

Evaluation: Child is relieved of pain during crisis; has no elevated temperature; has elastic skin turgor, moist mucous membranes, adequate fluid intake.

Goal 3: Parent/child at risk will receive screening and genetic counseling.

Plan/Implementation

- Teach parent about screening/diagnostic techniques
  - nonspecific screening tests for trait or disease: Sickledex
  - specific identification of trait and disease: Hgb electrophoresis ("protein fingerprinting") used if screening tests are positive
- Give information on available genetic counseling.

Evaluation: Parents receive screening and genetic counseling as indicated; demonstrate knowledge of transmission and implications for subsequent pregnancies.

□ Hemophilia

1. General Information

a. Definition, occurrence, and cause: hereditary coagulation defect, usually transmitted to affected male by female carrier through sex-linked recessive gene (see Figure 5.3), resulting in prolonged clotting time; most common type is hemophilia A-factor VIII deficiency; severity of the deficiency varies from mild to severe; at risk for acquired immune deficiency syndrome (AIDS) from contaminated blood products (see Table 5.9)

b. Medical treatment

1) replacement of factor VIII: transfusion of plasma, factor VIII concentrate, or cryoprecipitate to prevent bleeding episodes
2) additional treatment measures for more severe bleeding episodes
   a) immediate administration of factor VIII to control bleeding
   b) bedrest with covers off affected area to relieve pain; temporary immobilization of affected joints in a slightly flexed position with casts, splints, traction
   c) physical therapy to prevent contractures, beginning 48 hours after bleeding stops
   d) pain relief with sedatives/narcotics

2. Nursing Process

a. Assessment/Analysis

1) infant
   a) umbilical-cord hemorrhage
   b) hemorrhage following circumcision
2) any age
   a) hemarthrosis (bleeding into a joint space) is the most frequent site of bleeding; may result in crippling bony deformities
   b) epistaxis
   c) spontaneous hematuria

d) hemorrhage following tooth extraction or minor falls and cuts

3) diagnostic laboratory tests: only tests that measure clotting factors (e.g., PTT) are abnormal; platelet function tests (e.g., bleeding time) are normal

b. Plans, Implementation, and Evaluation

Goal 1: Parent/child will receive education to *prevent* bleeding, provide safety measures; will know how to treat minor bleeding episodes.

Plan/Implementation

- Prepare parents and child for home care and administration of factor VIII (where available)
  - teach about the disease
  - teach venipuncture procedure and how to monitor the transfusion
  - provide regular follow-up (family must be sufficiently motivated and stable to maintain a home-care program)
- Teach local treatment measures for minor bleeding episodes
  - apply direct pressure to site (10–15 minutes)
  - apply ice pack
  - immobilize and elevate affected part
- Teach safe administration of medication
  - give orally if possible
  - avoid injections; if necessary, after injection apply pressure until bleeding stops
- Avoid medications that increase bleeding (aspirin, phenacetin, phenothiazines, indomethacin [Indocin]).
- Institute dental precautions: soft toothbrush, Water Pik, good dental hygiene to avoid extractions.
- Encourage appropriate toys/games/sports
  - soft toys for infants
  - quiet activities, e.g., reading, swimming
  - avoid body-contact sports
  - careful handling of sharp objects
  - use of electric shavers (not razors)
- Use protective devices for young child: padded crib, playpen, side rails, protective padding and helmet for toddler.
- Teach to avoid overweight (causes strain on affected joints).
- Teach to wear Medic Alert identification.
- Inform appropriate school personnel.
- Avoid stressful situations (they increase susceptibility to bleeding).
- Seek emergency medical treatment in cases of uncontrolled bleeding.

Evaluation: Parent/child demonstrates ability to correctly manage home administration of factor VIII; states medication precautions, activities to avoid, and those that are permitted; parent provides appropriate protective devices at home; adequately cares for minor bleeding episodes (e.g., local pressure, ice pack); school personnel/friends are informed about child's condition and necessary restrictions/appropriate action during a bleeding episode.

Goal 2: Child/parent will receive emotional support.

Plan/Implementation

- Encourage realistic career goals.
- Allow child/family to discuss feelings and concerns about bleeding tendency and treatment, subsequent absences from school, reactions to peers, parental protectiveness.
- Encourage independence while maintaining safety.
- Refer to the local chapter of the National Hemophilia Foundation.

Evaluation: Child seeks independence within reasonable limits; asks questions about reactions of school friends; adolescent seeks out appropriate job opportunities.

References

Agamalian, B. (1986). Pediatric cardiac catheterization. *Journal of Pediatric Nursing 1*(2), 73–79.

Graber, H., & Balas-Stevens, S. (1984). A discharge tool for teaching parents to monitor infant apnea at home. *MCN: American Journal of Maternal/Child Nursing, 9*(3), 178–180.

Higgins, S., & Kashani, I. (1986). The cyanotic child: Heart defects and parental learning needs. *MCN: American Journal of Maternal/Child Nursing, 11*(4), 258–262.

Mott, S., Fazekas, N., & James, S. (1985). *Nursing care of children and families: A holistic approach.* Menlo Park, CA: Addison-Wesley.

Sacksteder, S., Gildea, J., & Dassey, C. (1978). Common congenital cardiac defects. *American Journal of Nursing, 78*, 266–277.

Sacksteder, S. (1978). Embryology and fetal circulation. *American Journal of Nursing, 78*, 262–265.

Scipien, G., et al. (1986). *Comprehensive pediatric nursing* (3rd ed.). New York: McGraw-Hill.

Servonsky, J., & Opas, S. (1987). *Nursing management of children.* Boston: Jones & Bartlett.

Shor, V. (1978). Congenital cardiac defects. *American Journal of Nursing, 78*, 256–261.

Swoiskin, S. (1986). Sudden infant death: Nursing care for the survivors. *Journal of Pediatric Nursing, 1*(1), 33–39.

Waechter, E., Phillips, J., & Holaday, B. (1985). *Nursing care of children* (10th ed.). Philadelphia: Lippincott.

Whaley, L., & Wong, D. (1986). *Nursing care of infants and children* (3rd ed.). St. Louis: Mosby.

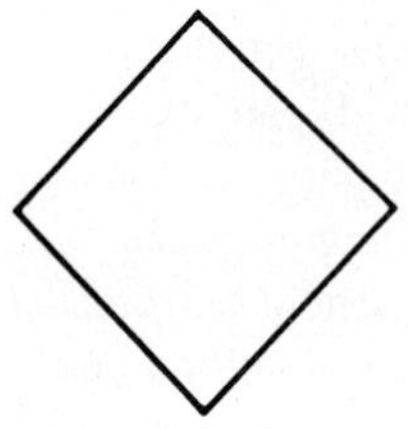

Nutrition and Metabolism

General Concepts

Overview/Physiology

1. Physiologic differences in infants and small children as compared with adults
   a. Greater proportion of body water, especially in extracellular space, until 2 years of age
   b. Water-turnover rate per unit of body weight is three times greater in infants
      1) higher metabolic rate
      2) functional immaturity of kidneys which impairs ability to conserve water
   c. Greater skin surface area in proportion to body weight; more susceptible to insensible water loss
   d. Greater gastrointestinal surface area; proportionately greater fluid loss from diarrhea
   e. Average daily water requirements are calculated according to child's weight
      1) 100 ml/kg for the first 10 kg of body weight
      2) 50 ml/kg for the next 10 kg of body weight
      3) 20 ml/kg for each additional kg

2. Digestive system
   a. High rate of peristalsis (increases susceptibility to diarrhea)
   b. Immature cardiac sphincter that relaxes easily
   c. Immature liver
   d. Low production of intestinal antibodies until 6–7 months of age
   e. Development of digestive processes is complete by toddlerhood

3. Endocrine system
   a. Functionally immature
   b. Blood sugar levels fluctuate
   c. Hormonal feedback mechanisms are not fully operational; infant is less able to tolerate stresses and metabolic demands of illness

Application of the Nursing Process to the Child with Problems of Nutrition and Metabolism

1. **Assessment/Analysis**
   a. Nursing history
      1) dietary-intake history: type, amount, frequency, tolerance
      2) vomiting or diarrhea: onset, severity, duration, description, precipitating factors, home management
      3) infant/child behavior: irritability, lethargy
      4) other signs and symptoms of illness such as fever, respiratory infection, abdominal pain
      5) frequency in voiding
      6) history of exposure to illness in family or community
      7) family history of hereditary disorders: cystic fibrosis, PKU, diabetes mellitus, cleft lip and palate, lactose intolerance
   b. Clinical appraisal
      1) general appearance: color, cry, behavior
      2) physical growth (refer to *Healthy Child* page 517)
      3) vital signs, presence of fever
      4) nutrition and hydration status, including signs of dehydration
         a) mild dehydration: weight loss of up to 5%
            - dry mucous membranes
            - poor tear production
            - decreased urine output with increased specific gravity
            - pallor
            - pulse normal or slightly increased
            - normal blood pressure
         b) moderate dehydration: weight loss between 5%–9%
            - very dry mucous membranes
            - poor skin turgor
            - pale to gray skin color
            - oliguria
            - tachycardia
            - slight decrease in BP

c) severe dehydration: weight loss between 10%–15%
- parched mucous membranes
- very poor skin turgor
- marked oliguria
- gray to mottled skin color
- severe tachycardia
- decreased blood pressure
- sunken eyes and fontanels
- tetany, convulsions

d) laboratory findings: elevated hematocrit and BUN

c. Diagnostic tests (refer to *Nursing Care of the Adult* page 202)

2. Analysis

a. Safe, effective care environment
1) potential for infection
2) potential for injury

b. Physiological integrity
1) fluid volume deficit
2) altered nutrition: less than body requirements
3) potential for aspiration

c. Psychological integrity
1) anxiety
2) self-esteem disturbance
3) fear

d. Health Promotion
1) altered family processes
2) altered growth and development
3) knowledge deficit

3. General Nursing Plan, Implementation, and Evaluation

Goal: Child will maintain fluid and electrolyte balance.

Plan/Implementation
- Administer fluids (PO, IV) as prescribed; usually includes sodium chloride and potassium replacement
  - use infusion pump to maintain accurate rate
  - restrain child as necessary to protect infusion site
  - observe infusion site for infiltration or redness, and report promptly
- Provide pacifier if infant is NPO.
- Administer electrolytes as prescribed (give potassium only when urinary output is adequate, i.e., 1–2 ml/kg/hour).
- Carefully monitor and record I&O (weigh diapers, indicate urine and stool output separately if possible).
- Monitor response to therapy (improved skin color and turgor, moist mucous membranes, stable vital signs, urine output within normal limits, urine specific gravity within normal limits, i.e., 1.005–1.025).
- Weigh child daily or every shift.
- Administer antiemetics as ordered.
- Gradually return to diet-for-age as tolerated.

Evaluation: Child regains and maintains fluid and electrolyte balance; shows no signs of dehydration, electrolyte, or acid-base imbalance; returns to usual diet without recurrence of vomiting or diarrhea.

Selected Health Problems Resulting in an Interference with Nutrition and Metabolism

☐ Vomiting and Diarrhea

1. General Information

a. Although vomiting and diarrhea are usually symptoms of other underlying problems or diseases, they are often the primary diagnosis in infants, because fluid and electrolyte imbalance can develop rapidly and become critical in a few hours.

b. Occurrence: these are very common health problems in infancy; younger infants and children who are debilitated, and those who are exposed to unsanitary environmental conditions are at greater risk of developing diarrhea

c. Causes
1) vomiting
a) gastrointestinal infection
b) allergy to formula, food, medications
c) emotional upsets
d) GI obstruction
e) toxin ingestion
f) increased intracranial pressure
g) overfeeding
h) diabetic ketoacidosis
i) migraine headaches
j) appendicitis
k) other infections (e.g., otitis media, meningitis, respiratory and urinary tract infections)

2) diarrhea (may be acute or chronic)
a) infection
- viruses, e.g., rotavirus (self-limiting)
- parasites, e.g., giardia
- enteropathic organisms such as

shigella, salmonella, *E. coli*, campylobacter

b) diet: formula or food allergy, high sugar or fat content, high bulk, overfeeding

c) emotional upsets

d) prolonged use of antibiotics (may destroy normal flora)

e) intestinal malabsorption

f) inflammatory bowel disease

g) extraintestinal: hepatic, pancreatic, thyroid disorders

h) ingestion of heavy metals such as lead and mercury

i) parenteral infections

d. Medical treatment: depends on severity of symptoms and degree of dehydration

1) medical intervention

a) bowel rest; IV and/or oral fluid and electrolyte replacement therapy; type and amount determined on basis of child's age, hydration status as determined by weight loss and lab values

b) antibiotic therapy for bacterial diarrhea

c) antiemetics, usually by rectal suppository

d) gradual reintroduction of solid foods

e) diagnosis and treatment of extraintestinal cause

2) surgical intervention for GI obstruction

2. Nursing Process

a. Assessment/Analysis

1) feeding technique and formula preparation (amount, type, formula reconstitution, position of infant, burping)

2) type of vomiting and/or diarrhea

a) vomiting

- *forceful* vomiting: evacuation of stomach contents; usually caused by overdistention from formula or air
- *projectile* vomiting: stomach contents propelled 2–3 feet from infant; indicates GI obstruction or increased intracranial pressure
- *regurgitation*: "spitting up" milk after feeding; smells sour; usually associated with rumination or gastroesophageal reflux

b) diarrhea

- *mild*: weight loss of 5% or less; stools are loose, runny, usually brown and brownish yellow
- *severe*: explosive, green watery stools, 10–12/day; weight loss 10% or more

3) character of vomitus or stool (ACCT)

a) *A*mount: measure or estimate

b) *C*olor/*C*onsistency

- vomitus
  - undigested food, uncurdled milk
  - sour milk curds
  - bile stained
  - blood tinged or coffee ground
- diarrhea
  - color (brown, green, yellow)
  - consistency (bulky, watery, runny, mucoid, bloody, seedy, pasty)

c) *T*ime

- frequency
- precedents (feeding, stimulants, emotional upsets)

4) diagnostic tests

a) stool pH and stool sugar with Clinitest

b) stool blood with guaiac or Hemoccult

c) stool sample for bacteria culture, ova and parasites

5) associated symptoms: anorexia, nausea, cramping, abdominal pain, fever, headache

6) signs of dehydration

7) change in acid-base balance

a) vomiting → loss of HCl → metabolic alkalosis

- compensation: kidneys conserve Na^+ and K^+, excrete HCO_3^-
- lab findings: urine pH greater than 7; serum pH greater than 7.43

b) diarrhea → metabolic acidosis

- compensation: respiratory hyperventilation (deep, rapid respirations)
- lab findings: urine pH less than 6; serum pH less than 7.33

b. Plans, Implementation, and Evaluation

Goal 1: Child's close contacts will be free from signs of infection.

Plan/Implementation

- Obtain stool culture to determine infecting organism.
- Isolate infant; use good handwashing technique; dispose of excreta and contaminated laundry appropriately.
- Teach parents protective measures.

- Administer antibiotics as ordered, observe for side effects.

Evaluation: Individuals involved with care of child, and other children in close proximity show no signs of spread of infection.

Goal 2: Child (with diarrhea) will maintain skin integrity.

Plan/Implementation
- Cleanse perineum and buttocks well after each stool.
- Expose to heat lamp or air (buttocks must be free of ointment before exposing to heat lamp).
- Apply ointment to protect skin.
- Take axillary temps to avoid stimulating peristalsis.

Evaluation: Child is free from skin breakdown; heals excoriated areas.

Goal 3: Child will maintain comfort and safety.

Plan/Implementation
- Position to prevent aspiration (on side or abdomen, or in infant seat).
- Give mouth care after vomiting and while NPO.
- If infant is NPO, offer pacifier to meet sucking needs.
- Change soiled clothing and linen immediately.
- Exercise restrained limbs.

Evaluation: Child is free from aspiration; rests and sleeps comfortably.

Goal 4: Child will resume diet for age without recurrence of vomiting or diarrhea.

Plan/Implementation
- Begin clear liquids such as noncarbonated soft drinks, Gatorade and half-strength flavored gelatin; use oral rehydration solutions (e.g., Pedialyte, Lytren, Reasol) for infants and young children.
- If vomiting, offer frequent small amounts (5–15 ml) depending on age every 20 minutes; increase the amount and intervals between feedings slowly.
- For diarrhea, offer large amounts of clear liquids at infrequent intervals.
- Discourage use of Popsicles and Kool-Aid as sole source of fluid replacement since they lack electrolytes.
- Limit apple juice.
- Discourage use of homemade electrolyte solutions.
- If infant is breast-feeding, continue and supplement with clear liquids.
- Add other liquids and solids gradually as tolerated.
- Encourage bananas, applesauce, strained carrots, and rice cereal.
- Discourage foods with high fat content.
- Add milk products last due to temporary lactose intolerance common after diarrhea.
- Switch to soy formula for 1–3 weeks if necessary

Evaluation: Child tolerates diet for age without recurrence of diarrhea or vomiting; gains or maintains present weight.

☐ Nonorganic Failure to Thrive

1. General Information

a. Definition: A syndrome used to describe infants and children who fail to gain weight as a result of psychosocial factors such as environmental deprivation; usually results from a disrupted relationship between child and primary care giver

b. Medical treatment

1) comprehensive diagnostic testing to rule out organic failure to thrive, which results from physical causes (e.g., malabsorption syndrome, gastroesophageal reflux, cystic fibrosis, genitourinary/cardiac defects, neurologic/endocrine disorders)

2) criteria used for diagnosis

a) absence of organic disease

b) weight below the 5th percentile with subsequent weight gain when nurtured

c) developmental lags that improve with stimulation

d) improvement in clinical signs of deprivation when nurtured

e) disruption in psychosocial environment

2. Nursing Process

a. Assessment/Analysis

1) infant

a) growth retardation: height and weight below 5th percentile

b) developmental delays: social, motor, language, cognitive

c) flat affect, withdrawn

d) feeding and elimination disorders

e) absence of stranger anxiety

f) avoids eye-to-eye contact

g) visually scans the environment

h) posture stiff or floppy

i) difficulty in feeding or eating (e.g.,

poor suck, anorexia, vomiting, rumination)
- j) slow in smiling or socially responding to others

2) parent
- a) handles infant only when necessary
- b) does not talk to, play with, or cuddle infant
- c) bothered by infant's sounds and smells
- d) holds infant away from body, no eye contact with infant
- e) responds inappropriately and inconsistently to infant's cues
- f) refers to infant as "bad" and "unloving"

b. Plans, Implementation, and Evaluation

Goal 1: Infant will show evidence of weight gain.

Plan/Implementation
- Calculate caloric requirements based on infant's weight: 115 calories/kg/day for the first year of life.
- Monitor I&O; describe frequency and precipitating events of any vomiting.
- Obtain daily weights and weekly length and head circumferences.
- Observe feeding patterns.
- Observe parent-infant interactions around feeding.

Evaluation: Infant shows steady weight gain, ingests and retains appropriate amount of nutrients necessary to meet caloric requirements.

Goal 2: Infant will show progression in development while hospitalized.

Plan/Implementation
- Utilize primary care givers.
- Hold, cuddle, talk to infant lovingly with reassurance to model for care givers.
- Monitor infant's response to care.
- Provide age-appropriate developmental and sensory stimulation.

Evaluation: Infant responds appropriately to developmental stimulation and nurturing; maintains eye contact; smiles; allows self to be held closely; demonstrates interest in environment.

Goal 3: Parents will show positive interaction with infant.

Plan/Implementation
- Welcome parents when visiting.
- Encourage parent participation in care, teaching as appropriate.
- Utilize anticipatory guidance re infant's capabilities, physical care, emotional needs (demonstrate by example).
- Encourage parents to express feelings about infant.
- Urge parents to talk to infant; point out positive responses.
- Identify stressors in family; refer to social services and family counseling as appropriate.
- Praise parents' involvement with child.
- Determine progress in parent-child relationship.
- Maintain a nonjudgmental attitude.

Evaluation: Parents provide some care to infant; hold, cuddle, and talk to infant; express feelings about infant.

Goal 4: Parent will participate in follow-up care after discharge.

Plan/Implementation
- Assess home environment.
- Refer to community resources (e.g., public health nurse, parent support group) as needed.
- Refer to agencies that can provide family counseling, financial assistance, e.g., WIC.
- Review infant's regimen with parent: nutrition, elimination, stimulation, etc.
- Arrange for return visit for infant to physician/ clinic.
- Review developmental milestones and age-appropriate stimulation.

Evaluation: Parent keeps all appointments including those with community resources, groups; infant continues weight gain and developmental progress.

☐ Pyloric Stenosis

1. General Information

a. Definition and occurrence: narrowing of the pylorus due to hypertrophy of circular muscle fibers; more commonly affects firstborn white males, 2 weeks to 3 months of age

b. Medical treatment
1) medical intervention
- a) barium swallow to confirm diagnosis
- b) IV fluids to hydrate and correct metabolic alkalosis
- c) nasogastric tube to decompress stomach

2) surgical intervention: Fredet-Ramstedt procedure (pylorotomy); hypertrophied muscle in *split down to but not through* submucosa, permitting pylorus to expand (if mucosa is cut, gastric contents will leak into peritoneum causing peritonitis)

2. Nursing Process

a. Assessment/Analysis

1) vomiting: amount, color, consistency, time
2) classic signs
   a) projectile vomiting (not bile stained since obstruction is above the duodenum)
   b) palpable, olive-size mass (usually in RUQ)
   c) observable left-to-right gastric peristaltic waves
3) metabolic alkalosis, caused by loss of HCl and K^+
4) signs and symptoms of food and fluid loss
   a) hunger after feeding
   b) weight loss, or failure to gain weight
   c) dehydration
   d) scanty, concentrated urine
   e) progressive constipation

b. Plans, Implementation, and Evaluation

Goal 1: Preoperatively, infant will regain/ maintain fluid and electrolyte balance.

Plan/Implementation
- Assess vital signs frequently.
- Assess signs of dehydration.
- Offer pacifier while NPO.
- Follow correct principles of IV fluid and electrolyte administration.
- Carefully monitor I&O and urine specific gravity.
- Weigh infant daily or every shift if condition warrants.
- Maintain nasogastric decompression as ordered.

Evaluation: Infant regains and maintains fluid and electrolyte balance; is free from signs of dehydration and metabolic alkalosis.

Goal 2: Postoperatively, infant will be free from vomiting and will ingest adequate nutrition.

Plan/Implementation
- Initiate glucose water or electrolyte solutions 4–6 hours post-op and gradually advance to full strength formula during 2nd post-op day.
- Give small frequent feedings; feed slowly.
- Burp every ½ oz; position on right side in semi-Fowler's position after feeding.
- Teach parent how to feed child; supervise as needed.
- Handle gently and minimally after feeding.
- Offer pacifier during period of restricted feeding.
- Keep accurate I&O.

Evaluation: Infant ingests adequate caloric and fluid intake; has no vomiting, no signs of dehydration; gains or maintains present weight.

Goal 3: Postoperatively, infant will be free from infection.

Plan/Implementation
- Observe operative site routinely for any drainage or signs of inflammation.
- Perform incision care/dressing change as ordered.
- Assess for signs of peritonitis (e.g., abdominal distention, fever, rigid abdomen, increased irritability, tachycardia, decreased or absent bowel sounds, rapidly thoracic breathing)

Evaluation: Infant remains afebrile, has soft abdomen, exhibits no signs of discomfort.

☐ Celiac Disease (Gluten Enteropathy)

1. General Information

a. Definition: a disease of unknown etiology characterized by the inability to tolerate gluten (one of the proteins found in wheat, rye, oats, and barley)

b. Occurrence: 21 in 100,000 live births; second leading cause of malabsorption in children; positive familial tendency

c. Pathophysiology: the ingestion of gluten results in the inability to fully digest gliadine (a fraction of gluten). Subsequently, there is an accumulation of the amino acid glutamine, which is toxic to the mucosal cells of the small intestine. This may lead to malabsorption of the following nutrients causing various complications:
   1) fats: steatorrhea, malnutrition
   2) proteins and carbohydrates: peripheral edema
   3) vitamin D and calcium: osteomalacia
   4) vitamin K: bleeding
   5) iron, folic acid, and vitamin B_{12}: anemia

d. Medical treatment
   1) Diagnosis
      a) positive fecal fat
      b) decreases in serum protein, prothrombin, folic acid, vitamin B_{12}, calcium
      c) anemia
      d) x-rays to determine bone age
      e) sweat test and pancreatic function tests (to rule out cystic fibrosis)
      f) improvement of clinical signs and symptoms after withdrawal of gluten from diet

g) bowel studies
h) peroral jejunal biopsy (diagnosis is confirmed when atrophic changes are seen in the mucosal wall)

2) dietary management
a) gluten-free diet
b) supplemental calories, vitamins, and iron
c) parenteral alimentation if malnourished

3) management during celiac crisis (acute episodes usually precipitated by gastrointestinal infection, dietary sources of gluten, and anticholinergic drugs)
a) IV fluids and electrolytes
b) albumin infusions (to prevent shock)
c) nasogastric decompression
d) corticosteroids (to decrease bowel inflammation)

2. Nursing Process

a. Assessment/Analysis

1) Clinical manifestations (highly variable)
a) chronic diarrhea (usually begins late in the first year of life)
b) failure to thrive
c) irritability
d) anorexia
e) vomiting
f) abdominal pain and distention
g) excessive appetite
h) rectal prolapse
i) peripheral edema
j) clubbing of fingers
k) wasting of muscles
l) excessive bruising

2) In celiac crisis
a) severe pale, bulky, foul-smelling stools
b) vomiting
c) signs of shock and metabolic acidosis
d) dependent edema

b. Plan, Implementation, and Evaluation

Goal 1: Child will remain free from injury during intestinal biopsy.

Plan/Implementation
- Prepare child and family for diagnostic procedure.
- Assess bleeding times and platelet count.
- Administer vitamin K prophylactically as ordered.
- Assess frequently following procedure for shock (early signs: tachycardia and signs of peripheral vasoconstriction; late signs: hypotension)

Evaluation: Child tolerates intestinal biopsy well, recovers free from signs of hemorrhage.

Goal 2: Child will adhere to nutritional management.

Plan/Implementation
- Assess family's understanding of disease process and need for gluten-free diet.
- Educate family regarding gluten-free foods; show parents how to read food labels (gluten is often listed as hydrolyzed vegetable protein).
- Encourage balanced diet with increased caloric intake; consult dietitian to help in meal planning.
- Reinforce to family the need for life-long dietary adherence.

Evaluation: Parents list elements of a gluten-free diet; child ingests only gluten-free, balanced meals.

Goal 3: Child will remain free of fluid and electrolyte imbalance during celiac crisis.

Plan/Implementation
- Monitor vital signs frequently.
- Assess for signs of shock and metabolic acidosis.
- Keep accurate I&O.
- Weigh child daily.
- Maintain nasogastric decompression as ordered.
- Administer corticosteroids, albumin, IV fluids, and electrolytes as ordered.
- Hematest all stools and nasogastric drainage.
- Educate family regarding precipitating factors of celiac crisis.

Evaluation: Child recovers from celiac crisis free from complications; achieves homeostasis.

□ Cleft Lip and Palate

1. General Information

a. Definition
1) *cleft lip*: incomplete fusion of facial process; may be small notch in the upper lip (incomplete) or extend to nasal septum and dental ridge (complete); may be unilateral or bilateral
2) *cleft palate*: fissures in soft and/or hard palate and alveolar (dental) ridge; may be midline, unilateral, or bilateral

b. Occurrence
1) cleft lip (with or without cleft palate): 1:1,000 live births, higher in males, whites, and Asians

2) cleft palate: 1:2,500, higher in females

c. Cause: often unknown, multifactorial inheritance, chromosomal abnormalities, maternal alcohol or drug ingestion, prenatal infection

d. Medical treatment: lip defect is surgically repaired between ages of 2 weeks–3 months so infant can suck properly and for cosmetic effect; repair of palate (Z-plasty) usually delayed until about 12–18 months of age to allow for bone growth and changes in contour of palate

2. Nursing Process

a. Assessment/Analysis

1) infant's ability to suck and swallow
2) parents' reaction to birth of an infant with a facial defect

b. Plans, Implementation, and Evaluation

Goal 1: Preoperatively, child will maintain adequate nutrition and will not aspirate fluids.

Plan/Implementation

- Feed slowly in upright position; use
  - soft nipple
  - special nipple (large opening)
  - red rubber catheter tubing attached to a LuerLock syringe (Brecht feeder)
  - cup for older infant with cleft palate
- Burp frequently.
- Rinse mouth with water after feedings to keep lip/palate cleansed.
- Teach parents how to feed and burp infant.
- Teach parents use and care of palate prosthesis.

Evaluation: Child ingests adequate fluids and calories; is free from aspiration and lip/palate infections.

Goal 2: Postoperatively, child will maintain a patent airway.

Plan/Implementation

- Observe for respiratory distress; assist in respiratory effort by repositioning child to facilitate breathing; aspirate oral secretions *gently*.
- Cleft palate: place in mist tent.
- Position infant to provide for drainage of mucus and to prevent trauma to suture lines
  - cleft lip repair: on side or in infant seat
  - cleft palate repair: on side or abdomen

Evaluation: Child has patent airway and adequate oxygenation; has no signs of respiratory distress.

Goal 3: Postoperatively, child will be free from trauma and infection of suture lines.

Plan/Implementation

- Minimize crying by holding and soothing infant as needed.
- Put elbow restraints on child; remove *one at a time* q2h for ROM exercises.
- Position as stated above.
- Maintain Logan bar on upper lip to decrease tension on suture line.
- Cleanse suture lines after feeding with sterile swabs and solution (usually diluted hydrogen peroxide) as ordered
  - for cleft lip repair: *roll* applicator without rubbing
  - for cleft palate repair: rinse mouth with sterile water after feeding
- Apply antibiotic ointment to lip suture line as prescribed.
- Encourage parents to stay with infant and participate in care.

Evaluation: Child has healing of suture lines without trauma and scarring associated with infection.

Goal 4: Postoperatively, child will ingest adequate nutrition.

Plan/Implementation

- Keep NPO initially, then introduce clear fluids in small amounts.
- Feed with medicine dropper, Brecht feeder (cleft lip), or cup (cleft palate); *no sucking*, straws, or spoons.
- While suture line heals, give soft diet; avoid hard food items, e.g., toast, cookies, potato chips.

Evaluation: Child takes food and fluids (appropriate for age); is free from choking or aspiration.

Goal 5: Child/parent will be referred for ongoing, long-term intervention and promotion of optimum development.

Plan/Implementation

- Teach parents signs of otitis media (fever, turning head to side, pulling at ear, discharge from ear, pain, crying); encourage parents to seek medical treatment for upper respiratory infections.
- Refer for regular evaluation of child's hearing, speech, and dental development.
- Assist parents to express feelings and concerns about defect and surgery.

- Refer parents to community resources
  - parent groups; local and state cleft palate associations
  - Crippled Children's Services, social services

Evaluation: Parents list early signs of ear infections and when to seek treatment; child has no permanent hearing loss; has age-appropriate language development, intelligible speech, normal tooth alignment; parent/child receive community support (emotional, financial, social).

☐ Congenital Hypothyroidism

1. General Information

a. Definition: congenital condition in which the fetal thyroid fails to develop, resulting in inadequate levels of T4 and other thyroid hormones in the fetus and newborn; also called cretinism; early diagnosis is essential to prevent mental retardation

b. Incidence: one of the most common endocrine problems of childhood; 1 in every 4,500 live births; twice as common in females as males; higher incidence in Down's Syndrome

c. Pathophysiology: thyroid hormones have a stimulating effect on metabolic rate, heat production, cardiac output, and growth of almost all tissues; lack of these hormones specifically affects brain, bone, and muscle growth in infants

d. Diagnosis

1) elevated serum TSH and decreased T4 levels in early days of life; screening is mandatory in most states

2) decreased uptake of radioactive iodine by thyroid after oral administration of isotope

e. Causes

1) hypoplasia or aplasia of thyroid gland

2) pituitary dysfunction

3) unresponsiveness of tissue to existing thyroid hormones

4) autoimmune destruction of the thyroid (juvenile hypothyroidism)

f. Medical treatment: thyroid replacement as soon as diagnosis is suspected

1) levothyroxine (Synthroid), 0.006 mg/kg/day or desiccated thyroid (Proloid), 4 mg/kg/day; adjusted according to clinical symptoms and T4 level

a) doses in children usually HIGHER than adult doses

b) given as a single dose in morning

c) replacement is a life-long necessity

2) side effects: dyspnea, tachycardia, fever, irritability, tremors, diarrhea, weight loss

2. Nursing Process

a. Assessment/Analysis

1) described as "good, quiet baby"

2) hoarse, weak cry

3) lethargy and excessive sleeping resulting in poor feeding

4) poor abdominal muscle tone; constipation

5) weak reflexes

6) large, protruding tongue

7) cold, mottled skin (hypothermia: 95°F or less)

8) delayed cognitive and motor development

9) delayed physical growth

10) prolonged physiologic jaundice

11) delayed passage of meconium

12) respiratory distress

13) see also "Hypothyroidism" page 222

b. Plans, Implementation, and Evaluation

Goal 1: Child's condition will be identified at the earliest possible stage.

Plan/Implementation

- Screen all children before discharge from the hospital or within first week of life.
- Be alert to earliest clinical manifestations and parental comments (e.g., "She is such a good baby, she hardly ever cries").
- Educate and support parents during diagnostic tests.

Evaluation: Infant is diagnosed within first several weeks of life; replacement therapy begins.

Goal 2: Parents will be prepared for home management to promote optimum development and relief of symptoms.

Plan/Implementation

- Provide information to family about condition.
- Encourage expression of concerns about child's behavior and development.
- If diagnosis is delayed, explore possible guilt feelings and discuss probability of mental retardation.
- Teach parents about medication administration, side effects, need for life-long administration
  - do not change brands without physician knowledge as hormone content varies
  - store in dry, dark place
  - measure pulse daily before administration (indication of drug effectiveness)
  - importance of regular, consistent administration of medication
  - if a dose is missed, give twice the dose the next day

– look for signs of overdose (e.g., dyspnea, fever, diaphoresis, irritability, rapid pulse)

- Teach parents how to measure pulse rate; consult physician if pulse is above normal range (see Table 5.1).
- Monitor child's growth and development periodically.
- Refer family to community support groups if needed.

Evaluation: Child is alert, active; grows normally; development continues within normal range; parent/child assumes self-care responsibility.

☐ Insulin-Dependent Diabetes Mellitus (IDDM: Type I)

1. General Information

a. Definition: metabolic disease of unknown inheritance mechanism that results in insulin deficiency because of reduction in pancreatic islet cell mass or destruction of islets and consequent alterations of carbohydrate, fat, and protein metabolism; also results in long-term alterations in vascular, nervous, renal, and ocular systems; damage to other organ systems may be related to degree of control of diabetes (see Table 5.20 for comparison with adult-onset diabetes)

b. Pathophysiology: refer to "Diabetes Mellitus" page 225

c. Medical treatment

1) medication

a) insulin therapy: human insulin usually recommended because of limited antigenicity, decreased dosage, increased solubility, and increased absorption

- dosage: 0.5–1.0 U/kg/day (usually in 2 divided doses)
- refer to Table 3.29

b) oral hypoglycemics: not used with children

2) meal plan: more flexible nutrition options than with adults; most commonly used are free (no concentrated sweets), exchange, and basic four food groups (usually 3 meals and 3 snacks/day); prudent fat intake

d. Modifying factors

1) puberty

a) onset complicates control by increasing insulin demands (growth is stimulated by gonadal steroids, which antagonize insulin action)

b) associated growth significantly increases caloric needs

2) exercise

a) reduces insulin requirements because glucose is catabolized without insulin during muscular activity

b) increases risk of insulin shock if diet isn't modified for vigorous exercise

3) illness and emotional disturbance

a) lessens ability to utilize glucose

Table 5.20 Comparison of Type 1 (insulin dependent) and Type 2 (non-insulin dependent) Diabetes Mellitus

	Type 1 (IDDM)	Type 2 (IDDM)
Characteristics		
Age of onset	Usually less than 20 years (Peaks: 5–7 years; puberty)	Usually over 35 years
Type of onset	Abrupt	Gradual
Nutritional status	Underweight	Overweight
Symptoms	Polydipsia, polyuria, polyphagia	May be none
Remission	Yes (honeymoon period)	No
Plasma insulin	Absent	Usually decreased
Management		
Medication	Insulin only	Oral hypoglycemics frequently used
Meal planning	Free or exchange	Exchange
Self-monitoring	Blood glucose monitoring preferred; when testing urine, use Clinitest; first voided specimen acceptable	Blood glucose monitoring preferred; when testing urine use Testape or Clinitest on second voided specimen
Hypoglycemia	Oral sugars and glucagon (for severe reactions)	Oral sugars only

b) requires increase in simple foods, decrease in fat
c) may increase insulin requirements because of decreased activity

2. Nursing Process

a. Assessment/Analysis

1) initial
   a) polydipsia, polyphagia, polyuria (bed-wetting): classic signs
   b) weight loss
   c) irritability, fatigue
   d) abdominal discomfort
   e) may be mistaken for influenza, gastroenteritis
   f) frequent infections, slow-to-heal skin injuries
2) often characterized by a remission or honeymoon period
   a) common in children with IDDM
   b) decreased amounts of insulin required
   c) occurs once, lasting a few weeks up to a year
3) diabetic ketoacidosis (DKA): polydipsia, polyphagia, polyuria, dehydration with possible hypovolemic shock, nausea and vomiting, acetone breath, Kussmaul's respirations, flushed dry skin (children who present with DKA for the first time often show signs of abdominal pain and rigidity, which may mimic appendicitis); refer to Table 3.31
4) hypoglycemia: irritability, trembling; apprehension; headache; hunger; blurred vision; mental confusion; sweating, pallor, seizures (more likely in infants and children); temper tantrums (common in toddlers)

b. Plan, Implementation, and Evaluation

Goal: Child/parent will be prepared for home management.

Plan/Implementation

- Teach blood glucose monitoring (preferred self-monitoring method)
  - finger stick technique
  - importance of exact timing
  - variation among different products (use same product for consistency and accuracy)
  - check expiration dates
  - 4 measurements per day (prior to each meal and bedtime snack)
  - interpretation of results
  - importance of record keeping
- Contact community resources for financial assistance as needed for home blood glucose monitoring
  - Medicaid coverage in some states
  - local diabetes associations
  - rentals available
  - private insurance
- Demonstrate urine testing for glucose and acetone (to be done if blood glucose level is greater than 240 mg); 2-to 5-drop Clinitest preferred; first-voided specimens used because of difficulty in obtaining second-voided specimens in children
- Teach insulin administration
  - knowledge of medication
  - proper mixing
  - injection technique
  - rotation of sites
  - use of insulin pump when indicated
- Involve dietitian with nutrition planning; adjust meal plans for activity and growth with periodic reassessment at least every 6 months
- Teach management of hyperglycemia
  - recognition of early signs and symptoms
  - importance of good control
  - food, activity, and insulin adjustment to improve control
- Teach management of hypoglycemia: ingest a rapidly absorbed glucose-containing food or liquid, such as 4 oz orange juice, 2 teaspoonfuls honey, 5–6 Life Savers (chewed), instant glucose, glucagon (for severe reactions).
- Demonstrate foot care: same as adult except bare feet acceptable.
- Prepare parents for developmental concerns with respect to management
  - for toddler and preschooler
    * finger sticks and injections (body integrity concerns)
    * need for control (autonomy)
    * finicky eating habits
    * how to recognize hypoglycemia
    * toilet training and urine testing
  - for school-age child
    * inform school, teacher, peers about symptoms/treatment
    * arrange to participate in gym and sports, adjusting medication as needed
    * problem solve to anticipate nutrition needs of lunches, parties, holidays
    * feelings of being different
  - for adolescent
    * discuss feelings/concerns about future: career, marriage, pregnancy

* acting out behaviors (anticipate and prevent)
* onset of puberty, changes in body image
* discuss the effects of drugs, alcohol, birth control pills on blood glucose levels

- Teach self-management as appropriate
  - at 6 or 8 years: assisting with urine tests, injections, diet selection, and blood glucose measurement
  - at 8 or 9 years: physical readiness; teach to do urine tests, injections, and blood glucose monitoring
  - at 12 to 13 years and beyond: cognitive readiness; teach meal planning, how to maintain food, activity, insulin balance
- Develop an exercise program that allows for optimal growth and development.
- Advise child and parents of need to obtain and wear medical-alert identification.

Evaluation: Child/parent incorporates necessary skills to daily routine; child does not have recurrent episodes of ketoacidosis or hypoglycemia; continues normal growth and development.

☐ Cystic Fibrosis

1. General Information

a. Definition: an inherited multisystem disorder characterized by widespread dysfunction of the exocrine glands (those whose secretions reach an epithelial surface, either directly or through a duct)

b. Cause and occurrence: autosomal recessive disorder (both parents are carriers: see Figure 5.3); most common genetic defect of caucasians; approximately 1 in 2,000 live births; 1 in 20 persons estimated to be a carrier

c. Pathosphysiology: abnormal secretion of thick tenacious mucous by the exocrine glands causes obstruction and results in varying degrees of pathology

1) *pulmonary effects*: depressed respiratory-cilia cells result in increased infection, bronchiole obstruction, and eventually pulmonary fibrosis; child ultimately develops chronic obstructive pulmonary disease; may progress to cor pulmonale; death can occur from respiratory infection or heart failure

2) *pancreas effects*: pancreatic fibrosis and eventual decrease of digestive enzymes (lipase, amylase, trypsin) resulting in severe malnutrition and failure to thrive; steatorrhea: fatty, bulky, foul-smelling stools that float because of undigested fat cells; also can affect pancreatic endocrine functions resulting in hyperglycemia, glucosuria, and ultimately requiring insulin replacement (risk of diabetes increases with age)

3) *salivary effects*: fibrosis and enlargement of glands caused by thickened secretions; elevated sodium and chloride in saliva

4) *sweat gland effects*: elevated sodium and chloride in sweat

5) *reproductive effects*

a) males: inability to produce sperm; the semen is thickened and tenacious; it plugs the duct in the testes, resulting in fibrosis; males are generally sterile but not impotent

b) females: difficult to conceive because cervical plug cannot be penetrated by normal sperm

6) *hepatic effects*: bile secreted by the liver to emulsify fat in the duodenum is thickened (inspissated) and may plug liver ductules, resulting in biliary cirrhosis and jaundice; can lead to esophageal varices; in newborn and infant, condition may be misdiagnosed as biliary atresia

d. Medical treatment

1) diagnostic testing

a) prenatal diagnosis: DNA analysis of chorionic villi samples; DNA or enzyme analysis of amniotic fluid samples

b) postnatal diagnosis: pilocarpine electrophoresis (sweat chloride test)

- normal sweat chloride values: less than 40 mEq/liter
- suggestive of CF: 40–60 mEq/liter
- diagnostic of CF: greater than 60 mEq/liter

2) medication

a) pancreatic enzymes by mouth (Pancrease, Cotazym-S: preparations that resist destruction by stomach acids)

b) fat soluble vitamins A, D, E, K in water-miscible form

c) "high dose" antibiotics for respiratory infections: penicillins and aminoglycosides (Ticarcillin, Colistin, Piperacillin, Tobramycin); *NOTE*: with aminoglycoside therapy, toxic effects include renal and ototoxicity

d) stool softeners, when necessary, for constipation
e) NaCl tablets added to diet in hot weather, during febrile illness, or strenuous activity; liberal dietary salt encouraged
f) oral iron supplements

3) oxygen therapy, aerosols, nebulizers, bronchodilators
4) percussion, postural drainage, and breathing exercises
5) sweat chloride testing or gene marker studies of other family members along with genetic counseling

2. Nursing Process

a. Assessment/Analysis

1) effects of mucous gland involvement
   a) dry, paroxysmal cough
   b) wheezing
   c) barrel-shaped chest as child grows older
   d) cyanosis and clubbing of fingers and toes due to hypoxia from chronic pulmonary disease
   e) thick, mucoid, tenacious pulmonary secretions expectorated following chest physical therapy
   f) since GI tract has a mucoid lining, newborn is at risk of meconium ileus (failure to pass meconium; impacted meconium causes bowel obstruction); older children are also at risk of bowel obstruction caused by fecal impactions
2) effects of pancreatic involvement
   a) abdominal distention
   b) ravenous appetite
   c) small stature
   d) delayed puberty
   e) decreased subcutaneous tissue
   f) pale, transparent skin
   g) easy fatigability
   h) malaise
   i) fatty, bulky, foul-smelling stools
   j) rectal prolapse
3) child tastes "salty" when kissed

b. Plans, Implementation, and Evaluation

Goal 1: Child will maintain effective airway clearance and remain free from pulmonary complications.

Plan/Implementation

- Teach parents how to administer nebulizer treatment with prescribed solution and carry out percussion and postural drainage at least twice daily, including on arising and at bedtime; discourage treatments immediately before or after meals
  - percussion and postural drainage are carried out before and after nebulizer treatment
  - nebulizer solution usually contains bronchodilators and saline; mucolytics rarely used
- Teach child and family correct administration of medications (antibiotics, bronchodilators, expectorants).
- Teach child breathing exercises (done after postural drainage).
- Encourage child to engage in physical activities (swimming, gymnastics, baseball).
- Teach child and family general health measures to prevent respiratory infections (e.g., immunizations on time, avoid crowds and people with URIs, prevent chilling, no smoking in the home, provide proper nutrition).
- Observe and record sputum amount, color, consistency.
- Review social implications of sputum by age
  - 2-year-olds and under cannot expectorate
  - socially unacceptable for older children to spit, especially for teenager with beginning sexual identity and relationships
  - review with older children how to take care of bad breath
  - if tetracycline given, warn that it stains teeth

Evaluation: Child and parents implement daily pulmonary therapies; child is free from respiratory infections or they are detected and treated early and vigorously; maintains optimal ventilation.

Goal 2: Child will maintain adequate nutritional and electrolyte intake.

Plan/Implementation

- Give pancreatic enzymes as ordered
  - dosage: individualized, 1–6 capsules/meal
  - side effects: nausea, vomiting, gastric irritation
  - just prior to meals, to assist digestion
  - do not crush enteric coated preparations
  - capsules may be opened and sprinkled on food
  - mix with pureed fruit for infants; older children can swallow capsules
  - antacid may be prescribed concurrently
  - monitor I&O, appetite, quality of stools, and weight
- Encourage intake of balanced nutrition high in

protein and carbohydrate (use supplements such as Carnation Instant Breakfast or Sustacal); give snacks with high food value preceded by appropriate amounts of enzymes (these children have additional protein and caloric requirements); fats should be unsaturated.

- Administer water-miscible vitamins daily.
- Encourage child to assume responsibility for healthy food selection.

Evaluation: Child's nutritional intake is adequate to meet growth needs.

Goal 3: Child and parents will learn to cope with the chronicity of cystic fibrosis.

Plan/Implementation

- Encourage and permit child/parents to express their feelings regarding diagnosis and its effects, and prognosis.
- Provide ongoing support and teaching as disease progresses.
- Encourage child to assume age-appropriate responsibility for care to increase feelings of control.
- Provide positive reinforcement to enhance child's self-esteem.
- Plan exercise program that allows for optimal growth and development.
- Refer for genetic counseling: essential for persons with CF and all family members.
- Support family in decision to seek genetic counseling.
- Refer to community support groups; Cystic Fibrosis Foundation.

Evaluation: Child and parents verbalize their feelings about the disease; show adaptive behaviors; and seek genetic counseling and community support groups.

References

Bishop, W.P., & Ulshen, M.H. (1988). Bacterial gastroenteritis. *Pediatric Clinics of North America, 35*(1), 69–87.

Brink, S.J. (1988). Pediatric, adolescent, and young-adult nutrition issues in IDDM. *Diabetes Care, 11*, 192–199.

Gavin, J.R. III. (1988). Diabetes and exercise. *American Journal of Nursing, 88*, 178–180.

Hoette, S. (1983). The adolescent with diabetes mellitus. *Nursing Clinics of North America, 18*, 763–776.

Hodges, L., & Parker, J. (1987). Concerns of parents with diabetic children. *Pediatric Nursing, 13*(1), 22–24, 68.

Krauser, K., & Madden, P. (1983). The child with diabetes mellitus. *Nursing Clinics of North America, 18*, 749–761.

Loman, D., & Galgani, C. (1984). Monitoring diabetic children's blood-glucose levels at home. *MCN: American Journal of Maternal/Child Nursing, 9*(3), 192–196.

Meyer, P.A. (1988). Parental adaptation to cystic fibrosis. *Journal of Pediatric Health Care, 2*(1), 20–28.

Mott, S., Fazekas, N., & James, S. (1985). *Nursing care of children and families: A holistic approach.* Menlo Park, CA: Addison-Wesley.

Scipien, G., et al. (1986). *Comprehensive pediatric nursing* (3rd ed.). New York: McGraw-Hill.

Servonsky, J., & Opas, S. (1987). *Nursing management of children.* Boston: Jones & Bartlett.

Stullenbarger, B., et al. (1987). Family adaptation to cystic fibrosis. *Pediatric Nursing, 13*(1), 29–37.

Vaughan, V., & Behrman, R. (1987). *Nelson's textbook of pediatrics* (13th ed.). Philadelphia: Saunders.

Waechter, E., Phillips, J., & Holaday, B. (1985). *Nursing care of children* (10th ed.). Philadelphia: Lippincott.

Whaley, L., & Wong, D. (1986). *Nursing care of infants and children* (3rd ed.). St. Louis: Mosby.

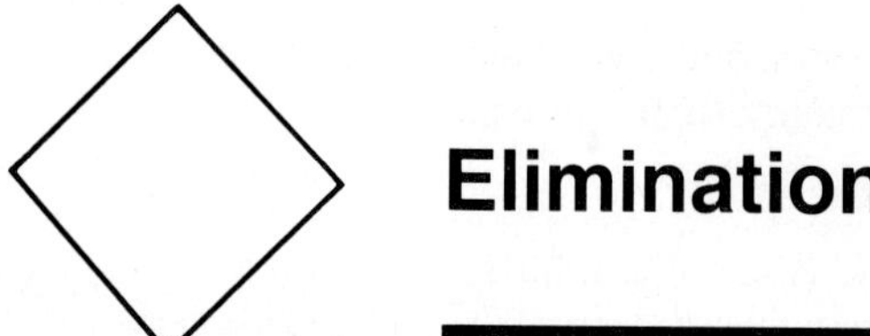

Elimination

General Concepts

Overview/Physiology

1. Urinary elimination
   a. Kidney development is not complete until approximately one year of age
   b. Immature functioning of nephrons; poor filtration and absorption during first year of life; ability to concentrate urine gradually increases during first year of life
   c. Urinary bladder is an abdominal organ during infancy; as pelvic shape changes, the bladder gradually settles and becomes a pelvic organ
   d. Average daily urine output
      1) newborn: 150–300 ml
      2) infant: 400–500 ml
      3) 1–6 years: 500–700 ml
      4) 6–15 years: 700–1,400 ml
2. Bowel elimination
   a. Large and small intestines serve as the major organs for detoxification during infancy while the liver and kidneys are maturing
   b. Development of digestive processes is complete by the early toddler years
3. Voluntary control of elimination
   a. Myelination of the spinal cord is complete by 18–24 months of age resulting in capacity for voluntary control of urinary and anal sphincters
   b. Bladder capacity increases (greater in girls than boys) as voluntary control is achieved

Application of the Nursing Process to the Child with Elimination Problems

1. **Assessment**
   a. Nursing history
      1) voiding patterns: day and night; frequency; color, clarity, estimated amount of urine output; recent changes or problems (e.g., nocturia, urgency, dysuria, infections)
      2) bowel elimination patterns: frequency, consistency, and color; recent changes or problems (e.g., diarrhea, constipation, abdominal cramping)
      3) alterations in elimination: neurogenic bowel and bladder, ostomy, enuresis, encopresis; problem management; medications (e.g., urinary antiseptics, laxatives, antidiarrheal drugs)
   b. Clinical appraisal
      1) observation of urine and stool
      2) palpation and auscultation of abdomen and bladder (normally nonpalpable), including bowel sounds (all quadrants)
   c. Diagnostic tests (refer to *Nursing Care of the Adult* page 236)
2. **Analysis**
   a. Safe, effective care environment
      1) potential for infection
      2) potential impaired skin integrity
   b. Physiological integrity
      1) activity intolerance
      2) potential fluid volume deficit/excess
      3) constipation
      4) altered patterns of urinary elimination
      5) altered tissue perfusion
   c. Psychological integrity
      1) body image disturbance
   d. Health promotion/maintenance
      1) altered family processes
      2) knowledge deficit
3. **General Nursing Plans, Implementation, and Evaluation:** see Selected Health Problems

Selected Health Problems Resulting in an Interference with Urinary or Bowel Elimination

☐ Hypospadias

1. **General Information**
   a. Definition: congenital abnormality in which urethral opening is located behind the glans penis or lies on ventral surface of penis; frequently associated with chordee, which results in a downward curve of penis
   b. Medical treatment

1) surgical intervention to provide normal function and appearance (usually 2–3 surgeries)
   a) urethroplasty: skin grafting to extend urethra and surgically reconstruct a new urinary meatus
   b) surgical release of chordee
2) circumcision is contraindicated, since foreskin may be needed for reconstructive surgery

2. Nursing Process

a. Assessment/Analyis

1) abnormal placement of urethral meatus
2) abnormal urine stream
3) associated problems
   a) chordee
   b) undescended testes

b. Plans, Implementation, and Evaluation

Goal 1: Child will maintain integrity of surgical repair.

Plan/Implementation

- Check pressure dressing for evidence of bleeding and to ensure intact dressing.
- Monitor function of urinary diversion apparatus (permits urine to bypass the operative site)
  - Foley catheter
  - suprapubic tube
  - perineal urethrotomy
- Check for adequate circulation to tip of penis.
- Observe for difficulties following catheter removal
  - inability to void
  - painful voiding (dysuria)
  - urinary tract infection
  - hematuria
  - frequency
- Prevent trauma to surgical site.

Evaluation: Child voids normally; maintains dry and intact surgical dressing and site.

Goal 2: Parents/child will experience minimal mutilation fears; will cope with altered body image.

Plan/Implementation

- Identify defect in infancy to allow complete surgical repair before 5–6 years of age (preferred age: 6–18 months).
- Encourage child to express mutilation fears through play before surgery.
- Reinforce that surgery is to repair anomaly child was born with and is not punishment for sex play or masturbation.
- Prepare parents/child for appearance after surgery.
- Encourage child to examine surgical site after repair to minimize castration anxiety.
- Encourage expression of parental concerns about child's future sexual functioning.

Evaluation: Parents/child discuss surgical outcome in positive terms; child expresses, through play, appropriate reasons for surgery.

☐ Urinary Tract Infection

1. General Information

a. Definition: bacteriuria with or without signs and symptoms of inflammation of the urinary bladder or kidneys, resulting in risk of renal damage

b. Incidence: 1%–2% of the childhood population; girls have a 10–30 times greater risk than boys (5% of girls have a urinary tract infection by age 18); peak age is 2–6 years

c. Predisposing factors
   1) poor hygiene, prolonged use of a single diaper (especially disposable diapers)
   2) tight-fitting clothing, e.g., blue jeans
   3) ureteral reflux caused by congenital malposition of ureters
   4) concurrent vaginitis or pinworms
   5) neurogenic bladder

d. Medical treatment
   1) antibiotic therapy: usually ampicillin, amoxicillin, or sulfonamides for short, intensive treatment, 10–14 days
   2) longer-term urinary antiseptic therapy: nitrofurantoin (Furadantin) or methenamine mandelate (Mandelamine) to maintain sterility of urine
   3) surgical correction of congenital malposition of ureters (ureteral reimplantation) to correct reflux

2. Nursing Process

a. Assessment/Analysis

1) frequency, urgency, dysuria, dribbling, enuresis
2) foul-smelling urine
3) lower abdominal pain
4) nausea, poor feeding, lethargy
5) fever, chills, flank pain (all usually indicate an acute infection of the upper urinary tract)

b. Plan, Implementation, and Evaluation

Goal 1: Child's urinary tract infection will be detected and treated early.

Plan/Implementation
- Ensure child receives annual routine urinalysis (especially girls, ages 2–6 years).
- Provide age-appropriate preparation of child for intrusive diagnostic tests (usually done under general anesthesia).
- Emphasize importance of full course of antibiotic therapy and continuing antiseptics even when child has no signs of infection.
- Emphasize necessity of follow-up urine culture after antibiotic therapy completed.

Evaluation: Child is free from urinary tract infection; has no recurrence.

Goal 2: Child and parents will be knowledgeable about prevention of urinary tract infection.

Plan/Implementation
- Teach good hygiene measures
  - wipe front to back
  - avoid bubble baths
  - wear loose-fitting clothing and cotton panties
- Caution child not to "hold" urine, but to void as soon as urge is felt.
- Teach child to empty bladder completely with each voiding.
- Advise an increase in daily fluid intake, especially fluids that acidify urine (e.g., apple and cranberry juice).

Evaluation: Child is free from urinary tract infection; uses appropriate hygiene measures; empties bladder with each voiding; child's daily fluid intake is adequate.

☐ Vesicoureteral Reflux (VUR)

1. General Information

a. Definition: retrograde flow of bladder urine into the ureters; increases the chance for infection

b. Causes

1) primary: results from congenitally abnormal insertion of the ureters into the bladder

2) secondary: occurs as a result of infection or a neurogenic bladder

c. Peak age: 46% of infants younger than 23 months with urinary tract infections and 9% of children 24–60 months of age with urinary tract infections exhibit VUR

d. Medical treatment

1) continuous low-dose antibiotic therapy (nitrofurantoin and trimethoprim-sulfamethoxazole)

2) frequent urine cultures

3) surgical intervention (ureteral reimplantation is the procedure of choice)

2. Nursing Process

a. Assessment/Analysis

1) reflux of urine into kidneys

2) chronic urinary tract infections

3) associated problems

b. Plans, Implementation, and Evaluation

Goal 1: Child will be free from infection.

Plan/Implementation
- Monitor vital signs.
- Encourage fluid intake.
- Monitor urine cultures.

Evaluation: Child is afebrile, has no complaints of dysuria.

Goal 2: Child will maintain integrity of surgical repair.

Plan/Implementation
- Check dressing for intactness and evidence of bleeding.
- Monitor function of urinary diversion apparatus (suprapubic catheter and left and right ureteral catheters or stent).
- Monitor separate outputs from each catheter (suprapubic catheter will contain gross blood immediately following surgery).
- Check bed cradle and 4-point restraints to prevent trauma.
- Hydrate with IV or oral fluids.
- Administer post-op antibiotics as ordered.
- Observe for difficulties following catheter removal (removed separately beginning on the 5th–10th day post-op).

Evaluation: The child has clean, dry wound; maintains patency of suprapubic catheter.

Goal 3: Child will not retain urine.

Plan/Implementation
- Encourage child to void in a continuous stream and to empty bladder completely.
- Observe and record amount, color, and frequency of each voided specimen.

Evaluation: Child empties bladder completely with each void.

Goal 4: Child and parents will understand methods to prevent problems.

Plan/Implementation
- Teach child and family correct administration of antibiotics.
- Teach regarding general health measures to prevent urinary tract infections. (e.g., no bubble baths, empty bladder completely).

Evaluation: Child and parents list and follow measures to prevent further infections.

☐ Nephritis

1. General Information

a. Definition: acute glymerulonephritis (AGN) is an immune complex disease that occurs as a reaction to the group A beta-hemolytic *streptococcus*. It causes inflammation and transient damage to the glomerulus. There is a latent period of 10–14 days between the streptococcal infection and the onset of symptoms.

b. Incidence: peak age is 6–7 years; history of URI, scarlet fever, or impetigo 1–3 weeks prior to the onset of symptoms; 2 times higher incidence in boys

c. Medical treatment

1) bedrest until hypertension and hematuria subside

2) medication

a) antibiotics (penicillin) to eradicate strep infection (indicated by an elevated antistreptolysin-O [ASO] titer)

b) antihypertensives and diuretics to control BP (diuretics are of limited value since they do not reach the distal tubules)

c) digitalis (with congestive heart failure)

d) anticonvulsants (with hypertensive encephalopathy)

3) diet

a) fluid restriction for cardiac failure or anuria

b) moderate sodium restriction

c) low potassium until urine output is normal

d) regular protein diet

2. Nursing Process

a. Assessment/Analysis

1) moderate edema

2) elevated BP

3) moderate proteinuria (rarely seen)

4) gross hematuria

5) elevated serum K^+

6) mild hypoproteinemia

7) elevated urine specific gravity

8) ASO titer

b. Plans, Implementation, and Evaluation

Goal 1: Child will be free from infection and hematuria.

Plan/Implementation
- Monitor temperature.
- Keep child away from infected persons.
- Administer antibiotics as ordered.
- Teach parents administration, action, and side effects of medications.
- Record frequency of urinary output; hematest each voided specimen.
- Measure I&O.
- Restrict fluids if anuria is present.

Evaluation: Child has vital signs and lab values within normal ranges; has normal urine output.

Goal 2: Child will regain/maintain good nutrition within dietary limitations.

Plan/Implementation
- Offer regular diet or low protein and low sodium diet if ordered.
- Offer small, frequent, attractive meals.
- Restrict fluids if anuria is present.
- Restrict high potassium foods during oliguria.

Evaluation: Child ingests a diet adequate for age.

Goal 3: Child will maintain normal tissue perfusion.

Plan/Implementation
- Monitor vital signs, especially BP.
- Monitor urinary output.
- Observe skin color.
- Assess changes in edema by weighing daily.
- Monitor arterial pulses.
- Administer antihypertensives as ordered.
- Keep environment calm.

Evaluation: Child is free from renal failure or cardiac decompensation; maintains BP within normal range.

Goal 4: Child and family will be prepared for home care.

Plan/Implementation
- Let family verbalize concerns.
- Refer to support groups as necessary.
- Teach the family about
  - urine testing

- side effects of drugs
- diet therapies

■ Plan follow-up care.
■ Culture throats of each family member for strep.

Evaluation: Child and family accurately describe discharge instructions in their own words.

☐ Nephrosis

1. General Information

a. Definition: a chronic condition characterized by glomerular membrane permeability to proteins, especially albumin; also called nephrotic syndrome

b. Causes
- **1)** idiopathic (80% of cases)
- **2)** congenital
- **3)** drug toxicity
- **4)** sequelae of various diseases

c. Peak age: 2–5 years; 60% are boys

d. Medical treatment
- **1)** activity as tolerated unless edematous, then bedrest
- **2)** medication
  - **a)** prednisone to reduce proteinuria and edema, to induce remission, to produce diuresis
    - ■ dosage is 2mg/kg/day until urine is free from protein
    - ■ side effects: immonosuppression, potassium loss, gastric ulcer, hypertension, growth failure, Cushing's syndrome
    - ■ nursing implications
      - taper dose gradually to avoid adrenal insufficiency
      - administer with meals or milk to minimize gastric irritation
      - monitor fluid balance
      - protect from infection
  - **b)** antibiotics to decrease risk of infection
  - **c)** IV salt-poor albumin during acute phase
- **3)** diet
  - **a)** fluid, sodium restriction if edema present
  - **b)** high protein, high potassium

2. Nursing Process

a. Assessment/Analysis
- **1)** insidious weight gain
- **2)** severe edema
  - **a)** periorbital, facial
  - **b)** generalized: feet, scrotal/labial, ascites
- **3)** respiratory difficulty due to pleural effusion
- **4)** oliguria, increased urine specific gravity
- **5)** massive proteinuria
- **6)** marked hypoproteinemia
- **7)** hyperlipidemia
- **8)** irritability
- **9)** increased susceptibility to infection
- **10)** anorexia
- **11)** diarrhea

b. Plans, Implementation, and Evaluation

Goal 1: Child will be free from infection, skin breakdown.

Plan/Implementation
■ Monitor vital signs and lab values.
■ Keep child away from infected persons.
■ Administer antibiotics as ordered.
■ Give medications by mouth if possible.
■ Teach parents administration, action, and side effects of medications.
■ Give good skin care.
■ Support edematous organs (utilize scrotal support if needed with pillows or a rolled towel).
■ Change body position often.
■ Cleanse edematous eyelids with saline wipes.
■ Place in a semi-Fowler's position to facilitate breathing.
■ Handle gently with any movement.

Evaluation: Child has intact skin; has normal vital signs, lab values.

Goal 2: Child will conserve energy and play quiet activities suitable for age.

Plan/Implementation
■ Balance rest and activities; maintain bedrest with edema.
■ Provide quiet activities for age.
■ Observe for fatigue.
■ Explain reasons for bedrest.

Evaluation: Child tolerates play activities without fatigue.

Goal 3: Child will maintain fluid balance.

Plan/Implementation
■ Measure I&O; weigh diapers.
■ Weigh and measure abdominal girth daily.
■ Assess changes in edema each shift.
■ Limit fluids if necessary.

Evaluation: Child has no generalized edema, increased abdominal girth; maintains urine output, balanced I&O.

Goal 4: Child will maintain nutritional intake.

Plan/Implementation
- Offer high-protein, high-carbohydrate, high-potassium diet.
- Restrict sodium intake if edematous.
- Serve small, frequent, attractive meals.

Evaluation: Child eats an adequate diet for age within dietary restrictions.

Goal 5: Child will accept body changes.

Plan/Implementation
- Provide feedback re body changes; reassure as needed.
- Encourage verbalization of feelings about body changes.
- Teach that changes are caused by medications and will diminish when medications are discontinued.

Evaluation: Child expresses feelings about body changes, capitalizes on positive aspects of self, looks forward to discontinuing medications.

Goal 6: Child and family will be prepared for home care.

Plan/Implementation
- Let family verbalize concerns.
- Refer to support groups as needed.
- Teach about
  - urine testing
  - side effects of drugs
  - prevention of infection
  - diet therapies
- Maintain follow-up contact with the family.

Evaluation: Child and family describe discharge instructions correctly.

☐ Lower GI Tract Obstruction

1. General Information

a. Definitions

1) *intussusception*: telescoping of one portion of intestine into another usually involving ileocecal valve, resulting in obstruction of blood supply with ischemia and death of telescoped portion; one of the most common causes of intestinal obstruction in infancy; most cases occur in children under 2 years of age; 3 times more common in boys; higher incidence in children with cystic fibrosis and celiac disease

2) *Hirschsprung's disease* (aganglionic megacolon): congenital absence of parasympathetic ganglia of distal colon and rectum, resulting in inadequate peristalsis; stool and flatus accumulate in colon proximal to defect, causing dilatation and hypertrophy of bowel; usually diagnosed in neonatal period or early infancy; 4 times more common in boys; higher incidence in children with Down syndrome

b. Medical treatment

1) *intussusception*

a) hydrostatic reduction with barium enema before bowel becomes necrotic

b) if bowel necrosis has occurred, surgical intervention: resection and anastomosis

2) *Hirschsprung's disease*

a) barium enema to aid diagnosis

b) rectal biopsy to confirm absence of ganglion cells

c) resection of aganglionic portion of bowel, temporary colostomy of sigmoid or transverse colon to rest bowel and restore nutritional balance; abdominal-perineal pull-through anastomosis at approximately 1 year of age

2. Nursing Process

a. Assessment/Analysis

1) *intussusception:* acute, recurrent, episodic, severe, colicky abdominal pain; "currant jelly" stools containing blood and mucus, caused by bowel gangrene (occurs about 12 hours after onset of abdominal pain); palpable sausage-shaped mass in right upper quadrant

2) *Hirschsprung's disease*

a) delayed passage of meconium in newborn; failure to thrive

b) chronic constipation

c) ribbonlike, foul-smelling stools

d) breath has foul odor

e) severe abdominal distention with shortness of breath

f) at risk for enterocolitis, which increases risk of fatality

3) both

a) bile-stained vomiting (the obstruction is below ampulla of Vater which empties bile into duodenum)

b) abdominal distention

b. Plans, Implementation, and Evaluation

Goal 1: Child will maintain adequate hydration and nutrition, and regain normal elimination.

Plan/Implementation

- Give IV fluids as ordered; hyperalimentation may be ordered for infants with Hirschsprung's disease.
- Usually keep NPO: give mouth care, pacifier.
- Keep accurate I&O; measure and record drainage (NG, colostomy); irrigate NG tube as ordered.
- Assess bowel sounds frequently.
- Take axillary temperature only.
- Gradually reintroduce feedings and return to normal diet post-op after NG tube has been removed and bowel sounds have returned.

Evaluation: Child is adequately hydrated (elastic skin turgor, moist mucous membranes, etc.), has adequate caloric intake; returns to normal diet without complications (e.g., vomiting); is free from abdominal distention and establishes normal bowel elimination postoperatively.

Goal 2: Child with colostomy/ileostomy will have intact, functioning stoma without irritation or infection.

Plan/Implementation

- Refer to "Mechanical Obstruction of the Colon" page 264.
- Instruct child/parent on stoma care
  - diaper only may be used in infants with sigmoid colostomy
  - select appliance that fits child's size, activity level, and development
  - use hypoallergenic supplies as children's skin tends to be more sensitive
  - encourage self-care
    - * by 6–7 years, should be able to remove and reapply pouch with assistance
    - * by 10–11 years, able to assume all responsibility
- Inspect stoma daily for redness, irritation, or breakdown.
- Do not submerge colostomy in bath water.
- Refer parents to local ostomy association for assistance and support.

Evaluation: Child has healthy, functioning stoma; becomes involved in developmentally appropriate self-care.

References

James, S., & Mott, S. (1988). *Child Health Nursing*. Menlo Park, CA: Addison-Wesley.

Marlow, D., & Redding, B. (1988). *Textbook of Pediatric Nursing* (6th ed.). Philadelphia: Saunders.

Servonsky, J., & Opas, S. (1987). *Nursing Management of Children*. Boston: Jones & Bartlett.

Scipien, G., et al. (1986). *Comprehensive Pediatric Nursing*. New York: McGraw Hill.

Siegel, S., et al. (1980). Urinary infections in infants and preschool children. *American Journal of the Disabled Child*, *134*, 369–372.

Smith, M., et al. (1987). *Child and Family*. New York: McGraw-Hill.

Whaley, L., & Wong, D. (1987). *Nursing Care of Infants and Children*. St. Louis, MO: Mosby.

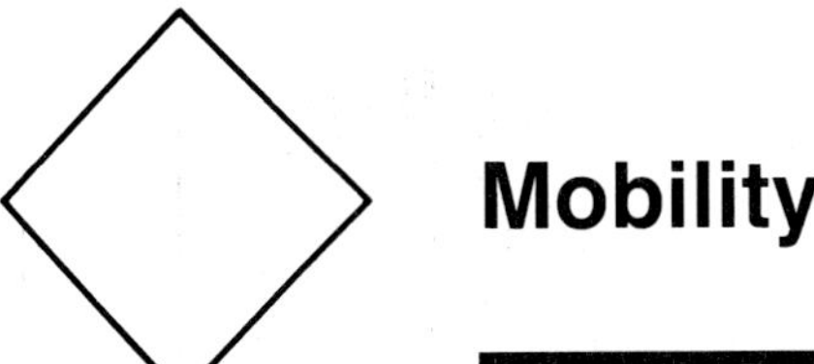

Mobility

General Concepts

Overview/Physiology

1. Skeletal maturation
   a. Accurate "bone age" is determined by x-ray of ossification centers
   b. Correlates closely with other measures of physiologic maturity (e.g., onset of menarche) rather than with height or chronologic age
   c. Complete when epiphysis fuses completely with diaphysis, usually 18–21 years of age (earlier in girls than boys)
2. Differences in children's skeletal system compared with the adults'
   a. Thick periosteum: stronger, more active osteogenic potential
   b. More plastic (pliable) bone: more porous, allows bending and buckling; this flexibility diffuses and absorbs a significant amount of the force of impact
   c. Rapid healing: decreases as child gets older (younger bones can be remolded more easily)
   d. Stiffness is unusual, even after lengthy immobilization

Application of the Nursing Process to the Child with an Interference with Mobility

1. **Assessment**
   a. Nursing injury
      1) development of motor skills: delays, recent changes or interferences
      2) signs and symptoms of current health problem: pain, altered structure or mobility
   b. Clinical appraisal
      1) muscle strength and symmetry
      2) balance, gait, and posture
      3) range-of-motion
      4) obvious structural deformities or functional deficits
   c. Radiologic tests of affected body part (refer to *Nursing Care of the Adult* page 294)
2. **Analysis**
   a. Safe, effective care environment
      1) potential for injury
      2) knowledge deficit
      3) potential for infection
   b. Physiological integrity
      1) potential for aspiration
      2) impaired physical mobility
      3) potential altered peripheral tissue perfusion
   c. Psychological integrity
      1) body image disturbance
      2) social isolation
      3) altered role performance
   d. Health promotion/maintenance
      1) altered growth and development
      2) diversional activity deficit
      3) bathing/hygiene self-care deficit
3. **General Nursing Plans, Implementation, and Evaluation**

Goal 1: Child's deformity will be detected and treated early.

Plan/Implementation
- Screen child for skeletal deformity
  - in newborn period for congenital clubfoot and congenital hip dysplasia
  - during preadolescence and adolescence for scoliosis
- Refer child with possible deformity for immediate treatment.
- Teach child/parents the importance of adhering to prescribed treatment plan to minimize or prevent serious, permanent deformity.
- Stress importance of continued follow-up care to prevent recurrence.

Evaluation: Child will maintain correct alignment of the affected body part during the period of treatment.

Goal 2: Child will maintain correct alignment of the affected body part during the period of treatment.

Plan/Implementation
- Teach child/parents prescribed exercises, application of splints or brace, cast care.

- Provide care for child in traction (see Table 5.21, Figure 5.4)
  - maintain traction apparatus (elastic bandages, splints, rings, ropes, pulleys, weights)
  - do *NOT* allow weights to rest on floor or bed
  - maintain correct body alignment
  - elevate head or foot of bed as needed to provide correct pull and countertraction
  - assess skin color, sensation, movement of extremity at least every 4 hours
- Provide care for child in cast
  - use palms of hands when handling wet cast
  - keep cast elevated and exposed to air to dry
  - "petal" cast edges (protects cast and skin); use waterproof adhesive tape petals (see Figure 5.5)
  - protect cast from being soiled with urine or stool (position child with buttocks lower than shoulders during toileting)
  - use Bradford frame for smaller children
  - provide toys too large to fit down cast
  - stay with child during mealtimes
  - observe for signs of impaired circulation and infection (fever, lethargy, foul odor), do *NOT* rely on child to verbalize discomfort; change position frequently; do *NOT* use abduction-stabilizer bar on hip spica as a handle for turning child

Evaluation: Child maintains correct alignment of affected body part; has permanent deformity prevented; child/parents provide appropriate care of child in cast, splint, or brace.

Goal 3: Child's skin integrity will be maintained during period of immobilization.

Plan/Implementation

- Assess for areas of skin breakdown.
- Change position frequently or encourage movement within limitations imposed by traction, cast, or brace to relieve pressure.
- Check pin sites (skeletal traction) for bleeding, redness, edema, infection.
- Provide pin care as needed.
- Monitor circulation of affected extremities (normal skin color, blanches easily, warm to touch, able to wiggle fingers and toes, peripheral pulses present).
- Give meticulous skin care to areas near edges of cast or in contact with brace or traction apparatus.

Evaluation: Child's skin integrity is maintained; circulation is maintained; child is free from skin breakdown/infection.

Goal 4: Child's developmental progress will be maintained during immobilization (brace, cast, or traction).

Plan/Implementation

- Provide age-appropriate stimulation, activity.

Table 5.21 Types of Traction

General	
Skin traction	Direct pull to skin surface and indirect pull to skeletal structures by means of adhesive strips or elastic bandage
Skeletal traction	Direct pull to skeletal structures by means of pin, wire, or tongs inserted into bone distal to fracture
Specific	
Bryant's traction	Unidirectional, lower extremity skin traction with child's hips flexed at 90° angle, knees extended, and legs and buttocks suspended
Buck's extension	Skin traction to lower extremity with hips and legs extended. Used mostly when short term traction is needed.
Russell traction	Two-directional, lower extremity skin traction with padded knee sling; immobilizes hip and knee in flexed position. One pull line is longitudinal; the other is perpendicular to leg. Traction pull is twice the amount of weight applied.
Balance suspension with Thomas ring splint and Pearson attachment	Two-directional, skin or skeletal traction that suspends leg with hip slightly flexed; Thomas ring circles uppermost portion of the thigh while Pearson attachment supports lower part of leg. Alignment is maintained even when child lifts off bed.
Halo-femoral traction	Metal rings (halo) are attached to the skull and pins are inserted into distal femur also. Progressive traction is applied upward to the halo and downward to the distal end of the femur, increasing weights twice daily until alignment is achieved.

Figure 5.4 Types of Traction

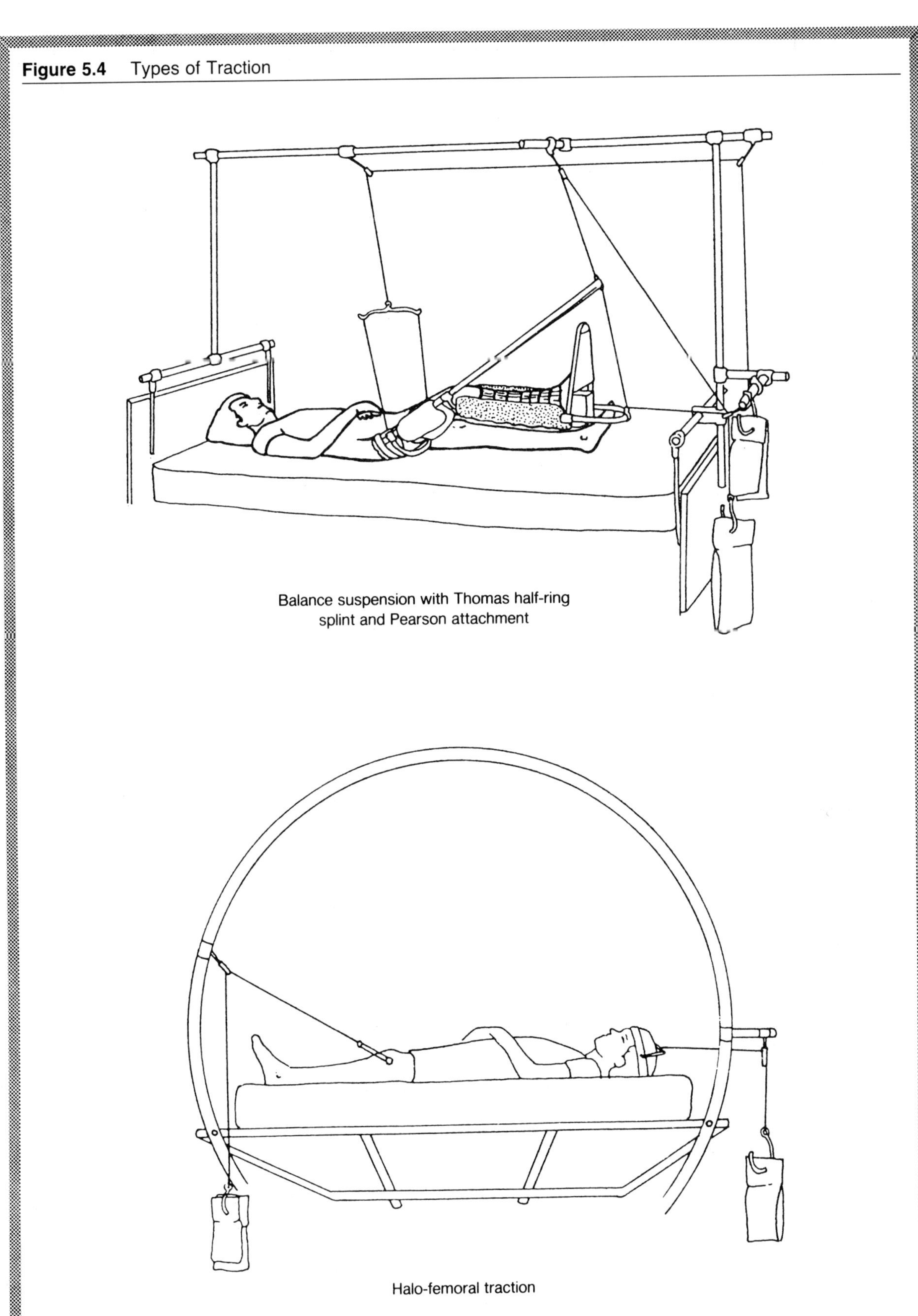

Balance suspension with Thomas half-ring splint and Pearson attachment

Halo-femoral traction

Figure 5.4 Continued

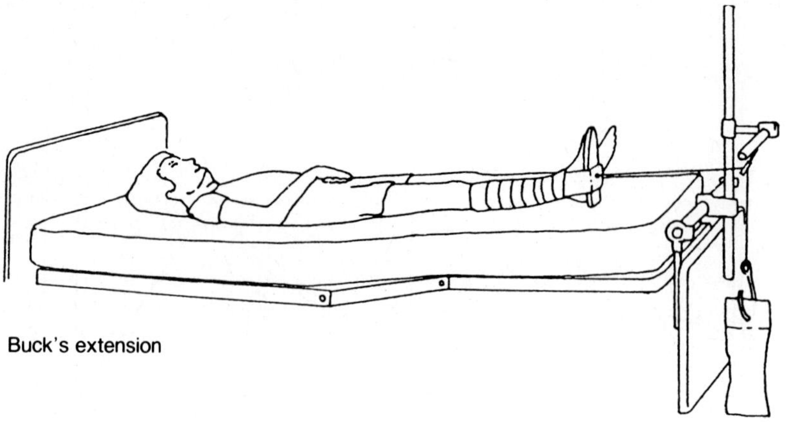

Buck's extension

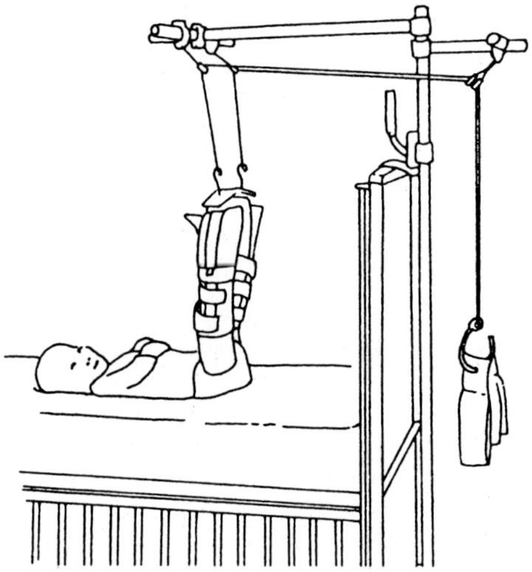

Bryant's traction

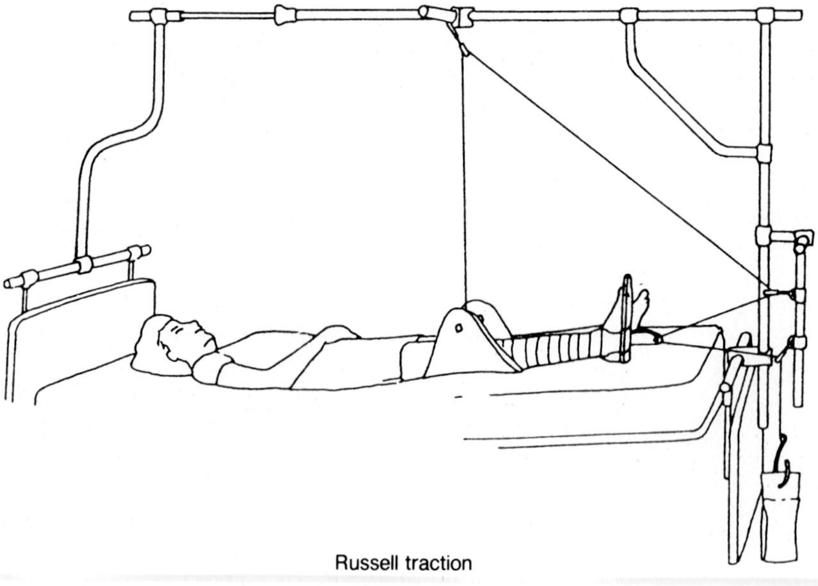

Russell traction

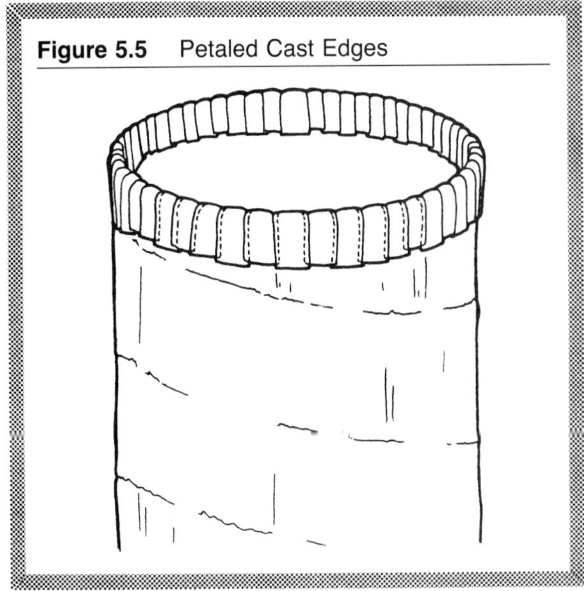
Figure 5.5 Petaled Cast Edges

- Encourage child to participate in own daily care and maintain control as much as possible.
- Provide for child to maintain educational progress while immobilized (hospital teacher, homebound teacher, daily contact with regular teacher).
- Arrange for and encourage interaction with peers, siblings if child is hospitalized or confined to home.

Evaluation: Child maintains developmental and educational progress while immobilized; has no developmental delays; participates in own care.

Selected Health Problems Resulting in an Interference with Mobility

☐ Congenital Clubfoot

1. General Information

a. Definition: congenital skeletal deformity of the foot. The most common type is talipes equinovarus (95% of cases), characterized by inversion and plantar flexion (directed inward and downward) of foot; may be unilateral or bilateral.

b. Incidence
  1) boys are affected twice as often as girls
  2) unilateral is slightly more common than bilateral
  3) frequency: 1:1,000 in general population

c. Medical treatment
  1) early correction: successive casts until foot is manipulated into an overcorrected position, followed by Denis Browne splint (metal crossbar with shoes on opposite feet) to maintain correction
  2) mild clubfoot: passive stretching exercises several times per day or a Denis Browne splint
  3) later correction in older child or for recurrent clubfoot: surgical intervention (tendon transfer, arthrodesis) followed by casting, corrective shoes

2. Nursing Process

a. **Assessment/Analysis:** differentiate true clubfoot from positional deformity
  1) true clubfoot cannot be passively manipulated into an overcorrected position
  2) positional deformity can be passively corrected or overcorrected

b. **Plans, Implementation, and Evaluation** (see General Nursing Plans page 605)

☐ Congenital Hip Dysplasia

1. General Information

a. Definitions
  1) *subluxation*: head of femur is partially displaced but remains in contact with acetabulum
  2) *complete dislocation of hip*: head of femur is completely displaced

b. Incidence
  1) 70% are female
  2) unilateral twice as common as bilateral
  3) frequency: 1 in 500
  4) highest incidence in Eskimo and American Indian cultures where infants are swaddled tightly; lowest incidence in cultures where infants are carried with legs abducted on mother's hip

c. Medical treatment
  1) newborn: double or tripole diapering
  2) infant: Frejka pillow splint, Von Rosen splint
  3) toddler: Bryant's or Russell traction, followed by hip spica cast or open reduction and casting
  4) preschooler: combination of traction, open reduction, osteotomy, tendonotomy, casting: more difficult to treat because of secondary changes in hip joint
  5) school age or older: total hip replacement when older; because of severe muscle shortening and bone deformity, may no longer be amenable to treatment

2. Nursing Process

a. Assessment/Analysis

1) *infant*
   a) limited abduction of affected hip
   b) wide perineum
   c) shortening of leg on affected side
   d) asymmetry of thigh and gluteal folds
   e) positive Ortolani's sign: clicking when leg abducted, caused by femoral head slipping over acetabulum
2) *older child*
   a) Trendelenburg's sign: when child stands on affected leg, pelvis tilts downward on unaffected side instead of upward
   b) limp on affected side
   c) flattening of buttock on affected side

b. Plans, Implementation, and Evaluation (see General Nursing Plans page 605)

☐ Legg-Calvé-Perthes Disease

1. General Information

a. Definition: self-limiting avascular necrosis of the femoral head; untreated, the head becomes flattened and deformed, resulting in permanent disability

b. Incidence
   1) onset usually between 3 and 11 years of age
   2) 4 times more common in boys
   3) usually unilateral; 15% bilateral
   4) possible familial tendency

c. Medical treatment: the earlier the age of onset, the better the results of treatment
   1) bedrest and skin traction to the limb during the painful initial period
   2) some weight bearing allowed after resolution of the initial stage of the disease; use of abduction braces, casts, or hip sling
   3) full weight bearing if no new dense areas develop in femoral head in 2 months
   4) surgical osteotomy of femur done if medical management is ineffective

2. Nursing Process

a. Assessment/Analysis

1) hip, groin or thigh pain
2) referred knee pain
3) limp
4) limited motion—abduction and internal rotation
5) atrophy of thigh muscles from disuse

b. Plans, Implementation, and Evaluation see General Nursing Plans page 605)

☐ Scoliosis

1. General Information

a. Definition: lateral curvature of the spine, which results in structural and functional alterations in spine, chest, and pelvis

b. Incidence
   1) 15% of children between ages 10–21 are affected
   2) 7 times more common in adolescent females
   3) 70% of cases are idiopathic (i.e., without apparent cause)

c. Medical treatment
   1) medical intervention
      a) exercises (for curvatures less than 20°)
      b) braces, casts, traction (for curvatures 20°–40°)
         - Milwaukee brace (most common, most effective)
         - Risser plaster jacket/cast
         - halofemoral or halopelvic traction (continuous or intermittent)
   2) surgical intervention: spinal fusion with Harrington rods, or Laque wires, Dwyer instrumentation, followed by application of body cast/brace (for curvatures greater than 40°)

2. Nursing Process

a. Assessment/Analysis

1) spinal curve may be obvious
2) elevated shoulder or hip
3) structural asymmetry (scapulae, waist, shoulders, breasts)
4) rib hump apparent when child bends at waist

b. Plans, Implementation, and Evaluation

Goal: Adolescent and family will adjust to lengthy treatment regimen.

Plan/Implementation
- Allow adolescent and parents to express feelings and concerns about long-term bracing or casting (6 months to 3 years for medical intervention)
- Help adolescent cope with altered body image
  - emphasize and enhance positive attributes (hair, makeup)
  - help with selection of attractive camouflage clothing

- encourage involvement in appropriate activities (choir, school clubs, etc.)

■ Demonstrate alternative ways of getting in and out of bed, dressing, etc.

■ Advise standing at drafting table or easel for homework.

■ Teach application and removal of brace (must wear 23 hours/day; remove for 1 hour for hygiene or swimming).

■ Teach adolescent to wear T-shirt under brace.

■ Check for loosening of brace; tighten as necessary.

■ Keep brace clean: wash plastic with soap and water, clean leather with saddle soap.

■ Provide for needs of adolescent following surgical intervention (spinal fusion)
- keep bed flat; logroll q2h
- assess circulatory and neurologic status in legs and feet
- administer analgesics for pain
- monitor incision sites for bleeding and signs of infection
- monitor respiratory status
- cough and deep breathe; use inspirometer

Evaluation: Child with scoliosis copes with treatment regimen and altered body image; recovers from surgery free from complications; is free from permanent disability.

☐ Osteomyelitis

1. General Information

a. Definition: rapid-onset bacterial infection of the bone and its marrow; metaphyseal area of the long bones in the arms and legs is affected; causes bone destruction and formation of abscesses; *Staphylococcus aureus* is causative organism in 80%–90% of cases

b. Incidence

1) most frequent in school-age children (5–14 years)

2) boys affected 2–3 times more often than girls

3) poor physical health, inadequate nutrition, and unsanitary environmental conditions are predisposing factors

c. Medical treatment

1) medical intervention

a) intravenous antibiotic therapy for 3–4 weeks; penicillin G (large doses) in conjunction with methicillin or oxacillin

b) bedrest with immobilization of affected extremity

c) splint or bivalved cast to immobilize affected extremity

2) surgical intervention: surgical drainage with insertion of polyethylene tubes in wound for antibiotic instillation

2. Nursing Process

a. Assessment/Analysis

1) fever

2) elevated pulse

3) localized tenderness, warmth, redness, and swelling over affected area of bone

4) limited, painful movement

5) diagnostic tests

a) elevated WBC count

b) positive blood and wound cultures

c) elevated ESR (erythrocyte sedimentation rate)

b. Plans, Implementation, and Evaluation

Goal 1: Child's wound will heal; child will recover from illness free from complications.

Plan/Implementation

■ Carefully administer prescribed antibiotics (IV, wound).

■ Provide wound care (irrigations, dressings, medications) as ordered.

■ Encourage a nutritious diet (high calorie, high protein).

■ Maintain immobilization (positioning, cast, splint).

Evaluation: Child's wound heals; has uneventful recovery.

Goal 2: Child will experience minimal pain/discomfort.

Plan/Implementation

■ Assist child to achieve comfortable positions while immobilized.

■ Check splint or cast for correct fit.

■ Provide age-appropriate diversional activities.

■ Administer prescribed analgesics as needed.

Evaluation: Child experiences minimal discomfort during period of treatment.

References

Davis, S., & Lewis, S. (1984). Managing scoliosis: Fashions for the body and mind. *MCN: American Journal of Maternal/Child Nursing*, 9(3), 186–187.

James, S., & Mott, S. (1988). *Child health nursing: Essential care of children and families*. Reading, MA: Addison-Wesley.

Mather, L.S. (1987). The secret to life in a spica. *American Journal of Nursing*, *87*, 56–58.

Mott, S., Fazekas, N., & James, S. (1985). *Nursing care of children and families: A holistic approach.* Menlo Park, CA: Addison-Wesley.

Muller, D. (1984). Harnessing babies' dysplastic hips. *American Journal of Nursing*, *84*, 1006–1008.

Scipien, G., et al. (1986). *Comprehensive pediatric nursing* (3rd ed.). New York: McGraw-Hill.

Servonsky, J., & Opas, S. (1987). *Nursing management of children.* Boston: Jones & Bartlett.

Waechter, E., Phillips, J., & Holaday, B. (1985). *Nursing care of children* (10th ed.). Philadelphia: Lippincott.

Whaley, L., & Wong, D. (1986). *Nursing care of infants and children* (3rd ed.). St. Louis: Mosby.

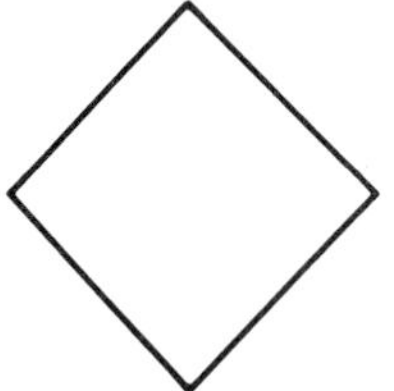

Cellular Aberration (Childhood Cancer)

General Concepts (see also *Nursing Care of the Adult* page 306)

Overview/Physiology

1. Cancer is the leading cause of death from disease between the ages of 3 and 15
   a. Leukemias and lymphomas account for over 40% of childhood malignancies
   b. Brain tumors account for 20% of childhood cancers
   c. Embryonal tumors (e.g., Wilms' tumor and neuroblastoma) and sarcomas account for another 20% of childhood malignancies
   d. The survival rate for childhood cancer has dramatically increased in the last two decades, especially for acute lymphocytic leukemia
2. Differences in childhood cancers as compared with adult cancers
   a. Higher incidence of embryonal tumors
   b. Occur more frequently in rapidly growing tissues, such as bone marrow
   c. Higher rate of metastasis
3. Medical treatment
   a. Surgery: excision of all or part of solid tumors; may only be palliative if cancer has metastasized; most successful with localized and encapsulated tumors
   b. Chemotherapy: administration of antineoplastic drugs
      1) classification
         a) cell-cycle specific: destroys cells in specific phases of cell division
            - most effective for rapidly growing cells
            - least toxic
            - examples: cytosine arabinoside, methotrexate
         b) cell-cycle nonspecific: destroys cells at any phase
            - most effective for slow-growing, solid tumors
            - examples: alkylating agents, hormones, antibiotics, nitrosureas
         c) cytotoxic action (see Table 5.22 for specific drugs)
            - alkylating agents: alkyl group; replaces hydrogen atom, causing cell to die
            - antimetabolites: similar to essential elements needed for cell growth, but in altered form; prevents synthesis of DNA or RNA
            - plant alkaloids: stop cell growth in metaphase
            - antitumor antibiotics: interfere with cell division by reacting with DNA and RNA
            - hormones, adrenocorticosteroids: depress mitosis of lymphoid cells; androgens and estrogens are used for breast and prostatic cancers, probably affecting growth regulation
            - miscellaneous agents: enzymes, such as L-asparaginase, hydroxyurea, nitrosureas; metals such as cis-platinum
      2) combination chemotherapy: two or more drugs used simultaneously; each drug has a different effect on cell growth; increases effectiveness, decreases resistance of cancer cells to drugs
   c. Irradiation: frequently used in childhood cancers as an adjunct to surgery and/or chemotherapy; may be curative or palliative

Application of the Nursing Process to the Child with Cancer

1. **Assessment**
   a. Nursing history (see *Nursing Care of the Adult* page 307)
   b. Clinical appraisal: physical findings will vary according to the type of cancer
   c. Diagnostic tests: same as for adult except that bone marrow aspiration is usually performed on the posterior iliac crest
2. **Analysis**
   a. Safe, effective care environment

Table 5.22 Commonly Used Chemotherapeutic Agents

Drug	Uses	Side Effects	Specific Nursing Concerns
Alkylating Agents			
	Hodgkin's and other lymphomas Leukemias Neuroblastomas Retinoblastomas Multiple myeloma	Nausea and vomiting Bone-marrow depression Alopecia	
Cyclophosphamide (Cytoxan)			Chemical cystitis may result; force fluids, report burning or hematuria.
Mechlorethamine nitrogen mustard, Mustargen)			Use immediately after reconstitution. Avoid vapors in eyes; if solution comes into contact with skin, flush with liberal amounts of water. Ensure IV is in place to prevent necrosis and sloughing.
Chlorambucil (Leukeran)			Side effects occur slowly and with high doses.
Cis-platinum			Toxic to kidneys and ears; can cause anaphylaxis. Hydrate well before and during treatment with IVs and mannitol. Monitor renal function and audiograms.
Antimetabolites			
	Acute lymphocytic leukemia, acute myelocytic leukemia, brain tumors, ovarian, breast, prostatic, testicular cancers	Mild to moderate nausea and vomiting Bone-marrow depression Stomatitis Dermatitis	
5-Fluorouracil (5FU, Adrucil)			Chronic nausea and vomiting with prolonged use. Check oral mucosa. If stomatitis and diarrhea are severe, stop drug. When outdoors, use sun screen.
Methotrexate (Mexate)			Toxic to liver, kidney. Avoid aspirin, sulfonamides, and tetracycline while on drug. Avoid vitamins containing folic acid. Leukovorin used as an antidote for high doses, "Leukovorin rescue."
6 Mercaptopurine (6-MP)			Give allopurinol concurrently to inhibit uric acid production from cell destruction, thus increasing drug's potency.
Cytosine arabinoside (Ara-C, Cytosar)			Crosses blood-brain barrier. May be hepatotoxic; monitor liver function.

Table 5.22 Continued

Drug	Uses	Side Effects	Specific Nursing Concerns
Plant Alkaloids	Acute lymphocytic leukemia, Hodgkin's, Wilms' tumor, sarcomas, breast cancer, testicular cancer	Minimal nausea and vomiting Alopecia Neurotoxic	
Vincristine (Oncovin)			Monitor for neurotoxicity: reflexes, weakness, parasthesias, jaw pain, constipation. Check IV placement to prevent cellulitis.
Vinblastine (Velban)			Headaches; less neurotoxic than vincristine.
Antitumor Antibiotics	Sarcomas, neuroblastoma, head and neck tumors, testicular, ovarian, breast cancer	Severe nausea and vomiting Stomatitis Diarrhea Bone-marrow depression	
Actinomycin D (Dactinomycin)			Used for Wilms' tumor; enhances effects of radiation (also increases toxicity). Extravasation can cause necrosis; maintain patent IV.
Doxorubicin hydrochloride (Adriamycin)			Monitor for cardiac dysrhythmias (cardiotoxicity is irreversible). Caution that urine turns red.
Hormones			
Adrenal cortical steroids Prednisone Dexamethosone (Decadron)	Leukemia, Hodgkin's, breast cancer, lymphomas, multiple myeloma, cerebral edema caused by brain metastasis	See Table 3.26.	See Table 3.26.
Androgens Testosterone (Oreton) Fluoxymesterone (Halotestin)	Breast cancer in postmenopausal women	Fluid retention Nausea Masculinization	Give low-salt diet; provide psychologic support for masculinization effects.
Estrogens Diethylstilbesterol (DES) Ethinyl estradiol (Estinyl)	Prostatic cancer, breast cancer that is estrogen-receptor-positive in postmenopausal women	Fluid retention Feminization Gynecomastia in males	Give low-salt diet; provide psychologic support to males experiencing feminization.
Antiestrogens Tamoxifen (Nolvadex)	Breast cancer; prostatic cancer	Hot flashes Generally mild nausea	
Miscellaneous Agents			
Enzymes L-asparaginase	Leukemias, Hodgkin's	Severe nausea and vomiting; fever Liver dysfunction Anaphylaxis	Monitor BUN and serum ammonia levels. Observe for allergic reaction (have epinephrine 1:1,000 at bedside).

1) potential for infection
2) potential for injury
3) impaired home maintenance management

b. Physiological integrity
1) pain
2) diarrhea, constipation
3) fluid volume deficit

c. Psychological integrity
1) fear
2) social isolation
3) ineffective individual coping

d. Health promotion/maintenance
1) knowledge deficit
2) altered parenting
3) altered growth and development

3. General Nursing Plans, Implementation, and Evaluation

Goal 1: Child/family will be prepared for diagnostic tests.

Plan/Implementation

- Provide age-appropriate explanation of procedure (what will happen, what it will feel like, what child is expected to do).
- Give parents option of staying with child during procedure so they can provide needed emotional support to child.
- Hold child firmly during procedure to facilitate needle insertion (e.g., bone-marrow aspiration, LP).
- Reassure child throughout procedure.
- After the procedure, provide child opportunities to express feelings (verbally, through therapeutic play).
- Provide positive feedback to child concerning child's cooperation during the procedure.

Evaluation: Child copes with diagnostic procedures; cooperates with procedure; expresses feelings during and after procedure.

Goal 2: Child/family will be prepared for surgery (refer to "Ill and Hospitalized Child" page 529).

Goal 3: Child/family will be prepared for chemotherapy.

Plan/Implementation

- Explain benefits of chemotherapy, using terms the child and family can understand.
- Reinforce physician's explanation of types of chemotherapy child will receive.
- Explain side effects that may occur and identify measures that will help lessen side effects
  - nausea and vomiting: administer antiemetics prior to chemotherapy
  - diarrhea: administer antispasmodics, adjust diet
  - anorexia: monitor weight; provide soft diet, small frequent feedings, favorite foods and liquids, give choices
  - stomatitis (see Goal 6)
  - alopecia: provide wig, scarf, hat as desired
  - fatigue: provide frequent rest periods, encourage quiet activities

Evaluation: Child/family list side effects; implement measures that minimize these effects and promote child's comfort.

Goal 4: Child/family will be prepared for radiation therapy.

Plan/Implementation

- Reinforce reasons for and benefits of radiation.
- Prepare for and manage side effects of radiation therapy.
  - nausea and vomiting: administer prescribed antiemetics as needed, bland diet, clear liquids
  - peeling skin: meticulous skin care; avoid direct exposure to sun; do not wash off skin markings (dark purple lines that define area to be irradiated)
  - risk of fracture: explain to child/family why child should avoid weight bearing; help plan to meet child's need for mobility through alternative means, such as crutches or stimulating activities while on bedrest
  - delays in physical development: discuss possible outcomes with parents and child (as appropriate) such as pathologic fractures, spinal deformities, growth retardation, sterility, delayed appearance of secondary sex characteristics, chromosomal damage

Evaluation: Child/family state reasons for radiation and knowledge of side effects that may occur.

Goal 5: Child will be free from infection.

Plan/Implementation

- Maintain reverse isolation, or private room with strict handwashing if child is severely immunosuppressed.
- Prevent contact with anyone with infection.
- Rinse mouth regularly before meals, after meals, and q4h (removes debris as a source for growth of bacteria and fungi).
- Administer antibiotics and observe for side effects.

- Take measures to prevent skin breakdown.
- Do not give immunizations until child's immune response is adequate.
- Permit return to school when WBCs approach normal level (2,000/mm^3).

Evaluation: Child is free from infections, such as URIs, thrush, pneumonia; has intact skin.

Goal 6: Child will receive care for ulcerations of mouth and rectal area.

Plan/Implementation

- Provide meticulous oral hygiene before/after meals.
- Offer mouthwash frequently; apply local anesthetic (viscous xylocaine) prn.
- Encourage fluids, nonirritating foods (soft foods, cool drinks).
- Avoid rectal temperatures/suppositories.
- Encourage sitz baths; offer pericare after voiding or BM.
- Expose ulcerated anal area to air and heat.

Evaluation: Child is free from increased ulceration; experiences healing of lesions in mouth and rectum.

Goal 7: Child will ingest foods and fluids to meet nutritional needs.

Plan/Implementation

- Rinse mouth before child eats.
- Offer small, frequent meals.
- Provide soft foods; permit favorite foods child tolerates.
- Use nutritional supplements.

Evaluation: Child ingests fluid and diet as prescribed, including own preferences.

Goal 8. Child's pain will be relieved and comfort promoted.

Plan/Implementation

- Administer nonnarcotic/narcotic analgesics as needed.
- Maintain comfortable body position, turning at least q2h and prn.
- Teach child to focus on TV, music, friend when having pain.
- Provide soothing skin care.

Evaluation: Child experiences relief of pain; is positioned comfortably in bed or chair.

Goal 9: Child's growth and development will be fostered throughout the course of illness and treatment.

Plan/Implementation

- Refer to "Healthy Child" page 517 for developmental needs appropriate to child's age.
- Encourage child to participate in self-care to the extent possible.
- Provide opportunities for child to exercise some control over daily routine (food choices, selection of play activities).
- Maintain child's educational progress as much as possible.
- Maintain child's contact with siblings and friends (through visiting, telephone calls, letters).

Evaluation: Child is free from significant developmental or educational delays; demonstrates age-appropriate skills and behaviors.

Goal 10: Child and family cope with the stresses of living with cancer and its treatment.

Plan/Implementation

- Encourage parents/family to continue to provide care of child as much as desired and possible.
- Encourage expressions of fear, feelings, concerns about cancer and its treatment.
- Refer to parent-support groups (Candlelighters, Compassionate Friends).
- Assess child's understanding of diagnosis and prognosis (see Table 5.23).

Table 5.23 The Child's Concept of Death

Infants and Toddlers

React more to pain and to parents' responses and behaviors than to probability of death; cannot verbalize their understanding; only understand "alive", not "dead"; may persist in ritualistic activities.

Preschool

Death is a kind of sleep, temporary; believe their own illness is punishment; fear painful procedures and being separated from parents.

School-age

6–7 years old: personify death, such as God, devil, "bogeyman"; fear the mutilation of death.

9–10 years old: similar to adult concept; understand death is eventually inevitable and irreversible; fear the unknown about death; need concrete explanations and a chance to share their fears and gain some control.

Adolescents

Have the most difficulty coping with death; have adult cognitive understanding but death is a threat to their identity; fear the physical changes of terminal illness.

- Help child express feelings through play and art.
- Encourage family to treat child as normally as possible (i.e., age-appropriate limit setting and enforcement, avoid excessive gifts or privileges).
- If child's condition becomes terminal, support family as they prepare for child's death; refer for home or hospice care, as appropriate and desired by family.

Evaluation: Child and family cope with child's illness and treatment; parents participate in community support groups as desired, express their fears and feelings about child's illness and prognosis.

Selected Health Problems Resulting From Cellular Aberration

☐ Leukemia

1. General Information

a. Definition: malignant neoplasm of unknown etiology that involves all blood-forming organs and is characterized by abnormal overproduction of immature forms of any of the leukocytes. Interferes with normal blood cell production resulting in decreased erythrocytes, decreased platelets.
   1) types
      a) lymphocytic: predominance of stem cells, lymphoblasts, usually known as acute lymphocytic leukemia (ALL); 80% of childhood leukemias are of this type
      b) myelogenous: predominance of monocytes and immature granulocytes (more common in adults); 10%–20% of childhood leukemias are myelogenous
   2) pathophysiology: leukemic cells proliferate and deprive normal blood cells of nutrients needed for metabolism
      a) anemia results from decreased red blood cell production, blood loss
      b) immunosuppression occurs from large numbers of *immature* white blood cells or profound neutropenia
      c) hemorrhage results from thrombocytopenia
      d) leukemic invasion of other organ systems occurs (extramedullary disease)
         - liver
         - spleen
         - lymph nodes
         - CNS
         - kidneys
         - lungs
         - gonads
      e) hyperuricemia may result after the start of chemotherapy when large numbers of cells are rapidly destroyed

b. Incidence
   1) most common childhood cancer
   2) peak age of onset is 2–5 years; more frequent in males
   3) 50% of children with ALL who are treated in major research centers live 5 years or longer

c. Medical treatment
   1) diagnostic measures
      a) bone-marrow aspiration
      b) lumbar puncture
      c) frequent blood counts
   2) chemotherapy—3 phases
      a) remission induction: to reduce leukemia-cell population and attain remission, usually with corticosteroids and vincristine
      b) consolidation (sanctuary): after remission is achieved, prophylactic treatment of the CNS, usually with intrathecal use of methotrexate
      c) maintenance course: to maintain remission, usually with combination drugs
   3) additional therapies
      a) radiation: irradiate cranium and spine as prophylaxis against CNS involvement
      b) bone-marrow transplantation

d. Prognosis: disease is characterized by remissions and exacerbations; outlook varies according to type of cell involved, response to treatment, age at diagnosis, initial WBC, and extent of involvement

2. Nursing Process

a. **Assessment/Analysis**
   1) bleeding tendencies
      a) petechiae often the first sign, due to low platelet count

   - **b)** hemorrhage (nose bleeds, gingival bleeding; intracranial hemorrhage in advanced disease)
- **2)** anemia: fatigue, pallor
- **3)** neutropenia: immunosuppression leads to secondary infection and fever, since cells are not capable of normal phagocytosis
- **4)** pain
   - **a)** abdomen: due to enlarged liver, spleen, lymph nodes, and other organs from cell infiltration
   - **b)** bones and joints
- **5)** anorexia and weight loss; ulcers of mucous membranes of GI tract
- **6)** vomiting and increased intracranial pressure from CNS involvement
- **7)** impaired kidney function
- **8)** emotional reaction, coping skills of parents, siblings, child, and significant extended-family members
- **9)** developmental/educational needs of child

b. Plans, Implementation, and Evaluation

Goal 1: Child will be free from hemorrhage.

Plan/Implementation
- Observe for epistaxis, gingival bleeding.
- Handle gently.
- Inspect skin and mucous membranes daily.
- Keep lips and nostrils clean and lubricated.
- Pad bed/crib to avoid trauma.
- Monitor blood work.

Evaluation: Child is free from bruises/bleeding from traumatic handling; has early signs of hemorrhage detected and reported.

Goal 2: Child will receive transfusions properly and safely.

Plan/Implementation
- Administer blood products properly
  - take baseline vital signs pretransfusion
  - check label with RN prior to transfusion for name, blood type, RH, hospital number, and physician's name
  - flush tubing with isotonic saline solution (hemolysis can occur if dextrose in line)
  - administer blood at room temperature within 4 hours of refrigeration
  - administer transfusion slowly to determine possible transfusion reaction, to prevent circulatory overload, and to protect small veins
  - stay with child for 1st 15 minutes; have parent or other adult stay with young child throughout transfusion
  - take vital signs q15min for 1st hour
  - do not give IV medications while blood is infusing
  - use blood filter
- Monitor intravenous transfusions
  - whole blood/packed cells (cannot be continuously maintained on transfusions since preservative in whole blood functions as anticoagulant)
  - platelets last 1–3 days; do not need to crossmatch for blood group or type but doing so decreases chance of immunization to another platelet group; spontaneous hemorrhage can occur at platelet levels below 20,000/mm^3
  - leukocytes last 2–3 days; need compatible donors; febrile responses (with moderate to severe chills) are common; give antihistamines or antipyretics as ordered
- Observe for complications/reactions to blood transfusions, e.g.
  - chills
  - fever (give antipyretic prn)
  - headache
  - apprehension (give sedatives prn)
  - pain in back, legs, or chest
  - hypotension (give IV fluids, vasopressors)
  - dyspnea (give O_2, bronchodilator [epinephrine] as ordered)
  - urticaria (give antihistamines prn)
- Promptly manage a transfusion reaction
  - stop the transfusion of blood
  - monitor vital signs
  - do not leave child alone
  - run IV fluids to maintain patency of the IV line
  - notify physician
  - return untransfused blood to blood bank

Evaluation: Child receives correct transfusion, is free from preventable complications (e.g., hemolysis); early signs of reaction (e.g., rash) are detected, and transfusion reaction is managed properly.

☐ Solid Tumors

1. General Information: see Table 5.24

2. Nursing Process: see Table 5.24

Table 5.24 Common Solid Tumor Cancers in Children

Definition	Assessment	Medical Treatment	Nursing Plan/Implementation
Brain Tumors			
Neoplasms in the cranium; most brain tumors in children are *infratentorial* (below the tentorium cerebelli), thus affecting the cerebellum and brain stem, making them less operable.	Signs of increased ICP: see Table 5.14.	Surgical excision to extent possible Irradiation Chemotherapy: methotrexate, vincristine	Perform frequent neurochecks. Institute seizure precautions. Post-op care: • Observe cranial dressing for drainage and record. • Reinforce but DO NOT CHANGE cranial dressing. • Position flat or on side with neck slightly extended. • Monitor fluid intake (IV, PO) carefully to prevent overload. • Avoid analgesics and sedatives that cause CNS depression. • Avoid coughing, straining, jarring movements.
Neuroblastoma			
Malignant embryonic abdominal tumor; most common in infancy	Abdominal mass that crosses midline Lymphadenopathy Urinary frequency or retention (pressure from tumor) Urine catecholamines (elevated)	Surgical excision and staging (to determine extent of other treatment and prognosis) Irradiation Chemotherapy	See General Nursing Plans page 616.
Wilms' Tumor			
Malignant embryonic tumor of kidney, usually encapsulated until late stages; 90% survival if detected while encapsulated; peak age of occurrence—3 years; more common in boys; increased incidence in siblings or twin; usually unilateral.	Palpable abdominal mass Abdominal distention Hypertension (excess renine secretion)	IVP Nephrectomy and adrenalectomy, staging (to determine treatment and prognosis) Irradiation Chemotherapy: actinomycin D, vincristine	• Handle carefully; DO NOT PALPATE ABDOMEN. • Monitor kidney function, e.g., I&O, urine specific gravity, BP.
Osteogenic Sarcoma			
Primary bone tumor, usually affecting distal femur or proximal tibia; most common in adolescent males.	Pain Localized swelling Limp or limited ROM	Amputation (above the knee or total hip disarticulation) Prophylactic lung irradiation Chemotherapy: doxorubicin, cisplatin, methotrexate with leukovorin rescue	• Post-op stump care (see *Nursing Care of the Adult* page 299). • Support coping responses in adjusting to loss of body part.

References

Bleyer, W. (1985). Cancer chemotherapy in infants and children. *Pediatric Clinics of North America, 32*, 554–557.

Krulik, T. (1988). *The child and family facing life threatening illness*. Philadelphia: Lippincott.

Maul, S. (1983). Childhood brain tumors: A special nursing challenge. *MCN: American Journal of Maternal/Child Nursing, 8*(4), 123–131.

Mott, S., Fazekas, N., & James, S. (1985). *Nursing care of children and families: A holistic approach*. Menlo Park, CA: Addison-Wesley.

Rose, M., & Thomas, R. *Children with chronic conditions*. Orlando, Florida: Grune & Stratton.

Scipien, G., et al. (1986). *Comprehensive pediatric nursing* (3rd ed.). New York: McGraw-Hill.

Servonsky, J., & Opas, S. (1987). *Nursing management of children*. Boston: Jones & Bartlett.

Thorne, S. (1985). The family cancer experience. *Cancer Nursing, 8*, 285–291.

Waechter, E., Phillips, J., & Holaday, B. (1985). *Nursing care of children* (10th ed.). Philadelphia: Lippincott.

Waskerwitz, M.J. (1985). An overview of cancer in children in the 1980s. *Nursing Clinics of North America. 20*, 5–30.

Whaley, L., & Wong, D. (1986). *Nursing care of infants and children* (3rd ed.). St. Louis: Mosby.

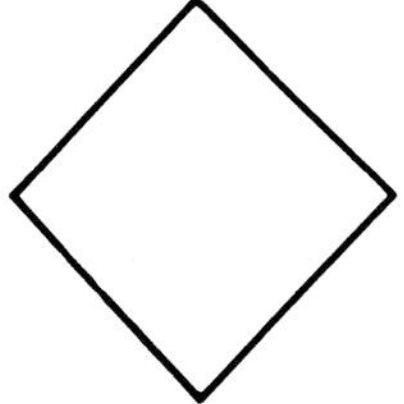

Reprints
Nursing Care of the Child

Reynolds, E., Ramenofsky, M. "The Emotional Impact of Trauma on Toddlers" 623

Rimar, J. "Shock In Infants and Children: Assessment and Treatment" 627

Meier, E. "Evaluating Head Trauma in Infants and Children" 635

Sheredy, C. "Factors to Consider when Assessing Responses to Pain" 639

The Emotional Impact Of Trauma On Toddlers

Reprinted from MCN: The American Journal of Maternal/Child Nursing, March/April, 1988

Attending to toddlers' emotional needs is as critical to their overall well-being as treating their physical wounds.

ELLEN A. REYNOLDS/MAX L. RAMENOFSKY

Multiple trauma is a term that evokes images of sudden, intense injury, rapid transport, resuscitative efforts by a team of health care professionals, multiple procedures, and an extended hospital stay. For the injured toddler, this stressful event occurs at a time of developmental transition. The toddler is starting to move from passivity to autonomy, is beginning to view himself as an individual person separate from his mother, and is learning to communicate with the world through language and other symbols.

Erik Erikson indicated that life is not only a sequence of developmental transitions, but of accidental crises as well (1). When one of these accidental crises occurs at a crucial stage of development, the effects may be severe. Such is the case when a toddler is hospitalized for trauma.

Toddlers (children between the ages of one and three) are at greater risk for permanent emotional problems related to the experience of hospitalization than any other developmental group (2). One- to four-year-olds comprise 31 percent of all pediatric trauma admissions (3). Because of the critical need for rapid, thorough diagnosis and treatment, especially with multitrauma patients, caregivers often neglect to consider the overwhelming emotional impact that trauma has on the child.

The Parent-Child Relationship

The toddler is in the process of individuation. After a successful attachment to the parent during the first year, the child is able to use the parent as a secure base from which to come and go, enabling him to deal with stresses as they arise. The security in this relationship comes from the sense of reliable accessibility provided by the parent. The child is likely to display intense proximity-seeking behaviors when he is separated from the parent, tired, in pain, or perceives threat (4).

Even in the most family-centered pediatric trauma centers, children are separated from their parents for a great deal of this critical time. From the time the paramedics arrive on the scene until the child is transported to an intensive care unit (ICU), there is little opportunity for parents to be with their child. For the conscious toddler, the combined experience of pain, unfamiliar surroundings, multiple strangers performing procedures, and the rapid sequence of invasive events is overwhelming. The child's natural instinct is to seek his attachment figure . . . the parent.

But, during the initial period of treatment, the child's parents are also experiencing the crisis. The child's injury, in all likelihood, was sudden and unexpected. The child's survival may be questionable and his parents may be confronting their own feelings of guilt for allowing the child to get hurt. The stress can alter the parents' usual responses to the toddler, causing the child further distress. One study demonstrated that parents in an emergency room did not function effectively in the parenting role due to their own helplessness, regression, and anxiety (5). The parents' anxiety may be unconsciously transmitted to the child.

Because of the physical unavailability of the parents caused by resuscitation and stabilization efforts, and because the parents may not be able to be emotionally supportive, the child may perceive his parents as having abrogated their role as protectors by allowing strangers to perform painful procedures. The toddler may experience a loss of trust in his parents and may demonstrate this by temporarily rejecting them. Two-year-old Jackie was hit by a car and spent eight days in a pediatric intensive care unit. During this time she was on a ventilator and received pancuronium (Pavulon) with sedation. For two days after extubation, she refused to look at her mother and rejected all of her mother's overtures of affection. Calmed by a nurse's explanation of what was going through

ELLEN A. REYNOLDS, R.N., M.S.N., *is pediatric trauma coordinator for the University of South Alabama Medical Center, Mobile, Alabama. She is a former staff nurse of the Emergency Medical Trauma Center, Children's Hospital National Medical Center, Washington, D.C.* MAX L. RAMENOFSKY, M.D., *is chief of the division of pediatric surgery, University of South Alabama Medical Center, chairman of the trauma committee of the American Pediatric Surgical Association, and co-principal investigator of the National Pediatric Trauma Registry, Department of Education Grant No. G008300042, Tufts-New England Medical Center and University of South Alabama. For reprints of this article, see the classified section.*

Jackie's mind, her mother was able to persist with her efforts to reassure Jackie. Jackie gradually became more responsive and had become her normal self a few days before she was discharged.

The Child's Developmental Phase

Cognitively, toddlers move through two sensorimotor stages and into the preconceptual stage within approximately two years of life. From 13 to 18 months, differentiation of self continues and memory begins to develop. By 18 to 24 months, egocentrism and magical thinking evolve. The rapid sequence of developmental events and the immaturity of his thought processes put the toddler at heightened risk for misinterpretation of treatment explanations, thus aggravating the emotional insult of the overall care.

For example, a toddler may interpret his hospitalization as a punishment for misbehavior, especially if he thinks his injury is the result of his own curiosity or exploration. Brief, simple explanations of procedures are easiest for toddlers to understand. A toddler cannot understand that a painful treatment will help him get better.

Following trauma, the toddler finds his expression of many of his newfound tasks and abilities restricted. A child who is just beginning to master verbal communication may suddenly find his skill thwarted by an endotracheal tube or tracheostomy. Restraints and traction may prevent him from dealing with the environment in his customary way. Generally, all aspects of autonomy have been taken away and the toddler finds himself again dependent on someone to feed, dress, and diaper him. In addition, body integrity may be of major concern to the toddler. Minor abrasions and lacerations may be more worrisome to him than is a less visible broken arm.

The Child's Past Experiences

Trauma is often the toddler's first introduction to the hospital. Well-child visits may have been the extent of the child's exposure to health care personnel. The most painful procedure he may have experienced may have been an immunization injection. While hospital tours and other types of preparation often help the older toddler cope with elective admission to a hospital, no such preparation precedes a traumatic admission. Therefore, the toddler has limited past experience on which he can draw to develop successful coping behaviors during hospitalization.

Extent of the Injury and Treatment

The severity of traumatic injuries runs the gamut from minor to life-threatening. Traumatic injuries tend to be painful and to require frequent diagnostic procedures for periodic reassessment. They also usually require some degree of immobilization, which in itself is stressful to a toddler.

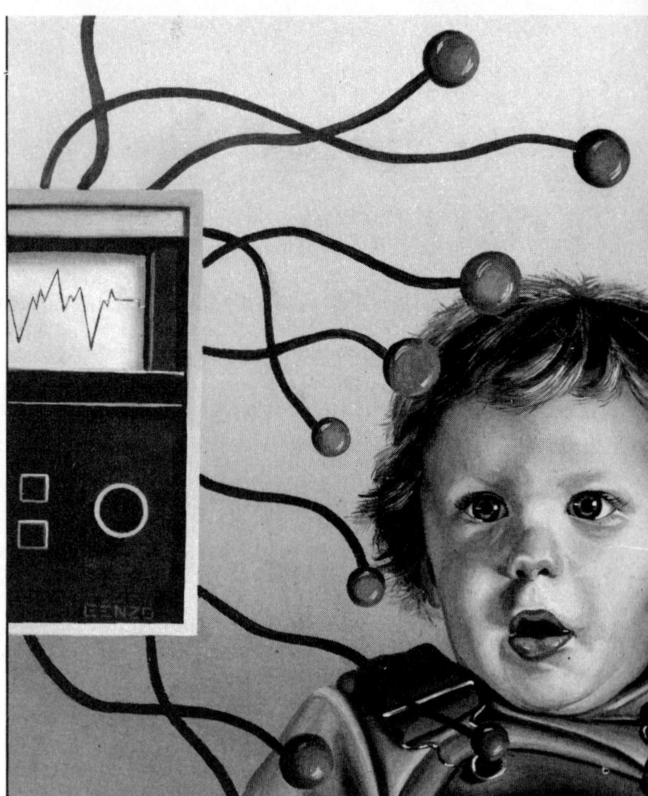

The toddler's tendency toward animism may lead the child to perceive machines as lifelike, frightening monsters.

A toddler who has suffered loss of consciousness prior to admission may be especially confused. Two-year-old Mia sustained a severe head injury and was comatose for several days. When she regained consciousness, she would stare out the window for long periods of time as if she was thinking. Finally, her mother asked her, "Mia, do you know why you are here?" Mia burst into tears and shook her head. Normal egocentrism and a tendency toward magical thinking, compounded by her coma, had made it difficult for her to understand what she'd been told and had made assessment of her comprehension difficult.

Invasive procedures, common elements of trauma care, are particularly threatening to the toddler. Blood drawing, tube insertions, and injections occur on a regular basis. Recollection of a painful event may cause anxiety over similar events. For example, the pain the toddler felt when a tourniquet was tightened may make him apprehensive about the inflation of a blood pressure cuff, a procedure that may not seem significantly different to the child. A toddler who sees a painful procedure performed on another child may become anxious about procedures to be performed on himself, due to his egocentrism.

In addition, because of the toddler's tendency toward animism, he may perceive machines and equipment as having lifelike qualities. The toddler may believe that he is about to be eaten by the computed tomography scanner or that alarms he hears are monsters trying to scare him.

The lengthy stay that trauma admission often entails causes stress for the toddler, too. Ritual and routine, so important in the toddler's life, are disrupted. Siblings may not be allowed to visit. Parents may not be able to room-in after the initial crisis is over, due to family and work responsibilities. As the child's immobility continues, his frustration will almost certainly increase.

Psychosocial Interventions

Equipped with knowledge of a toddler's developmental needs and the effects of hospitalization due to trauma, nurses can do a great deal to alleviate the child's resulting stress. First and foremost, parents must be included in the child's treatment and will need support throughout the hospitalization. Beginning with the initial resuscitation, parents of an injured child take on a new role. They will need information in order to successfully assume their new role and to cope accordingly. Questions regarding their child's injuries, treatment procedures and their outcomes, and prognostic indicators are uppermost in parents' minds and are to be answered as fully and truthfully as possible. From the time they enter the emergency room, through the completion of surgery, and until the child is released, they must be provided with frequent updates on their child's condition. As they become more comfortable in their new role, they will be better able to respond to their child's needs.

All toddlers need consistent parental presence (4,6,7). This need becomes even greater during stressful times such as hospitalization and is at its keenest during periods of highest stress such as when painful procedures are taking place. Preparing the parents by themselves ahead of time often enables them to work through their anxiety on their own, enabling them to provide greater support for the child. If possible, facilities should be made available to the parents so they can sleep in the hospital while their child is in the ICU.

With the multitude of disciplines involved in pediatric trauma care, every effort must be made to ensure a coordinated team approach. Often, this becomes the responsibility of the pediatric trauma coordinator or the child's primary nurse. She can see that duplication of special exams and tests is avoided and that specific hands-off times are scheduled and respected so that the toddler can have uninterrupted rest periods. If a child life specialist is available, she is to be included in the child's care as soon as possible.

With the wide range of developmental tasks characteristic of toddlers, it will take special effort for the nurse to correctly assess the patient's individual developmental level. Careful observation and taking a thorough history from the parents are the best ways to accomplish this. Questions such as "Is the child using words to convey needs?" and "Does he take a bottle or use a cup?" help pinpoint the child's developmental level. Hospitalization is not the time to introduce new routines such as toilet training, but encouraging the child to maintain established routines can give him a sense of control and mastery within the hospital environment. The child's nurse must understand that some regression is normal and convey her knowledge to the parents; regressive behavior is met with understanding, not punishment.

Recognizing the child's particular body image concerns will also facilitate treatment. For example, most toddlers are comforted by the application of an adhesive strip after a procedure, but this is not always the case. Two-year-old Bobby cried hysterically after blood drawing was over and a Band-Aid was put on. Observing the procedure one day, his mother remarked that Bobby had always been fearful of Band-Aids, preferring to be able to see his wounds. Bobby's crying decreased dramatically when his nurse applied site pressure for a longer time and left the Band-Aid off.

Involving the Child

Traumatic injuries and associated procedures are often extremely painful. Young children rarely fake or imagine pain, but because of their limited ability to communicate verbally, the nurse may find it difficult to assess the amount of the child's pain. His facial expressions, whether he is guarding himself, and whether he is crying are clues that the child feels pain. Maintenance of consistent medication schedules during the acute stages of trauma helps prevent pain from becoming unmanageable. Proper positioning, which also minimizes pain, is especially important for toddlers with head injuries, for whom the use of medications may be limited.

Children being pharmacologically paralyzed require particularly careful attention. Their pain is not affected by the drugs that paralyze their muscles, but the signs and signals of their pain will be masked. In such situations, the child's nurse has to rely on physiologic indicators such as elevated blood pressure, tachycardia, and diaphoresis to determine if the current pain control interventions are effective. Remember, too, that the paralyzed child may well be aware of and extremely frightened by his inability to move and communicate. Be sure to explain, comfort, and reassure the child throughout the period of paralysis.

If the child is in traction or on bedrest, efforts must be made to counteract the effects of immobility. Often the bed—traction and all—can be wheeled to the playroom or outdoors. Throwing games give toddlers a sense of mobility and can help them vent frustration.

When describing a procedure to the child, try to relate it to his past experience. Tamika, a 20-month-old, was terrified of blood drawing. But, her mother explained that Tamika had been fascinated by the wheal raised during a recent tine test for tuberculosis and had asked, "Bubble? Bubble?" during subsequent visits to the pediatrician. The next time the phlebotomist drew blood, she prefaced the stick by saying, "It's going to feel just like making the bubble." Tamika cooperated and showed no further signs of fear. Always give the child lots of reassurance after any procedure.

The toddler needs as much control of and independence in his care as possible. The nurse can make sure that all choices the child is given are acceptable options. A child's need for control is frequently expressed through negativism in eating behavior, which is of special concern when trying to maintain the high caloric intake required following multiple trauma. The issue can be minimized by creative nursing interventions. Parents can be asked to bring the child his favorite foods from home. A trip to the hospital cafeteria for a meal with siblings may be arranged. Maximizing the child's oral intake is preferable, but if nasogastric or parenteral supplements are necessary, make sure the child understands that the tube isn't a punishment for his not eating enough.

The toddler's need for reassurance and TLC throughout his hospitalization cannot be overemphasized. If resuscitation is needed, the presence of a single nurse who provides comfort and explanations will often decrease the child's physical resistance and crying. Ideally, one primary and one associate nurse will be assigned to the child. Encouraging parents to be with, hold, and touch their child fosters another source of comfort and reassurance for the child.

Interventions with the Parents in Mind

Providing support to the child's parents during trauma care is essential to their ability to support their critically injured child. Some suggestions that will help nurses see parents through this critical period are:

Encourage parents to verbalize their concerns. A nurse's warm, responsive approach and honest reassurance without raising false hopes will enable parents to share their thoughts and work through their fears (8).

Continue to provide information on the child's condition and treatment. Involve the parents in decision making whenever possible, giving them control in a situation in which they may otherwise feel themselves to be relatively helpless.

Help the parents develop their participation in their child's care to a level that is comfortable for them. Because parents are often torn between their desire to be there for their child and their discomfort with hospital equipment, they may need to be taught how to touch or hold their child. The child's nurse can provide options such as, "Would you like to bathe your child or hold her hand while I bathe her?"

Provide a comfortable environment for parents. A bedside chair, a pillow and blanket for sleeping, and a coffee pot in the waiting room are small amenities that can make a big difference in parents' perceptions of hospital staff support.

Making Trauma Less Traumatic

Regardless of the quality of nursing care and participation of the parents, hospitalization for trauma is frightening to children. No amount of nursing care can undo the event that caused the trauma to occur. But sensitive, thorough nursing care can alleviate the physical and emotional stresses prompted by the injury and ensure not only a successful physical recovery, but a successful emotional one as well. Nurses can effectively minimize the consequences of trauma that can haunt a toddler. In some cases, they can even help the child come away from the experience with a positive sense of mastery and accomplishment.

REFERENCES

1. ERIKSON, E. H. *Childhood and Society*. New York, W. W. Norton and Co., 1964.
2. ROBERTSON, JAMES. *Young Children in Hospital*. New York, Basic Books, 1969.
3. NATIONAL PEDIATRIC TRAUMA REGISTRY, DEPARTMENT OF EDUCATION. *Annual Report*. Presented to the American Pediatric Surgical Association, meeting held in Toronto, Canada, May 1986.
4. BOWLBY, JOHN. *Attachment and Loss*. New York, Basic Books, Vol.1, 1969, p. 259. (2nd ed. in 1983)
5. ROSKIES, E., AND OTHERS. Emergency hospitalization of young children: some neglected psychological considerations. *Med.Care* 13:570–581, July 1975.
6. FREUD, ANNA, ED. The role of bodily illness in the mental life of children. *Psychoanalytic Study of the Child* 7:69–80, 1952.
7. RUTTER, MICHAEL. Attachment and the development of social relationships. IN *Scientific Foundations of Developmental Psychiatry*, ed. by Michael Rutter. London, Heinemann Medical Books, 1980, (1987, text ed.)
8. CARNEVALE, F. A. Nursing the critically ill child: a responsive approach. *Focus Crit.Care* 12:10–13, Oct. 1985.

BIBLIOGRAPHY

BROOME, M. E. The child in pain: a model for assessment and intervention. *Crit.Care Q.* 8:47–55, June 1985.

ETZLER, C. A. Parents' reactions to pediatric critical care settings: a review of the literature. *Issues Compr.Pediatr.Nurs.* 7:319–331, June 1984.

LANNING, J. Pediatric trauma: emotional aspects. *AORN J.* 42:345–351, Sept. 1985.

LEWANDOWSKI, L. A. Psychosocial aspects of critical care. IN *Nursing Care of the Critically Ill Child: American Association of Critical Care Nurses*, ed. by M. F. Hazinski. St. Louis, C. V. Mosby Co., 1984.

WOLTERMAN, M. C., AND MILLER, M. Caring for parents in crisis. *Nurs.Forum* 22(1):34–37, 1985.

Shock In Infants And Children: Assessment And Treatment

Reprinted from MCN: The American Journal of Maternal/Child Nursing, March/April, 1988

As a youngster progresses through the phases of shock, his nurse must be ready to adjust care accordingly.

JOAN M. RIMAR

Because of the evolving nature of shock, nursing assessment and treatment of the various stages is a demanding, ongoing process. Signs and symptoms appear and disappear, and treatment is initiated, modified, or discontinued throughout the course of the illness. (Types of shock, their stages, and their symptoms were discussed in "Recognizing Shock Syndromes In Infants And Children," MCN, January/February 1988.) A child's ability to survive this fast-paced series of actions and reactions depends heavily on the services and skills of an astute, vigilant nurse.

Shock symptoms are caused by circulatory dysfunction and tissue oxygen and tissue nutrient deficits. Physical findings (temperature, skin color, etc.) and hemodynamic indices (blood pressure, central venous pressure, etc.) reflect the consequences of perfusion impairment on organ function and the child's general condition. Laboratory tests quantify the damage suffered.

Clinical Assessment

Impairment of peripheral circulation can be assessed by examination of the temperature, color, pulse, and capillary refill of the child's extremities. Normally, a child's extremities are warm and pink, with strong, equal pulses and brisk capillary refill. The child in shock, however, presents with cool and clammy skin, mottled or gray extremities, diminished pulses, and sluggish capillary refill, abnormalities primarily resulting from decreased cardiac output (CO) and increased systemic vascular resistance (SVR). However, septic shock, which in its early stage is associated with normal or increased CO, causes different initial signs and symptoms. Septic shock patients have warm and dry skin (they are often febrile) and they are well-perfused. They often look good despite the fact that they suffer from a life-threatening condition.

The circulatory dysfunction and depleted vascular volume characteristic of most shock syndromes are reflected in low blood pressure (BP), central venous pressure (CVP), and pulmonary capillary wedge pressure (PCWP)/left atrial pressure (LAP). Compensatory tachycardia can also occur and is often the first indicator of circulatory impairment. Again, the exception is septic shock. In the early stages of septic shock, and in cardiogenic shock, the CVP and PCWP/LAP are often normal or elevated.

Signs of dehydration also accompany these signs of hypovolemic shock. Skin turgor is poor, and the skin may remain "tented" when pinched. Mucous membranes are often dry, the fontanelle may be sunken, and daily weight may decrease.

Signs and symptoms of cerebral perfusion dysfunction are often subtle in the early stages of shock. The child's sensorium may be clouded, his response to stimuli may be poor, and he may be anxious, irritable, or lethargic. Infants frequently exhibit a weak cry and poor suck. As shock progresses, somnolence advances to obtundation.

In addition, arrhythmias, which impair cardiac

JOAN M. RIMAR, R.N., M.S.N., *is head nurse of the infant-toddler ward at Yale-New Haven Hospital in New Haven, Connecticut. To order reprints of this article, see the classified section.*

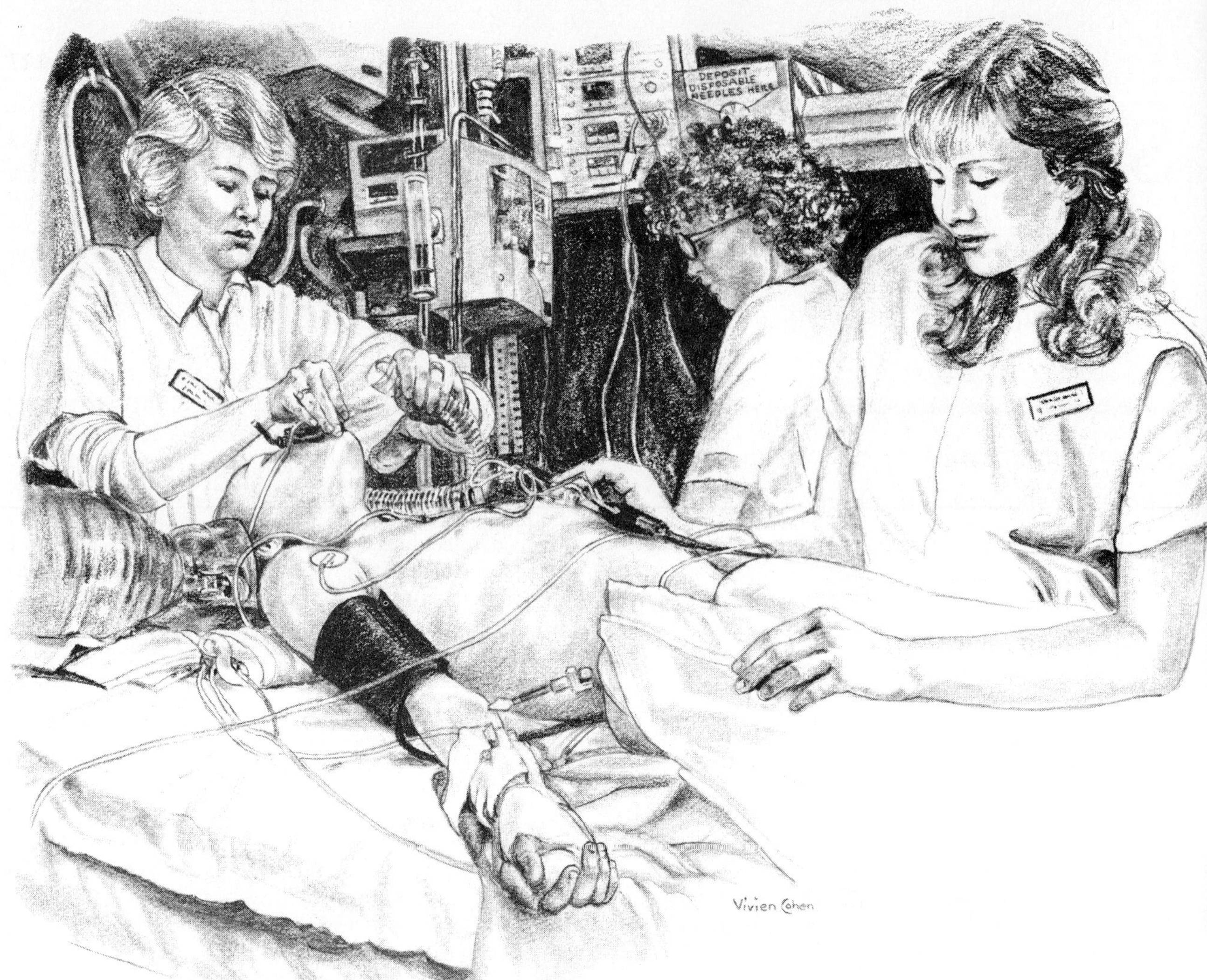

Because changes occur rapidly in shock and the effects of therapy must be evaluated quickly, continuous monitoring is an essential part of the treatment of an infant or child in shock.

function, are not uncommon in the presence of electrolyte imbalance, metabolic acidosis, and hypoxemia. All of these can occur in shock.

Even with normal or increased cardiac output, the child in shock may suffer myocardial injury. The reasons for the infarctions sustained by some patients in shock are not clear. Indications of damage to the heart muscle include S-T segment elevation on electrocardiogram (EKG) and abnormal cardiac enzyme values (creatine kinase-myocardial enzyme, or CK-MB) (1).

Urine output is an extremely important measurement when assessing infants and children in shock. Particularly in hypovolemic patients, output may decrease long before other signs of impaired tissue perfusion become evident. In general, urine output decreases when renal blood flow drops, and increases as flow increases. Renal blood flow, in turn, is dependent on cardiac output. Sudden drops in renal blood flow or pressure cause urine output to decrease and urine specific gravity to rise. Low urine output is <0.5–1.0 ml/kg/hour in infants and children and <1.0–2.0 ml/kg/hour in neonates. But, if the fall in renal blood pressure or flow is gradual, changes in urine output may appear slowly. In some patients with sepsis, urine output may initially be normal or increased, despite the relative hypovolemia associated with the condition (2).

Laboratory Evaluation

Laboratory tests are obtained as soon as possible after a child presents in shock. Further tests are acquired as dictated by the child's clinical condition. They are necessary in order to monitor a variety of potentially lethal conditions and irregularities that may be encountered in shock patients. Metabolic acidosis, hypoglycemia, electrolyte and coagulation abnormalities, infection, and renal failure are a few of these conditions.

Tests commonly obtained include: arterial and mixed venous blood gases; blood lactate; serum electrolytes, osmolality and glucose; coagulation studies; complete blood count with differential; creatinine and blood urea nitrogen; blood cultures; urinalysis; and urine sodium and osmolality. If the cause of shock is unclear, the possibility

Cardiovascular Drugs Used in the Treatment of Pediatric Shock

Drug	*Usual Intravenous Dose*	*Comments*
Isoproterenol	0.05–1.5 mcg/kg per min	Increases strength and rate of cardiac contraction. Dilates peripheral vessels. May increase myocardial work and oxygen consumption. May include arrhythmias.
Epinephrine	0.05–0.5 mcg/kg per min	At low doeses, increases strength and rate of cardiac contraction to moderate degree and causes systemic vascular resistance (SVR) to decrease slightly at low doses. At high doses, causes marked increase in strength and rate of cardiac contraction and severe vasoconstriction of peripheral vasculature (increased SVR). As epinephrine may decrease renal blood flow significantly, monitor urine output.
Dopamine	1–20 mcg/kg per min (higher doses may be used)	Effects vary with dose: low dose response primarily dopaminergic; mid-range cause moderate increase in heart rate and contractility; high doses (10–20 mcg/kg min) vasoconstriction predominates. May cause arrhythmias.
Dobutamine	2–15 mcg/kg per min (higher doses may be used)	Increases strength of cardiac contraction but causes minimal change in heart rate. On occasion, causes tachycardia and hypertension.
Amrinone	0.75 mg/kg initially; 5–10 mcg/kg per min (adult dose recommendation)	Increases strength of cardiac contraction and relaxes vascular smooth muscle, causing decreased afterload and preload. Clinical studies regarding use in children are ongoing.
Nitroprusside	0.5–10 mcg/kg per min	Dilates peripheral arteries and veins. May produce severe hypotension. Do not use in boluses. Immediate onset and short duration (2–4 sec) of action. Protect from light.
Phentolamine	1–20 mcg/kg per min	Dilates peripheral arteries and, to a lesser extent, veins. Also causes cardiac stimulation. May cause marked hypotension, tachycardia, and arrhythmias.
Hydralazine	0.1–0.5 mg/kg per dose every 3–6 hr	Primarily vasodilates peripheral arteries. Also maintains or increases renal and cerebral blood flow. May cause tachycardia.
Tolazoline	1–2 mg/kg initially; 1–2 mg/kg per hr	Decreases peripheral resistance and increases venous capacitance. Causes cardiac stimulation. Reduces pulmonary arterial pressure and resistance.

that it may be due to a drug overdose must be considered. Accordingly, blood and urine are screened, especially for barbiturates and major tranquilizers. Sequential chest x-rays will aid in the diagnosis of some complications of shock (pulmonary edema, for example) and facilitate evaluation of corresponding treatment.

Initial Treatment

Children in shock are often significantly hypotensive, obtunded, and require resuscitation. Immediate therapeutic goals at this time include establishment of a patent airway and maintenance of respiration and circulation while the underlying problem is assessed. Endotracheal intubation and mechanical ventilation with 100 percent oxygen is usually indicated. The heightened susceptibility of newborns to oxygen toxicity (particularly retrolental fibroplasia) must always be considered when determining inspired oxygen concentration for infants.

Emergency medications and fluids are given as soon as administration routes are available. The following routes (in the order of their desirability) are used for drug administration: central venous; peripheral venous/intraosseous (anterior tibial bone marrow); endotracheal; and intracardiac (3). Fluid boluses may be infused via any of the venous routes.

Two central lines (or one multilumen catheter) constitute optimal intravenous (IV) access. One of the central venous lines is used for pressure measurement and the other for infusion of drugs into the central circulatory system close to their sites of action (3). Because some drugs cause tissue necrosis when they infiltrate at peripheral sites, central infusion is preferable. Peripheral IV lines are inserted as they are required.

Monitoring

Continuous monitoring is essential in treating shock patients. Changes occur rapidly, and the effects of therapy must be evaluated quickly.

Cardiac function is followed in several ways. The EKG displays cardiac rate and rhythm. The arterial line measures systemic BP, including diastolic pressure (which reflects SVR), and pulse pressure (related to stroke volume). It also provides a way to obtain arterial blood for calculating the arteriovenous oxygen difference ($avDo_2$). The CVP line quantifies right ventricular preload and, in most children without right ventricular outflow obstruction, left ventricular preload, too. If necessary, a pulmonary artery catheter is inserted to measure left ventricular filling pressure. Cardiac output can be measured directly by using the pulmonary artery catheter and indirectly with the $avDo_2$. An echocardiogram will gauge left ventricular contractility and help determine whether a pericardial effusion is present (4).

Renal function and, indirectly, cardiac function are followed by monitoring urine output. A urinary drainage catheter and collection system is necessary for output measurement.

In addition, pulse oximeters or transcutaneous oxygen and carbon dioxide monitors help monitor respiratory function in infants and children.

Fluid Management

Fluid replacement is generally accepted as the most important immediate therapeutic goal in shock. Early correction of the volume deficit is necessary to increase CO (by increasing preload) and to reestablish the even distribution of microcirculatory flow. It also prevents later complications of shock such as acute renal failure. Improvement in pressure, flow, oxygen delivery, and oxygen consumption indicate successful fluid therapy (5).

Controversy exists, however, as to whether colloid or crystalloid distribution is best suited to fluid resuscitation; the literature is replete with apparently contradictory studies (6). Colloid usually refers to albumin, but also includes other prepared plasma fractions, synthetic plasma substitutes, whole blood, red blood cells, and fresh-frozen plasma. Normal saline and Ringer's lactate are the isotonic, crystalloid (electrolyte) solutions used for acute volume replacement in shock (7). More than twice as much crystalloid as colloid is necessary to achieve the same degree of hemodynamic stability (8).

Proponents of colloid use claim that colloids are more effective than crystalloids in achieving optimum hemodynamic and oxygen transport goals. They also cite the importance of colloids for maintaining plasma colloid osmotic pressure and minimizing interstitial edema (9). Prevention of interstitial edema, particularly in the lung, is important because accumulation of interstitial fluid (i.e. pulmonary edema) leads to deterioration in gas exchange (8).

Those who advocate crystalloid infusion argue that a balanced salt solution is all that is necessary to restore and maintain effective extracellular fluid volume (6). They also affirm that colloid therapy increases the risk of pulmonary edema in some patients (10). In addition, colloid is expensive and extremely difficult to titrate, making the possibility of fluid overload much greater than when crystalloid is used. Underreplacement is more likely to occur with crystalloid therapy.

In most clinical situations, theoretical considerations give way to practical concerns. A variety of volume expanders are usually employed, depending upon their availability and the kinds of losses the child has suffered. In a life-threatening situation, a balanced salt solution is probably the ideal infusate; it can be infused rapidly and is immediately available. The amount and rate of infusion depend on the child's condition; 10 ml/kg of estimated body weight of Ringer's lactate solution infused over several minutes is a reasonable starting point. A second bolus of the same amount is infused if there is no improvement in blood pressure or perfusion (11). The child is evaluated between boluses for the presence of pulmonary edema (4). If there continues to be no improvement in the child's condition, impaired myocardial function must be considered.

Blood is administered as soon as possible in order to replace whole-blood loss and correct anemia. If there is evidence of continued bleeding or consumption of clotting factors, fresh-frozen plasma should be given as well.

Efforts to improve cardiac output and tissue perfusion by volume augmentation when treating children with cardiogenic or septic shock must be carefully monitored (12). The volume of fluid that may be safely administered is contingent on cardiac competence. Routine measurement of CVP, pulmonary artery pressure, and PCWP enable early detection of cardiac decompensation and pulmonary edema and therefore provide an important guide for volume replacement (13).

Pharmacologic Management

If fluid therapy fails to improve the child's condition, a drug to enhance cardiovascular performance (see Cardiovascular Drugs Used in the Treatment of Pediatric Shock) is administered. Increasing the *inotropy* (strength) and/or *chronotropy* (rate) of cardiac contraction by continuous infusion of intravenous catecholamines (sympathomimetic amines) is particularly well-suited to this task. The rapid onset, controllable dosage, and ultrashort half-life of catecholamines make them effective for treating shock (11).

Epinephrine, dopamine, isoproterenol, and dobutamine are the most frequently used exogenous catecholamines. In general, epinephrine is used when the child is in cardiopulmonary arrest or arrest is imminent; dopamine is used for children with diminished urine output; isoproterenol is used when the child has bradycardia or acidemia; and dobutamine is used when the child has high ventricular filling pressures or as a substitute for isoproterenol when the child has tachycardia (4, 14). Frequently, more than one catecholamine is given at a time; finding the right doses and combinations may take a while. Because catecholamines increase myocardial oxygen consumption, signs of myocardial hypoxia or ischemia such as S-T segment and T-wave changes on the EKG may become apparent during administration.

Sympathomimetic amines stimulate alpha, beta, and dopaminergic receptors throughout the body causing a variety of effects. (See Adrenergic Receptors and Functions for a discussion of physiologic responses.) Isoproterenol is a pure beta agonist that increases heart rate and cardiac contractility and causes dilatation of skeletal muscle beds and a fall in SVR. This vasodilatation often reduces venous return to the heart, decreasing preload and stroke volume; therefore, hypovolemia must be corrected before initiating isoproterenol infusion and the child's CVP is to be followed closely during therapy.

Adequate oxygenation must be ensured for children receiving isoproterenol. Additionally, the lowest effective dose is used because the drug can induce severe cardiac arrhythmias such as ventricular tachycardia and fibrillation in hypoxic children (11). Isoproterenol is valuable for children with bradycardia or acidosis due to poor perfusion from vasoconstriction (4).

Epinephrine acts on both alpha and beta receptor sites. Its most pronounced action is on the beta receptors of the heart, vascular, and other smooth muscle. The drug increases the heart rate, BP (mainly systolic), and strength of ventricular contractions. Total peripheral resistance may be decreased, increased, or unaffected by epinephrine administration, depending on the ratio of alpha to beta activity in different vascular areas; the vasodilator effect usually predominates (16). High doses can increase resistance in the kidney and decrease renal blood flow to such an extent that irreversible renal failure develops. Epinephrine may be particularly helpful in septic shock and anaphylaxis when SVR is abnormally low (11).

Dopamine activates alpha and beta receptors in a dose-dependent fashion. At low doses (2–4 mcg/kg/minute), it causes a decrease in SVR and splanchnic and renal vasodilatation; the dopaminergic effect on the kidney results in increased urine output. It stimulates $beta_1$ receptors at moderate doses (5–8 mcg/kg/minute), and exhibits a moderate positive inotropic effect. At high doses ($>$ 10–15 mcg/kg/minute), dopamine is primarily an alpha agonist that causes renal vasoconstriction and increased SVR (11). Increased SVR will cause increased systemic afterload, which may diminish CO. When doses greater than 15 mcg/kg/minute are used, the child must be monitored for tachycardia, arrhythmias, and severe peripheral vasoconstriction.

Dobutamine, a synthetic catecholamine, is a $beta_1$ stimulant that increases cardiac contractility but causes only a slight increase in heart rate. The drug's opposing alpha and $beta_2$ effects on the peripheral vasculature minimize direct vascular activity, although SVR is usually decreased and minimal vasoconstriction is occasionally observed (16). Dobutamine has been found to be less effective in infants less than one year old than in older children (17).

Amrinone is a new, nonadrenergic, positive inotropic agent with vasodilator activity that is now undergoing research for use in children. Amrinone reduces afterload and preload by its direct relaxant effect on vascular smooth muscle. In children with depressed myocardial function, amrinone produces a prompt increase in CO (16).

Increased vascular resistance and consequent, increased ventricular afterload can result from activation of compensatory mechanisms and/or use of sympathomimetic agents in children who have shock. When an element of heart failure coexists with impeded ventricular outflow, the use of vasodilators, usually in combination with

Adrenergic Receptors and Functions

Receptor	*Site Of Action*	*Response*
Beta₁ (β_1)	Heart	cardioacceleration (sinoatrial and atrioventricular nodes), increased myocardial strength (atria and ventricles)
Beta₂ (β_2)	Peripheral vasculature: skeletal muscle	vasodilatation
	Lung	bronchodilatation
Alpha ($\propto$)	Heart: coronary circulation	vasoconstriction
	Lung	bronchoconstriction
	Peripheral vasculature: skin, mucosa, renal, splanchnic	vasoconstriction
Dopaminergic	Kidney	increased renal blood flow, increased urine output

Based on Crone, R.K., Acute circulatory failure in children, *Pediatr. Clin. North Am.* 27: 525–538, Aug. 1980 and Guyton, A. C., *Textbook of Medical Physiology*, 7th ed. Philadelphia, W. B. Saunders Co. 1986.

inotropic agents, is commonly indicated.

Vasodilators decrease ventricular afterload primarily by reducing impedance to left ventricular ejection (18). Afterload reduction may be accomplished with a direct vasodilator (nitroprusside sodium or hydralazine), a beta agonist (isoproterenol), or an alpha antagonist (phentolamine or tolazoline). All of these drugs, except hydralazine, are administered by continuous IV infusion. Hydralazine is given in single doses by slow intravenous push. Vasodilators can cause severe hypotension; hence, vasoconstricting agents, such as phenylephrine or norepinephrine, and fluid should be readily available (11).

Nitroprusside causes direct, balanced vasodilatation of peripheral veins and arteries. The subsequent fall in afterload and preload improves CO only when the effects of the drug that reduce outflow resistance predominate over the effects that reduce venous return (16). Filling pressures, therefore, must be at the upper limits of normal before nitroprusside infusion is begun (18). The dose range for the drug is 0.5–10 mcg/kg/minute for adults (19). However, manifestations of toxicity (headache, nausea, palpitations, hyperventilation, metabolic acidosis, and unexplained elevation of venous oxygen tension) have occurred at relatively low doses, leading some authors to suggest a maximum infusion rate of 4–8 mcg/kg/minute for adults and probably less for neonates and young children (20). Several precautions must be taken when the drug is administered: monitor serum levels of thiocyanate and cyanide, the toxic metabolites of nitroprusside; protect the 5 percent dextrose infusate containing the drug from light; and monitor BP continuously.

The alpha-adrenergic blocking agent phentolamine causes vasodilatation of peripheral veins and arteries. It dilates veins less effectively than does nitroprusside, resulting in a smaller reduction of left ventricular preload for a given reduction of afterload (18). Constraints to phentolamine use include its high cost and the large doses needed to maintain consistent vasodilatation.

Hydralazine exerts a peripheral vasodilating effect through direct relaxation of vascular smooth muscle, primarily arterial muscle, with little effect on venous beds. SVR decreases, but the change in filling pressure is minimal (16).

Tolazoline is a direct peripheral vasodilator with moderate alpha-adrenergic blocking activity. It decreases peripheral resistance, increases venous capacitance, and causes cardiac stimulation. In addition, tolazoline usually reduces pulmonary artery pressure and vascular resistance, which decreases right ventricular afterload and left ventricular preload. The use of epinephrine with large doses of tolazoline may cause epinephrine reversal, a further reduction of blood pressure that is followed by an exaggerated rebound (16).

Stimulation of peripheral $beta_2$ receptors by isoproterenol can enhance forward flow from the left ventricle by decreasing SVR. Other vasodilator drugs that are used occasionally in the treatment of shock include nitroglycerin, a potent venodilator that decreases preload, and captopril, an angiotensin-converting enzyme inhibitor that generally causes a decrease in both peripheral arterial pressure and resistance (16).

Other Pharmacologic Therapy

Acidosis depresses myocardial function, impairs ventilatory response, and renders sympathomimetic drugs ineffective. Therefore, when arterial blood pH is less than 7.20 and adequate ventilation has been established (i.e. the partial pressure of carbon dioxide is normal), correction with sodium bicarbonate is indicated (11). The initial dose is 1–2 mEq/kg given intravenously. Subsequent doses are titrated to the bicarbonate content of arterial blood.

Antibiotics are started as soon as possible if the etiology of shock is unknown or if infection is documented or suspected. Calcium replacement may be necessary because hypocalcemia occurs frequently in circulatory failure, especially after administration of large amounts of albumin, whole blood, or fresh-frozen plasma.

Recent evidence suggests that the release of endogenous opiate beta-endorphins during shock may contribute to hypotension. The opioid antagonist naloxone has been found to rapidly reverse hypotension secondary to endotoxin and blood loss in animals (22, 23). Naloxone has been used successfully in some children with septic shock who failed to respond to conventional therapy (24, 25). Further clinical trials are necessary, as response to naloxone therapy has been inconsistent and severe reactions may occur (26).

Similar variable results have been obtained with corticosteroid use in shock. In certain subgroups of septic shock patients, corticosteroids may improve short-term survival and instigate reversal of shock (27). Steroid administration is considered when adrenal insufficiency is suspected (4). Numerous other agents for the treatment of shock (particularly septic shock) are under investigation: endotoxin antiserum, anti-$complement_{5a}$ antibody, arachidonic acid inhibitors, fibronectin, toxic oxygen scavengers, and glucose-insulin-potassium (GIK) (28, 29).

Additional Therapies and Nutritional Support

The MAST (Military Anti-Shock Trousers) suit provides rapid redistribution of intravascular fluid. For children in hypovolemic shock, inflation

Potential Nursing Diagnoses for the Child in Shock*

- Airway clearance, ineffective
- Gas exchange, impaired
- Tissue perfusion, alteration in: cerebral, cardiopulmonary, renal, gastrointestinal, peripheral
- Cardiac output, alteration in: decreased
- Fluid volume deficit, actual or potential
- Infection, potential for
- Nutrition, alterations in: less than body requirements
- Body temperature, potential alteration in
- Hyperthermia
- Tissue integrity, impaired
- Skin integrity, impairment of: actual or potential
- Urinary elimination, alteration in patterns
- Bowel elimination, alteration in: constipation or diarrhea
- Self-care deficit: feeding, bathing/hygiene, toileting
- Comfort, alteration in: pain
- Sleep pattern disturbance
- Mobility, impaired physical
- Communication, impaired verbal
- Fear
- Anxiety
- Knowledge deficit
- Coping, ineffective family: compromised
- Family processes, alteration in
- Grieving, anticipatory

*Diagnostic categories approved by the North American Nursing Diagnosis (NANDA) Seventh National Conference

of the suit quickly "autotransfuses" the upper circulatory system with blood compressed from the venous beds in the abdomen and legs. Circulation to the brain and heart are thus preserved. There is concern, however, that inflation of the abdominal compartment may impair ventilation and cause respiratory acidosis by limiting diaphragmatic excursion. The MAST suit is not used to treat cardiogenic shock because it increases left ventricular afterload (7, 30).

Extracorporeal membrane oxygenation (ECMO), left ventricular assist devices, and intra-aortic balloon pumps have been used to treat shock in children, but further clinical experience and evaluation of their efficacy and indications for use are needed. Plasmapheresis (removal of the child's blood, separation of plasma, and reinjection of the packed cells in fresh plasma) and continuous arteriovenous hemofiltration (CAVH) have also been used to successfully treat septic shock (31–33). However, too few patients have received these treatments for their use to be recommended at this time.

Critically ill infants and children are particularly prone to malnutrition because of the nature and duration of their illnesses. Previously well-nourished infants and children will probably develop nutritional deficiencies after five to seven days of intensive care; infants and children who have been hospitalized for some time before the development of shock may already be malnourished (34). Parenteral or enteral nutritional support is initiated as soon as practical.

What Can Nurses Do?

The initial role of the nurse will vary depending on when in the course of shock she first encounters the child. In some cases, the nurse's primary role will be prevention of shock, particularly with children likely to develop septic shock. Septic shock may be avoided by reducing the potential for transmission and colonization of bacterial organisms by thorough handwashing, meticulous catheter and wound care, encouraging patients to do deep breathing exercises, and turning patients routinely (35). Nurses caring for infants and children at risk for sepsis must implement preventive measures immediately.

Prevention of shock is also possible for certain hospitalized infants and children with conditions that can lead to hypovolemia (vomiting and diarrhea, diabetes mellitus and insipidus, for example). Recording intake and output carefully, monitoring vital signs, and weighing patients frequently will enable the alert nurse to recognize deviations soon after they occur. She will then notify appropriate personnel.

The nurse's primary aim when treating the child with established shock is to increase tissue perfusion. Nursing care that facilitates this goal includes monitoring and interpreting indices that reflect circulatory adequacy, administering medical and nursing prescriptions for drugs and treatments, and monitoring and evaluating effects of interventions. Preventing complications and supporting the patient's family are other important aspects of good care.

Continuous assessment of cardiac, respiratory, neurologic, renal, hematologic, and integumentary function is essential. The importance and significance of information obtained from physical assessment, indwelling pressure lines, laboratory tests, and urinary drainage systems cannot be overemphasized. It is the nurse's responsibility to integrate and interpret this information to guide nursing care. She can also provide specific nursing interventions based on potential nursing diagnoses; see Potential Nursing Diagnoses for the Child in Shock.

Because the nurse is often the first person to encounter the data that may indicate an evolving problem, she may be the key to preventing the often lethal complications of shock. She ensures the minute to minute operation of equipment such as ventilators and medication infusions that will support system functions. It takes no more than an obstructed endotracheal tube or a kinked intravenous line to precipitate a crisis that will ultimately result in death.

The nurse can also play a valuable role by reducing the anxiety and fear that the infant or the child and his family will certainly experience. Hospital admission of almost any child causes strain, which is magnified when the child has a life-threatening condition (36). The strange environment, limitations on visiting, painful procedures, and the potential for death that accompany advanced shock are issues that must be addressed. The nurse must listen attentively and calmly to parents and explain policies, procedures, prognosis, and shock itself to them. Parents are to be encouraged to verbalize their questions, thoughts, and feelings and support personnel are to be involved.

For the child, relief from both physical and psychological pain through the use of potent analgesics such as intravenous morphine and antianxiety agents becomes important when comfort measures, distractions, etc., are unsuccessful or inappropriate. Family members can help themselves and the ill child by participating with him in active or passive play, as appropriate, and involving themselves in the activities of his daily life. They are never ushered from the bedside without good reason (37).

In these ways, a capable nurse can offset the extremely complicated and deadly progress of shock. Recognizing the child's condition early, diligently attending to the administration and evaluation of his treatment, and preventing the onset of common complications comprise a challenging and trying nursing role. Yet, the fulfillment of this role can decrease the degree of morbidity and increase the child's chance of survival, the most satisfactory outcome that can be achieved from the treatment of an infant or child in shock.

REFERENCES

1. McGRATH, R. B., AND REVTYAK, G. Secondary myocardial injury. *Crit.Care Med.* 12:1024–1026, Dec. 1984.
2. WILSON, R. F., ED. Shock. IN *Critical Care Manual: Principles and Techniques of Critical Care.* Kalamazoo, MI, Upjohn Co., 1977, pp. C1–C42.
3. Standards and guidelines for cardiopulmonary resuscitation (CPR) and emergency cardiac care (ECC). *JAMA* 255:2905–2992, June 6, 1986.
4. VARGO, T. Shock. IN *Life-threatening Episodes in Infants and Children: Cardiovascular Failure.* Kalamazoo, MI, Upjohn Co., 1984, pp. 5–10.
5. SHOEMAKER, W. C., AND HAUSER, C. J. Critique of crystalloid versus colloid therapy in shock and shock lung. *Crit.Care Med.* 7:117–124, Mar. 1979.
6. DODGE, C., AND GLASS, D. D. Crystalloid and colloid therapy. *Semin.Anesth.* 1:293–301, Dec. 1982.
7. SHINE, K. I., AND OTHERS. Aspects of the management of shock. *Ann.Intern.Med.* 93:723–734, Nov. 1980.
8. VIRGILIO, R. W., AND OTHERS. Balanced electrolyte solutions: experimental and clinical studies. *Crit.Care Med.* 7:98–106, Mar. 1979.
9. SHOEMAKER, W. C. Pathophysiology, monitoring, outcome prediction, and therapy of shock states. *Crit.Care Clin.* 3:307–357, Apr. 1987.
10. WEAVER, D. W., AND OTHERS. Pulmonary effects of albumin resuscitation for severe hypovolemic shock. *Arch.Surg.* 113:387–391, Apr. 1978.
11. CRONE, R. K. Acute circulatory failure in children. *Pediatr.Clin.North Am.* 27:525–538, Aug. 1980.
12. PERKIN, R. M., AND LEVIN, D. L. Shock in the pediatric patient: Part II: Therapy. *J.Pediatr.* 101:319–332, Sept. 1982.
13. WEIL, M. H., AND HENNING, R. J. New concepts in the diagnosis and fluid treatment of circulatory shock. *Anesth.Analg.* (Cleve) 58:124–132, Mar.–Apr. 1979.
14. CHERNOW, B., AND ROTH, B. L. Pharmacologic manipulation of the peripheral vasculature in shock: clinical and experimental approaches. *Circ.Shock* 18(2):141–155, 1986.
15. GUYTON, A. C. *Textbook of Medical Physiology.* 7th ed. Philadelphia, W. B. Saunders Co., 1986.
16. KASTRUP, E. K., AND OLAN, BERNIE, III, EDS. *Drugs Facts and Comparisons.* St. Louis, J. B. Lippincott Co., 1987.
17. PERKIN, R. M., AND OTHERS. Dobutamine: a hemodynamic evaluation in children with shock. *J.Pediatr.* 100:977–983, June 1982.
18. MASON, D. T. Afterload reduction and cardiac performance. Physiologic basis of systemic vasodilators as a new approach in treatment of congestive heart failure. *Am.J.Med.* 65:106–125, July 1978.
19. COLE, C. H., ED. *The Harriet Lane Handbook.* 10th ed. Chicago, Year Book Medical Publishers, 1984.
20. VESEY, C. J., AND COLE, P. V. Blood cyanide and thiocyanate concentrations produced by long-term therapy with sodium nitroprusside. *Br.J.Anaesth.* 57:148–155, Feb. 1985.
21. TRISSEL, L. A. *Handbook on Injectable Drugs.* 4th ed. Bethesda, MD, American Society of Hospital Pharmacists, 1986.
22. HOLADAY, J. W., AND FADEN, A. I. Naloxone reversal of endotoxin hypotension suggests a role of endorphins in shock. *Nature* 275:450–451, Oct. 5, 1978.
23. FADEN, A. I., AND HOLADAY, J. W. Opiate antagonists: a role in the treatment of hypovolemic shock. *Science* 205:317–318, July 20, 1979.
24. TIENGO, M. Naloxone in irreversible shock. (letter) *Lancet* 2:690, Sept. 27, 1980.
25. COCCHI, P., AND OTHERS. Naloxone in fulminant meningococcemia. (letter) *Pediatr.Infect.Dis.* 3:187, Mar.–Apr. 1984.
26. ROCK, P., AND OTHERS. Efficacy and safety of naloxone in septic shock. *Crit.Care Med.* 13:28–33, Jan. 1985.
27. SPRUNG, C. L., AND OTHERS. The effects of high dose corticosteroids in patients with septic shock. A prospective, controlled study. *N.Engl.J.Med.* 311:1137–1143, Nov. 1, 1984.
28. ZIMMERMAN, J. J., AND DIETRICH, K. A. Current perspectives on septic shock. *Pediatr.Clin.North Am.* 34:131–163, Feb. 1987.
29. BRONSVELD, W., AND OTHERS. Use of glucose-insulin-potassium (GIK) in human septic shock. *Crit.Care Med.* 13:566–570, July 1985.
30. CARTER, J. L., AND SMITH, B. L. Use of military antishock trousers: nursing implications. *Heart Lung* 11:422–425, Sept.–Oct. 1982.
31. SCHARFMAN, W. B., AND OTHERS. Plasmapheresis for meningococcemia with disseminated intravascular coagulation. (letter) *N.Engl.J.Med.* 300:1277–1278, May 31, 1979.
32. BJORVATN, B., AND OTHERS. Meningococcal septicaemia treated with combined plasmapheresis and leucapheresis or with blood exchange. *Br.Med.J.* 288:439–441, Feb. 11, 1984.
33. OSSENKOPPELE, G. J., AND OTHERS. Continuous arteriovenous hemofiltration as an adjunctive therapy for septic shock. *Crit.Care Med.* 13:102–104, Feb. 1985.
34. SEASHORE, J. H. Nutritional support of children in the intensive care unit. IN *Topics in Pediatric Critical Care,* ed. by R. I. Markowitz and R. S. Baltimore. New Haven, CT, The Yale Journal of Biology and Medicine, 1984, pp. 111–134.
35. KEELY, B. R. Septic Shock. *Crit.Care Q.* 7:59–67, Mar. 1985.
36. LEWANDOWSKI, L. Psychosocial aspects of pediatric critical care. IN *Nursing Care of the Critically Ill Child,* ed. by M. Hazinski. St. Louis, C. V. Mosby Co., 1984, p. 12.
37. RIMAR, J. M., AND OTHERS. Fulminant meningococcemia in children. *Heart Lung* 14:385–391, July 1985.

Evaluating Head Trauma In Infants And Children

Reprinted from MCN: The Journal of Maternal/Child Nursing, January/February 1983

Nurses can play a significant role in screening, evaluating, and managing this common injury.

ELLEN M. MEIER

Acute head trauma is an extremely common problem among children, accounting for nearly 250,000 hospital admissions annually. Many more cases are evaluated and released through emergency departments and outpatient clinics or over the telephone. Because the nurse may be responsible for eliciting all or part of the injured child's history, she must know what screening questions to ask and what complications to caution parents to watch for.

The child's history is all-important in determining whether the child requires immediate medical attention or can be kept at home for observation by the parents. The specific information needed includes when the injury occurred; how the injury occurred (for example, how far the child fell and to what type of surface); and how the child behaved immediately after the injury.

In addition, the nurse must ascertain whether the child experienced loss of consciousness or memory, vomiting, disorientation, confusion, lethargy, bleeding or cerebrospinal (CSF) fluid drainage from the nose or ears, or any lacerations. She must also determine whether the child has any preexisting illnesses, such as a seizure disorder, gait disturbance, or physical handicap. Since head trauma among infants and young children may be the result of child abuse, the nurse also evaluates the history in terms of the child's developmental ability, the likelihood of the injury occurring as described, and the presence of limb fractures or other associated injuries.

If the child is alert and mature enough, the nurse can obtain the history directly from him. If not, any observer of the injury can provide the necessary information. Frequently, the nurse can obtain the history over the telephone, thereby eliminating the need for a clinic or emergency room visit.

If the head injury was minimal and there was no loss of consciousness, bleeding, or disorientation, the child can be safely observed at home. However, if parents are hesitant about observing the child, the child should be seen and evaluated by a health care provider.

Many children have headaches or vomit once or twice during the first 24 hours following minor head trauma. Unless these symptoms are progressive or accompanied by increasing lethargy, they usually are of little concern.

Loss of consciousness, severe or progressive vomiting or headaches, amnesia, disorientation, seizures or weakness, bleeding or CSF drainage from the ears or nose, and any unusual changes in behavior, however, warrant immediate medical evaluation and follow-up. Depending on their severity, open wounds or lacerations may also need attention. Even if a wound is not serious, the child's immunization status must be determined.

While eliciting the child's history, the nurse often will realize that the injury could have been avoided had safety measures such as car seats or restraints been used. Since the injured child's parents probably are already feeling anxious or guilty about the incident, the nurse must be careful not to increase their guilt feelings, although she can tactfully give appropriate guidance on safety procedures and precautions.

When a Physical Examination Is Needed

Positive or focal (pointing to a localized area of injury within the central nervous system) neurological findings are rare in cases of simple head trauma. However, any child who has sustained a significant blow to the head, has lost consciousness, or has any suspicious symptoms needs a thorough general physical examination and a neurological examination.

MS. MEIER, R.N., M.N., *is the director of education and training for Kaiser Foundation Hospital in Panorama City, California. She is also a certified pediatric nurse practitioner.*

Signs of shock (increased pulse and decreased blood pressure) or increased intracranial pressure are important to watch for. Any abnormalities found during the physical and neurological examinations require further evaluation by a neurologist or neurosurgeon and possibly hospitalization of the child.

The entire body, including the mouth, neck, chest, abdomen, and extremities, must be examined for evidence of injury. The scalp must be inspected for depression or areas of soft spongy hematoma over a depressed skull facture. For infants, the anterior fontanelle must be assessed for evidence of fullness or bulging.

Transillumination of the skull can be performed to detect intracranial or extracranial fluid. Other physical findings indicating possible basal skull fracture are periorbital hemorrhage with bilateral black eyes (raccoon eyes), blood behind the eardrum (hemotympanum), bruising behind the ear (Battle's sign), and bleeding or CSF drainage from the ears or nose.

A thorough neurological examination includes an evaluation of the child's level of consciousness, orientation, memory, and motor abilities. Level of consciousness can range from agitated to alert to lethargic, stuporous, or comatose. Orientation and memory can be evaluated by having the child identify himself and his surroundings and relate the incident of the injury.

The eyes are an important element in the neurological examination. Pupil size and reactivity as well as extraocular movements can be evaluated to determine cranial nerve function. The fundi can be examined for papilledema and retinal hemorrhage. Retinal hemorrhages often accompany subdural hematomas in small infants who are held by their shoulders and shaken vigorously, a relatively common form of child abuse. The child who is alert can be tested for visual acuity and peripheral vision.

To evaluate the motor system, the child's gait and symmetry of muscle strength can be observed. Parasthesias or numbness should be assessed. For the older child, cerebellar function can be evaluated with the Romberg test or by heel-walking and toe-walking. Eliciting deep tendon reflexes and attempting to elicit Babinski's reflex (dorsiflexion and fanning of the toes by stroking the lateral sole, an abnormal finding in infants and children over the age of one year) completes the motor system examination.

When Diagnostic Studies Are Necessary

Routine skull films for minor head trauma yield few findings or results. Further, skull fracture alone does not necessarily indicate serious brain injury and does not change treatment plans, except for depressed and compound fractures, which require surgical correction. In a study of 354 infants and children who had skull roentgenography for head trauma, for example, only 4.2 percent had skull fracture and none had serious intracranial complications (1). Thus, unless there is significant reason to be suspicious of a pathological condition, routine skull films are unwise, especially in light of the ever-increasing concern about unnecessary exposure to radiation.

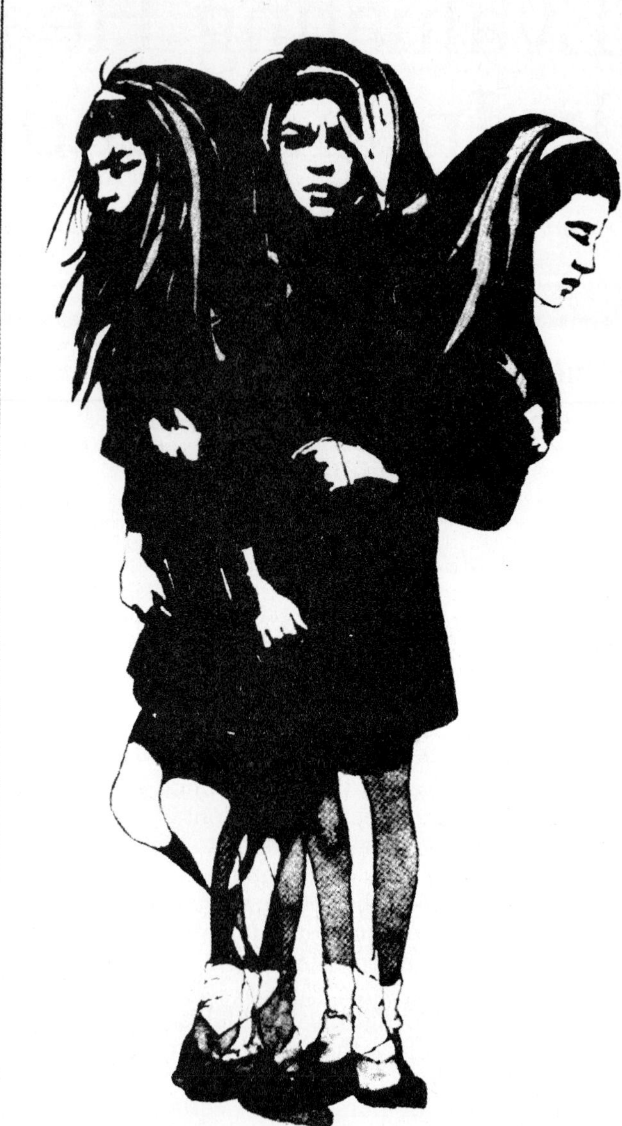

Evaluating all the symptoms accompanying head trauma is all-important in determining whether the child requires medical attention or can be kept at home for observation.

Criteria for determining when skull roentgenography is necessary were established in 1978 by Leon Phillips and modified in 1982 by John Leonidas and others (1,2). These criteria (listed in the table below) are useful to the nurse in the development of standardized procedures for the evaluation and management of head trauma. With such guidelines for the initiation of diagnostic studies, safe, high-quality health care can be provided without the expenditure of unnecessary time and money.

The availability of computerized transaxial tomography (CAT) scanning has greatly changed the role of radiology in the evaluation of head trauma. Intracranial hemorrhage and tissue structures are more clearly delineated by CAT scanning than by skull roentgenography. In addition, the CAT scan procedure is safe and painless and can be repeated to assess changing signs and symptoms. It is indicated for head trauma with localized or progressive signs or symptoms, although generally only after routine skull films have been obtained (3).

If head trauma is severe or there is injury to the neck, X-rays should also include anteroposterior and lateral views of the cervical spine. Because of the significance of spinal cord transection, cervical spine injury must be diagnosed as soon as possible. Lumbar puncture is not performed for head trauma unless central nervous system infection, such as meningitis, is suspected. It is contraindicated if intracranial pressure is increased or if a mass lesion is suspected (3).

Other diagnostic studies, such as subdural taps and ventricular drainage for subdural hematomas, may be necessary under selected and specific conditions. However, nurses usually are not involved in ordering or performing these studies.

PROPOSED CRITERIA FOR SKULL ROENTGENOGRAPHY FOR CHILDREN WITH HEAD TRAUMA*

Historical Criteria

- Age less than one year.
- Unconscious for more than five minutes.
- Gunshot wound or skull penetration.
- Previous craniotomy with shunting tube in place.

Physical Examination Criteria

- Palpable hematoma on scalp.
- Skull depression palpable or identified by probe in scalp laceration.
- Cerebrospinal fluid (CSF) discharge from ear or nose.
- Blood in middle ear.
- Battle's sign.
- Racoon eyes.
- Lethargy, coma, or stupor.
- Focal neurological signs.

*These criteria were established by John Leonidas and others and modified by Leon Phillips.

Differentiating Diagnoses

Minor head injury without positive history or physical examination findings is simply called head trauma or uncomplicated head trauma. Frequently, the diagnosis of concussion is made incorrectly. Concussion is defined as head injury followed by a period of unconsciousness (loss of awareness and responsiveness). The period of unresponsiveness may last from several seconds to several hours. If the injury was unwitnessed, the diagnosis of concussion is sometimes made if the child experiences retrograde or posttraumatic amnesia (3).

The diagnosis of skull fracture is made on the basis of radiologic findings. About 75 percent of skull fractures in children are linear fractures; other types include depressed, compound, and basal skull fractures. Although skull fracture does not warrant any specific management, it indicates that a significant injury occurred. Often, children with skull fractures are hospitalized for observation.

In addition to radiographic evidence, racoon eyes, hemotympanum, and Battle's sign are indications of basal skull fracture. Characteristic features of an occipital fracture are tachycardia, hypotension, and irregular respirations caused by brainstem compression. CSF rhinorrhea may indicate a fracture of the cribriform plate, whereas CSF otorrhea may indicate fracture of the petrous temporal bone (3).

Actual epidural or subdural hematomas are diagnosed by the child's history and physical examination findings, specifically those findings associated with increased intracranial pressure. They are also diagnosed by skull films, CAT scans, and special studies such as subdural taps.

Contusion of the brain is a bruising or crushing injury to the brain. It usually results from blunt trauma to the head and may be accompanied by skull fracture (3). Diagnosis is based on the presence of focal neurological signs, such as seizures, and is frequently confirmed by a CAT scan.

Superficial injuries to the head include scalp lacerations and hematomas. Often, a significant amount of scalp swelling follows head trauma, but it does not require treatment. Aspiration is of no benefit and just increases the risk of infection.

Scalp lacerations must be evaluated to determine whether sutures are required, and the child's tetanus status must always be determined. A fully immunized child with a minor scalp laceration need not receive tetanus toxoid or antitoxin. However, if an open scalp wound has been unattended for more than 24 hours, the child must receive both passive and active tetanus immunization even if he was fully immunized previously (4).

Most head injuries do not result in serious consequences. However, careful observation of the child during the first two days after a head injury is extremely important for recognizing complications. The following signs and symptoms must be reported and evaluated immediately:

- Persistent or progressive vomiting.
- Headache if it is long-lasting or increases in severity.
- Unusual drowsiness, confusion, irritability, or inability to awaken the child. (The child should be awakened every two hours for the first 24 hours following significant head trauma.)
- Convulsions or seizures.
- Dizziness, weakness, or numbness.
- Fever above 101°F.
- Visual disturbance or inequality of the pupil size.
- Clear fluid or blood coming from the nose or ears.

If you are uncertain or concerned about any of the above, call:

__________ at the following number __________

or return to ________________________________

Head trauma may be complicated by meningitis, especially when a child has a basal skull fracture. Signs and symptoms include fever, irritability, and meningeal irritation such as nuchal rigidity.

Other syndromes following head injury include posttraumatic epilepsy and transient posttraumatic blindness. These syndromes are dramatic but poorly understood. Posttraumatic blindness generally lasts minutes to hours. Seizures can occur up to one week following head trauma; between 20 percent and 25 percent of the children who experience head trauma have seizure disorders (5).

The Role of the Nurse

In dealing with head trauma, the nurse is primarily responsible for observation, guidance, and deciding whether the injury is severe enough to refer the child for consultation with a physician and perhaps with a neurologist or neurosurgeon. If the child is sent home, the nurse must give the parents or caretaker specific instructions as to what signs and symptoms require further evaluation. These can be printed on a sheet for the parents to take with them (see example above).

Most signs of significant injury will appear during the first 48 hours following the trauma. Since it is unrealistic to expect a child who has sustained a head injury to remain awake during this period when observation is critical, the nurse must reassure parents that there is no inherent danger in allowing the child to fall asleep. Children often are drowsy after the physical and emotional upheaval of head trauma. Awakening them for evaluation at two-hour intervals is sufficient and safe. The important issue is the child's overall level of consciousness.

When counseling over the telephone, the nurse can refer to the head injury sheet as she instructs parents about the signs of possible complications and when to seek further medical attention for the child. If an open wound has been sustained, the nurse must also determine the need for suturing and the child's immunization status. At no time should the nurse discourage parents from bringing in a child for evaluation by a health care professional if they are uneasy about observing the child at home.

Generally Favorable Prognosis

Only 5 percent to 10 percent of children who are hospitalized for head trauma show neurological signs and symptoms (6). Most who are hospitalized because of loss of consciousness or skull fracture recover completely within 24 to 48 hours. A small percentage experience seizures, motor deficits, or intellectual impairment.

In contrast to adults, children who experience head trauma continue to show improvement for more than three years following a comparable injury (7). Children with signs of severe injury also have a more favorable outcome than do adults with similar signs (8). Because of this prognosis, the child or infant who experiences head trauma should be evaluated and treated quickly and aggressively.

Nurses can play a significant role in the screening, evaluation, and management of this common and frightening injury. At the same time, they can promote health and safety procedures as well as plans for follow-up for the injured infant or child.

REFERENCES

1. LEONIDAS, J.C., AND OTHERS. Mild head trauma in children: when is a roentgenogram necessary. *Pediatrics* 69:139-143, Feb. 1982.
2. PHILLIPS, L.A. *A Study of the Effect of High Yield Criteria for Emergency Room Skull Radiography.* (DHEW Publ. (FDA) 78-8089) Washington D.C., U.S. Government Printing Office, 1978.
3. ROSMAN, N.P., AND OTHERS. Acute head trauma in infancy and childhood. Clinical and radiologic aspects. *Pediatr.Clin.North Am.* 26:707-736, Nov. 1979.
4. AMERICAN ACADEMY OF PEDIATRICS, Committee on Infectious Diseases. *Report.* 18th ed. Evanston, Ill., The Academy, 1977.
5. JENNETT, B. Trauma as a cause of epilepsy in childhood. *Dev.Med. Child Neurol.* 15:56-62, Feb. 1973.
6. DEANGELIS, CATHERINE. *Pediatric Primary Care.* 2nd ed. Boston, Little Brown and Co., 1979.
7. RICHARDSON, F. Some effects of severe head injury. A follow-up study of children and adolescents after protracted coma. *Dev.Med.Child Neurol.* 5:471-482, Oct. 1963.
8. OVERGAARD, J., AND OTHERS. Prognosis after head injury based on early clinical examination. *Lancet* 2:631-635, Sept. 22, 1973.

Factors To Consider When Assessing Responses To Pain

Reprinted from MCN: The American Journal of Maternal/Child Nursing, July/August 1984

CAROLYN SHEREDY

To assess pain, the nurse must be familiar not only with the physiology of pain but also with the person's general physical condition as well as the person's cultural and historical factors that contribute to pain. (See box for a discussion of the physiology of pain.) Systematic observation skills are extremely important (especially when assessing children under five or six years old) since behavioral cues often are the primary source of data. Increased irritability, restlessness, and lack of appetite are important indicators of pain, as are pulling, rubbing, and guarding certain body parts. Young children may become so preoccupied with pain that they begin to limit involvement and interactions with others in the environment.

Since children often mimic parents' responses to pain, interactions between parents and children need to be assessed. If a child is told by parents that "big boys (girls) don't cry," the child may deny or minimize the degree of pain in order to please the parents. Thus a child soon learns what is an acceptable or unacceptable attitude and response to pain.

Vital signs also are considered. Heart rate and respirations increase when a person experiences pain and should improve after measures are taken to relieve pain (such as, repositioning, medicating, and/or distracting). The intensity of pain and whether it increases, decreases, or remains the same is determined after pain relief is provided. Individuals in the school-age years and older are able to rate the intensity of pain on a scale of one to ten.

CAROLYN SHEREDY, R.N., B.S.N. is a clinical nurse at Group Health Association in Annandale, Virginia. At the time this article was written, she was a member of the p.r.n. staff at Children's Hospital National Medical Center in Washington, D.C.

A pain history is invaluable for assessing pain and evaluating pain-relief measures. Examples of variables affecting pain are listed in the table Variables Affecting Pain Responses. The nurse should consider not only physical, cultural, and historical factors that affect a person's response to pain but also the person's developmental level. The following discussion highlights the responses to pain of people at different developmental levels and some appropriate nursing interventions.

Infancy (birth to twelve months old). Infants usually indicate discomfort or pain through general body movements, changes in body state, stooling, hiccoughing, withdrawing the affected limb, and crying. Prolonged pain may lead to generalized body fatigue. Relief measures include removing the painful stimulus, if possible, as well as holding, touching, stroking, and providing a pacifier. Enabling the infant to assume a comfortable position also is helpful (see "The Neonate's Response to Pain" by Karen D'Apolito).

Toddler years (twelve months to three years old). Toddlers, like infants, may be unable to indicate the nature of pain in a meaningful manner. Language comprehension may be adequate, but the child may lack expressive language skills. Even if a toddler has mastered language skills, the unfamiliarity of the hospital may cause the child to be unusually silent or to regress in behavior. Often a toddler responds to pain through aggressive behavior such as biting, hitting, and temper tantrums or exhibits nonverbal cues such as clenching teeth, thumb sucking, or rocking.

A toddler's thinking basically is concrete and literal, and the toddler's concept of time is the present. Thus a toddler is unable to understand that "Mommy will come back" and needs to be familiarized with the hospital in order to reduce stress levels. Stress increases anxiety, which increases pain, which adds to the stress and anxiety that the toddler is experiencing. This cycle repeats itself unless the nurse intervenes.

Preschool years (three to five years old). The preschooler's greatest fear is of bodily injury. Placing a bandage over a cut or a scratch assures the child that his or her body will remain intact.

Because of increased maturity, the preschooler can verbalize fears and pains better than a toddler can. Also, the preschooler becomes adept at procrastination and believes that by saying "wait a minute" a painful procedure can be postponed or eliminated.

The preschooler's thinking is egocentric. All events and occurrences are believed to result from the child's own being. Consequently, hospitalizations may be viewed as a punishment. Parents may unknowingly reinforce this pattern of reasoning by saying, "If you aren't good, the nurse will give you a shot."

Prehospital visits familiarize the child with a new environment and reduce fearful misperceptions. Because fantasy and magical thinking are part of the preschooler's world, therapeutic play helps create a safe environment in which the child can work through feelings of fear, anger, or guilt about the trauma or pain.

Parents should be told how the child's developmental stage affects his or her response to pain and hospitalization. Often the child will cooperate with the nurse but exhibit aggressive behavior toward the parent. For example, a four year old may stoically receive an injection and then refuse a parent's comforting by turning over and hiding under a blanket.

VARIABLES AFFECTING PAIN RESPONSES

Variable	*Example*
Cultural background	An individual with an Oriental heritage may be stoic and not admit feeling pain.
Developmental level	Verbal communication in a toddler is inadequate.
Parents' attitudes	A parent may forewarn a child that an injection will or will not hurt.
Education (prehospital admission and preoperative teaching)	Fear of the unknown increases anxiety and pain.
Type of anesthesia	Local versus general.
Type of surgery performed	Cyst removal versus abdominal.
Nature of procedures	Intravenous insertion.
Frequency and duration of hospitalization	Repeated admission for renal dialysis.
Pain medication	Nurses may dispense medications conservatively because they fear addiction.
Parents' absence or presence	Pain increases in parents' absence because the child fears abandonment.
Nurses' attitudes	A nurse may draw conclusions about responses to pain on the basis of past experience or believe that an individual is "making a scene."

School-aged children (five to twelve years old). Because the school-aged child has a greater awareness of the body and internal organs, fear of bodily harm increases, and fear of death develops. However, a five year old's thinking is still concrete and animistic. Objects are defined in terms of their use and effects upon the child. Thus the child may believe that a needle used for an injection caused the original pain. When another child is seen crying during an examination, the child may believe that the examination will hurt him, too.

Reasoning begins to occur by the time children become seven years old. The concept of time also develops. Past and future have meaning. Thus the pain experience is time-limited.

Whereas younger school-aged children describe pain mostly in terms of physical aspects, older school-aged children include psychological components (1). Both hospitalized and nonhospitalized children can describe interventions for pain such as pain medication, rest or relaxation, and the presence of a sensitive person or stuffed animal.

School-aged children between ten and twelve years old may deny pain because of a desire to be brave. They may pretend that they are not in pain by reading or by watching television. However, no child should be without some kind of pain relief. A simple explanation that refusing pain relief does not indicate that a person is brave or strong often helps children acknowledge that they feel pain and convinces them that their responses to pain are not signs of weakness. In addition, providing pain-relief measures other than injections may encourage children to describe their responses to pain.

Adolescence (twelve to twenty years old). Adolescents may find the threat of illness or alteration of the body physically or psychologically disturbing because they fear loss of control. They may be able to accept intellectually the reasons for hospitalizations or illnesses but unable to accept emotionally the separation from family or friends. Moreover, adolescents frequently experience mood changes and extremes of behavior. Consequently, an adolescent may refuse pain medication during one shift but request it repeatedly during the next shift even though pain has not increased.

Understanding this phase of development is vital. The nurse needs to establish a trusting relationship in order to encourage the adolescent to share and discuss any fears and concerns.

Young adult (twenty years old and older). Young adults are affected more by sociocultural forces and value changes than by physical or cognitive development. The young adult has new roles of responsibility at work, home, and in society. Coping with these new changes can be a source of physical and psychological stress.

In this special series, the young adult being discussed is the childbearing woman. Her response to pain or discomfort may be influenced by cultural and psychosocial attitudes about pregnancy and motherhood. These factors as well as various comfort measures will be discussed in Part III of this series.

Summary. Knowledge of growth and development as well as the other factors discussed is needed in order to make an accurate evaluation of a person's responses to pain. The assessment of pain is an ongoing and at times difficult undertaking. However, the long-range benefit is a reduction in the psychological hurt that often accompanies physical pain.

THE PHYSIOLOGY OF PAIN

The perception of and response to pain are dependent upon the maturation of the central nervous system. When a painful stimulus is felt by an older child or an adult, two types of nerve fibers (A delta and C) transmit pain signals to the brain. These afferent (ascending to the brain) pain fibers carry pain impulses from free, specialized nerve endings that serve as pain sensors in the skin, muscles, blood vessels, and organs.

The pain impulses travel to the dorsal horns of the spinal cord, where a synapse occurs. The axons of the activated neurons cross to the opposite side of the spinal cord and travel to the thalamus via the spinothalamic tract and finally to the cortex (see figure).

Because myelinated A delta fibers transmit impulses more rapidly than unmyelinated C fibers, two types of pain sensation are felt after the onset of a painful stimulus. Sharp, pricking sensations are caused by stimula-

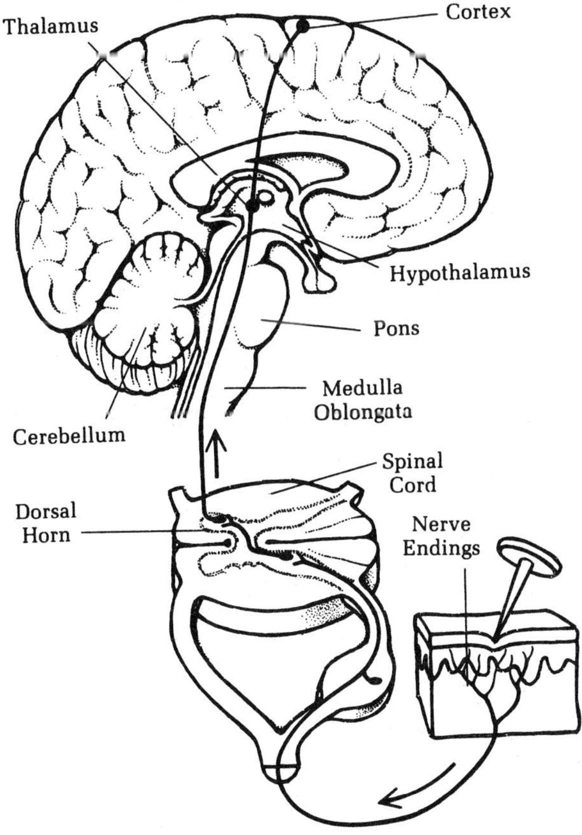

tion of A delta fibers, while prolonged, burning types of pain are caused by stimulation of unmyelinated C fibers. Activation of A delta fibers leads to a withdrawal response in the involved muscle or organ. The slow, burning sensation resulting from activation of C fibers tends to become more and more painful over time. This sensation causes the intolerable suffering of pain (2).

The sensation for chronic pain occurs in the medulla, reticular activating system, thalamus, hypothalamus, and other parts of the limbic system. As pain evolves from acute to chronic, different areas of the brain are involved in pain perception (3).

In addition to a sensory awareness of pain, visceral changes occur. They are caused by activation of the autonomic nervous system. Autonomic response fibers are located in the spinal cord, medulla, and midbrain. When a pain stimulus is received, blood pressure alterations, tachycardia, tachypnea, perspiration, or gastrointestinal disturbances may result. (For a detailed discussion of the infant's central nervous system, see "The Neonate's Response to Pain" by Karen D'Apolito.)

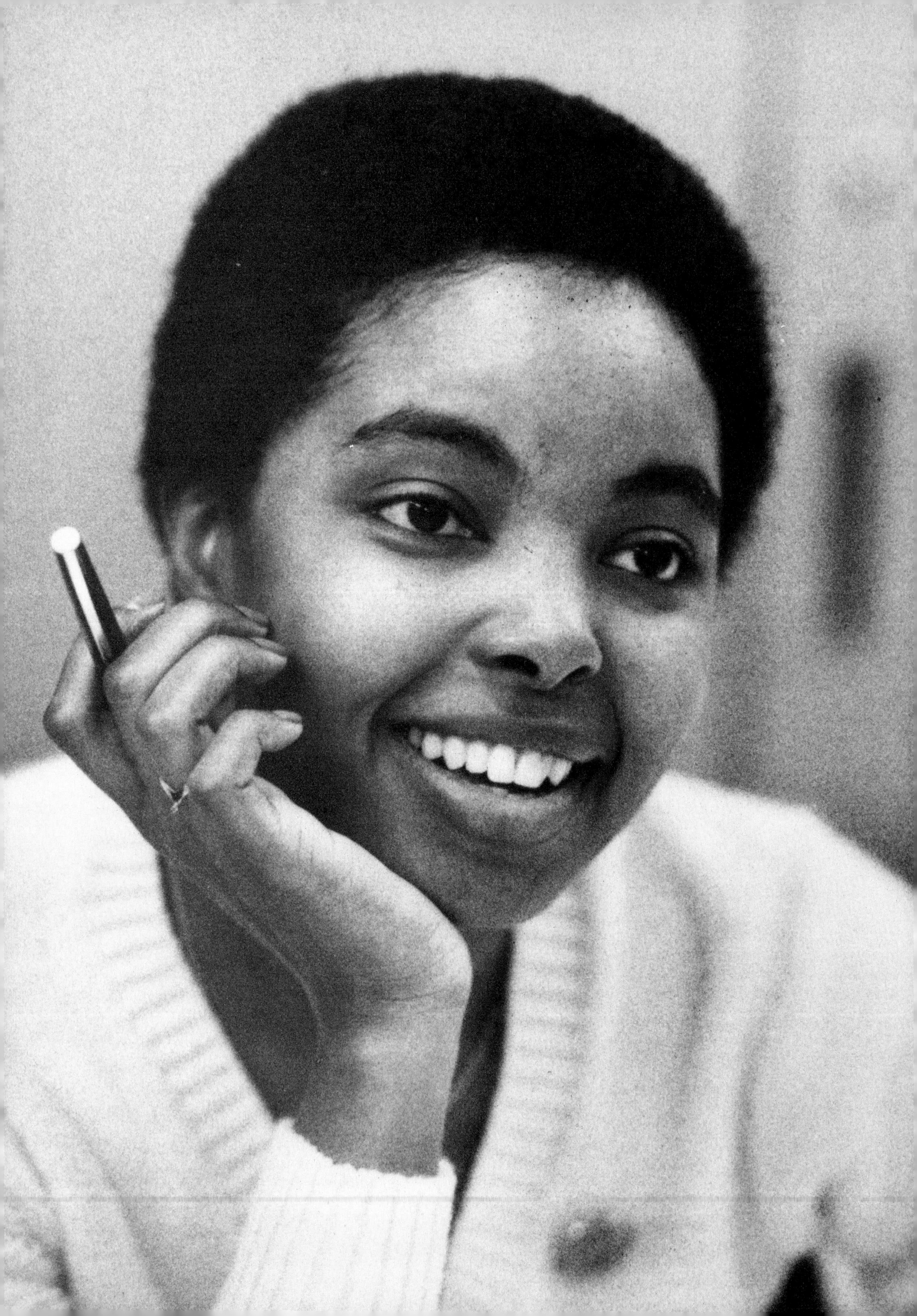

Questions and Answers

The questions and answers in this section have been organized in such a way as to stimulate the NCLEX-RN exam.

The 374 questions have been divided into four sections of 93 or 94 questions each. Each section tests your nursing knowledge in regard to care of the adult, the child, the childbearing family, and the client with psychosocial problems.

Instructions for Taking the Test

1. Review the information in Section One: Preparing for the NCLEX.
2. Time yourself, allowing one and one-half hours per section.
3. Read each question carefully and select *one* best answer to each question.
4. Do not leave questions blank, since you will not be penalized for random answers on the NCLEX-RN.
5. Score your exam using the answer key. Count any questions left unanswered as incorrect. A score of 75% (70 questions) or more correct answers per section is roughly equivalent to a passing grade.
6. Review the questions you answered incorrectly and restudy that specific material.

At the end of this section you will find information regarding the assignment of each question into Nursing Process and Client Need categories. These decisions were based on what the question tests and were made after consultation with the section coordinators and the National Council of State Boards of Nursing. You may use this information to determine if your incorrect answers reflect a weakness in a particular area. Remember, however, that NCLEX-RN is testing your abilities *to apply the steps of the nursing process*, not your ability to assign a category to an individual question.

Section 6: Questions and Answers (Sample NCLEX-RN Test) 643

Part One 645
Questions 645
Answers and Rationales 655
Part Two 663
Questions 663
Answers and Rationales 673
Part Three 681
Questions 681
Answers and Rationales 692
Part Four 700
Questions 700
Answers and Rationales 712
Nursing Process and Client Needs Categories 720
Appendix A 725
Approved Nursing Diagnoses from the North American Nursing Diagnosis Association, June 1988 725
Appendix B 727
Common Laboratory Values—Adult 727
Appendix C 729
Information for Foreign Nurse Graduates Who Wish to Practice in the United States 729
State Boards of Nursing 730
Index 733

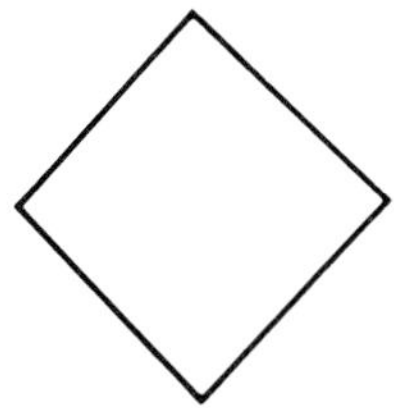

Sample Test Questions: Part One

The community health nurse makes a home visit to the Stephens family. Mona Stephens is a single mother with a 2½-year-old daughter, Vanessa, and a 3-week-old son, Burton. The family lives on public assistance and receives food stamps. Burton's formula is supplied by the WIC program.

1. The nurse would best initiate the visit with which remark?

○ **1.** "You look tired. Are you getting enough sleep?"
○ **2.** "Vanessa seems to like her new brother."
○ **3.** "Tell me what a typical day is like for the three of you."
○ **4.** "Are you having any trouble meeting your expenses?"

2. Ms. Stephens tells the nurse she is concerned about Burton's "throwing up. He does it every time he eats." What would be the nurse's best first response to further clarify this potential problem?

○ **1.** "About how much does he throw up each time, and what does it look like?"
○ **2.** "Are you burping him after every ounce?"
○ **3.** "Perhaps you aren't diluting his formula correctly. Let's check."
○ **4.** "Is he taking formula with iron?"

3. After ascertaining that Burton is experiencing normal newborn regurgitation, the nurse reassures his mother that newborns often experience this problem based on what knowledge?

○ **1.** The newborn's stomach capacity is very small.
○ **2.** It takes some time for the newborn to adjust to the formula's richness.
○ **3.** The lining of the newborn's stomach is easily irritated.
○ **4.** The cardiac sphincter between the esophagus and stomach is not fully matured.

4. The nurse has just finished talking with Ms. Stephens about accident prevention. Which of the following statements by the mother tells you the nurse's teaching was *not* effective?

○ **1.** "I can simply close the door to the bathroom and basement in order to keep Vanessa out."
○ **2.** "It's very important that my daughter not think of medicine as candy."
○ **3.** "I've put the poison control center phone number by all the phones in the house."
○ **4.** "You know, no matter how hard I try I just can't monitor everything she does."

5. The nurse makes a follow-up visit in 3 months. Which finding presents the greatest cause for concern?

○ **1.** Burton is taking 28 oz of formula daily along with 2 tbsp of cereal and pureed fruit twice daily.
○ **2.** Vanessa wets the bed 2 or 3 times a week.
○ **3.** Ms. Stephens says she is "always exhausted."
○ **4.** The only toys in the home are makeshift ones, such as shoe boxes, tissue paper, and pots and pans.

6. The nurse assesses Burton's development at this visit. He should be exhibiting which of the following behaviors?

○ **1.** Bears some weight on his legs.
○ **2.** Imitates speech sounds.
○ **3.** Sits with minimal support.
○ **4.** Uses a thumb-finger grasp.

Margaret Dunneden is a 40-year-old businesswoman who was admitted to the psychiatric unit 2 days ago for severe depression.

7. Mrs. Dunneden says to the nurse, "I'm terrible. I don't deserve to live." Which of the following responses by the nurse would be most appropriate?

- **1.** "Yes, it has occurred to us that you have that opinion of yourself."
- **2.** "If you continue to talk this way, I can't listen to you any more."
- **3.** "What has led you to think that you don't deserve to live?"
- **4.** "I don't think you're terrible. Don't you think you're liked here?"

8. When the nurse tells Mrs. Dunneden that he will be meeting with her for regular interviews, she says, "Why would you want to do that?" What would be the most therapeutic response?

- **1.** "I think you're worth the time and effort."
- **2.** "I have been assigned as your therapist."
- **3.** "You need to talk about your feelings."
- **4.** "You can't get better without help."

9. In planning Mrs. Dunneden's care, which of the following objectives is *first* priority?

- **1.** Promotion of self esteem.
- **2.** Establishment of the nurse-patient relationship.
- **3.** Promotion of expression of feelings.
- **4.** Protection from suicidal gestures.

10. Mrs. Dunneden tells the nurse she has just received a promotion and is in line for another significant advance in her company if she does as well in the new position as she did in the last. How is this information most likely related to her depression?

- **1.** Success can sometimes result in a depression.
- **2.** Depression includes grandiose delusions.
- **3.** This will help validate that she is not worthless.
- **4.** The promotion will give her a goal.

11. One day, the nurse notices Mrs. Dunneden sitting alone in the television lounge; and although the TV is on, she is not watching it. Which of the following would be the most therapeutic way to open a conversation with her?

- **1.** "What are you feeling?"
- **2.** "Do you like TV?"
- **3.** "Tell me how you're doing today."
- **4.** "You're not watching TV."

12. Instead of responding verbally, Mrs. Dunneden gets up and walks away. Which of the following is the most therapeutic thing for the nurse to do?

- **1.** Let her go.
- **2.** Follow her and encourage her to talk.
- **3.** Follow her and confront her avoidance behavior.
- **4.** Send another staff person to check on her.

13. One of the staff members reports that Mrs. Dunneden has been eating very little at meals. Which of the following is the most likely explanation of this behavior?

- **1.** It is a common side effect of antidepressants.
- **2.** The hospital food is probably unfamiliar to her.
- **3.** She is trying to get attention from the staff.
- **4.** It is part of her psychiatric problems.

14. Mrs. Dunneden begins to respond to her antidepressant trazodone HCl (Desyrel), and will continue to take it after she is discharged. Which of the following is the correct information to give her about her medication?

- **1.** It may be addicting and should be stopped as soon as she can tolerate being without it.
- **2.** Dizziness can be minimized by not taking the drug on an empty stomach.
- **3.** The drug may cause hypertension, and she should monitor her blood pressure.
- **4.** She should avoid foods such as aged cheeses and yogurt and products made with yeast, beer, and wine.

15. Mrs. Dunneden has become very involved in activities on the unit. She is talking to other clients and making plans to see all her family. She tells the nurse, "I don't know why I didn't do this before. I know everything will work out now." The nurse's most appropriate response would be

- **1.** "Are you making plans to harm yourself?"
- **2.** "I'm concerned that you are taking on too much too fast."
- **3.** "What is it that you are doing now?"
- **4.** "I'm glad to see that you've become interested in activities and people again."

16. Which of the following statements about suicide is accurate?

1. Suicide is the leading cause of death in this country among all age groups and among adolescents.
2. Depressed persons attempt suicide as an expression of anger.
3. Hospitalized persons rarely attempt suicide.
4. A person who talks about suicide will not attempt it.

17. When would you best begin preparing for the termination of your relationship with Mrs. Dunneden?

1. At your first meeting.
2. During the working phase.
3. After rapport has been established.
4. When her discharge date is set.

18. A few days before Mrs. Dunneden's scheduled discharge, the nurse finds her crying alone in her room. She says, "I just don't know if I'll be able to make it." What is the most therapeutic response?

1. "You're worried that you'll get depressed again."
2. "You won't be able to 'make' what?"
3. "You wouldn't be leaving if you couldn't make it."
4. "Everyone feels that way sometimes."

19. What is the most likely explanation for Mrs. Dunneden's behavior?

1. She is not ready for discharge.
2. She has become overly dependent on the hospital.
3. She is having a common reaction to discharge.
4. She needs to know the nurse still cares about her.

Alda Clark is a 75-year-old widow, who maintains her own residence. While cleaning the snow off her walk, she slipped and fell.

20. You notice Mrs. Clark is unable to move her left leg. Your first priority is to

1. Extend her leg into a normal position.
2. Try and reduce the fracture.
3. Elevate the extremity.
4. Treat her as if a fracture has occurred.

21. You suspect that Mrs. Clark fractured her left hip because of which of the following manifestations?

1. Edema around the site.
2. Internal rotation of the left hip.
3. Abduction of the left hip.
4. Shortened right leg.

22. Preparation of Mrs. Clark's skin before applying Buck's extension traction should include which of the following?

1. Surgical preparation of the area where pins will be inserted.
2. Close shaving of the leg with a safety razor.
3. Washing and drying of the skin.
4. Application of talc to area.

23. The diagnosis of extracapsular fracture of the left hip requiring internal fixation is made. The plan of care in the post-op course includes which of the following?

1. Sedation to reduce Mrs. Clark's pain.
2. Early ambulation with weight bearing on the left leg to prevent muscle atrophy.
3. Provisions for "log-rolling" Mrs. Clark.
4. Maintaining adduction of the left hip to prevent dislocation of the prosthesis.

24. Mrs. Clark has had osteoarthritis for years. She takes aspirin 600 mg q4h to relieve the pain. Side effects of aspirin are indicated by which of the following signs?

1. Urinary retention.
2. Bradycardia.
3. Tinnitus.
4. Diplopia.

25. Mrs. Clark expresses concern over her impending discharge. What would be the most effective intervention for Mrs. Clark?

1. Ask her what concerns her.
2. Discuss the possibility of placing her in a nursing home.
3. Teach her about hazards in her environment.
4. Have the social worker make a visit to Mrs. Clark's home.

Phillip Witten is employed as the manager of a real estate business. Subsequent to increasing pressures at work, hurried and irregular meals, and an unhappy home and family environment, Mr. Witten developed a duodenal ulcer.

26. The nurse knows that which of the following may be a manifestation of a duodenal ulcer?

1. Pain relieved by food ingestion.
2. Pain one-half hour after meals.
3. Vomiting.
4. Hematemesis.

27. Mr. Witten was placed on a bland diet regimen. Foods permitted on this diet include which one of the following?
   1. Creamed soup, pureed squash.
   2. Potato chips, whole wheat bread.
   3. Sponge cake, fried chicken.
   4. Bran muffins, unsalted butter.

28. Anticholinergic drugs are useful in the management of gastrointestinal problems such as Mr. Witten's duodenal ulcer. Which is their major action?
   1. Increase gastric motility.
   2. Reduce production of gastric secretions.
   3. Neutralize hydrochloric acid in the stomach.
   4. Absorb excess gastric secretions.

29. Mr. Witten has an order for antacids q2h. At 2:00 A.M. when the night nurse goes to his room to give him the antacid, he is asleep. What action is most appropriate?
   1. Wake him and give the medication.
   2. Let him sleep but wake him at 4:00 A.M. and give him a double dose of medicine.
   3. Let him sleep until he wakes up and then resume the antacid q2h.
   4. Wake him but give him a double dose of medicine so you do not have to wake him at 4:00 A.M.

30. Mr. Witten requires surgical intervention and has a gastric resection. Post-op nursing interventions include connecting his Salem sump tube to low continuous wall suction. If he starts to regurgitate, which action should the nurse take?
   1. Irrigate the tube with normal saline.
   2. Notify the physician.
   3. Switch the suction to low Gomco.
   4. Reposition the tube.

31. After his abdominal surgery, the nurse must be particularly conscientious in encouraging Mr. Witten to cough and deep breathe hourly for which of the following reasons?
   1. Marked changes in intrathoracic pressure will stimulate gastric drainage.
   2. The high, abdominal incision will lead to shallow breathing to avoid pain.
   3. The phrenic nerve has been permanently damaged during the surgical procedure.
   4. Deep breathing will prevent post-op vomiting and intestinal distention.

32. The nurse should be aware of potential complications after a total gastrectomy. For example, 2 months postoperatively, Mr. Witten sought help for complaints of dizziness, sweating, and tachycardia, which occurred 30 minutes after he ate. He also had lost 10 lb. Symptoms were probably due to which of the following?
   1. Pernicious anemia.
   2. Dumping syndrome.
   3. Recurrence of the ulcer at the incision.
   4. Pyloric stenosis.

Mark Parker, 3 years old, has Down syndrome. During a routine clinic visit, Mrs. Parker relates to the nurse that her husband is being transferred to another city. She is very concerned about the effect this move will have on Mark.

33. Which of the following suggestions should receive the highest priority when discussing the move with Mrs. Parker?
   1. Adhere to Mark's daily routine as much as possible during and after the move.
   2. Include Mark in all the family discussions concerning the move.
   3. Have Mark stay with relatives until the move is complete.
   4. Enroll Mark in a special day-care program as soon as possible.

34. Mrs. Parker is also concerned about Mark's weight. "He is so much smaller than other children his age." The nurse's response should be based on the knowledge that
   1. Mark needs more fluids and calories than the average 3-year-old.
   2. The height and weight of children with Down syndrome is usually below chronologic norms.
   3. Mrs. Parker should discuss this concern with Mark's pediatrician.
   4. Mark's growth will "catch up" in a few years.

35. Which of the following childhood problems poses the most serious threat to Mark's health?
   1. Conjunctivitis.
   2. Milk allergy.
   3. Chickenpox.
   4. Bronchitis.

36. A comprehensive preschool stimulation program has been planned for Mark according to his abilities. The primary goal of this program is which of the following?
- **1.** Mark will improve his muscle tone.
- **2.** Mark will achieve an optimal developmental level.
- **3.** Mark's family will be involved in his care.
- **4.** Mark will be ready to enter first grade at age 6.

37. Which of the following actions is likely to have the greatest impact on Mark's learning outcomes during the preschool stimulation program?
- **1.** Giving Mark's parents written instructions explaining the learning activities.
- **2.** Observing Mark's parents carrying out Mark's learning plan.
- **3.** Explaining the activities to Mark while they are being performed to increase his understanding.
- **4.** Praising Mark for his accomplishments and cooperation with the learning activities.

Thirteen-year-old Darren has hemophilia, and has recently been diagnosed with acquired immune deficiency syndrome (AIDS) resulting from contaminated blood products. Darren is currently free from infectious disease.

38. Darren has been hospitalized for hemarthrosis of his left elbow. He is complaining of severe elbow pain. In addition to placing Darren on bedrest, the nurse should
- **1.** Apply a heating pad to Darren's left elbow.
- **2.** Give Darren aspirin gr X PO.
- **3.** Gently perform passive range-of-motion exercises to Darren's left elbow.
- **4.** Elevate and immobilize Darren's left elbow in a flexed position.

39. The nurse plans to obtain a nursing history from Darren and his mother. No direct body contact with Darren will be necessary during this time. Since Darren has AIDS, the nurse should take which precautions?
- **1.** Wear a mask only.
- **2.** Put on a mask and gown.
- **3.** Wear a mask, gown, and gloves.
- **4.** No special precautions are needed.

40. A nursing student on Darren's unit tells the nurse she has a cousin with hemophilia and wants to know how the disease is inherited. The nurse explains that a female is usually the carrier of the disease, and when she marries a male who is free of the disease, the risk to their offspring for each pregnancy is what?
- **1.** All female children will be carriers of hemophilia.
- **2.** All male children will have the disease.
- **3.** Half the male children will have hemophilia.
- **4.** Half the female children will have hemophilia.

41. While Darren is on bedrest, which activity should the nurse *not* include as part of Darren's nursing care plan?
- **1.** Reading the daily newspaper.
- **2.** Playing Nerf basketball with his older brother.
- **3.** Watching his favorite football team on television.
- **4.** Playing chess with his father.

Ann Cooper, aged 28, was referred to the infertility clinic after 6 years of unsuccessful attempts to conceive. She and her husband, Tim, wish to exhaust all possibilities before applying to a community adoption agency.

42. After taking a complete health history from both partners, the nurse prepares them for further assessments. Which of the following fertility tests are generally suggested at the time of the initial visit?
- **1.** Testicular biopsy and culdoscopy.
- **2.** Laparoscopy and hormonal studies.
- **3.** Huhner test and thyroid screening.
- **4.** Semen analysis and cervical mucus observation.

43. After several months of consultation, the cause of infertility still has not been established. Mr. Cooper expresses his frustration that so little specific information has been given. Which of the following statements by the nurse is most appropriate?
- **1.** "I know you want a family, but these tests take time."
- **2.** "Your doctor is a very competent infertility specialist."
- **3.** "It is hard when you don't know which one of you is at fault."
- **4.** "Feeling frustration is understandable; let's discuss it."

44. The physician completes all tests and finds no physical reason for the inability of Mrs. Cooper to conceive. He prescribes the drug clomiphene citrate (Clomid) and will continue with hormonal studies. The couple should be aware that a side effect of this therapy may be

○ **1.** Uterine fibroids.
○ **2.** Multiple gestation.
○ **3.** Hypertension.
○ **4.** Transitory depression.

45. Several months after initiating Clomid therapy, the couple visit the clinic for confirmation of pregnancy. The physician estimates that Mrs. Cooper is approximately 8 weeks pregnant, and the couple is delighted. In setting a goal for antepartal care, which of the following is a priority?

○ **1.** Mother will adhere to regular clinic visit schedule.
○ **2.** Father will participate in each prenatal class.
○ **3.** Couple will practice exercises each day.
○ **4.** Mother will rest for 30 minutes daily.

46. In the 10th week of pregnancy, Mrs. Cooper experiences scant vaginal bleeding for several days. Urine HCG levels remain elevated, and the physician believes that there is no imminent risk of abortion. As the couple prepare to return home, which of the following must be included in teaching?

○ **1.** "Please call if you experience abdominal pain or cramping."
○ **2.** "Notify the doctor if you are nauseated or if you vomit."
○ **3.** "If you are very tired, please let us know."
○ **4.** "Report any signs of urinary frequency."

47. An ultrasound examination is scheduled at the next visit, in the 12th week of pregnancy. What is the chief purpose of this test?

○ **1.** Measure biparietal diameters.
○ **2.** Identify potential problems.
○ **3.** Confirm fetal viability.
○ **4.** Assess placental function.

48. The pregnancy advances without complications, and Mrs. Cooper keeps all clinic appointments faithfully. After an examination in the 32nd week, she discusses her concerns and discomforts. Mrs. Cooper reports occasional nightmares about labor and delivery. The nurse listens to her feelings and understands that this experience

○ **1.** Is common with a history of infertility.
○ **2.** Is unique to a primigravida.
○ **3.** May indicate deep psychologic problems.
○ **4.** Is quite usual in the third trimester.

49. The Coopers plan on a birthing-room delivery. Their Lamaze classes include an orientation to the unit and a tour of the nursery, in addition to the usual content and practice sessions. Which of the following statements following delivery indicates that the couple learned from the classes?

○ **1.** Breathing and relaxation techniques were used effectively.
○ **2.** Early mother-father-infant bonding was initiated.
○ **3.** No analgesics were requested during the first stage of labor.
○ **4.** Father remained supportive throughout the labor and delivery.

50. A 7-lb daughter was put to breast within an hour of birth. The nursing student asks the benefit of early nursing. The staff nurse explains that the chief reason for early breast-feeding is to

○ **1.** Enhance closeness to the newborn.
○ **2.** Promote uterine contraction.
○ **3.** Meet the nutritional needs of the infant.
○ **4.** Stimulate meconium passage.

51. On the infant's admission to the newborn nursery, a gestational assessment is performed. Which of the following observations indicates that the newborn is probably full term?

○ **1.** Apgar scores of 9 and 10 at 1 and 5 minutes.
○ **2.** Good reflex responses.
○ **3.** Many sole creases present.
○ **4.** Birth weight at 50th percentile.

52. While assessing the Cooper infant, the nurse notes that the newborn sneezes frequently and appears to be a nose breather. What is the correct analysis of these data?

○ **1.** There may be a respiratory problem.
○ **2.** Further assessment is indicated.
○ **3.** The environment may be cold.
○ **4.** These are normal responses.

53. The infant looks directly at her mother while breast-feeding and seems to react to voices of both the parents. Mr. Cooper asks the nurse if their daughter can see and hear. Which of the following responses is most accurate?

○ **1.** "We think that the newborn can see light and hear loud sounds."
○ **2.** "Research has shown that close-up vision and hearing are present."
○ **3.** "The newborn only appears to respond to sensory stimuli."
○ **4.** "It is impossible to determine this in the first days of life."

54. During the first 2 days of rooming-in, Mrs. Cooper is taught many aspects of newborn care. On the day of discharge, she is observed feeding and handling the baby. Which of the following actions best indicates that Mrs. Cooper has learned safe handling of her daughter?

1. The infant is placed on her right side after the feeding.
2. Breast-feeding is managed comfortably and effectively.
3. The diaper area is cleansed after passage of a stool.
4. The mother handles the baby gently while dressing her.

55. The father asks you about laboratory charges for PKU screening, and questions the need for the test. The nurse understands that PKU testing is valuable because

1. It identifies newborns with chromosomal abnormalities.
2. Routine screening tests meet state laws.
3. A rare metabolic disorder can be detected.
4. Autoimmune adaptation is evaluated.

Judy Rogers is a 25-year-old, Type I insulin-dependent diabetic. She works as a bookkeeper and has a young son. She has maintained fairly good diabetic control until recently and is now being admitted for reevaluation. Her insulin routine has been 22 units of NPH plus 5 units of regular insulin daily. She takes her insulin each morning at 7 o'clock.

56. Which piece of subjective data obtained on the nurse's admission assessment indicates a potentially serious problem with Mrs. Rogers' self-care management?

1. "I'm not getting as much sleep as I used to. Tommy seems to wake up at least once every night."
2. "I've been promoted at work, but the new job has more responsibility."
3. "I can't seem to find the time for morning urine tests anymore."
4. "I'm careful about never skipping meals, but I frequently have to eat breakfast at our 10 A.M. coffee break."

57. Since Mrs. Rogers takes NPH insulin, the nurse reinforces her knowledge of a proper diet by testing her understanding of the importance of snacks at which time of day?

1. Midmorning.
2. Midafternoon.
3. Early evening.
4. Bedtime.

58. Mrs. Rogers administers her insulin in 2 injections. What is the most accurate evaluation of this routine?

1. This is the only safe method because NPH should never be mixed with any other form of insulin.
2. This is the preferred method because it prevents mistakes in dosage.
3. There are no real advantages or disadvantages to administering the insulin in 1 or 2 injections.
4. Accurately mixing the 2 insulins in one injection means that injection sites can be used less frequently.

59. Which statement indicates that Mrs. Rogers rotates injection sites appropriately?

1. "I use each site only once a month."
2. "I can give myself my insulin with either hand."
3. "I alternate daily between sites on my thighs and upper arms."
4. "I can use sites on my arms, thighs, stomach and buttocks for injections."

Two-month-old Evan Martin was born with a unilateral complete cleft lip, and is 12 hours post-op surgical repair of the lip. His mother is staying in his hospital room.

60. Evan is acting fussy and starts to cry softly. The nurse should

1. Encourage Evan's mother to hold and rock him.
2. Give Evan his pacifier and rub his back.
3. Sedate Evan with diphenhydramine hydrochloride (Benadryl) elixir 2.5 mg.
4. Allow Evan to cry to facilitate lung inflation.

61. Evan's oral feedings of 4 to 6 ounces of infant formula every 4 or 5 hours are to be resumed. The nurse should teach Mrs. Martin to feed Evan using what method?

1. A bottle with a soft nipple.
2. A small paper cup.
3. A syringe with catheter tubing.
4. Nasogastric gavage.

62. While feeding Evan, Mrs. Martin asks the nurse, "Why do you think this happened to Evan?" The nurse should reply

1. "Cleft lip probably runs in your family."
2. "Sometimes it's hard to know why these things happen."
3. "Did you have any infections or take any drugs while you were pregnant?"
4. "What thoughts do you have about why it happened?"

63. Evan is seen for follow-up in the pediatric clinic 3 weeks after his surgery. What is the most crucial indicator of successful treatment of Evan's defect?

- **1.** Evan's suture line is clean and well healed.
- **2.** Evan's parents say they are "thrilled with how he looks now."
- **3.** Evan is making cooing and babbling sounds.
- **4.** Evan is now sleeping through the night.

Oscar Brown, aged 37, has had a cough and fatigue for several weeks. A sputum culture is positive for Mycobacterium tuberculosis.

64. Which of the following best prevents the transfer of the tuberculosis organism?

- **1.** Having Mr. Brown cover his nose and mouth with double-ply tissue when he coughs or sneezes.
- **2.** Instructing Mr. Brown's family in effective hand washing.
- **3.** Having Mr. Brown's laundry disinfected after use.
- **4.** Having Mr. Brown's dishes sterilized after use.

65. Mr. Brown and his family ask many questions when first told about his diagnosis of active tuberculosis, e.g., "How did this happen? What can we do? What will happen?" The nurse's best response might be which of the following?

- **1.** "Mr. Brown probably contracted tuberculosis from another person with tuberculosis."
- **2.** "Mr. Brown will be given medication and be treated at home."
- **3.** "You need not be concerned; tuberculosis is curable."
- **4.** "You seem very worried about the tuberculosis. What concerns you most?"

66. The definitive test for the diagnosis of tuberculosis is

- **1.** A positive PPD skin test.
- **2.** A positive sputum culture.
- **3.** Abnormal findings on chest x-ray.
- **4.** Abnormal results of a pulmonary function test.

67. Screening a population for tuberculosis with tuberculin skin testing is an example of

- **1.** Primary health promotion.
- **2.** Secondary health promotion.
- **3.** Tertiary health promotion.
- **4.** Primary prevention.

Harry Collins, a 39-year-old draftsman for a small engineering firm, came to the mental health center at the insistence of his wife. In his leisure time, Mr. Collins designs household gadgets. Mr. Collins has the persistent belief that someone is attempting to steal his designs. His attempts to prevent this are interfering with his marital relationship and with other social relationships. He has installed an elaborate alarm system in their home and spends hours finding places to hide his designs. He refuses to attend social functions because "someone will steal his ideas." Other than self-imposed isolation from his co-workers, he has no difficulties at work. He completes his work on time and is respected by colleagues as a hard worker.

68. Mr. Collins' symptoms are delusions of

- **1.** Grandeur.
- **2.** Persecution.
- **3.** Reference.
- **4.** Religiosity.

69. The nurse who takes Mr. Collins' admission history understands that his delusion is related to

- **1.** A desire for attention.
- **2.** Anger at his employer.
- **3.** Fear of losing control.
- **4.** Low self-esteem.

70. Mr. Collins is given a diagnosis of chronic paranoia. Based on this, the nurse would expect Mr. Collins to have

- **1.** Hallucinations.
- **2.** Hostility.
- **3.** Impaired intellectual functioning.
- **4.** Poor reality testing in all areas.

71. Which of the following problems is also true of Mr. Collins?

- **1.** Attention-getting behavior related to mistrust of others.
- **2.** Decreased intellectual functioning.
- **3.** Impaired marital relationship caused by suspiciousness.
- **4.** Paranoia.

72. Initial plans for Mr. Collins would best include

- **1.** Allowing Mr. Collins to initiate relationships and activities.
- **2.** A one-to-one relationship initiated by the nurse.
- **3.** Participation in a competitive sport.
- **4.** Participation in an occupational-therapy group.

73. Mr. Collins attends his first group-therapy session the second day of hospitalization. He leaves in the middle of the session and tells his nurse, "They don't know what they're doing in there. They're all crazy. I won't go to those meetings." The nurse's most appropriate action would be to

○ **1.** Develop a one-to-one relationship with Mr. Collins before he begins group therapy again.
○ **2.** Explain the benefits of group therapy in helping Mr. Collins overcome his delusions.
○ **3.** Insist that Mr. Collins return to the group session immediately.
○ **4.** Tell Mr. Collins that he is excluded today but must return to group therapy tomorrow.

74. All of the following nursing actions will be important in developing a one-to-one relationship with Mr. Collins *except*

○ **1.** Accurate and honest communications.
○ **2.** Clearly stated mutual expectations.
○ **3.** Confrontation regarding delusions.
○ **4.** Consistency in keeping appointments.

75. Mr. Collins has been hospitalized for a week. He still talks at length about the measures he can take to protect his designs. The nurse's most appropriate action is to

○ **1.** Involve Mr. Collins in an activity on the unit.
○ **2.** Listen attentively and encourage further discussion.
○ **3.** Tell Mr. Collins his plans are unnecessary.
○ **4.** Tell Mr. Collins she is aware of his actions.

76. Which of the following is the best indicator that Mr. Collins is improving?

○ **1.** He attends occupational therapy.
○ **2.** He attends to his personal hygiene and grooming.
○ **3.** He freely discusses his attempt to protect his designs.
○ **4.** He discusses feelings of anxiety with the nurse.

Sixteen-month-old Mi Lin Ngyen and her family moved to the US from Southeast Asia 1 month ago. Mi Lin and her parents visit the pediatric clinic for the first time.

77. Which of the following is *least* important for the nurse to consider when initiating interaction with Mi Lin?

○ **1.** Developmental level.
○ **2.** Racial heritage.
○ **3.** Cultural experiences.
○ **4.** Inability to comprehend English.

78. To gain Mi Lin's trust and cooperation, the nurse should first

○ **1.** Offer Mi Lin a toy to play with.
○ **2.** Pick Mi Lin up and hug her warmly.
○ **3.** Use a puppet to "talk" to Mi Lin.
○ **4.** Establish a positive interaction with Mi Lin's parents.

79. The nurse measures Mi Lin's length and weight and finds she is below the 5th percentile for both. A nutritional history reveals Mi Lin's caloric and nutrient intake is consistent with recommended guidelines. Which of the following interpretations is most valid?

○ **1.** Growth norms are based on American children, who tend to be larger on the average.
○ **2.** Mi Lin's parents may not have been truthful concerning her intake.
○ **3.** A hormone deficiency may be causing a growth lag.
○ **4.** Mi Lin may not be getting adequate activity and exercise.

80. When preparing to administer Mi Lin's DTP booster, the nurse should

○ **1.** Allow Mi Lin to play with a syringe for a few minutes.
○ **2.** Talk in a soothing tone to Mi Lin while her mother holds her firmly in her lap, and proceed quickly.
○ **3.** Explain to Mi Lin that she must "get a shot so you won't get sick."
○ **4.** Secure the assistance of at least 1 other nurse to help restrain Mi Lin.

Kathy Smith, 5 years old, has been admitted with a diagnosis of noncommunicating hydrocephalus secondary to postmeningitis adhesions.

81. What was probably the earliest manifestation of increased intracranial pressure that Kathy exhibited?

○ **1.** Early morning headache.
○ **2.** Clumsy gait.
○ **3.** Projectile vomiting.
○ **4.** Papilledema.

82. Following insertion of a ventriculoperitoneal shunt, the nurse should plan for Kathy to be placed in what position?

○ **1.** Semi-Fowler's on the operative side.
○ **2.** Semi-Fowler's on the unoperative side.
○ **3.** Flat on the operative side.
○ **4.** Flat on the unoperative side.

83. Post-op, which of the following findings is the most reliable indicator of a change in Kathy's intracranial pressure?
- ○ **1.** Change in sensorium.
- ○ **2.** Tachycardia.
- ○ **3.** Nausea and vomiting.
- ○ **4.** Pulmonary rales.

84. The physician has ordered Kathy's shunt to be pumped 4 times every shift. When preparing Kathy for this procedure, the nurse should
- ○ **1.** Explain to Kathy how it will feel when the shunt is pumped.
- ○ **2.** Tell Kathy why the shunt has to be pumped.
- ○ **3.** Remind Kathy to be brave so she will get well soon.
- ○ **4.** Ask Kathy to close her eyes and relax so it will be over quickly.

Julio Cortez, aged 47, is admitted from the ER with severe substernal chest pain. A diagnosis of acute myocardial infarction is made. He is in severe pain and is cold, clammy, and dyspneic.

85. All of the following interventions are important. Which should be done first?
- ○ **1.** Administer oxygen.
- ○ **2.** Place in semi-Fowler's position.
- ○ **3.** Institute complete bed rest.
- ○ **4.** Administer morphine by slow IV push.

86. Mr. Cortez is started on heparin therapy. You tell Mr. Cortez he is receiving heparin to
- ○ **1.** Thin his blood.
- ○ **2.** Slow the clotting of his blood.
- ○ **3.** Stop his blood from clotting.
- ○ **4.** Dissolve the clot in his heart.

87. Mr. Cortez begins to have blood in his stool and has episodes of epistaxis. In view of this development, which drug would you have available?
- ○ **1.** Vitamin C (ascorbic acid).
- ○ **2.** Vitamin K (AquaMEPHYTON).
- ○ **3.** Protamine sulfate.
- ○ **4.** Calcium chloride.

88. Mr. Cortez suffers congestive heart failure and is given digitalis. Which of the following indicates a toxic effect of digitalis?
- ○ **1.** Hypokalemia.
- ○ **2.** Tachycardia.
- ○ **3.** Nausea and vomiting.
- ○ **4.** Gynecomastia.

89. With left-sided congestive heart failure, which of the following symptoms is most expected?
- ○ **1.** Nocturnal dyspnea.
- ○ **2.** Sacral edema.
- ○ **3.** Oliguria.
- ○ **4.** Anorexia.

90. Mr. Cortez is advised to eliminate foods high in cholesterol from his diet. This means he should avoid eggs and
- ○ **1.** Liver.
- ○ **2.** Yogurt.
- ○ **3.** Chicken.
- ○ **4.** Corn oil.

Three-year-old Nicole Lyon's mother brings her to the emergency room because Nicole ate "half a bottle of my acetaminophen tablets 15 minutes ago."

91. The nurse ascertains that the bottle originally contained 100 tablets. The nurse's first action should be what?
- ○ **1.** Have Nicole drink an 8-oz glass of milk.
- ○ **2.** Give Nicole 30 ml of syrup of Ipecac followed by a glass of water.
- ○ **3.** Insert a nasogastric tube and administer activated charcoal.
- ○ **4.** Obtain a brief history of events leading up to the ingestion from Mrs. Lyon.

92. Nicole is admitted to the pediatric unit for observation. Which laboratory findings should the nurse monitor most closely for changes in Nicole's health status?
- ○ **1.** Hemoglobin and hematocrit.
- ○ **2.** White blood cell count and differential.
- ○ **3.** Blood gases (pO_2, pCO_2, and pH).
- ○ **4.** Serum transaminase levels (SGOT and SGPT).

93. Nicole is receiving N-acetylcysteine (Mucomyst) as an antidote to the acetaminophen. To make the drug more palatable for Nicole to drink, the nurse should mix the drug with what fluid?
- ○ **1.** Water.
- ○ **2.** Orange juice.
- ○ **3.** Milk.
- ○ **4.** Flavored milkshake.

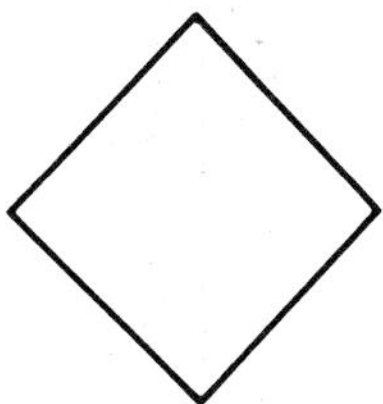

Correct Answers and Rationales: Part One

1. **#3.** This opening statement allows the nurse to gain an overall perspective of family functioning, yet is specific enough to focus the response (as opposed to, "Tell me how you are doing"). The other choices focus narrowly on one aspect, which might be appropriate as the visit proceeds, but are haphazard initial questions. Also, two of them (#1 and #4) require only a "yes" or "no" response and thus do not encourage disclosure by the client. THERAPEUTIC USE OF SELF/ PSYCHOSOCIAL, MENTAL HEALTH, PSYCHIATRIC PROBLEMS
2. **#1.** The nurse's first response should be to clarify and validate the problem by gathering additional information. Option #2 might be asked as the nurse proceeds to narrow the scope of the cause. #3 is likely to make the parent feel defensive, and #4 is irrelevant, since research does not implicate iron as a cause of regurgitation or vomiting. HEALTHY CHILD/ CHILD
3. **#4.** The young infant's cardiac sphincter is not yet fully matured and as a result often relaxes, allowing regurgitation of stomach contents. Although the newborn's stomach capacity is small, it is not the size per se, but the weak cardiac sphincter that precipitates spitting up. There is no scientific basis to support options #2 or #3. NORMAL NEWBORN/ CHILDBEARING FAMILY
4. **#1.** Usually by 2 years, the toddler can turn knobs and open doors; simply closing the door is not enough; the door should be locked and all harmful substances placed in a locked cabinet. Parents need to be told that medicine should not be treated as candy, the Poison Control Center number should be easily accessible and no matter how hard they try, they cannot watch their children all the time. Accidents will happen. HEALTHY CHILD/ CHILD
5. **#3.** Although tiredness is a common complaint of mothers of small children, Ms. Stephens' feeling "exhausted" may indicate anemia or poor coping. This needs to be further investigated. Although Burton does not need solids at his age, his caloric intake is within recommended ranges. Bed-wetting is not considered unusual in children of Vanessa's age, and she may still be adjusting to her new brother. These homemade toys provide appropriate developmental stimulation for Ms. Stephens' children. HEALTHY CHILD/CHILD
6. **#1.** Burton should be bearing some weight on his legs when held upright. Inability to do so may indicate a neuromotor delay. The other skills are too advanced for Burton's age. HEALTHY CHILD/CHILD
7. **#3.** This is the only response that recognizes and acknowledges the client's perception of her situation and that encourages her to explore it with the nurse. This response is therapeutic and conveys respect for the client's point of view and a desire to help her learn to cope with her problems. It promotes a relationship of trust. Option #1 is slightly sarcastic and #2 makes a listening relationship contingent on the patient's behavior. Option #4 contradicts the patient's ideas. THERAPEUTIC USE OF SELF/ PSYCHOSOCIAL, MENTAL HEALTH, PSYCHIATRIC PROBLEMS
8. **#3.** This option focuses on the client's needs without challenging the client. #1 reassures a client of his/her worth, but does not provide information necessary to set tone for nurse-client relationship. #2 presents factual information but does not focus on client needs or the purpose of nurse-client relationship. #4 challenges the client and does not focus on needs. THERAPEUTIC USE OF SELF/ PSYCHOSOCIAL, MENTAL HEALTH, PSYCHIATRIC PROBLEMS

9. **#4.** 50%–80% of all suicides are committed by depressed persons. Mrs. Dunneden is a high suicide risk and she has already expressed she doesn't desire to live anymore and may, therefore, have a plan. While Options #1, #2, and #3 are good objectives of care, they are not the first priority at this time. THERAPEUTIC USE OF SELF/ PSYCHOSOCIAL, MENTAL HEALTH, PSYCHIATRIC PROBLEMS

10. **#1.** Success can cause depression in some persons because of a fear of failure, which will lead to a loss of self-esteem. The promotion will increase stress and responsibility. Option #2 is not correct because there is no indication of delusions and #3 may lead to argument over worth. ELATED-DEPRESSIVE BEHAVIOR/ PSYCHOSOCIAL, MENTAL HEALTH, PSYCHIATRIC PROBLEMS

11. **#3.** Encourage the client to talk by using general, open-ended questions. Option #1 is too vague and #4 does not encourage the patient to talk. The TV is not the concern. THERAPEUTIC USE OF SELF/ PSYCHOSOCIAL, MENTAL HEALTH, PSYCHIATRIC PROBLEMS

12. **#2.** Stay with her to demonstrate caring. Encourage her to talk but do not push or confront her. Options #1 and #4 may be interpreted by the patient as a lack of caring. In this initial, early phase, confrontation might be destructive to the relationship. THERAPEUTIC USE OF SELF/PSYCHOSOCIAL, MENTAL HEALTH, PSYCHIATRIC PROBLEMS

13. **#4.** Anorexia is a common occurrence in depressed clients but is not a common side effect of antidepressants. Hospital food usually meets patient needs. There has been no indication that she desires staff attention. ELATED-DEPRESSIVE BEHAVIOR/ PSYCHOSOCIAL, MENTAL HEALTH, PSYCHIATRIC PROBLEMS

14. **#2.** The most common side effect of Desyrel is dizziness. Antidepressants are not addicting. #3 and #4 are common for MAO inhibitors. ELATED-DEPRESSIVE BEHAVIOR/ PSYCHOSOCIAL, MENTAL HEALTH, PSYCHIATRIC PROBLEMS

15. **#3.** Further assessment is necessary to determine if the client is suicidal or is making realistic plans and taking positive steps to become reinvolved with her environment. #1 is a possibility, however, more information is necessary before asking this direct question. #2 and #4 do not encourage further exploration of the client's actions and feelings and cut off communication about plans for self. ELATED-DEPRESSIVE BEHAVIOR/PSYCHOSOCIAL, MENTAL HEALTH, PSYCHIATRIC PROBLEMS

16. **#2.** Suicide is an act of self-punishment, of anger directed toward the self. The suicidal person is depressed, feels guilty, condemns self, and directs anger inward. Suicide is not the leading cause of death in all persons. Hospitalized patients and those who talk of suicide are vulnerable. ELATED-DEPRESSIVE BEHAVIOR/PSYCHOSOCIAL, MENTAL HEALTH, PSYCHIATRIC PROBLEMS

17. **#1.** Preparing for termination begins with the inception of the therapeutic relationship. Introduction of termination at any of the other times listed would disrupt the complete process of the relationship. THERAPEUTIC USE OF SELF/PSYCHOSOCIAL, MENTAL HEALTH, PSYCHIATRIC PROBLEMS

18. **#1.** Reflection will encourage the client to discuss her fears. Option #2 is too direct and does not acknowledge underlying concerns. #3 minimizes fear and closes off exploration of feelings and planning coping methods upon discharge. #4 fails to recognize client as an individual and is an attempt at unrealistic reassurance. THERAPEUTIC USE OF SELF/ PSYCHOSOCIAL, MENTAL HEALTH, PSYCHIATRIC PROBLEMS

19. **#3.** Clients often become anxious near discharge and reexperience symptoms they may not have shown for some time. There has been no data given to indicate that she is ready for discharge or that she is overly dependent. Crying is unlikely to be directly related to the nurses caring for her. ANXIOUS BEHAVIOR/ PSYCHOSOCIAL, MENTAL HEALTH, PSYCHIATRIC PROBLEMS

20. **#4.** The diagnosis has not been confirmed; you only suspect a fractured hip. Never attempt to reduce a fracture, or extend or elevate the extremity. You may cause more damage. ACTIVITY AND REST/ADULT

21. **#3.** Fractured hips present with abduction of the affected extremity and movement away from the main axis of the body. There is also external rotation of the hip and the leg is shortened. It is difficult to assess edema at this point. ACTIVITY AND REST/ADULT
22. **#3.** Washing and drying of the skin aids in securing the traction. Buck's traction does not involve the insertion of pins. Polyhealthy skin, i.e., without abrasions, tolerates skin traction well. MOBILITY/CHILD
23. **#3.** When the client is moved, she needs to be "log-rolled" with abductor splint or pillows between her legs. Abduction of the affected leg is to be maintained at all times. Sedation is not equivalent to pain relief and does not relieve pain. Early ambulation is advocated, however no weight bearing is allowed on the operated side. ACTIVITY AND REST/ADULT
24. **#3.** Doses of aspirin sufficient to relieve pain may cause tinnitus. The other side effects listed are not characteristic of aspirin. SURGERY/ ADULT
25. **#1.** Additional information is needed from Mrs. Clark regarding her concerns. The other choices *may* be appropriate but clarification regarding the patient's concerns is needed first. THERAPEUTIC USE OF SELF/ PSYCHOSOCIAL, MENTAL HEALTH, PSYCHIATRIC PROBLEMS
26. **#1.** Manifestations of a duodenal ulcer include: pain relieved by food ingestion, pain occurring 1–4 hours after eating, and melena. Vomiting and hematemesis are characteristic of gastric ulcers. NUTRITION AND METABOLISM/ADULT
27. **#1.** All fried foods and whole grains are prohibited on a bland diet. NUTRITION AND METABOLISM/ADULT
28. **#2.** Anticholinergic drugs block the effect of acetylcholine at receptor sites thereby reducing the production of gastric secretions. NUTRITION AND METABOLISM/ADULT
29. **#1.** Antacids are given to coat the ulcer to protect it from irritation. To be effective, they must be given on time. NUTRITION AND METABOLISM/ADULT
30. **#2.** Irrigation is contraindicated after gastric surgery, unless ordered, to avoid trauma to the surgical site. Salem sumps are repositioned after gastric surgery *only* by the physician. Repositioning can cause disruption of the suture line. Gomco suction is contraindicated because it is intermittent suction; to be effective, the Salem tube requires continuous suction. NUTRITION AND METABOLISM/ADULT
31. **#2.** After abdominal surgery, the client is at greatest risk for pulmonary complications. Therefore, encourage him to take deep breaths at least hourly. The other statements listed are not true. SURGERY/ADULT
32. **#2.** These are signs and symptoms of late dumping syndrome. Rapid emptying of the stomach contents into the intestine leads ultimately to a hypoglycemic reaction that causes the symptoms. NUTRITION AND METABOLISM/ADULT
33. **#1.** Maintaining consistency in Mark's environment is the single most effective way to promote a sense of security and continuity during the move. #2 is unrealistic in view of Mark's age and limitations. #3 and #4 may increase Mark's fear by adding more change in his life. ILL AND HOSPITALIZED CHILD/ CHILD
34. **#2.** Children with Down syndrome are smaller in size than their healthy age mates and will continue to be as they grow older. There are no data to suggest that Mark's fluid and caloric intake is inadequate. Referral of this mother's concern to the pediatrician is inappropriate since it is within the scope of nursing practice. SENSATION, PERCEPTION, PROTECTION/ CHILD
35. **#4.** Respiratory infections are common in children with Down syndrome and account for high morbidity. The hypotonicity of the chest and abdominal muscles is a major predisposing factor to respiratory infections. SENSATION, PERCEPTION, PROTECTION/CHILD
36. **#2.** The priority goal of caring for a child with any form of retardation is to promote optimal development. Options #1 and #3 are important goals, but are not as crucial as the broader goal of maximizing development. #4 may be unrealistic because of the mental retardation that accompanies Down syndrome. SENSATION, PERCEPTION, PROTECTION/ CHILD

37. **#4.** While all the options are necessary in a comprehensive preschool stimulation program, motivating the child to want to learn is the critical factor. This is best accomplished through praising the child's accomplishments. This option is also helpful in promoting self esteem. SENSATION, PERCEPTION, PROTECTION/CHILD
38. **#4.** During a bleeding episode involving a joint, the joint should be elevated and immobilized in a flexed position to minimize further bleeding and decrease pain. Heat will cause vasodilation and aggravate the bleeding episode. Ice packs, which promote vasoconstriction, should be applied to the elbow instead. Aspirin is contraindicated for the child with hemophilia because it interferes with platelet function. Range-of-motion exercises may cause further trauma to the joint during a bleeding episode. OXYGENATION/CHILD
39. **#4.** AIDS is transmitted in body secretions such as urine, stool, blood, and saliva. As long as the nurse does not have direct body contact with Darren, no special precautions are needed. SENSATION, PERCEPTION, PROTECTION/CHILD
40. **#3.** When a female carrier of hemophilia has children fathered by a male who is free of the disease, the risk to their offspring (*with each pregnancy*) is as follows: half the males will have hemophilia (XrY), half the males will be normal (XY), half the females will be carriers of the hemophilia gene (XrX), and half the females will be normal (XX). OXYGENATION/CHILD
41. **#2.** Playing Nerf basketball would be contraindicated for Darren because it would require him to move his elbow, which should remain immobilized while he is on bedrest to prevent further bleeding. The other activities are age appropriate and acceptable in terms of his treatment plan. HEALTHY CHILD/CHILD
42. **#4.** While the other tests may be performed later, they are involved or invasive. Semen analysis is a simple assessment. Cervical mucus consistency changes during the menstrual cycle, and gives clues to ovulation. FEMALE REPRODUCTIVE ANATOMY AND PHYSIOLOGY/CHILDBEARING FAMILY
43. **#4.** This response indicates understanding of common feelings about infertility and is considered therapeutic communication as it encourages further discussion. While options #1 and #2 are true, neither is helpful to the father. Option #3 blocks communication by introducing the concept of blame. THERAPEUTIC USE OF SELF/ PSYCHOSOCIAL, MENTAL HEALTH, PSYCHIATRIC PROBLEMS
44. **#2.** Clomid, a drug frequently prescribed to correct infertility, increases the risk of ovarian cysts and multiple births. None of the other choices is correct. FEMALE REPRODUCTIVE ANATOMY AND PHYSIOLOGY/ CHILDBEARING FAMILY
45. **#1.** The priority goal for any pregnant client is compliance with regular prenatal care. ANTEPARTAL CARE/CHILDBEARING FAMILY
46. **#1.** If the client experiences contractions, cramping, or more bleeding, she may be experiencing a miscarriage. The other symptoms listed are common in the first trimester and need not be reported. ANTEPARTAL CARE/CHILDBEARING FAMILY
47. **#3.** At this time in pregnancy, when the client has a history of bleeding, the test is performed to confirm fetal viability. Biparietal diameters are a useful assessment between 18 and 24 weeks gestation. Neither option #2 nor #4 is accurate. ANTEPARTAL CARE/ CHILDBEARING FAMILY
48. **#4.** These fears and dreams are common, especially in the last trimester. There is no higher incidence with infertility or in a first pregnancy. ANTEPARTAL CARE/ CHILDBEARING FAMILY
49. **#1.** The focus of Lamaze classes is the practice of breathing, relaxation, and conditioned responses for use during labor. While it is positive that bonding and support were noted, these are not criteria for evaluation of learning. Requests for analgesia during labor do not influence successful outcome of delivery of Lamaze couples. ANTEPARTAL CARE/ CHILDBEARING FAMILY

50. #1. While uterine contractions are stimulated by lactation, the major reason for initiating nursing soon after delivery is to promote closeness. Nutritional needs are minimal at this time. Breast-feeding has no specific effect on meconium passage, which normally occurs within the first 24 hours. POSTPARTAL CARE/CHILDBEARING FAMILY

51. #3. This is the only assessment that refers to gestational age. Apgar scores measure immediate adaptations to extrauterine life; birth weight is not necessarily related to length of gestation; reflexes may be good in some infants who were born before term. NORMAL NEWBORN/CHILDBEARING FAMILY

52. #4. These are normal responses. NORMAL NEWBORN/CHILDBEARING FAMILY

53. #2. Studies indicate that sensory development at birth is quite good. This response is more specific than option #1. NORMAL NEWBORN/CHILDBEARING FAMILY

54. #1. A newborn should be positioned on the abdomen or right side after feeding to prevent aspiration of milk or mucus. The other behaviors are appropriate, but do not evaluate *safe* care. NORMAL NEWBORN/ CHILDBEARING FAMILY

55. #3. While state laws do require PKU screening, the most appropriate response gives the major purpose of the test. The PKU test is specific for one inherited metabolic disorder rather than for vague chromosomal abnormalities. NORMAL NEWBORN/ CHILDBEARING FAMILY

56. #4. This is a potentially serious problem because she takes her insulin at 7 A.M. but does not eat until 10 A.M. Regular insulin's onset is 1 hour and it peaks in 2–4 hours. NUTRITION AND METABOLISM/ADULT

57. #2. Peak action for NPH is 8–12 hours after administration. Since she takes her insulin at 7 A.M. and the NPH peak action will be from 3 P.M. to 7 P.M. If she eats a snack between 3 and 4 P.M., she will cover the beginning peak time of the NPH. NUTRITION AND METABOLISM/ADULT

58. #4. NPH and regular insulin may be mixed. Accurately and consistently drawing up insulin, whether mixed or not, is the key to preventing mistakes in dosage. There is no need for 2 injections and this gives the patient more sites for rotation, decreasing the incidence of lipohypertrophy. NUTRITION AND METABOLISM/ADULT

59. #1. No injection site should be used more than once per month. While the other statements are all correct to some degree, this statement tells you the exact, correct information. NUTRITION AND METABOLISM/ADULT

60. #1. Sucking and crying are contraindicated post-op in infants who have had a cleft lip repair because of potential damage to the repair. Sedation with Benadryl is indicated only if Evan becomes very restless or agitated and is unable to be calmed by other measures such as holding, stroking, rocking. Allowing Evan's mother to hold and rock him also involves her directly in his care and, thus, increases her sense of control. NUTRITION AND METABOLISM/CHILD

61. #3. A syringe fitted with soft catheter tubing will allow Evan's mother to feed him adequate amounts of formula to the side and back of his mouth and prevent Evan from sucking, which may injure the lip repair. Evan should not be allowed to suck from a nipple in the post-op period because of possible damage created by tension on the suture line. Evan is too young to be able to drink from a cup; additionally, placement of the cup to his lips may stimulate his suck reflex or directly irritate the suture line. There is no reason to institute nasogastric feedings when a less invasive method, effective in providing adequate nutrition, is available. NUTRITION AND METABOLISM/CHILD

62. #4. This reply allows the nurse to ascertain what Mrs. Martin believes to be the cause of Evan's defect, and what specific concerns or unanswered questions about the cause she may have. The nurse can then further validate the mother's concerns before responding with information or appropriate supportive comments. Although cleft lip is known to be transmitted multifactorially, thus increasing the possibility of occurrence in families with a history of the defect, option #1 has not been validated and is not responsive to the mother's concern. Option #2 ignores Mrs. Martin's feelings in the situation. Teratogens, such as viruses or drugs, may also cause cleft lip, but option #3 is worded as a closed question and does not address the mother's question. NUTRITION AND METABOLISM/CHILD

63. **#1.** The goal of surgical repair of cleft lip is to achieve primary closure of the defect to ensure adequate nutrition through normal sucking, and to minimize scarring for cosmetic reasons. A clean, well-healed suture line indicates that Evan has the capacity to suck, and that he will have minimal scarring. Although it is important for the parent-infant relationship that Evan's parents are pleased with the repair, Evan's physiologic needs are more crucial when evaluating treatment outcomes. Options #3 and #4 illustrate typical development progress for a 3-month-old, and do not provide direct evidence of goal achievement. NUTRITION AND METABOLISM/CHILD
64. **#1.** Tuberculosis is an airborne disease transmitted by droplet nuclei. The patient should cover his nose and mouth with double-ply tissues when he coughs or sneezes; his bare hand will not stop the droplets. Proper handwashing removes the tubercle bacilli from the hands but eliminating droplet transmission best prevents the transfer of the disease. No special laundry or dishwashing techniques are needed. OXYGENATION/ADULT
65. **#4.** The multiple questions suggest anxiety and fear. #4 encourages Mr. Brown and his family to express their feelings. The other options, while factually correct, will probably not allay anxiety and imply that the nurse knows what is bothering Mr. Brown and his family. ANXIOUS BEHAVIOR/PSYCHOSOCIAL, MENTAL HEALTH, PSYCHIATRIC PROBLEMS
66. **#2.** A positive sputum culture for acid-fast bacilli confirms the diagnosis of active tuberculosis. A positive PPD indicates exposure to the tubercule bacillus, but not necessarily the presence of active disease. Abnormal findings on a chest x-ray or pulmonary function tests are not definitive for a diagnosis of tuberculosis. Skin testing, chest x-ray, and pulmonary function tests must all be confirmed by a positive sputum culture. OXYGENATION/ADULT
67. **#2.** The goal of tuberculin skin testing is the early diagnosis and treatment of tuberculosis, i.e., secondary health promotion. Primary health promotion and primary prevention aim at preventing the occurrence of a disease. Tertiary health promotion aims at preventing the complications of a disease. HEALTHY ADULT/ADULT
68. **#2.** Delusions of persecution are defined as false beliefs that oneself has been singled out for harassment. Delusions in this situation do not relate to ideas of superiority (#1), or focus on the self (#3) or on religious ideation (#4). GLOSSARY/PSYCHOSOCIAL, MENTAL HEALTH, PSYCHIATRIC PROBLEMS
69. **#4.** Content of the delusion serves to build up the person's self-esteem. Insufficient data are given to support the other choices. Delusions of persecution are not usually attributed to the behavior patterns described in options #1, #2, and #3. SUSPICIOUS BEHAVIOR/ PSYCHOSOCIAL, MENTAL HEALTH, PSYCHIATRIC PROBLEMS
70. **#2.** Persons with paranoid ideation have underlying hostility. There is no evidence of hallucinations. Intellectual functioning appears intact. Reality testing remains intact in paranoid clients except for the area related to the delusion. SUSPICIOUS BEHAVIOR/ PSYCHOSOCIAL, MENTAL HEALTH, PSYCHIATRIC PROBLEMS
71. **#3.** Mr. Collins has marital problems because of his behavior. There is no evidence that his behavior is attention seeking and his intellectual functioning is not disturbed. Paranoia is a medical diagnosis, not a nursing diagnosis. SUSPICIOUS BEHAVIOR/PSYCHOSOCIAL, MENTAL HEALTH, PSYCHIATRIC PROBLEMS
72. **#2.** Interventions would begin with one-to-one activities. Socialization is increased gradually. The client will need assistance to develop a relationship. Participation in demanding group activities may seem threatening. SUSPICIOUS BEHAVIOR/PSYCHOSOCIAL, MENTAL HEALTH, PSYCHIATRIC PROBLEMS
73. **#1.** Involve the suspicious client in group activity and relationships gradually. Begin by developing a one-to-one relationship; involve others slowly. Options #2, #3, and #4 do not allow for this gradual involvement. SUSPICIOUS BEHAVIOR/PSYCHOSOCIAL, MENTAL HEALTH, PSYCHIATRIC PROBLEMS
74. **#3.** Do not argue with the client about delusions. Consistency and clarity will enhance development of trust and are crucial in developing a relationship. THERAPEUTIC USE OF SELF/PSYCHOSOCIAL, MENTAL HEALTH, PSYCHIATRIC PROBLEMS

75. #1. Maintain a focus on reality without demeaning the client or becoming involved in arguments. Options #2 and #3 may lead to an argument. Option #4 shows a condescending attitude by the nurse and is not therapeutic. SUSPICIOUS BEHAVIOR/PSYCHOSOCIAL, MENTAL HEALTH, PSYCHIATRIC PROBLEMS

76. #4. The goal for a suspicious client is to recognize and express the anxiety that causes the delusion. No disruption of work or self-care abilities has been indicated. Discussion of delusions would indicate no change. SUSPICIOUS BEHAVIOR/PSYCHOSOCIAL, MENTAL HEALTH, PSYCHIATRIC PROBLEMS

77. #2. Although Mi Lin's racial heritage is an important factor to consider when assessing growth and physical health status, it has little bearing on how the nurse would approach Mi Lin in a clinical situation, whereas the other factors listed are essential in guiding the nurse's interaction with Mi Lin. HEALTHY CHILD/CHILD

78. #4. At this age, it is best to allow the child to make the first move. Establishing interaction with Mi Lin's parents first gives Mi Lin time to size the nurse up and see that her parents demonstrate trust in the nurse. The other nursing actions may be perceived as direct threats by Mi Lin, because of her language barrier and developmental level. HEALTHY CHILD/CHILD

79. #1. Asian children are shorter and weigh less, on the average, than American children, on whom growth norms are usually based. Even though the graphs have been recently revised to be more representative of children from varying backgrounds, the nurse should always consider the child's family heritage when evaluating variances from normal. No information has been provided to support any of the other options. HEALTHY CHILD/CHILD

80. #2. It is best to have a parent assist with holding the child during a briefly painful procedure, such as an immunization, if possible. Proceeding quickly is the desirable approach with a child this age for a procedure that will be over quickly. Prolonged explanations only increase the child's anxiety and, in Mi Lin's case, would not be understood because she does not speak English. She may be given the needleless syringe to play with *following* the injection. ILL AND HOSPITALIZED CHILD/CHILD

81. #1. Early morning headaches are frequently the earliest sign of increased intracranial pressure. The other manifestations are later signs of increased ICP. SENSATION, PERCEPTION, PROTECTION/CHILD

82. #4. Positioning the patient flat on the unoperative side will prevent pressure on the shunt valve and allow for gradual drainage of the spinal fluid. The other positions would place additional pressure on the shunt. SENSATION, PERCEPTION, PROTECTION/CHILD

83. #1. The primary indicator of changing intracranial pressure is a change in sensorium or level of consciousness. SENSATION, PERCEPTION, PROTECTION/CHILD

84. #1. Six-year-olds are in the preoperational stage of cognitive development and are most concerned about what sensations they will feel when facing an unfamiliar experience. Kathy would have difficulty understanding why the shunt must be pumped and, in any event, why is not as important as what or how. Option #3 and #4 do not actively involve Kathy in the experience or give her any sense of control, and will probably increase her fear and lessen her cooperation. ILL AND HOSPITALIZED CHILD/CHILD

85. #4. Relief of pain is the priority goal for a client with a myocardial infarction. All the interventions may be carried out, but relief of pain is first. OXYGENATION/ADULT

86. #2. Anticoagulant therapy is used to prolong, not prevent clotting. Anticoagulants have no thrombolytic (clot dissolving) action. "Blood thinner" is a term commonly used by lay persons for anticoagulants, but actually anticoagulants have no effect on hemoconcentration. OXYGENATION/ADULT

87. #3. Protamine sulfate is the antidote for heparin. Vitamin K is the antidote for *oral* anticoagulants. Neither vitamin C nor calcium chloride act as an antidote against anticoagulant drugs. OXYGENATION/ADULT

88. #3. Digitalis toxicity is manifested by gastrointestinal upset. Bradycardia, not tachycardia, is a side effect that may or may not indicate toxicity. Hypokalemia potentiates the effects of digitalis, but is not a toxic effect. Gynecomastia is an uncommon side effect. OXYGENATION/ADULT

89. #1. Left-sided congestive heart failure causes pulmonary congestion and symptoms. Oliguria, while present in both right-sided and left-sided congestive heart failure, is primarily a symptom of right-sided failure. Sacral edema and anorexia occur with right-sided congestive heart failure. OXYGENATION/ADULT

90. #1. Organ meats are high in cholesterol. Chicken and yogurt are low in cholesterol. Vegetable oils such as corn oil have no cholesterol. OXYGENATION/ADULT

91. #2. Use of syrup of Ipecac in age-appropriate dosage is the safest, most effective emergency treatment of accidental ingestion of all substances *except* hydrocarbons or caustics. The priority goal is to empty the potentially toxic acetaminophen from the stomach. Having the child drink milk may cause more rapid absorption of the tablets. Gastric lavage with administration of activated charcoal should be carried out *after* gastric emptying. Option #4 would waste valuable time and allow greater amounts of the acetaminophen to be absorbed. The history may be obtained during or immediately following administration of the syrup of Ipecac. SENSATION, PERCEPTION, PROTECTION/CHILD

92. #4. Acetaminophen is potentially toxic to the liver. Serum transaminase (SGOT and SGPT) levels should be closely monitored every 24 hours for 3 to 5 days following the ingestion to detect hepatic damage. Acetaminophen toxicity is not reflected by any of the other laboratory findings listed. SENSATION, PERCEPTION, PROTECTION/CHILD

93. #2. Orange juice will help disguise the taste of Mucomyst, whereas water will not. Milk products may interfere with the absorption of the Mucomyst and are, therefore, not recommended. SENSATION, PERCEPTION, PROTECTION/CHILD

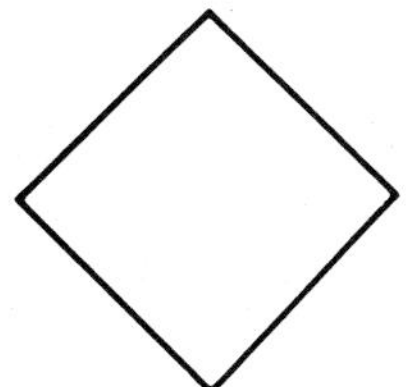

Sample Test Questions: Part Two

Josephine Harrod has been admitted to the hospital with hepatitis Type A.

94. Which of the following precautions is *inappropriate* to include in Mrs. Harrod's care?
- ○ **1.** Stool and needle isolation.
- ○ **2.** Special care of linens and food.
- ○ **3.** Use of a gown and gloves during client contact.
- ○ **4.** Reverse isolation.

95. Several months following her hospitalization for hepatitis, Mrs. Harrod reentered the hospital with complaints indicative of cholecystitis and cholelithiasis. Because she has an existing jaundice, which of the following tests should be performed prior to surgery?
- ○ **1.** Lee-White clotting time.
- ○ **2.** Bleeding time.
- ○ **3.** Prothrombin time.
- ○ **4.** Circulation time.

96. For which post-op complication is Mrs. Harrod at risk after gallbladder surgery?
- ○ **1.** Atelectasis.
- ○ **2.** Pneumonia.
- ○ **3.** Hemorrhage.
- ○ **4.** Thrombophlebitis.

97. Following surgery, Mrs. Harrod has a nasogastric tube in place with an order to irrigate it prn. What is the rationale for irrigating a post-op client's nasogastric tube?
- ○ **1.** To remove secretions from the stomach.
- ○ **2.** To decrease abdominal distention.
- ○ **3.** To minimize bleeding.
- ○ **4.** To maintain patency of the tube.

Barbara Tilson developed insulin-dependent diabetes at age 11. She is now 21; diet and insulin were balanced during this, her first pregnancy. A healthy 10-lb girl is delivered in the birthing room at 38 weeks of gestation.

98. When caring for Baby Girl Tilson in the delivery room, what is the priority nursing action?
- ○ **1.** Ensure proper identification.
- ○ **2.** Establish a warm environment.
- ○ **3.** Maintain a patient airway.
- ○ **4.** Facilitate parental bonding.

99. Considering the maternal history, which of the following goals is critical during the first hours of newborn care?
- ○ **1.** Hydration will be adequate.
- ○ **2.** Temperature will be maintained in the normal range.
- ○ **3.** Nutrition will be maintained.
- ○ **4.** Blood sugar will remain normal.

100. Mother and newborn will be sent home in 48 hours. Both appear to be adapting to breast-feeding. In preparing Mrs. Tilson for discharge you include infant-care teaching. Which of the following indicates the nurse understands the needs of the newborn with a diabetic mother?
- ○ **1.** "Observe the baby after feedings as asphyxia is a common problem."
- ○ **2.** "Watch the baby for signs of hypoglycemia in the first few weeks."
- ○ **3.** "Visit the pediatrician regularly throughout childhood because diabetes is hereditary."
- ○ **4.** "Supplement breast-feedings with skim milk to control weight."

101. The nurse reviews diabetic teaching with Mrs. Tilson, including manifestations of hypoglycemia. It is suggested that she immediately drink orange juice if she experiences
- ○ **1.** Nausea and vomiting, flushed dry skin.
- ○ **2.** Increased temperature, pulse, perspiration.
- ○ **3.** Polyuria, thirst, and dry skin.
- ○ **4.** Hunger, dizziness, clammy skin.

102. At the postpartum check-up, diabetic teaching is reinforced, with emphasis on hygiene and foot care. Which of the following practices indicates that further teaching is needed?
- ○ **1.** Nails are trimmed straight across.
- ○ **2.** Shoes fit well and give support.
- ○ **3.** Feet are bathed and inspected daily.
- ○ **4.** Hot Epsom salt soaks are used for painful corns.

103. Diet management for the breast-feeding diabetic focuses on an increase in
- **1.** Saturated fats, vitamin C, and fibers.
- **2.** Potassium, protein, and iodine.
- **3.** Fluids, simple sugars, and iron.
- **4.** Calcium, protein, and complex carbohydrates.

Allen Spinet, 23 years old, was injured in an automobile accident.

104. Of the following sequences, which would be the most appropriate in the immediate post-trauma minutes?
- **1.** Control the hemorrhage; establish an open airway; stabilize the fractured vertebrae; splint the fractured leg.
- **2.** Establish an open airway; control the hemorrhage; stabilize the fractured vertebrae; splint the fractured leg.
- **3.** Establish an open airway; stabilize the fractured vertebrae; control the hemorrhage; splint the fractured leg.
- **4.** Establish an open airway; control the hemorrhage; splint the fractured leg; stabilize the fractured vertebrae.

105. Which is the most important intervention in treating hemorrhage?
- **1.** Allay apprehension.
- **2.** Give oral fluids.
- **3.** Prevent chilling, but do not overheat.
- **4.** Restore blood volume.

106. Shock causes which of the following?
- **1.** A pO_2 greater than 80 mm Hg.
- **2.** A pH less than 7.34.
- **3.** A pCO_2 less than 45 mm Hg.
- **4.** A decrease in capillary permeability.

107. If cardiopulmonary resuscitation were performed on Mr. Spinet by 2 persons, which of the following ratios of cardiac compression to pulmonary ventilation would be used?
- **1.** 1:1.
- **2.** 5:1.
- **3.** 15:2.
- **4.** 20:2.

108. Effective cardiopulmonary resuscitation would be best indicated by which sign?
- **1.** Palpable carotid pulse.
- **2.** Dilated pupils.
- **3.** Easily blanched nail beds.
- **4.** Normal skin color.

109. Mr. Spinet is conscious and is bleeding from a compound fracture of the right leg. The adequacy of his general tissue perfusion can be determined by the assessment of all of the following except one. Which of the following is *incorrect*?
- **1.** Urinary output.
- **2.** Blood pressure.
- **3.** Level of consciousness.
- **4.** Skin color.

110. Mr. Spinet has been admitted to the ICU. He has a mean blood pressure of 90. He is on nitroprusside drip and an epinephrine drip with orders to keep blood pressure at a mean of 80. What is the most appropriate action?
- **1.** Decrease nitroprusside.
- **2.** Increase nitroprusside.
- **3.** Decrease epinephrine.
- **4.** Increase epinephrine.

111. What is the primary objective of therapy for Mr. Spinet's shock?
- **1.** Maintain adequate blood pressure.
- **2.** Improve tissue perfusion.
- **3.** Maintain adequate vascular tone.
- **4.** Improve kidney function.

112. Mr. Spinet's injuries include a skull fracture. One of the goals of care for him is to observe for increasing intracranial pressure. Increased intracranial pressure would be indicated by which signs?
- **1.** Increased pulse rate and increased blood pressure.
- **2.** Increased pulse rate and decreased blood pressure.
- **3.** Decreased pulse rate and increased blood pressure.
- **4.** Decreased pulse rate and decreased blood pressure.

113. In addition, which of the following would best indicate increased intracranial pressure?
- **1.** BP change from 110/80 mm Hg to 140/50 mm Hg.
- **2.** Pulse change from 78/minute to 92/minute.
- **3.** Respirations change from 16/minute to 26/minute.
- **4.** Change in level of consciousness from stupor to drowsy and restless.

Mr. "X" was admitted to the psychiatric unit without an awareness of who he was or where he lived. He has no evidence of a head injury or psychosis.

114. Mr. X is diagnosed as suffering a dissociative reaction. He probably has this as a reaction to which of the following?

○ **1.** A life-threatening situation.
○ **2.** An unresolved conflict.
○ **3.** A frustrating experience.
○ **4.** Taking the NCLEX examination.

115. Mr. X is using which of the following defense mechanisms?

○ **1.** Regression.
○ **2.** Denial.
○ **3.** Rationalization.
○ **4.** Repression.

116. Mr. X is hospitalized on a psychiatric unit. The therapeutic milieu will focus on which of the following?

○ **1.** Encouraging him to remember what happened to him.
○ **2.** Keeping him from other clients until staff is more certain of who he is.
○ **3.** Expecting him to be involved in daily activities on the unit as he is able.
○ **4.** Administering electroconvulsive therapy (ECT) to help him became aware of the conflict and deal with it.

John David Jankowski, 14 months old, is scheduled for palliative surgery for tetralogy of Fallot. His mother is staying in his hospital room until he is taken to surgery.

117. When reviewing John David's pre-op lab reports, the nurse should be most concerned about which value?

○ **1.** White blood cell count 14,000/mm^3.
○ **2.** Hematocrit 52%.
○ **3.** Serum pH 7.33.
○ **4.** Platelets 220,000/mm^3.

118. The surgeon plans to anastomose John David's left subclavian artery to his pulmonary artery. Mrs. Jankowski asks the nurse to explain the reason for this temporary palliative surgery. The nurse should reply

○ **1.** "The surgery will increase the amount of blood that flows through John David's lungs, so his body gets more oxygen."
○ **2.** "This procedure will change the direction of blood flow in his heart so his skin color will be less blue."
○ **3.** "The pressure on the heart chamber that pumps blood to the body will be relieved."
○ **4.** "The surgery will allow John David to grow and develop like a normal child."

119. Which activity would be most appropriate for John David preoperatively?

○ **1.** A play stethoscope.
○ **2.** A push-pull toy.
○ **3.** A shape sorter.
○ **4.** A toy trumpet.

120. John David is playing beside his mother's chair when he starts to investigate the contents of her purse. When Mrs. Jankowski takes her purse away from him, John David begins to cry, then screams, stomps his feet, and starts to gasp. Which action should the nurse take?

○ **1.** Allow Mrs. Jankowski to handle the situation.
○ **2.** Distract John David with one of his favorite toys.
○ **3.** Advise Mrs. Janowski to "be as easy as possible on him" until after surgery.
○ **4.** Hold John David in a squatting position.

Janice Carter is in the 37th week of pregnancy. Her husband calls the physician to report that his wife awakened in the middle of the night, lying in a pool of bright red blood.

121. The onset of third-trimester painless bleeding is usually a sign of potential

○ **1.** Abruptio placentae.
○ **2.** Placenta previa.
○ **3.** Incomplete abortion.
○ **4.** Ectopic pregnancy.

122. Mrs. Carter is admitted to the labor room. Which of the following is contraindicated during the admission assessment?

○ **1.** Vaginal examination.
○ **2.** X-ray pelvimetry.
○ **3.** Type and crossmatch.
○ **4.** Perineal prep.

123. Mrs. Carter is worried about her condition, and about her 2-year-old twins at home. Mr. Carter asks you if he should remain with Mrs. Carter or return home to check on the children and their teenaged sitter. Which response indicates an understanding of their feelings at this time?

○ **1.** "You would feel more secure if you checked on your family."
○ **2.** "Your wife is well cared for her. You may go home for a while."
○ **3.** "You really belong here, now. Call home and check on the children."
○ **4.** "Why not ask your wife what she feels would be best for her?"

124. An ultrasound confirms that the placenta totally covers the cervical os. Mrs. Carter is prepared for a cesarean birth. In addition to providing emotional support, preparation for the client includes all *except*
- **1.** Type and crossmatch.
- **2.** Insertion of Foley catheter.
- **3.** Skin prep and shave.
- **4.** Tap-water enema.

125. Mrs. Carter will receive a spinal anesthetic. As she signs the consent forms, she asks about the possibility of postanesthetic headaches. An appropriate response is
- **1.** "Headaches rarely occur, and are usually mild."
- **2.** "Medication is available to counteract headaches, and is given as needed."
- **3.** "If there is an allergy to the agent used, headaches may occur."
- **4.** "This problem may be prevented by keeping the bed flat."

126. Baby Carter, 6 lb 4 oz, is delivered by cesarean section, and appears to be in stable condition. Mrs. Carter's blood loss during delivery was 1,200 ml. She receives 2 units of whole blood. While she is in the recovery room, several changes in her condition are noted. Which assessment should be reported to the physician immediately?
- **1.** Pulse changes from 88 to 120; she is restless.
- **2.** Blood pressure is stable at 100/80; she appears pale.
- **3.** Temperature rises to 100.2°F; her mouth is dry.
- **4.** Lochia rubra noted; she seems to be in pain.

127. An IV of 1,000 ml of 5% dextrose in saline with 10 units of Pitocin is ordered. The solution is to infuse in 6 hours. Drop factor is 10. At what rate should the IV infuse?
- **1.** 2.7 drops per minute.
- **2.** 3.7 drops per minute.
- **3.** 27 drops per minute.
- **4.** 37 drops per minute.

128. In evaluating Mrs. Carter's response to Pitocin, which observation indicates a potential problem?
- **1.** Fundus is firmly contracted.
- **2.** Urinary output is 20/ml/hour.
- **3.** IV is infusing well.
- **4.** Slight cramps are reported.

Loretta Neter, a 22-year-old woman, is admitted to an inpatient psychiatric unit. Paralysis developed in her right arm, for which no physical cause can be found. The admitting diagnosis is conversion reaction.

129. Miss Neter is using which of the following defense mechanisms?
- **1.** Reaction formation and projection.
- **2.** Suppression and compensation.
- **3.** Isolation and undoing.
- **4.** Repression and displacement.

130. Miss Neter tends to focus on her paralysis in her interactions with others by asking for help, even for things she can do herself, and by talking about how she feels about having a paralyzed arm. Which of the following interventions would be most appropriate when dealing with this dynamic?
- **1.** Allow the client to discuss her symptoms to help relieve her anxiety.
- **2.** Encourage the client to get involved in activities on the unit and to discuss other topics.
- **3.** Insist that the client not discuss her paralysis or receive help from others to force her to learn new ways of handling anxiety.
- **4.** Insist she discuss her physical symptoms with the nurses and the physician only, not with friends and family.

131. One day Miss Neter says to the nurse, "I suppose you think I'm faking my paralysis." Which of the following would be the best nursing response?
- **1.** "Yes, I think you could move your arm if you chose to do so."
- **2.** "I think you know that there is no physical cause for your paralysis."
- **3.** "I believe you are presently unable to move your arm, regardless of the cause."
- **4.** "I believe your paralysis is physical and that you may have been misdiagnosed."

132. Miss Neter's comment is most likely due to which of the following explanations?
- **1.** She is having auditory hallucinations.
- **2.** She is having paranoid delusions.
- **3.** She is seeking reassurance.
- **4.** She is lonely.

Three-month-old Pedro Cruz is seen in the pediatric clinic for well baby care. During this visit, the physician diagnoses congenital hypothyroidism.

133. When explaining the diagnosis to Mr. and Mrs. Cruz, the nurse should describe which findings as characteristic of congenital hypothyroidism?
○ **1.** Hyperirritability, prominent nasal bridge.
○ **2.** Tachycardia, small oral cavity.
○ **3.** Constant hunger, runny stools.
○ **4.** Inactivity, mottled skin.

134. Pedro is placed on levothyroxine (Synthroid) 25 mcg per day. The nurse should provide which instruction to Pedro's parents?
○ **1.** The medication should be given until symptoms subside, then gradually discontinued.
○ **2.** Pedro can be expected to lose some weight as he adjusts to the medication.
○ **3.** The medication should be administered as a single morning dose.
○ **4.** Constipation may develop, and indicates toxicity.

Janie Olivera, age 5 years, has just been diagnosed with acute lymphoblastic leukemia. She has been admitted to the pediatric unit for induction chemotherapy.

135. In assessing the Oliveras' response to Janie's diagnosis, the nurse should initially expect which parental reaction?
○ **1.** Expressing feelings of guilt and remorse.
○ **2.** Hoping that the diagnosis is wrong.
○ **3.** Making frequent demands on the staff.
○ **4.** Asking about unconventional types of treatment.

136. Which of the following behaviors would best indicate to the nurse that Janie is adequately prepared for bone-marrow aspiration? Janie
○ **1.** Explains that her healthy blood cells are sick and need special medicine.
○ **2.** Tells her mom that she likes her nurse and wants to play after the test.
○ **3.** Willingly allows the nurse to take her to the treatment room.
○ **4.** Tells her dolls that she has to have a needle in her hip to test her blood.

137. A chemotherapeutic regimen of vincristine and prednisone has been initiated for Janie. The nurse should report which of the following reactions to the physician?
○ **1.** Petechiae appear on Janie's chest and face.
○ **2.** Janie vomits two times after breakfast.
○ **3.** Janie complains of tingling in her fingers and toes.
○ **4.** Janie develops small ulcerations on her lips.

138. Janie is receiving a unit of packed cells intravenously. Which intravenous solution would be appropriate to use to flush the tubing prior to initiating the transfusion?
○ **1.** Lactated Ringer's solution.
○ **2.** 5% dextrose in water.
○ **3.** 5% dextrose in one-quarter normal saline.
○ **4.** Hyperalimentation solution.

139. Janie is also receiving radiation therapy. Mr. Olivera says he has heard that there are serious side effects, and asks the nurse what these are. Which one of the following is *not* a side effect of radiation therapy?
○ **1.** Delays in physical development.
○ **2.** Susceptibility to bone fractures.
○ **3.** Early onset of secondary sex characteristics.
○ **4.** Possible damage to chromosomes.

140. Janie is crying softly and says she is "hurting." Janie's pulse rate is elevated. Which of the following protocols would be most effective when administering Janie's pain medication?
○ **1.** Give when she becomes restless and is unable to sleep.
○ **2.** Give on a preventive schedule after assessing her pain responses.
○ **3.** Give whether Janie or her parents request it be given.
○ **4.** Give every 3 to 4 hours around the clock.

141. Mrs. Olivera tells the nurse that Janie is supposed to receive a DTP and TOPV booster before she starts kindergarten this year, and asks when she should take Janie to the health department to receive these. Which response by the nurse is accurate?
○ **1.** "We can give it before she leaves the hospital."
○ **2.** "Wait until a week or so before she starts school."
○ **3.** "When her white blood cell count returns to a normal level."
○ **4.** "Because of her diagnosis, Janie won't ever be able to be immunized again."

Olivia Carnelli, aged 76, is scheduled for a right modified mastectomy tomorrow.

142. Preoperatively, you would discuss post-op
○ **1.** Skin grafting.
○ **2.** *Peau d'orange* skin changes.
○ **3.** Treatment of intraductal edema.
○ **4.** Use of a HemoVac.

143. During a discussion with Mrs. Carnelli about the surgical skin prep she will receive, the nurse notices that Mrs. Carnelli seems close to tears. What would be the nurse's most appropriate response?

- **1.** "I'll stop this discussion for a while."
- **2.** "You must pay close attention to what I'm saying."
- **3.** "You seem close to tears, can you tell me what you're feeling?"
- **4.** Continue on with the explanation.

144. When Mrs. Carnelli returns from surgery, she is monitored for signs and symptoms of hemorrhage. In addition to assessing her vital signs, the nurse should

- **1.** Ask her if her back feels wet.
- **2.** Assess her level of consciousness.
- **3.** Observe the amount of drainage in the HemoVac.
- **4.** Visually check under her back for drainage.

145. Which of the following plans would be most likely to meet Mrs. Carnelli's learning needs for discharge planning?

- **1.** Provide written materials for her to read during the day.
- **2.** Offer brief, frequent one-to-one sessions.
- **3.** Teach her during a single session taking a sufficient amount of time to provide complete factual material.
- **4.** Have her join a group session with peers; use charts, several speakers, and handouts.

146. The nurse discusses ways of minimizing lymphedema with Mrs. Carnelli. Which of the following statements indicates a need for more teaching?

- **1.** "I'll avoid any constriction around my arm."
- **2.** "I'll make sure I drink plenty of fluids."
- **3.** "I'll sleep with my arm elevated on pillows."
- **4.** "I'll keep my right arm elevated as much as possible during the day."

147. Before Mrs. Carnelli is discharged the nurse would expect her to

- **1.** Be able to explain incision care.
- **2.** Have adapted to her altered body image.
- **3.** Have completed the grieving process.
- **4.** Have received an order for a Jobst pressure machine.

Mrs. Keller brings her son, Jermaine, who just turned 5, to the pediatrician's office for a complete health appraisal prior to his entering kindergarten next month.

148. The nurse should focus part of the assessment on Jermaine's achievement of psychosocial tasks. At this age, Jermaine should be trying to accomplish a sense of

- **1.** Autonomy.
- **2.** Identity.
- **3.** Mastery.
- **4.** Initiative.

149. The nurse evaluates Jermaine's readiness to attend kindergarten. Jermaine should be able to

- **1.** Tie his shoelaces.
- **2.** Count to 20.
- **3.** Tell time on a clock.
- **4.** Print his name.

150. Part of the assessment of Jermaine includes vision screening using the Snellen E chart to test for visual acuity. Jermaine's results are 20/30 vision in both eyes. Which action should the nurse take?

- **1.** Rescreen Jermaine immediately.
- **2.** Rescreen Jermaine in 2 weeks.
- **3.** Refer Jermaine to an opthalmologist for a complete eye exam.
- **4.** Explain to Jermaine and his mother that his vision is normal.

151. While conducting vision screening, the nurse should also screen Jermaine for

- **1.** Strabismus.
- **2.** Diplopia.
- **3.** Papilledema.
- **4.** Pupil reactivity.

152. Jermaine's height is at the 50th percentile. His weight is at the 90th percentile. A nutritional history reveals that Jermaine's diet is very high in carbohydrates and fats. The nurse helps Jermaine's mother develop a plan to ensure Jermaine gets the nutrients he needs without overeating. This diet should provide Jermaine with approximately how many calories per day?

- **1.** 1,200.
- **2.** 1,700.
- **3.** 2,400.
- **4.** 2,800.

153. Treatment of Jermaine's overweight would best include

- **1.** A planned program of activity and exercise.
- **2.** A daily appetite suppressant.
- **3.** Large doses of supplemental vitamins.
- **4.** Withholding all sweets.

154. Jermaine returns for a follow-up visit in 6 months. Which of the following best indicates Jermaine is progressing satisfactorily with his nutritional plan?

○ **1.** Jermaine has lost 5 lb.
○ **2.** Jermaine's daily intake has been 300 calories less than recommended.
○ **3.** Jermaine's weight is now in the 75th percentile.
○ **4.** Jermaine has stopped craving junk food.

Gloria Rock, age 31, gravida 5, para 4, has just delivered her fifth son following a 2-hour labor. The baby weighs 9 lb 10 oz.

155. Based on the data given, a potential problem for Mrs. Rock is

○ **1.** Thrombophlebitis.
○ **2.** Postpartal hemorrhage.
○ **3.** Puerperal infection.
○ **4.** Urinary retention.

156. One day postpartum, Mrs. Rock complains that excessive perspiring kept her awake at night. She is worried that there is a problem. An appropriate response is

○ **1.** "IV fluids administered during labor sometimes cause sweating."
○ **2.** "Maybe you drank too much fluid during the day."
○ **3.** "Fluids that were retained during pregnancy are normally lost."
○ **4.** "You may be experiencing signs of infection."

157. Mrs. Rock comments, "I hope this is our last baby because we can't afford any more." The nurse's best response would be

○ **1.** "Discuss this with your physician at your postpartum check-up."
○ **2.** "You need not worry until you quit breast-feeding."
○ **3.** "Let's talk about birth-control methods."
○ **4.** "Perhaps the social worker can help you."

158. Mrs. Rock goes home from the hospital and returns to the clinic for measurement of a diaphragm. The nurse explains to Mrs. Rock that this type of contraception is effective only if the device is used properly. The teaching has been effective if Mrs. Rock reports

○ **1.** Using K-Y jelly as a lubricant.
○ **2.** Removing the device 6 hours after coitus.
○ **3.** Storing it in a jar of alcohol.
○ **4.** Wearing the diaphragm for 1–2 days.

Otis O'Shea, aged 28, is admitted to the hospital after becoming embroiled in an argument with the police during a routine traffic check. His admitting diagnosis is paranoid schizophrenia.

159. As the nurse is orienting Mr. O'Shea to the unit, he states, "They can't arrest me, I'm J. Paul Getty, and I don't have to fool with inconsequential people like the police." Which of the following would be the best initial response?

○ **1.** "Can't arrest you?"
○ **2.** "What made you so angry, Mr. O'Shea?"
○ **3.** "This is your room, Mr. O'Shea."
○ **4.** "Your record indicates your name is Otis O'Shea."

160. The defense mechanism being used by Mr. O'Shea is which of the following?

○ **1.** Denial.
○ **2.** Fantasy.
○ **3.** Introjection.
○ **4.** Projection.

161. The physician leaves orders for Mr. O'Shea to have haloperidol (Haldol) 75 mg qid. Which of the following would be the most appropriate action for the nurse to take?

○ **1.** Call the physician; the dose is too low.
○ **2.** Call the physician; the dose is too high.
○ **3.** Call the physician; Haldol is not effective for paranoid schizophrenia.
○ **4.** Administer the drug; the medication and dose are appropriate.

162. Shortly after admission, Mr. O'Shea is seen ordering the other clients around. What action should the nurse best take?

○ **1.** Confront him with his behavior on a one-to-one basis.
○ **2.** Encourage other clients to confront him in a group meeting.
○ **3.** Seclude him.
○ **4.** Spend more time with him on a one-to-one basis.

163. Shortly after breakfast one morning the nurse hears Mr. O'Shea talking loudly and notes that he is beginning to pace in the hall. What would be the best initial action for the nurse to take?

○ **1.** Tell him, "Let's have a cup of coffee and talk about what's making you angry."
○ **2.** Offer him a prn medication for agitation.
○ **3.** Suggest that he use the punching bag.
○ **4.** Isolate him before he hurts someone on the unit.

164. Mr. O'Shea has not had a bowel movement for 6 days. This is most likely related to which of the following?
- **1.** His decreased activity level.
- **2.** Lack of fiber in his diet.
- **3.** A side effect of Haldol.
- **4.** Constriction of the bowel as a result of tension.

165. Mr. O'Shea has a great deal of difficulty making decisions. This is most likely the result of which of the following?
- **1.** Autism.
- **2.** Mixed feelings.
- **3.** Ambivalence.
- **4.** Apathy.

166. When Mr. O'Shea's behavior becomes more appropriate the nurse decides to include him in the preparation for the next unit party. Which of the following would be the most appropriate activity for him?
- **1.** Assign him to the entertainment committee.
- **2.** Ask him to take charge of making the coffee and seeing that the pot is kept filled.
- **3.** Put him in charge of the clean-up committee.
- **4.** Ask him to arrange for the pizza to be delivered.

167. Mr. O'Shea has an erratic employment history and is at present unemployed. He is planning to secure a job before discharge. What nursing action would be the most useful?
- **1.** Help him read the want ads.
- **2.** Role play the job interview with him.
- **3.** Refer him for vocational testing.
- **4.** Encourage him to write a resume.

13-year-old Tim McMichael is brought to the emergency department by his camp leader. During a summer overnight youth campout, Tim's kerosene lamp overturned and ignited his sleeping bag. Tim's shirt sleeve caught fire when he tried to put out the fire. He has second degree burns of his right hand and forearm.

168. Immediate care of the burn wound should include
- **1.** Immersing Tim's hand and forearm in cool water.
- **2.** Applying ice packs to the injury.
- **3.** Pulling adherent charred clothing from the burn wounds.
- **4.** Covering the burn with cortisone cream.

169. Tim's immunization history indicates that he has received all childhood immunizations according to the recommended schedule. At this time, tetanus prophylaxis for Tim should include
- **1.** Tetanus toxoid.
- **2.** Tetanus immune globulin.
- **3.** Tetanus toxoid and tetanus immune globulin.
- **4.** No additional protection.

170. After cleansing and debridement of the wound, the physician decides to apply silver sulfadiazine (Silvadene) and cover the wound with a bulky gauze dressing. The primary advantage of the closed method used to treat Tim's burn is that it
- **1.** Protects the wound from further injury.
- **2.** Minimizes fluid loss from the burn surface.
- **3.** Alleviates pain caused by exposure of the wound to air.
- **4.** Prevents contractures of the hand and wrist.

171. Tim's parents come to take him home. The nurse is teaching them how to change his dressing. Which discharge instruction should the nurse include in the teaching plan?
- **1.** The silver sulfadiazine cream will be painful when first applied to the burn.
- **2.** Tim should return to the laboratory each day to have his blood pH monitored.
- **3.** Old cream should be removed by soaking the wound in warm, soapy water.
- **4.** The silver sulfadiazine cream may cause a change in color of adjacent healthy skin.

172. Which of the following foods should the nurse suggest Tim eat most often during the next several weeks?
- **1.** Meats, citrus fruits, and milk.
- **2.** Vegetables, cheese, and yogurt.
- **3.** Breads, cereals, and pastas.
- **4.** Milkshakes, salads, and soups.

173. Tim returns for follow-up. His wound is healing well. Which behavior indicates that Tim may be having difficulty coping with his burn injury?
- **1.** Asks when he can begin playing football again.
- **2.** Says he is not interested in girls.
- **3.** Refuses to wear short-sleeve shirts.
- **4.** Is quiet and nontalkative during the office visit.

174. The nurse observes that Tim has mild acne, and that the lesions are especially noticeable on his forehead and chin. When asked if he would like some suggestions to help clear up the lesions, Tim nods. The nurse should suggest that Tim

- ○ **1.** Use a commercial sunlamp for 5 minutes daily.
- ○ **2.** Wear an absorbent headband during exercise or hot weather.
- ○ **3.** Purchase an over-the-counter product that contains benzoyl peroxide.
- ○ **4.** Avoid chocolate, fried foods, and iodized salt.

Jeff Tate, 34 years old, presents to the health clinic complaining of urinary burning, frequency, and urgency; hematuria; fever and chills. Lab tests on a clean catch urine reveal RBCs and WBCs: too many to count, numerous hyaline casts, and bacteria greater than 100,000/ml. A physical exam reveals extreme costovertebral angle (CFA) tenderness. Mr. Tate is diagnosed as having pyelonephritis, and he is admitted to the hospital.

175. The most important blood test of kidney filtration ordered for Mr. Tate would be

- ○ **1.** Glucose.
- ○ **2.** Electrolytes.
- ○ **3.** Creatinine.
- ○ **4.** BUN.

176. An intravenous pyelogram (IVP) is ordered for Mr. Tate. Which of the following would be the most important for the nurse to do the night before the IVP?

- ○ **1.** Give a cathartic and enemas to cleanse the bowel.
- ○ **2.** Instruct the client to be NPO after midnight.
- ○ **3.** Identify by history any client allergies to medicines or foods.
- ○ **4.** Teach the client that x-rays will be taken at multiple intervals.

177. Mr. Tate is placed on a regimen of a sulfonamide antibiotic (Bactrim). As a nurse, you know which of the following to be true concerning this drug?

- ○ **1.** It is metabolized by the liver and excreted through the bile.
- ○ **2.** It produces a false-negative glucose on urine tests.
- ○ **3.** It is more soluble in acidic urine.
- ○ **4.** It can crystalize in the urine if fluid intake is insufficient.

178. Upon Mr. Tate's discharge, the physician wants him to maintain his urine in a more acidic state by eating an acid-ash diet. Which of the following foods would you teach the client can be unrestricted in his diet?

- ○ **1.** Milk.
- ○ **2.** Carrots.
- ○ **3.** Grape-Nuts.
- ○ **4.** Dried apricots.

179. Which of the following interventions would be a priority in discharge teaching for Mr. Tate?

- ○ **1.** Drink at least 3–4 liters of fluid/day.
- ○ **2.** Take sitz baths 3–4 times/day for urethral burning.
- ○ **3.** Void immediately after sexual intercourse.
- ○ **4.** Avoid exposure to persons with upper respiratory infections.

180. After 3 weeks, Mr. Tate returns to the ER with severe, sharp, deep lumbar pain radiating to his right side. A repeat IVP reveals a kidney stone in the right ureter at the bifurcation of the iliac vessel. Upon his admission to the hospital, which of the following goals would take initial priority in this client's nursing care?

- ○ **1.** Client will decrease risk of future kidney stones.
- ○ **2.** Client will be prepared for possible urinary tract surgery.
- ○ **3.** Client will be free from discomfort of kidney stones.
- ○ **4.** Client will have fluid intake of 3–5 liters/day.

Carol Clay, G1 PO, is being admitted to the hospital in labor. She has had regular prenatal care, attended prenatal classes with her husband, and had an uncomplicated pregnancy.

181. Which of the following observations would be the most reliable guide to assess Mrs. Clay's progress in labor?

- ○ **1.** Contractions that are getting more intense.
- ○ **2.** Breathing that is becoming more rapid.
- ○ **3.** Progressive dilatation of the cervix.
- ○ **4.** Increased vaginal discharge (or rupture of membranes).

182. Mrs. Clay ambulates with her husband. Which of the following would warrant bedrest or further evaluation of her condition?

○ **1.** Contractions that are intense and last 60 seconds.
○ **2.** Progressive sarcal discomfort during contractions.
○ **3.** Rapid, shallow respirations during contractions.
○ **4.** A desire to defecate at the peak of contractions.

183. Mrs. Clay's blood pressure is monitored every 2 hours. Blood pressure is recorded in between contractions because

○ **1.** Assessing during contractions gives erratic readings.
○ **2.** Monitoring blood pressure during contractions is inaccurate.
○ **3.** Taking blood pressure during contractions distracts the client from breathing patterns.
○ **4.** Maintaining the arm in position during contractions is difficult for the client.

184. In early labor, the fetal heart tones are auscultated at regular intervals. The most appropriate time to listen to FHT is

○ **1.** During contractions.
○ **2.** Between contractions.
○ **3.** Soon after contractions.
○ **4.** During and soon after contractions.

Virginia Ryan calls the adolescent mental health clinic worried about her 16-year-old daughter, Kathleen. She tells the nurse that Kathleen is obsessed about dieting and exercising even though she seems healthy and has not lost any weight.

185. Mrs. Ryan says her daughter eats very well but spends more and more time in the bathroom after meals. Kathleen denies anything is troubling her. The nurse's initial response to Mrs. Ryan would be

○ **1.** "She's a typical teenager, gobbling her food and then shutting herself off in a room."
○ **2.** "It sounds as if Kathleen is anorexic."
○ **3.** "Are you worried Kathleen may have an eating disorder?"
○ **4.** "Let's figure out if she's depressed."

186. Kathleen's symptoms suggest she is

○ **1.** Depressed.
○ **2.** Anorexic.
○ **3.** A chemical abuser.
○ **4.** Bulimic.

187. Mrs. Ryan brings Kathleen into the emergency room the next day because Kathleen has admitted to her she has been abusing laxatives and diet pills. The first goal of treatment will be to

○ **1.** Help Kathleen develop insight into her behavior.
○ **2.** Promote Kathleen's acceptance of herself and body.
○ **3.** Promote adequate nutritional intake and retention of food.
○ **4.** Help her develop realistic expectations for dieting, exercising.

Correct Answers and Rationales: Part Two

94. **#4.** The hepatitis type A virus is spread via contact with oral and respiratory secretions, feces, and serum from an infected person. NUTRITION AND METABOLISM/ADULT

95. **#3.** Jaundice is a sign of obstructive disease (i.e., obstruction of the bile duct, possibly from a gallstone). Prothrombin, a protein produced by the liver, is used in the clotting of blood. Its production depends on adequate intake and absorption of vitamin K. Obstruction of the bile flow may impair absorption. Prolonged prothrombin time may lead to hemorrhage. The Lee-White clotting time is a relatively insensitive test for coagulation; bleeding time only measures the initial phase of hemostasis. NUTRITION AND METABOLISM/ADULT

96. **#1.** Because of the high incision and upper abdominal pain, the post op client resists coughing and deep breathing and is likely to develop atelectasis. SURGERY/ADULT

97. **#4.** Irrigation maintains the patency of the tube, which will also accomplish options #1 and #2. NUTRITION AND METABOLISM/ADULT

98. **#3.** Although all are appropriate interventions, the priority is to establish and maintain a patent airway. INTRAPARTAL/CHILDBEARING FAMILY

99. **#4.** The plan is based on an understanding that in the first hours after delivery, excess insulin may lead to hypoglycemia. Brain damage will result if low blood sugar is not corrected. Assessment of glucose level is done frequently. If low, early feeding is essential. Hydration is not critical in the first hours of life. All newborns need an environment that conserves body temperature. HIGH-RISK NEWBORN/CHILDBEARING FAMILY

100. **#3.** The teaching for this mother must include emphasis on regular pediatric care, considering the possibility of inherited tendency to diabetes. Asphyxia is a potential problem for a diabetic's newborn in the immediate delivery process. Skim milk is never suggested for a newborn. Risk of hypoglycemia passes after initial adaptation to feedings. HIGH-RISK NEWBORN/CHILDBEARING FAMILY

101. **#4.** The release of epinephrine in response to an abnormal drop in blood-sugar level results in dizziness and trembling. Hunger is characteristic of hypoglycemia. The other symptoms are manifestations of acidosis or infection. NUTRITION AND METABOLISM/ADULT

102. **#4.** Evaluation of the care of feet indicates that the client needs further teaching if hot Epsom salt soaks are being used. This solution is drying and could burn the feet. Daily washing of the feet prevents skin breakdown. NUTRITION AND METABOLISM/ADULT

103. **#4.** Protein and calcium are needed to meet lactation needs. Complex carbohydrates provide fiber and enhance blood sugar control. Saturated fats should be reduced for diabetics. Increased potassium is not recommended, as it may be a factor in hypoglycemia. Simple sugars may lead to blood glucose imbalance. POSTPARTAL CARE/CHILDBEARING FAMILY

104. **#2.** An open airway is the first priority following trauma. Control of hemorrhage is second. Stabilization of the fractured vertebrae takes precedence over splinting of the leg. OXYGENATION/ADULT

105. **#4.** Primary intervention with hemorrhage includes measures to stop bleeding and restore blood volume in order to prevent irreversible shock. The other interventions are appropriate but of secondary importance. OXYGENATION/ADULT

106. **#2.** Shock causes metabolic acidosis (a pH less than 7.34). Tissue metabolism continues so that large amounts of acid are emptied and accumulate in the stagnant blood. With progressive tissue hypoxia, anaerobic metabolism produces nonvolatile lactic acid, which further increases the acidosis. Shock also produces hypoxia (pO_2 less than 80 mm Hg); hypercapnia (pCO_2 greater than 45 mm Hg); and an increase in capillary permeability. OXYGENATION/ADULT

107. #2. According to the American Heart Association, the 2 rescuer CPR compression-ventilation ratio is 5:1 with a 1 to 1½ second pause for ventilation. 15:2 is the recommended compression-ventilation ratio for 1 rescuer CPR. The compression rate for either 1 or 2 rescuer CPR is 80–100 per minute. 1:1 or 20:2 compression-ventilation ratios are not recommended. OXYGENATION/ADULT

108. #1. A palpable carotid pulse would be the best indicator of adequate sternal compression. It is a better indicator of effective CPR than skin color. Easily blanched nail beds and dilated pupils indicate inadequate perfusion. Some emergency drugs alter pupil reaction (e.g., atropine). OXYGENATION/ADULT

109. #4. Alterations in skin color may result from changes in vasomotor tone yet give little indication of perfusion of the vital organs. Options #1, #2, and #3 are reliable indicators of vital tissue perfusion. OXYGENATION/ADULT

110. #3. Doing either #2 or #3 would bring the BP down; but since vasoconstriction causes other problems, you would want to decrease the epinephrine rather than increase the nitroprusside. Options #1 and #4 would cause BP to rise further. OXYGENATION/ADULT

111. #2. All are goals of treatment, but tissue perfusion must be improved to prevent irreversible damage and death of tissues. If tissue perfusion improves, the other goals will be accompanied secondarily. OXYGENATION/ADULT

112. #3. Cerebral pressure rises as a result of tissue injury, edema, and hypoxia. BP increases in response to the hypoxic stimulation of the vasomotor center. Pulse rate slows as blood pressure increases. SAFETY AND SECURITY/ADULT

113. #1. A widening pulse pressure is characteristic of increasing intracranial pressure, also pulse rate decreases, respirations decrease, and level of consciousness decreases. SAFETY AND SECURITY/ADULT

114. #2. Dissociative reactions are hysterical reactions characterized by bizarre behavior in which the client splits off one portion of his conscious mind from the whole when that represents some major, otherwise unresolvable, conflict. This is a neurotic rather than psychotic reaction. Life-threatening experiences and frustrations can upset the psychologic equilibrium of some persons, but it is unlikely that they would precipitate an event of the magnitude of dissociative reaction. ANXIOUS BEHAVIOR/PSYCHOSOCIAL, MENTAL HEALTH, PSYCHIATRIC PROBLEMS

115. #4. Repression is the unconscious involuntary forgetting of unacceptable or painful thoughts, impulses, feelings, or acts. A dissociative reaction is the unconscious use of repression to forget events that may cause persons to recall painful material. Options #1, #2, and #3 do not play a significant part in a dissociative reaction. Regression involves returning to an earlier level of emotional development and organization; someone practicing denial treats obvious reality factors as though they do not exist. Rationalization is an attempt to justify feelings. GLOSSARY/PSYCHOSOCIAL, MENTAL HEALTH, PSYCHIATRIC PROBLEMS

116. #3. Mr. X will best be helped by decreased anxiety and active involvement. The focus is on reality-based milieu activities. The staff relates to him within the reality of the situation (i.e., relationships and day-to-day activities of the milieu). ECT would not help because it is believed that ECT helps seal off, rather than increase awareness of, unconscious conflicts. THERAPEUTIC USE OF SELF/PSYCHOSOCIAL, MENTAL HEALTH, PSYCHIATRIC PROBLEMS

117. #2. The child with cyanotic heart disease is prone to polycythemia (an increase in circulating red blood cells), which leads to a rise in hematocrit. Normal hematocrit values for a child are 32%–47%. All other values are within normal limits. OXYGENATION/CHILD

118. #1. The purpose of palliative surgery for the child with tetralogy of Fallot is to increase the pulmonary blood flow, which increases the amount of oxygenated blood to the tissues. The procedure will not affect the intracardiac shunting of blood from right to left or provide enough oxygen to his tissues to allow for normal development. In tetralogy of Fallot, the pressure is increased in the right ventricle (not the left) because of the pulmonary stenosis. OXYGENATION/CHILD

119. #3. The shape sorter is age appropriate (toddlers are interested in how things fit together, such as different shapes into their respective slots) and is a quiet activity. A priority goal preoperatively is to minimize the workload of the heart. The push-pull toy and the toy trumpet will increase the oxygen demands and, therefore, cardiac workload. A play stethoscope is too advanced for John David (it is an appropriate toy for a preschooler). HEALTHY CHILD/CHILD

120. #4. Gasping indicates that John David is at risk for having an anoxic spell and should be placed in a knee-chest (squatting) position to increase the blood flow to his heart, lungs, and brain. Although options #1 and #2 are appropriate responses for handling toddlers' temper tantrums, in this instance, John David's physiologic needs take priority over his developmental needs. Encouraging Mrs. Jankowski to set few limits is not in John David's best interests developmentally. OXYGENATION/CHILD

121. #2. Low implantation of the placenta causes painless bleeding in the third trimester. Abruptio placentae often is accompanied by pain or tenderness. Ectopic pregnancy and abortion occur earlier in pregnancy. ANTEPARTAL CARE/CHILDBEARING FAMILY

122. #1. A vaginal examination is contraindicated for this client, because it might stimulate contractions and increase the risk of placental delivery. The other options if ordered may be safely done. ANTEPARTAL CARE/ CHILDBEARING FAMILY

123. #4. Since the mother is worried, her feelings should be considered. The nurse appropriately suggests shared decision-making. INTRAPARTAL CARE/CHILDBEARING FAMILY

124. #4. All of these are part of preparation for cesarean birth except an enema, which could stimulate contractions and cause bleeding. INTRAPARTAL CARE/CHILDBEARING FAMILY

125. #4. The bed will be kept flat for 8–12 hours after use of spinal anesthetic to minimize the possibility of headaches. While it is true that medication is available, the chief focus of teaching is on position. POSTPARTAL CARE/ CHILDBEARING FAMILY

126. #1. Rapid pulse and apprehension are signs of shock. Other observations listed are normal at this time. POSTPARTAL CARE/ CHILDBEARING FAMILY

127. #3. With a drop factor of 10 drops/ml; the desired rate is 27 drops/minute. INTRAPARTAL CARE/CHILDBEARING FAMILY

128. #2. Pitocin has an antidiuretic effect in addition to stimulating contractions and causing cramps. Urinary output must be carefully monitored. Less than 30–50 ml per hour is cause for concern and should be reported. The medication may be discontinued. INTRAPARTAL CARE/CHILDBEARING FAMILY

129. #4. She is repressing conflicting feelings that she unconsciously believes she cannot handle and displaces the resulting anxiety into the physical symptom of paralysis. In this way, her focus is on the paralysis. As a result, she is relieved of the need to deal with the original conflict. Suppression is a conscious mechanism; and if she were using suppression, she would consciously know that her paralysis was an emotional response and it would be within her conscious control. Reaction formation expresses feelings opposite to those being experienced. Projection ascribes to another person or object the unacceptable thoughts and feelings. Compensation is substituting an unattainable goal for another to make up for a real or imagined inadequacy. Isolation is blocking the feelings associated with an unpleasant, threatening situation or thought. Undoing cancels the effect of another response just made. GLOSSARY/PSYCHOSOCIAL, MENTAL HEALTH, PSYCHIATRIC PROBLEMS

130. #2. It is important to encourage her to give up the symptom by not focusing on it. However, since the symptom is a method she uses to relieve anxiety, staff members need to help her find new ways of relieving anxiety before she will give up her present method of relieving it. However, one cannot force a person to learn new ways of handling anxiety that come out of the unconscious. Since her symptoms unconsciously control the anxiety, discussion alone would not relieve the symptoms. It is inappropriate to focus on physical symptoms as they are of unconscious origin. ANXIOUS BEHAVIOR/PSYCHOSOCIAL, MENTAL HEALTH, PSYCHIATRIC PROBLEMS

131. #3. This is the response that demonstrates the nurse's understanding of the pain the symptom is causing the client and its reality to her. Options #1 and #2 contradict the client's behavior. Option #4 would promote doubt in competence of staff and is untrue. ANXIOUS BEHAVIOR/PSYCHOSOCIAL, MENTAL HEALTH, PSYCHIATRIC PROBLEMS

132. #3. The client is seeking reassurance about the origin of her symptoms. This client is not psychotic and loneliness, though painful, does not cause the dramatic unconscious behavior/ symptoms described. ANXIOUS BEHAVIOR/ PSYCHOSOCIAL, MENTAL HEALTH, PSYCHIATRIC PROBLEMS

133. #4. The infant with congenital hypothyroidism is inactive (often described as a good, quiet baby) and undemanding. The disease is also characterized by mottling of the skin, constipation, a large protruding tongue, and a flattened nasal bridge. NUTRITION AND METABOLISM/CHILD

134. #3. Thyroid replacement should be given as a single morning dose throughout the child's lifetime. Diarrhea, tachycardia, and weight loss indicate toxicity. NUTRITION AND METABOLISM/CHILD

135. #2. The initial response to diagnosis of a life-threatening illness is shock, disbelief, and hope that "it's not real." Frequent demands and feelings of guilt and remorse characterize later stages of the grieving process. Asking about unconventional treatments should alert the nurse to be concerned that the parents may not understand the meaning of the diagnosis. LOSS, DEATH AND DYING/ PSYCHOSOCIAL, MENTAL HEALTH, PSYCHIATRIC PROBLEMS

136. #4. Option #1 indicates some understanding of the disease, but not the bone-marrow procedure. #2 and #3 reflect adaptation to hospitalization. #4 indicates that Janie comprehends what will happen to her during the procedure. ILL AND HOSPITALIZED CHILD/CHILD

137. #3. Petechiae result from the leukemic process. Vomiting and stomatitis are expected side effects of chemotherapy. Vincristine causes neurotoxic responses, such as numbness and tingling, jaw pain, and constipation, which should be reported because they may indicate toxicity. CELLULAR ABERRATION/CHILD

138. #1. When administering blood products, only saline solutions or solutions that don't contain any dextrose or glucose should be used. Dextrose and glucose solutions (hyperalimentation solutions contain hypertonic glucose concentrations) will cause hemolysis of the blood cells. CELLULAR ABERRATION/ CHILD

139. #3. Radiation therapy may cause delayed onset of puberty, delays in physical growth, pathologic bone fractures, and chromosomal damage because of its effects on normal cells. CELLULAR ABERRATION/CHILD

140. #2. Pain control is best achieved on a preventive schedule after assessing the time period that a particular dosage is effective for the child and the child's general pain responses. This prevents fluctuation in pain threshold levels. Waiting until the child becomes restless and unable to sleep will lessen the effectiveness of analgesia when given. Pain medications should not be given more often than every 3 to 4 hours, but giving them that often round the clock may not be necessary for a particular child. ILL AND HOSPITALIZED CHILD/ CHILD

141. #3. Immunosuppression is a contraindication for giving immunizations. Immunizing a child who is immunosuppressed can lead to overwhelming infection and death. As soon as the child's white blood cell count is normal, the DPT and TOPV boosters may be given since the child's immune system can respond normally. CELLULAR ABERRATION/CHILD

142. #4. Postoperatively, Mrs. Carnelli will probably have a HemoVac in place. Skin grafting is associated with the more extensive, Halsted radical mastectomy. *Peau d'orange* change in skin is a pre-op assessment parameter, noted on self-breast examination. CELLULAR ABERRATION/ADULT

143. #3. Acknowledging what the patient is feeling encourages verbalization about the feeling. #1 avoids an opportunity for further discussion. #2 is too demanding and does not acknowledge what the patient is feeling. #4 avoids even observation of client's feelings. INTRODUCTION/PSYCHOSOCIAL, MENTAL HEALTH, PSYCHIATRIC PROBLEMS

144. #4. Drainage is drawn to the back of the dressing by gravity. Unless her back is checked for drainage, Mrs. Carnelli may hemorrhage significantly without its being detected. Alterations in level of consciousness are associated with decreased oxygenation resulting from a number of factors. She would have to lose a significant amount of blood before her state of consciousness would be altered. CELLULAR ABERRATION/ADULT

145. #2. This best allows the nurse to assess understanding of material and provides an opportunity to adapt to the patient's concentration span. Option #1 is not best with this age group since they may have trouble with written content or may not be motivated to read. #3 and #4 may overtax the client and do not allow feelings about the surgery and diagnosis to be expressed. Option #4 is more appropriate with 20 to 30 year olds. HEALTHY ADULT/ADULT

146. #2. The patient should decrease her intake of sodium and liquids. This response indicates she needs additional teaching. CELLULAR ABERRATION/ADULT

147. #1. Prior to discharge, Mrs. Carnelli should be able to explain incision care. Adapting to an altered body image takes weeks or months, as does the grieving process. The latter may even be delayed two or three months. A Jobst pressure machine is used only if other methods for preventing lymphedema are ineffective. CELLULAR ABERRATION/ADULT

148. #4. The psychosocial task at this age is accomplishment of a sense of initiative. Autonomy is the toddler's major task, identity the adolescent's. Mastery is important throughout childhood but is most characteristic of the school-age child. HEALTHY CHILD/CHILD

149. #2. The average 5-year-old can count to 20, recite the alphabet, and recognize most colors. It is not until about age 6 that children can print their names. At age 7, children can tell clock time and tie their shoelaces. HEALTHY CHILD/CHILD

150. #4. These results are normal; 20/20 or 20/30 vision is considered within normal limits at this age, because visual acuity may not be fully developed. HEALTHY CHILD/CHILD

151. #1. Strabismus is a common health problem that must be detected early to prevent amblyopia. The other options are used to assess neurologic status. HEALTHY CHILD/CHILD

152. #2. Recommended caloric intake at this age is approximately 1,700 calories/day. HEALTHY CHILD/CHILD

153. #1. A carefully planned program of diet and exercise that meets the child's continued needs for growth is essential. Focus should be on slowing weight gain to allow height to catch up over a period of several months, rather than trying to have the child lose weight. Appetite suppressants are without merit in the treatment of childhood overweight and obesity. Large doses of vitamins are unnecessary, if the child is eating a well-balanced diet, and may actually be harmful to the child. Withholding all sweets is unrealistic and may lead to cheating. The child should be helped to change his eating habits without the recognition that an occasional sweet treat is acceptable. NUTRITION AND METABOLISM/CHILD

154. #3. Because of slowing of Jermaine's weight gain, his weight is now only one standard deviation from his height. Weight loss and caloric restriction are not desired outcomes. Jermaine may not be craving junk food, but this option doesn't give you enough information to evaluate his progress (e.g., he may not be eating junk food, but his caloric intake may be as high as previously if he is substituting other foods). NUTRITION AND METABOLISM/CHILD

155. #2. The uterine muscle may contract poorly due to overdistension from a large baby and several past pregnancies. Rapid labor may delay involution as well. While the other complications may occur, they are not specific in this case. POSTPARTAL CARE/CHILDBEARING FAMILY

156. #3. Fluid shifts during the postpartal period cause a normal diaphoresis and diuresis. Intake is related to urinary output, but options #1 and #2 are not accurate. While hormones dramatically affect adaptation after delivery, this symptom alone does not suggest infection. POSTPARTAL CARE/CHILDBEARING FAMILY

157. #3. This is the best option, and is an appropriate way to initiate teaching. Breast-feeding is not a means of contraception. Delaying a discussion until the check-up may lead to another pregnancy. POSTPARTAL CARE/CHILDBEARING FAMILY

158. #2. This describes the proper time for removal of a diaphragm. Spermicidal, not K-Y jelly, should be used. Alcohol rapidly dries rubber and reduces effectiveness. While a cervical sponge may be left in place for 1–2 days, a diaphragm should be removed 6 hours after intercourse.

159. #3. This response keeps the interaction reality oriented. #1 and #2 probe into the client's delusion. #4 may provoke an argument. WITHDRAWN BEHAVIOR/ PSYCHOSOCIAL, MENTAL HEALTH, PSYCHIATRIC PROBLEMS

160. #4. Projection is unconsciously attributing one's own unacceptable qualities and emotions to others. He is saying, "I'm not inconsequential. They are." #1, #2, and #3 are not found in this clinical situation. GLOSSARY/PSYCHOSOCIAL, MENTAL HEALTH, PSYCHIATRIC PROBLEMS

161. #2. The maximum therapeutic dose for Haldol is 100 mg daily. WITHDRAWN BEHAVIOR/ PSYCHOSOCIAL, MENTAL HEALTH, PSYCHIATRIC PROBLEMS

162. #4. The suspicious, hostile, or aggressive client should be worked with initially, and probably for an extended time, on a one-to-one basis. This will allow a trusting relationship to develop. #1 and #2 will provoke anger and hostility and will reinforce defenses. Option #3 isolates the client and may also reinforce defenses and perpetuate the delusional system. SUSPICIOUS BEHAVIOR/PSYCHOSOCIAL, MENTAL HEALTH, PSYCHIATRIC PROBLEMS

163. #1. Intervene while the client is still able to talk about feelings. Option #2 will not allow the client the opportunity to learn to deal with negative feelings. #3 also will not allow the client to learn verbal methods of dealing with anger. #4 is not justified by his behavior at this time. SUSPICIOUS BEHAVIOR/ PSYCHOSOCIAL, MENTAL HEALTH, PSYCHIATRIC PROBLEMS

164. #3. Constipation is a side effect of Haldol. #1, #2, and #4 can cause constipation, but no data have been given to support them. WITHDRAWN BEHAVIOR/ PSYCHOSOCIAL, MENTAL HEALTH, PSYCHIATRIC PROBLEMS

165. #3. Ambivalence is the coexistence of 2 opposing feelings toward another person, object, or idea. Although the term "mixed feelings" is sometimes used, ambivalence is the proper term. Extreme withdrawal (autism) and low level of interest in or response to surroundings (apathy) have not been described. GLOSSARY/PSYCHOSOCIAL, MENTAL HEALTH, PSYCHIATRIC PROBLEMS

166. #2. Put the suspicious, hostile, aggressive client in charge of things, not people. Option #2 is the only response that meets that criterion. #1, #3, and #4 will subject this client to the stress of relating to people, especially in situations of authority. SUSPICIOUS BEHAVIOR/PSYCHOSOCIAL, MENTAL HEALTH, PSYCHIATRIC PROBLEMS

167. #2. This allows the client to practice verbally what he is going to say before he is in the actual situation (one that is likely to be stressful). Options #1, #3, and #4 may also be useful; but with Mr. O'Shea's employment history, vocational counseling, a resume, and the want ads are less likely to be useful than learning to deal with stressful situations. WITHDRAWN BEHAVIOR/ PSYCHOSOCIAL, MENTAL HEALTH, PSYCHIATRIC PROBLEMS

168. #1. Emergency care of a burn wound such as this involves dousing or immersing the injury in cool water to prevent further thermal damage. Ice packs or ice water can cause further damage to the injured tissue and are contraindicated. Adherent clothing should never be pulled from a burn injury because of the possibility of damaging remaining tissue. Covering the burn with any kind of substance (cream, margarine, ointments) can trap heat and also cause further damage and increase the risk of infection. SENSATION, PERCEPTION, PROTECTION/ CHILD

169. #1. Because Tim's wound is not tetanus prone (i.e., does not involve muscle tissue, not contaminated with saliva or excrement, less than 24 hours old), and he has received a full series of primary immunizations with his last booster less than 10 years ago (between 4 and 6 years of age) but more than 5 years ago, he needs tetanus toxoid (given in the form of Td). Tetanus immune globulin (passive immunity) is indicated only if the previous immunization history is unknown or uncertain, or the burn wound is tetanus prone (i.e., burn wounds that involve muscle tissue or are highly contaminated). SENSATION, PERCEPTION, PROTECTION/CHILD

170. #2. The major advantage of the closed method is to minimize fluid lost from the burn surface by applying gentle pressure to the burn wound. Use of Silvadene will also reduce the possibility of wound infection. Although the dressing will protect the wound and reduce pain, these are not the primary reasons for using this method. Wrapping the wound will partially immobilize the hand and wrist and, therefore, may increase the possibility of contracture. SENSATION, PERCEPTION, PROTECTION/CHILD

171. #3. Removal of old cream is essential in keeping the wound clean and ensuring that newly applied cream is effective in reducing the chance of bacterial contamination. The wound should be cleansed with warm sudsy water (using a soap like Ivory flakes or Dreft, *not* a detergent). Silvadene is not painful when applied and does not interfere with acid-base or electrolyte balance. Silver nitrate, not Silvadene, may cause skin discoloration when used to treat burn wounds. SENSATION, PERCEPTION, PROTECTION/CHILD

172. #1. The burn-injured client needs large amounts of protein and vitamin C for wound healing. Meats and milk are high in protein, and citrus fruits are high in vitamin C. SENSATION, PERCEPTION, PROTECTION/CHILD

173. #3. Refusal to wear short-sleeve shirts in the summer indicates that Tim may be trying to hide his burn injury from himself and others and, therefore, may need help in coping with this body change. Asking about resumption of physical activity is a healthy sign. Many teenage boys this age are not yet interested in girls, and adolescents are often quiet and nontalkative in unfamiliar situations or with adults. LOSS, DEATH AND DYING/ PSYCHOSOCIAL, MENTAL HEALTH, PSYCHIATRIC PROBLEMS

174. #3. Acne is caused by sebum blocking skin pores and is most effectively treated by adequate daily cleansing, followed by application of anti-acne product that contains benzoyl peroxide, a peeling and drying agent. Use of a headband during exercise or hot weather can cause secretions to be retained, with further blockage of skin pores. There is no evidence that chocolate, iodine, or greasy foods contribute to acne. Use of ultraviolet light should be reserved for severe cases of acne and done under the supervision of a physician. SENSATION, PERCEPTION, PROTECTION/ CHILD

175. #3. This is a specific measurement to determine kidney function, primarily glomerular filtration. Creatinine is produced at a constant rate; it is not reabsorbed and is only minimally secreted. BUN is less reliable because urea, after being filtered, is reabsorbed back into renal tubular cells. Additionally, urea production varies according to liver function and protein intake and breakdown. The test for serum glucose is used to screen for disorders of metabolism. Electrolyte studies are not specific to kidney filtration. ELIMINATION/ADULT

176. #3. The dye used for an IVP is iodine based and can cause a severe allergic reaction (anaphylaxis) in sensitive individuals. Food allergies to shellfish can indicate an iodine allergy, because shellfish are high in iodine content. The other options should be done; but because of the possible danger to the client, the allergy history takes priority. ELIMINATION/ ADULT

177. **#4.** Sulfonamides dissolve well in urine and are excreted unchanged in the urine; therefore they are excellent for treating urinary tract infections. However, if fluid intake is not sufficient, the drug can crystalize, resulting in renal toxicity. While on the drug regimen, intake should be sufficient to maintain a urine output of at least 1 liter/day. Sulfonamides are metabolized by the liver and excreted via the kidneys, may produce a false positive glucose on urine tests, and are more soluble in alkaline urine. ELIMINATION/ADULT

178. **#3.** Whole grains are unrestricted in an acid-ash diet. Carrots and dried apricots are not allowed and only 1 pint of milk is allowed daily. NUTRITION AND METABOLISM/ ADULT

179. **#1.** A high urine output helps flush out bacteria from the urinary tract and maintain a low urine osmolarity. Encourage clients to void every 2 to 3 hours during the day and 1 to 2 times during the night. Sitz baths are helpful during an acute episode but are not a priority of discharge planning. Voiding after intercourse is recommended for women who have repeated urinary tract infections. Avoidance of exposure to respiratory infections would be highly desirable if the client was showing signs and symptoms of renal failure. At this point, Mr. Tate is not in this category. ELIMINATION/ ADULT

180. **#3.** All of these goals are worthwhile and will need to be met prior to discharge; however, because of the severity of the renal colic, option #3 must be the first priority. Only then can the client respond to teaching and begin taking increased fluids. Morphine may have to be given for the pain, depending upon the severity. IV fluids may have to be started to increase intake initially. ELIMINATION/ ADULT

181. **#3.** Cervical dilatation is the most reliable index of the progress of labor. Other options may or may not indicate true progress. #1 is possible with hypertonic dysfunction, #2 could be related to anxiety, and #4 can occur at any time and may not relate to progress. INTRAPARTAL CARE/CHILDBEARING FAMILY

182. **#4.** This symptom is related to sacral pressure and progression into the second stage of labor. The other options do not warrant further evaluation as long as the client is comfortable ambulating. INTRAPARTAL CARE/ CHILDBEARING FAMILY

183. **#2.** Blood pressure rises during contractions and, therefore, gives an inaccurate reading. Option #1 is incorrect as erratic could mean increasing or decreasing. Options #3 and #4 may be true but are not valid reasons. INTRAPARTAL CARE/CHILDBEARING FAMILY

184. **#4.** To assess for late decelerations it is necessary to listen during and soon after contractions. Early fetal distress would be completely missed if option #2 were followed. INTRAPARTAL CARE/CHILDBEARING FAMILY

185. **#3.** From the signs Mrs. Ryan describes, it is evident she suspects Kathleen has an eating problem. But the lack of weight loss does not seem to fit with what she knows, so she's not sure. Option #3 verbalizes the implied question Mrs. Ryan seems to be asking as well as gets to the point of her daughter having an eating disorder, which the symptoms support. Option #1 and #2 are wrong because Kathleen is showing typical symptoms of bulimia. Option #4 may be true, but the central problem is the eating disorder, bulimia. ANXIOUS BEHAVIOR/PSYCHOSOCIAL, MENTAL HEALTH, PSYCHIATRIC PROBLEMS

186. **#4.** Kathleen is showing the classic signs of bulimia and the ones that differentiate it from anorexia (healthy appearance, normal weight, furtive trips to the bathroom after meals). Options #1, #2, #3 are wrong for the symptoms presented. ANXIOUS BEHAVIOR/ PSYCHOSOCIAL, MENTAL HEALTH, PSYCHIATRIC PROBLEMS

187. **#3.** Initially Kathleen will show some of the physical effects of long-term vomiting and use of laxatives. Options #1, #2, and #4 are also good objectives of care, but are secondary to stabilizing her food retention and intake. ANXIOUS BEHAVIOR/PSYCHOSOCIAL, MENTAL HEALTH, PSYCHIATRIC PROBLEMS

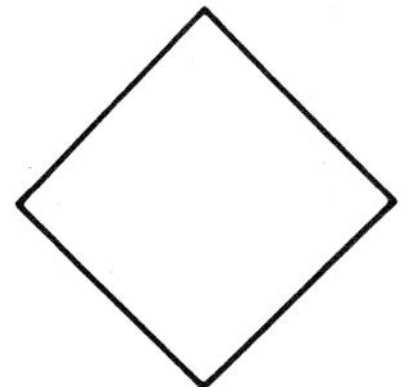

Sample Test Questions: Part Three

Carol Perez, 21 years old, is in acute renal failure following a large loss of blood from injuries she received in a car accident. Her 24-hour urine output is 275 ml. Her serum BUN is 90 mg/100 ml and her serum creatinine is 7.2 mg/100 ml.

188. During the oliguric phase of acute renal failure, which of the following would be an appropriate nursing intervention?

○ **1.** Increase dietary sodium and potassium.
○ **2.** Restrict fluid to 1,500 ml daily.
○ **3.** Weigh client 3 times weekly.
○ **4.** Provide a low protein, high carbohydrate diet.

189. Mrs. Perez fails to respond to therapy to correct her acute renal failure. She goes into chronic renal failure with the prospect of having to start dialysis or have a kidney transplant. Which of the following indicators would you expect to see in Mrs. Perez as the renal failure becomes more severe?

○ **1.** Anemia.
○ **2.** Hypokalemia.
○ **3.** Diaphoresis.
○ **4.** Hypotension.

190. In planning Mrs. Perez's diet, which of the following food sources would be the best source of high biologic-value protein?

○ **1.** Bananas.
○ **2.** Asparagus.
○ **3.** Eggs.
○ **4.** Mushrooms.

191. While waiting for a suitable transplant kidney to be identified, Mrs. Perez has to begin dialysis. An arteriovenous (AV) fistula is created for hemodialysis. As a nurse, you understand that one major complication you must observe for following an AV fistula is

○ **1.** Rejection of the silastic cannula connecting the artery and vein.
○ **2.** Accidental dislodgment of the cannula with resulting hemorrhage.
○ **3.** Thrombosis of the artery and vein site.
○ **4.** Cardiac irritation caused by the cannula's insertion.

192. Nursing assessment of the access site to the AV fistula would best include

○ **1.** Taking blood pressures in the affected arm to monitor the presence of good circulation.
○ **2.** Make sure the color of the blood in the fistula is bright, cranberry red.
○ **3.** Checking skin temperatures and pulses proximal to the fistula to assess circulation.
○ **4.** Palpating the access site for a thrill to assess circulation.

193. While waiting for the AV-fistula site to mature for hemodialysis, Mrs. Perez is maintained using peritoneal dialysis. During peritoneal dialysis, the nurse notes a retention of 600 ml of dialysate fluid after draining the periotoneal cavity. The initial response of the nurse would best be to

○ **1.** Infuse an additional 1,400 ml of fresh dialysate and continue with dialysis.
○ **2.** Have the client turn from side to side to help localize fluid to promote drainage.
○ **3.** Check vital signs to assess whether a fluid overload is occurring.
○ **4.** Notify the physician of the fluid retention.

194. Today Mrs. Perez will undergo hemodialysis for the first time. Which of the following interventions, if implemented, would be most likely to help her avoid disequilibrium syndrome?

○ **1.** Withhold her antihypertensive medications.
○ **2.** Dialyze her for a short period of time.
○ **3.** Dialyze her in a sitting position.
○ **4.** Withhold protein from her diet.

195. While waiting for a compatible kidney for transplant, Mrs. Perez will be discharged home. Because of the distance of the hemodialysis center from her home, the physician decides to maintain her with continuous ambulatory peritoneal dialysis (CAPD). When educating Mrs. Perez about CAPD, the top priority is to teach her

- **1.** Sterile technique to help prevent peritonitis.
- **2.** To maintain a more liberal protein diet.
- **3.** To maintain a daily written record of blood pressure and weight.
- **4.** To continue regular medical and nursing follow-up.

196. Mrs. Perez returns to the hospital for a kidney transplant. Which of the following interventions would do the most to help prevent transplant rejection?

- **1.** Transfusion of 4 units of typed and cross-matched blood.
- **2.** Administration of prophylactic antibiotics.
- **3.** Hemodialysis until the transplant begins to function.
- **4.** Administration of immunosuppressive drugs.

Chris and Jack O'Neal delayed childbearing for several years. After a year of planning, the O'Neals conceive. During her pregnancy, Mrs. O'Neal is carefully monitored because of a history of cardiac surgery as a child.

197. An internist follows her condition periodically during pregnancy, and shares information with the obstetrician and primary nurse. The chief potential problem for this client during the third trimester is

- **1.** Premature delivery.
- **2.** Cardiac decompensation.
- **3.** Dehydration.
- **4.** Infection.

198. Mrs. O'Neal develops severe hypertension, experiences headaches, and is hospitalized. She is given IV magnesium sulfate to prevent convulsions. In evaluating the client's response to therapy, which effect is expected?

- **1.** Muscle cramps.
- **2.** Hyperreflexia.
- **3.** Polyuria.
- **4.** Central nervous system depression.

199. Mr. O'Neal stays with his wife all through labor. Which of the following statements made by him would best indicate that he understands his role during labor?

- **1.** "I should take my coffee break soon, as Chris will need me with her in transition."
- **2.** "I will be able to leave Chris around lunch time, as she will prefer the professional care as the pain gets intense."
- **3.** "My presence distracts her and she tries to talk to me instead of resting between contractions."
- **4.** "Transition is a hard time and she is getting very irritable. I will take my break now and be back to help her to push."

200. Mrs. O'Neal's condition is stabilized, and she delivers an 8-lb son. The infant has an initial axillary temperature of 96°F. If the infant is cold stressed and is not warmed immediately, the nurse would initially observe

- **1.** Shivering.
- **2.** Cyanosis.
- **3.** Respiratory rate increase.
- **4.** Irritability.

201. Baby Boy O'Neal appears pink and active, but slight grunting on expiration is noted when using the Silverman-Anderson scale. What additional assessments are indicated?

- **1.** Heart rate.
- **2.** Chest movements.
- **3.** Blood gases.
- **4.** Color.

202. While performing a physical assessment of Baby Boy O'Neal, a swelling is observed on the side of the infant's head. This swelling is soft, does not pulsate or bulge when the infant cries, and does not cross suture lines. The parents ask about the mass. The problem is most likely

- **1.** Intracranial hemorrhage.
- **2.** Cephalhematoma.
- **3.** Caput succedaneum.
- **4.** Hydrocephalus.

203. Mrs. O'Neal holds her baby on the first day of rooming-in. Which of the following behaviors could indicate potential problems with early attachment?

- **1.** Mrs. O'Neal complains of episiotomy pain while sitting with her infant.
- **2.** She appears discouraged with early breast-feeding attempts.
- **3.** There is little attempt to touch or speak to the alert newborn.
- **4.** When the infant is quiet, Mrs. O'Neal often naps.

204. On her third postpartum day, Mrs. O'Neal is found crying and expresses inadequacy in meeting her baby's needs. The nursing student asks about this behavior. The nurse suggests that Mrs. O'Neal is probably experiencing

- **1.** Postpartum blues.
- **2.** Normal taking-in behavior.
- **3.** Abnormal bonding.
- **4.** Early psychotic depression.

205. Two weeks have elapsed. Mrs. O'Neal is breast-feeding. What is a goal of care at this time?

- **1.** Mother will limit nursing to 20-to 30-minute periods.
- **2.** Parents will supplement feedings with bottle once daily.
- **3.** Mother will reduce caloric intake to prepregnancy amount.
- **4.** Couple will alternate night feedings.

Roger Caine, a 30-year-old insurance salesman, was awarded an expense-paid Caribbean cruise for his outstanding sales record. While on his trip, he became restless and overactive. He insisted on eating every meal at the captain's table. He danced until the wee hours and was up early, ready to go. He talked fast and behaved grandiosely. Upon arrival in New York, he spent money excessively. He demanded a luxurious hotel suite and loudly berated the hotel manager because no luxurious hotel suite was available. Shortly thereafter, he was admitted to a hospital with a diagnosis of manic-depression. At the hospital, history taking revealed he had been hospitalized 2 years earlier for depression.

206. When it's time for lunch, Mr. Caine tells you he's too busy. He says he has an impending multimillion-dollar deal he has to negotiate and he has people to call and see. The nurse's best response would be

- **1.** "Visiting hours aren't until 4:00 P.M., so you can't see anyone now."
- **2.** "When you're finished, please come to the dining room to eat."
- **3.** "Mr. Caine, you need to eat now. I'll go with you to help you."
- **4.** "If you don't eat now, we'll need to put you in the seclusion room."

207. Which of the following actions must be *avoided* to ensure effective intervention with Mr. Caine's manipulative or demanding behavior?

- **1.** Give a short, clear definition of limits that will be set.
- **2.** Consistently enforce the limits that were set.
- **3.** Allow some leeway when limits are violated.
- **4.** Hold frequent staff conferences to ensure cohesiveness and consistency in carrying out the plan of care.

208. Which of the following should be considered first when planning Mr. Caine's physical care?

- **1.** Mr. Caine will be overly concerned about cleanliness.
- **2.** Mr. Caine is an adult who needs to be given autonomy in his care.
- **3.** Mr. Caine needs more knowledge about his illness.
- **4.** Mr. Caine may disregard his physical needs.

209. Mr. Caine is to be maintained on a regimen of lithium carbonate. What is the therapeutic blood level for lithium?

- **1.** 0.8–2.6 mEq/l.
- **2.** 0.8–1.5 mEq/l.
- **3.** 1.6–2.4 mEq/l.
- **4.** 2.9–3.2 mEq/l.

210. Mr. Caine should be observed for side effects of lithium. Which of the following is *not* an expected side effect?

- **1.** Nausea and sluggish feeling.
- **2.** Muscle weakness.
- **3.** Thirst and polyuria.
- **4.** Diffuse rash.

211. Mr. Caine has difficulty sleeping. He rarely sleeps more than 3 hours at a time. All of the following might alleviate his insomnia *except* one. Which one?

- **1.** Provide an evening of quiet activity.
- **2.** Give him a warm drink at bedtime.
- **3.** Administer a sedative for sleep.
- **4.** Encourage him to take a cool shower before retiring.

Antoinette Davis, a newborn, has meningomyelocele. She is being transferred directly from the delivery room to a special care unit.

212. The nurse should place Antoinette in which position?

- **1.** Semi-Fowler's.
- **2.** Supine.
- **3.** On her side.
- **4.** Prone.

213. Mr. and Mrs. Davis have consented to surgical closure of Antoinette's defect. Prior to surgery, the defect should be

- **1.** Covered with dry sterile dressings.
- **2.** Left open to the air.
- **3.** Covered with sterile saline soaks.
- **4.** Covered with gauze impregnated with petroleum jelly.

214. Twenty-four hours before surgery, Antoinette develops a fever. She is fussy, irritable, and refuses her formula. Which nursing measure should the nurse carry out first?

- **1.** Examine the meningomyelocele sac.
- **2.** Contact Antoinette's physician.
- **3.** Place Antoinette in strict isolation.
- **4.** Ask Mrs. Davis to feed Antoinette.

215. While caring for Antoinette postoperatively, which nursing action should receive the highest priority?

- **1.** Maintain her legs in abduction.
- **2.** Measure her head circumference daily.
- **3.** Provide tactile and verbal stimulation.
- **4.** Change her position frequently.

216. Antoinette is receiving ampicillin 75 mg IV every 6 hours. When reconstituted with sterile saline, the vial contains 125 mg per 1.2 ml. The nurse should administer what amount of the solution in the drip chamber?

- **1.** 0.60 ml.
- **2.** 0.72 ml.
- **3.** 0.84 ml.
- **4.** 1.00 ml.

217. The physician has also prescribed phenytoin (Dilantin) elixir 20 mg PO BID for Antionette. The drug comes in a concentration of 30 mg per 4 ml. The nurse should administer what amount?

- **1.** 0.67 ml.
- **2.** 1.5 ml.
- **3.** 2.6 ml.
- **4.** 3.0 ml.

218. Which potential problem presents the most serious threat to Antoinette's long-term management?

- **1.** Flexion contractures of the hips.
- **2.** Frequent colds.
- **3.** Constipation.
- **4.** Recurrent urinary tract infection.

Henry Duboff, a 50-year-old white man, awakes in the middle of the night with severe dyspnea, bilateral basilar rales, and expectoration of frothy, blood-tinged sputum. He is brought to the hospital by the paramedics in congestive heart failure complicated by pulmonary edema.

219. Dyspnea is a characteristic sign of left-sided congestive heart failure. This is primarily the result of which mechanism?

- **1.** Accumulation of serous fluid in alveolar spaces.
- **2.** Obstruction of bronchi by mucoid secretions.
- **3.** Compression of lung tissue by a dilated heart.
- **4.** Restriction of respiratory movement by ascites.

220. Edema caused by right-sided congestive heart failure tends to be which of the following?

- **1.** Painful.
- **2.** Dependent.
- **3.** Periorbital.
- **4.** Nonpitting.

221. What is the optimal bed position for the client with congestive heart failure?

- **1.** Position of comfort, to relax the client.
- **2.** Semi-recumbent, to ease dyspnea and metabolic demands of the heart.
- **3.** Sims, to decrease danger of pulmonary edema.
- **4.** Dorsal recumbent, to decrease edema formation in the extremities.

222. Respirations of the client with congestive heart failure are usually of which kind?
- ○ **1.** Rapid and shallow.
- ○ **2.** Deep and stertorous.
- ○ **3.** Rapid and wheezing.
- ○ **4.** Biot's

223. How do rotating tourniquets relieve the symptoms of acute pulmonary edema?
- ○ **1.** Cause vasoconstriction.
- ○ **2.** Cause vasodilation.
- ○ **3.** Decrease the amount of circulating blood.
- ○ **4.** Increase the amount of circulating blood.

224. When tourniquets are applied to extremities to relieve the symptoms of pulmonary edema, one tourniquet should be rotated, in order, on a regular basis. How often are they rotated?
- ○ **1.** Every 5 minutes.
- ○ **2.** Every 10 minutes.
- ○ **3.** Every 15 minutes.
- ○ **4.** Every 20 minutes.

225. When Mr. Duboff is admitted to CCU, his ECG shows changes indicative of an anterior myocardial infarction. Which criteria should the nurse monitor to assess his cardiac status?
- ○ **1.** ECG changes, serum enzymes, and leg cramps.
- ○ **2.** Chest pain, ECG changes, and serum enzymes.
- ○ **3.** Chest pain, ECG changes, and serum creatinine.
- ○ **4.** ECG changes, serum electrolytes, and blood urea nitrogen.

226. Mr. Duboff continues to have ventricular dysrhythmias even though he is being treated with lidocaine (Xylocaine). His second hospital day, he goes into a cardiac arrest. Which of these responses by the nurse would be appropriate initially?
- ○ **1.** Open his airway.
- ○ **2.** Start chest compression.
- ○ **3.** Check his carotid pulse.
- ○ **4.** Put him on a hard surface.

227. Mr. Duboff has been resuscitated with success and is transferred to the medical floor 4 days postarrest. At this time, he is scheduled for a cardiac catheterization. The nurse emphasizes to him that during the procedure he will be
- ○ **1.** Heavily sedated and will not be able to move.
- ○ **2.** Under a general anesthetic and unconscious.
- ○ **3.** Awake, not sedated, and asked to remain still.
- ○ **4.** Awake, mildly sedated, and asked to change his position.

228. The information gathered from the left cardiac catheterization will include all but one of the following. Which one is *incorrect*?
- ○ **1.** Patency of the coronary arteries.
- ○ **2.** Status of collateral circulation.
- ○ **3.** Patency of the pulmonary artery.
- ○ **4.** Perfusion of the myocardium.

229. Post-cardiac catheterization, in what position will Mr. Duboff be placed?
- ○ **1.** Supine with affected leg extended.
- ○ **2.** Supine with affected leg flexed.
- ○ **3.** Side lying with both legs flexed.
- ○ **4.** Any position he desires.

Jo Ellen Baxter, a 50-year-old with a diagnosis of chronic, undifferentiated schizophrenia, is hospitalized on a surgical unit for an appendectomy.

230. The day after surgery, Mrs. Baxter tells the nurse that she feels creatures eating away at her abdomen. What is the first thing the nurse needs to do?
- ○ **1.** Request an increase in her phenothiazines to control the psychosis.
- ○ **2.** Talk with her more often to help control her stress level.
- ○ **3.** Assess for possible abdominal pains.
- ○ **4.** Request an order for benztropine (Cogentin) to control her extrapyramidal symptoms.

231. The care needs of a chronic schizophrenic client are best reflected in which of the following statements?
- ○ **1.** Have a different staff member care for her each day to avoid intimacy.
- ○ **2.** Have one staff member care for her as much as possible to increase trust.
- ○ **3.** Have one staff member care for her and remain with her the entire shift to increase intimacy and closeness.
- ○ **4.** There is no need to be concerned about the assignment, since Mrs. Baxter will not know the difference.

232. Oral antibiotics are started. Mrs. Baxter has been taking her phenothiazines at home reliably for years. Which of the following is the most appropriate nursing intervention?

- ○ **1.** Set up a plan to describe to Mrs. Baxter the cause of her problem, the effects of her body, and physiologic changes caused by her disease.
- ○ **2.** Tell her how often to take the medication and have her do it a few times while in the hospital.
- ○ **3.** Insist she not be discharged until the course of the medication has been given.
- ○ **4.** Request a home health nurse come into her home and give her the medication.

233. While you are talking to Mrs. Baxter one day, she tells you that the "creatures from Odum have just left my room." The creatures from Odum are probably which of the following?

- ○ **1.** The result of an extrapyramidal reaction.
- ○ **2.** A response to a phobic fear of being alone.
- ○ **3.** A symbol from her autistic world.
- ○ **4.** An example of flight-of-ideas.

234. Which of the following is the most appropriate nursing response to Mrs. Baxter's statement about the creatures from Odum?

- ○ **1.** Acknowledge that the creatures have special meaning for Mrs. Baxter.
- ○ **2.** Suggest a variety of interpretations of the creatures for Mrs. Baxter.
- ○ **3.** Tell Mrs. Baxter to call you the next time she sees them.
- ○ **4.** Tell her you don't like to talk about creatures.

Justine Turner, 10 years old, has had insulin-dependent diabetes mellitus (IDDM) since age 5. She is seen with her father in the diabetics clinic for a routine follow-up.

235. Which statement made by Justine to the nurse indicates that Justine has achieved developmentally appropriate self-management of her diabetes?

- ○ **1.** "My mom does my urine tests most of the time."
- ○ **2.** "I give my injections but Dad checks to be sure I do it right."
- ○ **3.** "I'm not allowed to help with my finger sticks yet."
- ○ **4.** "I decide what I want to eat and when."

236. Justine tells the nurse, "I'm on our school's soccer team now. We just started practice, and we sure do a lot of running." What changes in Justine's control of her diabetes should be expected as a result?

- ○ **1.** Decreased insulin requirements.
- ○ **2.** Increased insulin requirements.
- ○ **3.** Decreased risk of insulin shock.
- ○ **4.** Increased risk of ketoacidosis.

237. As Justine enters early adolescence, which area is most important for the nurse to prepare Justine and her family for?

- ○ **1.** A rapid gain in weight.
- ○ **2.** Changes in diet and insulin requirements.
- ○ **3.** The need to limit physical activity.
- ○ **4.** A switch to oral hypoglycemics.

238. Two weeks later, Justine is admitted to the hospital in diabetic ketoacidosis. Which manifestation should the nurse expect to observe?

- ○ **1.** Seizures, trembling.
- ○ **2.** Pallor, sweating.
- ○ **3.** Vomiting, dry mucous membranes.
- ○ **4.** Hunger, diplopia.

239. During the hospitalization, which of the following is most likely to be a major concern for Justine?

- ○ **1.** Placement in unfamiliar surroundings.
- ○ **2.** Fear of painful treatments.
- ○ **3.** Absence from school and social activities.
- ○ **4.** Worry over restricted mobility.

John Coates, 15 years old, was admitted to a psychiatric unit 2 weeks ago because his adolescence had been turbulent. His relationships with peers have been troubled. He goes to occupational therapy and becomes angry during the group activity.

240. When John returns to the unit, he says that the occupational therapists don't like him. John is probably experiencing which one of the following?

- ○ **1.** Trying to avoid OT because he is shy.
- ○ **2.** Feeling threatened by the group.
- ○ **3.** Feeling angry with a group member.
- ○ **4.** Being annoyed by the occupational therapists.

241. What is a more appropriate plan for John?
- ○ **1.** Require that he attend OT so that he will learn to adjust.
- ○ **2.** Tell him he cannot go to OT until he learns to act properly.
- ○ **3.** Put him in group therapy instead.
- ○ **4.** Have him work alone with an occupational therapist for awhile.

Eight-year-old Chad Fredricks is brought to the emergency room by his mother. He has multiple bruises over his entire body and a fractured right arm. His mother states he was playing with his wagon and fell on his right arm. The mother describes him as a "troublemaker" and a bad kid. He is not crying and refuses to speak to the nurse or his mother. The nurse thinks that Chad may be a victim of child abuse.

242. All but one of the following reasons make the nurses suspicious. Which is the one *exception*?
- ○ **1.** The multiple bruises do not fit the description of the accident.
- ○ **2.** The mother identifies him as a bad child.
- ○ **3.** Chad does not turn to his mother for solace.
- ○ **4.** Chad, by playing with a wagon, shows regression or retarded development for an 8-year-old.

243. Mrs. Fredricks is advised that Chad will need to have his arm set and placed in a cast; then he will be hospitalized for further asseessment and treatment. She is questioned about her methods of disciplining Chad. She responds angrily by saying, "Of course, I spank him. He's such a troublemaker; he does things purposely to upset me. He's so ungrateful. Sometimes I feel overwhelmed by it all, but I do not abuse him. I'm not overly violent. I hit him only when he asks for it." The nurse knows that Mrs. Fredricks is probably doing which of the following?
- ○ **1.** Lying to the hospital personnel to protect herself; she knows she's abusive.
- ○ **2.** Telling the truth and it is someone else who hits the child.
- ○ **3.** Is not aware of the fact that her behavior is abusive.
- ○ **4.** Descipling the child appropriately, since he seems to have a behavior problem.

244. The nurse realizes that the hospital has certain legal responsibilities in Chad's case. All of the following should be done *except* which one?
- ○ **1.** Document all bruises and cuts; include their placement and size.
- ○ **2.** Chart interaction patterns between Chad and his mother.
- ○ **3.** Document staff perceptions of the relationship between Chad and his mother.
- ○ **4.** Report to the state child-welfare agency.

245. The nurse needs to understand that parents who abuse their children
- ○ **1.** Frequently do not know or are unable to ask for help until after they have felt overwhelmed by problems.
- ○ **2.** Plan ahead as to when and how to abuse their children.
- ○ **3.** Rarely were abused themselves; so they do not recognize the problem until it is too late.
- ○ **4.** Usually are not concerned about their abusive actions.

246. After providing for physical care of the hospitalized abused child, the nurse needs to give priority to play activities that encourage the child to
- ○ **1.** Describe details of the traumatic events.
- ○ **2.** Maintain control over his feelings, e.g., games that are quiet or include many rules.
- ○ **3.** Be distracted from unpleasant experiences.
- ○ **4.** Share feelings of joy, anger, fear, or loneliness.

247. The nurse assigned to Chad recognizes her own negative feelings towards Mrs. Fredricks. The nurse's best action would be to
- ○ **1.** Continue to care for Chad and relate to the mother during visiting hours and not share feelings with other staff, since they might be influenced by negativism.
- ○ **2.** Be open with the mother about feelings, e.g., saying, "I can help you more if I am honest with you."
- ○ **3.** Ask other nurses to discuss the case over lunch to reduce guilt feelings about disliking the mother.
- ○ **4.** Discuss feelings with the head nurse, along with details of the care plan, asking for evaluation of the nursing care for the client and her mother, and discussing implications of reassignment to another case.

248. Interventions to assist Mrs. Fredricks best include which of the following?

- ○ **1.** Techniques to handle angry behavior before it goes out of control.
- ○ **2.** Encouragement that the problems of parents lessen as a child grows older.
- ○ **3.** Opportunities to discuss how child abuse started in the family.
- ○ **4.** Discussions on how parents can make children follow rules.

249. The nurse will know Mrs. Fredricks is responding to treatment when Mrs. Fredricks takes which of the following steps?

- ○ **1.** Decides to place Chad for adoption.
- ○ **2.** Begins to talk more realistically about Chad's mistakes.
- ○ **3.** Talks about her own frustrations and anxieties.
- ○ **4.** Realizes that her needs are secondary to Chad's.

250. Another good indicator of progress for both the child and the mother is which of the following?

- ○ **1.** Both sleep and eat well and carry out daily activities with no thoughts about past abusive behavior.
- ○ **2.** They rarely encounter frustrating conflicts.
- ○ **3.** When frustrated by Chad, Mrs. Fredricks uses 1 or 2 of the alternatives to physical punishment she has learned.
- ○ **4.** The mother has planned many separate activities for herself and Chad so they have much less time together.

Lan Yang, aged 60, undergoes a total laryngectomy for cancer of the larynx. He returns from surgery with a laryngectomy tube and an NG tube.

251. In the immediate post-op period, Mr. Yang requires both nasopharyngeal suctioning and suctioning through the larngectomy tube. Which of the following should the nurse do when performing these procedures?

- ○ **1.** Use a clean suction setup each time.
- ○ **2.** Apply constant suction.
- ○ **3.** Suction the laryngectomy tube, then the nose.
- ○ **4.** Lubricate the catheter with a petroleum jelly.

252. The nasogastric tube is used to provide Mr. Yang with fluids and nutrients for approximately 10 days for which of the following reasons?

- ○ **1.** To prevent pain while swallowing.
- ○ **2.** To prevent contamination of the suture line.
- ○ **3.** To decrease need for swallowing.
- ○ **4.** To prevent aspiration.

253. When should Mr. Yang best start speech rehabilitation?

- ○ **1.** When he leaves the hospital.
- ○ **2.** When esophageal suture line is healed.
- ○ **3.** Three months after surgery.
- ○ **4.** When he regains all his strength.

A 28-year-old neighbor, Lucia Ortega, is in the second month of pregnancy and feels fairly well. While giving a history, she talks about her job in a small animal hospital, where she is a helper to the veterinarian. She plans to continue working during the pregnancy.

254. Which of the following tasks should the nurse suggest Mrs. Ortega assign to a high school student who helps part time?

- ○ **1.** Operating a computer to prepare weekly statements.
- ○ **2.** Preparing the surgical suite for minor procedures.
- ○ **3.** Handling rabies and distemper vaccines and syringes.
- ○ **4.** Administering antibiotic ear drops to small animals.

255. Mrs. Ortega takes home a small abandoned kitten who appears to be in good condition. What teaching is most appropriate at this time?

- ○ **1.** ''Realize that the kitten may be jealous of your infant.''
- ○ **2.** ''Ask your husband if he will care for the litter box.''
- ○ **3.** ''Check to see if you and your husband have any allergies.''
- ○ **4.** ''Be sure to keep the animal indoors at all times.''

256. Several weeks later, Mrs. Ortega develops vague flulike symptoms. Which of the following statements by the client indicates she has learned what was taught at the early antepartal visits?

○ **1.** "I know I shouldn't take any over-the-counter remedies now."
○ **2.** "I feel so tired all the time; so I must need the rest."
○ **3.** "I urinate frequently, so I probably am drinking too many fluids."
○ **4.** "Between the morning sickness and the flu, I'll be happy to lose weight."

257. It is established that Mrs. Ortega's symptoms are caused by toxoplasmosis. As the pregnancy advances, the physician is concerned that fetal growth is not appropriate for gestation. Which of the following tests would best provide information about the development of the fetus?

○ **1.** Urine estriol.
○ **2.** Amniocentesis.
○ **3.** Ultrasound.
○ **4.** Nonstress test.

258. Suspicions are confirmed, and the couple is told that it appears the fetus suffers from intrauterine growth retardation. The physician spends much time with them, drawing sketches of the placenta and the fetus. As the nurse talks with them afterward, Mrs. Ortega begins to cry. "I don't think I can cope with a retarded baby." Which response is most appropriate?

○ **1.** "Perhaps you were not listening to the doctor's explanation."
○ **2.** "Are there other retarded children in either family?"
○ **3.** "There are many resources available to help you."
○ **4.** "Let's talk about what the doctor said to us all."

259. A 5-lb infant is delivered vaginally at 39 weeks. Apgar socres are 9 and 10 at 1 and 5 minutes. The newborn appears active, wide-eyed, and alert. There was slight meconium staining of the placenta and cord. What analysis is justified?

○ **1.** The baby may have suffered chronic hypoxia.
○ **2.** It appears that the baby's condition is normal.
○ **3.** Assessments indicate good adaptation.
○ **4.** This child may have been somewhat premature.

260. Although the Ortega infant appears to behave normally, it is observed that the child occasionally cries, then appears to quiet himself and fall asleep. What is the best explanation of this behavior?

○ **1.** The baby's needs have not been met.
○ **2.** This is normal, expected behavior.
○ **3.** The central nervous system may be immature.
○ **4.** The newborn is not able to deal with frustration.

261. Which of the following is most important in the discharge teaching plan for the Ortega infant?

○ **1.** Parents will keep pediatric clinic appointments.
○ **2.** Mother will feed the newborn every 2 to 3 hours.
○ **3.** Mother will weigh the child daily.
○ **4.** Father will participate in care daily.

The admission of Sam Levitt to a young-adult psychiatric unit was precipitated by his attempts to beat up his father. A history of episodic agitation and aggressive behavior for many months preceded this event.

262. The admitting nurse would best give priority attention to which one of the following areas?

○ **1.** The client's thoughts about being harmed by others.
○ **2.** His thoughts of harming other persons at a future time.
○ **3.** Thought patterns that are disconnected and unrelated.
○ **4.** Thoughts that describe false, fixed beliefs.

263. When the unit becomes especially active and noisy with visitors and newly admitted persons, Mr. Levitt is most likely to

○ **1.** Insist in a loud voice that a staff member escort him to the canteen immediately.
○ **2.** Retreat to his room for an extra nap.
○ **3.** Initiate a pool game with another client and play to win.
○ **4.** Engage a staff person in a heated discussion about patient-government activities.

264. A priority nursing goal for Mr. Levitt on admission is to assist him to
- ○ **1.** Discuss childhood situations in which he lashed out at persons in order to increase his self-understanding.
- ○ **2.** Participate in a variety of physical activities in order to dissipate his destructive feelings.
- ○ **3.** Talk at length about his deep-seated anger in order to reduce the chance he will strike out again.
- ○ **4.** Make plans to reapply for admission to the community college he had attended.

265. Mr. Levitt was found pacing, striking his fists in the air, and cursing another client named Mrs. Sanders. The nurse would best say
- ○ **1.** "Mr. Levitt, stop cursing at Mrs. Sanders. I will stay and help you control yourself."
- ○ **2.** "You must feel very angry. Maybe you should calm down."
- ○ **3.** "Mr. Levitt, Mrs. Sanders did nothing to upset you; so please stop threatening her."
- ○ **4.** "Mr. Levitt, calm down. You can get rid of all this energy in the gym this afternoon. Come and eat breakfast now."

266. When Mr. Levitt's father escorts his son to the unit following the son's first weekend pass from the inpatient setting, the nurse speaks to them together. The nurse's most important focus is
- ○ **1.** How both the father and son felt about the weekend.
- ○ **2.** What activities they did that were satisfying to both.
- ○ **3.** How frequently, if at all, Mr. Levitt lost control.
- ○ **4.** What events occurred that indicated progress in Mr. Levitt's ability to refrain from threatening behavior.

267. A long-term indicator of Mr. Levitt's progress will be his
- ○ **1.** Ability to move from verbal to physical activities when he senses increased anger.
- ○ **2.** Deliberate actions to engage in several community activities separate from his family.
- ○ **3.** Assuming responsibility to be punctual for all therapy sessions.
- ○ **4.** Willingness to admit that he has a bad temper and that he must do something about it.

When Edward Barden, a 37-year-old construction worker, is admitted to the nursing unit, he tells you that he has pain radiating down his right leg.

268. Which of the following is *not* appropriate to include in the assessment?
- ○ **1.** Activities that occur prior to the pain.
- ○ **2.** What relieves the pain.
- ○ **3.** How he carries out activities of daily living.
- ○ **4.** How he got to the hospital.

269. Mr. Braden is scheduled for a myelogram. Which of the following nursing care considerations is best included in the postprocedure care?
- ○ **1.** Keep the client in bed for 6–8 hours.
- ○ **2.** Allow the client to go to the bathroom as soon as he gets back to his room in order to excrete the dye.
- ○ **3.** Limit fluids.
- ○ **4.** Provide heavy sedation for his spinal headache.

270. The myelogram indicates that Mr. Barden has a ruptured intervertebral disk at L4-5 and is scheduled for a laminectomy. What does the nurse include in the pre-op teaching?
- ○ **1.** Post-op "log-rolling."
- ○ **2.** Getting out of bed the third post-op day.
- ○ **3.** Activities to be avoided after discharge.
- ○ **4.** Use of a turning frame.

271. In the immediate post-op period, Mr. Barden complains of a severe headache, numbness and tingling in his feet. What is the nurse's first action?
- ○ **1.** Notify the physician at once.
- ○ **2.** Medicate him for the discomfort.
- ○ **3.** Explain that this is normal.
- ○ **4.** Compare this numbness and tingling with his pre-op neurologic assessment data.

Mrs. Jan Tiplady is seen in the obstetric clinic to confirm a suspected pregnancy. Her history reveals that she has 2 children at home, both born at 40 weeks of gestation. She delivered a stillborn at 36 weeks.

272. Which of the following is a correct determination of Mrs. Tiplady's obstetric statistics?
- ○ **1.** T3, P0, A0, L2.
- ○ **2.** T2, P1, A0, L2.
- ○ **3.** T2, P0, A1, L2.
- ○ **4.** T3, P0, A1, L2.

273. Upon assessment, these signs and symptoms are found to be present in Mrs. Tiplady. Which of the following is a correctly identified sign of pregnancy?

- ○ **1.** Amenorrhea: probable.
- ○ **2.** Chadwick's sign: probable.
- ○ **3.** Urine human chorionic gonadotropin (HCG): positive.
- ○ **4.** Nausea and vomiting: presumptive.

274. Blood is drawn on Mrs. Tiplady for hemoglobin and hematocrit. The results are compared with the CBC done 6 months prior to conception. Because of the normal physiologic changes occurring during pregnancy, the nurse can expect to find

- ○ **1.** An increase in the hematocrit.
- ○ **2.** A decrease in the hematocrit.
- ○ **3.** An increase in the hemoglobin to meet the requirements of the fetus.
- ○ **4.** No change in the blood levels since the body will maintain homeostasis.

275. At a clinic visit in the tenth week, Mrs. Tiplady relates to the nurse that her pregnancy was planned. However, she finds herself questioning whether this was realistic, with 2 preschoolers at home. Which of the following responses by the nurse is most appropriate?

- ○ **1.** "Perhaps you should explore the possibility of terminating the pregnancy."
- ○ **2.** "It's normal to feel ambivalent. Let's talk about it."
- ○ **3.** "Once you feel the life within you, these feelings will subside."
- ○ **4.** "I can arrange an appointment for counseling if you wish."

276. Mrs. Tiplady reveals that she had experienced bladder infections with her past pregnancies. The nurse explains to the client that

- ○ **1.** Many women have a hereditary predisposition to bladder infection in pregnancy.
- ○ **2.** Pregnancy predisposes a woman to bladder infections because of dilatation of the ureters and decreased bladder tone.
- ○ **3.** Although bladder infections occur frequently in pregnancy, they are of little consequence.
- ○ **4.** Clients are generally placed on prophylactic antibiotics when such a history exists.

277. The nurse provides nutritional counseling for Mrs. Tiplady. Since the client does not like to drink milk, which of the following would best meet her need for calcium?

- ○ **1.** Nuts, sardines.
- ○ **2.** Yogurt, cheese.
- ○ **3.** Meat, leafy vegetables.
- ○ **4.** Custard, dried fruits.

278. In the 16th week, Mrs. Tiplady phones the clinic to report symptoms of frequency and burning on urination. Which of the following statements indicates she learned from the early discussion of bladder infection?

- ○ **1.** "I realize the frequency is due to pressure of the uterus on the bladder."
- ○ **2.** "I have noticed mild symptoms for the last 10 days."
- ○ **3.** "I called immediately. I understand this can be serious."
- ○ **4.** "I refilled my prescription for antibiotics from last year."

Carla Davis comes to the emergency room by herself and tells the admitting nurse that she has been raped.

279. Which of the following is the first action the nurse would take?

- ○ **1.** Determine Miss Davis's most immediate concern and needs.
- ○ **2.** Encourage Miss Davis to report the rape to the police.
- ○ **3.** Identify Miss Davis's support network and contact them.
- ○ **4.** Perform a vaginal examination.

280. Miss Davis tearfully tells the nurse, "It's all my fault. I should never have gone shopping this evening and it wouldn't have happened." The most appropriate response is

- ○ **1.** "Do you usually go shopping alone in the evening?"
- ○ **2.** "It is understandable that you feel very upset now; as time goes on you'll feel less uncomfortable about going out alone."
- ○ **3.** "It would be better to take someone with you in this neighborhood."
- ○ **4.** "You did not cause this to happen; the person who raped you is responsible."

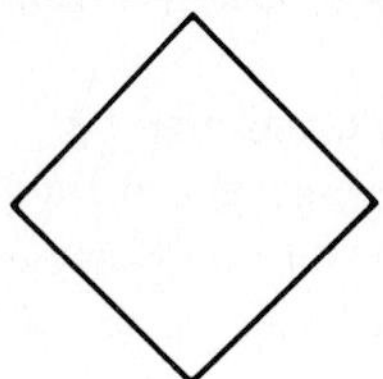

Correct Answers and Rationales: Part Three

188. #4. Nitrogenous waste products from protein metabolism result in an elevation of BUN; therefore, a low protein diet is needed. The protein given should be of high biologic value (i.e., contain all essential amino acids). A high carbohydrate diet will help reverse gluconeogenesis. The client should be weighed daily. Intake is calculated on urine output plus 500–1,000 ml of insensible water loss every 24 hours. Her potassium is already elevated; therefore, the diet should be restrictive of potassium and may even require the administration of ion-exchange resins such as Kayexalate. ELIMINATION/ADULT

189. #1. Anemia occurs in chronic renal disease because renal erythropoietin production is decreased and the bone marrow is depressed by the increasing uremia. Because of the decreased ability of the kidneys to excrete waste products and maintain normal fluid and electrolyte balance, hyperkalemia and hypertension develop. The stimulation of the renin-angiotension mechanism also contributes to the hypertension. The skin becomes very dry because the sweat glands atrophy. ELIMINATION/ADULT

190. #3. Milk, meats, fish, and eggs are considered the best sources of high biologic-value protein. Some vegetables have all of the essential amino acids but are not consistently the best sources. In contrast, fruits are poor sources of high biologic-value protein. ELIMINATION/ ADULT

191. #3. An AV fistula is an *internal* access created by a side-to-side or end-to-end anastomosis of an adjacent vein and artery. This results in an enlarged vein because of the high pressure in the artery. The resulting vessel provides an easy access for venipuncture. Thrombosis at this site can be a major complication. Rejection does not occur, because no foreign material is involved. Dislodgment is not a problem, because the fistula is internal. (An AV *shunt* is external.) Cardiac irritation is a problem with subclavian catheters used for temporary access for hemodialysis. ELIMINATION/ADULT

192. #4. The presence of a bruit and a thrill indicates good circulation. Skin temperatures and pulses should be assessed *distal* to the fistula. Blood pressure and venipunctures should never be done in the affected limb in order to help promote the longevity of the fistula. Since an AV fistula is *internal*, it is not possible to assess the color of the blood. ELIMINATION/ADULT

193. #2. Any fluid retention greater than 300 ml needs to be assessed prior to continuing with dialysis. Turning the client from side to side may help drain the remaining dialysate thereby eliminating the need for contacting the physician. Vital signs must be monitored at frequent intervals throughout the dialysis. ELIMINATION/ADULT

194. #2. Disequilibrium syndrome is believed by some to be caused by too rapid or excess fluid removal from the circulatory system. Dialysis for a short time (2 to 4 hours) and at a reduced rate of blood flow is effective in decreasing occurrence and severity. ELIMINATION/ ADULT

195. #1. The most common recurring problem with peritoneal dialysis is peritonitis; therefore, education on proper techniques to help decrease its occurrence should take priority. All the other listed interventions are also important and should be included in the teaching. ELIMINATION/ADULT

196. #4. The main defense against transplant rejection is immunosuppressive drugs (e.g., azathioprine [Imuran], prednisone). This therapy is begun prior to surgery and continues following surgery. It is important for the client not to discontinue this drug therapy unless instructed to do so by a physician, and then the reduction is done slowly over an extended period of time. Immunosuppressive drugs increase the patient's susceptibility to infection. ELIMINATION/ADULT

197. **#2.** This is a period of maximum cardiac output, and as a result, cardiac decompensation may occur. The other potential problems are not necessarily associated with cardiac disease. ANTEPARTAL CARE/CHILDBEARING FAMILY

198. **#4.** Magnesium sulfate is a central nervous system depressant. The client must be closely observed for profound symptoms such as diminished respiratory rate. Muscle cramps indicate toxic effects of the drug; hyperstimulation of reflexes may indicate impending seizure. Anuria is sometimes observed in such a patient. ANTEPARTAL CARE/CHILDBEARING FAMILY

199. **#1.** The most needed time for the husband's presence is during transition. The other options show a lack of understanding of the client's needs during labor. INTRAPARTAL CARE/ CHILDBEARING FAMILY

200. **#3.** Cold stress increases metabolic efforts; respiratory distress can result. Cyanosis is a late change. A newborn does not shiver to maintain body temperature. NEWBORN CARE/ CHILDBEARING FAMILY

201. **#2.** All are important assessments of respiratory function, but only breathing movements are part of the Silverman-Andersen scale. HIGH-RISK NEWBORN/ CHILDBEARING FAMILY

202. **#2.** Cephalhematoma is an effusion of blood between the bone and the periosteum. This problem resolves shortly after birth. Intracranial hemorrhage is a life-threatening occurrence. Hydrocephalus requires close monitoring and intervention. NEWBORN CARE/ CHILDBEARING FAMILY

203. **#3.** Talking to the infant in the first 24 hours is part of early bonding. Since this is the first day, she may need more time to get acquainted with the newborn. It is normal to feel discouraged with initial feeding; this is not likely to indicate attachment problems. POSTPARTAL CARE/CHILDBEARING FAMILY

204. **#1.** Fatigue and hormone changes cause this behavior. If the behavior is prolonged beyond 6 weeks, there may be a serious psychologic problem. The client is in the "taking hold" phase of adaptation. POSTPARTAL CARE/ CHILDBEARING FAMILY

205. **#1.** Mastitis can occur 2 to 3 weeks after delivery as organisms enter through a traumatized nipple; thus, nursing periods should be limited and breasts alternated. In early breast-feeding, supplemental feedings should be infrequent. The nursing mother should not attempt weight reduction. POSTPARTAL CARE/CHILDBEARING FAMILY

206. **#3.** When a person is in the manic phase of bipolar disorder he tends to disregard physical needs and he needs clear, concise, firm, and explicit directions to meet these needs. Option #1 evades the issue of taking care of his physical needs. Option #2 is too passive and left on his own, he won't come. Option #3 is too premature and punitive. ELATED-DEPRESSIVE BEHAVIOR/PSYCHOSOCIAL, MENTAL HEALTH, PSYCHIATRIC PROBLEMS

207. **#3.** Manipulative and/or demanding behavior of the manic client is most effectively controlled by limit setting that is clearly spelled out to him, is fair, and is consistently enforced. Leeway when limits are violated may only increase pathologic behavior. Since his behavior often provokes staff anger, staff-client arguments and rejection of the client are common. This reaffirms the client's feelings of rejection. It is important to note that only frequent staff conferences and staff planning can provide a therapeutic plan of care and the support for staff, which is essential if they are to give the needed care. ELATED-DEPRESSIVE BEHAVIOR/PSYCHOSOCIAL, MENTAL HEALTH, PSYCHIATRIC PROBLEMS

208. **#4.** A manic client will often disregard the basic needs of eating, sleeping, bowel/bladder control, etc., so nurses need to carefully monitor all physical needs. Options #1, #2, and #3 generally are not true during the acute phase of mania. ELATED-DEPRESSIVE BEHAVIOR/PSYCHOSOCIAL, MENTAL HEALTH, PSYCHIATRIC PROBLEMS

209. **#2.** Lithium toxicity is closely related to serum lithium levels and can occur at doses close to therapeutic levels. Adverse reactions are seldom encountered at levels below maximum therapeutic levels, except in clients sensitive to lithium. ELATED-DEPRESSIVE BEHAVIOR/ PSYCHOSOCIAL, MENTAL HEALTH, PSYCHIATRIC PROBLEMS

210. #4. Options #1 through #3 are clinical signs of toxicity that must be detected and reported to the physician immediately. ELATED-DEPRESSIVE BEHAVIOR/PSYCHOSOCIAL, MENTAL HEALTH, PSYCHIATRIC PROBLEMS

211. #4. This would stimulate the client, not sedate him. Activities that decrease stimuli may help counteract insomnia. Rest and sleep are vital for the manic client, because hyperactivity may lead to dangerous exhaustion. ELATED-DEPRESSIVE BEHAVIOR/PSYCHOSOCIAL, MENTAL HEALTH, PSYCHIATRIC PROBLEMS

212. #4. Antoinette must be kept in the prone position to reduce tension on and prevent trauma to the sac. The spine and semi-Fowler's position would place tension on the sac. The side-lying position is difficult to maintain in a newborn. SENSATION, PERCEPTION, PROTECTION/CHILD

213. #3. Before surgical closure of the sac, it is important to prevent drying of the sac so the fragile tissue does not tear and allow cerebrospinal fluid to leak, increasing the risk of meningitis. Sterile saline soaks help to prevent drying. Dry sterile dressings or leaving the sac open to the air is advocated only if surgery is to be delayed. Petroleum jelly gauze is contraindicated in either case. SENSATION, PERCEPTION, PROTECTION/CHILD

214. #1. An elevated temperature accompanied by behavioral changes may be an early sign of infection. Any leak, abrasion, or tear of the meningomyelocele sac would further support the possibility of infection (e.g., meningitis). Assess the sac before notifying the physician. Isolation precautions should be instituted to protect the other babies and would be appropriate once the sac has been assessed. While Mrs. Davis might help calm Antoinette, it is not appropriate until the nursing assessment is complete. SENSATION, PERCEPTION, PROTECTION/CHILD

215. #2. While all these nursing actions would be appropriate, measuring head circumference daily is essential. Hydrocephalus is a common complication of meningomyelocele. The primary sign of hydrocephalus in infants is head enlargement. Any change in the size of the infant's head can be assessed with daily measurements. SENSATION, PERCEPTION, PROTECTION/CHILD

216. #2. The equation should be set up with 125 mg per 1.2 ml = 75 mg per X ml. Thus, 125X = 1.2 multiplied by 75, which becomes 125X = 90.90 divided by 125 = 0.72. Therefore, the nurse should administer 0.72 ml as the correct dose. ILL AND HOSPITALIZED CHILD/CHILD

217. #3. The equation is set up with 30 mg per 4 ml = 20 mg per X ml. Thus, 30X = 20 multiplied by 4, which becomes 30X = 80. 80 divided by 30 = 2.6. Therefore, the nurse should administer 2.6 ml as the correct dose. ILL AND HOSPITALIZED CHILD/CHILD

218. #4. Renal problems present a major threat to the life of the child with spina bifida as well as to her self-image and willingness to become involved with activities and individuals outside the home. The other areas may become problematic but are generally not life threatening. SENSATION, PERCEPTION, PROTECTION/CHILD

219. #1. Left-sided congestive heart failure causes pulmonary circulatory congestion, which reduces the diffusion of O_2 and CO_2 across the alveolar membrane. The resultant hypoxia causes dyspnea. Options #2, #3, and #4 may be present with congestive heart failure, but they are not the primary cause of the dyspnea. OXYGENATION/ADULT

220. #2. Because of gravity, dependent edema occurs in right-sided congestive heart failure. Cardiac failure edema is also painless and pitting. It does not involve the face. OXYGENATION/ADULT

221. #2. The client with congestive heart failure can breathe with more ease in a Fowler's or semi-Fowler's position. Maximal lung expansion is permitted, because there is full expansion of the rib cage and there is less upward pressure from the abdominal organs on the diaphragm. OXYGENATION/ADULT

222. #1. Respirations in congestive heart failure are rapid and shallow because of the pulmonary circulatory congestion. Deep, stertorous, wheezing, or Biot's respirations are not characteristic of congestive heart failure. OXYGENATION/ADULT

223. #3. Rotating tourniquets used in pulmonary edema decreases (not increases) venous return to the right side of the heart. The reduced blood volume decreases the pulmonary circulatory congestion and pulmonary edema. Rotating tourniquets produce neither vasoconstriction nor vasodilation. OXYGENATION/ADULT

224. **#3.** Rotation every 15 minutes ensures that the venous return of a single extremity is occluded for no more than 45 minutes. Shorter or longer periods of venous occlusion are not recommended. OXYGENATION/ADULT

225. **#2.** Chest pain, ECG changes, and serum enzymes best indicate the status of a post-myocardial infarction client. All will show definite changes as the infarction process evolves. Leg cramps and changes in serum electrolytes, serum creatinine, and blood urea nitrogen are not indicators of cardiac status following an infarction. OXYGENATION/ADULT

226. **#1.** The first step in a cardiac arrest is to ensure the client has an open airway. The second priority is to establish breathing. The third priority is to establish cardiac function. OXYGENATION/ADULT

227. **#4.** During a cardiac catheterization, the client may be asked to make verbal responses, change position, and cough and deep breathe. In order to do this, the client will be only mildly sedated. OXYGENATION/ADULT

228. **#3.** A left-sided cardiac catheterization will show coronary artery patency and perfusion of the myocardium. A left-sided cardiac catheterization will not demonstrate any pathologic condition in the right side of the heart or the pulmonary artery. OXYGENATION/ADULT

229. **#1.** During the left-sided cardiac catheterization, the catheter is introduced into the femoral artery of the leg. Postcatheterization, the client is cautioned to keep the affected leg extended (not flexed) to avoid any increase in pressure at the puncture site. OXYGENATION/ADULT

230. **#3.** Chronic schizophrenics will sometimes incorporate pain into their delusional system. Option #1 may be needed but only after assessment of the behavior is completed. Although talking is important, the abdominal pains take priority. The symptom described is not an extrapyramidal reaction. WITHDRAWN BEHAVIOR/PSYCHOSOCIAL, MENTAL HEALTH, PSYCHIATRIC PROBLEMS

231. **#2.** Sameness will increase trust in Mrs. Baxter, but intimacy will frighten her and cause her to withdraw more into herself. A wide variety of caretakers will only increase confusion and reduce trust. Option #3 has advantages but may be overpowering to this client. WITHDRAWN BEHAVIOR/PSYCHOSOCIAL, MENTAL HEALTH, PSYCHIATRIC PROBLEMS

232. **#2.** Lengthy explanations will be too confusing. Rather tell her how to take the drugs and show her, and she will probably be as reliable with them as she has been with phenothiazines. It is better to return the client to her usual environment than hold her in the hospital for the needs described. Reliable self-administration is better than forced dependency. WITHDRAWN BEHAVIOR/PSYCHOSOCIAL, MENTAL HEALTH, PSYCHIATRIC PROBLEMS

233. **#3.** The creatures are part of her hallucinatory world into which she withdraws at times. Hallucinations as described are not usually associated with extrapyramidal reactions, nor is hallucinatory activity viewed as phobic or as flight-of-ideas. WITHDRAWN BEHAVIOR/PSYCHOSOCIAL, MENTAL HEALTH, PSYCHIATRIC PROBLEMS

234. **#1.** This statement acknowledges the importance of the hallucination for Mrs. Baxter without undermining her need for the symptom; it also does not indicate that the nurse regards the hallucination content as real. Interpretation is not usually a part of nursing practice. Option #3 supports her hallucination. Option #4 is not sensitive to the client's needs. WITHDRAWN BEHAVIOR/PSYCHOSOCIAL, MENTAL HEALTH, PSYCHIATRIC PROBLEMS

235. **#2.** The 10-year-old should be involved in all aspects of managing her diabetes, but still requires supervision and support by an adult. Options #1 and #3 indicate overinvolvement of the parents, while option #4 indicates the parents are not providing adequate supervision. A 10-year-old is not yet capable of full self-management. ILL AND HOSPITALIZED CHILD/CHILD

236. **#1.** Exercise reduces insulin requirements since glucose can be utilized without insulin during periods of muscular activity. There is an increased risk of insulin shock if nutrition is not modified to reflect changes in caloric requirements during exercise. The risk of hyperglycemia is lowered as a result of exercise. NUTRITION AND METABOLISM/ CHILD

237. **#2.** The effect of changes in puberty on dietary and insulin management should be anticipated and discussed with the pre-adolescent and her family. Rapid weight gain is unexpected in adolescents with IDDM, and they cannot be maintained on oral hypoglycemics at any point in their lives. Physical activity should be encouraged. NUTRITION AND METABOLISM/CHILD

238. **#3.** Ketoacidosis is manifested by nausea, vomiting, acetone breath, flushing, dry skin and mucous membranes, and dehydration. The other manifestations are commonly seen with hypoglycemia. NUTRITION AND METABOLISM/ADULT

239. **#3.** The school-age child is developmentally concerned with a sense of industry, which is accomplished through peer interactions and school activities. Fear of painful procedures characterizes preschoolers. The school-age child has little difficulty adjusting to new environments. Justine's activity should not be restricted; therefore, restricted mobility will not be a concern. ILL AND HOSPITALIZED CHILD/CHILD

240. **#2.** He is probably indicating his discomfort with the group. Perhaps projection is the main defense mechanism used in this situation. There is no evidence that John is shy nor that he is angry with any one group member; likewise there is no evidence that the therapists annoy him. THERAPEUTIC USE OF SELF/ PSYCHOSOCIAL, MENTAL HEALTH, PSYCHIATRIC PROBLEMS

241. **#4.** He will have the benefit of OT without feeling threatened by the group. Requiring attendance may be useful in the future, but interpersonal group skills are best learned gradually. Withholding the OT experience will not facilitate his learning. Group therapy is an entirely different experience than OT. THERAPEUTIC USE OF SELF/ PSYCHOSOCIAL, MENTAL HEALTH, PSYCHIATRIC PROBLEMS

242. **#4.** While a symptom of child abuse is that the child exhibits behavior not appropriate to age, playing with a wagon is appropriate for an 8-year-old. Options #1, #2, and #3 are classic behaviors found in abusive relationships. SOCIALLY MALADAPTIVE BEHAVIOR/ PSYCHOSOCIAL, MENTAL HEALTH, PSYCHIATRIC PROBLEMS

243. **#3.** Some abusive parents do not see their behavior as inappropriate. They may have been abused as children and so raise their children as they were raised. None of the behaviors in #1, #2, and #4 are characteristics of abusive parents' actions. SOCIALLY MALADAPTIVE BEHAVIOR/PSYCHOSOCIAL, MENTAL HEALTH, PSYCHIATRIC PROBLEMS

244. **#3.** The nurse documents behaviors and factual information, which may become evidence. Ideas about what might have happened are not the hospital staff's responsibility to report. Accurate documentation and reporting is required and in the best interest of parent and child. SOCIALLY MALADAPTIVE BEHAVIOR/ PSYCHOSOCIAL, MENTAL HEALTH, PSYCHIATRIC PROBLEMS

245. **#1.** Complex, lifelong dynamics of being abused or unable to handle frustration leave the parent overwhelmed by problems. The parent loses control and the ability to change the behavior. Abuse is usually impulsive, not planned. Abusers are frequently the abused of past years. Usually the parent is concerned about actions but out of control. SOCIALLY MALADAPTIVE BEHAVIOR/ PSYCHOSOCIAL, MENTAL HEALTH, PSYCHIATRIC PROBLEMS

246. **#4.** Recovery for the abused child can be facilitated by the freedom to express emotion in a caring, safe environment. Although sharing details and gaining emotional control are important to the healing process, the expression of emotion is a priority if therapeutic interventions are to be successful. SOCIALLY MALADAPTIVE BEHAVIOR/ PSYCHOSOCIAL, MENTAL HEALTH, PSYCHIATRIC PROBLEMS

247. #4. Negative feelings toward abusing parents are not uncommon, and the nurse can handle them professionally by discussing them with the head nurse. Carrying burdens alone does not promote mental health, but the mother should not be burdened with rejection. Staff discussions might be helpful but violation of professional confidentiality is possible. SOCIALLY MALADAPTIVE BEHAVIOR/ PSYCHOSOCIAL, MENTAL HEALTH, PSYCHIATRIC PROBLEMS

248. #1. Effective control of anger is important in order to reduce abuse. Problems of child raising tend to increase with the child's age, the complexity of child abuse does not allow for finding a starting point, and focusing on making children follow rules usually reflects negative feelings rather than fosters a positive environment. SOCIALLY MALADAPTIVE BEHAVIOR/PSYCHOSOCIAL, MENTAL HEALTH, PSYCHIATRIC PROBLEMS

249. #3. In discussing her own feelings, Mrs. Fredricks can learn how to control stress more effectively. Options #1, #2, and #4 are inappropriate because they focus on Chad rather than herself and the interaction. SOCIALLY MALADAPTIVE BEHAVIOR/ PSYCHOSOCIAL, MENTAL HEALTH, PSYCHIATRIC PROBLEMS

250. #3. This indicates learning alternatives to anger and harmful punishment, which are significant aspects of nursing interventions for the abusive parent. #1 does not indicate changes in behavior patterns when frustrated or angry. #2 is a positive change, but, again, does not indicate constructive coping during frustration. #3 indicates avoidance rather than successful coping. SOCIALLY MALADAPTIVE BEHAVIOR/ PSYCHOSOCIAL, MENTAL HEALTH, PSYCHIATRIC PROBLEMS

251. #3. The laryngectomy tube enters directly into the trachea; it should be suctioned first with sterile equipment. Sterile technique is used to prevent lower airway infections by the introduction of bacteria into the trachea. The nose requires clean technique and can be suctioned with the same catheter after the trachea is suctioned. Intermittent, not constant, suction is used. Only a sterile water-soluble lubricant is used for the catheter. Oil-based lubricants, such as petroleum jelly, can cause pneumonia if aspirated into the lower airway. OXYGENATION/ADULT

252. #2. The NG tube is used primarily to prevent food and fluid from contaminating the pharyngeal and esophageal suture line during healing. Swallowing may also be reduced, but it is not the primary reason for the use of the NG tube. OXYGENATION/ADULT

253. #2. Speech rehabilitation can be started as soon as the esophageal suture line has healed. Time of healing is determined on an individual basis. OXYGENATION/ADULT

254. #3. This is a task that poses potential danger to a pregnant woman in the first trimester. There would appear to be no risks with the other tasks. ANTEPARTAL CARE/ CHILDBEARING FAMILY

255. #2. There is danger in handling cat litter, so this is an essential aspect of teaching. ANTEPARTAL CARE/CHILDBEARING FAMILY

256. #1. This response indicates she has learned *essential* content of antepartal teaching. Rest is always important; but first trimester fatigue is related to hormone changes. The pregnant woman should drink 6 to 8 glasses of fluids daily. Weight should be maintained in early pregnancy to provide for fetal growth. ANTEPARTAL CARE/CHILDBEARING FAMILY

257. #3. An ultrasound examination would provide information on the fetal development. Estriol and nonstress tests indicate placental-fetal well-being, while the aminocentesis may provide a variety of information from genetic information to extent of lung development. ANTEPARTAL CARE/CHILDBEARING FAMILY

258. #4. This best meets the couple's needs. Apparently they have misunderstood the physician's explanation. Time to discuss feelings should be provided. ANTEPARTAL CARE/CHILDBEARING FAMILY

259. #1. The signs indicate hypoxia. While the Apgar score is normal, the deprivation of nutrients and oxygen in utero causes retarded intrauterine growth. NEWBORN CARE/ CHILDBEARING FAMILY

260. #2. The newborn has the ability to calm itself and go into a quiet sleep state. NEWBORN CARE/CHILDBEARING FAMILY

261. #1. Since the baby was exposed to infection and deprived of nutrients and oxygen during pregnancy, it is essential to monitor health and growth throughout infancy and childhood. Feeding frequently may depend on volume ingested. A weekly assessment of weight gain is sufficient. NEWBORN CARE/ CHILDBEARING FAMILY

262. #2. The nurse would give priority to collecting data relevant to the known past history. The safety of others takes precedence over thought disorders described in options #3 and #4. Client's fears of being harmed can be worked with at a later time. SOCIALLY MALADAPTIVE BEHAVIOR/ PSYCHOSOCIAL, MENTAL HEALTH, PSYCHIATRIC PROBLEMS.

263. #1. The high-activity milieu may precipitate a sense of losing control in angry clients. Likewise, they rarely can give to others, or sustain interaction. Seeking self-centered attention from staff might be viewed as a plea for help. It is the most likely action of this client under the circumstances. The desire for extra sleep is unlikely, as is initiation of interaction in a game requiring competition and concentration. It is also unlikely that he would be concerned with the world outside himself. SOCIALLY MALADAPTIVE BEHAVIOR/ PSYCHOSOCIAL, MENTAL HEALTH, PSYCHIATRIC PROBLEMS

264. #2. Only after anger is constructively released can the client focus on specific feelings and self-understanding. Future plans, although important, cannot be realistically developed until anger is reduced. Retrospective understanding requires that present feelings be relieved *first*. SOCIALLY MALADAPTIVE BEHAVIOR/PSYCHOSOCIAL, MENTAL HEALTH, PSYCHIATRIC PROBLEMS

265. #1. To disrupt angry outbursts, get the client's attention by using his name. Give firm, simple directions. Stay with client in order to help him gain internal control. Options #2, #3, and #4 are examples of weakly stated interventions that delay action or do not provide structure. SOCIALLY MALADAPTIVE BEHAVIOR/ PSYCHOSOCIAL, MENTAL HEALTH, PSYCHIATRIC PROBLEMS

266. #4. It is important to learn about situations that the potentially violent person has handled well. This information can disclose strengths and give the nurse a chance to give positive reinforcement and assess the effects of hospitalization. The feelings in options #1 and #2 are of secondary importance to control of violent behavior. Option #3 does not focus exclusively on negative behavior. SOCIALLY MALADAPTIVE BEHAVIOR/ PSYCHOSOCIAL, MENTAL HEALTH, PSYCHIATRIC PROBLEMS

267. #2. The ability to extend relationships beyond the family indicates developing security and independence. It also dilutes the intense family situations that often precipitate violence. Although the behaviors in options #1, #3, and #4 are positive, they do not suggest as high a level of significant behavioral change. SOCIALLY MALADAPTIVE BEHAVIOR/ PSYCHOSOCIAL, MENTAL HEALTH, PSYCHIATRIC PROBLEMS

268. #4. The mode of transportation to the hospital is not significant as part of your initial assessment. The other assessments listed are pertinent to the client's admitting complaint. ACTIVITY AND REST/ADULT

269. #1. Bedrest is necessary for 6 to 8 hours to prevent a spinal headache. Although the client may need to void, he cannot get out of bed. Fluids are to be encouraged for rehydration and replacement of cerebrospinal fluid and to minimize postlumbar puncture headache. Only mild sedation is required for a spinal headache. If an oil-based dye was used, the head of the bed is elevated postprocedure to prevent the dye from coming into contact with the meninges and causing irritation. If a water-based dye was used, the bed may be kept flat. ACTIVITY AND REST/ADULT

270. #1. Postoperatively, the patient is turned as a unit, i.e., logrolled. A turning frame is used if the patient has a fusion. The patient will be out of bed on the first or second post-op day. Activities to be avoided after discharge would be included in discharge instructions. ACTIVITY AND REST/ADULT

271. **#4.** Post-op numbness and tingling should be compared to the patient's pre-op neurologic assessment data. If the patient had no numbness and tingling preoperatively, or if it is more severe, the nurse notifies the physician. Sensory manifestations may be due to inflammatory changes and will be temporary. However, they always must be assessed. ACTIVITY AND REST/ADULT

272. **#2.** This item requires correct identification of terms used in a TPAL chart; analysis of data in the history leads to the only correct response. T = term births (2 pregnancies carried to 40 weeks gestation); P = premature births (the stillborn delivered at 36 weeks gestation is considered a premature birth); A = abortion history (the client has no history of abortions, since all pregnancies extended beyond 20 weeks); L = number of living children (2 living children). ANTEPARTAL CARE/ CHILDBEARING FAMILY

273. **#4.** Morning sickness is correctly classified as a "presumptive sign." Amenorrhea and Chadwick's sign are also presumptive signs of pregnancy. Urine positive for HCG is a probable sign of pregnancy (95%–98% accuracy). ANTEPARTAL CARE/ CHILDBEARING FAMILY

274. **#2.** There is an increase in both plasma and cells during pregnancy. However, the increase in plasma is greater than the increase in red blood cells. This results in a hemodilution of blood causing a fall in the hematocrit. This is referred to as the normal physiologic anemia of pregnancy. ANTEPARTAL CARE/ CHILDBEARING FAMILY

275. **#2.** Ambivalence is a normal psychologic reaction during the first trimester. In communicating therapeutically, it is important to relate to the client that such feelings are frequently experienced. The nurse should allow the client to ventilate her feelings in regard to this. The other options do not encourage the client to share feelings; rather they immediately suggest an alternative or focus on long-term changes. ANTEPARTAL CARE/ CHILDBEARING FAMILY

276. **#2.** Increasing progesterone levels during pregnancy result in smooth muscle relaxation leading to dilatation of the ureters, especially the right, and decreased bladder tone. Urinary stasis is thus created, contributing to bladder infections. Bladder infection during pregnancy can lead to serious complication for both mother and fetus. If an infection occurs, antibiotics may be prescribed. However, use of such medication as a preventive is never suggested because of the teratogenic potential. ANTEPARTAL CARE/CHILDBEARING FAMILY

277. **#2.** Cheese and yogurt are both good substitutes for milk. Other sources of calcium include some fish, including sardines, ice cream, and dried beans. While leafy vegetables and grains contain calcium, recent research indicates that it is poorly absorbed. ANTEPARTAL CARE/CHILDBEARING FAMILY

278. **#3.** This reflects an understanding of potential risks. While bladder pressure causes frequency in the first and third trimesters, burning is never expected. Since the remaining options indicate delayed or self-treatment, they are incorrect. ANTEPARTAL CARE/ CHILDBEARING FAMILY

279. **#1.** This is a nonjudgmental, empathetic intervention. It allows the client to begin to reestablish a sense of control that was lost when she was raped. #2 presents the nurse's viewpoint and can impede the client's independent decision-making. #3 and #4 are important but should be done when client is ready. SOCIALLY MALADAPTIVE BEHAVIOR/PSYCHOSOCIAL, MENTAL HEALTH, PSYCHIATRIC PROBLEMS

280. **#4.** Reinforce the responsibility of the rapist, not the victim. Recognize that victims feel guilt, but do not reinforce those guilt feelings. #1 does not acknowledge the client's feelings and may be interpreted by client as reinforcement of them. #2 offers reassurance but does not address guilt feelings. #3 would reinforce guilt feelings. SOCIALLY MALADAPTIVE BEHAVIOR/ PSYCHOSOCIAL, MENTAL HEALTH, PSYCHIATRIC PROBLEMS

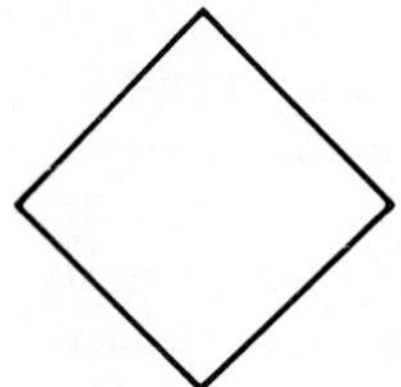

Sample Test Questions: Part Four

A new client, John Small, has been admitted to a 20-bed psychiatric unit of a university hospital. He was brought in by the police after getting in a fight and tearing up a bar. He is 6 ft 3 in tall and weighs 275 lb. At the present time, he is pacing in the unit recreation room, mumbling. His jaws are tight and his hands are clenched. Other clients are afraid of him and are trying to avoid him by going to their rooms.

281. Which of the following would the nurse best use initially in an attempt to prevent a crisis on the unit?

○ **1.** Keep the other clients away and observe Mr. Small's behavior until he calms down.
○ **2.** Place Mr. Small in seclusion immediately and then help him to verbally express his anger.
○ **3.** Approach Mr. Small on a one-to-one basis and offer him a prn medication immediately.
○ **4.** Approach Mr. Small on a one-to-one basis, help him identify his anger, and offer him alternatives.

282. The milieu (environment) is a very important tool in working with an angry client. The environment may be therapeutic or nontherapeutic. Which of the following descriptions suggests an environment that would be most helpful in preventing a crisis for Mr. Small?

○ **1.** Body bags, large outside grounds, art activities, and a variety of places for Mr. Small to be alone.
○ **2.** Many programmed activities that encourage him to become involved in his own goals and treatment.
○ **3.** Setting firm, clear rules and limits.
○ **4.** Freedom for him to determine his own privileges.

283. Mr. Small continues to exhibit increasing signs of anxiety. He is shouting at and threatening the nurse and other clients. The nurse would take all of the following actions *except*

○ **1.** Offer Mr. Small a chance to dice the carrots for the salad being served at dinner.
○ **2.** Call a crisis team that could, if necessary, quickly subdue Mr. Small.
○ **3.** Prepare Mr. Small a prn medication and a seclusion room with restraints.
○ **4.** Keep the other clients away from Mr. Small.

284. Mr. Small continues to become more agitated, and he attempts to hit another client. The nurse decides that he needs to be placed in seclusion with full, leather restraints. Which one of the following interventions would *not* be utilized when restraining a client?

○ **1.** Have an established team that can move as quickly as possible.
○ **2.** Remove the glasses and jewelry of staff and the client to prevent Mr. Small from destroying anything.
○ **3.** Identify for Mr. Small the positive behaviors the staff expects from him.
○ **4.** Utilize more staff and security guards whenever possible as members of the team.

285. Mr. Small has been out of seclusion for several hours. He is expressing that his rights have been violated and he demands to leave the hospital. The law includes several important provisions that apply to seclusion, restraints, and medication. Which one of the following statements would *not* apply in this situation?

○ **1.** Mr. Small can refuse to be placed in seclusion and restraints.
○ **2.** He can refuse to take his medication.
○ **3.** He can be retained in the hospital against his will if he is admitted by the state under an emergency or involuntary admission.
○ **4.** Mr. Small is entitled to legal counsel to discuss his future plans and concerns.

286. Mr. Small expresses concern about others knowing all about his "private life and behavior." Provisions have been made in the law to speak to his concerns. Which one of the following would *not* pertain to his concern?

- ○ **1.** Clients should have access to phones where others cannot hear conversations.
- ○ **2.** Information in clinical records should not be a part of the public record.
- ○ **3.** Information cannot be released without the client's consent.
- ○ **4.** Staff must include specific information in a separate document that is not part of the hospital record.

287. The timing of interventions for angry, aggressive behavior is best when the intervention occurs

- ○ **1.** Before the initial anxiety is converted to aggressive behavior.
- ○ **2.** After the aggressive act has occurred.
- ○ **3.** During the aggressive act.
- ○ **4.** After the initial anxiety.

Seven-month-old Maria Juarez has a congenitally dislocated right hip.

288. The nurse should expect to note which finding when assessing Maria?

- ○ **1.** Easily abducted right hip.
- ○ **2.** Lengthening of the right leg.
- ○ **3.** Severe pain on hip movement.
- ○ **4.** Widening of the perineum.

289. Maria has been fitted with a von Rosen splint. During a home visit to evaluate the effectiveness of teaching Maria's parents how to care for Maria during the treatment period, which outcome demonstrated by the parents indicates they understand the seriousness of Maria's defect?

- ○ **1.** Her parents apply and remove the splint correctly.
- ○ **2.** The Juarezes keep Maria in the splint at all times except when she is being bathed.
- ○ **3.** Mr. and Mrs. Juarez change Maria's position at least every 2 hours.
- ○ **4.** The parents provide age-appropriate sensorimotor activities and stimulation for Maria.

The labor-room nurse is monitoring the induction of labor for a primigravida, Mary Albert, who has failed to progress in labor over 24 hours.

290. In evaluating the action of the medication oxytocin (Pitocin) which of the following indicates an adverse effect?

- ○ **1.** A contraction lasting over 120 seconds.
- ○ **2.** A decrease in blood pressure.
- ○ **3.** Urinary output of 100 ml per hour.
- ○ **4.** Increasing intensity of contractions.

291. The induction stimulates regular contractions and Mrs. Albert is now in active labor. She expresses concern about her ability to behave as she would wish during the remainder of labor. Which of these nursing interventions would be most supportive?

- ○ **1.** Acknowledge that responses are often influenced by culture.
- ○ **2.** Inform her that medication is available if she needs it.
- ○ **3.** Instruct the client in relaxation and breathing exercises.
- ○ **4.** Reassure her that she is accepted regardless of behavior.

292. While monitoring fetal heart rate responses to contractions, the following assessment is made: a fetal heart rate deceleration of uniform shape begins just as the contraction is under way and returns to the baseline at the end of the contraction. Which of the following nursing interventions is appropriate?

- ○ **1.** Administer O_2.
- ○ **2.** Turn the mother on her left side.
- ○ **3.** Notify the physician.
- ○ **4.** Continue observations of labor.

293. Mrs. Albert delivers a 7-lb daughter. One-half hour after delivery, the fundus is firm, 1 inch below the umbilicus; lochia is rubra; client complains of thirst; there are slight tremors of lower extremities. Analysis of this data suggests

- ○ **1.** Impending shock.
- ○ **2.** Circulatory overload.
- ○ **3.** Sub-involution.
- ○ **4.** Normal postpartum adaptation.

294. Two hours postdelivery, Mrs. Albert complains of severe perineal pain. Which nursing action is a priority?

- ○ **1.** Administer prescribed pain medication.
- ○ **2.** Initiate sitz baths.
- ○ **3.** Inspect the perineum.
- ○ **4.** Teach perineal muscle exercises.

295. Which of the following nursing assessments suggests bladder distension 6 hours after delivery?

- **1.** Poor abdominal muscle tone.
- **2.** Increased lochia rubra with clots.
- **3.** Hard, contracted uterus.
- **4.** Uterus soft to the right of midline.

Juanita Sanchez, aged 78, has been living with her daughter since her husband's death 5 years ago. She has become increasingly forgetful and unable to care for herself. She wanders away from home frequently and is argumentative, because of organic brain syndrome. The family has decided to place Mrs. Sanchez in a nursing home.

296. Based on the diagnosis of organic brain syndrome, nursing assessment of Mrs. Sanchez would most likely reveal which of the following intellectual changes?

- **1.** Decreased ability to handle anxiety.
- **2.** Disorientation to time and place.
- **3.** Emotional lability.
- **4.** Paranoid ideation.

297. Mrs. Sanchez becomes more confused after she has been admitted to the nursing home. Which of the following actions would be most helpful to decrease her confusion?

- **1.** Assist Mrs. Sanchez with all activities of daily living.
- **2.** Find out from the family what her usual daily routine is and follow it as closely as possible.
- **3.** Restrict visitors during the first 2 weeks, so she can adjust to the nursing home.
- **4.** Wait for the confusion to decrease as Mrs. Sanchez adjusts to her new environment.

298. Mrs. Sanchez's increased confusion is probably caused by

- **1.** Anger at her daughter.
- **2.** Decreased personal space.
- **3.** Increased brain deterioration.
- **4.** Unfamiliar surroundings.

299. Mrs. Sanchez frequently wanders from her room into other clients' rooms or out to the street. The most effective nursing intervention would be to

- **1.** Accompany Mrs. Sanchez when she wanders and guide her to her room or the dayroom.
- **2.** Ask Mrs. Sanchez to explain why she cannot remain in her room or public areas.
- **3.** Confine Mrs. Sanchez to her room, because she gets lost too frequently.
- **4.** Restrain Mrs. Sanchez in her chair; so she will not disturb others or become lost.

300. Mrs. Sanchez repeatedly attempts to leave the nursing home stating, "My husband is waiting at home for me. I have to leave work now." The nurse's most appropriate response is

- **1.** "He knows you're staying here tonight; come back in now."
- **2.** "Mrs. Sanchez, you know you retired 13 years ago and your husband is dead."
- **3.** "You can't leave now; you have to stay here."
- **4.** "Your husband died 5 years ago, and you're in the nursing home now."

301. Mrs. Sanchez's daughter states that Mrs. Sanchez had lost 11 lb in the past 3 months. Which of the following would be the most appropriate nursing intervention to ensure adequate nutrition?

- **1.** Feed Mrs. Sanchez when she does not finish her meal.
- **2.** Give Mrs. Sanchez 6 small feedings during the day.
- **3.** Tell Mrs. Sanchez that she will be tube-fed if she does not eat.
- **4.** Observe Mrs. Sanchez's eating and weigh her before developing a plan.

302. Which of the following will be most effective in assisting Mrs. Sanchez to maintain a reality orientation?

- **1.** Call Mrs. Sanchez by name and identify yourself each time you enter her room.
- **2.** Encourage Mrs. Sanchez to spend her time watching television in her room.
- **3.** Plan a different schedule of activities every day to prevent boredom.
- **4.** Rotate staff assignments so she will know each staff member.

303. Mrs. Sanchez is most likely to demonstrate which of the following?
- **1.** Decreased attention span and ability to learn new things.
- **2.** Equal recall of both recent and past events.
- **3.** Increased ability to adapt to change in her environment.
- **4.** Increased interest in hygiene and grooming.

304. The nurse notes that Mrs. Sanchez frequently confabulates when asked about her everyday activities. She does this in order to
- **1.** Fill in memory gaps.
- **2.** Get attention from the nurse.
- **3.** Increase her attention span.
- **4.** Prevent regression.

305. The night nurse reports that Mrs. Sanchez is very confused, is in and out of bed, and makes multiple requests for assistance throughout the night. Which of the following nursing actions would most effectively lessen her confusion?
- **1.** Alter her bedtime routine to increase physical activity.
- **2.** Give her a detailed explanation of her need for adequate rest.
- **3.** Turn on night-lights in her bedroom and bathroom.
- **4.** Give her a sedative to help her sleep.

306. Mrs. Sanchez has difficulty deciding what to wear in the morning. The most effective nursing intervention would be to
- **1.** Give her as much time as she needs to make her own decision.
- **2.** Help her select an outfit and get dressed.
- **3.** Lay out her clothes each morning before she awakens.
- **4.** Tell her she must hurry or she will miss breakfast.

307. Mrs. Sanchez tells her daughter not to visit since she does not care enough to let her own mother stay at home. The daughter tells the nurse, "I don't know what to do. Mother's so angry she doesn't want to see me. But I had to do something. We couldn't take care of her anymore." The nurse's most appropriate initial response would be
- **1.** "Wait a few days and she'll get over this."
- **2.** "She'll be OK once she gets settled here; don't worry."
- **3.** "You feel guilty about leaving your mother here."
- **4.** "This is a very difficult time for you and your mother."

308. The daughter asks if she should come back the next day to visit. The nurse's most appropriate response would be
- **1.** "Come back tomorrow; your interest is important for your mother."
- **2.** "Is there anyone else who could visit your mother?"
- **3.** "Wait until your mother calls you to say she wants to see you."
- **4.** "Your mother will be busy with the staff and clients. She won't miss you if you don't come."

309. An hour after her daughter leaves, Mrs. Sanchez tells the nurse, "I haven't seen my daughter in days. Something must be wrong." The nurse's most appropriate response would be
- **1.** "Are you afraid she won't come back to visit you?"
- **2.** "I'm sure you'll hear from her again soon."
- **3.** "You're confused; she was here earlier tonight."
- **4.** "Your daughter was here before dinner this evening."

310. Which of the following would be most helpful in providing ongoing care for Mrs. Sanchez?
- **1.** Follow her usual routine as much as possible.
- **2.** Involve her in all unit activities to decrease her loneliness.
- **3.** Provide one-to-one teaching sessions to help her understand her limitations.
- **4.** Adhere strictly to the unit's routine.

Eleven-year-old Gail is hospitalized with rheumatic fever with carditis and polyarthritis. She also has Sydenham's Chorea.

311. Which of the following is true concerning rheumatic fever?
- **1.** It is usually associated with glomerulonephritis.
- **2.** Symptoms disappear shortly after the fever abates and the temperature returns to normal.
- **3.** The child should resume normal activities as soon as she feels well.
- **4.** It usually follows a strep infection.

312. In planning your nursing care, you note that Gail is on bedrest. What is the rationale for this?
- **1.** To help the pain of the arthritis that accompanies the disease.
- **2.** To minimize the effects of the carditis.
- **3.** So other children will not see Gail's choreiform movements.
- **4.** To help alleviate the febrile effects of the disease.

313. Which of the following is likely to be the major psychologic stressor of Gail's illness and hospitalization?
- **1.** Fear of painful procedures.
- **2.** Separation from her family.
- **3.** Activity restriction.
- **4.** Worry about possible outcomes.

314. Which of the following children should the nurse select as Gail's roommate?
- **1.** Seven-year-old Susan who also has rheumatic fever.
- **2.** Ten-year-old Amy with insulin-dependent diabetes.
- **3.** Thirteen-year-old Sharon with sickle cell vaso-occlusive crisis.
- **4.** Twelve-year-old Evelyn with fever of unknown origin.

315. Which of the following activities is most appropriate for Gail?
- **1.** Listening to records and the radio.
- **2.** Watching television.
- **3.** Playing Ping-Pong in the game room.
- **4.** Crocheting a small afghan.

316. Gail's blood tests show the following results. Which is the most indicative of an improvement in her condition?
- **1.** Positive C-reactive protein.
- **2.** White blood cell count of 11,000.
- **3.** Decreased erythrocyte sedimentation rate (ESR).
- **4.** Elevated antistreptolysin O (ASO) titer.

317. Gail is readmitted to the hospital 2 months later for a cardiac catheterization. When preparing Gail for the procedure, the nurse should take into account which of the following?
- **1.** Concrete explanations and experiences will be most meaningful.
- **2.** Gail is likely to misinterpret the procedure as punishment for previous misbehavior.
- **3.** Gail should be given a full verbal explanation of the procedure using correct medical terminology.
- **4.** Gail should be allowed to make all decisions concerning her care.

Elizabeth Johnson, 21, delivered her first child this morning, after a long and difficult labor, with the fetus in posterior position.

318. Which of the following behaviors is common during this time of restoration and is characteristic of "taking-in"?
- **1.** Showing an interest in newborn care.
- **2.** Asking if "rooming-in" can begin immediately.
- **3.** Talking constantly about the labor and delivery.
- **4.** Experiencing mild transient feelings of depression.

319. In evaluating Mrs. Johnson's condition on the day after delivery, which finding suggests normal reproductive adaptation?
- **1.** Fundus firm, 1 cm below the umbilicus.
- **2.** Scant lochia serosa.
- **3.** Moderate breast engorgement.
- **4.** Perineal sutures healed.

320. On the third day after delivery Mrs. Johnson complains of breast engorgement. Her 6 lb infant sucks briefly, then sleeps when put to breast. An appropriate plan is the client will
- **1.** Restrict intake of fluids until engorgement is relieved.
- **2.** Use ice packs on breasts just prior to nursing.
- **3.** Pump or express milk when the baby does not empty breasts.
- **4.** Discontinue breast-feeding temporarily until the newborn is alert.

321. Mrs. Johnson asks if breast-feeding will change the shape of her breast. Which of the following is an appropriate response?

- ○ **1.** "Yes, the shape of your breast may be affected if the baby is allowed to nurse too vigorously."
- ○ **2.** "Breast-feeding does not affect the shape of the breast. However, wearing a proper breast support is important."
- ○ **3.** "If you breast-feed for more than 6 months, the shape of the breast will change."
- ○ **4.** "Breast-feeding may change the shape of the breast, however, this shouldn't be the most important consideration."

322. Prior to discharge, both Mr. and Mrs. Johnson attend several classes on infant care. Which statement by the new father indicates he has a realistic understanding of newborn behavior?

- ○ **1.** "I hope we can get him on a schedule of 2 naps and a full night's sleep."
- ○ **2.** "I don't want him to be spoiled, so he'll learn quickly not to cry for attention."
- ○ **3.** "If we can get him on a schedule for feedings, he'll nurse better."
- ○ **4.** "It looks like the next weeks will be mostly feeding, changing, and caring for baby."

323. At the postpartum clinic visit, Mrs. Johnson seems very discouraged about breast-feeding. She says, "Neither baby Tim nor I seem to be successful at this breast-feeding. Maybe it's because I am so small." The nurse's response to the mother is based on the understanding of which of the following?

- ○ **1.** Hormone levels may vary in individual women.
- ○ **2.** Desire to breast-feed affects milk production.
- ○ **3.** Primigravidas are usually apprehensive about feeding.
- ○ **4.** Breast size is not a factor in volume of milk produced.

Twenty-two-month-old Katie is admitted to the pediatric unit with acute laryngotracheobronchitis.

324. When a nursing history is taken, Katie's mother tells the nurse that Katie is toilet-trained. Which additional information is the most important for the nurse to ascertain?

- ○ **1.** The age at which Katie began toilet training.
- ○ **2.** Katie's toilet habits and routine at home.
- ○ **3.** Katie's mother's understanding of the possibility of regression in Katie's toileting habits while she is hospitalized.
- ○ **4.** Katie's willingness to accept help from the nursing staff with her toileting needs.

325. Developmentally, Katie should exhibit which of the following behaviors?

- ○ **1.** Dress and undress herself without help.
- ○ **2.** Share her toys with other children.
- ○ **3.** Speak in 5-to 6-word sentences.
- ○ **4.** Feed herself well with a spoon.

326. Katie has an IV of 500 ml of 5% dextrose in 0.25% normal saline ordered to infuse over 8 hours. The nurse should set the microdrip regulator to infuse at a rate of how many drops per minute?

- ○ **1.** 21.
- ○ **2.** 30.
- ○ **3.** 63.
- ○ **4.** 125.

327. Katie is in a croup tent with compressed air. Nursing care of Katie should include which measure?

- ○ **1.** Explain to her why she must stay in the tent.
- ○ **2.** Restrict her fluid intake to no more than 32 oz a day.
- ○ **3.** Administer a cough suppressant to control her cough.
- ○ **4.** Change her wet bed linens frequently.

328. Chest percussion and postural drainage are prescribed four times a day for Katie. When should the nurse plan to carry out Katie's chest therapy?

- ○ **1.** Just before Katie eats and at bedtime.
- ○ **2.** Halfway between mealtimes and at bedtime.
- ○ **3.** Upon arising and 1 hour after meals.
- ○ **4.** During intervals between Katie's naps.

329. Following chest percussion and postural drainage, which finding indicates that the treatment has not been entirely effective?

- ○ **1.** Inspiratory stridor.
- ○ **2.** Rales and rhonchi.
- ○ **3.** Suprasternal retractions.
- ○ **4.** Harsh metallic cough.

330. Katie is hospitalized for 4 days. Katie's parents visit every evening but are unable to stay with her overnight. Which behavior is Katie most likely to demonstrate when separating from her parents?

- ○ **1.** Readily seeks comfort from the nurse.
- ○ **2.** Sucks her thumb, whines, and curls up in a corner of her crib.
- ○ **3.** Cries loudly and tries to cling to her parents.
- ○ **4.** Waves and blows them a kiss.

331. When planning care for the hospitalized toddler whose mother can not room-in, which nursing action would be most appropriate?

- ○ **1.** Encourage the mother to leave an article of her clothing.
- ○ **2.** Assign the toddler a roommate close in age to keep him/her company.
- ○ **3.** Inform the mother that toddlers handle separation easily.
- ○ **4.** Suggest that mother limit visits to reduce the toddler's separation anxiety.

332. When Katie is discharged, which instruction to Katie's parents is not appropriate?

- ○ **1.** Katie may show some regression in her behavior for a few weeks.
- ○ **2.** Katie should not be separated from her parents for lengthy periods of time until she feels secure again.
- ○ **3.** Katie should be allowed to sleep with her parents for a few nights until she readjusts to being home.
- ○ **4.** Katie's parents should reinstate limits that were in effect prior to her hospitalization.

Stanley Brown, a 50-year-old man who has been a heavy smoker for the past 20 years, is admitted to the hospital with a diagnosis of emphysema with right lower lobe pneumonia. Upon his arrival at the medical floor, the nurse carries out the assessment, which is as follows: extremely dyspneic, ashen in color, perspiring profusely, very agitated, and coughing up large amounts of tenacious white sputum. Mr. Brown's orders include stat blood gases; O_2 at 2 liters; aminophylline IV drip; sputum for C&S; start ampicillin (Polycillin) 1 gm after sputum is obtained.

333. All of the following information is provided by Mr. Brown. What probably precipitated his emphysema flare-up?

- ○ **1.** He wore a new cotton suit 2 days ago.
- ○ **2.** He smoked more cigarettes than usual 3 days ago.
- ○ **3.** He went bowling last week.
- ○ **4.** He has had a cold for the past week.

334. What is the expected action of aminophylline?

- ○ **1.** Increase the production of sputum.
- ○ **2.** Relax the bronchial muscle.
- ○ **3.** Promote sleep and relieve anxiety.
- ○ **4.** Liquefy tenacious sputum.

335. To detect a common side effect of aminophylline, the nurse should assess Mr. Brown for the possible development of which symptom?

- ○ **1.** Generalized dermatitis.
- ○ **2.** Hematuria.
- ○ **3.** Urinary retention.
- ○ **4.** Tachycardia.

336. Mr. Brown's blood-gas results demonstrate a pH of 7.37, pO_2 of 65 mm Hg, and a pCO_2 of 50 mm Hg. On the basis of this information, which statement is most justified?

- ○ **1.** Mr. Brown has acute respiratory insufficiency and needs to have his O_2 turned up to 8 liters.
- ○ **2.** Mr. Brown has acute pulmonary failure and needs to be placed on a ventilator.
- ○ **3.** Mr. Brown has adapted to his high level of arterial CO_2 and is in chronic respiratory acidosis.
- ○ **4.** Mr. Brown demonstrates chronic respiratory acidosis and will soon display neurologic changes.

337. Mr. Brown produces sputum, which is sent to the lab for culture and sensitivity. Then, IV ampicillin (Polycillin) is started. You know that this drug belongs to the penicillin family of antibiotics and that the pencillins, among all the antimicrobials, are most often responsible for which of the following?

- ○ **1.** Anaphylaxis.
- ○ **2.** Urinary retention.
- ○ **3.** Nausea and vomiting.
- ○ **4.** Gastric perforation.

338. Mr. Brown does not improve. On the third day post-hospital admission, his temperature is 103.4°F (39.7°C), he has right-sided chest pain and decreased right-sided chest excursion. A portable chest x-ray reveals further extension of his pneumonia with a spontaneous pneumothroax. Mr. Brown is informed by Dr. Stone that a chest tube must be inserted immediately. To assist Mr. Brown to comply with this procedure, which of the following pieces of information does the nurse need to have in order to be of most help in answering his questions?

- ○ **1.** The pneumothorax is caused by disruption in the integrity of the pleura.
- ○ **2.** A rib has fractured and is causing changes in thoracic pressures.
- ○ **3.** Air has collected in the mediastinal space.
- ○ **4.** The pneumothorax is caused by the accumulation of pus in the lung tissue.

339. Mr. Brown asks the nurse how the chest tube will help him to breathe with greater ease. Which of the following responses by the nurse would be *incorrect*?

- ○ **1.** The chest tube will allow for the drainage of fluid and air from the pleural space.
- ○ **2.** The chest tube will aid in reestablishing positive pressure in the pleural space.
- ○ **3.** The chest tube will aid in reexpansion of the lung.
- ○ **4.** The chest tube will aid in reestablishing negative pressure in the pleural space.

340. After the chest tube is inserted and connected to the Pleur-evac, Mr. Brown wants to know why there are water "bubbles" in the water-seal container. Which of these responses by the nurse would be best?

- ○ **1.** "You should ask your doctor for more information."
- ○ **2.** "It indicates that the system is working correctly."
- ○ **3.** "Oh! don't worry about it. I am taking good care of you."
- ○ **4.** "It indicates that your lung has not fully expanded."

341. Mr. Brown progresses well. One week post-op, his chest tube is removed. Mr. Brown tells the nurse he realizes proper nutrition is very important for his future health, but he just does not have much of an appetite. Which of these responses by the nurse would be most helpful?

- ○ **1.** Eat 3 large meals a day that are high in carbohydrate.
- ○ **2.** Eat 3 large meals a day that are high in protein.
- ○ **3.** Eat 6 small meals a day that are high in carbohydrate.
- ○ **4.** Eat 6 small meals a day that are high in protein.

342. When Mr. Brown is discharged, he and his wife are referred to the Visiting Nurse Association. Mr. Brown and his wife will more readily accept aid from this organization if which of the following is noted?

- ○ **1.** The need that they think they have for such help.
- ○ **2.** The enthusiasm of the nurse who plans their care.
- ○ **3.** The availability of the help.
- ○ **4.** The willingness of Mrs. Brown to accept the help.

Michael Lamaroux, a 34-year-old construction worker, is admitted to a medical-surgical unit following an auto accident for treatment of fractured femurs and his right hip. He had been drinking and hit another car. Although Mr. Lamaroux's blood-alcohol level is high, he insists that he only had 1 beer. He is to have surgery for reduction of his fractured hip.

343. He tells his nurse that he is especially sensitive to pain and has used Percodan for headaches in the past. What is the best initial statement the nurse can make?

- ○ **1.** "Do you have any medications with you that were not prescribed by a physician?"
- ○ **2.** "Be sure not to take any medications except what we give you for pain."
- ○ **3.** "Have you ever felt like you needed medication to help you get through the day?"
- ○ **4.** "I need you to make a verbal contract with me right now that you will not take any medication except what is ordered for you at this time. Other drugs may interfere with your anesthesia tomorrow."

344. In order for withdrawal symptoms to occur in a person with a substance use disorder, which of the following is *not* necessary?

1. Physiologic dependence.
2. Marked tolerance.
3. Diminished intake.
4. Cessation of intake.

345. Which of the following ego-defense mechanisms is a top and continuing priority in dealing with alcoholic clients?

1. Dependency.
2. Denial.
3. Paranoia.
4. Projection.

346. Of all the following approaches to the treatment of alcoholism, which has been found to be the most effective to date?

1. Membership in Alcoholics Anonymous.
2. Family-systems approach.
3. Treating the alcoholism as a chronic disease.
4. Individual psychotherapy.

347. Following inpatient treatment for his fractures and for his substance abuse, Mr. Lamaroux agress to involve himself in therapy. Which of the following would have the *least* influence on the structure of family-therapy sessions?

1. Genetic factors and chronic disease effects of alcoholism.
2. History of alcoholism in other family members and the previous generation.
3. Over-and underfunctioning within the family.
4. How closeness and distance are dealt with in the family.

348. Which of the following interventions would be the nurse's highest priority in the detoxification stage of alcoholism?

1. Confront manipulative behavior designed to gain access to alcohol.
2. Administer vitamin B supplements knowing that alcoholism has resulted in a severe depletion.
3. Report potassium level of 1.4 mEq/liter.
4. Provide ample opportunities to decrease social isolation and improve social skills.

349. As Mr. Lamaroux progresses in his treatment he remarks to the nurse, "I'm no good. My drinking has almost destroyed everything I value most." Which response from the nurse would be most helpful?

1. "What did you do that was so bad?"
2. "Yes, it's time you stopped drinking."
3. "Have you been to this stage of treatment before?"
4. "It sounds like you're feeling guilty about your drinking."

350. In revising the goals, the nurse writes, "Client will decrease drug-seeking, manipulative, and acting-out behavior." Which of the following nursing orders is *not* appropriate for the updated care plan in light of Mr. Lamaroux's drug and alcohol problems?

1. Set firm and consistent limits.
2. Clearly define acceptable and unacceptable behavior.
3. Hold a care conference to assure that entire staff adopt a consistent approach to client's behavior.
4. Provide a high level of sympathy and empathy for his difficulties.

Sylvia Marlin, a 28-year-old newlywed, is admitted to the hospital with an enlarged thyroid gland.

351. In taking a nursing history, which of the following is considered a risk factor in the development of cancer of the thyroid?

1. A diet low in iodine.
2. A diet high in iodine.
3. A history of high doses of vitamin D.
4. A history of irradiation of the head or neck.

352. In carrying out an initial and daily assessment of a client with thyroid enlargement, the nurse will carefully observe for which of the following?

1. Difficulty in swallowing or breathing.
2. Excessive saliva production.
3. Muscle twitching.
4. Tingling around the lips.

353. In addition to having an enlarged thyroid gland, Mrs. Marlin has been experiencing symptoms suggestive of hyperthyroidism. What might these symptoms include?

- ○ **1.** Fatigue, weight gain, dry skin, cold intolerance.
- ○ **2.** Decreased pulse rate, slurred speech, constipation, cold intolerance.
- ○ **3.** Nervousness, weight loss, tachycardia, heat intolerance.
- ○ **4.** Abdominal pain, diarrhea, fatty food intolerance, heat intolerance.

354. Mrs. Marlin's laboratory workup will probably indicate which of the following?

- ○ **1.** Deficiency of serum T_3 and/or T_4.
- ○ **2.** Increased levels of serum T_3 and/or T_4.
- ○ **3.** Deficiency of serum TSH.
- ○ **4.** Increased levels of serum ACTH.

355. A serious form of hyperthyroidism results in a condition known as what?

- ○ **1.** Myxedema.
- ○ **2.** Cretinism.
- ○ **3.** Graves' disease.
- ○ **4.** Addison's disease.

356. Mrs. Marlin's hyperfunctioning thyroid results in exophthalmos. Nursing interventions specific for this problem should include which of the following?

- ○ **1.** Frequent mouth care using a soft toothbrush and normal saline mouthwash.
- ○ **2.** A private room with decreased environmental stimulation and light.
- ○ **3.** Lubricating eye drops and instructions to blink at regular intervals.
- ○ **4.** Frequent monitoring of vital signs and body temperature.

357. Mrs. Marlin's diagnosis workup includes a radioactive iodine (RAI) uptake. In preparing the patient for this procedure, what should the nurse do?

- ○ **1.** Take a history of all recent medications and x-ray examinations.
- ○ **2.** Place the client on a low sodium diet for 3 days prior to the test.
- ○ **3.** Prepare the client for isolation using radiation precautions.
- ○ **4.** Instruct the client in 24-hour urine collection techniques.

358. To inhibit thyroid hormone synthesis, Mrs. Marlin is given propylthiouracil (PTU). In reviewing this medication with her prior to discharge, the nurse would include all of the following *except* which one?

- ○ **1.** Report weight loss and increased pulse rate.
- ○ **2.** Report fever, sore throat, rash.
- ○ **3.** Take the drug once daily at the same time each day.
- ○ **4.** Some weight gain is to be expected.

359. Antithyroid drug therapy has proved to be ineffective. Mrs. Marlin is readmitted to the hospital for thyroidectomy. Prior to thyroidectomy, an iodine solution has been administered for several weeks in order to decrease the vascularity and size of the thyroid gland. When giving an iodine solution, the nurse should do which of the following?

- ○ **1.** Give the drug on an empty stomach to speed its rate of absorption.
- ○ **2.** Dilute the drug in fruit juice, milk, or water.
- ○ **3.** Avoid giving the drug with milk or antacids.
- ○ **4.** Avoid giving the drug at bedtime.

360. Prior to her surgery, Mrs. Marlin acquires coryza, stomatitis, and swollen salivary glands. What should the nurse do?

- ○ **1.** Put the patient in protective isolation.
- ○ **2.** Isolate the client from other pre-op clients.
- ○ **3.** Evaluate the client's diet for excessive iodine intake.
- ○ **4.** Hold the iodine solution and report the client's symptoms.

361. Post-op care of the client following thyroidectomy includes which of the following?

- ○ **1.** Keep the head of the bed flat to prevent neck flexion.
- ○ **2.** Avoid coughing and deep breathing to prevent injury to the suture line.
- ○ **3.** Restrict ambulation until the suture line is healed.
- ○ **4.** Check the back of the neck and upper part of the back when assessing the dressing.

362. Following thyroidectomy, the nurse frequently assesses the client's voice and ability to speak. What is the nurse trying to evaluate?

- ○ **1.** Changes in level of consciousness.
- ○ **2.** Recovery from anesthesia.
- ○ **3.** Injury to the parathyroid gland.
- ○ **4.** Spasm or edema of vocal chords.

363. Mrs. Marlin begins to experience respiratory distress. A check of the surgical dressing reveals it to be tight about her neck with a small amount of bloody drainage. What should the nurse do?
- ○ **1.** Administer oxygen at 2 liters via nasal prongs.
- ○ **2.** Reinforce the dressing and notify the doctor.
- ○ **3.** Loosen the dressing and notify the doctor.
- ○ **4.** Place the client in low-Fowler's position and notify the doctor.

364. The nurse will instruct Mrs. Marlin to avoid which of the following activities for several weeks following a thyroidectomy?
- ○ **1.** Turning the head.
- ○ **2.** Sitting in a chair.
- ○ **3.** Brushing the teeth.
- ○ **4.** Side-lying position.

365. The nurse observes Mrs. Marlin for injury to the parathyroid gland as a result of her surgery. Which of the following indicates parathyroid damage?
- ○ **1.** Vague abdominal pain.
- ○ **2.** Nausea and vomiting.
- ○ **3.** Decreased serum calcium.
- ○ **4.** Decreased serum phosphorus.

366. Treatment of parathyroid hormone deficiency can be expected to include which of the following?
- ○ **1.** Thyroid preparations.
- ○ **2.** Digitalis.
- ○ **3.** Calcium gluconate.
- ○ **4.** High phosphorus diet.

367. Following a total thyroidectomy, what should the nurse teach the client?
- ○ **1.** Take thyroid medication daily for the rest of life.
- ○ **2.** Thyroid medication will be prescribed for 1–2 years.
- ○ **3.** Restrict sea food, iodized salt, and green vegetable intake.
- ○ **4.** Take iodine solution daily for the rest of life.

Seven-year-old Kenisha Collins has acute post-streptococcal nephritis.

368. The nurse makes a home visit to monitor Kenisha's response to treatment. Which of the following is it necessary for the nurse to include when evaluating Kenisha?
- ○ **1.** Blood pressure measurement.
- ○ **2.** Auscultation of breath sounds.
- ○ **3.** Urine test for sugar and acetone.
- ○ **4.** Abdominal circumference measurements.

369. Which of Kenisha's meals reported by her mother indicates that Mrs. Collins does not fully understand Kenisha's dietary restrictions?
- ○ **1.** Fried chicken, mashed potatoes, green beans, apple juice.
- ○ **2.** Broiled fish, macaroni salad, applesauce, grape juice.
- ○ **3.** Scrambled eggs, bacon, muffin with jelly, orange juice.
- ○ **4.** Grilled cheese sandwich, carrots, fruit cocktail, milk.

370. Mrs. Collins asks the nurse if Kenisha will "probably end up on one of those kidney machines." The nurse's reply should be based on the knowledge that Kenisha will most likely
- ○ **1.** Return to normal renal functioning.
- ○ **2.** Develop acute renal failure, requiring dialysis.
- ○ **3.** Develop chronic renal failure, necessitating a kidney transplant.
- ○ **4.** Have numerous recurrences of the disease.

David James is a 31-year-old married man with two children. He is a devout Catholic. He has been diagnosed with leukemia and the disease has been treated with drug therapy for 2½ years. Mr. James has been admitted to the hospital with pneumonia and has been placed in protective isolation.

371. Mr. James has told the nurses that he knows he is going to die, but that is all he has said about it. He talks about his disease in clinical terms to the nurses, never about his own experiences. One day he comments to his primary nurse, "I am so worried." The best response from the nurse is
- ○ **1.** "It must frighten you to know you are dying."
- ○ **2.** "It must make you very uncomfortable."
- ○ **3.** "Have you shared these feelings with your family?"
- ○ **4.** "Tell me exactly what things are worrying you."

372. Which of the following interventions would be most significant in helping Mr. James cope with this death?

○ **1.** Distract him by initiating conversation that does not deal with his disease.

○ **2.** Encourage him to reach out and spend more time with his wife and children.

⊗ **3.** Listen and allow Mr. James to reminisce about his life.

○ **4.** Help him spend most of his time sleeping.

373. Mr. James tells the nurse he does not want his wife and children to know that he is dying. What would be the most helpful response?

○ **1.** "They would not want you to upset yourself by worrying about them."

⊗ **2.** "You are concerned that they will be upset?"

○ **3.** "I think we should talk about something less stressful for you."

○ **4.** Sit quietly and say nothing.

374. Which of the following interventions is the most effective in helping Mrs. James and her two children deal with Mr. James's impending death?

○ **1.** Try to keep all of the family members at the same stage in the grieving process.

⊘ **2.** Encourage the family members to verbalize their anger, sadness, and guilt to the nurse.

○ **3.** Encourage the family members to spend as much time as possible at the hospital, even if they are just sitting in the waiting room.

○ **4.** Encourage the family members to cry, but not in the presence of Mr. James.

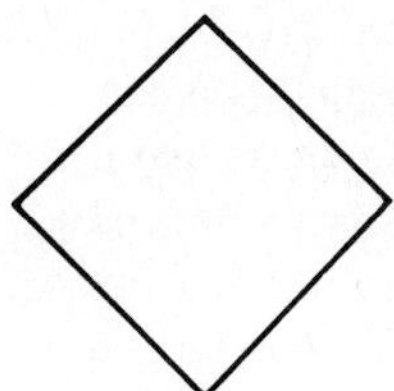

Correct Answers and Rationales: Part Four

281. #1. Many clients interpret the nurse's entering "their space" as a threat, and Mr. Small is exhibiting signs of increased anxiety. His history indicates that he has utilized violent, aggressive behavior in response to increased anxiety. The nurse and the client do not have an established nurse-client relationship, and the nurse has not assessed his behavior and responses to others. Therefore, the nurse should reduce the environmental stimuli and assess his response to the decrease. Seclusion is a last resort to assist clients to control behavior. The one-to-one attempt may be viewed as violation of personal space and behavioral distractions should be employed before medications if possible. Option #4 is not appropriate because at this stage of acting out, clients usually are unable to make decisions or identify anger. SOCIALLY MALADAPTIVE BEHAVIOR/ PSYCHOSOCIAL, MENTAL HEALTH, PSYCHIATRIC PROBLEMS

282. #3. Mr. Small is having difficulty maintaining self-control. Clear, firm limits will reduce his anxiety by providing a sense of control. Rules provide a sense of security until the client can provide his own controls. An expansive environment does not provide controls needed and Mr. Small is not ready to develop his own treatment plan or determine his own needs. SOCIALLY MALADAPTIVE BEHAVIOR/ PSYCHOSOCIAL, MENTAL HEALTH, PSYCHIATRIC PROBLEMS

283. #1. The client is showing signs of escalating anxiety. He has a history of doing harm to others. The nurse needs to offer simple, limited, alternative behaviors without providing the client access to any weapons that could be used to do harm to himself or others. Nursing intervention with the angry patient is best done with a team and preparation for this client's care is in order for his protection. It is appropriate to help the client avoid altercations when possible. SOCIALLY MALADAPTIVE BEHAVIOR/PSYCHOSOCIAL, MENTAL HEALTH, PSYCHIATRIC PROBLEMS

284. #3. When a client is placed in seclusion, communication should be kept simple and aimed at helping the client understand that the staff is assuming control until he can control his own behavior. When the staff is placing the client in restraints, his anxiety level will be raised and his hearing will become more selective. Expectations should be communicated at a time when the client's anxiety is lower. Options #1, #2, and #4 are all measures directed at staff and client safety. SOCIALLY MALADAPTIVE BEHAVIOR/ PSYCHOSOCIAL, MENTAL HEALTH, PSYCHIATRIC PROBLEMS

285. #1. Client's rights are addressed in state laws. State laws have statutes to include the conditions under which restraints can be used. Mr. Small's aggressive, violent behavior supports the need to protect others. Options #2, #3, and #4 all reflect state laws or patient rights applicable in this situation. LEGAL ASPECTS/PSYCHOSOCIAL, MENTAL HEALTH, PSYCHIATRIC PROBLEMS

286. #4. The law does deal with confidentiality concerns of clients. Limiting the documentation of staff is in violation of the portion of most state laws that indicates the record must contain specific data. Options #1, #2, and #3 address laws protecting client confidentiality. LEGAL ASPECTS/PSYCHOSOCIAL, MENTAL HEALTH, PSYCHIATRIC PROBLEMS

287. #1. Anger is cyclic. Once the client works out his anger and frustration in an aggressive act, he feels guilty and needs to justify and explain his behavior. While his anxiety is temporarily decreased, he experiences a decrease in self-esteem, which further increases the anxiety and can result in more acting-out behavior. The best intervention is to stop the anger cycle before it begins. Options #2, #3, and #4 reflect the later aspects of the anger cycle when intervention is more difficult. SOCIALLY MALADAPTIVE BEHAVIOR/ PSYCHOSOCIAL, MENTAL HEALTH, PSYCHIATRIC PROBLEMS

288. **#4.** The findings of congenital dislocated hip include *limited abduction* of the affected hip, *shortening* of the leg on the affected side, and widening of the perineum caused by the head of the femur slipping out of the acetabulum. The infant rarely experiences pain in the affected hip. MOBILITY/CHILD

289. **#2.** All of these outcomes are desirable, but the parents' compliance with keeping Maria in her splint at all times except bathtime is the most crucial indicator that they understand the possible consequences of not adhering to the treatment plan. MOBILITY/CHILD

290. **#1.** If contractions exceed 90 seconds in duration, there is a danger of ruptured uterus. Adverse blood pressure changes with Pitocin are seen in hypertension. A desired effect is increased strength and frequency of contractions. INTRAPARTAL CARE/CHILDBEARING FAMILY

291. **#4.** Acceptance is needed in time of stress, as the woman seeks to maintain control. INTRAPARTAL CARE/CHILDBEARING FAMILY

292. **#4.** This is a normal occurrence. Continue to observe fetal heart rate and contractions. INTRAPARTAL CARE/CHILDBEARING FAMILY

293. **#4.** These are normal adaptations. POSTPARTAL CARE/CHILDBEARING FAMILY

294. **#3.** Such pain may be associated with the development of a hematoma. Assessment should precede intervention. Comfort measures may follow. POSTPARTAL CARE/CHILDBEARING FAMILY

295. **#4.** A full bladder displaces the uterus and prevents contraction. Suggest that the client void and reassess fundus and lochia. POSTPARTAL CARE/CHILDBEARING FAMILY

296. **#2.** This is the only symptom listed that is indicative of a problem with intellectual function. Options #1, #3, and #4 indicate changes in emotional functioning. CONFUSED BEHAVIOR/PSYCHOSOCIAL, MENTAL HEALTH, PSYCHIATRIC PROBLEMS

297. **#2.** A familiar, established routine decreases confusion and the demands on the client's coping mechanisms. Efforts should be made to follow previous dependence, #3 would lead to increased feelings of isolation. Waiting will not lessen the confusion. CONFUSED BEHAVIOR/PSYCHOSOCIAL, MENTAL HEALTH, PSYCHIATRIC PROBLEMS

298. **#4.** Admission to a care facility often exacerbates symptoms because of the new environment. Although options #1, #2, and #3 are important considerations, it is unlikely they ''cause'' the confusion as it is described in this situation. CONFUSED BEHAVIOR/PSYCHOSOCIAL, MENTAL HEALTH, PSYCHIATRIC PROBLEMS

299. **#1.** Personal attention and assistance for client's safety will enhance feelings of securit Confinement and restraints increase feelings of hopelessness and inadequacy, which may lead to increased confusion. These clients will not be able to explain their behavior, and requests for such explanations may increase argumentativeness. CONFUSED BEHAVIOR/PSYCHOSOCIAL, MENTAL HEALTH, PSYCHIATRIC PROBLEMS

300. **#4.** This provides reality orientation without degrading or arguing with the client. Inaccurate information confuses the client further. Option #2 does not tell the client where she is now and verbal constraints may confuse the client. CONFUSED BEHAVIOR/PSYCHOSOCIAL, MENTAL HEALTH, PSYCHIATRIC PROBLEMS

301. **#2.** Provide smaller meals that require less attention to complete. The other choices would decrease independence, threaten the client, or allow the problem to continue. CONFUSED BEHAVIOR/PSYCHOSOCIAL, MENTAL HEALTH, PSYCHIATRIC PROBLEMS

302. **#1.** Identify yourself to avoid misidentification and call the client by name to reinforce her sense of identity. Option #2 would decrease her interaction with others, possibly increasing confusion. Options #3 and #4 provide an inappropriate degree of stimulation. CONFUSED BEHAVIOR/PSYCHOSOCIAL, MENTAL HEALTH, PSYCHIATRIC PROBLEMS

303. **#1.** Decreased ability to learn because of decreased attention span are characteristics of organic brain syndrome. Recent and remote memory changes are variable. As memory changes occur, the person will have more difficulty adapting to change and attending to usual activities of daily living. CONFUSED BEHAVIOR/PSYCHOSOCIAL, MENTAL HEALTH, PSYCHIATRIC PROBLEMS

304. **#1.** Confabulation involves using old memories or inventing information to fill in memory gaps about present experiences. There is no evidence of a special need to gain attention. Confabulation does not increase attention span or prevent regression. CONFUSED BEHAVIOR/PSYCHOSOCIAL, MENTAL HEALTH, PSYCHIATRIC PROBLEMS

305. **#3.** Avoiding shadows and darkness will help decrease her disorientation. Maintain her usual bedtime routine; alterations may only increase restlessness. These clients will not understand or remember explanations. Sedatives often increase activity and confusion in the elderly. CONFUSED BEHAVIOR/PSYCHOSOCIAL, MENTAL HEALTH, PSYCHIATRIC PROBLEMS

306. **#2.** Provide assistance and direction with activities of daily living as needed. Giving her time will not increase her decisiveness or lesson confusion. Laying out her clothes makes the decision for her and decreases independence. Rushing her will increase confusion. CONFUSED BEHAVIOR/PSYCHOSOCIAL, MENTAL HEALTH, PSYCHIATRIC PROBLEMS

307. **#4.** Assist family members to explore their feelings. Maintaining family contact is necessary for orientation and self-identity. Reassurance will not help family members deal with feelings or the situation. There is insufficient evidence to justify an inference of guilt. THERAPEUTIC USE OF SELF/ PSYCHOSOCIAL, MENTAL HEALTH, PSYCHIATRIC PROBLEMS

308. **#1.** Assist with feelings and client situations so family members will not withdraw from the client. Encourage regular visits. Options #2, #3, and #4 tend to separate family and client rather than to enhance their feelings at this difficult time. CONFUSED BEHAVIOR/ PSYCHOSOCIAL, MENTAL HEALTH, PSYCHIATRIC PROBLEMS

309. **#4.** Provide concrete information that reinforces reality without emphasizing the client's deficits. Probing for feelings increases confusion and argumentativeness in these clients. CONFUSED BEHAVIOR/ PSYCHOSOCIAL, MENTAL HEALTH, PSYCHIATRIC PROBLEMS

310. **#1.** Decreasing the number of adjustments needed in a new environment lessens confusion. Do not overstimulate or confront clients with deficits. Provide for individualization of care instead of rigid routines. CONFUSED BEHAVIOR/ PSYCHOSOCIAL, MENTAL HEALTH, PSYCHIATRIC PROBLEMS

311. **#4.** Two possible sequelae of a strep infection are rheumatic fever and glomerulonephritis, but the two do not necessarily occur in conjunction with each other. OXYGENATION/CHILD

312. **#2.** The major sequela of rheumatic fever is heart damage, particularly scarring of the mitral valve. Bedrest is recommended for the client with carditis to minimize metabolic needs and ease the work load of the heart.

313. **#2.** All are potential stressors, but the school-age child is especially vulnerable to the loss of control that results from decreased and restricted mobility. Gail is old enough to understand and accept explanations of possible outcomes, reasons for hospitalization, and procedures such as venipuncture, but is likely to be easily frustrated by bedrest requirements. ILL AND HOSPITALIZED CHILD/CHILD

314. **#2.** Seven-year-old Susan is somewhat young to be the best choice, even though she has the same health problem. Because Gail has carditis, she should not be placed with Sharon; Gail had a recent strep infection and Sharon's condition may be aggravated by exposure to a potential source of infection. On the other hand, Evelyn has a fever, which may indicate a concurrent infection to which Gail should not be exposed. Amy is the best choice, because she is close enough in age, has no infectious condition, and, like Gail, has a chronic illness. OXYGENATION/CHILD

315. **#4.** Gail is on bedrest with bathroom privileges and cannot go to the playroom. Listening to records and watching television are passive activities. Crocheting requires minimal exertion, does not involve the large joints which may be painful, and also fosters Gail's feelings of accomplishment. ILL AND HOSPITALIZED CHILD/CHILD

316. **#3.** A decreasing ESR indicates a decrease in the body's inflammatory response. The WBC is slightly elevated; a positive C-reactive protein indicates continued inflammation; the elevated ASO titer indicates a recent strep infection. OXYGENATION/CHILD

317. #3. Gail is able to cognitively understand full explanations using correct terminology. Such explanations also consider her emotional needs and foster feelings of control. However, while she should be included in making decisions that affect her, she is not legally able to give consent for or refuse necessary care. Concrete thinking and misunderstanding of the causes of illness characterize the younger child. HEALTHY CHILD/CHILD

318. #3. There is a need during this phase to integrate the experience of delivery into reality. An interest in rooming-in and care usually follow in 2–3 days. POSTPARTAL CARE/ CHILDBEARING FAMILY

319. #1. This indicates normal uterine involution. At this stage lochia should be rubra. Serosa is a sign that the cervix is blocked, probably by clots. Engorgement and healing do not occur this early. POSTPARTAL CARE/ CHILDBEARING FAMILY

320. #3. Complete emptying of the breasts is important for the comfort of the mother. Engorgement is a normal physiologic process. The newborn should be stimulated to suck. Restriction of fluids to less than 6–8 glasses daily is not appropriate. Ice packs may relieve discomfort between feedings but may reduce flow of milk as blood vessels, ducts constrict. POSTPARTAL CARE/CHILDBEARING FAMILY

321. #2. The shape of the breast will not be changed by breast-feeding. The bra will prevent breakdown of breast musculature and provide comfort. POSTPARTAL CARE/ CHILDBEARING FAMILY

322. #4. The newborn sleeps more than 20 hours daily, nurses every 2 to 3 hours, urinates often, and has frequent stools. New parents will find their lives dramatically changed. The newborn will feed on demand in the first weeks, and parents cannot ''schedule'' naps or feedings. The father's comment on crying indicates a lack of understanding of the newborn's need to communicate and need for love. NEWBORN CARE/CHILD BEARING FAMILY

323. #4. Breast size is not a factor in volume of milk produced. This mother needs support and teaching. POSTPARTAL CARE/ CHILDBEARING FAMILY

324. #2. Although all these pieces of information may be important and may be ascertained at some point during Katie's hospital stay, the nurse must know Katie's usual patterns in order to develop an appropriate care plan to meet Katie's toileting needs. ILL AND HOSPITALIZED CHILD/CHILD

325. #4. Dressing without supervision, sharing with other children, and using complete sentences are characteristics of preschoolers, not toddlers. Katie should have learned to use a spoon well by 18 months of age. HEALTHY CHILD/ CHILD

326. #3. When a microdrip is used for an intravenous infusion, the number of ml per hour is equal to the number of drops per minute. Therefore, the nurse should divide the total amount of 500 ml by 8 hours to determine the amount per hour to be infused. This amount equals 63 ml per hour; therefore, the microdrip regulator should be set at 63 drops per minute. ILL AND HOSPITALIZED CHILD/CHILD

327. #4. Bed linens should be changed frequently to prevent chilling and promote comfort. Cough suppressants are contraindicated, and children with croup need a liberal fluid intake because of the possibility of dehydration secondary to increased sensible fluid loss. Katie is too young to comprehend an explanation of why she must stay in the tent. OXYGENATION/CHILD

328. #1. Chest therapy in a child with a respiratory infection should be carried out just prior to mealtimes so the airway is cleared and Katie will be able to eat without tiring. Chest therapy should also be done at bedtime to facilitate sleep by helping Katie breathe more easily. Chest therapy after meals may cause Katie to vomit. Trying to schedule the treatment around Katie's naptimes is inefficient and too unpredictable. OXYGENATION/CHILD

329. #2. Chest therapy is carried out to keep the lower airway passage clear, and to facilitate drainage of lower airway secretions. Inspiratory stridor, suprasternal retractions, and a harsh metallic cough indicate upper airway involvement and are not used to evaluate the effectiveness of chest percussion and drainage. The presence of rales and rhonchi indicates that the lower airway passages are still congested and, therefore, the treatment has not been completely effective. OXYGENATION/CHILD

330. **#3.** Protest behavior most characterizes the toddler's separation from parents. Despair or detachment behavior is unlikely to appear when hospitalization is short, especially when parents visit daily. ILL AND HOSPITALIZED CHILD/CHILD

331. **#1.** Of all the age groups, toddlers handle separation and hospitalization very poorly. If a mother cannot room in, the next best thing is an article of clothing to remind the child of the mother. ILL AND HOSPITALIZED CHILD/ CHILD

332. **#3.** Allowing Katie to sleep with her parents may increase Katie's insecurity and reinforces dependency (not autonomy) since this was not part of her routine prior to hospitalization. HEALTHY CHILD/CHILD

333. **#4.** Respiratory infections, such as flu or colds, are the most common cause of exacerbations in clients with emphysema (chronic obstructive pulmonary disease [COPD]). Health teaching for clients with COPD includes instructions on how to prevent respiratory infections and directions to seek early treatment of respiratory infections that do occur. OXYGENATION/ADULT

334. **#2.** Aminophylline has a beta-adrenergic effect that results in the relaxation of bronchial muscle. Aminophylline has no mucolytic or sedative effects. OXYGENATION/ADULT

335. **#4.** Tachycardia and palpitations are common side effects of aminophylline because it stimulates the cardiac muscle. Other side effects include GI upset, urinary frequency, nervousness, and insomnia. OXYGENATION/ ADULT

336. **#3.** A normal pH with elevated pCO_2 indicates chronic respiratory acidosis. Clients with chronic COPD adjust to the high level of arterial CO_2, and signs of neurologic involvement are usually not present. Oxygen is always administered in low concentrations (1–2 liter/min) in the presence of hypercapnia and hypoxia because of the danger of CO_2 narcosis and respiratory failure. OXYGENATION/ ADULT

337. **#1.** Among the antimicrobial drugs, penicillins are most often responsible for anaphylaxis because of their allergic properties. Persons known to be allergic to one penicillin preparation should not be given any form of the drug. OXYGENATION/ADULT

338. **#1.** Disruption in the integrity of the pleura allows air from the lung to enter the pleural (not mediastinal) space. In this case, there is no rib involvement. OXYGENATION/ADULT

339. **#2.** The primary purpose of a chest tube is to reestablish subatmospheric (negative) pressure in the pleural space by the removal of air and fluid. This allows reexpansion of the lung. OXYGENATION/ADULT

340. **#4.** Correct information allays anxiety. Option #4 is the most accurate and is more specific than option #2. Options #1 and #3 do not answer the client's question. When the lung is fully expanded, the bubbling will cease. In a chest drainage system, connected to suction, continuous bubbling in the second bottle indicates normal functioning. OXYGENATION/ADULT

341. **#3.** Clients with emphysema may not be able to tolerate eating large meals; they might tolerate frequent small meals better. Also their need for carbohydrates is increased due to the increased energy expended for the work of breathing. OXYGENATION/ADULT

342. **#1.** The willingness to accept professional help depends upon the need as the client and family see it. All the other factors are important also, but first the client and family must want the service. THERAPEUTIC USE OF SELF/ PSYCHOSOCIAL, MENTAL HEALTH, PSYCHIATRIC PROBLEMS

343. **#3.** This response encourages the client to discuss his feelings and can provide important clues to what is troubling him or what has been difficult for him. THERAPEUTIC USE OF SELF/PSYCHOSOCIAL, MENTAL HEALTH, PSYCHIATRIC PROBLEMS

344. **#4.** Even diminished intake can lead to withdrawal symptoms. Cessation is not a prerequisite to their occurrence. SUBSTANCE USE DISORDER/PSYCHOSOCIAL, MENTAL HEALTH, PSYCHIATRIC PROBLEMS

345. **#2.** The alcoholic client's denial of problems is evidenced by recognition that something is wrong, but denying that medical, emotional, or social problems are related to the consumption of alcohol. #1 and #4 may be seen, but are not the priority for developing nursing care. Once the problem of denial is addressed, dependency and projection will decrease. #3, paranoia, is not a defense mechanism. SUBSTANCE USE DISORDER/ PSYCHOSOCIAL, MENTAL HEALTH, PSYCHIATRIC PROBLEMS

346. #1. The lowest rate of recidivism has been shown for those alcoholic clients who become involved with AA. Peer support and networking has more success than family or individual therapy or the chronic disease approach. Alcoholics Anonymous may be used in combination with these treatment approaches. SUBSTANCE USE DISORDER/PSYCHOSOCIAL, MENTAL HEALTH, PSYCHIATRIC PROBLEMS

347. #1. Although genetic factors and chronic disease effects are important, options #2 through #4 are important areas to explore and focus upon in the family-therapy sessions. SUBSTANCE USE DISORDER/PSYCHOSOCIAL, MENTAL HEALTH, PSYCHIATRIC PROBLEMS

348. #3. In the detoxification stage of alcoholism the body chemistry changes can be rapid and severe. Sodium potassium level changes are especially vulnerable because of vomiting and fluid shifts. The heart, already burdened by the process of detoxification, is especially sensitive to low potassium levels. Option #1 is important but not as dangerous a problem. #2 is true but is not an immediate concern. #4 is a priority at a later stage. SUBSTANCE USE DISORDER/PSYCHOSOCIAL, MENTAL HEALTH, PSYCHIATRIC PROBLEMS

349. #4. The patient needs to do his own evaluating as to his readiness to change direction. The nurse serves best by helping him to clarify his thoughts and feelings. #2 is judgmental and insensitive. The timing belongs to the patient. #3 is inconsequential in light of the patient's remarks. #1 might be appropriate but #4 is more geared to the feeling level of the statement. SUBSTANCE USE DISORDER/PSYCHOSOCIAL, MENTAL HEALTH, PSYCHIATRIC PROBLEMS

350. #4. Too much sympathy and empathy reinforce the client's view of himself as a victim of alcohol, drugs, or other people. The client will not accept responsibility for himself, nor will he be able to break through his denial if a high level of sympathy and empathy is given. The client would then manipulate his nurse and avoid dealing with his problems. Options #1, #2, and #3 are critical to setting the stage for the client to work on his problems. The client needs to internalize limits. SUBSTANCE USE DISORDER/PSYCHOSOCIAL, MENTAL HEALTH, PSYCHIATRIC PROBLEMS

351. #4. While a dietary deficiency of iodine may cause goiter and hypothyroidism, dietary iodine is not now considered a risk factor in the development of thyroid cancer. However, a history of irradiation of head, neck, or chest (e.g., for acne, enlarged thymus or tonsils, Hodgkin's disease) is strongly associated with the development of thyroid cancer. High doses of vitamin D are used to treat hypoparathyroidism. NUTRITION AND METABOLISM/ADULT

352. #1. An enlarged thyroid may encroach on organs in close proximity. Swallowing and breathing are usually the first functions to be affected. Muscle twitching and tingling around the lips would be the result of parathyroid involvement. NUTRITION AND METABOLISM/ADULT

353. #3. Options #1 and #2 suggest hypofunction of the thyroid gland. The symptoms listed in option #4 are not, as a group, specific for thyroid dysfunction. NUTRITION AND METABOLISM/ADULT

354. #2. Primary thyroid hyperactivity is characterized by elevations in serum triiodothyronine (T_3) and/or thyroxine (T_4). Secondary hyperthyroidism, caused by malfunction of the pituitary gland, is characterized by an overproduction of thyroid-stimulating hormone (TSH). Serum ACTH levels remain unaffected unless hyperpituitarism is involved. NUTRITION AND METABOLISM/ADULT

355. #3. Graves' disease is hyperthyroidism accompanied by goiter and/or exophthalmos. It is thought to be autoimmune in nature because of the presence of long-acting thyroid stimulators (LATS) in the blood of many, but not all, affected persons. Myxedema is caused by hypofunction of the thyroid; cretinism is caused by congenital hypothyroidism. Addison's disease is caused by adrenocortical hypofunction. NUTRITION AND METABOLISM/ADULT

356. #3. Exophthalmos is characterized by bulging eyes. To prevent drying of the overly exposed eyeballs, lubricating eye drops, such as methylcellulose drops, are frequently prescribed. In addition, self-lubrication and protection through regular blinking are encouraged. While not specific to exopthalmos, placement of clients in areas of low environmental stimuli in order to decrease adrenergic activity and frequent monitoring of vital signs for changes are considered important aspects of the nursing care plan. NUTRITION AND METABOLISM/ADULT

357. #1. Results of the test are affected by the client's intake of iodides (in medications or x-ray contrast media) and thyroid hormones. Proper interpretation of results requires this information be noted on laboratory slips. This test does not involve a 24-hour urine collection. Rather, the thyroid is scanned and the amount of radioactivity is determined. The patient is not placed in isolation. NUTRITION AND METABOLISM/ADULT

358. #3. Propylthiouracil should be taken every 8 hours to ensure adequate levels over a 24-hour period. Too low a dosage will be evidenced by a return of weight loss and rapid pulse rate. A serious side effect of this drug is agranulocytosis, evidenced by indications of infection (fever, sore throat, or rash). In returning to a euthyroid state, the client can be expected to regain previously lost weight. NUTRITION AND METABOLISM/ADULT

359. #2. To disguise the salty taste and to decrease gastric irritation, iodine solutions should be well diluted in a full glass of fruit juice, milk, or water and administered after meals and at bedtime. NUTRITION AND METABOLISM/ADULT

360. #4. These symptoms are indicative of iodine poisoning (iodism). The nurse's first action should be to discontinue iodine therapy and report the client's signs and symptoms to the physician. A secondary consideration is to explore additional sources of iodine in the diet (e.g., iodized salt, seafood, vegetables grown near the seaside). Isolation of the client is not required, and symptoms will subside with adjustment of iodine intake. NUTRITION AND METABOLISM/ADULT

361. #4. Hemorrhage is a serious complication following thyroidectomy. Because of gravity, drainage may not be visible along the suture line on the anterior neck dressing, but rather at the back of the neck and upper part of the back. The preferred position for the post-thyroidectomy client is semi-Fowler's with good neck support. Turning, coughing, and deep breathing as well as early ambulation can be accomplished while the head and neck are supported in a neutral position. NUTRITION AND METABOLISM/ADULT

362. #4. Increasing hoarseness post-thyroidectomy may indicate injury to the recurrent laryngeal nerve or swelling in the area of the glottis. Parathyroid injury will be evidenced by muscular tingling or twitching. NUTRITION AND METABOLISM/ADULT

363. #3. Respiratory distress and a tightening neck dressing may indicate hemorrhage into tissues or increasing edema in the neck area. Loosening the dressing to prevent further tracheal compression should be the nurse's first action. Reinforcement of the dressing would only increase tracheal compression. High-Fowler's position alone will not decrease swelling; the dressing must also be loosened. NUTRITION AND METABOLISM/ADULT

364. #1. Sitting in a chair, brushing the teeth, and lying on one's side may all be accomplished without the flexion, extension, or rotation of the neck that should be avoided in the early post-op period because of the strain this places on the suture line. The client must be instructed to turn the whole body, not just the head during this time. NUTRITION AND METABOLISM/ADULT

365. #3. Injury to the parathyroid gland would be accompanied by decreased serum calcium, elevated serum phosphorus, painful muscle spasms, tingling around the lips, and numbness of the fingertips. NUTRITION AND METABOLISM/ADULT

366. #3. The treatment of choice, both on an emergency and long-term basis, is the administration of calcium gluconate. Thyroid preparations have no influence on parathyroid functioning. Digitalis is a cardiotonic and requires normal levels of calcium to produce desired effects. Since phosphate levels increase in hypoparathyroid conditions, dietary phosphorus would be contraindicated. NUTRITION AND METABOLISM/ADULT

367. **#1.** Following total removal of the thyroid gland, the client must take thyroid medication daily for the rest of life to supply the hormones essential for maintenance of body metabolism. Since the thyroid hormones themselves are taken, dietary iodine is no longer needed to support their synthesis within the body. Dietary iodine need not be advised or restricted. NUTRITION AND METABOLISM/ADULT

368. **#1.** Elevated blood pressure is one of the primary manifestations of poststreptococcal nephritis and should be monitored on a regular basis. Return of the blood pressure to normal indicates the disease process is resolving. The edema associated with this disease affects the face and extremities, not the abdomen, so it is not necessary to measure abdominal girth. The urine should be checked for specific gravity, protein, and blood. Although assessment of breath sounds is an important part of evaluating general health status, it is not essential in this case. ELIMINATION/CHILD

369. **#3.** The child with poststreptococcal nephritis needs a diet with normal protein, moderate sodium restriction, and low potassium. This meal is high in sodium (bacon) and high in potassium (orange juice) and, therefore, indicates the mother does not clearly understand the diet or the importance of the restrictions. ELIMINATION/CHILD

370. **#1.** Fewer than one-quarter of the children with poststreptococcal nephritis develop chronic renal failure. Recurrences are very rare. With proper treatment, these children return to normal renal functioning within 3 to 4 weeks. ELIMINATION/CHILD

371. **#2.** This response acknowledges empathy and encourages further expression of feeling. #1 is too confrontive, too fast. #3 cuts off communication of feelings between client and nurse. #4 is too demanding of information and cuts off spontaneous discussion of feelings by the client. LOSS, DEATH, DYING/ PSYCHOSOCIAL, MENTAL HEALTH, PSYCHIATRIC PROBLEMS

372. **#3.** Terminally ill clients need to review their lives to explore the meaning their lives have had. #1 and #4 reinforces denial and nonacceptance of the inevitable. Withdrawal from relationships normally occurs among the terminally ill. LOSS, DEATH, DYING/ PSYCHOSOCIAL, MENTAL HEALTH, PSYCHIATRIC PROBLEMS

373. **#2.** Verbalize implied feelings, give the client permission to discuss feelings, and assist the client to work through the denial stage. Options #1 and #3 cut off communication. Silent support is important but is not appropriate when the client is demonstrating a need to talk and is asking for information. LOSS, DEATH, DYING/PSYCHOSOCIAL, MENTAL HEALTH, PSYCHIATRIC PROBLEMS

374. **#2.** Verbal expression of grief facilitates mourning. Option #1 is too controlling, does not permit individual needs of family members in dealing with their grief. #3 discourages family members from taking care of themselves and could hamper the family grieving process. #4 does not facilitate the family's communication about the grieving process. LOSS, DEATH, DYING/PSYCHOSOCIAL, MENTAL HEALTH, PSYCHIATRIC PROBLEMS

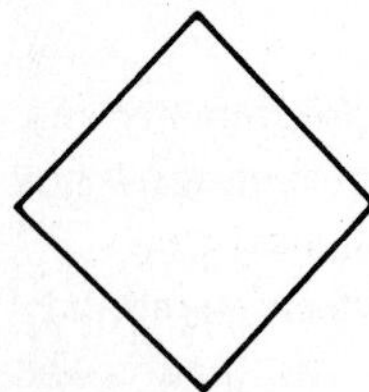

Nursing Process and Client Needs Categories

AS = Assessment
AN = Analysis
PL = Plan
IM = Implementation
EV = Evaluation

E = Safe, Effective Care Environment
PS = Physiological Integrity
PC = Psychological Integrity
H = Health Promotion and Maintenance

	Nursing Process	Client Needs
1.	AS	PC
2.	AS	E
3.	AN	PS
4.	EV	H
5.	AN	H
6.	AS	H
7.	IM	PC
8.	IM	PC
9.	PL	PC
10.	AN	PC
11.	IM	PC
12.	IM	PC
13.	AN	PC
14.	IM	H
15.	IM	PC
16.	AN	PC
17.	PL	E
18.	IM	PC
19.	AN	E
20.	AN	PS
21.	AS	PS
22.	IM	E
23.	PL	PS
24.	AS	PS
25.	IM	PC
26.	AS	PS
27.	AN	E
28.	AS	PS
29.	IM	PS
30.	EV	PS
31.	AN	PS
32.	EV	PS
33.	PL	PC
34.	AN	H
35.	AN	H
36.	PL	H
37.	EV	H
38.	AN	E

	Nursing Process	Client Needs
39.	IM	E
40.	AS	PS
41.	IM	E
42.	AS	H
43.	IM	PC
44.	IM	E
45.	PL	H
46.	IM	PS
47.	AS	PS
48.	AN	PC
49.	EV	PC
50.	IM	H
51.	AN	PS
52.	AN	PS
53.	IM	H
54.	EV	E
55.	AS	H
56.	AS	E
57.	AN	H
58.	EV	E
59.	EV	E
60.	IM	E
61.	IM	E
62.	IM	PC
63.	EV	H
64.	IM	E
65.	IM	H
66.	AN	H
67.	AS	H
68.	AN	PC
69.	AN	PC
70.	AS	PC
71.	AS	PC
72.	PL	E
73.	IM	PC
74.	IM	PC
75.	IM	PC
76.	EV	PC

	Nursing Process	Client Needs
77.	AS	PC
78.	IM	PS
79.	AN	PC
80.	IM	PC
81.	AS	PS
82.	PL	E
83.	EV	PS
84.	IM	PC
85.	IM	PS
86.	IM	PS
87.	AN	E
88.	AS	PS
89.	AS	PS
90.	AN	H
91.	IM	E
92.	AN	PS
93.	IM	E
94.	IM	PS
95.	IM	PS
96.	AN	PS
97.	AN	PS
98.	IM	E
99.	PL	E
100.	EV	H
101.	IM	E
102.	EV	E
103.	IM	PS
104.	PL	PS
105.	IM	PS
106.	AN	PS
107.	IM	PS
108.	EV	PS
109.	AS	PS
110.	IM	PS
111.	PL	PS
112.	AS	PS
113.	AS	PS
114.	AN	PC
115.	AN	PC
116.	PL	E
117.	AN	PS
118.	IM	PS
119.	IM	H
120.	IM	E
121.	AN	PS
122.	IM	E
123.	IM	PC
124.	IM	E
125.	IM	H
126.	AS	PS
127.	IM	PS
128.	EV	PS

	Nursing Process	Client Needs
129.	AN	PC
130.	IM	PC
131.	IM	PC
132.	AN	PC
133.	AS	PS
134.	IM	E
135.	AN	PC
136.	EV	PC
137.	AN	E
138.	IM	PS
139.	AN	PS
140.	IM	E
141.	IM	E
142.	IM	PS
143.	IM	PC
144.	IM	E
145.	IM	H
146.	EV	PS
147.	EV	E
148.	AS	PC
149.	AS	H
150.	AN	H
151.	AS	H
152.	IM	H
153.	PL	PS
154.	EV	PS
155.	AN	PS
156.	IM	H
157.	IM	PC
158.	EV	H
159.	IM	PC
160.	AN	PC
161.	IM	E
162.	IM	E
163.	IM	E
164.	AN	PS
165.	AN	PC
166.	IM	E
167.	IM	H
168.	IM	E
169.	IM	H
170.	IM	PS
171.	PL	E
172.	PL	PS
173.	EV	PC
174.	PL	PS
175.	PL	PS
176.	EV	E
177.	AS	PS
178.	IM	H
179.	IM	H
180.	PL	PS

	Nursing Process	Client Needs
181.	AS	PS
182.	AS	E
183.	IM	E
184.	AS	PS
185.	IM	PC
186.	AN	PC
187.	PL	PC
188.	IM	PS
189.	AS	PS
190.	PL	E
191.	AS	PS
192.	AS	E
193.	IM	PS
194.	IM	E
195.	IM	H
196.	IM	E
197.	AN	PS
198.	EV	E
199.	EV	PC
200.	AS	PS
201.	AN	E
202.	AS	H
203.	AN	H
204.	AN	PC
205.	PL	H
206.	IM	PC
207.	IM	E
208.	AN	PC
209.	AS	PS
210.	AS	PS
211.	IM	E
212.	IM	E
213.	IM	E
214.	AN	E
215.	IM	E
216.	IM	PS
217.	IM	PS
218.	AN	PS
219.	AS	PS
220.	AS	PS
221.	IM	PS
222.	AS	PS
223.	AS	PS
224.	IM	E
225.	AS	PS
226.	IM	PS
227.	IM	E
228.	AS	E
229.	PL	PS
230.	IM	E
231.	IM	PC
232.	IM	H

	Nursing Process	Client Needs
233.	AN	PC
234.	IM	PC
235.	EV	PC
236.	AN	PS
237.	PL	PS
238.	AS	PS
239.	AS	PC
240.	AN	PC
241.	PL	E
242.	AS	PC
243.	AN	PC
244.	IM	E
245.	AN	PC
246.	PL	PC
247.	IM	PC
248.	IM	PC
249.	EV	PC
250.	EV	PC
251.	IM	E
252.	PL	E
253.	IM	H
254.	AN	H
255.	IM	H
256.	EV	H
257.	AS	PS
258.	IM	PC
259.	AN	PS
260.	AN	PC
261.	PL	H
262.	AS	E
263.	AS	PC
264.	PL	PC
265.	IM	E
266.	PL	PC
267.	EV	PC
268.	AS	E
269.	IM	E
270.	IM	E
271.	EV	E
272.	AS	H
273.	AN	PS
274.	AS	PS
275.	IM	PC
276.	IM	H
277.	IM	H
278.	EV	E
279.	PL	PC
280.	IM	PC
281.	IM	E
282.	IM	E
283.	IM	E
284.	IM	E

	Nursing Process	Client Needs
285.	AN	PC
286.	AN	PC
287.	IM	PC
288.	AS	PS
289.	EV	H
290.	AN	E
291.	IM	E
292.	IM	E
293.	AN	PS
294.	PL	E
295.	AN	E
296.	AS	PC
297.	IM	E
298.	AN	PC
299.	IM	PC
300.	IM	E
301.	IM	E
302.	IM	PC
303.	AS	PC
304.	AN	PC
305.	IM	PC
306.	IM	H
307.	IM	PC
308.	IM	H
309.	IM	PC
310.	PL	PC
311.	AS	PS
312.	PL	E
313.	PL	PS
314.	PL	H
315.	IM	E
316.	EV	PS
317.	AN	PS
318.	AN	PC
319.	AS	PS
320.	PL	E
321.	IM	E
322.	EV	H
323.	IM	H
324.	AS	H
325.	AS	H
326.	IM	E
327.	IM	E
328.	PL	E
329.	EV	PS

	Nursing Process	Client Needs
330.	AS	PS
331.	PL	PS
332.	PL	PS
333.	AS	E
334.	AS	PS
335.	AS	PS
336.	AN	PS
337.	AS	PS
338.	AS	PS
339.	AS	E
340.	AS	E
341.	IM	H
342.	AN	H
343.	IM	E
344.	AN	PC
345.	AN	PC
346.	PL	PC
347.	AN	PC
348.	PL	PS
349.	IM	PC
350.	IM	E
351.	AS	PS
352.	AS	PS
353.	AS	PS
354.	AS	PS
355.	AS	PS
356.	IM	E
257.	PL	E
358.	IM	H
359.	IM	E
360.	IM	E
361.	IM	PS
362.	EV	PS
363.	IM	PS
364.	IM	H
365.	AS	PS
366.	PL	PS
367.	IM	H
368.	EV	PS
369.	AN	PS
370.	EV	PS
371.	IM	PC
372.	IM	PC
373.	IM	H
374.	IM	PC

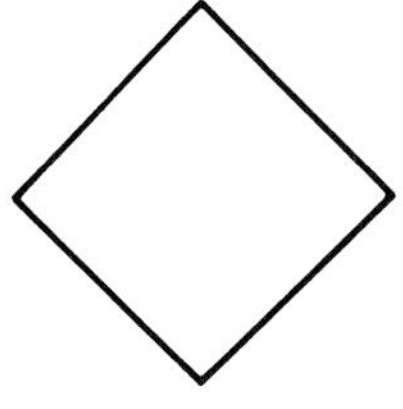

Appendix A

Approved Nursing Diagnoses from the North American Nursing Diagnosis Association, June 1988

Exchanging
Altered nutrition: more than body requirements
Altered nutrition: less than body requirements
Altered nutrition: potential for more than body requirements
Potential for infection
Potential altered body temperature
Hypothermia
Hyperthermia
Ineffective thermoregulation
Dysreflexia
Constipation
Perceived constipation
Colonic constipation
Diarrhea
Bowel incontinence
Altered patterns of urinary elimination
Stress incontinence
Reflex incontinence
Urge incontinence
Functional incontinence
Total incontinence
Urinary retention
Altered tissue perfusion (specify type: renal, cerebral, cardiopulmonary, gastrointestinal, peripheral)
Fluid volume excess
Fluid volume deficit (1)
Fluid volume deficit (2)
Potential fluid volume deficit
Decreased cardiac output
Impaired gas exchange
Ineffective airway clearance
Ineffective breathing pattern
Potential for injury
Potential for suffocation
Potential for poisoning
Potential for trauma
Potential for aspiration
Potential for disuse syndrome
Potential impaired skin integrity
Impaired skin integrity
Impaired tissue integrity
Altered oral mucous membrane

Communicating
Impaired verbal communication

Relating
Impaired social interaction
Social isolation
Altered role performance
Altered parenting
Potential altered parenting
Sexual dysfunction
Altered family processes
Parental role conflict
Altered sexuality patterns

Valuing
Spiritual distress

Choosing
Ineffective individual coping
Impaired adjustment
Defensive coping
Ineffective denial
Ineffective family coping: disabling
Ineffective family coping: compromised
Family coping: potential for growth
Noncompliance
Decisional conflict
Health seeking behaviors

Moving
Impaired physical mobility
Activity intolerance
Fatigue
Potential activity intolerance
Sleep pattern disturbance
Diversional activity deficit
Impaired home maintenance management
Altered health maintenance
Feeding self care deficit
Impaired swallowing
Ineffective breastfeeding
Bathing/hygiene self care deficit
Dressing/grooming self care deficit

Toileting self care deficit
Altered growth and development
Perceiving
Body image disturbance
Self esteem disturbance
Chronic low self esteem
Situational low self esteem
Personal identity disturbance
Sensory/perceptual alterations (specify) (visual, auditory kinesthetic, gustatory, tactile, olfactory)
Unilateral neglect
Hopelessness
Powerlessness
Knowing
Knowledge deficit
Altered thought processes
Feeling
Pain
Chronic pain
Dysfunctional grieving
Anticipatory grieving
Potential for violence: self-directed or directed at others
Post-trauma response
Rape-trauma syndrome
Rape-trauma syndrome: compound reaction
Rape-trauma syndrome: silent reaction
Anxiety
Fear

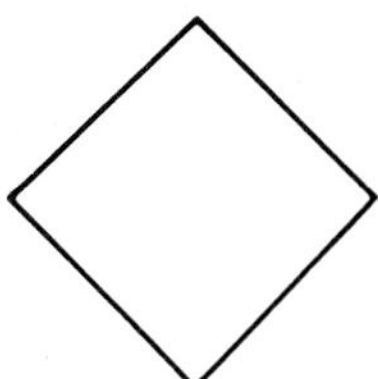

Appendix B
Common Laboratory Values—Adult[a]

	Conventional	SI Units
Hematologic Tests		
Hematocrit	Male: 42%–54%	0.42–0.54
	Female: 38%–46%	0.38–0.46
Hemoglobin	Male: 14–18 gm/100 ml	8.1–11.2 mmol/L
	Female: 12–16 gm/ml	7.4–9.9 mmol/L
Red Blood Cells	4.2–6.2 million/mm^3	4.2–6.2 × 10^{12}/L
White Blood Cells	5,000–10,000/mm^3	5–10 × 10^9/L
Platelets	150,000–350,000/mm^3	150–350 × 10^9/L
Erythrocyte Sedimentation Rate	Male: 0–10 mm/hour	0–10 mm/hour
	Female: 0–20 mm/hour	0–20 mm/hour
Prothrombin Time	<2 seconds deviation from control	<2 seconds deviation from control
Partial Thromboplastin Time	25–38 seconds	25–38 seconds
Blood Chemistry Tests		
Acid Phosphatase[b]	Male: 0.13–0.63 sigma units/ml	36–175 nmol. sec^{-1}/L
	Female: 0.01–0.56 sigma units/ml	2.8–156 nmol. sec^{-1}/L
Alkaline Phosphatase[b]	13–39 units/L	217–650 nmol. sec^{-1}/L
Albumin	3.5–5.0 g/100 ml	35–50 g/L
Ammonia	12–55 mcmol/L	12–55 mcmol/L
Amylase[b]	4–25 units/ml	4–25 arb. units
Bilirubin	Direct:	
	up to 0.4–1.5 mg/100 ml	up to 7 mcmol/L
	Total:	
	up to 1.0 mg/100 ml	up to 17 mcmol/L
Calcium	8.5–10.5 mg/100 ml	2.1–2.6 mmol/L
CO_2	24–30 mEq/L	24–30 mmol/L
Chloride	100–106 mEq/L	100–106 mmol/L
Cholesterol	120–200 mg/100 ml	3.1–5.69 mmol/L
Creatine Kinase[b]	Male: 17–148 units/L	238–2467 nmol sec^{-1}/L
(Creatine Phosphokinase)	Female: 10–79 units/L	167–1317 nmol sec^{-1}/L
Creatinine	0.6–1.5 mg/100 ml	53–133 mcmol/L
Globulin	2.3–3.5 g/100 ml	23–35 g/L
Glucose	70–110 mg/100 ml	3.9–5.6 mmol/L
Iron	50–150 mcg/L	9.0–26.9 mcmol/L
Iron-binding Capacity	250–410 mcg/100 ml	44.8–73.4 mcmol/L
Lactic Dehydrogenase[b]	45–90 units/L	750–1,500 nmol sec^{-1}/L
Lipase[b]	2 units/ml or less	up to 2 arb. units
Lithium	0.5–1.5 mEq/L	0.5–1.5 mEq/L
O_2 Saturation	96%–100%	0.96–1.00
PCO_2	35–45 mm Hg	4.7–6.0 kPa
pH	7.35–7.45	7.35–7.45
PO_2	75–100 mm HG	10–13.3 kPa

	Conventional	SI Units
Potassium	3.5–5.0 mEq/L	3.5–5.0 nmol/L
Protein	6.0–8.4 g/100 ml	60–84 g/L
SGOT[b]	7–27 units/L	117–450 nmol sec^{-1}/L
SGPT[b]	1–21 units/L	17–350 nmol sec^{-1}/L
Sodium	135–145 mEq/L	135–145 nmol/L
Triglycerides	40–150 mg/100 ml	0.4–1.5 g/L
Urea Nitrogen	8–25 mg/100 ml	2.9–8.9 nmol/L
Uric Acid	3–7 mg/100 ml	0.18–0.42 mmol/L

Reference: Tilkian, S., Conover, M., and Tilkian, A. (1987). *Clinical implications of laboratory tests, 4th ed.*, St. Louis, MO: Mosby.

[a]Normal value ranges will vary from laboratory to laboratory.

[b]Enzyme value ranges may vary widely from laboratory to laboratory. Any actual patient result must be compared with laboratory standards for accurate evaluation.

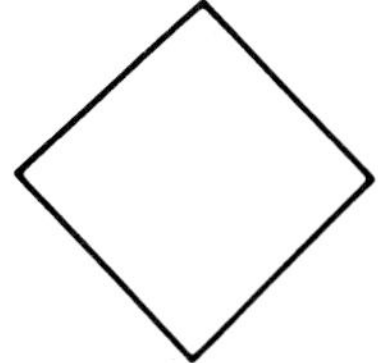

Appendix C

Information for Foreign Nurse Graduates Who Wish to Practice in the United States

Nursing practice in the United States is regulated by each state through its Nurse Practice Act and the State Board of Nursing (or State Board of Nurse Examiners). These licensing laws and appointed boards establish the qualifications for obtaining a license in the state, as well as the grounds for denying a license to an applicant or suspending a nurse's license. Of particular significance is the board's role in defining the scope of nursing practice in a particular state. Qualifications for obtaining a license generally include:

- graduation from an accredited nursing education program
- a satisfactory score on the National Council Licensure Examination (NCLEX) or Canadian Nursing Association Testing Service (CNATS)
- submission of a completed application form with specified fee

Foreign nurse graduates must also obtain an H1 visa, which is a temporary working visa granted to individuals who are not seeking permanent residency in the United States. To obtain an H1 visa, a foreign nurse graduate must have a certificate issued by the U.S. Commission on Graduates of Foreign Nursing Schools (CGFNS). This requirement also applies to Canadian nurses who want to obtain a license in Indiana, Montana, South Dakota, and Washington state. The CGFNS certificate is awarded for successful scores on an examination. This multiple-choice examination is intended to screen foreign nurse graduates and evaluate their understanding of written English and medical terminology, as well as their basic nursing knowledge. The CGFNS examination is given twice a year in sites throughout the world. To take this examination, the foreign nurse graduate must submit a completed application form and $95 (U.S.) three months before the examination is held, i.e., 1 January for the April exam and 1 July for the October exam. The CGFNS address is 3624 Market St., Philadelphia, PA 19104.

After obtaining a CGFNS certificate, the employing hospital will file for an H1 visa on behalf of the foreign nurse. The Bureau of Immigration and Naturalization Service returns the visa to the hospital who will send it to the nearest U.S. embassy for delivery to the nurse. Because this visa restricts the holder to working at only one hospital in the U.S., a new H1 visa must be obtained if the nurse wishes to work in another hospital or health care facility. Prior to coming to the U.S., the nurse should write to the appropriate State Board for information about obtaining a license and for an application to take the NCLEX at the next available opportunity. The foreign nurse graduate may then move to the U.S. and practice nursing, usually with some restrictions, until the next NCLEX examination is given. While the NCLEX examination is identical throughout the states, each state grants a license (that is the designation "Registered Nurse") based on the individual's score.

The NCLEX is a two-day long, multiple-choice examination that evaluates a nurse's ability to systematically analyze and conceptualize nursing care utilizing the scientific method of problem solving commonly called the Nursing Process. Successfully obtaining a minimum score on the examination enables the recipient to obtain a license to practice nursing in that state. Generally, once a license is obtained in one state, other states will recognize that license and grant their state license by endorsement. A nurse who wishes to relocate or move to another state (remember that a new H1 visa is required) should contact the State Board of Nursing of the prospective employer's state prior to the anticipated move to inquire about obtaining a license by endorsement. Requirements for licensure by endorsement vary and may change periodically, so it is important to obtain the most current information from the individual State Board of Nursing.

The H1 visa may be extended annually for a total of five years. A resident alien who wishes to remain in the U.S. beyond this period must apply for permanent residency.

A WORD FOR CANADIAN NURSES

Like the U.S., each Canadian province has its own nurse practice act and laws that vary slightly from province to province. All provinces, except Prince Edward Island and Ontario, require nurses to join the provincial nursing association to obtain a license. The provincial nursing association requires successful completion of the CNATS. Several U.S. states also accept the CNATS, thus exempting those Canadians who wish to practice in those states from taking the NCLEX. Those states include:

Alabama
Alaska
Arizona
Arkansas
California
Delaware
Georgia
Idaho
Kentucky
Maine
Mississippi
Missouri
New Mexico
North Dakota
Ohio
Pennsylvania
Rhode Island
Tennessee
Utah
Wisconsin

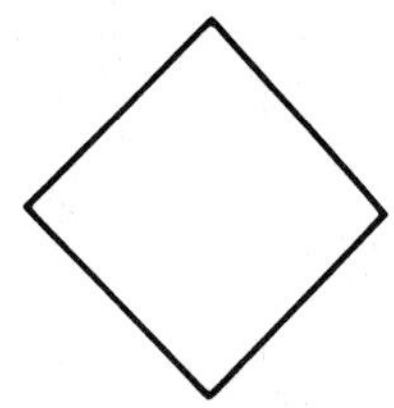

State Boards of Nursing

Shirley J. Dykes, Exec. Off.
Board of Nursing
500 Eastern Blvd., Suite 203
Montgomery, AL 36117 Tel.: (205) 261-4060

Gail McGuill, RN, Exec. Sec.
Alaska Board of Nursing
3601 C St., Suite 7222
Anchorage, AK 99503 Tel.: (907) 561-2878

E. B. U. Malae, RN, Sec.
Health Services Regulatory Board
LBJ Tropical Medical Center
Pago Pago, American Samoa 96799

F. Roberts, Exec. Dir.
Arizona State Board of Nursing
5050 W. 19 Ave., Suite 103
Phoenix, AZ 85015 Tel.: (602) 255-5092

June Garner, Exec. Dir.
Arkansas State Board of Nursing
Univ. Towers Bldg., Suite 800
Little Rock, AR 72204 Tel.: (501) 371-2751

Dr. Catherine Puri, Exec. Off.
Board of Registered Nursing
1030 13th St., Suite 200
Sacramento, CA 95814 Tel.: (916) 324-2715

Mrs. Karen Brunley, Prog. Admin.
Colorado State Board of Nursing
1525 Sherman St., Room 132
Denver, CO 82003 Tel.: (303) 866-2451

Dr. Marie Hilliard, Exec. Off.
Department of Health Services
150 Washington St.
Hartford, CT 06106 Tel.: (203) 566-1041

Rosalee J. Seymor, Exec. Dir.
Delaware Board of Nursing
O'Neill Bldg., P.O. Box 1401
Dover, DE 19901 Tel.: (302) 736-4522

Ms. Barbara Hagens, Pres.
District of Columbia Board of Nursing
614 H St. N.W.
Washington, DC 20013 Tel.: (202) 727-7468

Mrs. Judie K. Ritter, Exec. Dir.
Florida State Board of Nursing
111 E. Coastline Dr.
Jacksonville, FL 30303 Tel.: (904) 359-6339

Mrs. Carolyn Hutcherson, Exec. Dir.
Georgia Board of Nursing
166 Pryor St., S.W.
Atlanta, GA 30334 Tel.: (404) 656-3949

Teofila P. Cruz, Adm.
Guam Board of Nurse Examiners
P.O. Box 2816
Agana, Guam 96910 Tel.: (671) 724-2950

Jerold Sakoda, Exec. Sec.
Hawaii Board of Nursing
Box 3469
Honolulu, HI 96801 Tel.: (808) 548-3086

Mrs. Phyllis Sheridan, RN, Exec. Dir.
Idaho State Board of Nursing
700 West State St.
Boise, ID 83720 Tel.: (208) 334-3110

Judy Otto, Nursing Ed. Coord.
Department of Registration and Education
320 W. Washington St.
Springfield, IL 62786 Tel.: (217) 782-4385

Barbara Powers, Adm.
Indiana State Board of Nursing
1 American Sq., Box 82067, Rm. 1020
Indianapolis, IN 46282 Tel.: (317) 232-2960

Ann E. Mowery, Exec. Dir.
Iowa Board of Nursing
1223 E. Court Ave.
Des Moines, IA 50319 Tel.: (515) 281-4828

Dr. Lois Rich-Scibetta, RN, Exec. Admin.
Kansas State Board of Nursing
900 S.W. Jackson Landon St. Bldg.
Topeka, KS 66612-1256 Tel.: (913) 296-3782

Sharon M. Weisenbeck, Exec. Dir.
Kentucky Board of Nursing
4010 Dupont Cir., Suite 430
Louisville, KY 40207 Tel.: (502) 897-5143

Miss Merlyn Maillian, RN, Exec. Dir.
Louisiana State Board of Nursing
907 Pere Marquette Bldg.
New Orleans, LA 70112 Tel.: (504) 568-5464

Jean C. Carson, Exec. Dir.
Maine State Board of Nursing
295 Water St.
Augusta, ME 04330 Tel.: (207) 289-5324

Donna Dorsey, Exec. Dir.
Maryland Board of Nursing
201 W. Preston St.
Baltimore, MD 21201 Tel.: (301) 225-5880

Mary H. Snodgrass, Exec. Sec.
Board of Registration in Nursing
100 Cambridge St., Rm. 150
Boston, MA 02202 Tel.: (617) 727-9967

Elizabeth Jensen, Nsg. Consultant
Michigan Board of Nursing
P.O. Box 30018, 611 West Ottawa
Lansing, MI 48909 Tel.: (517) 332-1197

Joyce M. Schowalter, Exec. Dir.
Minnesota Board of Nursing
2700 University Ave., W. 108
Minneapolis, MN 55414 Tel.: (612) 642-0577

W. Ray Cleere, Commissioner Higher Ed.
Mississippi Board of Nursing
135 Bounds St., Suite 101
Jackson, MS 39206 Tel.: (601) 982-6611

Florence McGuire, RN, Exec. Dir.
Missouri State Board of Nursing
3523 N. Ten Mile Dr., P.O. Box 656
Jefferson City, MO 65101 Tel.: (314) 751-2334

Phyllis M. McDonald, Exec. Sec.
Montana State Board of Nursing
1424 Ninth Ave.
Helena, MT 59620-0407 Tel.: (406) 444-4279

Dr. Charlene Kelly, Assoc. Dir.
Bureau of Examining Bd., NE Dept. of Health
P.O. Box 95007
Lincoln, NE 68509 Tel.: (402) 471-2115

Lonna Burress, Exec. Dir.
Nevada State Board of Nursing
1280 Terminal Way, Room 116
Reno, NV 89502 Tel.: (702) 786-2778

Mrs. Martha Ginty, Exec. Dir.
State Board of Nursing
Dept. of Ed.—101 Pleasant St.
Concord, NH 03301 Tel.: (603) 271-2323

Sr. Teresa L. Harris, Exec. Dir.
New Jersey Board of Nursing
1100 Raymond Blvd., Room 319
Newark, NJ 07102 Tel.: (201) 648-2570

Nancy L. Twigg, Exec. Dir.
New Mexico Board of Nursing
4125 Carlisle N.E.
Albuquerque, NM 87107 Tel.: (505) 841-6524

Dr. Melene A. Megel, Exec. Sec.
New York State Board for Nursing
The Cultural Center, Room 3013
Albany, NY 12230 Tel.: (518) 474-3843

Carol A. Osman, Exec. Dir.
Board of Nursing
P.O. Box 2129
Raleigh, NC 27602 Tel.: (919) 828-0470

Karen MacDonald, Exec. Dir.
North Dakota Board of Nursing
7th St., South Arbor Ave.
Bismarck, ND 58501 Tel.: (701) 224-2974

Miss Rosa Lee Weinert, Exec. Dir.
State Board of Nursing Education
and Nurse Registration
65 S. Front St., Room 509
Columbus, OH 43215 Tel.: (614) 466-3947

Ms. Sulinda Moffett, Exec. Dir.
Board of Nurse Registration
and Nursing Education
2915 N. Classen Blvd.
Oklahoma City, OK 73106 Tel.: (405) 525-2076

Dorothy J. Davy, Exec. Dir.
Oregon State Board of Nursing
1400 S.W. 5th Ave., Room 904
Portland, OR 97201 Tel.: (503) 229-6149

Miriam H. Lima, Exec. Sec.
Pennsylvania State Board of Nursing
P.O. Box 2649
Harrisburg, PA 17105 Tel.: (717) 783-7142

Luz Villafane, Supervisor
Accreditation and Development
for Schools of Nursing
Council on Higher Education of PR
Rio Piedras, PR 00933 Tel.: (809) 758-3350

Bertha Mugurdichian, RN, Dir.
Board of Registration in Nursing
75 Davis St., Room 104
Providence, RI 02908-2488 Tel.: (401) 277-2827

Mrs. Renatta Loquist, Exec. Dir.
State Board of Nursing for South Carolina
1777 St. Julia Pl., Suite 102
Columbia, SC 29204-2488 Tel.: (803) 737-6594

Carol A. Stuart, Exec. Sec.
South Dakota Board of Nursing
304 S. Phillips Ave., Suite 205
Sioux Falls, SD 57102 Tel.: (605) 334-1243

Elizabeth J. Lund, RN, Exec. Dir.
Tennessee Board of Nursing
283 Plus Park Blvd.
Nashville, TN 37217 Tel.: (615) 367-62644

Margaret L. Rowland, Exec. Dir.
Texas Board of Nurse Examiners
1300 E. Anderson Ln., Bldg. C-225
Austin, TX 78752 Tel.: (512) 835-4880

Ann G. Peterson, Exec. Sec.
Utah State Board of Nursing
160 E. 300 South, Box 45802
Salt Lake City, UT 84145 Tel.: (801) 530-6789

Executive Director
Vermont Board of Nursing,
Licensing and Registration Div.
109 State St.
Montpelier, VT 05602 Tel.: (802) 468-5611

Juanita Molloy, RN, Exec. Sec.
Virgin Islands Board of Nurse Licensure
P.O. Box 7309
St. Thomas, VI 00801 Tel.: (809) 776-7397

Mrs. Corinne F. Dorsey, RN, Exec. Dir.
Virginia State Board of Nursing
1601 Rolling Hills Dr.
Richmond, VA 23229 Tel.: (804) 662-9909

Constance E. Roth, RN, Exec. Dir.
Washington State Board of Nursing
P.O. Box 9012
Olympia, WA 98504 Tel.: (206) 459-1923

Miss Garnette Thorne, RN, Exec. Dir.
Board of Examiners for Registered Nurses
922 Quarrier St., Suite 309
Charleston, WV 25301 Tel.: (304) 348-3596

Ramona Weakland Warden, Director
Wisconsin State Bureau of Health Service Prof.
P.O. Box 8935
Madison, WI 53708-8935 Tel.: (608) 266-0072

Mrs. Joan Bouchard, RN, Exec. Dir.
State of Wyoming Board of Nursing
2301 Central Ave., Barrett Bldg.
Cheyenne, WY 82002 Tel.: (307) 777-7601

INDEX

Abduction, definition of, 293
Abortion, 404
Abruptio placentae, *407*, 407-408
Absence seizure, 561
AC-A, 85
Acceptance, as stage of mourning, 31
Accident prevention, 519-520, 522, 524, 525, 645 [1-6]
Acetaminophen, 161, 321, 322t
  poisoning, 546t, 654 [91-93]
Acetazolamide, 287t
Acetohexamide, 227t
Acetophenazine, 75t, 119
Acetylcysteine, 187t, 654 [93]
Acetylsalicylic acid, 301t
Achromycin. *See* Tetracycline
Acid-base balance, 233
Acne vulgaris, 544t, 671 [174]
Acquired immunedeficiency syndrome, 315-316, 543t, 649 [38-41]
  of newborn, 473-474
  during pregnancy, 414
Acromegaly, 219
Acting-out behavior. *See* Socially maladaptive behavior
Actinomycin D, 615t
Activase. *See* Tissue plasminogen activator
Activity and rest, 293-305
Activity therapy, 76
Acute lymphocytic leukemia, 618-619, 667 [135-141]
Adapin. *See* Doxepin
Addiction, definition of, 91
Addison's disease, 225
Adduction, definition of, 293
Adenoidectomy, 537
Adenosine diphosphate, 201
Adenosine triphosphate, 201
Adhesions, postmeningitis, 653
Adjuvant therapy, definition of, 306
Adolescence
  concept of death during, 617t
  contraception in, 505
  hospitalization during, 530
  occupational therapy during, 686-687 [240-241]
  pain responses in, 641
  pregnancy during, 416-417, 500-505
  psychosocial development in, 17t
  stages of, 501
Adrenal glands, 218
  hyperfunction of, 223-225
  hyposecretion of, 225
Adrenalin. *See* Epinephrine
Adrenocorticotropic hormone, 217t
Adriamycin. *See* Doxorubicin hydrochloride
Adrucil. *See* 5-Fluorouracil
Adult
  healthy, 151-155
  pain responses of, 641
  psychosocial development of, 16-19, 17t-18t
Advil. *See* Ibuprofen
Aerosporin. *See* Polymixin
Affect, definition of, 91
Affective disorders, 50-61
  depression, 53-58
  elation and hyperactive behavior, 58-61
  medications for, 51t-52t
  nursing process for, 32-33
Aggressive behavior, 62-71, 689 [262-267], 700-701 [281-287]. *See also* Socially maladaptive behavior
Aging. *See* Edlerly
Agoraphobia, 40
Agranulocytosis, 122
Airbron. *See* Acetylcysteine
Akathisia
  antipsychotic-induced, 113-114, 125
  definition of, 91, 113
  treatment of, 114
Akinesia, due to antipsychotics, 112
Akinetic seizure, 561
Akineton. *See* Biperiden hydrochloride
Al-Anon, 85
Alateen, 85
Alcohol
  addiction of newborn, 472-473
  antipsychotics and, 120t
  lithium and, 104
Alcoholics Anonymous, 85
Alcoholism, 83-87, 143, 707-708 [351-354]
  definition of, 83
  epidemiology of, 84
  lithium for, 101
  nursing process, 85-87
  stages of, 86
  treatment of, 84-85
  withdrawal symptoms, 84
Aldactone. *See* Spironolactone
Aldomet. *See* Methyldopa
Aldosterone, 217t, 236
Alka-2. *See* Calcium carbonate
Alkylating agents, 614t
Allergies, to foods, 518-519
Allopurinol, 303t
Alpha-fetoprotein, 403
Alphamul. *See* Castor oil
AlternaGel. *See* Aluminum hydroxide
Alu-Cap. *See* Aluminum hydroxide
Aluminum carbonate, 207t
Aluminum hydroxide, 207t
Alveolus, 163
Alzheimer's disease, 48-49
Amantadine, 282t
  for parkinsonism, 112, 113
Ambenonium chloride, 286t
Ambivalence, 74
  definition of, 91
  of self-destructive persons, 139
Amblyopia, 537
Aminophylline, 187t, 569t
Amitriptyline, 51t, 124, 327
Ammonium chloride, 187t
Amniocentesis, 402
Amniotic fluid, 394-395
  analysis of, 402-403, 403t
  embolism, 440
Amobarbital, 131-132, 134
Amoxapine, 124
Amoxicillin, 189t
  for otitis media, 536
Amoxil. *See* Amoxicillin
Amphetamines
  abuse of, 88, 89t
  lithium and, 104
Amphojel. *See* Aluminum hydroxide
Ampicillin, 189t
  for otitis media, 536
Amputation, 299-300
Amrinone, 629t, 631
Amylase, 217t
Amyotrophic lateral sclerosis, 284-285
Amytal. *See* Amobarbital
Anacin-3. *See* Acetaminophen
Anal fissure, 266-267
Analgesics, 161t, 320-329
  anticonvulsants, 327
  antihistamines, 327
  caffeine, 327
  for children, 328
  dextroamphetamine, 327
  drugs to avoid, 327-328
  for elderly, 328-329
  during labor, 424-426
  narcotic, 321-327, 322t-323t
    continuous administration of, 324
    dose and time course of, 324-325
    physical dependence on, 325-326
    psychological dependence on, 326-327
    routes of administration, 324
    side effects of, 325
    tolerance to, 325
  nonnarcotic, 321, 322t
  phenothiazines, 327
  placebos and, 328
  stepwise use of, 329
  steroids, 327
  tricyclic antidepressants, 327
Anatomy
  female reproductive, 383-385, *384*
  male reproductive, *254*
Androgens, 217t
Anectine. *See* Succinylcholine
Anemia
  in dialysis patient, 360
  iron-deficiency, 579-580
  peptic ulcer disease and, 209
  during pregnancy, 413
  sickle cell, 580-582
Anesthesia
  antipsychotics and, 120t

Page numbers in *italics* denotes figures; those followed by "t" denotes tables. Numbers within brackets indicate questions.

---

complications of, 160t
during labor and delivery, 426
lithium and, 104
stages of, 159t
types of, 160t
Angel dust, 88, 89t
Anger, 700-701 [281-287]
as stage of mourning, 30
Angina pectoris, 171-173, *172*, 173t
Angiography
cardiac, 167-168
hepatic, 203
renal, 240
Angiotensin, 236
Anorexia nervosa, 43, 672 [185-187]
Antabuse. *See* Disulfiram
Antacids, 207t
Antianxiety agents, 40, 41t, 130-135. *See also* Sedative-hypnotics
Antibiotics, 189t, 288t
antitumor, 615t
Anticholinesterase agents, 285, 286t
Anticoagulants, 176t
Anticonvulsants, 327, 410t
antipsychotics and, 120t
Antidepressants, 51t-52t, 124, 327
antipsychotics and, 120t
lithium and, 104
Antidiarrheals, 260t
Antidiuretic hormone, 217t
Antiemetics, 310t, 325
Antiestrogens, 615t
Antiflatulent, 207t
Antigout drugs, 303t
Antihistamines, 41t, 135, 327
Antihypertensives, 180t-181t
lithium and, 104
Antiinflammatory agents, 288t, 301t, 321, 322t
lithium and, 104
Antimanic agent. *See* Lithium
Antimetabolites, 614t
Antineoplastic agents, 613, 614t-615t
Antiparkinsonian agents, 112-113, 282t
Antipsychotics, 75t, 116-123, 125
classification of, 116-117, 119t
contraindications to, 118
drug interactions with, 120t
extrapyramidal side effects of, 111-115, 125
akathisia, 113-114
classes of, 111
dyskinesias and dystonias, 113
nursing implications of, 115
parkinsonism, 111-113
tardive dyskinesia, 114
treatment of, 114-115
indications for, 116, 125
lithium and, 103-104
misconceptions about, 122-123
other side effects of, 76t, 120-122, 125
patient teaching about, 122-123
in pregnancy, 118
properties of, 117
for rapid neuroleptization, 119-120
selection of, 117-118
usage guidelines for, 118-119
AntiRh O (D) gamma globulin, 444t
Antiseizure agents, 562t
Antisocial behavior, 70-71
Antituberculosis drugs, 191t
Anuria, 359
Anxiety, 36-46
anorexia nervosa, 43
anticipatory, 36
bulimia, 43-44
causes of, 36
conversion disorders, 45
definition of, 36, 91
diagnosis of, 37
dissociative reactions, 41-42
levels of, 36-37
manifestations of, 37t
nursing process for, 37-40
obsessive-compulsive disorders, 42-43
phobias, 40-41
post-traumatic stress disorders, 46
psychosomatic disorders, 44-45
stress management techniques, 39t-40t
tranquilizers for, 40, 41t
Aorta, coarctation of, *574*, 575
Apgar score, 463-464, 464t, 650 [51]
Aphasia, 271
Apresoline. *See* Hydralazine
Ara-C. *See* Cytosine arabinoside
Artane. *See* Trihexyphenidyl
Arterial blood gases, normal
in adults, 168
in children, 566t
Arterial insufficiency, 183-185, *184*
Arteriography, cerebral, 272-273
Arteriosclerosis obliterans, 183
Arthritis, 300-302
Arthroplasty, 300
Ascites, 215-216
Asendin. *See* Amoxapine
L-Asparaginase, 615t
Aspirin, 161, 301t, 321, 322t, 647 [24]
poisoning, 546t
Asthma, 185, 569t, 569-571
Atarax. *See* Hydroxyzine
"Athlete's foot", 545t
Ativan. *See* Lorazepam
Atrial septal defect, 572, *573*, 575
Atropine sulfate, 170t, 287t
Attention deficit disorder, 556
Audiogram, 273
Aureomycin. *See* Tetracycline
Auscultation
of abdomen, 201
of fetal heart. *See* Fetal heart rate monitoring
of heart, 165, *165*
Autism, 73
definition of, 91
Autonomic dysreflexia, 280-281
in spinal cord-injured person, 369-370
Autonomic nervous system, 269
in spinal cord-injured person, 369-370
Autosomal dominant diseases, *581*
Autosomal recessive diseases, *581*
Azathioprine, 253t
Azulfidine. *See* Sulfasalazine

Babinski's reflex, 458, 636
Baciguent. *See* Bacitracin ophthalmic ointment
Bacitracin, 189t
Bacitracin ophthalmic ointment, 288t
Bactrim. *See* Co-trimoxazole
Balance suspension, 606t, *607*
Barbiturates, 131-132, 134t, 327-328
abuse of, 88, 89t, 143
antipsychotics and, 120t
classification of, 131
disadvantages of, 131-132
tolerance to, 132
usage guidelines for, 132
Bargaining, as stage of mourning, 30
Barium enema, 258
Bartholin's glands, 384
Basajel. *See* Aluminum carbonate
Basal body temperature, *386*
Battle's sign, 636-637
Behavior. *See also* specific behaviors
anxious, 36-46
confused, 48-49, 126-129
elated-depressive, 50-61
frightened, 129
socially maladaptive, 62-69
substance use disorders, 81-90
suspicious, 70-71
theories of, 21, 22t
withdrawn, 72-80
Behavior modification, 26
Benadryl. *See* Diphenhydramine
Benign prostatic hypertrophy, 254-256
Benzodiazepines, 41t, 131-133, 327
abuse of, 88, 89t
advantages of, 132
disadvantages of, 132
indications for, 133
preoperative, 133
Benzquinamide, 310t
Benzthiazide, 180t
Benztropine mesylate, 282t
for dystonias, 113
for parkinsonism, 112, 113
Beprenorphine, 161
Beta-blockers, 135, 173t, 287t
Beta-Chlor. *See* Chloral betaine
Betamethasone valerate, 226t
Bilirubin, 467-468
jaundice and, 506-507
metabolism of, 506, *507*
Billroth I and II procedures, 206
Biopsy
colonic, 258
endometrial, 386t
renal, 240-241
Biperiden hydrochloride, 113
Bipolar disorder, 55, 59, 683-684 [206-211]
lithium for, 101, 683 [209-210]
Birth. *See* Labor and delivery
Birth injuries, 474-475
Birthmarks, 455
Bisacodyl, 260t
Bishydroxycoumarin, 176t
Bismuth subsalicylate, 260t
Bladder, 232
cancer of, 244-245
neurogenic, in spinal cord-injured person, 367
Blefcon. *See* Sulfacetamide sodium
Blood, 164
Blood chemistry values, adult, 727-728
Blood pressure
high, 182-183
of newborn, 458
in pregnancy, 492-493
variations in vascular system, 162, *164*
Blood urea nitrogen, 239
Body image, 18-19
Body surface area estimation, 534t
Bones, 293
Bowel elimination, 257-267
alterations in, 259-261
in children, 598
management in dialysis patient, 359-360
problems affecting, 258-267. *See also*

Colon problems
  in spinal cord-injured person, 367
Brain, 268, *278*
  contusion of, 275, 637
  tumors of, 620t
Brain scan, 272
Brainstem, 268
Braxton Hicks' contractions, 390
Breast, 385
  cancer of, 313-315
  postpartum changes in, 442
  self-examination of, 309, 389
Breast-feeding, 460, 465, 705 [333-335]
  jaundice and, 468, 507-509
Breathholding, 561
Breathing, normal, 163-164
Breech birth, 419
Bretylium tosylate, 170t
Bretylol. *See* Bretylium tosylate
Brevital. *See* Methohexital
Bromocriptine mesylate, 445t
Bronchial asthma, 185, 569t, 569-571
Bronchiolitis, 568, 568t
Bronchitis, chronic, 185
Bronchodilators, 187t, 569t
Bronchopulmonary dysplasia, 568-569
Bryant's traction, 606t, *608*
Buck's traction, 606t, *608*
Buerger's disease, 183
Bulimia, 43-44
Buminal. *See* Phenobarbital
Buprenex. *See* Buprenorphine
Buprenorphine, 323t
Burns, 548-553, 549t, *550*, 670 [168-173]
  classification of, 548, *550*
  nursing process for, 551-553
  treatment of, 549-551
Butabarbital, 131-132, 134
Butaperazine, 119
Butazolidin. *See* Phenylbutazone
Butisol. *See* Butabarbital
Butorphanol, 161, 323t
"Butterfly" rash, 302
Butyrophenones, 75t

Caffeine, 327
Calan. *See* Verapamil
Calcitonin, 217t
Calcium, in spinal cord-injured person, 369
Calcium carbonate, 207t
Calcium channel blockers, 173t
Calcium chloride, 170t
Calculi, urinary, 243-244
Canadian nurses, 729-730
Cancer, 306-315
  bladder, 244-245
  brain, 620t
  breast, 313-315
  cervical, 312-313
  in children, 613-620
  classification of, 307
  colonic, 265-266
  endometrial, 313
  Hodgkin's disease, 311-312, 312t
  laryngeal, 196-198, 688 [251-253]
  leukemia, 618-619
  lung, 195-196
  neuroblastoma, 620t
  nursing process for, 307-311
  osteogenic sarcoma, 620t
  pain of, 320
  prostatic, 256-257
  terminology of, 306
  warning signs of, 307
  Wilms' tumor, 620t
Candidiasis, 542t
Cannabinoids, 328
Cantor tube, 265
Capreomycin, 191t
Captopril, 632
Caput succedaneum, 456
Carbacel. *See* Carbachol
Carbachol, 287t
Carbamazepine, 327, 562t
Carbidopa-levodopa, 282t
Carbonic anhydrase inhibitors, 287t
Carcinoembryonic antigen, 307
Carcinoma, definition of, 306
Cardase. *See* Ethoxzalamide
Cardiac catheterization
  in adults, 167-168, 685 [227-229]
  in children, 571t
Cardiac glycosides, 179t
Cardilate. *See* Erythrityl tetranitrate
Cardiopulmonary arrest, 169
Cardiopulmonary resuscitation, 169, 664 [107-108]
Cardiovascular system, 162-185. *See also* Oxygenation problems
  of children, 565
  normal, 152, 162, *163*
  in pregnancy, 392, 412-413
Cardizem. *See* Diltiazem
Carphenazine, 75t, 119
Cartilage, 293
Cascara, 260t
Cas-Evac. *See* Cascara
Cast care, 296-297, 606, *609*
Castor oil, 260t
Cataracts, 286-289
Catatonic schizophrenia, 80t
Celiac disease, 589-590
Central nervous system, 268
Cepastat. *See* Capreomycin
Cephalexin, 189t
Cephalohematoma, 456
Cephalothin, 189t
Cephulac. *See* Lactulose
Cerebellum, 268
Cerebral palsy, 557-558
Cerebrovascular accident, 277-279, *278*
Cervical cancer, 312-313
Cervical cap, 387t
Cervical os, incompetent, 404-405
Cervix, involution of, 441
Cesarean birth, *438*, 438-439
  vaginal delivery after, 439
Chadwick's sign, 390, 393
Chemotherapy, 308, 613, 614t-615t
  MOPP, 311
Chest tubes, 193-195, *194-195*, 331-350, 707
  bottle systems for, *334*, 334-335
  design of, 331
  disposable unit systems for, 335, *335*
  functions of, 333
  gravity systems vs. systems on suction, 333
  patient effects of changes in, 340-342
  problems with, 336-339
  proximal vs. distal ends of, 336
  recognizing malfunctions in, 348-350
  repairing malfunctions in, 342-348
  substances evacuated by, 333
  suction source for, 336
Chickenpox, 539
Childbearing, 649-651 [42-55]. *See also* Newborn
  antepartal care, 383-417. *See also* Pregnancy
  intrapartal care, 419-440. *See also* Labor and delivery
  long-term problems due to, 451-452
  postpartal care, 441-452. *See also* Postpartum period
  preparation for, 400t
Children, 517-642
  abuse of, 687-688 [242-250]
  burns of, 548-553, 549t, *550*, 670 [168-173]
  cancer of, 613-620
    brain tumors, 620t
    leukemia, 618-619
    neuroblastoma, 620t
    nursing process for, 613-618
    osteogenic sarcoma, 620t
    Wilms' tumor, 620t
  cardiac catheterization in, 571t
  cardiovascular problems of, 571-579
    congenital heart disease, 572-578, *573-574*
    nursing process for, 571-572
    rheumatic fever/rheumatic heart disease, 578-579
  cognitive development of, 517, 520-525
  communicable diseases of, 538-541
  death and dying of
    child's concept of, 617t
    nursing process, 34-35
    responses to death, 31
  developmental/neurological disabilities of, 553-564
    attention deficit disorder, 556
    cerebral palsy, 557-558
    Down syndrome, 556-557
    hydrocephalus, 558-559, 559t
    meningitis, 563-564
    mental retardation, 555t, 555-556
    nursing process for, 553-555
    seizure disorders, 560-563, 562t
    spina bifida, 559-560
  drug doses for, 534t
  elimination problems of, 598-604
    hypospadias, 598-599
    lower GI tract obstruction, 603-604
    nephritis, 601-602
    nephrosis, 602-603
    nursing process for, 598
    urinary tract infection, 599-600
    vesicoureteral reflux, 600-601
  emotional impact of trauma on, 623-626
  growth and development of
    adolescent, 524-525
    infant, 517-520
    newborn, 454-475. *See also* Newborn
    preschooler, 522-523
    school age, 523-524
    toddler, 520-522
  head injury in, 635-638. *See also* Head injury
  hematologic problems of, 579-583
    hemophilia, 582-583
    iron-deficiency anemia, 579-580
    nursing process for, 579
    sickle cell anemia, 580-582
  hematology values in, 566t
  hospitalization of, 529-534
  isolation procedures for, 540t
  language development of, 517-518, 521, 522

medication and temperature guide for, 532t-533t
musculoskeletal problems of, 605-611
clubfoot, 609
congenital hip dysplasia, 609-610
Legg-Calvé-Perthes disease, 610
nursing process for, 605-609
osteomyelitis, 611
scoliosis, 610-611
nursing process for, 525-527
nutrition and metabolism problems of, 584-597, 668-669 [152-154]
celiac disease, 589-590
cleft lip and palate, 590-592
congenital hypothyroidism, 592-593
cystic fibrosis, 595-597
diabetes mellitus, 593t, 593-595, 686 [235-239]
nonorganic failure to thrive, 587-588
nursing process for, 584-585
pyloric stenosis, 588-589
vomiting and diarrhea, 585-587
oxygenation in, 565-583
pain responses of, 328, 639-641
physical restraints for, 532t
play of, 518, 521-523
poisoning of, 545-548, 546t-547t
psychosocial development of, 17t, 517, 520, 522-524
respiratory problems of, 565-571
bronchial asthma, 569t, 569-571
bronchiolitis, 568, 568t
bronchopulmonary dysplasia, 568-569
epiglottitis, 568, 568t
laryngotracheobronchitis, 568, 568t
nursing process for, 565-567
spasmodic croup, 568, 568t
sudden infant death syndrome, 567-568
schizophrenia in, 80t
sensory problems of, 534-538, 668 [150-151]
nursing process for, 534
otitis media, 534-537
strabismus, 537-538
tonsillectomy and adenoidectomy, 537
sexually transmitted diseases in, 541, 542t-543t
shock in, 627-634. *See also* Shock
skin problems of, 543-545, 544t-545t
Chlamydial infection, 543t
Chloral betaine, 134
Chloral hydrate, 133, 134t
abuse of, 89t
Chlorambucil, 614t
Chlordiazepoxide, 132-133, 134t
abuse of, 88, 89t
Chlordiazepoxide-amitriptyline, 51t
Chloride balance, 232
Chloroprothixene, 75t
Chlorothiazide, 180t
Chlorotrianisene, 445t
Chlorphenoxamine hydrochloride, 113
Chlorpromazine, 75t, 116-123, 125, 327
lithium and, 103-104
side effects of, 115
Chlorpropamide, 227t
Chlorprothixene, 119
Cholangiogram, 202
Cholecystitis, 210-211, 663 [95-96]
Cholecystogram, 202
Cholecystokinin, 200t
Cholelithiasis, 210-211
Cholesterol, 654 [90]
content of foods, 177t
Choline magnesium trisalicylate, 321, 322t
Cholinergic crisis, 286
Chordee, 599
Chorea, 578
Chorionic villus sampling, 402
Chronic obstructive pulmonary disease, 184-188
Chvostek's sign, 223
Cigarette smoking, antipsychotics and, 120t
Cimetidine, 207t
Cinobac. *See* Cinoxacin
Cinoxacin, 241t
CircOlectric bed, 280
Circulatory problems, 183-185, *184*
Circumcision, 465
Cirrhosis, 213-214
Cis-platinum, 614t
Citrucel. *See* Methylcellulose
Clark's rule, 534t
Cleft lip and palate, 590-592, 651-652 [60-63]
Clinoril. *See* Sulindac
Clonazepam, 327, 562t
Clonopin. *See* Clonazepam
Clorazepate, 134t
abuse of, 88, 89t
Clubfoot, 609
Coarctation of aorta, *574*, 575
Cocaine, 88, 89t, 142-145, 328
behavior of users of, 144
detoxification from, 143
lithium and, 104
misconceptions about, 486
motivations for treatment, 144-145
physical effects of, 144
popularity of, 142
prenatal use of, 484-489
caring for users, 487-489
effects on newborn, 486-487
pharmacology of, 484-486
postpartum care, 489
pregnancy complications due to, 486
users of, 145
Codeine, 161, 322t
abuse of, 87-88, 89t
Cogentin. *See* Benztropine mesylate
Cognitive development, 16, 18-19, 517, 520-525
Colace. *See* Docusate sodium
Colchicine, 303t
Colectomy, 263-264
Colistin, 189t
Collagen disease, 302
Colon, 257
Colon problems, 258-267
alteration in bowel elimination, 259-261
colon cancer, 265-266
hemorrhoids/anal fissure, 266-267
Hirschsprung's disease, 603-604
inflammatory bowel disease, 261-263
intussusception, 603-604
mechanical obstruction of colon, 264-265
nursing process for, 258-259
total colectomy with ileostomy, 263-264
Colonoscopy, 258
Color exchange, 109, 110
Coly-Mycin. *See* Colistin
Coma, diabetic, 230t, 230-231
Committment procedure, 28
definition of, 91
Communication
of self-destructive persons, 139-140
test items on, 7-8, 8t
therapeutic, 15, 22-24, 24t
Compazine. *See* Prochlorperazine
Compensation, definition of, 21
Complete blood count, normal, 168, 202
Computerized axial tomography, 272
Concussion, 275
Condom, 388t
Condylomata, 415
Confabulation, definition of, 91
Conflict, definition of, 91
Confusion, 48-49, 126-129, 702-703 [296-310]
definition of, 48, 91
factors associated with, 128
factors contributing to, 127, 129
management of, 128
nursing process for, 48-49
reduction of, 126-127
syndromes of, 48
Congenital anomalies, 474-475
Congenital heart disease, 572-578, *573-574*
Congenital hypothyroidism, 592-593, 667 [133-134]
Congestive heart failure, 178-182, 654 [88-89], 684-685 [219-222]
definition of, 178
drug therapy for, 179t-181t
left- vs. right-sided, 178, 179t
Conjunctivitis, chemical, 456
Constipation, 259-261
in dialysis patient, 359
during pregnancy, 397
Contraception, 387t-388t, 669 [155-158]
for adolescent, 505
Contraction stress test, 401
Contusion, cerebral, 275, 637
Conversion, definition of, 21
Conversion disorders, 45, 666 [129-132]
Coombs' test, 468
Corrosive substance ingestion, 547t
Cortef. *See* Hydrocortisone
Corticosteroids, 226t, 327, 569t, 632
Cortisone acetate, 288t
Co-trimoxazole, 241t
Cough medications, 187t
Cough reflex, 457
Coumadin. *See* Warfarin sodium
Countertransference, definition of, 91
Covert, definition of, 91
Crack, 142-145. *See also* Cocaine
Cranioplasty, 276
Craniotomy, 276
Creatinine clearance, 239
Cretinism, 222
"Crib death", 567-568
Crisis intervention therapy, 25-26
definition of, 91
for suicide prevention, 141
Crohn's disease, 261-263
Croup, 568, 568t
Crutches, 295
Crutchfield tongs, 365, *365*
Crystapen. *See* Penicillin
Crystodigin. *See* Digitoxin
Culdocentesis, 483
Culdoscopy, 386t
Cultural/ethnic issues, 20
Cushing's syndrome, 223-224
Cyclophosphamide, 614t

Cycloplegics, 287t
Cycloserine, 191t
Cyclosporin, 253t
Cycrimine hydrochloride, 113
Cystic fibrosis, 595-597
Cystitis, 242-243
  postpartal, 450
Cystocele, 451
Cystography, 240
Cystoscopy, 240
Cytomegalovirus infection, 415
Cytomel. *See* Liothyronine
Cytosar. *See* Cytosine arabinoside
Cytosine arabinoside, 614t
Cytoxan. *See* Cyclophosphamide

Dactinomycin. *See* Actinomycin D
Daily fetal movement counting, 400
Dalmane. *See* Flurazepam
Daranide. *See* Dichlorphenamide
Daricon. *See* Oxyphencyclimine
Darvon. *See* Propoxyphene
Datril. *See* Acetaminophen
Daxolin. *See* Loxapine
Deafness, 271
Death and dying, 32-35, 710-711 [375-378]
  child's concept of, 617t
  nursing process
    for adults, 32-34
    for children, 34-35
  responses to
    children's, 31
    client's, 32
    nurse's, 32
Decadron. *See* Dexamethasone
Decerebrate posturing, 272, *273*
Decorticate posturing, 272, *272*
Decubitus ulcers, 367-368, *368*
Dedilanid. *See* Lanatoside C
Defense mechanisms, 21-22
Dehydration, 234t
Deladumone OB, 445t
Delirium tremens, 84, 87
  definition of, 91
Deltasone. *See* Prednisone
Delusions, 73, 652-653 [68-76]
  definition of, 91
  nursing process for, 78-79
Demerol. *See* Meperidine
Denial
  definition of, 21
  as stage of mourning, 30
Denis Browne splint, 609
Dental care, for children, 521, 524
Denver Developmental Screening Test, 553
Depakene. *See* Sodium valproate
Depersonalization, 73-74
  definition of, 91
Depression, 53-58, 646-647 [7-19]
  causes of, 53-54
  definition of, 53
  drug therapy for. *See* Antidepressants
  neurotic, 54
  nursing process for, 55-58
  postpartum, 450, 451t
  psychotic, 54
    agitated, 54-55
    bipolar, 55
    retarded, 55
  reactive, 54
  seasonal affective disorder, 54
  as stage of mourning, 30-31
  suicide risk, 55-56, 56t
  transitory, 54
Dermatitis, atopic, 544t
Desipramine, 124, 327
Desyrel. *See* Trazodone
Dexamethasone, 226t, 327, 615t
Dexedrine. *See* Dextroamphetamine
Dextroamphetamine, 325, 327
Dextrostix, 461
Diabeta. *See* Glyburide
Diabetes insipidus, 220
Diabetes mellitus, 225-231, 651 [56-59]
  in children, 593-595, 686 [235-239]
  exercise and, 356-358
  insulin dependent, 593t
  non-insulin dependent, 593t
  in pregnancy, 410-412, 663 [98-103]
Diabetic exchange lists, 229t
Diabinese. *See* Chlorpropamide
Diagnostic and Statistical Manual of Mental Disorders classification, 15
  of alcohol abuse, 85
  of anorexia nervosa, 43
  of confused behavior, 48
  of conversion disorders, 45
  of depressive disorders, 54-55
  of dissociative reactions, 42
  of drug abuse, 88
  of elation and hyperactive behavior, 58-59
  of obsessive-compulsive disorders, 42
  of paranoia, 70
  of phobias, 41
  of post-traumatic stress disorder, 45
  of psychosomatic disorders, 44
  of socially maladaptive behavior, 62, 63, 66
  of withdrawn behavior, 76
Dialose. *See* Docusate potassium
Dialysis, *249*, 249-252, 681-682 [191-195]
  bowel management during, 359-360
  hemodialysis, 251-252
  peritoneal, 249-250
Diamox. *See* Acetazolamide
Diaphragm, contraceptive, 387t
Diarrhea, 259-261
  in children, 585-587
Diazepam, 41t, 132-133, 134t, 562t
  abuse of, 88, 89t
Dibenzoxanzephines, 75t
Dichlorphenamide, 287t
Dicumarol. *See* Bishydroxycoumarin
Diet. *See also* Nutrition
  after myocardial infarction, 175, 177t
  cholesterol content of foods, 177t
  diabetic exchange lists, 229t
  for dialysis patient, 359-360
  high fiber/roughage, 210t
  low-fat, 210t
  low-protein, 247t
  low-residue, 263t
  postoperative, 160t
  potassium content of foods, 182t
  during pregnancy, 397-398, 398t-399t
  in pregnancy, 493
  sodium content of foods, 177t
  for spinal cord-injured person, 369
Diethylstilbestrol, 615t
Differentiation, definition of, 306
Diflunisal, 161t
Digestive enzymes, 200t
Digestive problems
  cholecystitis/cholelithiasis, 210-211
  cirrhosis, 213-214
  diverticulosis/diverticulitis, 209-210
  gastritis, 205-206
  hepatitis, 212-213
  hiatal hernia, 205
  pancreatitis, 211-212
  peptic ulcer, 206-209
  in pregnancy, 392
Digestive tract, 199-201
Digitalis, 179t, 654 [88]
Digitoxin, 179t
Digoxin, 179t
  lithium and, 104
Dihydroindolones, 75t
Dilantin. *See* Phenytoin
Dilaudid. *See* Hydromorphone
Diltiazem, 173t
Dimenhydrinate, 310t
Diphenhydramine, 135
  for dystonias, 113
Diphenidol, 310t
Diplopia, 537
Discipline, of toddler, 521-522
Disipal. *See* Orphenadrine hydrochloride
Displacement, definition of, 21
Dissociation, definition of, 21
Dissociative reaction, 41-42, 665 [114-116]
Disulfiram, 87
Disulfiram, lithium and, 104
Diuretics
  lithium and, 104
  osmotic, 246t
  potassium-sparing, 180t
  potent, 180t
  thiazide, 180t
Diuril. *See* Chlorothiazide
Diverticulosis/diverticulitis, 209-210
Dobutamine, 170t, 629t, 631
Dobutrex. *See* Dobutamine
Docusate calcium, 260t
Docusate potassium, 260t
Docusate sodium, 260t
Dolobid. *See* Diflunisal
Dolophine. *See* Methadone
Dopamine, 170t, 629t, 631
Doriden. *See* Glutethimide
Double bind, definition of, 91
Down syndrome, 457, 556-557, 648-649 [33-37]
Doxepin, 51t, 124, 327
Doxorubicin hydrochloride, 615t
Dramamine. *See* Dimenhydrinate
Drugs. *See also* specific drugs and drug classes
  abuse of. *See* Substance abuse disorders
  analgesics, 161t, 320-329
  antacids, 207t
  antianxiety agents, 40, 41t
  antibiotics, 189t, 288t
  anticholinesterase agents, 286t
  anticoagulants, 176t
  anticonvulsants, 410t
  antidepressants, 51t-52t, 124
  antidiarrheals, 260t
  antiemetics, 310t
  antiflatulent, 207t
  antigout, 303t
  antihistamines, 135
  antihypertensives, 180t-181t
  antiinflammatory agents, 288t, 301t, 321, 322t
  antimanic, 41t, 51t-52t, 59, 101-105, 125
  antineoplastic agents, 613, 614t-615t

antiparkinsonian, 112-113, 282t
antipsychotics, 75t-76t, 111-123, 125
antiseizure agents, 562t
antituberculosis agents, 191t
barbiturates, 131-132, 134t
beta-blockers, 135, 287t
bronchodilators, 187t, 569t
carbonic anhydrase inhibitors, 287t
cardiac glycosides, 179t
corticosteroids, 569t
cough medications, 187t
cycloplegics, 287t
diuretics, 246t
emergency, 170t
expectorants, 569t
histamine receptor blocking agents, 207t
hypoglycemics, 227t
immunosuppressants, 253t
lactation suppressants, 445t
laxatives, 260t-261t
miotics, 287t
sedative-hypnotics, 130-135
steroids, 226t
thrombolytic, 176t
tocolytic agents, 435, 436t
uterine smooth muscle stimulants, 431t
Ducolax. *See* Bisacodyl
Dumping syndrome, 209
Dwyer instrumentation, 610
Dying. *See* Death and dying
Dymelor. *See* Acetohexamide
Dysarthria, 271
Dyskinesia, 113
Dyspnea, 684 [219]
Dysreflexia, autonomic, 280-281
in spinal cord-injured persons, 369-370
Dystocia, 432-434
Dystonia
definition of, 91
due to antipsychotics, 113, 125

Ear, 270
Echocardiography, 167
Eclampsia, 408-410, 409t
Ectopic pregnancy, 405, *405*, 479-483
causes of, 480
conditions mimicking, 481
counseling for, 480, 483
diagnosis of, 481-483
incidence of, 480
surgery for, 483
Eczema, 544t
Edecrin. *See* Ethacrynic acid
Edema
in pregnancy, 496
pulmonary, 685 [223-224]
Edrophonium chloride, 285, 286t
Ego, definition of, 91
Elastic bandages, 299
Elation, 58-61. *See also* Mania
Elavil. *See* Amitriptyline
Elderly
healthy, 153-154
psychosocial development of, 18t, 19
Electrocardiogram, 167, *167*
Electroconvulsive therapy, 50, 57
Electroencephalogram, 273
Electrolyte imbalance, 234t-236t
Elimination
of adult, 232-267
of children, 598-604
Embolism
amniotic fluid, 440
pulmonary, 192-193, 448
Emergency drugs, 170t
Emete-Con. *See* Benzquinamide
Emotional development, 18-19
Emphysema, 185, 706-707 [345-350]
Encephalopathy, hepatic, 216
Endocrine problems
adrenal hyperfunction, 223-225
adrenal hyposecretion, 225
diabetes mellitus, 225-231
hyperparathyroidism, 222-223
hyperpituitarism, 219-220
hyperthyroidism, 220-222
hypoparathyroidism, 223
hypopituitarism, 220
hypothyroidism, 222
Endocrine system, 216-219
Endometrial cancer, 313
Endoscopy, 203
Enemas
barium, 258
for dialysis patients, 360
Ephedrine, 187t
Epidural hematoma, 275
Epiglottitis, 568, 568t
Epilepsy, 560-563
Epinephrine, 170t, 187t, 217t, 569t, 629t, 631
Episiotomy, 436, *437*
Epistaxis, 291-292
Epson salt. *See* Magnesium citrate
Epstein's pearls, 457
Equanil. *See* Meprobamate
Ergonovine maleate, 431t
Ergotrate. *See* Ergonovine maleate
Erikson's developmental stages, 371-372, 374
Erythema marginatum rheumaticum, 578
Erythema toxicum, 455
Erythrityl tetranitrate, 173t
Erythroblastosis fetalis, 468
Erythropoietin, 236
Eserine. *See* Physostigmine salicylate
Esidrix. *See* Hydrochlorothiazide
Eskalith. *See* Lithium
Esophageal varices, 214-215
Estinyl. *See* Ethinyl estradiol
Estrogen, 217t, 385
Estrogen replacement therapy, 385
Ethacrynic acid, 180t
Ethambutol, 191t
Ethchlorvynol, 133, 134t
abuse of, 88
Ethinyl estradiol, 615t
Ethionamide, 191t
Ethnicity, 20
Ethopropazine hydrochloride, 113
Ethosuximide, 562t
Ethoxzalamide, 287t
Exanthema subitum, 539
Excretory urogram, 239
Exercise
for diabetics, 356-358
for dialysis patients, 360
Exhibitionism, 65
Exna. *See* Benzthiazide
Expectorants, 187t, 569t
Extension, definition of, 293
Extracorporeal membrane oxygenation, 633
Extrapyramidal reaction
to antipsychotics, 111-115, 125
definition of, 91
Eye, 269, *270*

Factor VIII deficiency, 582-583
Failure to thrive, nonorganic, 587-588
Fallopian tube, 384
Fallot's tetralogy, *574*, 575-576, 665 [117-120]
Family planning methods, 387t-388t
Family therapy, 16, 26
definition of, 91, 92
Family violence, 63-66
Fantasy, definition of, 22
Fear, definition of, 36
Febrile seizure, 561
Feldene. *See* Piroxicam
Femoral-head prosthesis, 298
Fenoprofen, 161, 321, 322t
Fertility assessment, 386t
Fertilization, 385
Fetal alcohol syndrome, 473
Fetal blood sampling, 424
Fetal death, 498-499
Fetal heart rate monitoring, 400-401, 421-422, *421-423*, 422t, 424t, 428, *429*, 672 [184]
Fibroids, uterine, 452
Fiflunisal, 321, 322t
Fixation, definition of, 22
Flexion, definition of, 293
Flight of ideas, definition of, 91-92
Floropryl. *See* Isoflurophate
Fludrocortisone acetate, 288t
Fluid imbalance, 234t
in shock, 630
Fluophenazine, 75t
5-Fluorouracil, 614t
Fluoxetine, 51t
Fluoxymesterone, 615t
Fluphenazine, 119, 125, 327
extrapyramidal side effects of, 115
Flurazepam, 134t
Follicle-stimulating hormone, 217t
Fontanels, 456, *456*
Food allergies, 518-519
Food groups, 152t
Foreign nurses, 729-730
Foster frame, 280
Fractures, 295-297
of hip, 297-299
Fredet-Ramstedt procedure, 588
Frejka pillow splint, 609
Friedman curve, 433, *434*
Frightened behavior, 129
Full-body relaxation, 106-107, 110
Furadantin. *See* Nitrofurantoin
Furosemide, 180t

Gagging reflex, 458
Gallbladder, 199
Gantrisin. *See* Sulfisoxazole
Gastrectomy, 648 [30-32]
Gastrin, 199, 200t
Gastritis, 205-206
Genetic transmission, *581*
Genital warts, 415
Genitourinary system, normal, 152-153
Gentamicin, 189t
Geramycin. *See* Gentamicin
Geriatrics. *See* Elderly
German measles, 539
Gestational age, 460-463, *461*
Glans clitoris, 383
Glaucoma, 290-291
Glipizide, 227t
Glomerulonephritis, acute, 601-602

Glucagon, 217t
Glucocorticoids, 217t
Glucose, urinary, 238
Glucose monitoring, 228
Glucotrol. *See* Glipizide
Gluten enteropathy, 589-590
Glutethimide, 133, 134t
  abuse of, 88, 89t
Glyburide, 227t
Gonorrhea, 542t
  during pregnancy, 414
Goodell's sign, 390
Gouty arthritis, 300-302
Grand mal seizure, 561
Grasp reflexes, 458
Graves' disease, 220-222
Grief, 475
  definitions of, 30
  stages of, 30-31, 370
  unresolved, 30, 97-100
Group psychotherapy, 16, 26, 652-653 [72-73]
Growth hormone, 217t
Guaifenesin, 187t, 569t
Guanethidine, 180t
  antipsychotics and, 120t

Haldol. *See* Haloperidol
Hallucinations, 73, 129
  definition of, 92
  nursing process for, 78-79
Hallucinogens, 88, 89t
Halo-femoral traction, 606t, *607*
Halo fixation, 365, *365*
Haloperidol, 75t, 116-123, 125
  extrapyramidal side effects of, 115
  lithium and, 103-104
Halotestin. *See* Fluoxymesterone
Hand-foot syndrome, 582
Harrington rods, 610
Head injury, 275-276
  in children
    diagnostic studies for, 636-637
    differential diagnosis of, 637-638
    history taking, 635
    manifestations of, 635
    nurse's role for, 638
    physical exam for, 635-636
    prognosis of, 638
    sequellae of, 638
  in infants and children, 635-638
Health
  characteristics of, 151
  definition of, 151
Health promotion, levels of, 151
Healthy adult, 151-155
  elderly, 153-154
  nursing process for, 154-155
  young and middle-aged, 151-153
Hearing, 270, 271, 526
Heart
  auscultation of, 165, *165*
  normal, 162, *163*
Heart disease
  congenital, 572-578, *573-574*
  rheumatic, 578-579
Heat loss, of newborn, 459, 464, 466-467
Hegar's sign, 390
Heimlich's maneuver, 169
Hematologic values
  adult, 727
  child, 566t
Hematoma
  epidural, 275
  postpartal, 448
  subdural, 276
Hemodialysis, 251-252
Hemoglobin S, 580
Hemophilia, 582-583, 649 [38-41]
Hemopneumothorax, 332-333
Hemorrhage, 664 [104-105]
  cerebral, 275-276
  postpartal, 447-448
  subconjunctival, 456
Hemorrhoids, 266-267
  during pregnancy, 397
Hemotympanum, 636-637
Heparin sodium, 176t, 654 [86]
Hepatic encephalopathy, 216
Hepatitis, 212-213
  during pregnancy, 415
  type A, 663 [94-97]
Hernia, hiatal, 205
Herniated nucleus pulposus, 302-305
Heroin, 87-88, 89t, 143, 323t, 328-329
Herpes simplex virus infection, 542t
  during pregnancy, 415
Hiatal hernia, 205
Hiccoughing reflex, 458
Hip
  congenital dislocation of, 609-610, 701 [288-289]
  fracture of, 297-299, 647 [20-25]
  subluxation of, 609-610
Hiprex. *See* Methanamine hippurate
Hirschsprung's disease, 603-604
Histamine receptor blocking agents, 207t
Hodgkin's disease, 311-312, 312t
Homan's sign, 443, 452
Homatropine, 287t
Hormones, 217t
  gastrointestinal, 200t
Hostile-aggressive behavior, 66-67
Human chorionic gonadotropin
  assays of, 482
  in ectopic pregnancy, 481-482
Human immunodeficiency virus, 315-316, 543t
Human needs, categories of, 5t, 5-6
Hyaline membrane disease, 435, 469-470, *470*
Hydatidiform mole, *405*, 405-406
Hydralazine, 180t, 629t, 632
  antipsychotics and, 120t
Hydramnios, 474
Hydrobromide, 287t
Hydrocarbon ingestion, 547t
Hydrocephalus, 558-559, 559t, 653-654 [81-84]
Hydrochloric acid, 199
Hydrochlorothiazide, 180t
  antipsychotics and, 120t
Hydrocortisone, 226t, 569t
Hydrodiuril. *See* Hydrochlorothiazide
Hydromorphone, 89t, 161, 323t
  abuse of, 87-88
Hydrops fetalis, 468
Hydroxyzine, 41t, 135, 325, 327
Hymen, 383
Hyperactive behavior, elation and, 58-61
Hyperbilirubinemia, 467, 506-510
  breast-feeding and, 507-509
  obstetric interventions and, 508
  treatment of, 509-510
Hypercalcemia, 235t
Hypercapnia, 184
Hyperemia gravidarum, 414
Hyperglycemia, due to antipsychotics, 122
Hyperkalemia, 235t
Hyperkinesis, 556
Hypermagnesemia, 236t
Hypernatremia, 234t
Hyperparathyroidism, 222-223
Hyperphosphatemia, 359
Hyperpituitarism, 219-220
Hypertension, 182-183
  pregnancy-induced, 408-410, 409t, 490-497
    causes of, 492
    management of, 496-497
    monitoring for, 492-496
    pathology associated with, 490-492
    patients at risk for, 496
Hyperthyroidism, 220-222, 708-710 [355-371]
Hypocalcemia, 235t, 359
Hypoglycemia, 230t, 230-231, 594
  neonatal, 471-472
Hypoglycemics, 227t
Hypokalemia, 235t
Hypomagnesemia, 236t
Hyponatremia, 234t
Hypoparathyroidism, 223
Hypopituitarism, 220
Hypospadias, 598-599
Hypothalamic crisis, 122
Hypothermia, of newborn, 459, 464, 466-467
Hypothyroidism, 222
  congenital, 592-593, 667 [133-134]
Hypoxemia, 184
Hysterosalpingogram, 386t

Ibuprofen, 161, 301t, 321, 322t
Icterus neonatorum, 455-456
Id, definition of, 92
Idealization, definition of, 21
Ideas of reference, definition of, 22, 92
Identification, definition of, 21
Ileal conduit, 245
Ileostomy, 263-264
Illusion, 129
  definition of, 92
Imipramine, 51t, 124, 327
Immobilization complications, 297
Immunizations, for children, 519, 520t
Immunosuppressive drugs, 253t
Imodium. *See* Loperamide
Impetigo contagiosa, 544t
Impulsivity, 60
Imuran. *See* Azathioprine
Incompetence
  competency hearings, 28
  definition of, 92
Inderal. *See* Propranolol
Indocin. *See* Indomethacin
Indomethacin, 301t
  lithium and, 104
Infant, 517-520. *See also* Newborn
  accident prevention for, 519-520
  concept of death, 617t
  growth and development of, 517-518
  head injury in, 635-638
  hospitalization of, 529
  immunizations for, 519, 520t
  nutrition for, 518-519, 519t
  pain responses of, 639
  sleep pattern of, 519
  sudden death of, 567-568
Infantile spasm, 561
Infections

of newborn, 472
during pregnancy, 414-416
puerperal, 448-449
Infertility, 649-650 [42-45]
Inflammatory bowel disease, 261-263
INH. *See* Isoniazid
Insanity, definition of, 29
Insight, definition of, 92
Insulin, 217t, 227t, 651 [56-59]
Interpersonal, definition of, 92
Intracranial pressure, increased, 558-559, 559t, 664 [112-113]
Intracranial surgery, 276-277
Intradural block, 426
Intraocular pressure, 290-291
Intrapsychic, definition of, 92
Intrauterine device, 387t
Intravenous pyelogram, 239
Intravenous therapy, calculating rates for, 160t
Introjection, definition of, 21
Intropin. *See* Dopamine
Intussusception, intestinal, 603-604
Iodine, radioactive, 221
Iron-deficiency anemia, 579-580
Ismelin. *See* Guanethidine
Isocarboxazid, 51t, 124
Isoflurophate, 287t
Isoimmunization, 443-444, 444t, 467, *467*
Isolation
definition of, 21
procedures for, 540t
Isometric exercises, 293
Isoniazid, 191t
Isoproterenol, 187t, 629t, 631
Isopto carbachol. *See* Carbachol
Isordil. *See* Isosorbide dinitrate
Isosorbide dinitrate, 173t
Isoxuprine, 435
Isuprel. *See* Isoproterenol

Jacksonian seizure, 561
Jaundice
breast-feeding associated, 507-509
breast milk, 468, 507-509
cholestatic, due to antipsychotics, 122
neonatal, 455-456, 458, 467-468
pathologic, 467, 506-510
physiologic, 467
"Jock itch", 545t
Joints, 293

Kanamycin, 189t, 191t
Kantrex. *See* Kanamycin
Kaopectate, 260t
Kaposi's sarcoma, 315
Kegel exercises, 452
Kemadrin. *See* Procyclidine hydrochloride
Kenalog. *See* Triamcinolone acetate
Kernicterus, 467-468
Ketoacidosis, 230t, 230-231
Ketones, urinary, 238
Kidney, 232, *233*
acute failure of, 245-247, 681-682 [188-196]
of child, 598
chronic failure of, 247-249
transplantation of, 252-254, 681-682 [191-196]
Korsakoff's syndrome, 48

Labia majora, 383
Labia minora, 383
Lability, definition of, 92
Labor and delivery, 419-440, 650 [48-50], 671-672 [181-184], 701-702 [290-295]
analgesia during, 424-426
anesthesia during, 426
cesarean birth, *438*, 438-439
episiotomy during, 436, *437*
fetal heart rate during, 421-422, *421-423*, 422t, 424t
high risk, 431, 665-666 [121-128], 682-683 [199-201]
nursing process during, 426-431
onset of, 421
presentation in, 419, *420*
problems during
amniotic fluid embolism, 440
dystocia, 432-434
emergency birth, 435-436
premature labor, 434-435
uterine rupture, 439-440
signs of labor, 420
stages and phases of, 425t
true vs. false labor, 420
use of forceps during, 436-437
uterine contractions during, 424, *426*
vacuum extraction, 437-438
vaginal delivery after cesarean birth, 439
Laboratory values, adult, 727-728
Laceration
cerebral, 275
perineal, 437
scalp, 637
Lactation, 442
suppression of, 445t
Lactulose, 261t
Laminectomy, 303, 690 [270-271]
Lanatoside C, 179t
Language development, 517-518, 521, 522
Lanoxin. *See* Digoxin
Lanugo, 455
Laparoscopy, 386t, 483
Large bowel. *See* Colon
Larodopa. *See* Levodopa
Laryngeal cancer, 196-198, 688 [251-253]
Laryngitis, acute spasmodic, 568, 568t
Laryngotracheobronchitis, 568, 568t, 705-706 [336-344]
Lasix. *See* Furosemide
Latent, definition of, 92
Laxatives, 260t-261t, 325
for dialysis patient, 360
Lead poisoning, 547t
Lecithin/sphingomyelin ratio, 402
Legal issues, of psychiatric nursing, 28-29
Legg-Calvé-Perthes disease, 610
Leopold's maneuver, 427, *427*
Leukemia, 618-619, 667 [135-141]
LeVeen shunt, 215
Level of consciousness, 271
Levodopa, 282t
antipsychotics and, 120t
Levo-Dromoran. *See* Levorphanol
Levoprome. *See* Methotrimeprazine
Levorphanol, 161, 323t
Levothyroxine, 222, 592, 667 [134]
Librium. *See* Chlordiazepoxide
Lice, 545t
Licensure exam. *See* NCLEX-RN
Lidocaine, 170t
Lidone. *See* Molindone
Life-cycle stages, 17t-18t, 21
Life expectancy, 151
Life span, 151
Ligaments, 293
Limbitrol. *See* Chlordiazepoxide-amitriptyline
Limit setting, definition of, 92
Liothyronine, 222
Lipase, 199, 217t
Lithane. *See* Lithium
Lithium, 41t, 51t-52t, 59, 101-105, 125, 683 [209-210]
contraindications to, 104t-105t
drug interactions with, 103-104
indications for, 101
long-term effects of, 103
patient teaching about, 104-105
in pregnancy, 104-105
side effects and toxicity of, 102t, 102-103, 125
usage guidelines for, 101-102
Lithobid. *See* Lithium
Lithonate. *See* Lithium
Lithotabs. *See* Lithium
Liver
angiography of, 203
biopsy of, 204
cirrhosis, 213-214
complications of disease of, 214-216
hepatitis, 212-213
Liver function studies, 202
Lochia, 441, 442t
Lomotil, 260t
Loose associations, 74
definition of, 92
Loperamide, 260t
Lorazepam, 41t, 134t
Loss. *See also* Death and dying
adaptive responses to, 30
definition of, 30
nursing process for, 31-32
physical, 31-32
psychologic, 32
Loxapine, 75t, 119, 125
Loxitance. *See* Loxapine
Loxitane. *See* Loxapine
LSD, 88, 89t
Ludiomil. *See* Maprotiline
Luekeran. *See* Chlorambucil
Lumbar puncture, 272
Lung, 162
cancer of, 195-196
fetal maturity of, 402
normal, 152
Lupus, 302
Luque wires, 610
Luteinizing hormone, 217t
Lymphoma, 311-312
Lysergic acid diethylamide, 88, 89t

Macrodantin. *See* Nitrofurantoin
Magaldrate, 207t
Magnesium citrate, 261t
Magnesium hydroxide, 207t, 261t
Magnesium sulfate, 261t, 410t, 435
Major tranquilizers. *See* Antipsychotics
Mandelamine. *See* Methenamine mandelate
Mania, 58-61
acute, 58
delirious, 59
mild, 58
nursing process for, 59-61
Manic-depression, 55, 59
Manipulation, definition of, 92
Mannitol, 246t

Mantoux test, 190
Maprotiline, 51t, 124
Marijuana, 89t, 328
Marplan. *See* Isocarboxazid
Massage, 293
Mastectomy, 313, 667-668 [142-147]
Mastitis, 449-450
McDonald procedure, 404
McDonald's rule, 396, 396t
Mean arterial pressure, 162
Mechlorethamine nitrogen mustard, 614t
Meconium-aspiration syndrome, 469
Medrol. *See* Methylprednisolone acetate
Melanocyte-stimulating hormone, 217t
Mellaril. *See* Thioridazine
Meningitis, 563-564
Meningocele, 559
Meningomyelocele, 559, 684 [212-218]
Menopause, 385, 389
Menstrual cycle, 385
Mental health nursing. *See* Psychiatric nursing
Mental Health Systems Act (1980), 28
Mental retardation, 555t, 555-556. *See also* Down syndrome
Mental status examination, definition of, 92
Meperidine, 161, 322t, 323t, 325
  abuse of, 87-88, 89t
  antipsychotics and, 120t
Meprobamate, 41t, 133, 134t
  abuse of, 88, 89t
6-Mercaptopurine, 614t
Merital. *See* Nomifensine
Mescaline, 88, 89t
Mesoridazine, 119
Mestinon. *See* Pyridostigmine bromide
Metabolic acidosis, 586
Metabolic alkalosis, 586
Metabolism, 200-201. *See also* Nutrition
Metamucil. *See* Psyllium hydrophilic
Metastasis, definition of, 306
Methadone, 89t, 161, 323t
Methanamine hippurate, 241t, 242
Methaqualone, 133, 134t
  abuse of, 89t
Methazolamide, 287t
Methenamine mandelate, 599
Methergine. *See* Methylergonovine maleate
Methicillin, 189t
Methohexital, 134
Methotrexate, 614t
Methotrimeprazine, 327
Methylcellulose, 260t
Methyldopa, 180t
Methylergonovine maleate, 431t
Methylphenidate, 89t, 556
Methylprednisolone, 226t, 569t
Methyprylon, 133, 134t
Metoclopramide, 310t
Mexate. *See* Methotrexate
Micronase. *See* Glyburide
Milia, 455
Milieu, definition of, 92
Milieu therapy, 26, 50
  for withdrawn behavior, 74-76
Military Anti-Shock Trousers (MAST), 632-633
Milk of Magnesia. *See* Magnesium hydroxide
Miller-Abbott tube, 265
Miltown. *See* Meprobamate
Milwaukee brace, 610
Mineral oil, 261t
Mineralocorticoids, 217t
Minimal brain dysfunction, 556
Minocin. *See* Minocycline
Minocycline, 189t
Miostat. *See* Carbachol
Miotics, 287t
Moban. *See* Molindone
Modified autogenic relaxation, 107, 110
Mogadon. *See* Nitrazepam
Molindone, 75t, 119, 125
Mongolian spots, 455
Monilial infection, during pregnancy, 415
Monoamine oxidase inhibitors, 51t
  lithium and, 104
Mons pubis, 383
MOPP chemotherapy, 311
Morning sickness, 391, 397
Moro reflex, 458
Morphine, 323t
  abuse of, 87-88, 89t
  lithium and, 104
Motrin. *See* Ibuprofen
Mourning, 475. *See also* Grief
  definition of, 30
  stages of, 30-31
Mucomyst. *See* Acetylcysteine
Multiple gestation, 416
Multiple sclerosis, 283-284
Mumps, 539
Muscle relaxants, lithium and, 104
Muscle spasms, in spinal cord-injured person, 368-369
Musculoskeletal problems
  amputation, 299-300
  arthritis, 300-302
  of children, 605-611
  collagen disease, 302
  congenital clubfoot, 609
  congenital hip dysplasia, 609-610
  fractures, 295-297
  herniated nucleus pulposus, 302-305
  Legg-Calvé-Perthes disease, 610
  nursing process for, 293-295
  osteomyelitis, 611
  in pregnancy, 391-392
  scoliosis, 610-611
  in spinal cord-injured person, 367-369
Musculoskeletal system, 293
  of adult, 152
  of child, 605
Music, for relaxation, 109
Mustargen. *See* Mechlorethamine nitrogen mustard
Myambutol. *See* Ethambutol
Myasthenia gravis, 285-286
Myciguent. *See* Neomycin sulfate
Myelogram, 294, 690 [269-270]
Mylicon. *See* Simethicone
Myocardial infarction, 173-177, *174-175*, 175t-177t, 654 [85-90]
  blood tests for, 175t
  definition of, 173
  diet after, 175, 177t
  drug therapy for, 176t
  enzyme patterns after, *175*
Mysoline. *See* Primidone
Mytelase. *See* Ambenonium chloride
Myxedema, 222

Naegele's rule, 395t
Nafcillin, 189t
Nalbuphine, 161, 323t
Nalfon. *See* Fenoprofen
Naloxone, 326, 632
Naprosyn. *See* Naproxen
Naproxen, 161t, 301t, 321, 322t
Narcissism, definition of, 92
Narcotic abuse, 87-88, 89t
Nardil. *See* Phenelzine
Nasal surgery, 291
Natural family planning, 388t
Navane. *See* Thiothixene
NCLEX-RN
  communication test items on, 7-8, 8t
  format of, 4-6
    categories of human needs, 5t, 5-6
    nursing process, 4, 4t
  keys to success on, 6-9, 10t
    affective, 9
    cognitive, 6t, 6-9
  preparing for, 3-6
  scoring of, 6
Necrotizing enterocolitis, neonatal, 470-471
Nembutal. *See* Pentobarbital
Neologism, definition of, 92
Neomycin, 189t, 288t
Neoplasia. *See* Cancer
Neoplasm, definition of, 306
Neostigmine bromide, 286t, 287t
Neostigmine methylsulfate, 286t
Nephrectomy, 243
Nephritis, 601-602, 710 [372-374]
Nephrolithotomy, 243
Nephron, 232, *233*
Nephrosis, 602-603
Neptazane. *See* Methazolamide
Nervous system, 268-269
Nervous system problems
  acute head injury, 275-276
  amyotrophic lateral sclerosis, 284-285
  cerebrovascular accident, 277-279, *278*
  intracranial surgery, 276-277
  multiple sclerosis, 283-284
  myasthenia gravis, 285-286
  Parkinson's syndrome, 281-283
  spinal cord injury, 279-281, 280t
Neuroblastoma, 620t
Neuroleptics. *See* Antipsychotics
Neurologic examination, 271
Neurologic functioning, normal, 152-153
Neuromuscular blockade, during labor and delivery, 426
Neurosis, definition of, 92
Newborn, 454-475, 517-520, 645 [1-6], 650-651 [50-59], 682-683 [201-203]
  acquired immunedeficiency syndrome in, 473-474
  bathing of, 465
  birth injuries/congenital anomalies of, 474-475
  body features of, 455-457
  characteristics of, 454-455
  cocaine-exposed, 486-487
  drug/alcohol addiction of, 472-473
  gestational age of, 460-463, *461*
    large-for-gestational-age, 463
    postmature, 462-463
    premature, 460-462
    small-for-gestational-age, 463
  high-risk, 466
  hypoglycemia in, 471-472
  hypothermia in, 464, 466-467
  infections of, 472
  jaundice of, 467-468
  necrotizing enterocolitis in, 470-471

nursing process for, 463-466
parental reaction to sick/disabled/malformed infant, 475
reflexes of, 458
respiratory distress syndrome in, 435, *470*, 3669-470
systems adaptations of, 458-460, *459*
Nifedipine, 173t
Nipple-stimulation contraction test, 401
Nipride. *See* Nitroprusside
Nitrates, 173t
Nitrazepam, 134t
Nitro-Bid. *See* Nitroglycerin
Nitrofurantoin, 241t, 599
Nitroglycerin, 173t, 632
Nitrol. *See* Nitroglycerin
Nitroprusside, 181t, 629t, 632
Noctec. *See* Chloral hydrate
Noludar. *See* Methyprylon
Nolvadex. *See* Tamoxifen
Nomifensine, 124
Non-Hodgkin's lymphoma, 311
Nonorganic failure to thrive, 587-588
Nonstress testing, 400-401
Norepinephrine, 217t
Norpramin. *See* Desipramine
Nortriptyline, 124
Nose, 270
Nose surgery, 291
Nosebleed, 291-292
Nubain. *See* Nalbuphine
Nucleus pulposus, herniated, 302-305
Numorphan. *See* Oxymorphone
Nurse-client relationship, 22-24
characteristics of, 22-23
communication skills in, 24t
phases of, 23-24
purpose of, 22
therapeutic, 15, 23
Nursing diagnoses, 725-726
Nursing process, 4, 4t
client needs categories and, 720-723
Nutrition
for adult, 153t
basic food groups, 152t
for children
adolescent, 525
infant, 518-519, 519t
newborn, 460, 465-466
preschooler, 523
school age, 524
toddler, 521
human vs. cow's milk, 460t
during pregnancy, 397-398, 398t-399t
for spinal cord-injured person, 366
total parenteral, 351-355

Obsessive-compulsive disorders, 42-43
Obstruction, colonic, 264-265
Occupational therapy, 76, 686-687 [240-241]
Oliguria, 359
Oncovin. *See* Vincristine
Opiate abuse, 87-88
Opium, 87-88, 89t
Optimil. *See* Methaqualone
Oral contraceptives, 387t
Oretic. *See* Hydrochlorothiazide
Oreton. *See* Testosterone
Organic brain syndrome, 103
Orientation, definition of, 92
Orinase. *See* Tolbutamide
Orphenadrine hydrochloride, 113
Orthostatic hypotension, 121
Osmitrol. *See* Mannitol
Osteoarthritis, 300-302
Osteogenic sarcoma, 620t
Osteomyelitis, 611
Osteoporosis, 389t
Osteotomy, 300
Otitis media, 534-537
Ovary, 384
Overhydration, 234t
Overt, definition of, 92
Ovulation, 385
Oxacillin, 189t
Oxazepam, 41t, 134t
abuse of, 88, 89t
Oxycodone, 161, 322t
Oxygenation, extracorporeal membrane, 633
Oxygenation problems, 162-198. *See also* specific disorders
angina pectoris, 171-173, *172*, 173t
cardiopulmonary arrest, 169
chest tubes and chest surgery, 193-195, *194-195*
of children, 565-583
bronchial asthma, 569t, 569-571
bronchiolitis, 568, 568t
bronchopulmonary dysplasia, 568-569
congenital heart disease, 572-578, *573-574*
epiglottitis, 568, 568t
laryngotracheobronchitis, 568, 568t
nursing process for, 565 567, 571-572
rheumatic fever/rheumatic heart disease, 578-579
spasmodic croup, 568, 568t
sudden infant death syndrome, 567-568
chronic obstructive pulmonary disease, 184-188
circulatory problems, 183-185, *184*
congestive heart failure, 178-182
diagnostic tests for, *166-167*, 166-168
hypertension, 182-183
laryngeal cancer, 196-198
lung cancer, 195-196
myocardial infarction, 173-177, *174-175*, 175t-177t
nursing process for, 164-169
pacemaker, 177-178
pneumonia, 188, 190
pulmonary embolus, 192-193
shock, 170-171
in spinal cord-injured person, 366
tuberculosis, 190-191
Oxymorphone, 161, 323t
Oxyphencyclimine, 210
Oxytocin, 217t, 433, 433t, 666 [127-128], 701 [290-291]
Oxytocin challenge test, 401

Pacemakers, 177-178
Pagitane. *See* Cycrimine hydrochloride
Pain
acute, 320
analgesia for, 320-329. *See also* Analgesics
cancer, 320
child responses to, 328
chronic, 320
definition of, 320
physiology of, 641
prostaglandin E_2 and, 321
psychiatric disorders and, 328
responses to, 639-641
Palliation, definition of, 306
Pamelor. *See* Nortriptyline
Panadol. *See* Acetaminophen
Pancreas, 199, 218
Pancreatic function studies, 202
Pancreatitis, 211-212
Pancuronium, lithium and, 104
Panic, 36-37
Papanicolaou test, 309, 389, 389t
Para-aminosalicylic acid, 191t
Paracervical block, 426
Paragoric, 260t
Paral. *See* Paraldehyde
Paraldehyde, 133, 134t
Paralysis. *See* Spinal cord injury
Paranoia, 70-71, 652-653 [68-76]
Paranoid, definition of, 92
Paranoid schizophrenia, 80t, 669-670 [159-167]
Paraplegia, *362*. *See also* Spinal cord injury
Parasympathetic nerves, 269, 269t
Parathormone, 217t
Parathyroid glands, 218
Parenteral nutrition, total, 351-355
Parest. *See* Methaqualone
Parkinsonism, 281-283
drug therapy of, 112-113
due to antipsychotics, 111-113, 125
vs. schizophrenia, 112
Parlodel. *See* Bromocriptine mesylate
Parnate. *See* Tranylcypromine
Parotitis, 539
Parsidol. *See* Ethopropazine hydrochloride
Patent ductus arteriosus, *573*, 575
Pavulon. *See* Pancuronium
PCP, 88, 89t
Pediculosis, 545t
Pelvic inflammatory disease, 480, 483
Pelvic measurements, 383
Pelvis, female, 383
Penfluridol, 119
Penicillin, 189t
Pentaerythritol tetranitrate, 173t
Pentafin. *See* Pentrerythritol tetranitrate
Pentazocine, 161, 322t, 323t, 325
Pentobarbital, 131-132, 134
Pentothal. *See* Thiopental
Pentritol. *See* Pentrerythritol tetranitrate
Pepsin, 199
Peptic ulcer disease, 206-209, 647-648 [26-32]
Pepto-Bismol. *See* Bismuth subsalicylate
Peridural block, 426
Perineum
laceration of, 437
postpartum healing of, 441, 443
Peripheral nervous system, 268
Peripheral vascular disease, 183-185, *184*
Peritoneal dialysis, 249-250
Peritrate. *See* Pentrerythritol tetranitrate
Permitil. *See* Fluophenazine
Perphenazine, 75t, 119, 125, 310t
extrapyramidal side effects of, 115
Personality, definition of, 92
Petit mal seizure, 561
Phenazopyridine hydrochloride, 241t
Phenelzine, 124
Phenergan. *See* Promethazine
Phenobarbital, 131-132, 134, 562t
abuse of, 89t
Phenothiazines, 75t, 116-123, 327

Phenoxene. *See* Chlorphenoxamine hydrochloride
Phentolamine, 629t, 632
Phenylbutazone, 301t, 303t
  lithium and, 104
Phenylketonuria, 465, 651 [59]
Phenytoin, 327, 562t
Pheochromocytoma, 223-225
Phlebothrombosis, 183
Phobia, 40-41
  definition of, 92
Phototoxicity, due to antipsychotics, 122
Physostigmine salicylate, 287t
Pigmentary retinopathy, 122
Pigmentation, due to antipsychotics, 122
Pilocarpine hydrochloride, 287t
Pimozide, 119
Pinworms, 543, 545
Piperacetazine, 119
Piperazines, 119
Piperidines, 119
Piroxicam, 301t
Pitocin. *See* Oxytocin
Placenta, 391
  assessing function of, 402
  retained fragments of, 447
Placenta previa, *406*, 406-407
Placidyl. *See* Ethchlorvynol
Plant alkaloids, 615t
Pleur-evac system, 193, *195*, 335, *335*, 707
Pneumonia, 188, 190
  pneumocystis carinii, 315
  in spinal cord-injured person, 366
Pneumothorax, 332-333, 707 [350]
  tension, 193, 333
Poisoning, 545-548, 546t-547t, 654 [91-93]
Polycillin. *See* Ampicillin
Polycythemia, 508
Polymixin, 189t, 288t
Post-traumatic stress disorders, 46
Postpartum period, 441-452, 645 [1-6], 683 [203-205], 703-704 [318-335]
  care of adolescent mother in, 500-505
  maternal psychologic adaptation during, 442-443, 443t
  nursing process during, 443-447
    for high-risk client, 446-447
  problems during
    cystitis, 449-450
    hematoma, 448
    hemorrhage, 447-448
    mastitis, 449-450
    psychological maladaptations, 450, 451t
    puerperal infection, 448-449
    pulmonary embolus, 448
  restoration to pregravid status during, 441-442
Postural hypotension, 369
Posturing, 272, *272-273*
Potassium
  balance of, 232-233
  food content of, 182t
Potassium iodide, 187t
Prazepam, 134t
Prednisone, 226t, 615t
Preeclampsia, 408-410, 409t, 490-497
Pregnancy, 390-417, 650 [45-49], 690-691 [272-278]
  of adolescent, 416-417
  anticipatory guidance during, 396-397
  antipsychotics in, 118
  bleeding in, 665-666 [121-128]
  body system changes in, 390-392
  cocaine use during, 484-489
    pharmacology of, 484-486
  danger signals of, 396
  diagnostic tests during, 400-403
  discomforts of, 397
  ectopic, 405, *405*, 479-483. *See also* Ectopic pregnancy
  fetal development in, 394
  high-risk, 399-403, 682-683 [197-198]
  lithium in, 104-105
  management of, 395
  multiple gestation, 416
  nursing process during, 395-399
  paternal reactions to, 393
  problems during
    abortion, 404
    abruptio placentae, *407*, 407-408
    anemia, 413
    cardiac disorders, 412-413
    diabetes, 410-412, 663-664 [98-103]
    fetal death, 498-499
    hydatidiform mole, *405*, 405-406
    hyperemia gravidarum, 414
    hypertension, 408-410, 409t, 490-497
    incompetent cervical os, 404-405
    infections, 414-416
    placenta previa, *406*, 406-407
    toxoplasmosis, 688-689 [254-261]
  psychosocial adaptations in, 392-393
  sibling reactions to, 393
  signs and symptoms of, 393-394
Preludin, 89t
Preschooler
  concept of death of, 617t
  healthy, 522-523
  hospitalization of, 529-530
  pain responses of, 640
Primidone, 562t
Pro-Banthine. *See* Propantheline
Procainamide, 170t
Procaine, 189t
Procardia. *See* Nifedipine
Prochlorperazine, 119, 310t, 327
Proctoscopy, 258
Procyclidine hydrochloride, 282t
  for parkinsonism, 113
Progesterone, 217t
Projection, definition of, 22
Proketazine. *See* Carphenazine
Prolactin, 217t
Prolapse, uterine, 451-452
Prolixin. *See* Fluphenazine
Promethazine, 135
Pronestyl. *See* Procainamide
Propantheline, 210
Propoxyphene, 322t
Propranolol, 135, 173t, 180t, 221
Propylthiouricil, 221
Prostaglandin E_2, 321
Prostaphlin. *See* Oxacillin
Prostate
  benign hypertrophy of, 254-256
  cancer of, 256-257
Prostatectomy, 255t, *256*
Prostigmin. *See* Neostigmine methylsulfate
Protein, urinary, 238
Proteinuria, in pregnancy, 496
Protriptyline, 124
Prozac. *See* Fluoxetine
Psychiatric nursing
  definition of, 15
  interpersonal relationships in, 15-16
  legal issues of, 28-29
    civil admission procedures, 28
    competency hearings, 28
    criminal procedures, 28-29
    judicial precedents, 29
    nurse's role, 29
  nurse-client relationship, 22-24, 24t
  nursing process, 24-25
  practice locations of, 16
  practice of, 15
  roles of, 16
  scope of profession, 15
  terminology of, 91-93
  treatment modalities of, 25-26
Psychoanalysis, definition of, 92
Psychodrama, definition of, 92
Psychodynamics, definition of, 92
Psychogenic, definition of, 92
Psychomotor seizure, 561
Psychosis. *See also* Withdrawn behavior
  atypical, 80t
  brief reactive, 80t
  definition of, 92-93
  postpartum, 450
Psychosocial assessment, 25
Psychosocial development, 16-20, 17t-18t, 371-372, 374
Psychosomatic disorders, 44-45
Psychotherapy, 50
  definition of, 25, 93
  group, 16, 26
  individual, 16
Psyllium hydrophilic, 210, 260t
Puberty, 524-525
Pudendal block, 426
Puerperal infection, 448-449
Pulmonary edema, 685 [223-224]
Pulmonary embolus, 192-193
  postpartal, 448
Pulmonary function tests, 166, *166*
Pulmonic stenosis, *574*, 575
Purified protein derivative (PPD) test, 190
Purodigin. *See* Digitoxin
Pyelogram
  intravenous, 239
  retrograde, 239-240
Pyelolithotomy, 243
Pyelonephritis, 242-243, 671 [175-180]
Pyloric stenosis, 588-589
Pyloroplasty, 206
Pylorotomy, 588
Pyrazinamide, 191t
Pyridium. *See* Phenazopyridine hydrochloride
Pyridostigmine bromide, 286t

Quaalude. *See* Methaqualone
Quadriplegia, *362*. *See also* Spinal cord injury
Queckenstedt's test, 272, 365
Questions and answers, 643-719
Quide. *See* Piperacetazine

Raccoon eyes, 636-637
Radiation therapy, 307-311, 613, 616
Radical mastectomy, 313
Range-of-motion exercises, 293
Ranitidine, 207t
Rape, 65-66, 691 [279-280]
Rationalization, definition of, 21
Rau-sed. *See* Reserpine
Raynaud's disease, 183
Raynaud's phenomenon, 302

Reach-to-Recovery, 315
Reaction formation, definition of, 21
Reality, definition of, 93
Rectal examination, 309
Rectocele, 451
Reed-Sternberg cells, 311
Reflexes, of newborn, 458
Regional enteritis, 261-263
Reglan. *See* Metoclopramide
Regression
  definition of, 22
  in spinal cord-injured person, 371
Regurgitation, 586
Relaxation techniques, 106-110
  behavioral manifestations of, 107
  body postures for, 108
  characteristics of, 106
  cognitive manifestations of, 107
  color exchange, 109, 110
  ending of, 109-110
  full-body relaxation, 106-107, 110
  modified autogenic relaxation, 107, 110
  music, 109
  physiologic manifestations of, 107
  sensory pacing, 107, 109, 110
  ten-second methods, 109
Renal disorders, due to lithium therapy, 103
Renal failure
  acute, 245-247, 681-682 [188-196]
  chronic, 247-249
  fluid restriction in, 359
Renin, 236
Repoise. *See* Butaperazine
Repression, definition of, 21
Reproductive system
  normal female, 383-385, *384*
  normal male, *254*
  in pregnancy, 390-391
Reserpine, 180t
Reserpoid. *See* Reserpine
Respiratory distress syndrome of newborn, 435, 469-470, *470*
Respiratory system, 162, 162-164. *See also* Oxygenation problems
  of children, 565
Restraints, pediatric, 532t
Retinal detachment, 289-290
Retinopathy, pigmentary, 122
Retrograde pyelogram, 239-240
Retrovir. *See* Zidovudine
Reye's syndrome, 539
Rh sensitization, 443-444, 444t, 467, *467*
Rheumatic fever, 578-579, 703-704 [311-317]
Rheumatic heart disease, 578-579
Rheumatoid arthritis, 300-302
RhoGAM, 443-444, 444t, 468
Rifadin. *See* Rifampin
Rifampin, 191t
Rigidity
  cogwheel, 103, 112
  lead-pipe, 112
Ringworm, 545t
Rinne test, 273, 526
Riopan. *See* Magaldrate
Risser plaster jacket, 610
Ritalin. *See* Methylphenidate
Ritodrine, 435, 436t
Robitussin. *See* Guaifenesin
Rocky Mountain spotted fever, 539
Romberg test, 636
Rooting reflex, 458
Roseola, 539
Rubella, 539
  during pregnancy, 414-415
Rule of nines, 548, *550*
Russell traction, 606t, *608*

Sadomasochism, 65
Safety and security, 268-292
  nursing process for, 270-275
Saint Vitus' dance, 578
Salicylate poisoning, 546t
Saliva, 199
Sandimmune. *See* Cyclosporine
Sandril. *See* Reserpine
Sarcoma
  definition of, 306
  Kaposi's, 315
Scabies, 542t
Scalp laceration, 637
Scarlet fever, 539
Schilling's test, 203-204
Schizoaffective disorders, 80t
  lithium for, 101
Schizophrenia, 72-80, 685-686 [230-234]. *See also* Withdrawn behavior
  catatonic, 80t
  childhood, 80t
  paranoid, 80t, 669-670 [159-167]
  undifferentiated, 80t
Schizophreniform disorders, 80t
Schizophrenogenic, definition of, 93
School age child
  concept of death of, 617t
  healthy, 523-524
  hospitalization of, 530
  pain responses of, 640-641
School phobia, 524
Scoliosis, 610-611
Seasonal affective disorder, 54
Secobarbital, 131-132, 134
  abuse of, 89t
Seconal. *See* Secobarbital
Secretin, 200t
Sedative-hypnotics, 130-135, 327-328
  antihistamines, 135
  barbiturates, 131-132
  beta-blockers, 135
  classification of, 131
  contraindications to, 133-135
  indications for, 130-135
  nonbarbiturate-nonbenzodiazepine compounds, 133
  side effects of, 131, 133
  tolerance to, 131
  usage guidelines for, 133
  withdrawal from, 131
Seizure disorders, 560-563, 562t
  due to antipsychotics, 121
Self-help groups, 26
Senna, 260t
Senokot. *See* Senna
Sensory pacing, 107, 109, 110
Septra. *See* Co-trimoxazole
Serax. *See* Oxazepam
Serentil. *See* Mesoridazine
Seromycin. *See* Cycloserine
Serpasil. *See* Reserpine
Serum placental lactogen, 402
Sex hormones, 217t
Sex-linked recessive diseases, *581*
Sexual acting out, 67-70
Sexuality, 19-20
  antipsychotics and sexual functioning, 121
  causes of role dissatisfaction, 19
  definitions of, 19
  factors affecting functioning, 19-20
Sexually transmitted diseases, 541, 542t-543t
  during pregnancy, 414
Sheehan's syndrome, 220
Shirodkar procedure, 404
Shock, 170-171, 664 [106-111]
  in children, 627-634
    clinical assessment of, 627-628
    drug therapy for, 629t, 630-632
    drugs for, 629t
    extracorporeal membrane oxygenation for, 633
    fluid management in, 630
    initial treatment of, 629
    lab evaluation of, 628-629
    MAST suit for, 632-633
    monitoring of, *628*, 629-630
    nurse's roles for, 633-634
    nursing diagnoses for, 633t
Shock therapy. *See* Electroconvulsive therapy
"Shrinker sock", 299
Shunt, ventriculoperitoneal, 653-654 [81-84]
SIADH, 219-220
Sickle cell anemia, 580-582
Sigmoidoscopy, 258
Significant others, definition of, 93
Silverman-Anderson scale, 469, *470*
Simethicone, 207t
Sims-Huhner test, 386t
Sinemet. *See* Carbidopa-levodopa
Sinequan. *See* Doxepin
Skeletal traction, 606t
Skene's ducts, 384
Skin problems, 543-545, 544t-545t
Skin traction, 606t
Skull fracture, 635-638, 664 [112-113]
Sleep
  of infant, 519
  of preschooler, 523
Small bowel secretions, 199
Sneezing reflex, 458
Snellen test, 273
Social phobia, 40-41
Socially maladaptive behavior, 62-71, 689-690 [262-267], 700-701 [281-287]
  antisocial behavior, 70-71
  family violence, 63-66
  hostile-aggressive behavior, 66-67
  nursing process for, 62-63
  sexual acting out, 67-70
Sociotherapy, 16
Sodium
  balance of, 232
  food content of, 177t
Sodium bicarbonate, 170t, 207t, 632
Sodium valproate, 327, 562t
Solacen. *See* Tybamate
Solu-Cortef. *See* Hydrocortisone
Solu-Medrol. *See* Methylprednisolone
Somnos. *See* Chloral hydrate
Sopor. *See* Methaqualone
Sorbitrate. *See* Isosorbide dinitrate
Spectinomycin, lithium and, 104
Spermicides, 388t
Spina bifida, 559-560
Spinal cord, 260
Spinal cord injury, 279-281
  acute care of, 362-363, 365-367
  autonomic nervous system disturbances

with, 369-370
  decubitus ulcers with, 367-368, *368*
  maintaining elimination in, 366-367
  maintaining hydration and nutrition in, 366
  maintaining respiratory function in, 366
  management of, i, 365
  metabolic disturbances with, 369
  movement control and, 280t
  muscle spasms with, 368-369
  neurogenic bowel and bladder with, 367
  patient transfer after, *361*, 361-362
  psychological care for, 370-377
    developing autonomy, 375-376
    developing initiative, 376-377
    developing trust, 372-375
    developmental stages, 371-372, 374
  stabilization of, 364-365
  types of, 363, *363-364*
Spinal fusion, 303
Spinal shock, 366
Spironolactone, 180t, 215
Sprain, definition of, 293
SSKI, 569t
Stadol. *See* Butorphanol
Staphcillin. *See* Methicillin
State nursing boards, 731-733
Status epilepticus, 561
Stelazine. *See* Trifluoperazine
Stepping reflex, 458
Sterilization, 388t
Steroids, 226t
Stillbirth, 498-499
Stimulant abuse, 88, 89t
Stomach secretions, 199
Stone disease, 243-244
Stool softeners, 360
Stool tests, 202, 258
Stork bite, 455
STP, 88
Strabismus, 537-538
Strain, definition of, 293
Streptase. *See* Streptokinase
Streptococcal infection, during pregnancy, 414
Streptokinase, 176t
Streptomycin, 189t, 191t
Stress. *See also* Anxiety
  management of, 39t-40t
  post-traumatic stress disorders, 46
Stress ulcer, 281, 367
Stressor, definition of, 93
Stretching reflex, 458
Stroke, 277-279, *278*
Stryker frame, 280
Stuttering, 522
Subaortic stenosis, *574*, 575
Subdural hematoma, 276
Sublimation, definition of, 21
Substance abuse disorders, 81-90, 707-708 [351-354]
  alcoholism, 83-87
  amphetamines and cocaine, 88
  barbiturates, 88
  definition of, 81
  drug use assessment, 488
  hallucinogens, 88
  of health professionals, 82
  neonatal addictions, 472-473
  nursing process, 82-83
  opiates, 87-88
  overdose of, 89t
  during pregnancy, 484-489
  substance dependence, 81-82
  vs. substance use, 81
  withdrawal from, 89t
Substitution, definition of, 21
Succinylcholine, lithium and, 104
Sucking reflex, 458
Sudden infant death syndrome, 567-568
Suicide, 136-141, 646-647 [16]
  assessing potential for, 56, 76, 137-141
  case study of, 137-139
  characteristics of victims of, 139-140
  crisis intervention techniques, 141
  methods of, 56t
  nursing process for, 56
  persons at risk for, 55
Sulfacetamide sodium, 288t
Sulfasalazine, 241t
Sulfisoxazole, 241t
Sulindac, 301t
Sundowning, 129
Superego, definition of, 93
Suppression, definition of, 21
Surfak. *See* Docusate calcium
Surgery, 157-161
  common complications of, 157
  discharge planning, 160
  factors affecting response to, 157
  operative care, 160
  postoperative care, 159-160
  preoperative care, 157-158
Surmontil. *See* Trimipramine
Suspicious behavior, 70-71
  nursing process for, 70
  paranoia, 70-71
Swallowing reflex, 458
Sydenham's chorea, 578
Symbolization, definition of, 21
Symmetrel. *See* Amantadine
Sympathetic nerves, 269, 269t
Syncope, in spinal cord-injured person, 369
Syndrome of inappropriate secretion of antidiuretic hormone, 219-220
Synovectomy, 300
Synthroid. *See* Levothyroxine
Syphilis, 542t
  during pregnancy, 414
Systemic lupus erythematosus, 302

Tace. *See* Chlorotrianisene
Tagamet. *See* Cimetidine
Talwin. *See* Pentazocine
Tamoxifen, 615t
Taractan. *See* Chlorprothixene
Tardive dyskinesia, 114, 125
  definition of, 93
Tegretol. *See* Carbamazepine
Tendon transplant, 300
Tendons, 293
Tensilon. *See* Edrophonium chloride
Tension pneumothorax, 193, 333
Terbutaline, 435
Terramycin. *See* Tetracycline
Testes, undescended, 599
Testosterone, 217t, 615t
Tetracycline, 189t, 288t
  lithium and, 104
Tetrahydrocannabinol, 328
Tetralogy of Fallot, *574*, 575-576, 665 [117-120]
Theophylline, 187t, 569t
Therapeutic relationships, 15, 22-24
Therapist, definition of, 93
Thermoregulation, of newborn, 459, 464, 466-467
Thiethylperazine, 310t
Thiopental, 134
Thioridazine, 75t, 116-123, 125
  side effects of, 115
Thiothixene, 75t, 119, 125
Thioxanthenes, 75t, 119
Thomas half-ring splint, 606t, *607*
Thorazine. *See* Chlorpromazine
Throat, 270
Thrombolytic drugs, 176t
Thrombophlebitis, 183-185
Thyroid gland, 218
Thyroid hormones, 217t
Thyroidectomy, 221, 709-710 [363-371]
Thyrotoxicosis, 220-222
Thyrotropic hormone, 217t
Tigan. *See* Trimethobenzamide
Timolol maleate, 287t
Timoptic. *See* Timolol maleate
Tindal. *See* Acetophenazine
Tinea, 545t
Tissue plasminogen activator, 176t
Tocolytic agents, 435, 436t
Toddler, 520-522, 653 [77-80]
  accident prevention for, 522
  concept of death of, 617t
  dental care for, 521
  discipline of, 521-522
  emotional impact of trauma on, 623-626
  growth and development of, 520-521
  hospitalization of, 529
  nutrition for, 521
  pain responses of, 639-640
  toilet training of, 521
Tofranil. *See* Imipramine
Toilet training, 521
Tokodynamometer, 422
Tolazamide, 227t
Tolazoline, 629t, 632
Tolbutamide, 227t
Tolinase. *See* Tolazamide
Tonic neck reflex, 458
Tonsillectomy, 537
TORCH, 414, 472
Torecan. *See* Thiethylperazine
Total parenteral nutrition, 351-355
Tourniquets, *181*, 685 [223-224]
Toxemia of pregnancy, 408-410, 409t
Toxoplasmosis, 414
  in pregnancy, 688-689 [254-261]
Traction, types of, 606t, *607-608*
Transderm-Nitro. *See* Nitroglycerin
Transference, definition of, 93
Transplantation, kidney, 252-254
Transposition of great vessels, *574*, 576
Tranxene. *See* Clorazepate
Tranylcypromine, 124
Tranzene, 41t
Trauma, 664 [104-113]
  emotional impact on toddlers, 623-626
  head, 275-276. *See also* Head injury
    in infants and children, 635-638
Trazodone, 124, 646 [14]
Trecator-C. *See* Ethionamide
Trendelenburg's sign, 610
Triamcinolone acetate, 226t
Trichomoniasis, 542t
  during pregnancy, 415
Triclofos, 134
Triclos. *See* Triclofos
Trifluoperazine, 75t, 116-123, 125

extrapyramidal side effects of, 115
Trifluopromazine, 119
Trihexyphenidyl, 282t
for parkinsonism, 113
Trilafon. *See* Perphenazine
Trilisate. *See* Choline magnesium trisalicylate
Trimethobenzamide, 310t
Trimipramine, 124
Triplets, 416
Trisomy 21, 556-557, 648-649 [33-37]
Trousseau's sign, 223
Trypsin, 217t
Tubal ligation, 388t
Tuberculosis, 190-191, 652 [64-67]
during pregnancy, 415
Tuinal abuse, 89t
Tums. *See* Calcium carbonate
Twins, 416
Tybamate, 133, 134t
Tybatran. *See* Tybamate
Tylenol. *See* Acetaminophen

Ulcerative colitis, 261-263
Ulcers
decubitus, 367-368, *368*
peptic, 206-209, 647-648 [26-32]
stress, 281, 367
Ultrasonic transducer, 422
Ultrasonography, during pregnancy, 401-402, 482
Unconscious, definition of, 93
Undoing, definition of, 21
Unipen. *See* Nafcillin
Ureter, 232
Ureterolithotomy, 243
Ureterostomy, cutaneous, 245
Urethra, 232
Urethritis, nongonococcal, 414
Urinalysis, 237-239
to assess placental functioning, 402, 403t
Urinary diversion, 245
Urinary excretion, 233
Urinary system, 232-242
of newborn, 459-460
Urinary tract infection, 242-243
of children, 599-600
during pregnancy, 415
Urinary tract problems
acute renal failure, 245-247
bladder cancer, 244-245
chronic renal failure, 247-249
dialysis, *249*, 249-252
drug therapy for, 241t
kidney transplantation, 252-254
nursing process for, 236-242
in pregnancy, 392
with spinal cord injury, 366-367
urinary calculi, 243-244
Uterine smooth muscle stimulants, 431t
Uterus, 384
contractions during labor, 424, *426*
dysfunction of, in labor, 432, 432t
endometrial cancer, 313
fibroid tumors of, 452
involution of, 441
prolapse of, 451-452
rupture of, 439-440

Vagina, 385
Vaginal sponge, 387t
Vagotomy, 206
Valisone. *See* Betamethasone valerate
Valium. *See* Diazepam
Valproic acid, 327, 562t
Varicella zoster, 539
Varices, esophageal, 214-215
Varicose ulcers, 183, 185
Varicose veins, 183-185
during pregnancy, 397
Vasectomy, 388t
Vasodilan. *See* Isoxuprine
Vaso-occlusive crisis, 580, 582
Velban. *See* Vinblastine
Venous insufficiency, 183-185, *184*
Ventricular septal defect, *573*, 575
Ventriculoperitoneal shunt, 653-654 [81-84]
Verapamil, 170t, 173t
Vernix caseosa, 455
Verstran. *See* Prazepam
Vesicoureteral reflux, 600-601
Vesprin. *See* Triflupromazine
Vinblastine, 615t
Vincristine, 615t
Violent behavior, 62-71. *See also* Socially maladaptive behavior
Vision, 269, *270*, 271
Vision problems, 668 [150-151]
cataracts, 286-289
glaucoma, 290-291
retinal detachment, 289-290
strabismus, 537-538
Vistaril. *See* Hydroxyzine
Vivactil. *See* Protriptyline
Vomiting
in children, 585-587
forceful, 586
pernicious, of pregnancy, 414
projectile, 586
Von Rosen splint, 609, 701 [289]
Vontrol. *See* Diphenidol
Voyeurism, 65

Walking reflex, 458
Warfarin sodium, 176t
Warts, genital, 415
Water balance, 232
Weber test, 273, 526
Weight
gain in pregnancy, 493
postpartum loss, 442
Whisper test, 273
Wilms' tumor, 620t
Withdrawal
from alcohol, 84
definition of, 22
from drugs, 89t
Withdrawn behavior, 72-80
causes of, 72
definition of, 72
management of, 74-75
manifestations of, 72-74
behavioral, 72-73
psychologic, 73-74
sociologic, 74
medications for, 74, 75t
nursing process for, 76-79
types of, 80, 80t
Word salad, definition of, 93

X-linked diseases, *581*
Xanax, 41t
Xylocaine. *See* Lidocaine

Yawning reflex, 458
Young's rule, 534t

Zantac. *See* Ranitidine
Zarontin. *See* Ethosuximide
Zelmid. *See* Zimelidine
Zidovudine, 315
Zimelidine, 51t
Zyloprim. *See* Allopurinol